Rush University Medical Center

REVIEW OF SURGERY

Rush University Medical Center

REVIEW OF SURGERY

SIXTH EDITION

Jonathan A. Myers MD
Professor of Surgery
Director of Clinical Operations
Department of Surgery
Rush University Medical Center
Chicago, IL, USA

Minh B. Luu MD
Associate Professor of Surgery
Associate Residency Program Director
Department of Surgery
Rush University Medical Center
Chicago, IL, USA

Keith W. Millikan MD
Professor and Senior Vice-Chair of Surgery
Department of Surgery
Rush University Medical Center
Chicago, IL, USA

Bruce A. Orkin MD
Professor of Surgery
Department of Surgery
Rush University Medical Center
Chicago, IL, USA

Steven D. Bines MD
Associate Professor of Surgery
Department of Surgery
Rush University Medical Center
Chicago, IL, USA

Edie Y. Chan MD
Assistant Professor of Surgery
Department of General Surgery, Division of Transplantation
Program Director, Residency Program, Department of Surgery
Rush University Medical Center
Chicago, IL, USA

Edward F. Hollinger MD PhD
Assistant Professor of Surgery, Assistant Attending
Department of Surgery, Section of Abdominal Transplant, Rush University Medical Center
Chicago, IL, USA

For additional online content visit ExpertConsult.com

ELSEVIER Edinburgh London New York Oxford Philadelphia St Louis Sydney 2018

ELSEVIER

First edition 1988
Second edition 1994
Third edition 2000
Fourth edition 2007
Fifth edition 2011
Sixth edition 2018

Notices

Knowledge and best practice in this field are constantly changing. As new research and experience broaden our understanding, changes in research methods, professional practices, or medical treatment may become necessary.

Practitioners and researchers must always rely on their own experience and knowledge in evaluating and using any information, methods, compounds, or experiments described herein. In using such information or methods, they should be mindful of their own safety and the safety of others, including parties to whom they have a professional responsibility.

With respect to any drug or pharmaceutical products identified, readers are advised to check the most current information provided (i) on procedures featured or (ii) by the manufacturer of each product to be administered to verify the recommended dose or formula, the method and duration of administration, and contraindications. It is the responsibility of practitioners, relying on their own experience and knowledge about their patients, to make diagnoses, to determine dosages and the best treatment for each individual patient, and to take all appropriate safety precautions.

To the fullest extent of the law, neither the Publisher nor the authors, contributors, or editors assume any liability for any injury and/or damage to persons or property as a matter of products liability, negligence or otherwise, or from any use or operation of any methods, products, instructions, or ideas contained in the material herein.

ISBN: 978-0-323-48532-6
eBook ISBN: 978-0-323-54959-2

The Publisher's policy is to use paper manufactured from sustainable forests

Printed in China
Last digit is the print number: 9 8 7 6 5 4 3 2 1

Content Strategist: Michael Houston/Russell Gabbedy
Content Development Specialist: Nani Clansey
Project Manager: Dr. Atiyaah Muskaan
Design: Miles Hitchen
Illustration Manager: Emily Costantino
Marketing Manager: Melissa Fogarty

LIST OF CONTRIBUTORS

Shabirhusain S. Abadin, MD
Endocrine and General Surgeon
John H. Stroger, Jr. and Provident Hospitals of Cook County
Associate Program Director - Endocrine Surgery Fellowship
John H. Stroger, Jr. Hospital and North Shore University
Assistant Clinical Professor in Surgery
Rush University Medical Center
Chicago, IL, USA

Chetan V. Aher, MD
Assistant Professor of Surgery
Division of General Surgery
Vanderbilt University Medical Center
Nashville, TN, USA

Elizabeth Aitcheson, MD
Resident
Department of Surgery
Rush University Medical Center
Chicago, IL, USA

Samer Al-Khudari, MD, FACS
Assistant Professor
Head & Neck Oncology and Microvascular Reconstruction
Medical Student Director
Department of Otorhinolaryngology-Head & Neck Surgery
Rush University Medical Center
Chicago, IL, USA

Gillian Alex, MD
Resident
Department of Surgery
Rush University Medical Center
Chicago, IL, USA

Robin A. Alley, MD
Assistant Professor of Clinical Surgery
Department of General Surgery
University of Illinois College of Medicine
Peoria, IL, USA

Anuja K. Antony, MD, MPH, FACS
Associate Professor
Medical Director
Director of Breast Reconstruction
Department of Plastic Surgery
Rush University Medical Center
Chicago, IL, USA

Andrew T. Arndt, MD
Assistant Professor
Department of Thoracic and Cardiac Surgery
Rush University Medical Center
Chicago, IL, USA

Nasim T. Babazadeh, MD
Resident
Department of Surgery
Rush University Medical Center
Chicago, IL, USA

Steven D. Bines, MD
Associate Professor of Surgery
Department of Surgery
Rush University Medical Center
Chicago, IL, USA

Joseph Broucek, MD
Chief Administrative Resident
Department of Surgery
Rush University Medical Center
Chicago, IL, USA

Richard W. Byrne, MD
The Roger C. Bone, MD, Presidential Professor, Department of Neurosurgery, Rush Medical College
Professor, Department of Neurosurgery
Medical Director, University Neurosurgery
Rush University Medical Center
Chicago, IL, USA

Edie Y. Chan, MD
Associate Professor of Surgery
Department of Surgery
Rush University Medical Center
Chicago, IL, USA

Bill Chiu, MD
Assistant Professor of Surgery
Section of Pediatric Surgery
Department of Surgery
Rush University Medical Center
Chicago, IL, USA

Jose R. Cintron, MD, FACS, FASCRS
Chairman, Division of Colon and Rectal Surgery
John H. Stroger Hospital of Cook County
Associate Professor of Surgery
University of Illinois College of Medicine
Chicago, IL, USA

Rebecca A. Deal, MD
General Surgery Resident
Department of Surgery
Rush University Medical Center
Chicago, IL, USA

Joseph Durham, MD
Chief, Division of Vascular Surgery
John H. Stroger Hospital of Cook County
Chicago, IL, USA

Brett Fair, MD
Resident
Department of Surgery
Rush University Medical Center
Chicago, IL, USA

Erin C. Farlow, MD
Vascular Surgeon
Department of Surgery
Cook County Health and Hospitals System
Chicago, IL, USA

Vidyaratna A. Fleetwood, MD
Resident
Department of Surgery
Rush University Medical Center
Chicago, IL, USA

Charles Fredericks, MD
Resident
Department of Surgery
Rush University Medical Center
Chicago, IL, USA

Alfred Guirguis, DO, MPH
Assistant Professor of Obstetrics and Gynecology
Rush University Medical Center
Chicago, IL, USA

Samir K. Gupta, MD, FACS
Assistant Professor of Surgery
Section Chief, Acute Care Surgery and Surgical Critical Care
Department of Surgery
Medical Director, SICU
Rush University Medical Center
Chicago, IL, USA

Jamie Harris, MD
Resident
Department of Surgery
Rush University Medical Center
Chicago, IL, USA

Edward F. Hollinger, MD, PhD
Assistant Professor of Surgery
Surgical Director of Renal Transplant
Department of Surgery
Rush University Medical Center
Chicago, IL, USA

Richard A. Jacobson, MD
Resident
Department of Surgery
Rush University Medical Center
Chicago, IL, USA

Lia Jordano, MD
Resident
Department of Surgery
Rush University Medical Center
Chicago, IL, USA

Vicky Kang, BS
Medical Student
Rush Medical College
Rush University Medical Center
Chicago, IL, USA

Justin M. Karush, DO
Assistant Professor of Surgery
Department of Cardiovascular and Thoracic Surgery
Rush University Medical Center
Chicago, IL, USA

Richard Keen, MD
Chairman, Department of Surgery
Cook County Health and Hospitals System
Chicago, IL, USA

Christopher Knapp, MD
Resident
Department of Surgery
Rush University Medical Center
Chicago, IL, USA

Ryan C. Knoper, MD
Resident
Department of Surgery
Rush University Medical Center
Chicago, IL, USA

Michelle A. Kominiarek, MD, MS
Associate Professor
Department of Obstetrics and Gynecology
Northwestern University Feinberg School of Medicine
Chicago, IL, USA

James Kong, MD
Fellow
Department of Plastic & Reconstructive Surgery
Rush University Medical Center
Chicago, IL, USA

Katherine Kopkash, MD
Assistant Professor of Surgery
Director of Oncoplastic Breast Surgery
Department of Surgery
Rush University Medical Center
Chicago, IL, USA

John C. Kubasiak, MD
Resident
Department of Surgery
Rush University Medical Center
Chicago, IL, USA

MacKenzie Landin, MD
Resident
Department of Surgery
Rush University Medical Center
Chicago, IL, USA

Minh B. Luu, MD
Associate Professor of Surgery
Associate Residency Program Director
Department of Surgery
Rush University Medical Center
Chicago, IL, USA

Andrea Madrigrano, MD
Assistant Professor
Department of Surgery
Rush University Medical Center
Chicago, IL, USA

Kristine Makiewicz, MD
General Surgery Resident
Department of Surgery
Rush University Medical Center
Chicago, IL, USA

Thomas A. Messer, MD
Trauma & Burn Surgeon, John H. Stroger Hospital of Cook County
Assistant Professor, Rush University Medical Center
Chicago, IL, USA

Keith Millikan, MD, FACS
Professor and Senior Vice-Chair of Surgery
Department of Surgery
Rush University Medical Center
Chicago, IL, USA

Jonathan A. Myers, MD
Professor of Surgery
Director of Clinical Operations
Department of Surgery
Rush University Medical Center
Chicago, IL, USA

M. Caroline Nally, MD
Resident
Department of Surgery
Rush University Medical Center
Chicago, IL, USA

Philip Omotosho, MD
Chief, Division of Minimally Invasive & Bariatric Surgery
Director of Quality & Clinical Effectiveness
Department of Surgery, Rush University Medical Center
Chicago, IL, USA

Donnamarie Packer, MD
Resident
Department of Surgery
Rush University Medical Center
Chicago, IL, USA

Peter Papagiannopoulos, MD
Resident
Department of Otorhinolaryngology-Head & Neck Surgery
Rush University Medical Center
Chicago, IL, USA

Purvi P. Patel, MD
Surgical Critical Care Fellow
Department of Surgery
University of Nevada School of Medicine
Las Vegas, NV, USA

Srikumar Pillai, MD
Associate Professor
Department of Surgery, Rush Medical College
Division Chief, Pediatric Surgery, Department of Surgery
Rush University Medical Center
Chicago, IL, USA

Samer R. Rajjoub, MD
Attending, Endocrine and General Surgery
Palos Health
Clinical Assistant Professor of Surgery
Department of Surgery
Loyola University Medical Center
Maywood, IL, USA

Ruta Rao, MD
Associate Professor of Medicine
Director, Coleman Comprehensive Breast Clinic
Director, Hematology & Oncology Fellowship Program
Rush University Medical Center
Chicago, IL, USA

Emilie Robinson, MD
Resident
Department of Surgery
Rush University Medical Center
Chicago, IL, USA

David M. Rothenberg, MD, FCCM
The Max S. Sadove Professor of Anesthesiology
Vice-Chair, Academic Affairs, Department of Anesthesiology
Associate Dean, Academic Affiliations
Rush University Medical Center
Chicago, IL, USA

Scott W. Schimpke, MD
Resident
Department of Surgery
Rush University Medical Center
Chicago, IL, USA

Christopher W. Seder, MD
Assistant Professor of Surgery
Associate Program Director, Cardiovascular and Thoracic Surgery Residency
Department of Cardiovascular and Thoracic Surgery
Rush University Medical Center
Chicago, IL, USA

Ami N. Shah, MD, FACS, FAAP
Division of Pediatric Surgery, Department of Surgery, Rush University Medical Center
Director of Pediatric Trauma, John H. Stroger Hospital
Chicago, IL, USA

Behnoosh Shayegan, MD
Assistant Professor
Department of Anesthesiology
Rush University Medical Center
Chicago, IL, USA

Neha Sheng, MD
Vascular Surgeon
Department of Surgery Cook County Health and Hospitals System
Chicago, IL, USA

Shauna M. Sheppard, MD
Rush Surgery Class of 2019
Rush University Medical Center
Chicago, IL, USA

Marc Singer, MD
Assistant Professor
Department of Surgery
Rush University Medical Center
Chicago, IL, USA

Nicole Siparsky, MD, FACS
Assistant Professor of Surgery
Rush University Medical Center
Department of Surgery
Section of Surgical Critical Care & Acute Care Surgery
Chicago, IL, USA

Adam P. Smith, MD
Neurological Surgery
Rocky Mountain Brain & Spine Institute
Denver, CO, USA

Jill Smolevitz, MD
Resident
Department of Surgery
Rush University Medical Center
Chicago, IL, USA

Jennifer D. Son, MD
Department of Surgery
Rush University Medical Center
Chicago, IL, USA

Tara Spivey, MD
Resident
Department of Surgery
Rush University Medical Center
Chicago, IL, USA

John F. Tierney, MD
Resident
Department of Surgery
Rush University Medical Center
Chicago, IL, USA

Michael Tran, MD
Resident
Department of Surgery
Rush University Medical Center
Chicago, IL, USA

Benjamin R. Veenstra, MD
Assistant Professor of Surgery
Associate Clerkship Director
Department of Surgery
Division of MIS and Bariatrics
Rush University Medical Center
Chicago, IL, USA

Thomas R. Witt, MD
Associate Professor of Surgery
Rush University Medical Center
Chicago, IL, USA

James R. Yon, MD
Trauma and Acute Care Surgery
Swedish Medical Center
Englewood, CO, USA

Shannon Zielsdorf, MD
Resident
Department of Surgery
Rush University Medical Center
Chicago, IL, USA

FOREWORD

The 6th edition of the *Rush University Medical Center Review of Surgery* is dedicated to our current and former General Surgery residents who have been an integral part of our program since the book's inception in 1988. This book is intended to address the needs of those preparing for the board examination as well as those who need to maintain an up to date knowledge for the maintenance of certification examination. We thank all of you for motivating us to become better surgeons and for helping us to deliver the best care for our patients. We hope you benefit from this book.

DEDICATIONS

This book is dedicated to my wife, Beth, and my children, Jack and Megan, for their ongoing love and support and keeping me focused on the important things in life.
Jonathan A. Myers, MD

To my lovely wife, Kristin, and our twins, Henry and Emma.
Minh B. Luu, MD

To my parents, John and Joan, for making it all possible.
To my wife, Janet, for her never-ending understanding and support of my career.
To my children, Keith, Michael, Kyle, Kameron, Samantha, and John, for inspiring my optimism for the future.
Keith W. Millikan, MD

To my wonderful and supportive wife, Ethel Seltzer, and our children, Roxanne, Daniel, David, Peter, and Nora.
Bruce A. Orkin, MD

For SAKER5
Steven D. Bines, MD

To my parents, Ed and Lois, my wife, Michelle, and my children, Andrew, David, and Luke.
Edward F. Hollinger, MD, PhD

PREFACE

The editors of the *Rush University Medical Center Review of Surgery* are pleased to present the 6th edition of this book.

This edition includes 35 chapters divided into 9 sections. Four chapters that were deemed less relevant to board preparation were eliminated, and several sections were reconfigured. All remaining chapters were updated and enhanced to impart the most up-to-date knowledge to the reader. Each subject was once again based on current practice and referenced with widely read textbooks of surgery.

Contributions for this text were solicited from more than 60 active clinicians, all presently or formerly affiliated with Rush University. Topics cover current knowledge in the rapidly evolving field of medicine, incorporating surgical care, basic science, patient safety, core competencies, and multispecialty disease-driven care.

We are confident that the 6th edition of the *Rush University Medical Center Review of Surgery* will continue to provide a basis for the reader to gain the knowledge needed in general surgery and associated specialties and serve as a primer to those preparing for certification exams.

ACKNOWLEDGMENTS

The editors wish to recognize the achievements of the outstanding group of contributors whose efforts were invaluable to the completion of this book. The associate editors provided tremendous energy in selecting authors, maintaining deadlines, and delivering stellar work.

This edition could not have been completed without the tireless work of Kathy Martin, who led the charge to piece together all components of this text and seamlessly coordinate our efforts. Thank you to Skye Unrein and Shannon Patrick for their administrative assistance and to the excellent staff at Elsevier for their direction.

We would not be here today were it not for the groundwork laid by former editors of the previous editions of this book including Steven Economou, Daniel Deziel, Thomas Witt, Theodore Saclarides, Edgar Staren, Richard Prinz, Walter McCarthy, and Linnea Hauge. Finally, a heartfelt thanks to Jose Velasco, the 5th edition senior editor, for his mentorship and guidance on this project.

HOW TO USE

The topics in the 6th edition have been divided into 35 chapters, split into 9 sections, which should facilitate a review of the material for certification, or maintenance of certification, in general surgery.

Each section contains a variable number of chapters, encompassing questions, and the corresponding comments and references attached to each question. Most questions are followed by one or more references that link them to a relevant textbook and to selected articles. Authors sought evidence-based material as appropriate. A select best answer format is utilized. At the end of each question, a letter indicates the preferred answer, followed by comments elaborating on the topic. A list of references is included at the end of each chapter.

Words and phrases appearing in boldface type within the text indicate links to facilitate a search of the material to be reviewed.

TABLE OF CONTENTS

SECTION I

SURGICAL FUNDAMENTALS

CHAPTER 1

PHYSIOLOGIC RESPONSE TO INJURY

Gillian Alex, M.D., and Ami Shah, M.D.

1. Cytokines involved in the initial proinflammatory response include all of the following except:

A. Interleukin-6

B. Interleukin-10

C. Tumor necrosis factor-α

D. Interleukin-1

E. Interleukin-8

ANSWER: B

COMMENTS: The complement cascade is the earliest humoral system activated in response to injury. C3a and C5a, the biologically active anaphylatoxins, induce the release of proinflammatory cytokines. Tumor necrosis factor-α (TNF-α) and interleukin-1 (IL-1) are the key mediators of this cascade. IL-6 induces T and B cells, and IL-8 recruits and activates inflammatory cells at the site of injury. IL-10, in contrast, is one of the key mediators of the antiinflammatory response and acts to inhibit the aforementioned cytokines.

Ref.: 1

2. Which of the following is true regarding the role of TNF-α release in the inflammatory response?

A. It can be effectively blocked by anti–TNF-α antibodies to halt systemic inflammatory response syndrome (SIRS).

B. It does not have any beneficial effects in the early phases of the inflammatory response.

C. It is primarily from leukocytes.

D. It promotes polymorphonuclear (PMN) cell adherence and further cytokine release.

E. It is always deleterious.

ANSWER: D

COMMENTS: TNF-α is a vital component of the early inflammatory response, especially locally, at the site of injury. It is released when the biologically active anaphylatoxins C3a and C5a are stimulated by the humoral system. Infusion of low doses of TNF-α in rats simulates the septic response, resulting in fever, hypotension, fatigue, and anorexia. TNF-α promotes adherence of PMN cells to endothelium, production of prostaglandins by fibroblasts, and activation of neutrophils and stimulates the release of multiple other cytokines from lymphocytes. TNF-α becomes deleterious when the proinflammatory stimuli are unchecked, leading to cellular damage and multiorgan system failure. TNF-α is released by macrophages and natural killer cells, but not leukocytes. Trials involving anti–TNF-α antibodies (NORASEPT, INTERSEPT) have not shown statistically significant improvement in patient outcomes.

Ref.: 1

3. A 56-year-old female is admitted to the intensive care unit (ICU) with a diffuse axonal injury after a motor vehicle crash. The nursing staff notices coffee ground material coming from her orogastric tube. What is the best intervention to prevent this complication?

A. Enteral feeding

B. Oral sucralfate

C. Oral proton pump inhibitor (PPI)

D. Intravenous (IV) H_2 blocker

E. IV PPI drip

ANSWER: D

COMMENTS: Stress-related gastritis can cause clinically significant bleeding in up to 5%–10% of ICU patients; therefore stress ulcer prophylaxis is now routinely administered in the ICU. Ulcers and bleeding are thought to be secondary to mucosal damage caused by low-flow states and subclinical hypoperfusion to the gastric mucosa. Patients with the following criteria should receive stress ulcer prophylaxis:

- coagulopathy defined as platelets < 50,000 cells per mcl (microliter); INR > 1.5; or PTT > two times the normal reference range
- mechanical ventilation > 48 h
- history of gastrointestinal ulcer or bleed
- traumatic brain/spinal cord injury or burn
- two or more of the following minor criteria:
  - Sepsis
  - ICU admission
  - Occult gastrointestinal bleed > 6 days
  - Glucocorticoids > 250 mg

Clinical data suggest that if enteral access is possible,the best agent is an oral PPI. If enteral access is not feasible, an IV PPI or H_2 antagonist is an alternative. IV PPIs are costly, so most centers favor an IV H_2 antagonist. Sucralfate has been studied and is effective in protecting against stress gastritis, but a disadvantage is its interference with the absorption of other medications such as antibiotics, warfarin, and phenytoin. Previously, it was thought that the use of H_2 blockers was associated with nosocomial pneumonia because of gastric bacterial colonization and subsequent aspiration. However, more recent trials have not demonstrated any difference between other protective agents and H_2 receptor antagonists in the rate of ventilator-associated pneumonia. Antacids have not shown efficacy in preventing stress-related mucosal lesions in the ICU patients and are not considered as appropriate prophylactic agents.

Ref.: 2

4. A 64-year-old male with severe pancreatitis is transferred to the ICU from an outside hospital. A report is given to the nurse that the patient has received "large-volume resuscitation." Upon reaching the ICU, he is afebrile, tachycardic to 127, and has a BP of 120/60 mmHg. His abdomen is tense and full; he has a Foley in place but no urine in the bag. You suspect abdominal compartment syndrome (ACS). What is the mechanism of his oliguria?

A. Extrinsic compression of abdominal organs on the kidneys, leading to reduced GFR
B. Elevated renal venous pressure, leading to reduced GFR
C. Decreased arterial flow to the kidney, leading to reduced glomerular filtration rate (GFR)
D. Extrinsic compression of the ureters, causing an obstructive oliguric renal failure
E. Compression of the bladder, causing an obstructive oliguric renal failure

ANSWER: B

COMMENTS: Intraabdominal hypertension can be defined as intraabdominal pressure greater than or equal to 20 cm H_2O. ACS occurs in the setting of intraabdominal hypertension and evidence of abdominal hypoperfusion. ACS reduces the GFR secondary to elevated renal venous pressure and causes oliguria. Other physiologic derangements that can be seen are elevation of the diaphragms impeding oxygenation and ventilation raising the central intrathoracic, venous, and intracranial pressures. All of these issues can be treated with decompressive laparotomy. Decompressive laparotomy should be employed as a treatment for ACS when there is evidence of end-organ dysfunction.

Ref.: 2

5. For the patient in Question 4, which of the following parameters would necessitate a decompressive laparotomy for treatment?

A. Peak airway pressures of 30 mmHg
B. Systemic vascular resistance of 1400 dyn/s/cm^5
C. Pulmonary capillary wedge pressure of 18 mmHg
D. Urine output of 0 ml
E. Requirements of Fraction of inspired oxygen $(FiO)_2$ of 80% with positive end-expiratory pressure (PEEP) of 12

ANSWER: D

COMMENTS: Decompressive laparotomy should be performed only when there is evidence of end-organ dysfunction. Of all the answer choices provided, only decreased urine output indicates end-organ dysfunction. The rest of the parameters may be seen in ACS but do not indicate organ damage secondary to ACS; however, laparotomy would improve all of the parameters above.

Ref.: 2

6. A patient is brought to the emergency department after being found unresponsive. Electroencephalography (EEG) indicates status epilepticus. A potential secondary clinical consequence is:

A. Meningitis
B. Hypothermia
C. Myoglobinuria
D. Cerebrovascular accident
E. Hypoglycemia

ANSWER: C

COMMENTS: Status epilepticus is an entity that should be considered in any patient with recurrent or persistent seizure activity or in those who do not wake up after seizure activity. One of the potential systemic complications is rhabdomyolysis, which would result in myoglobinuria, elevated serum creatinine kinase, and pigmented granular urinary casts. The other options are potential primary causes of seizure activity. Rhabdomyolysis is a direct result of muscle injury and can be caused by prolonged seizure activity; major trauma; drug overdose; vascular embolism; extremity compartment syndrome; malignant hyperthermia; neuroleptic malignant syndrome; myositis; severe exertion; alcoholism; and medications such as statins, macrolide antibiotics, and cyclosporine.

Ref.: 2

7. Euthyroid sick syndrome is diagnosed in a patient in the surgical ICU. All of the following are part of this clinical phenomenon except:

A. The patient behaves as though clinically hypothyroid
B. Normal or decreased total serum thyroxine (T_4) level
C. Increased serum reversed triiodothyronine (rT_3) level
D. Decreased thyroid stimulating hormone (TSH) level
E. Decreased total serum T_3 level

ANSWER: A

COMMENTS: The hallmark of this diagnosis is that the patient behaves neither clinically hypothyroid nor hyperthyroid. The other choices are the expected laboratory findings in patients with this syndrome. Referred to alternatively as euthyroid sick syndrome, low T_3 syndrome, low T_4 syndrome, and nonthyroidal illness, considerable debate exists regarding whether this syndrome represents a pathologic process or an adaptive response to systemic illness that allows the body to lower its tissue energy requirements. In light of this controversy, no consensus has been reached on how to treat this entity or whether any treatment at all is necessary. Because the interpretation of thyroid function tests in critically ill patients is complex, these tests should not be done in an ICU setting unless a thyroid disorder is strongly suspected.

Ref.: 2

8. Acute respiratory distress syndrome (ARDS) develops in an acutely injured patient. If an alveolar biopsy specimen were taken within the first 24 h, the histologic examination would demonstrate:

A. Influx of protein-rich fluid and leukocytes
B. Preservation of type II pneumocytes
C. Bacterial colonization
D. Alveolar hemorrhage
E. High levels of collagen and fibronectin

ANSWER: A

COMMENTS: ARDS involves three distinct phases. The early, exudative phase is characterized by disruption of the alveolar epithelium with an influx of protein-rich fluid and leukocytes. Type II pneumocytes are damaged, and therefore surfactant production is halted. The second fibroproliferative phase includes the arrival of mesenchymal cells that produce collagen and fibronectin. The third, or resolution, phase involves gradual remodeling and clearance of edema.

Ref.: 2 and 3

9. An obese patient with a body mass index (BMI) of 50 underwent a laparoscopic gastric bypass. Because of a technical difficulty in the case, the procedure lasted for 8 h. The patient was doing well postoperatively until 4 h, when the nurse noted a change in the urine color from yellow to dark brown. She also reported that the patient's urine output decreased and his creatinine increased from 1.0 to 1.5. Which test would confirm the cause of these findings?

A. Renal ultrasound

B. Haptoglobin

C. Serum creatinine kinase

D. Complete blood count

E. Urine electrolytes

ANSWER: C

COMMENTS: Rhabdomyolysis can occur postoperatively in obese patients whose back and buttock muscles were compressed against the operating table for a prolonged time. Preventive measures include the use of larger tables to better distribute body weight, effective padding at all pressure points, intraoperative changing of patient position, and limitation of operative times. Physicians should have a high index of suspicion for rhabdomyolysis in this patient population so that early recognition and treatment can prevent the potentially devastating consequence of acute renal failure (ARF) in this already high-risk group. Creatinine kinase should be measured in any patient complaining of muscle pain or in whom dark urine, oliguria, or rising plasma creatinine develops.

Ref.: 4

10. The **primary** algorithm to treat the patient in Question 9 includes all of the following except:

A. Loop diuretics

B. Mannitol

C. Aggressive intravenous fluid resuscitation

D. Sodium bicarbonate

E. Serial basic metabolic panels

ANSWER: A

COMMENTS: The goal of the treatment algorithm for rhabdomyolysis is to prevent ARF. The cause of rhabdomyolysis-induced ARF is multifactorial and includes hypovolemia, ischemia, direct tubule toxicity caused by the heme pigment in myoglobin, and intratubular obstruction by casts. Treatment of rhabdomyolysis is to induce prompt polyuria with sufficient intravenous fluid resuscitation to produce 1.5 to 2 mL/kg/h of urine. Concurrently, urine alkalinization with a goal urine pH greater than 6.5 should be instituted with sodium bicarbonate to prevent precipitation of casts and obstruction of nephrons. Mannitol may also act as a free radical scavenger in addition to a diuretic, although this is somewhat controversial. Loop diuretics can be used as an alternative if brisk urine output cannot be achieved with the aforementioned measures, but they have the disadvantage of acidifying the urine.

Ref.: 4

11. An 82-year-old female with multiple prior abdominal surgeries presents with a small bowel obstruction. She undergoes an exploratory laparotomy with an extensive lysis of adhesions for 7 h. She receives 2 L of crystalloid during the case and has 200 cc of urine output. Her creatinine increases by 0.6 mg/dL the next day. All of the following are appropriate treatments except:

A. Rule out causes of outflow obstruction

B. Recheck hemoglobin

C. Calculate fractional excretion of sodium (FeNa)

D. Give a bolus of fluid

E. Start vasopressors for a mean arterial pressure (MAP) goal of 65 mmHg

ANSWER: E

COMMENTS: The most common cause of postoperative acute kidney injury (AKI) is renal hypoperfusion secondary to hypovolemia. Nephrogenic injury in patients with hypovolemia occurs when the renal arteries constrict in response to increased levels of epinephrine, angiotensin II, and vasopressin and the nephrons receive inadequate delivery of oxygen. The goal of the treatment is to quickly reverse shock and restore renal blood flow. The primary treatment is always intravenous fluid resuscitation. Active bleeding and obstruction should be ruled out. FeNa should be calculated to confirm your cause. Vasopressors should be avoided whenever possible because the resultant vasoconstriction may exacerbate the ischemic insult to the kidneys.

Ref.: 4

12. A 52-year-old diabetic male presents to the emergency department with chest pain, diaphoresis, and an elevated troponin. He is taken to the cardiac catheterization lab. Which of the following is true of contrast-induced AKI (CIAKI)?

A. It is the most common form of iatrogenic AKI in hospitalized patients.

B. CIAKI is characterized by oliguria.

C. Evidence of CIAKI occurs within 6 to 24 h of contrast administration.

D. The creatinine returns to normal within 1 month of insult for most patients.

E. The 1-year mortality associated with CIAKI is $< 5\%$.

ANSWER: A

COMMENTS: CIAKI is the most common cause of iatrogenic AKI in hospitalized patients. It generally presents as a nonoliguric injury, with an increase in creatinine seen 48 to 72 h after the dye load was administered. Patients' creatinine returns to baseline within 7 to 10 days. The 1-year associated mortality is 30%.

Ref.: 5

13. Which of the following interventions reduces the likelihood of CIAKI?

A. *N*-acetylcysteine administration before giving the dye load

B. A one-time dose of prednisone 40 mg before administration of dye load

C. 0.9% normal saline for 12 h before and after giving the dye load

D. 0.45% normal saline for 12 h before and after giving the dye load

E. 1 L bolus of 0.9 normal saline at the time of giving the dye load

ANSWER: C

COMMENTS: The pathogenesis of CIAKI is primarily an ischemic form of injury caused by the vasoconstrictive properties of contrast media. In addition, contrast media can potentially have direct toxic effects on endothelial cells and renal tubules. Patients with diminished renal vasodilatory capacity (i.e., diabetic nephropathy) have an increased risk of CIAKI. Hydration is the only intervention proven to prevent CIAKI, with oral hydration more efficient than PO. Randomized controlled trials have found a small superiority in treatment, with 0.9% over 0.45% saline. There have also been multiple smaller studies demonstrating that 12 h of rehydration before and after dye load is more beneficial than a single bolus before the contrast load. *N*-acetylcysteine has been used for the prevention of CIAKI, with mixed results in the literature. However, due to the low cost and low side-effect profile, some authors still advocate its use.

Ref.: 5

14. A 47-year-old male with Crohn's colitis maintained on 40 åmg prednisone daily for the past year presents for elective colectomy. The procedure was uncomplicated, and he was adequately resuscitated. In the postanesthesia care unit (PACU) the patient is noted to be febrile and hypotensive with MAPs in the 50s. What is your next step in management?

A. IV dobutamine

B. Hydrocortisone

C. 1 unit of packed red blood cells

D. Antibiotics

E. Epinephrine

ANSWER: B

COMMENTS: The patient in the above scenario has been exposed to prolonged steroids and, as a result, has relative adrenal insufficiency. These patients may experience shock when they do not receive glucocorticoid replacement during times of relative corticoid and mineralocorticoid deficiencies. Signs and symptoms of acute insufficiency include fever, nausea, vomiting, refractory hypotension, and lethargy. Intravenous volume replacement with isotonic fluids and immediate IV steroid treatment with hydrocortisone are essential.

Ref.: 6

15. You are called by a PACU nurse for a patient who just underwent an elective splenectomy for idiopathic thrombotic purpura. The patient is afebrile, tachycardic, and hypotensive. What is your next step in management?

A. Check hemoglobin

B. IV fluid resuscitation

C. Electrocardiogram

D. Antibiotics

E. Start vasopressors

ANSWER: A

COMMENTS: Anytime a patient in the immediate postoperative period becomes unstable, evaluation for bleeding is critical. Hemoglobin should be checked, and if necessary, the patient should be returned to the operating room. The other steps may ultimately be required; however, bleeding must be ruled out first.

Ref.: 6

16. Which of the following metabolic changes occur during times of physiologic stress?

A. Increase in growth hormone (GH) release

B. Increase in TSH

C. Increased levels of T4 and T3

D. Initial insulin increase and then suppression

E. Increase in cortisol excretion

ANSWER: E

COMMENTS: There are many metabolic changes in times of stress. Cortisol is a major effector of metabolism and is the main hormone increased in the stress response. Cortisol inhibits growth hormone (GH) release, decreasing GH levels. Insulin-like growth factor levels are decreased in these times as well. Injury decreases TSH and conversion of T4 into T3, resulting in decreased levels of both T4 and T3. There are two patterns of insulin release, initial suppression followed by elevated release but increased peripheral resistance, leading to hyperglycemia.

Ref.: 6

17. Which of the following patients most likely has sepsis and should have prompt evaluation for transfer to an ICU?

A. A 27-year-old female after lithotripsy for nephrolithiasis who is afebrile with a heart rate (HR) of 102, BP 90/40 mmHg, altered mental status, and white blood cell (WBC) count of 9

B. A 72-year-old male with pancreatitis and a temperature of 102 degrees Farenheit, HR 110 beats/min, BP 110/60 mmHg, and WBC count of 14 cells per mcl

C. A 53-year-old female at postoperative day 0 from a colon resection who is tachycardic to 120 s and requires intubation in the PACU

D. An 84-year-old nursing home resident with a urine culture positive for Proteus spp.

E. An 18-year-old male who presented with a gangrenous appendicitis, is now at postoperative day 0 from a laparoscopic appendectomy, and is febrile to 103 and tachycardic to 130 s with BP of 140/70

ANSWER: A

COMMENTS: In 2016, the consensus guidelines on the definitions of sepsis and septic shock were revised for the first time since 2001. The aim of the consensus committee was to change the definitions to reflect the change in understanding of the pathophysiology and natural history of sepsis. The committee defined sepsis as a life-threatening organ dysfunction caused by dysregulated host responses to infection. The prior definition of sepsis included two or more SIRS criteria plus a possible source of infection. SIRS may reflect a host response that is merely adaptive; therefore the old definition did not adequately identify all patients who may benefit from intensive therapies. Through examination of large data sets, the quick sepsis-related organ failure assessment (qSOFA) was developed to help promptly identify patients with suspected infection who are likely to have a prolonged ICU stay or die in the hospital. Criteria for the qSOFA are altered mental status, respiratory rate > 22/min, or systolic BP < 100 mmHg. Patients who screen positive warrant a higher level of care and intervention. Of the patients listed above, only patient A meets the criterion for qSOFA. While several of the others may meet criteria based on the former definition of sepsis, their conditions may be physiologic responses to injury and not suggestive of impending life-threatening injury and therefore do not need intensive monitoring.

Ref.: 7

18. Which of the following is the best parameter for monitoring septic shock?

A. Central venous pressure (CVP)

B. Vasopressor requirement

C. Urine output

D. Serum lactate

E. Mental status changes

ANSWER: D

COMMENTS: Septic shock is a subset of sepsis in which underlying circulatory and cellular/metabolic abnormalities are profound enough to substantially increase mortality. Patients with septic shock can be identified with a clinical construct of sepsis with persistent hypotension requiring vasopressors to maintain a MAP > 65 mmHg and a serum lactate level > 2 mmol/L despite adequate volume resuscitation. With these criteria, hospital mortality is in excess of 40%. Serum lactate is a good indicator of global perfusion. By definition, patients with sepsis suffer global hypoperfusion. CVP is often unreliable and can be affected by patient positioning, catheter positioning, and other physiologic derangements. Vasopressor requirements are often needed in septic shock to help improve perfusion but cannot be used as a direct measure of perfusion. Oliguria and altered mental status are signs of end-organ damage.

Ref.: 7

19. All of the following are negative outcomes that have been directly associated with perioperative hypothermia except:

A. Coagulopathy

B. Wound infections

C. Nosocomial pneumonia

D. Myocardial ischemia

E. Delayed wound healing

ANSWER: C

COMMENTS: Preservation of normothermia in surgical patients is important and is one of the goals of the Surgical Care Improvement Project (SCIP). Hypothermia results in peripheral vasoconstriction, which leads to decreased subcutaneous oxygen tension and antibiotic delivery. Both neutrophil activity and leukocyte chemotaxis are impaired. All of these sequelae give rise to an increased incidence of wound infections. Globally reduced enzyme function leads to coagulopathy. Collagen cross-linking and therefore wound healing is affected by hypothermia. An increased risk for myocardial ischemia in patients with known coronary artery disease has been associated with hypothermic states. There has not been a direct correlation between the development of nosocomial pneumonia and hypothermia. The SCIP measures aim to achieve a target temperature of 36.0°C in perioperative patients using active warming methods.

Ref.: 8

20. An obese 21-year-old male suffers multiple fractures and a liver injury; 21 days later, he develops acute dyspnea, diaphoresis, and desaturates to 86% at room air. A computed tomography (CT) of the chest is positive for pulmonary embolus. All of the following are risk factors for venous thromboembolic events except:

A. Severity of injury

B. BMI

C. Smoking

D. Pelvic fractures

E. Hypertriglyceridemia

ANSWER: E

COMMENTS: Venous thromboembolic disease (VTE), which can manifest as deep venous thrombus (DVT) or pulmonary embolism (PE), is common and can have serious or fatal consequences. Risk factors for VTE frequently encountered by surgeons include increased severity of injury, increased BMI, history of smoking, intraabdominal cancers, pelvic fractures or surgery, lithotomy positioning, and operative times longer than 2 h. Hypertriglyceridemia and hypercholesterolemia have been examined as risk factors for VTE, but no statistically significant association has been established.

Ref.: 2, 9

21. Which of the following patients should receive prolonged prophylaxis (28 days) for VTE?

A. Female with a newly diagnosed DVT in her right popliteal vein

B. Male with chronic pulmonary embolus who undergoes a laparoscopic cholecystectomy

C. Female with gastric cancer who undergoes a total gastrectomy

D. Female with uterine fibroids undergoing total abdominal hysterectomy

E. Female with breast cancer undergoing bilateral mastectomy

ANSWER: C

COMMENTS: Continued prophylaxis after surgery should be based on the assessment of risk of VTE. In patients with abdominal cancer, VTE is an important cause of death. About 29% of patients with abdominal cancer will develop a complication of VTE during their disease course. Continuing chemical prophylaxis for 28 days postoperatively decreases the incidence of thromboembolic events and has a risk reduction of >50% in mortality, which persists for greater than 3 months. Patients A and B both require therapeutic treatment and not prophylaxis.

Ref.: 9

22. Which of the following is a contraindication to enteral feeding?

A. Ileus

B. Small bowel anastomosis

C. Hemodynamic instability requiring vasopressors

D. Pancreatitis

E. Pneumonia

ANSWER: C

COMMENTS: Enteral feeding should be initiated early in the course of critical illness or injury. The intestine plays a role in digestion and absorption of nutrients and acts as a barrier to enteric flora, preventing host invasion by microorganisms or their toxins. This intestinal barrier can be impaired during critical illness, making patients susceptible to bacterial translocation. Enteral feeding is protective against microvilli atrophy and impairment of the intestinal barrier. Patients can and should be fed in all of the scenarios above with the exception of hemodynamic instability. In times of global hypoperfusion there is a risk of intestinal ischemia caused by enteral feedings. Patients with pancreatitis may receive enteral feedings; however, postpyloric feedings are preferred.

Ref.: 10

23. A patient with a previous history of ischemic bowel requiring extensive bowel resection, now with only 100 cm of bowel remaining and dependent on total parenteral nutrition (TPN), presents to your office complaining of hair loss, rash on the extremities, and dry skin. Which nutrient deficiency is this patient most likely suffering from?

A. Copper

B. Selenium

C. Vitamin D

D. Essential fatty acids

E. Zinc

ANSWER: D

COMMENTS: Short gut as a result of small bowel loss and or dysfunction of the remaining bowel is characterized by malabsorption of nutrients, diarrhea, and weight loss. Essential fatty acids are not part of TPN formulas, and deficiency causes dermatitis, diarrhea, alopecia, patchy red areas on the skin, brittle nails, easy bruising, bleeding tendencies, and delayed wound healing.

Ref.: 11

24. Strategies that have been suggested to decrease the risk for postoperative pulmonary complications include all of the following except:

A. Routine nasogastric tube decompression

B. Lung expansion maneuvers

C. Preoperative smoking cessation

D. Postoperative epidural anesthesia

E. Use of intraoperative short-acting neuromuscular blocking agents

ANSWER: A

COMMENTS: Postoperative pulmonary complications include atelectasis, pneumonia, prolonged mechanical ventilation, bronchospasm, and exacerbation of the underlying lung disease. Aggressive pulmonary toilet, smoking cessation, epidural analgesia, and minimal neuromuscular blockade have been shown to be effective means of reducing postoperative respiratory complications. In contrast, because systemic reviews have found that routine use of nasogastric decompression increases pulmonary complications, nasogastric tubes should be used postoperatively only when specifically indicated for the operative procedure. An early postoperative fever is most likely due to atelectasis causing a respiratory shunt secondary to alveolar collapse. This results in varying degrees of hypoxemia. Persistent collapse leaves alveoli prone to bacterial colonization. Aggressive pulmonary toilet with incentive spirometry, forced coughing, and frequent turning is the best prevention.

Ref.: 12

25. A patient with resolving ARDS requires a tracheostomy. The family wants to know the benefit of early tracheostomy compared with prolonged intubation. Which of the following is correct?

A. There is no difference in overall mortality between patients receiving prolonged endotracheal (ET) intubation and those receiving tracheostomy.

B. There is increased sedation and pain requirement with a surgically placed tracheostomy.

C. There is an increased risk of pneumonia with ET intubation.

D. There is a decrease in the time required for mechanical ventilation with tracheostomy.

E. ICU stays are the same for both ET intubation and tracheostomy.

ANSWER: A

COMMENTS: There is no mortality difference between patients receiving prolonged endotracheal intubation and those receiving a tracheostomy. Patients with a tracheostomy do have shorter stays in the ICU and decreased sedation and pain requirements. There are equivocal rates of pneumonia and days requiring mechanical ventilation in both tracheostomy and ET intubation.

Ref.: 13

REFERENCES

1. O'Leary PJ, Tabuenca A. *The Physiologic Basis of Surgery*. 4th ed. Philadelphia, PA: Lippincott Williams & Wilkins; 2008.
2. O'Keefe G. Critical care and postinjury management. In: Mulholland MW, Lillemoe KD, Doherty GM, Maier RV, Simeone DM, Upchurch GR, eds. *Greenfield's Surgery: Scientific Principles & Practice*. 5th ed. Philadelphia, PA: Lippincott Williams & Wilkins; 2011.
3. The ARDS. Definition Task Force. Acute respiratory distress syndrome. *JAMA*. 2012;307(23):2526–2533.
4. Mullins RJ. Acute renal failure. In: Cameron JL, ed. *Current Surgical Therapy*. 9th ed. Philadelphia, PA: Mosby; 2008.
5. Weisbord SD, Palevsky PM. Strategies for the prevention of contrast-induced acute kidney injury. *Curr Opin Nephrol Hypertens*. 2010; 19(6):539–549.
6. Olson JA, Scheri RP. Adrenal gland. In: Mulholland MW, Lillemoe KD, Doherty GM, Maier RV, Simeone DM, Upchurch GR, eds. *Greenfield's Surgery: Scientific Principles & Practice*. 5th ed. Philadelphia, PA: Lippincott Williams & Wilkins; 2011.
7. Singer M, Deutschman CS, Seymour CW, et al. The third international consensus definitions for sepsis and septic shock (sepsis-3). *JAMA*. 2016;315(8):801–810.
8. Thomsen RW, Martinez EA, Simon BA. Perioperative care and monitoring of the surgical patient: evidence-based performance practices. In: Cameron JL, ed. *Current Surgical Therapy*. 9th ed. Philadelphia, PA: CV Mosby; 2008.

9. Bergqvist D, Agnelli G, Cohen AT, et al. Duration of prophylaxis against venous thromboembolism with enoxaparin after surgery for cancer. *N Eng J Med*. 2002;346(13):975–980.
10. McClave SA, Taylor BE, Martindale RG, et al. Guidelines for the provision and assessment of nutrition support therapy in the adult critically ill patient: Society of Critical Care Medicine (SCCM) and American Society for Parenteral and Enteral Nutrition (ASPEN). *J Parenter Enteral Nutr*. 2016;40(2):159–211.
11. Keating KP, Marshall W. Nutritional support in the critically ill. In: Cameron JL, ed. *Current Surgical Therapy*. 9th ed. Philadelphia, PA: CV Mosby; 2008.
12. Mendez-Tellez PA, Dorman T. Postoperative respiratory failure. In: Cameron JL, ed. *Current Surgical Therapy*. 9th ed. Philadelphia, PA: CV Mosby; 2008.
13. Andriolo BNG, Andriolo RB, Saconato H, Atallah AN, Valente O. Early versus late tracheostomy for critically ill patients. *Cochrane Database Syst Rev*. 2015; Issue 1. DOI:10.1002/14651858.CD007271.pub2?

CHAPTER 2

WOUND HEALING AND CELL BIOLOGY

Steven D. Bines, M.D.

1. Which of the following statements regarding the role of collagen in wound healing is true?
   A. Collagen synthesis in the initial phase of injury is the sole responsibility of endothelial cells.
   B. Net collagen content increases for up to 2 years after injury.
   C. At 3 weeks after injury, more than 50% of the tensile strength of the wound has been restored.
   D. Tensile strength of the wound increases gradually for up to 2 years after injury; however, it generally reaches a level of only about 80% of that of uninjured tissue.
   E. Tensile strength is the force necessary to reopen a wound.

ANSWER: D

COMMENTS: Synthesis of collagen by fibroblasts begins as early as 10 h after injury and increases rapidly; it peaks by day 6 or 7 and then continues more slowly until day 42. Collagen continues to mature and remodel for years. Its solubility in saline solution and the thermal shrinkage temperature of collagen reflect the intermolecular cross-links, which are directly proportional to collagen age. After 6 weeks, there is no measurable increase in the net collagen content. However, synthesis and turnover are ongoing for life. Historical accounts of sailors with scurvy (with impaired collagen production) who experienced reopening of previously healed wounds illustrate this fact. Tensile strength correlates with the total collagen content for approximately the first 3 weeks of wound healing. At 3 weeks, the tensile strength of the skin is 30% of normal. After this time, there is a much slower increase in the content of collagen until it plateaus at about 6 weeks. Nevertheless, tensile strength continues to increase because of intermolecular bonding in collagen and changes in the physical arrangement of collagen fibers. Although the most rapid increase in tensile strength occurs during the first 6 weeks of healing, there is a slow gain for at least 2 years. Its ultimate strength, however, never equals that of the unwounded tissue, with a level of just 80% of the original skin strength being reached. Tensile strength is measured as the load capacity per unit area. It may be differentiated from burst strength, which is the force required to break a wound (independent of its area). For example, in wounds of the face and back, burst strength is different because of differences in skin thickness, even though tensile strength may be similar. Corticosteroids affect wound healing by inhibiting fibroblast proliferation and epithelialization. The latter effect can be reversed by the administration of vitamin A.

Ref.: 1–3, 6

2. A 34-year-old man sustained a gunshot wound to his abdomen that necessitated exploratory laparotomy and small bowel resection. Two weeks after the initial operation, he was reexplored for a large intraabdominal abscess. Which of the following will result in the most rapid gain in strength of the new incision?
   A. A separate transverse incision is made.
   B. The midline scar is excised with a 1-cm margin.
   C. The midline incision is reopened without excision of the scar.
   D. The midline incision is left to heal by secondary intention.
   E. The rate of gain in strength is not affected by the incision technique.

ANSWER: C

COMMENTS: When a normally healing wound is disrupted after approximately the fifth day and then reclosed, the return of wound strength is more rapid than that with primary healing. This is termed the secondary healing effect and appears to be caused by the elimination of the lag phase present in normal primary healing. If the skin edges more than about 7 mm around the initial wound are excised, the resulting incision is through essentially uninjured tissue, so accelerated secondary healing does not occur.

Ref.: 2, 3, 6

3. A 29-year-old black woman is scheduled for incision and drainage of a breast abscess that has recurred three times despite ultrasound-guided needle drainage. The patient has a history of keloid formation and is concerned about an unsightly scar on her breast. Which of the following statements concerning wound healing is true?
   A. Keloids contain an overabundance of fibroblasts.
   B. A hypertrophic scar extends beyond the boundaries of the original wound.
   C. Improvement is usually seen with keloid excision followed by intralesional steroid injection.
   D. An incision placed perpendicular to the lines of natural skin tension will result in the least obvious scar.
   E. Hypertrophic scars occur most commonly on the lower extremities.

ANSWER: C

COMMENTS: Keloids are caused by an imbalance between collagen production and degradation. The result is a scar that extends beyond the boundaries of the original wound. The absolute number of fibroblasts is not increased. Treatment of keloids is difficult. There is often some improvement with excision and intralesional steroid injection. If this technique is not successful, excision and radiation treatment can be used. Hypertrophic scars contain an overabundance of collagen, but the dimensions of the scar are confined to the boundaries of the original wound. Hypertrophic scars are often seen in the upper part of the torso and across flexor surfaces. Scar formation is affected by multiple factors, including the patient's genetic makeup, wound location, age, nutritional status, infection, tension, and surgical technique. In planning for surgical incisions, an effort to parallel natural tension lines will promote improved wound healing.

Ref.: 2, 3, 6

4. A 30-year-old man is scheduled for definitive management of his open wounds after undergoing embolectomy and fasciotomies on his left lower extremity. Which of the following statements is true regarding the use of split- and full-thickness skin grafts?

A. A split-thickness skin graft undergoes approximately 40% shrinkage of its surface area immediately after harvesting.

B. A full-thickness skin graft undergoes approximately 10% shrinkage of its surface area immediately after harvesting.

C. Secondary contraction is more likely to occur after adequate healing of a full-thickness skin graft than after adequate healing of a split-thickness skin graft.

D. Sensation usually returns to areas that have undergone skin grafting.

E. Skin grafts may be exposed to moderate amounts of sunlight without changing pigmentation.

ANSWER: D

COMMENTS: Skin grafts are considered to be full thickness when they are harvested at the dermal–subcutaneous junction. Split-thickness skin grafts are those that contain epidermis and variable partial thicknesses of the underlying dermis. They are usually 0.018 to 0.060 inch in thickness. Cells from epidermal appendages deep to the plane of graft harvest resurface on the donor site of a split-thickness skin graft in approximately 1 to 3 weeks, depending on the depth. The donor site requires a moist environment to promote epithelialization, and such an environment is maintained by using polyurethane or hydrocolloid dressings. Because a full-thickness graft removes all epidermal appendages, the defects must be closed primarily. When a skin graft is harvested, there is immediate shrinkage of the surface area of the graft. This process, known as primary contraction, is due to recoil of the elastic fibers of the dermis. The thicker the skin graft, the greater the immediate shrinkage, with full-thickness grafts shrinking by approximately 40% of their initial surface area and split-thickness grafts shrinking by approximately 10% of their initial surface area. Shrinkage must be considered when planning the amount of skin to harvest for covering a given wound size. Secondary contraction occurs when contractile myofibroblasts in the bed of a granulating wound interact with collagen fibers to cause a decrease in the wound's surface area. Secondary contraction is greater in wounds covered with split-thickness grafts than in those covered with full-thickness grafts. The amount of secondary contracture is inversely proportional to the amount of dermis included in the graft rather than the absolute thickness of the graft. Dermal elements hasten the displacement of myofibroblasts from the wound bed.

Sensation may return to areas that have been grafted if the bed is suitable and not significantly scarred. Although sensation is not completely normal, it is usually adequate for protection. This process begins at about 10 weeks and is maximal at 2 years. Skin grafts appear to be more sensitive than the normal surrounding skin to melanocyte stimulation during exposure to ultraviolet sunlight. Early exposure to sunlight after grafting may lead to permanently increased pigmentation of the graft and should be avoided. Dermabrasion or the application of hydroquinones may be beneficial in reducing this pigmentation.

Ref.: 2, 3, 6

5. A 21-year-old graduate student has a large hypertrophic scar on the lower part of her face. The patient had sustained a laceration on her face 2 years previously after hitting her face on the side of a swimming pool. Which of the following statements regarding scar revision is true?

A. Scar maturation refers to the change in size of the wound in the first 1 to 2 months.

B. Scar revision should have been performed in the first 3 months after injury to minimize fibrosis.

C. Revision should be performed earlier in children than in adults.

D. It corrects undesirable pigmentation.

E. Scar revision should be delayed for approximately 1 year to allow maturation.

ANSWER: E

COMMENTS: Changes in pliability, pigmentation, and configuration of a scar are known as scar maturation. This process continues for many months after an incision; therefore it is generally recommended that revision not be carried out for approximately 12 to 18 months because natural improvement can be anticipated within this period. In general, scar maturation occurs more rapidly in adults than in children. Most erythematous scars show little improvement after revision; therefore scar revision should not be undertaken for correction of undesirable scar color alone.

Ref.: 2, 3, 6

6. A 68-year-old diabetic man undergoes a below-knee amputation. The patient's postoperative course is complicated by severe depression and anorexia. Before discharge, the patient is started on a multivitamin regimen. Which of the following statements regarding wound healing is true?

A. Vitamin A is needed for hydroxylation of lysine and proline in collagen synthesis.

B. High doses of vitamin C improve wound healing.

C. Vitamin E is involved in the stimulation of fibroplasia, collagen cross-linking, and epithelialization.

D. Zinc deficiency results in delayed early wound healing.

E. Iron deficiency has been linked to defects in long-term wound remodeling.

ANSWER: D

COMMENTS: Vitamin A is involved in the stimulation of fibroplasia and epithelialization. Although there has been no conclusive evidence of its efficacy in humans, in animal studies vitamin A has been shown to reverse the inhibitory effects of glucocorticoids in the inflammatory phase of wound healing and epithelialization.

Vitamin C is a necessary cofactor in the hydroxylation and cross-linking of lysine and proline in collagen synthesis. Deficiencies in vitamin C (scurvy) can lead to the production of inadequately hydroxylated collagen, which either degrades rapidly or never forms proper cross-links. Doses higher than physiologic doses do not improve wound healing. Vitamin E is applied to wounds and incisions by many patients, but there is no evidence to support the role of vitamin E in wound healing. Large doses of vitamin E have been found to inhibit wound healing. Zinc is a necessary cofactor of RNA and DNA polymerase, and deficiencies have been linked to poor early wound healing. Iron (specifically, the ferrous iron) is necessary for converting hydroxyproline to proline. However, chronic anemia and iron deficiency have not been linked to delayed or impaired wound healing.

Ref.: 2, 3, 6

7. Which of the following statements regarding wound epithelialization is true?

A. Integrins act as a key modulator of the interaction between epithelial cells and the surrounding environment.

B. Structural support and attachment between the epidermis and dermis are provided by tight cell junctions.

C. Early tensile strength of the wound is a direct result of collagen deposition.

D. A reepithelialized wound develops hair follicles and sweat glands like those seen in the normal skin.

E. Contact inhibition can prevent collagen deposition and result in a chronic (nonhealing) wound.

ANSWER: A

COMMENTS: Migration of epithelial cells is one of the earliest events in wound healing. Shortly after injury and during the inflammatory phase, basal epithelial cells begin to multiply and migrate across the defect, with fibrin strands being used as the support structure. Integrins are the main cellular receptors involved in epithelial migration; they act as sensors and integrators between the extracellular matrix and the epithelial cell cytoskeleton. Tight junctions within the epithelium contribute to its impermeability, whereas the basement membrane contributes to structural support and attachment of the epidermis to the dermis. Surgical incisions seal rather promptly and after 24 h are protected from the external environment. Early tensile strength is a result of blood vessel ingrowth, epithelialization, and protein aggregation. After covering the wound, the epithelial cells keratinize. The reepithelialized wound has no sweat glands or hair follicles, which distinguishes it from the normal skin. Control of the cellular process during wound epithelialization is not completely understood, but it appears to be regulated in part by contact inhibition, with growth being arrested when two or more similar cells come into surface contact. Derangements in the control of this process can result in epidermoid malignancy. Malignancy is more frequently observed in wounds resulting from ionizing radiation or chemical injury, but it can occur in any wound when the healing process has been chronically disrupted. For example, squamous cell carcinoma may develop in patients with chronic burn wounds or osteomyelitis (Marjolin's ulcer).

Ref.: 2, 4–6

8. In DNA replication, what type of mutation is specifically associated with the generation of a stop codon?

A. Point mutation

B. Missense mutation

C. Nonsense mutation

D. Frameshift mutation

E. Neutral mutation

ANSWER: C

COMMENTS: A change in a single base pair is known as a point mutation. A single amino acid change resulting from a point mutation is known as a missense mutation. A missense mutation may cause changes in the structure of the protein that lead to altered biologic activity. Nonsense mutations occur if a point mutation results in the replacement of an amino acid codon with a stop codon. Nonsense mutations lead to premature termination of translation and often result in the loss of encoded protein. Frameshift mutations occur when a few base pairs are added or deleted and lead to the introduction of unrelated amino acids or stop codons. A neutral mutation occurs when the change results in the substitution of a different but chemically similar amino acid. Frequently, the amino acids are similar enough that little or no change occurs in the resultant protein.

Ref.: 7

9. Which of the following is correct regarding cell signaling?

A. Cytokines are exclusively peptide mediators.

B. Autocrine mediators are secreted by a cell and act on adjacent cells of a different type.

C. Cytokines are usually produced by cells specialized for only that purpose.

D. The effects of hormones are generally local rather than global.

E. Growth factors are frequently mediated by second messenger systems such as diacylglycerol (DAG) and cyclic adenosine monophosphate (cAMP).

ANSWER: E

COMMENTS: Cytokines are proteins, glycoproteins, or peptides that bind to target cell surface receptors to stimulate a cellular response. They are important mediators of wound healing. Cytokines can reach target cells by paracrine, autocrine, or intracrine routes. Paracrine mediators are produced by one cell and act on an adjacent target cell. Autocrine mediators are secreted by a cell and act on cell surface receptors on the same cell. Intracrine mediators act within a single cell. Hormones are released by cells and act on a distant target (endocrine route). Although the distinction between cytokines and hormones has blurred, in general, hormones are secreted from specialized glands (e.g., insulin, parathyroid hormone) and cytokines are secreted by a wide variety of cell types. Hormones typically induce body-wide effects, whereas the effects of cytokines may be more localized (e.g., wound healing at the site of an injury). Generally, growth factors are named according to their tissue of origin or their originally discovered action. Growth factors interact with specific membrane receptors to initiate a series of events that ultimately lead to stimulation of cell growth, proliferation, or differentiation. The intermediate events activate a variety of second messenger systems mediated by agents such as inositol 1,4,5-triphosphate (IP_3), DAG, and cAMP.

Ref.: 7–9

10. A 25-year-old man presents to the office with complaints of contracture of his left index finger after a burn injury. Which of the following statements is true about growth factors?

A. Epidermal growth factor (EGF) stimulates the production of collagen.

B. Vascular endothelial growth factor (VEGF) and platelet-derived growth factor (PDGF) both stimulate angiogenesis by binding to a common receptor.

C. Fibroblast growth factor (FGF) stimulates wound contraction.

D. Transforming growth factor-β (TGF-β) is stored in endothelial cells.

E. Tumor necrosis factor-α (TNF-α) inhibits angiogenesis.

ANSWER: C

COMMENTS: EGF was the first cytokine described. It is a potent mitogen for epithelial cells, endothelial cells, and fibroblasts. EGF stimulates the synthesis of fibronectin, angiogenesis, and collagenase activity. PDGF is released from the alpha granules of platelets and is responsible for the stimulation of neutrophils and macrophages and for increasing the production of TGF-β. PDGF is a mitogen and chemotactic agent for fibroblasts and smooth muscle cells and stimulates angiogenesis, collagen synthesis, and collagenase activity. VEGF is similar to PDGF but does not bind to the same receptors. VEGF is mitogenic for endothelial cells. Its role in promoting angiogenesis has led to an interest in anti-VEGF therapies for cancer. FGF has acidic and basic forms whose actions are identical but whose strengths differ (basic FGF is 10 times stronger than acidic FGF). FGF is mitogenic for endothelial cells, fibroblasts, keratinocytes, and myoblasts; stimulates wound contraction and epithelialization; and induces the production of collagen, fibronectin, and proteoglycans. It is an important mediator of angiogenesis. TGF-β is released from the alpha granules of platelets and has been shown to regulate its own production in an autocrine manner. TGF-β stimulates fibroblast proliferation and the production of proteoglycans, collagen, and fibrin. It is an important mediator of fibrosis. Administration of TGF-β has been suggested as an approach to reduce scarring and reverse the inhibition of wound healing by glucocorticoids. TNF-α is a mitogen for fibroblasts and is produced by macrophages. It stimulates angiogenesis and the synthesis of collagen and collagenase.

Ref.: 3, 6, 10, 11

11. An 85-year-old nursing home patient is found to have a worsening stage III sacral pressure ulcer. The ulcer is debrided and tissue for culture obtained. Tissue cultures reveal 10^8 organisms per gram of tissue after operative debridement. What is the next most appropriate step in the management of the patient's wound?

A. Muscle flap coverage

B. Wound vacuum-assisted closure (VAC)

C. Intravenous antibiotics

D. Repeat debridement

E. Debridement with immediate application of a split-thickness skin graft

ANSWER: D

COMMENTS: The National Pressure Ulcer Advisory Panel has recommended a staging system for pressure sores that is useful in planning treatment. Stage I is represented by the presence of nonblanching erythema of intact skin. Stage II is characterized by partial-thickness skin loss involving the epidermis or dermis. Clinically, the ulcer is manifested as a blister, abrasion, or shallow crater. Stage III is full-thickness skin loss with involvement of the underlying subcutaneous tissue. Stage III wounds may extend down to but not through the underlying fascia. Stage IV represents full-thickness skin loss with extensive destruction or tissue necrosis of underlying structures, which may include muscle and bone. Studies have shown that wounds with quantitative cultures revealing more than 10^6 organisms per gram of tissue that undergo reconstruction with skin or even muscle flaps have a significantly greater risk for complications, including infection, accumulation of fluid, and wound dehiscence. Similarly, a skin graft is unlikely to survive in an environment with such a high bacterial inoculate. Negative-pressure wound therapy, such as with the wound VAC system, involves the use of a sponge and an occlusive dressing connected to a suction apparatus in a closed system. In patients with large wounds, a wound VAC may serve as a bridge to reduce the wound size for definitive reconstruction. It has been shown to be effective in reducing wound edema, controlling wound drainage, encouraging diminution of wound size, and facilitating the formation of granulation tissue. Although studies have shown that wound VAC therapy may reduce bacterial counts over time, the most appropriate management of such patients is repeat debridement of the wound. Intravenous antibiotics may be recommended to treat the underlying osteomyelitis.

Ref.: 2, 3, 6, 12

12. A 45-year-old woman undergoes bilateral transverse rectus abdominis muscle (TRAM) breast reconstruction after modified radical mastectomy. The patient is scheduled for postoperative radiation therapy and is concerned that this will affect her wound-healing ability. Which of the following statements regarding wound healing in this patient is true?

A. Denervation has a profound effect on wound contraction and epithelialization.

B. A bacterial count of 1000 organisms per square centimeter retards wound healing.

C. Chemotherapy beginning 10 to 14 days after primary wound closure has little effect on the final status of a wound.

D. Tissue ischemia is the main component of tissue damage after irradiation.

E. Postoperative radiation therapy should be delayed for at least 4 to 6 months after surgery to decrease the incidence of wound complications.

ANSWER: C

COMMENTS: Denervation has no effect on wound contraction or epithelialization. Flap wounds in paraplegics heal satisfactorily when other factors, such as nutrition and temperature, are controlled. Subinfectious bacterial levels appear to accelerate wound healing and the formation of granulation tissue. However, when the level reaches 10^6 organisms per square centimeter of wound, healing is delayed because of decreased tissue oxygen pressure, increased collagenolysis, and a prolonged inflammatory phase. Various chemotherapeutic agents affect wound healing. Most antimetabolic agents (e.g., 5-fluorouracil) do not delay wound healing, although agents such as doxorubicin have been shown to delay wound healing. When chemotherapy begins 10 to 14 days after wound closure, little effect is noted on its final status despite a demonstrable early retardation in the wound strength. Tissue ischemia may not be the primary factor involved in chronic wound-healing problems associated with irradiation. Such problems are most likely related to changes within the nuclei and concomitant cytoplasmic malformation. To decrease wound complications, it is usual to delay surgery until at least 3 to 4 weeks after full-dose irradiation and to avoid radiation therapy for at least 3 to 4 weeks after surgery.

Ref.: 2–4, 6, 13

13. A 46-year-old man is evaluated shortly after undergoing radiation therapy and chemotherapy for primary laryngeal cancer. He also gives a history of long-term steroid use for rheumatoid arthritis. The patient complains of a chronic, nonhealing wound on his neck, just over his right clavicular head. Which statement regarding the treatment of this wound is true?

A. The wound should be treated with compression dressings.

B. The wound should be treated with injected steroids.

C. The patient should start taking vitamin A, and the wound should bc covered with antimicrobial dressings.

D. The patient should start taking vitamin C, and the wound should be kept open to air.

E. The wound should be excised and a skin graft applied.

ANSWER: C

COMMENTS: Radiation results in progressive endarteritis obliterans and microvascular damage to the skin, which leads to skin ischemia and fibrotic interstitial changes. This leaves wounds in the skin particularly prone to infection. The use of antimicrobial dressings capable of maintaining a moist environment is ideal for these wounds. Research also supports the use of hyperbaric oxygen and growth factors to promote wound healing. Patients taking steroids should receive daily vitamin A supplements. Wounds in these patients show decreased rates of angiogenesis, collagen deposition, and cellular proliferation. Wounds should be kept free of bacterial contamination.

Ref.: 11, 14

14. A 25-year-old ballet dancer with a history of anorexia nervosa arrives at the emergency department with right lower quadrant pain. After an appendectomy, a wound infection at the surgical site requires debridement. The patient is placed on an antibiotic regimen, and the wound is packed with wet-to-dry dressings. Regarding wound healing and malnutrition, which of the following statements is true?

A. Hypoproteinemia leads to decreased levels of arginine and glutamine, which are essential in wound healing.

B. Cell membranes rapidly become dehydrated in the absence of vitamin E, resulting in delayed wound healing.

C. Zinc is essential to the fibroblast's ability to cross-link collagen.

D. Vitamin D serves an immunomodulatory role in wound healing.

E. The patient should be treated with high-dose vitamin C, vitamin A, and zinc.

ANSWER: D

COMMENTS: Adequate amounts of protein, carbohydrates, fatty acids, and vitamins are essential for wound healing. Hypoproteinemia results in decreased delivery of the essential amino acids used in the synthesis of collagen. Carbohydrates and fats provide energy for wound healing, and in their absence, proteins are rapidly broken down. Fatty acids are vital components of cell membranes. Vitamin C is a cofactor for hydroxylation of lysine and proline during collagen synthesis, and its deficiency leads to decreased collagen cross-linking by fibroblasts. Vitamin C is also effective in providing resistance to infection. Vitamin A is essential for normal epithelialization, proteoglycan synthesis, and enhanced immune function. Vitamin D is required for normal calcium metabolism, but it is also involved in promoting immune function in the skin. Vitamin E has not been shown to play a role in wound healing. Zinc deficiency leads to a deficient formation of granulation tissue and inhibition of cellular proliferation. Increased administration of vitamins and minerals does not accelerate wound healing and often has a deleterious effect.

Ref.: 2, 15

15. Which of the following statements regarding second messenger systems is true?

A. Most receptor proteins (such as G proteins) are completely extracellular.

B. Both the "first messenger" and "second messenger" mediators of cell signaling function within the cell cytoplasm.

C. Adenylate cyclase stimulates the conversion of cAMP to adenosine triphosphate (ATP).

D. IP_3 generally increases cytoplasmic calcium concentrations.

E. IP_3 and DAG together lead to inactivation of protein kinase C.

ANSWER: D

COMMENTS: The thyrotropin (TSH) receptor is a $G_{\alpha s}$ receptor found mainly on the surface of thyroid follicular cells. When activated, it stimulates increased production of thyroxine (T_4) and triiodothyronine (T_3).

Several families of receptor proteins have been identified. The most common is the G protein (guanine nucleotide–binding protein) family, a subset of guanosine triphosphatase (GTPase) enzymes. All G protein–coupled receptors have characteristic seven transmembrane domains. Binding of an extracellular ligand causes a conformational change in the receptor that allows it to exchange guanosine diphosphate (GDP) for guanosine triphosphate (GTP) on the intracellular portion of the G protein. The intracellular portion of the "large" (heterotrimeric) G protein–coupled receptor consists of three subunits, G_α, G_β, and G_γ. Other "small" (monomeric) G protein receptors have only a homologue of the G_α portion. There are several important subsets of the "large" G protein receptors, and they are classified according to the specific intracellular pathway that is activated.

$G_{\alpha s}$ stimulates membrane-associated adenylate cyclase to produce cAMP from ATP. cAMP is a second messenger that activates protein kinase A, which results in the phosphorylation of downstream targets. $G_{\alpha s}$ ligands include adrenocorticotropic hormone (ACTH), calcitonin, glucagon, histamine (H_2), TSH, and many others. $G_{\alpha i}$ inhibits the production of cAMP from ATP. $G_{\alpha i}$ ligands include acetylcholine (M_2 and M_4), dopamine (D_2, D_3, and D_4), and histamine (H_3 and H_4). $G_{\alpha q}$ activates phospholipase C, which cleaves phosphatidylinositol 4,5-bisphosphate (PIP_2) into IP_3 and DAG. IP_3 mediates the release of calcium from intracellular reservoirs, such as the endoplasmic reticulum (ER), sarcoplasmic reticulum (SR) in muscle, and mitochondria. IP_3 and DAG together work to activate protein kinase C, which can modulate membrane permeability and activate gene transcription. $G_{\alpha q}$ ligands include histamine (H_1), serotonin (5-HT_2), and muscarinic receptors.

The most well-known "small" G protein receptors are the Ras family GTPases. The Ras receptors influence a wide variety of processes in the cell, including growth, cellular differentiation, and cell movement.

Ref.: 7, 8, 16

16. Inflammatory breast cancer is diagnosed in a 36-year-old woman. A decision is made to treat the patient with radiation, along with paclitaxel and doxorubicin. Which of the following statements regarding cellular motility and contractility is true?

A. Actin fibers are found mainly in muscle cells.

B. The interactions between actin and myosin that underlie the contraction of skeletal muscle require calcium but not ATP.

C. Intermediate filaments extend from the centrosome to the nucleus.

D. The proteins kinesin and dynein are required for directional transport of cellular components along the microtubules.

E. The microtubules used to form the spindle apparatus are synthesized de novo before each mitosis.

ANSWER: D

COMMENTS: The cytoskeleton provides the structural framework for the cell. It is composed of three main types of protein polymers: actin filaments, intermediate filaments, and microtubules. Actin filaments are found in nearly all types of cells. They form a cortical layer beneath the plasma membrane of most cells, the stress fibers of fibroblasts, and the cytoskeleton of microvilli of intestinal epithelial cells. In muscle cells, the interaction between the heads of myosin (thick filaments) and actin (thin filaments) requires hydrolysis of ATP to separate the filaments at the end of the power stroke. Calcium and troponin C (an actin-associated protein) are also required to expose the binding site for myosin on the actin filament. Intermediate filaments are a heterogeneous group of proteins that extend from the nucleus to the cell surface. They interact with other cytoskeletal filaments and binding proteins to produce their effects.

Microtubules arise from the centrosome, with the cell's microtubule-organizing center being located near the nucleus. Microtubules are in a constant dynamic equilibrium between assembly and disassembly. Movement of cellular components, such as vacuoles, along the microtubules requires ATP and either of two associated proteins: kinesin for movement away from the centrosome and dynein for movement toward it. Cilia and flagella contain columns of doublet microtubules in a 9–2 arrangement (nine doublets in a circle surrounding two central doublets). Movement is accomplished when the doublets slide along each other in a process mediated by dynein and fueled by hydrolysis of ATP. Microtubules also play an important role in cell division. Assembly of the mitotic spindle involves replication and splitting of the microtubule-organizing center into the two spindle poles and reorganization of the cytoskeletal microtubules to form the spindle apparatus.

Ref.: 8, 16

17. Regarding chemotherapeutic agents, which of the following statements is true?

A. Paclitaxel is a manmade taxane first manufactured in the polycarbon industry.

B. Taxanes unwind DNA thus preventing transcription.

C. Vinca alkaloids inhibit cell division by disrupting the mitotic spindle.

D. Doxirubicin intercalates between DNA base pairs thus disrupting transcription.

E. Taxanes impair the progression of topoisomerase ii.

ANSWER: C

COMMENTS: Taxanes function as mitotic inhibitors by inhibiting depolymerization of the mitotic spindle, which results in a "frozen" mitosis. Paclitaxel is a natural taxane that prevents depolymerization of cellular microtubules. The vinca alkaloids (e.g., vinblastine, vincristine) also inhibit cell division but by disrupting the mitotic spindle. Doxorubicin (Adriamycin) intercalates between DNA base pairs and impairs the progression of topoisomerase ii, which unwinds DNA for transcription.

Ref.: 8, 16

18. A 27-year-old woman sustains an incomplete T10 spinal cord injury after falling off a horse. The patient is given 30 mg/kg of methylprednisolone. Which of the following is true regarding steroid hormones and their receptors?

A. Steroid hormones are synthesized from proteins.

B. In the bloodstream, steroid hormones often dimerize to facilitate transport.

C. Steroid hormone receptors are found only in the cytoplasm.

D. Heat shock proteins (HSPs) are usually associated with cytosolic steroid hormone receptors.

E. Binding of the steroid hormone to a receptor induces a second messenger cascade to alter cellular metabolism.

ANSWER: D

COMMENTS: Steroid hormones are synthesized from cholesterol. Their lipophilic nature allows them to cross cell membranes easily. Steroid hormones can be divided into five groups based on their receptors: glucocorticoids, mineralocorticoids, androgens, estrogens, and progestogens. In the bloodstream, steroid hormones are generally bound to specific carrier proteins such as sex hormone–binding globulin or corticosteroid-binding globulin. Receptors for steroid hormones are most commonly located in the cytosol, although they are also found in the nucleus and on the cell membrane. After binding to the steroid hormone, steroid receptors often dimerize. For many cytosolic steroid receptors, binding of the ligand induces a conformational change and releases HSPs. Nuclear steroid receptors are not generally associated with HSPs. HSPs themselves have several roles, including functioning as intracellular chaperones for other proteins, serving as transcription factors, and facilitating antigen binding. They may also serve as targets for therapeutics. Ultimately, the activated steroid receptor must enter the nucleus to serve as a transcription factor for augmentation or suppression of the expression of particular genes. The resulting messenger RNA leaves the nucleus for the ribosomes, where it is translated to produce specific proteins.

Ref.: 16

19. A 55-year-old man with a history of hepatitis C cirrhosis has complaints of nausea, fever, and progressive lethargy. Part of his evaluation includes an assessment of his hepatitis C viral load. Which of the following tests would be most useful in assessing his hepatitis C viral load?

A. Western blot

B. Gel electrophoresis

C. Fluorescence microscopy
D. Polymerase chain reaction (PCR)
E. Expression cloning

ANSWER: D

COMMENTS: Western blot is a technique used to detect specific proteins in a sample. An antibody to the protein of interest is used as a probe. Gel electrophoresis is a method for separating proteins or nucleic acids according to their size, mass, or composition. It is based on the differential rate of movement of the molecules of interest through a gel when an electric field is applied. PCR is a technique by which DNA may be massively amplified. Primers or oligonucleotides are synthesized to complement one strand of the DNA to be amplified. Amplification involves three temperature-cycled steps: (1) heating for separation (denaturation) of the double-helix structure into two single strands, (2) cooling for hybridization of each single strand with its primer (annealing), and (3) heating for DNA synthesis (elongation). The steps are repeated with exponential amplification of the DNA of interest. When RNA is used, reverse transcriptase is employed initially to transcribe the RNA to DNA before amplification. Quantitative PCR can be used in real time to measure the starting concentration of DNA or RNA in a sample, for example, the amount of hepatitis C RNA in a blood sample. With expression cloning, DNA coding for a protein of interest is cloned into a plasmid (extrachromosomal DNA molecule) that can be inserted into a bacterial or animal cell. The cell expresses the protein, which allows the production of sufficient amounts for study. Fluorescence microscopy is performed by labeling a component of interest in a sample with a molecule that absorbs light at one wavelength and emits at another (fluorescence).

Ref.: 16

20. A 56-year-old man underwent total thyroidectomy for papillary cancer. On the first postoperative day, the patient complains of circumoral tingling and muscle weakness. Which of the following statements regarding the electrical properties of cell membranes is not true?

A. Ions flow through hydrophilic channels formed by specific transmembrane proteins.
B. Lipids provide the ability to store electric charge (capacitance).
C. Active pumps maintain the ionic gradients necessary for a resting membrane potential.
D. Initiation of an action potential depends on voltage-gated channels.
E. Large numbers of sodium ions rush in during the initial phase of a nerve action potential.

ANSWER: E

COMMENTS: This patient has clinical findings associated with hypocalcemia. Specific transmembrane proteins provide hydrophilic paths for the ions (primarily Na^+, K^+, Ca^{2+}, and Cl^-) involved in electrical signaling. The amino acid sequence in specific regions of these proteins determines the selectivity for ions. The lipid component of the plasma membrane provides the capability of storing electric charge (capacitance), and the protein component provides the capability of resisting electric charge (resistance). Establishment and maintenance of a resting cell membrane potential require the separation of charge maintained by membrane capacitance, selective permeability of the plasma membrane, concentration gradients (intracellular versus extracellular) of the permeant ions, and impermeant intracellular anions. Active pumping by the sodium [sodium-potassium adenosine triphosphatase (Na^+, K^+-ATPase)] or calcium pumps generally maintains the ionic concentration gradients. Action potentials are regenerative (self-sustaining) transient depolarizations caused by the activation of voltage-sensitive sodium and potassium channels. Only a small volume of Na^+ is necessary to initiate an action potential. In fact, the amount of Na^+ that flows into a typical nerve cell during an action potential would change the intracellular Na^+ concentration by only a few parts per million.

Ref.: 16, 17

21. Which cell junction acts as a transmembrane linkage without an intracellular communication function?

A. Tight junction
B. Gap junction
C. Desmosome
D. Connexon
E. All of the above junctions have an intracellular communication function

ANSWER: C

COMMENTS: Any patient undergoing abdominal surgery will sustain a certain amount of capillary leakage. A proposed mechanism involves increased release of nitric oxide (NO), which causes vasodilation in precapillary cells and vasoconstriction in postcapillary cells, ultimately resulting in increased third-spacing of fluids. There are three major types of cell junctions: gap junctions, desmosomes, and tight junctions. Gap junctions are the most common and function primarily in intercellular communication and cellular adhesion. The connection between cells maintained by a gap junction is not particularly stable; it depends on a variety of complexes on each cell but not on connecting proteins (hence the term gap). Gap junctions serve as a pathway of permeability between cells for many different molecules weighing up to 1000 daltons. Connexons are protein assemblies formed by six identical protein subunits. They span the intercellular gap of the lipid bilayer to form an aqueous channel connecting the bilayers. Desmosomes function as cellular adhesion points but do not provide a pathway of communication. They are linked by filaments that function as transmembrane linkers, but desmosomes are not points of true cell fusion. Tight junctions, in contrast, are true points of cell fusion and are impermeable barriers. They prevent leakage of molecules across the epithelium in either direction. They also limit the movement of membrane proteins within the lipid bilayer of the plasma membrane and therefore maintain cells in a differentiated polar state.

Ref.: 16, 18

22. A 42-year-old woman with a history of end-stage renal disease is being evaluated for cadaveric renal transplantation. Which of the following statements regarding cell surface antigens is true?

A. Cell surface antigens are generally glycoproteins or glycolipids.
B. Histocompatibility antigens are not cell surface antigens.
C. ABO antigens are glycoproteins.
D. ABO antibodies are present at birth.
E. Human leukocyte antigen (HLA) has an extracellular hydrophobic region and an intracellular hydrophilic region.

ANSWER: A

COMMENTS: Cell surface antigens are generally glycoproteins or glycolipids that are anchored to either a protein or a lipid. Common examples include the ABO blood group antigens and the histocompatibility antigens. Antigens of the ABO system are glycolipids whose oligosaccharide portions are responsible for the antigenic properties. The structures of the blood group oligosaccharides occur commonly in nature and lead to the stimulation needed to produce anti-A or anti-B antibodies after a few months of life. HLA antigens are two-chain glycoproteins that are anchored in the cell membrane at the carboxyl terminal. These antigens contain an extracellular hydrophilic region, a transmembrane hydrophobic region, and an intracellular hydrophilic region. This transmembrane structure allows extracellular signals to be transmitted to the interior of the cell.

Ref.: 19

23. Regarding chemical messengers, which statement is true?

A. They depend on cell surface–bound proteins to exert their effect.

B. They are limited to intracellular receptors to exert their effect.

C. First messengers bind directly to DNA to begin the protein synthesis process.

D. Extracellular ligands are termed the "second messengers."

E. Extracellular ligands are termed the "first messengers."

ANSWER: E

COMMENTS: Chemical messengers can influence intracellular physiology via several mechanisms. Some ligands, such as acetylcholine (binding to the nicotinic cholinergic receptor) or norepinephrine (binding to the potassium channel in cardiac muscle), directly bind to ion channels in the cell membrane to alter their conductance. Some lipid-soluble messengers, such as steroid and thyroid hormones, enter the cell and bind to nuclear or cytoplasmic receptors, which then bind to DNA to increase transcription of selected mRNA. Many other extracellular messengers bind to the extracellular portion of transmembrane receptor proteins to trigger the release of intracellular mediators. The extracellular ligands are termed as the "first messenger," whereas the intracellular mediators are "second messengers." Examples of second messengers include IP_3, DAG, calcium, and cAMP.

Ref.: 18, 20

24. A 67-year-old man undergoes revascularization of his right lower extremity after sustaining thrombosis secondary to a popliteal artery aneurysm. Shortly after surgery, a compartment syndrome of the affected limb develops and is attributed to reperfusion injury. Research suggests that ER stress may be responsible for apoptosis after ischemia. Which of the following statements regarding the ER is not true?

A. Rough ER is a primary site of lipid synthesis.

B. Smooth ER plays an important role in the metabolism of drugs.

C. Ribosomes attached to the rough ER manufacture proteins for use within the cell.

D. SR is found mainly in epithelial cells.

E. SR plays an important role in gluconeogenesis.

ANSWER: B

COMMENTS: The ER is part of a network that includes mitochondria, lysosomes, microbodies, the Golgi complex, and the nuclear envelope. This network forms an intracellular circulatory system that allows vital substrates to reach the interior of the cell for transportation and assembly. There are two types of ER. Rough ER is coated with ribosomes and functions as the site of synthesis of membrane and secreted proteins. Other ribosomes that circulate freely in the cytoplasm synthesize proteins destined to remain within the cell. Smooth ER plays a major role in metabolic processes, including the synthesis of lipids and steroids, metabolism of carbohydrates (especially gluconeogenesis), drug detoxification, and molecular conjugation. Smooth ER contains the enzyme glucose-6-phosphatase, which converts glucose-6-phosphate to glucose during gluconeogenesis. Cells that synthesize large amounts of protein for export have abundant rough ER, whereas cells that produce steroids (e.g., those in the adrenal cortex) generally have smoother ER. The smooth ER is continuous with the nuclear envelope. The SR is a distinct type of smooth ER found in striated and smooth muscles. The SR contains large stores of calcium, which it sequesters and then releases when the cell is stimulated. The release of calcium from the SR plays a major role in excitation–contraction coupling, which allows muscle cells to convert an electric stimulus to a mechanical response.

Ref.: 18, 20

25. Which of the following statements regarding lysosomes is true?

A. Primary lysosomes usually contain extracellular material targeted for digestion.

B. Lysosomal enzymes work effectively in the acidic pH of the cytoplasm.

C. Serum levels of lysosomal acid phosphatases may have prognostic value in diseases such as prostate cancer.

D. Lysosomal storage diseases such as Tay-Sachs result from unregulated activity of lysosomal enzymes.

E. To better isolate their hydrolytic enzymes, lysosomes are resistant to fusion with other cell membranes.

ANSWER: C

COMMENTS: Lysosomes are membrane-bound organelles that contain acid hydrolases. Heterolysosomes are involved in the endocytosis and digestion of extracellular material, whereas autolysosomes are involved in digestion of the cell's own intracellular material. Primary lysosomes are formed by the addition of hydrolytic enzymes (from the rough ER) to endosomes from the Golgi complex. Combining a primary lysosome with a phagosome creates a phagolysosome. Lysosomal enzymes are hydrolases that are resistant to autolysis. They function best in the acidic milieu of the lysosome; the slightly alkaline pH of the surrounding cytosol helps protect the cell from injury if the lysosome leaks. Acid phosphatase is a marker enzyme for lysosomes. Different forms of acid phosphatases are found in lysosomes from various organs, and serum levels may be indicative of specific diseases (for example, prostatic acid phosphatase may have prognostic significance in prostate cancer).

One of the distinguishing characteristics of lysosomal membranes is their ability to fuse with other cell membranes. Lysosomal membranes have a high proportion of lipids in a micellar configuration, primarily because of the presence of the phospholipid lysolecithin. This increased micellar configuration facilitates fusion of the lysosome membrane with the phagosome membrane for digestion and with the plasma membrane for secretion. Steroids are thought to work partially by stabilizing lysosomal membranes, thereby inhibiting membrane fusion and enzyme release. Lysosomes may engage in autophagocytosis, which is thought to be important for cell turnover, cell remodeling, and tissue changes. Several lysosomal storage diseases, such as Tay-Sachs, Gaucher, and Pompe disease, are caused by inactive or missing lysosomal digestive proteins. These genetic diseases lead to the accumulation of normally degraded substrates within the cell.

Ref.: 18, 20

26. A 56-year-old man is transferred from the county jail with complaints of hemoptysis, fever, and chills. The patient had undergone left lower lobectomy 6 years ago for an isolated lung nodule. Chest radiography on admission shows a lesion in the left upper lobe that is concerning for tuberculosis. The cell wall of *Mycobacterium tuberculosis* prevents lysosomes from fusing with phagosomes, which contributes to its tendency to lead to granuloma formation. Which of the following statements regarding endocytosis is not true?

A. Phagocytosis refers to engulfment of particulate matter.

B. Pinocytosis refers to the engulfment of soluble material.

C. Only specialized cells of the immune system are capable of endocytosis.

D. Opsonins increase the likelihood of phagocytosis by binding to the antigen.

E. Antibodies and complement fragments can serve as opsonins.

ANSWER: C

COMMENTS: All cells are capable of endocytosis, which is the process of internalizing extracellular molecules by engulfing the molecule within the cell membrane. Pinocytosis (cell drinking) is the engulfment of soluble material. Phagocytosis (cell eating) is the process by which cells ingest solids. For cells of the immune system, such as macrophages, dendritic cells, and polymorphonuclear leukocytes, phagocytosis is particularly important in recognizing and combating pathogens. In phagocytosis the cell membrane surrounding the engulfed material pinches off and forms a vesicle called phagosome. The phagosome maintains the material separate from the cytosol of the cell. The phagosome fuses with a lysosome, which leads to degradation of the engulfed material. Degradation can be oxygen dependent (by the production of reactive oxygen species) or oxygen independent (generally by proteolytic enzymes and cationic proteins).

Typically, both the target (antigen) and the phagocyte are negatively charged. This limits their ability to come into close proximity. Opsonins are molecules that act to enhance phagocytosis. Opsonization occurs when antigens are bound by antibody or complement molecules (or both). Phagocytic cells express receptors (Fc, CR1) that bind opsonin molecules (antibody, C3b), which greatly increases the affinity of the phagocyte for the antigen. Phagocytosis is an unlikely event if the antigen is not opsonized.

Ref.: 7, 20

27. For tumors with a high mitotic index indicative of active growth, which portion of the cell cycle in the actively dividing cells is most sensitive to ionizing radiation?

A. S phase

B. M phase

C. G_1 phase

D. G_2 phase

E. All phases are equally radiosensitive.

ANSWER: B

COMMENTS: The primary mechanism by which ionizing radiation induces cell death is direct or indirect injury to DNA. Ionizing radiation can cause lethal damage (damage that cannot be repaired; for example, most double-strand DNA breaks) or sublethal damage (damage that can be repaired if conditions are correct; for example, most single-strand DNA breaks). Factors that increase the cell's ability to repair damage make it less sensitive to ionizing radiation. The cell division cycle is divided into four distinct phases. Replication of DNA occurs in the synthesis (S) phase, whereas nuclear division and cell fission occur in the mitotic (M) phase. The intervals between these two phases are called the gap (G) phases. Cells in the M phase (mitosis) have the least capability to repair sublethal damage and hence are the most radiation sensitive. Cells in the S phase have the most capability of repairing damage and consequently are the most radiation resistant. Resting cells (G_0) are less sensitive to radiation injury than cells that are actively dividing (and proceeding through the cell cycle). Cancer cells are generally less differentiated (with less ability to repair DNA damage) and more rapidly dividing than normal tissue. The fact that tumor cells are usually more sensitive to radiation than the surrounding normal tissue is an important determinant of the utility of radiation therapy.

Ref.: 21

28. Which of the following statements regarding oxidative phosphorylation and mitochondria is true?

A. Glycoproteins are transported into the mitochondrial matrix to facilitate oxidative phosphorylation.

B. The citric acid cycle takes place within the inner mitochondrial membrane.

C. Oxidative phosphorylation via ATP synthase converts adenosine diphosphate (ADP) to ATP.

D. Electrochemical (proton) gradients provide the energy to power chemosmotic production of ATP.

E. Mitochondrial DNA is almost exclusively paternally derived.

ANSWER: D

COMMENTS: Metabolic substrates such as fats, proteins, and glycoproteins are converted to fatty acids and pyruvate and transported into mitochondria. Within the mitochondrial matrix, they are metabolized by the citric acid (Krebs) cycle to produce the reduced forms of nicotinamide adenine dinucleotide (NADH) and flavin adenine dinucleotide ($FADH_2$). The reducing power of these substrates fuels transfer of electrons from electron donors to receptors as oxidative phosphorylation. The resultant high-energy electrons pass along the electron transport chain and release the energy used to move protons across the inner mitochondrial membrane to generate potential energy in the form of electrical and pH gradients. ATP synthase uses the energy obtained from allowing protons to flow down this gradient to synthesize ATP from ADP. This process is called chemosmosis. Three ATP molecules are generated for each mole of oxygen consumed. Mitochondrial DNA is transmitted only from the mother because sperm contains few mitochondria. During sepsis, inhibited mitochondrial function as a result of hypoxia or other mediators of sepsis has been postulated to contribute to organ injury through accelerated oxidant production and thus promotion of cell death.

Ref.: 22

29. A 26-year-old with a history of type 2 neurofibromatosis is scheduled to undergo resection of an acoustic neuroma. The *NF2* gene is located on the long arm of chromosome 22. Which of the following statements regarding chromosomes is not true?

A. The nucleus contains the entire cellular DNA.

B. Histones compact and organize the DNA strands.

C. Interactions between DNA and proteins expose specific genes and control their expression.

D. During mitosis, the spindle apparatus attaches to the chromosome at the centromere.

E. Telomeres maintain chromosomal length through the replication cycles.

ANSWER: A

COMMENTS: Chromosomes are formed by the combination of double-stranded helical DNA with histones and other proteins. The interactions between DNA and proteins stabilize the chromosomal structure. Most cellular DNA is located in the nucleus, although a small portion is found in the mitochondria. Each chromosomal double helix contains approximately 108 base pairs. There are several levels of organizational restructuring, from DNA and histones binding to form chromatin all the way to the complex folded structure of the chromosome itself. To express a gene, that portion of the chromosome must be unfolded and unwrapped to expose the DNA double helix. Gene expression is regulated by the binding of nonchromosomal proteins, called transcription factors, to specific regions of the DNA (enhancer and promoter sequences). Several distinct regions of chromosomes are identifiable: the origins of replication (sites of initiation of DNA synthesis), the centromere (site of spindle attachment during mitosis), and telomeres (specialized end structures that maintain the length of the chromosome through replication cycles).

Ref.: 23

30. Which enzyme is responsible for the catalysis of deoxynucleoside triphosphates into DNA?

A. DNA helicase

B. DNA ligase

C. DNA polymerase

D. DNA primase

E. All of the above

ANSWER: C

COMMENTS: DNA polymerases are enzymes that catalyze the assembly of deoxynucleoside triphosphates into DNA. There are several types of DNA polymerases. DNA polymerase III promotes DNA elongation by nucleotide linkage, whereas DNA polymerase I functions to fill gaps and repair DNA. DNA helicase is the enzyme involved in unwinding the double-stranded DNA into individual strands before replication, transcription, or repair. DNA primase catalyzes the formation of RNA primers used to initiate DNA synthesis. DNA ligase joins the DNA fragments generated by the degradation of RNA primers.

Ref.: 23

31. Which of the following statements regarding protein synthesis is not true?

A. Transcription of messenger RNA occurs in the nucleus.

B. Messenger RNA moves from the nucleus to the cytoplasm and attaches to free ribosomes in the cytoplasm.

C. The enzyme RNA polymerase catalyzes the transcription of messenger RNA from DNA.

D. Introns are placed into the DNA transcript by splicing.

E. Posttranslational processing includes glycosylation and enzymatic cleavage.

ANSWER: D

COMMENTS: The sequence of nucleotides in DNA determines the amino acid sequence of the protein. Protein synthesis involves (1) transcription of messenger RNA from the gene that codes for the protein, (2) translation of the messenger RNA into a protein, and (3) posttranslational processing of the protein, which may involve enzymatic cleavage or glycosylation of the protein. Transcription takes place in the nucleus, whereas translation and posttranslational processing occur in the rough ER, Golgi complex, or free ribosomes in the cytoplasm. Transcription of messenger RNA from DNA occurs by the assembly of complementary base pairs on the DNA template one nucleotide at a time. This step is catalyzed by the enzyme RNA polymerase. Eukaryotic genes are interrupted by noncoding regions called introns. Introns are removed from the RNA transcript by splicing. The resulting messenger RNA is moved to the cytoplasm in which it binds to ribosomes to begin translation. The initial step in protein synthesis is attachment of the messenger RNA to a ribosome that is preloaded with transfer RNA that recognizes the start codon (three bases) AUG and thus sets the reading frame for the translation. Subsequent binding of aminoacyl–transfer RNA to the ribosomes that match the three-nucleotide codons specifying each amino acid results in peptide synthesis as the ribosome moves along the messenger RNA molecule. The first portion of the protein that is synthesized is an amino-terminal leader called the signal peptide. At this stage, the ribosome becomes attached to the rough ER. As translation continues, the signal peptide is inserted into the rough ER membrane by another transmembrane protein and later cleaved as the peptide elongates.

Ref.: 24

32. Which of the following methods is most useful for determining the RNA content of a sample?

A. Southern blotting

B. Northern blotting

C. Western blotting

D. PCR

E. None of the above

ANSWER: B

COMMENTS: Blotting is a method used to study macromolecules (DNA, RNA, or proteins) separated by gel electrophoresis (usually by size) and transferred onto a carrier (technically, the transfer is the "blot"). The macromolecules can then be visualized by specific probes or staining methods. A Southern blot is used for detection of specific DNA sequences. A Northern blot performs the same function but for RNA or mRNA samples. A Western blot is used to detect specific proteins in a sample, with an antibody to the protein of interest being used as a probe. An Eastern blot is a modification of the Western blot technique that is used to detect posttranslational modification of proteins. There are several other modifications of the technique; for example, Southwestern blotting is used to detect DNA-binding proteins. The origin of the nomenclature is derived from the Southern blot, which is named after its inventor biologist Edwin Southern.

Ref.: 24

33. The three phases of wound healing, in order, are:

A. Inflammation, proliferation, and maturation

B. Inflammation, proliferation, and contraction

C. Eschar formation, inflammation, and maturation

D. Fibrous exudate, granulation, and epithelialization

E. Coagulation, granulation, and epithelialization

ANSWER: A

COMMENTS: Wound healing is broken down into three phases: inflammation, proliferation, and maturation. There are many events associated with these phases, and taken together, they describe a continuous process where many events occur simultaneously. The inflammatory phase starts immediately after the injury occurs and lasts up to 72 h. After the injury, there is a transient period (about 10 min) of vasoconstriction followed by active vasodilation. These events are mediated by substances released secondary to the local tissue injury. Vasoactive components such as histamine cause brief periods of vasodilation and increased vascular permeability. The kinins (bradykinin and kallidin) are released by the enzymatic action of kallikrein, which is formed after activation of the coagulation cascade. These components, in addition to those of the complement system, stimulate the release of prostaglandins (particularly PGE_1 and PGE_2), which work in concert to maintain more prolonged vessel permeability not only of capillaries but also of larger vessels. In addition, these substances, particularly the complement component C5a and platelet-derived factors such as PDGF, act as chemotactic stimuli for neutrophils to enter the wound. Although neutrophils can phagocytize bacteria from a wound, the results of studies involving clean wound healing show that healing can proceed normally without them. Monocytes, however, must be present for normal wound healing because in addition to their role in phagocytosis, they are required to trigger a normal fibroblast response. The later phases of wound healing include the proliferative or regenerative phase and the remodeling phase. The proliferative phase is marked by the appearance of fibroblasts in the wound, which leads to the formation of granulation tissue. The remodeling (maturation) phase involves an increase in wound strength secondary to collagen remodeling and lasts up to 1 year after the initial injury. The three main phases of wound healing may occur sequentially or simultaneously.

Ref.: 25

34. Which of the following statements regarding wound healing is true?

A. Granulation tissue results from the cross-linking of coagulation debris.

B. Fibroblasts migrate to the acute wound after the appearance of granulation tissue.

C. Myoepithelial cell–derived growth factors cause fibroblast differentiation.

D. It is during the proliferative phase that the scaffolding for tissue repair is laid.

E. Mucopolysaccharide levels peak 6 weeks after injury.

ANSWER: D

COMMENTS: After the acute effects of inflammation begin to resolve, the proliferative phase of healing begins. It is during this phase of wound healing that the scaffolding for tissue repair is created because of angiogenesis, fibroplasia, and epithelialization. The formation of granulation tissue characterizes this phase. Granulation tissue is composed of a capillary bed; fibroblasts; macrophages; and loosely arranged hyaluronic acid, collagen, and fibronectin. The collagen in the granulation tissue is produced by fibroblasts. The fibroblasts themselves dedifferentiate from nearby mesenchymal cells. The time taken by these cells to become collagen-producing fibroblasts is 3–5 days. This period is known as the lag phase. Tensile strength correlates with the total collagen content for approximately the first 3 weeks of wound healing. At 3 weeks, the tensile strength of the skin is 30% of the normal. It plateaus at about 6 weeks. Simultaneously, macrophages and platelets produce cytokines and growth factors that stimulate fibroblast production. Collagen synthesis peaks at 4 weeks and then enters a phase of collagen maturation that can continue for months. During the maturation phase, glycoprotein and mucopolysaccharide levels decrease and new capillaries regress and disappear.

Ref.: 25

35. How does von Willebrand factor VIII affect coagulation during the inflammatory phase of wound healing?

A. Von Willebrand factor causes platelets to adhere to intact endothelium.

B. Integrin receptors require von Willebrand factor as a coenzyme.

C. Von Willebrand factor stimulates megakaryocytes to produce platelets.

D. Platelet-collagen contact requires von Willebrand factor VIII.

E. Von Willebrand factor VIII facilitates collagen cross-linking.

ANSWER: D

COMMENTS: Platelets delivered to the wound perform several acts that result in platelet plug formation. The first act is adherence to damaged endothelium. This is mediated by a number of platelet and integrin receptors. Platelet activation requires contact with exposed type IV and V collagen from the damaged capillary endothelium. This initial contact requires von Willebrand factor VIII. The factor is synthesized in megakaryocytes and endothelial cells.

Ref.: 25

36. Regarding polymorphonucleocytes (PMN) and macrophages, which statement is true?

A. PMNs are essential for wound healing.

B. Macrophages are essential for wound healing.

C. Both PMNs and macrophages are essential for wound healing.

D. M1 macrophages predominate in the proliferative phase.

E. Macrophages are phenotypically stable.

ANSWER: B

COMMENTS: PMNs mediate wound inflammation but are not essential for wound healing. Macrophages are able to replace their antimicrobial role. Sterile wounds heal normally without PMNs. However, macrophages are crucial to wound healing. They appear 24 to 48 h after injury and are derived from migrating monocytes initially attracted to the wound.

The macrophage exhibits two different phenotypes, and they are differentiated by their method of activation. A macrophage stimulated by lipopolysaccharide INF gamma becomes an M1 macrophage. These macrophages release TMF-alpha, NO, and interleukin (IL)-6. M2 macrophages are activated by IL-4 and IL-13; they suppress inflammatory reactions and play a role in wound healing and angiogenesis. In the inflammatory phase of wound healing, M1 macrophages predominate. In the proliferative phase, M2 macrophages predominate.

***Ref.*:** 25

REFERENCES

1. Alarcon LH, Fink MP. Mediators of the inflammatory response. In: Townsend CM, Beauchamp RD, Evers BM, et al., eds. *Sabiston Textbook of Surgery: The Biological Basis of Modern Surgical Practice*. 18th ed. Philadelphia: WB Saunders; 2008.
2. Ethridge RT, Leong M, Phillips LG. Wound healing. In: Townsend CM, Beauchamp RD, Evers BM, et al., eds. *Sabiston Textbook of Surgery: The Biological Basis of Modern Surgical Practice*. 18th ed. Philadelphia: WB Saunders; 2008.
3. Fine NA, Mustoe TA. Wound healing. In: Mulholland MW, Lillemoe KD, Doherty GM, et al., eds. *Greenfield's Surgery: Scientific Principles and Practice*. 4th ed. Philadelphia: Lippincott Williams & Wilkins; 2006.
4. Simmons RL, Steel DL. *Basic Science Review for Surgeons*. Philadelphia: WB Saunders; 1992.
5. Gupta S, Lawrence WT. Wound healing normal and abnormal mechanisms and closure techniques. In: O'Leary JP, Tabuenca A, eds. *The Physiologic Basis of Surgery*. 4th ed. Philadelphia: Lippincott Williams & Wilkins; 2008.
6. Barbul A, Efron DT. Wound healing. In: Brunicardi FC, Andersen DK, Billiar TR, et al., eds. *Schwartz's Principles of Surgery*. 9th ed. New York: McGraw-Hill; 2010.
7. Ko TC, Evers BM. Molecular and cell biology. In: Townsend CM, Beauchamp RD, Evers BM, et al., eds. *Sabiston Textbook of Surgery: The Biological Basis of Modern Surgical Practice*. 18th ed. Philadelphia: WB Saunders; 2008.
8. Williams JA, Dawson DC. Cell structure and function. In: Mulholland MW, Lillemoe KD, Doherty GM, et al., eds. *Greenfield's Surgery: Scientific Principles and Practice*. 4th ed. Philadelphia: Lippincott Williams & Wilkins; 2006.
9. Rosengart MR, Billiar TR. Inflammation. In: Mulholland MW, Lillemoe KD, Doherty GM, et al., eds. *Greenfield's Surgery: Scientific Principles and Practice*. 4th ed. Philadelphia: Lippincott Williams & Wilkins; 2006.
10. Peacock Jr EE. Symposium on biological control of scar tissue. *Plast Reconstr Surg*. 1968;41:8–12.
11. Barbul A. Immune aspects of wound repair. *Clin Plast Surg*. 1990; 17:433–442.
12. Galiano RD, Mustoe TA. Wound care. In: Aston S, Seasley R, Thorne C, eds. *Grabb and Smith's Plastic Surgery*. 6th ed. Philadelphia: Lippincott-Raven; 2007.
13. Basson MD, Burney RE. Defective wound healing in patients with paraplegia and quadriplegia. *Surg Gynecol Obstet*. 1982;155:9–12.
14. Gurtner GC. Wound healing: normal and abnormal. In: Aston S, Seasley R, Thorne C, eds. *Grabb and Smith's Plastic Surgery*. 6th ed. Philadelphia: Lippincott-Raven; 2007.
15. Martindale RG, Zhou M. Nutrition and metabolism. In: O'Leary JP, Tabuenca A, eds. *The Physiologic Basis of Surgery*. 4th ed. Philadelphia: Lippincott Williams & Wilkins; 2008.
16. Reeves ME. Cell biology. In: O'Leary JP, Tabuenca A, eds. *The Physiologic Basis of Surgery*. 4th ed. Philadelphia: Lippincott Williams & Wilkins; 2008.
17. Transport across cell membranes. In: Lodish H, Berk A, Zipursky SL, et al., eds. *Molecular Cell Biology*. New York: Scientific American Books; 1999.
18. Biomembranes and the subcellular organization of eukaryotic cells. In: Lodish H, Berk A, Zipursky SL, et al., eds. *Molecular Cell Biology*. New York: Scientific American Books; 1999.
19. Protein sorting, organelle biogenesis and protein secretion. In: Lodish H, Berk A, Zipursky SL, et al., eds. *Molecular Cell Biology*. New York: Scientific American Books; 1999.
20. The dynamic cell. In: Lodish H, Berk A, Zipursky SL, et al., eds. *Molecular Cell Biology*. New York: Scientific American Books; 1999.
21. Radiosensitivity and cell age in the mitotic cycle. In: Hall EJ, Amato JG, eds. *Radiobiology for the Radiologist*. 6th ed. Philadelphia: Lippincott Williams & Wilkins; 2005.
22. Cellular energetics, glycolysis, aerobic oxidation and photosynthesis. In: Lodish H, Berk A, Zipursky SL, et al., eds. *Molecular Cell Biology*. New York: Scientific American Books; 1999.
23. DNA replication, repair and recombination. In: Lodish H, Berk A, Zipursky SL, et al., eds. *Molecular Cell Biology*. New York: Scientific American Books; 1999.
24. Recombinant DNA and genomics. In: Lodish H, Berk A, Zipursky SL, et al., eds. *Molecular Cell Biology*. New York: Scientific American Books; 1999.
25. Townsend C, Beauchamp RD, Evers BM, et al. Chapter 6. Wound Healing. In: *Sabiston Textbook of Surgery*. New York: Elsevier; 2016:130–162.

CHAPTER 3

HEMOSTASIS AND TRANSFUSION

Richard A. Jacobson, M.D., and Erin C. Farlow, M.D.

1. Which of the following is an antifibrinolytic agent used in regular clinical practice?
    A. Unfractionated heparin (UFH)
    B. Tranexamic acid (TXA)
    C. Protamine sulfate
    D. Tissue plasminogen activator (tPA)
    E. Plasminogen activator inhibitor-1 (PAI-1)

ANSWER: B

COMMENTS: This question aims to delineate the processes of clot formation and breakdown, or coagulation and fibrinolysis. Fibrinolysis is the process of active clot breakdown. The fibrinolytic system is regulated by activators and inhibitors of its principal protease plasminogen, the inactive form of active plasmin. Plasmin(ogen) activity becomes deranged in certain states such as major trauma and sepsis, both of which lead to hyperfibrinolysis, or excessive breakdown of newly formed clot, leading to excessive blood loss. This state has a similar presentation to, but is clinically and therapeutically distinct from, coagulopathy, which is a derangement in the ability to primarily form a clot.

UFH is a glycosaminoglycan used in clinical practice to promote the activity of the anticoagulant protein antithrombin III against thrombin and factor Xa. Its principal use is in therapeutic anticoagulation and venous thromboembolism (VTE) prophylaxis. Protamine sulfate is a protein that binds heparin and neutralizes its anticoagulant activity, often used to reverse supratherapeutic doses of UFH. Neither UFH nor protamine sulfate has a significant direct impact on fibrinolysis. tPA is a profibrinolytic agent sometimes used in the clinical management of acute vascular occlusion. It promotes intravascular clot breakdown, and its effect would be the opposite of what is desired in a hyperfibrinolytic state. PAI-1 is an endogenous antifibrinolytic protein that is not currently used in clinical practice.

TXA is an exogenous lysine analogue that competitively inhibits the conversion of plasminogen into active plasmin; thus it is antifibrinolytic. In trauma patients with hemodynamically significant hemorrhage, administration of TXA (1-g IV bolus followed by 1-g IV infusion over 8 h) within 3 h of injury has been shown to decrease the overall mortality and mortality secondary to bleeding without an increase in vascular occlusive events. There was no benefit from the administration of TXA beyond 3 h postinjury.

Ref.: 1, 2

2. Placement of an inferior vena cava (IVC) filter in patients with proximal lower extremity deep-vein thrombosis (DVT) is indicated in each of the following scenarios except:
    A. Known large esophageal varices
    B. Pulmonary embolus despite therapeutic anticoagulation
    C. High-risk sonographic appearance of the proximal DVT
    D. Recurrent unprovoked DVT
    E. Severe congestive heart failure

ANSWER: D

COMMENTS: Mesh filters placed percutaneously in the infrarenal IVC can prevent lower extremity venous thromboses from embolizing to the lungs. Use and complications of these filters have increased substantially over the last decade. While older model filters are permanent, more recently developed filters may be safely removed or left in place. Once a patient is safely anticoagulated, it is recommended that retrievable filters be removed. As a practical matter, retrieval rates in temporary filters are historically low and long-term filter placement is associated with complications such as filter migration, caval thrombosis, and IVC perforation. Indications for IVC filter placement include a proximal lower extremity DVT plus (1) any absolute contraindication to anticoagulation (A), (2) pulmonary embolism (PE) that occurrs while a patient is therapeutically anticoagulated (B), (3) high-risk sonographic appearance of the thrombus such as a free-floating leading edge or iliocaval DVT (relative indication), and (4) low cardiopulmonary reserve (relative indication), in which case PE could be hemodynamically catastrophic. IVC filter placement in patients without acute DVT, but a high risk of developing provoked DVT with absolute contraindications to anticoagulation, such as brain or spinal cord trauma, is a topic of active debate. In patients who may safely and effectively undergo conventional anticoagulation, IVC filter placement is of no benefit.

The first-line treatment of an unprovoked proximal vein (popliteal, femoral, or iliac) DVT is anticoagulation for 3 to 12 months unless otherwise contraindicated. Specific anticoagulation regimens vary by institution and clinical setting. Recurrent provoked DVT is treated with longer-term anticoagulation but is not an indication for IVC filter placement.

Ref.: 3–5

3. Dosing for therapeutic anticoagulation of which of the following modalities is least affected by renal impairment?
    A. Warfarin
    B. Low-molecular-weight heparin

C. UFH

D. Rivaroxaban (Xarelto)

E. Dabigatran (Pradaxa)

ANSWER: C

COMMENTS: Kidney disease in itself is a risk factor for both thrombotic and adverse bleeding events. Uremic patients demonstrate impaired platelet adhesion and aggregation that present as increased risk of clinical bleeding and laboratory elevation of bleeding time. These abnormalities are frequently correctable with the administration of desmopressin (DDAVP), which acts to increase the release of factor VIII:von Willebrand factor (vWF) from endothelial cells.

Therapeutic anticoagulation in patients with chronic or acute kidney disease requires particular consideration. Rivaroxaban, dabigatran, and low-molecular-weight heparin demonstrate impaired clearance in both acute and chronic kidney disease. Use of these medications even for prophylactic anticoagulation in patients with severe renal disease is associated with bleeding complications, and while not absolutely contraindicated, alternative methods should be considered. Warfarin is cleared primarily by the cytochrome P450 system, which causes therapeutic liability secondary to hepatic dysfunction or drug–drug interactions. However, indirect effects of kidney failure consistently increase warfarin sensitivity and require dose titration and frequent monitoring. UFH is cleared mainly by the reticuloendothelial system except at high doses when unbound molecules are renally cleared. This generally does not require dose adjustments, but monitoring with serial activated partial thromboplastin time (aPTT) is indicated as in patients without renal dysfunction.

Ref.: 6

4. Which of the following statements about resuscitation for hemorrhagic shock is true?

A. Blood products should be used as the initial resuscitative fluid in hemodynamically unstable patients.

B. A balanced transfusion ratio (1:1:1) between packed red blood cells (PRBCs), fresh-frozen plasma (FFP), and platelets (PLTs) reduces the severity of coagulopathy in hemorrhagic shock.

C. Patients with circulating factor levels 50% of the normal will show clinically impaired hemostasis.

D. Addition of TXA to massive transfusion protocols comes with an increased risk of thrombotic complications.

E. Albumin-containing solutions have a proven mortality benefit over crystalloid fluids in the resuscitation of hypovolemic shock.

ANSWER: B

COMMENTS: Previous theories of intravenous fluid resuscitation relied heavily upon crystalloid fluids to bolster blood volume and pressure. However, recent studies such as the Prospective, Observational, Multicenter, Major Trauma Transfusion (PROMMTT) and Pragmatic, Randomized Optimal Platelet and Plasma Ratios (PROPPR) have changed this practice. These studies were grounded in findings from battlefield transfusion studies showing decreased mortality in patients transfused with whole blood when components such as PRBCs and FFP were unavailable. The theory is that aggressive resuscitation with crystalloid fluids exacerbates the consumptive coagulopathy of trauma (clotting factors are used up in achieving systemic hemostasis) with an iatrogenic dilutional coagulopathy. Thus crystalloid-resuscitated patients initially responded hemodynamically but were coagulopathic and continued to bleed.

The PROMMTT trial first showed that patients who received higher ratios of platelets and plasma to FFPs had reduced all-cause mortality in the first 24 h following injury. These results were sustained at 30 days postinjury. The PROPPR trial refined these findings and showed superior outcomes with a 1:1:1 ratio of PRBC:FFP:PLT compared with a 1:1:2 ratio. The data trended toward significance in 24-h and 30-day mortality but was underpowered.

Ref.: 7, 8

5. A unit of blood could be transfused most rapidly through which of the following vascular access catheters?

A. A 7-Fr, 16-cm, triple-lumen catheter in the right internal jugular vein (lumens: 16, 18, 18 gauge)

B. A 7-Fr, 30-cm, triple-lumen catheter in the right internal jugular vein (lumens: 16, 18, 18 gauge)

C. An 18-gauge catheter peripherally inserted into the cephalic vein at the wrist

D. A 16-gauge, 3-cm peripheral IV in the right antecubital fossa

E. An 18-gauge, 3-cm peripheral IV in the right antecubital fossa

ANSWER: D

COMMENTS: Steady flow through a vascular catheter (and any rigid tube including blood vessels as well for that matter) is governed by the Hagen-Poiseuille equation, $Q = (\pi \Delta P r^4)/8\ \mu L$, where Q = flow rate, P = the driving pressure gradient, r = radius of the tube (catheter), μ = viscosity of the fluid in question (PRBCs), and L = length of the tube (catheter). Radius of the catheter is the most important determinant of the flow rate, as it is raised to a power of four. In two catheters with identical radii, flow rates will be higher in the shorter of the two. Therefore when rapid transfusion is needed, faster flows can be obtained with larger-bore, shorter catheters, meaning that central lines are inferior to large-bore peripheral IVs for initial resuscitation.

Ref.: 9

6. Transfusion of a unit of PRBCs into a hemodynamically stable patient with hemoglobin 7.5 g/dL does which of the following?

A. Increases systemic oxygen delivery (DO_2)

B. Increases tissue extraction of oxygen

C. Increases systemic oxygen uptake (VO_2)

D. Increases arterial O_2 saturation (Sao_2)

E. Decreases venous O_2 saturation (Svo_2)

ANSWER: A

COMMENTS: Multiple well-designed studies have shown that overuse of RBC transfusions in the critical care setting leads to poor outcomes. The findings of these studies can be summed up as "a risk to multiple organ systems without a physiologic benefit." Increasing circulating hemoglobin concentration through PRBC transfusion serves to increase systemic oxygen delivery (DO_2), which is determined by cardiac output and arterial oxygen concentration. This does not, however, lead to an increase in VO_2. Animal and human studies have shown that the increase in oxygen delivery with RBC transfusions is accompanied by a proportional decrease in tissue oxygen extraction, leading to no net change in systemic oxygen utilization. These studies were the basic science grounding for the 1999 Trial of Transfusion Requirements in Critical Care (TRICC) trial, which showed decreased mortality in the euvolemic intensive care unit (ICU) patients who were treated with a restrictive transfusion threshold [hemoglobin (Hb) < 7] compared with those treated with a liberal transfusion threshold (Hb < 10).

Ref.: 10

7. Impaired platelet aggregation in uremia is responsive to all of the following except:

A. Hemodialysis

B. Cryoprecipitate

C. DDAVP

D. Platelet transfusion

E. Desmopressin

ANSWER: D

COMMENTS: The uremic patient will have clinically and biochemically evident impaired platelet adhesion. In the lab, this presents as an increased bleeding time. This occurs as a result of increased circulating levels of prostacyclin and altered binding to exposed vWF on the vascular endothelium. This generally becomes clinically evident in patients with a creatinine level above 6.7 mg/dL. At this level, upper gastrointestinal (GI) bleeding is a major cause of mortality.

Hemodialysis can correct uremic bleeding in many patients. Beyond that, the vasopressin analogue desmopressin (DDAVP) acts to stimulate the release of circulating vWF and corrects impaired adhesion. If bleeding persists, cryoprecipitate can be utilized as it contains vWF, thus directly increasing circulating levels. Transfusion of platelets is not appropriate unless absolute counts are critically low, as the transfused platelets will show the same poor aggregative qualities as those already in circulation.

Ref.: 11

8. Which of the following is most indicative of heparin-induced thrombocytopenia (HIT) in a patient undergoing an elective procedure without a past medical history?

A. Platelet counts falling by 50% by postoperative day 7 to a nadir of 100K

B. Platelet counts falling over 90% by postoperative day 7 to a nadir of 5K

C. Platelet counts falling by 50% by postoperative day 3 to a nadir of 40K

D. Low levels of serotonin release in response to therapeutic heparin exposure in laboratory assays

E. Negative enzyme-linked immunosorbent assay (ELISA) for antiplatelet factor 4 immunoglobulins

ANSWER: A

COMMENTS: The temporal course and magnitude of thrombocytopenia are essential to evaluation for HIT. Falling platelet counts in the first 3 days following a patient's initial exposure to heparin generally resolve spontaneously without discontinuation of heparin and are not clinically significant. True HIT is immune mediated. Thus clinical and laboratory manifestations usually occur for a minimum of 4 days after initial exposure. Given the nature of immune reactions, this time frame is invalid if the patient has been exposed to heparin at any time in the 3 months prior to his or her most recent exposure. Absolute counts generally do not fall below 20,000 and are usually between 50 and 150,000 in true HIT. Thus other etiologies should be considered if thrombocytopenia is severe. Despite low platelet counts, HIT is a hypercoagulable state secondary to deranged platelet degranulation and frequently presents with thrombosis, more commonly in the venous system.

HIT is not a dose-dependent reaction—patients with heparin-locked peripheral IVs have essentially the same risk as those on an UFH drip. Thus at the first suspicion of HIT, all heparin-containing medications should be discontinued and the appropriate serum assays sent. A serotonin release assay will show exaggerated release in response to physiologic doses of heparin and a diminished response at supratherapeutic concentrations. Serum ELISA for antiplatelet factor 4 antibodies will be positive. The risk of developing HIT is lower with low-molecular-weight heparins than with UFH. Once the diagnosis is confirmed, patients should be started on therapeutic levels of direct thrombin inhibitors such as argatroban to prevent additional thrombosis.

Ref.: 12

9. Which of the following is not a proven etiology of disseminated intravascular coagulation (DIC)?

A. Gram-negative sepsis

B. Trauma

C. Retained products of conception

D. Malignancy

E. Supratherapeutic UFH drip

ANSWER: E

COMMENTS: DIC is a chain reaction. An initial inflammatory or traumatic insult leads to systemic activation of the coagulation system, which in turn leads to increased systemic inflammation, and so on. Patients will present clinically with bleeding from mucosal surfaces and IV access sites secondary to a consumptive coagulopathy. In addition, systemic microvascular thrombosis often causes multisystem organ dysfunction. Lab studies will show elevated international normalized ratio, prolonged aPTT, low fibrinogen, and elevated D-dimer. Of the answer choices, all but a supratherapeutic heparin drip include an instigating inflammatory response that drives the coagulation–inflammatory cycle that creates DIC. When patients with these conditions become coagulopathic, DIC should be suspected. Unfortunately, no specific treatment has been shown to correct DIC. Procoagulants such as clotting factor concentrates "feed the fire" so to speak and further drive the coagulation–inflammatory cycle. Management of suspected DIC is limited to source control and supportive care.

Ref.: 13

10. Which of the following is false regarding the factor V Leiden mutation?

A. Both heterozygous and homozygous mutations are associated with increased rates of VTE.

B. Carriers with provoked DVTs are generally managed with the same therapeutic regimen as noncarriers.

C. The hypercoagulable state associated with the mutation is readily detectable on standard clinical coagulation assays as a shortened prothrombin time (PT).

D. Although the structural mutation is on factor V, it impacts the functional activity of activated protein C.

E. Roughly 5% of the American population is heterozygous, with the highest prevalence in Caucasians.

ANSWER: C

COMMENTS: Factor V Leiden is a mutation that alters the cleavage target of activated protein C. Protein C is activated by thrombin with its cofactor thrombomodulin and proceeds to cleave and inactivate the procoagulant factor V. Patients with the mutation resist cleavage and show increased thrombin generation and clotting compared with the general population. In normal hemostasis, the concept of autoregulation dictates that anticoagulant proteins such as protein C are activated in conjunction with procoagulants to prevent runaway clotting and end the process of hemostasis. Patients with the factor V Leiden mutation are deficient in this crucial anticoagulant pathway and thus are prone to thrombosis.

The condition is most prevalent in Caucasians, and both heterozygotes and homozygotes are at increased risk for venous thrombosis. Odds ratios calculated from retrospective studies are 4.9 and 20.0 for any VTE in heterozygotes and homozygotes, respectively. Although carriers are at a higher risk than the general population, DVT and PE are generally not treated differently in the acute setting or for long term in these patients.

Ref.: 14

11. Heparin acts principally through which mechanism?

A. Indirect inhibition of factors II and X through antithrombin III activation

B. Direct inhibition of thrombin

C. Direct degradation of cross-linked fibrin clots

D. Inhibition of platelet aggregation

E. Inhibition of platelet adhesion to exposed tissue collagen during primary hemostasis

ANSWER: A

COMMENTS: Heparin is a polysaccharide molecule that is both produced endogenously and administered either subcutaneously or intravenously. Its principal mechanism of action is to serve as a scaffold between the anticoagulant protein antithrombin III and its targets, thrombin and factor X. In the presence of heparin, antithrombin III acts to inactivate its targets at a rate roughly three orders of magnitude higher than it does in the absence of heparin. Single-nucleotide polymorphisms in the heparin-binding domain of antithrombin III have been identified in the general population and help explain the clinical observation that patients require various amounts of heparin to achieve therapeutic anticoagulation. Direct thrombin inhibitors such as argatroban inhibit thrombin activity outside of the antithrombin pathway—for this reason, traditional dose monitoring techniques such as aPTT are ineffective. Both direct thrombin inhibitors and heparin serve to prevent the formation of blood clots. Fibrinolytic agents such as tPA and urokinase lead to plasmin-mediated degradation of existing fibrin clots. While heparin can, in fact, alter platelet function through minor pathways, this is not its principal mechanism of action. Clopidogrel acts to irreversibly inhibit platelet aggregation through inhibition of adenosine diphosphate (ADP) binding to its surface receptor. Aspirin irreversibly inhibits cyclooxygenase 1 (COX-1), preventing platelet generation of prothrombotic thromboxane A2.

Ref.: 15

12. Gelatin sponge (Gelfoam), oxidized cellulose (Surgicel), fibrin sealants (Tisseel, Evicel), and topical thrombin all have what in common?

A. They are grossly resorbable.

B. They have intrinsic hemostatic activity.

C. They are derived from human tissue.

D. They should be used for definitive control of anastomotic bleeding.

E. They directly generate fibrin clots.

ANSWER: A

COMMENTS: Topical hemostatic agents are useful adjuncts in the cessation of tissue surface bleeding. They are derived from human, plant, or animal tissue and may or may not have intrinsic hemostatic activity. The agents that are intrinsically hemostatic (Tisseel, Evicel, and topical thrombin) directly lead to generation of fibrin clots on the surfaces to which they are applied. Others (Gelfoam, Surgicel) have an indirect mechanism and provide a scaffold for hemostasis on a cut tissue edge. In any case, anastomotic or pulsatile bleeding should be definitively controlled with suture ligation or other means.

Ref.: 9

13. Which of the following is most clearly diagnostic for lower extremity DVT in an ICU patient?

A. Venous duplex study with incompressibility and sluggish flow through the external iliac vein

B. Venous duplex study with incompressibility and sluggish flow through the great saphenous vein below the knee

C. Computed tomography (CT) of the lower extremities with a thrombus in the external iliac

D. Elevated circulating D-dimer

E. Unilateral leg swelling

ANSWER: A

COMMENTS: Hospitalized patients, particularly those in the ICU, are predisposed to venous thromboembolic events. Risk factors include recent surgery or trauma (particularly to the central nervous system), active or occult malignancy, acute illness, prior VTE, mechanical ventilation, and immobility. Many times patients lie with silent DVTs that first present as symptomatic pulmonary emboli. Early detection and appropriate intervention are essential to prevent such events.

Virtually all patients with the risk factors listed above will have an elevated circulating D-dimer, as any active fibrinolysis will raise the level of circulating fibrin split products. Thus the specificity and positive predictive value of this test are unacceptably low in the postsurgical and critical care setting. Duplex ultrasound looks at the compressibility of a vein and flow. Incompressibility and sluggish flow indicate thrombosis. Clinically relevant DVTs that carry the risk of PE are limited to thromboses of the deep veins above the knee. CT scans of the lower extremities may raise suspicion for a DVT; however, the follow-up duplex result makes the diagnosis.

Ref.: 9

14. The following groups of patients have a biochemically evident hypercoagulable state along with increased incidence of clinically relevant VTE except:

A. Patients with sickle cell anemia

B. Children with essential hypertension

C. Patients with solid-organ malignancy

D. Diabetics

E. Smokers

ANSWER: B

COMMENTS: The incidence of VTE is low in children compared with that in adults. This is attributable to distinct dynamics of the hemostatic and fibrinolytic systems in children and adults. Most recent studies point to two principal differences: increased efficiency of the fibrinolytic system in children and lower circulating levels of fibrinogen. Put simply, these differences lead to equally effective hemostasis without thrombosis in children compared with adults. For this reason, VTE prophylaxis is not recommended in childhood. The hemostatic system in children has been described as a juvenile protective factor against VTE, and further research is warranted into pathways that would make the hemostatic system in adults behave more like it does in children. Every other answer choice listed describes a patient group at increased risk for VTE compared with the general population.

Ref.: 16

15. In patients with acute DVT, treatment with novel anticoagulants compared with vitamin K antagonists such as Coumadin showed:

A. Higher incidence of DVT recurrence
B. Lower incidence of PE
C. Higher incidence of significant bleeding complications
D. Lower incidence of significant bleeding complications
E. Lower incidence of all-cause mortality

ANSWER: D

COMMENTS: Novel anticoagulants such as dabigatran (Pradaxa) and rivaroxaban (Xarelto) are the cause of significant anxiety in the surgical world due to the lack of effective reversal agents. However, the broad view of anticoagulation with these agents helps explain their popularity. At this point, multiple studies have shown that a broad group of novel anticoagulants, including rivaroxaban, dabigatran, apixaban, and edoxaban, are associated with similar rates of recurrent VTE, fatal PE, and overall mortality compared with traditional vitamin K antagonists such as warfarin, along with a significantly lower incidence of major bleeding. Bleeding in patients receiving warfarin was attributed to labile pharmacodynamics, leading to supratherapeutic anticoagulation.

Currently, anticoagulation with Coumadin is familiar to surgeons and the most easily reversible modality, but data from the medical world and consumer preference (most of these drugs do not require routine dose monitoring) suggest that these agents will become progressively more popular. Further research into reversal agents for novel anticoagulants is absolutely essential, and surgeons should stay abreast of developments on this front.

Ref.: 17, 18

16. Which of the following coagulation assays is used clinically to detect a hyperfibrinolytic state?

A. PT
B. aPTT
C. Bleeding time
D. Thromboelastography
E. Activated clotting time

ANSWER: D

COMMENTS: Traditional coagulation assays such as PT and aPTT were designed for accurate dosing of anticoagulant medications. While they give some insight into patients' global coagulation status, they were not intended for this purpose and did not approach the complete picture of a patient's propensity to bleed or clot. Thromboelastography is an old test that has recently been put to new clinical use in trauma patients. It is capable of detecting a hyperfibrinolytic state and the bleeding propensity through the percent lysis parameter or a variation of it. This information is useful in determining the appropriateness of antifibrinolytic therapy and correlates well with injury severity scores and the magnitude of the systemic inflammatory response. No test used in clinical practice can detect a hypercoagulable state and thrombosis risk with good sensitivity.

Ref.: 19

17. Which of the following does not assist in hemostasis of massively bleeding trauma patients?

A. Permissive hypotension
B. Crystalloid resuscitation
C. Active warming
D. Recombinant factor VII
E. Balanced transfusion ratio (platelets:FFP:PRBC)

ANSWER: B

COMMENTS: In massively bleeding patients, three important factors are perfusion of vital organs, control of bleeding, and regulation of the propensity to bleed. Trauma patients, particularly those with blunt trauma, have an intrinsic coagulopathy that can worsen with misguided resuscitation. The traditional practice of aggressive crystalloid resuscitation achieves the first goal at the expense of the other two. This is because infusion of large amounts of intravascular fluid decreases circulating concentrations of clotting factors, leading to dilutional coagulopathy, and excessive perfusion pressure leads to clot dislocation. In patients with hemorrhagic shock, fluid-based resuscitation with a mean arterial pressure (MAP) goal of 50 mmHg decreases bleeding and increases long-term survival compared with patients who received fluids with a MAP goal of 65. Severe derangements in body temperature alter the dynamics of the hemostatic system and can cause coagulopathy. Recombinant factor VII has been shown to decrease hemorrhagic mortality in specific subsets of patients in the setting of trauma. Both whole-blood transfusions and balanced transfusion ratios have been shown to decrease blood product requirements and attenuate coagulopathy in hemorrhagic shock.

Ref.: 20, 21

18. The overall incidence, in terms of events per units transfused, of transfusion-related acute lung injury (TRALI) is closest to:

A. 1 in 10
B. 1 in 100
C. 1 in 1000
D. 1 in 10,000
E. 1 in 100,000

ANSWER: D

COMMENTS: While uncommon, TRALI is the leading cause of transfusion-related deaths. In order to have a proper index of clinical suspicion, physicians ordering transfusions should be familiar with the relative rates of complications. Broadly, 1 in 100 patients will experience urticaria; 1 in 1000 will develop anaphylaxis; and 1 in 10,000 will experience TRALI. Hepatitis B virus is transmitted in less than 1 in 200,000 units transfused and is by far the most frequently transmitted viral pathogen in blood products.

TRALI usually appears within the first hour after a transfusion begins. It presents with fever, respiratory distress, and, eventually, diffuse infiltrates seen on chest films. On the first suspicion of TRALI, the transfusion should be stopped and supportive care initiated. Broadly, TRALI is treated in a similar fashion to ARDS.

Ref.: 9

19. A patient with previously unrecognized gram-negative sepsis begins to bleed from peripheral IV catheter sites and is noted to have prolonged PT and aPTT along with a fibrinogen of 120 mg/dL. The most effective treatment for this patient's coagulopathy is:

A. IV antibiotics and fluid resuscitation

B. PRBC transfusion

C. Desmopressin

D. FFP

E. All of the above

ANSWER: A

COMMENTS: In DIC, the mainstays of treatment are supportive care and control of the inflammatory instigator. This patient has gram-negative sepsis, a known cause of DIC, and should be treated for that first and foremost. If the infection is not controlled, the coagulopathy will run rampant and the patient will bleed despite efforts to correct the coagulopathy, which is a secondary outcome of the underlying sepsis. If patients become critically deficient in platelets (<10,000/μL per microliter), they should be given supplemental platelets; however, the response will almost always be less than expected, secondary to ongoing consumption. Fibrinogen levels should be monitored and replenished with cryoprecipitate if they fall below 100 mg/dL.

Ref.: 13

20. Which of the following is false about fibrinogen?

A. Circulating levels are on average higher in children than in adults.

B. It is a scaffold for infiltration of inflammatory cells into a healing wound.

C. Circulating levels decrease in direct proportion to the total blood loss in hemorrhage.

D. Pure fibrinogen may be delivered to bleeding patients as a reconstituted solution.

E. It is a negative acute-phase reactant.

ANSWER: E

COMMENTS: Platelets are the brick and fibrinogen is the mortar of hemostasis. In acute bleeding, fibrinogen is generally the first factor to become critically depleted through volume loss, consumption, and dilutional mechanisms. Circulating levels are generally twice as high in adults as they are in children. Outside of its hemostatic function, fibrin is intrinsically inflammatory. Targets on its gamma chain attract inflammatory cells to sites of injury and are an essential part of the healing process in multiple organ systems. Recent trials show that lyophilized fibrinogen has great promise as a hemostatic agent. These powdered formulations are much better suited to long-term storage and do not require thawing and warming as blood products do.

The acute-phase response induces the up- or downregulation of over 1000 hepatic genes in response to interleukin (IL)-6, tumor necrosis factor, and IL-1 beta released from the site of injury. Most clotting factors are positive acute-phase reactants, meaning that production rises in times of stress. Other proteins, including albumin, are negative acute-phase reactants.

Ref.:22

21. With regard to normal hemostasis, which of the following statements is true?

A. Vascular disruption is followed by vasoconstriction mediated by vasoactive substances released by activated platelets.

B. Platelet adhesion is mediated by fibrin monomers.

C. The intact endothelial surface supports platelet adhesion and thrombus formation.

D. Heparin inhibits ADP-stimulated platelet aggregation.

E. A prolonged bleeding time may be due to thrombocytopenia, a qualitative platelet defect, or reduced amounts of vWF.

ANSWER: E

COMMENTS: Blood fluidity is maintained by the action of inhibitors of blood coagulation and by the nonthrombogenic vascular surface. Three physiologic reactions mediate initial hemostasis following vascular injury: (1) the vascular response (vasoconstriction) to injury; (2) platelet activation, adherence, and aggregation; and (3) generation of thrombin with subsequent conversion of fibrinogen into fibrin. Injury exposes subendothelial components and induces vasoconstriction independent of platelet participation (answer A), which results in decreased blood flow but an increase in local shear force. Within seconds, platelets are activated by the increase in shear force and adhere to exposed subendothelial collagen by a mechanism dependent on the participation of vWF (answer B). Adhesion stimulates the release of platelet ADP, thereby mediating the recruitment of additional platelets. Fibrinogen binds to activated platelet receptors, and platelet aggregation follows to create a primary hemostatic plug (answer B; adhesion and aggregation are distinct processes). The intact endothelium is antithrombotic (answer C). Formation of the plug requires calcium and magnesium and is not affected by heparin (answer D). Bleeding time measurements reflect the time that it takes to form this platelet plug. A reduction in platelet number or function, loss of vascular integrity, or a reduction in the amount or function of vWF may prolong the bleeding time.

Ref.: 23

22. With regard to drug effects and platelet function, which of the following statements is true?

A. Vasodilators such as prostaglandin E1 (PGE1), prostacyclin (PGI2), theophylline, and dipyridamole elevate cyclic adenosine monophosphate (cAMP) levels and block platelet aggregation.

B. Aspirin and indomethacin interfere with platelet release of ADP and inhibit aggregation.

C. Furosemide competitively inhibits PGE2.

D. The effect of aspirin is reversible in 2 to 3 days.

E. Aspirin will decrease platelet counts, but bleeding time is unchanged.

ANSWER: A

COMMENTS: Aspirin, indomethacin, and most other nonsteroidal antiinflammatory drugs (NSAIDs) are inhibitors of prostaglandin synthesis. They block the formation of PGG2 and PGH2 from platelet arachidonic acid and, as a result, inhibit platelet aggregation. PGI2, PGE1, and thromboxane A2 stimulate cAMP production, whereas dipyridamole and theophylline derivatives block its degradation. Aspirin inhibits thromboxane production, acetylates fibrinogen, interferes with fibrin formation, and makes fibrin susceptible to accelerated fibrinolysis. The effect of aspirin begins within 2 h, is irreversible, and lasts the 7- to 9-day life span of affected platelets. The clinical result is increased bruising and bleeding and increased risk of surgical bleeding. Platelet counts are normal, but the bleeding time is prolonged. Furosemide competitively inhibits ADP-induced platelet aggregation and reduces the response of platelets to PGG2. Furosemide may also cause thrombocytopenia. A wide variety of drugs inhibit platelet function.

Ref.: 24

23. With regard to measurement of bleeding times, which of the following statements is true?

A. Spontaneous bleeding may occur with platelet counts higher than 15,000/μL.

B. Platelet counts higher than 150,000/μL exclude the possibility of a primary hemostatic disorder.

C. Bleeding time is a predictor of surgical bleeding.

D. Platelet counts higher than 50,000/μL are usually associated with a normal bleeding time and adequate surgical hemostasis.

E. Normal bleeding time excludes von Willebrand disease as a potential factor affecting surgical hemostasis.

ANSWER: D

COMMENTS: The bleeding time is a crude measure of platelet function, number of platelets, or both. The normal value is 3 to 9 min and implies normal platelet function and counts greater than 50,000/μL. Spontaneous bleeding rarely occurs when the platelet count is greater than 10,000/μL. The bleeding time is prolonged in patients with normal platelet counts in whom qualitative abnormalities are present as a primary platelet disorder or one secondary to drugs, uremia, or liver disease or in those who have thrombasthenia or a variety of other defects in platelet function. Patients with defective platelets or capillaries; those with von Willebrand disease; and those with a history of recent ingestion of aspirin, NSAIDs, antibiotics (penicillins and cephalosporins), and a wide variety of miscellaneous drugs also have prolonged bleeding times. False-negative (normal) bleeding times are frequently due to the technical difficulty of performing the test and its lack of sensitivity. For example, only 60% of patients with von Willebrand disease have a prolonged bleeding time. Other tests of platelet function include assessment of platelet aggregation in response to a variety of agonists.

Ref.: 25

24. With regard to classic hemophilia (hemophilia A), which of the following statements is true?

A. The incidence in the general population is 1 in 1000.

B. A given patient's baseline factor VIII or IX level may fluctuate with stress.

C. Muscle compartment bleeding is the most common orthopedic problem.

D. Factor VIII replacement therapy is required before any elective surgery.

E. Therapy with cryoprecipitate plasma is free of risk for hepatitis.

ANSWER: D

COMMENTS: The incidence of classic hemophilia, the most common form of hemophilia, is 1 in 5000 males. Bleeding in patients with hemophilia usually appears during early childhood. Hemarthrosis is the most common orthopedic problem. Epistaxis, hematuria, and intracranial bleeding may occur. Equinus contracture, Volkmann's contracture of the forearm, and flexion contracture of the elbows or knees are sequelae of these bleeding episodes. Retroperitoneal or intramural intestinal bleeding may produce abdominal symptoms. The level of factor VIII or IX in plasma (which tends to remain stable throughout life) determines the tendency to bleed. Spontaneous bleeding is frequent in patients with severe disease, defined as less than 1% (of normal) factor VIII or IX activity. Bleeding typically occurs with trauma in patients with moderately severe disease, defined as 1%–5% factor activity. In patients with mild hemophilia A or B, defined as 6%–25% factor activity, bleeding typically occurs only with major trauma or surgery. The factor VIII or IX level must be raised to at least 30% to achieve hemostasis and to control minor hemorrhage. A level of approximately 50% is required to control joint and muscle bleeding, whereas a level of 80%–100% is necessary to treat life-threatening hemorrhage (central nervous system, retroperitoneal, or retropharyngeal bleeding) and to prepare patients for elective surgery. After elective surgery, levels of 25% should be maintained for at least 2 weeks. Transmission of hepatitis or human immunodeficiency virus, the development of neutralizing antibodies, and qualitative platelet dysfunction are possible complications of factor replacement therapy. Appropriate replacement includes infusions of factor VIII and factor IX. These products are available in both recombinant and highly purified concentrates that are virally inactivated. Cryoprecipitate is not an optimal replacement therapy for factor VIII and vWF, does not contain factor IX, and is associated with a risk of viral transmission.

Ref.: 26

25. A 12-year-old boy with known factor VIII deficiency has a painful, swollen, immobile right knee. The clinician suspects hemarthrosis. Therapeutic options include which of the following?

A. Immediate aspiration and compression dressings to prevent cartilage necrosis

B. Compression dressings and immobilization to prevent further bleeding

C. Immediate aspiration after appropriate factor VIII replacement therapy

D. Initial trial of factor VIII therapy, compression dressings, cold packs, and rest followed by active range-of-motion exercises

E. None of the above

ANSWER: D

COMMENTS: Treatment of hemarthrosis is aimed at preventing chronic synovitis and degenerative arthritis. Early, intensive factor VIII therapy is critical for limiting the extent of hemorrhage. Factor VIII replacement therapy is most effective when initiated before swelling of the joint capsule. Frequently, replacement therapy is initiated before the onset of any objective physical findings, when the patient perceives only subtle signs of joint hemorrhage. Factor VIII therapy, joint rest, compression dressing, and cold packs constitute the usual initial therapy. Aspiration is to be avoided. The goal of treatment of hemarthrosis is maintenance of range of motion. Active range-of-motion exercises should begin 24 h after factor VIII therapy. Compression and cold packs should be continued for 3 to 5 days.

Ref.: 26

26. With regard to von Willebrand disease, which of the following statements is true?

A. It is more common than hemophilia.

B. It is best treated with cryoprecipitate plasma.

C. Factor VIII levels are constant over time in a given patient.

D. Bleeding after elective surgery is rare.

E. All types of von Willebrand diseases can be effectively treated with desmopressin

ANSWER: A

COMMENTS: von Willebrand disease is the most common congenital bleeding disorder, with 1% of the population being affected. The prevalence of patients with symptomatic bleeding is approximately 1 in 1000. Most patients have mild disease unless challenged by trauma or surgery. von Willebrand disease is associated with a variable deficiency of both vWF and factor VIII. A platelet defect is also present in most patients. The severity of coagulation abnormalities varies from patient to patient and from time to time for a given patient. In all but 1%–2% of patients, the bleeding manifestations are milder than in classic hemophilia patients. In the same group of patients with type 3 von Willebrand disease, bleeding is more severe than in hemophilia patients. Bleeding is treated with desmopressin (DDAVP), which induces the release of vWF from storage sites in endothelial cells and platelets. The effect of DDAVP is rapid, with maximal procoagulant effects being reached in 1 to 2 h. The effects dissipate quickly (within 12 to 24 h) thus necessitating repeated dosing. When more than two or three doses of DDAVP are given, the effects may diminish or are absent. DDAVP is most effective for type 1 disease and is not effective for type 3 disease. Because of a risk for thrombocytopenia, DDAVP is specifically contraindicated in type 2B disease but may be effective in other forms of type 2 disease. In type 3 and most type 2 von Willebrand diseases, specific vWF replacement product should be administered.

Ref.: 27

27. With regard to polycythemia vera, which of the following statements is not true?

A. Spontaneous thrombosis is a complication of polycythemia vera.

B. Spontaneous hemorrhage is a possible complication of polycythemia vera.

C. The reason for bleeding is a deficit in platelet function.

D. A hematocrit of less than 48% and a platelet count of less than 400,000/μL are desirable before an elective operation is performed on a patient with polycythemia vera.

E. Postoperative complication rates may be as high as 60%.

ANSWER: E

COMMENTS: Patients with untreated polycythemia vera are at a high risk for postoperative bleeding or thrombosis. The complication rate is highest with uncontrolled erythrocytosis. Increased viscosity and platelet count, along with a tendency toward stasis, may explain the spontaneous thrombosis seen in patients with polycythemia vera. Patients most likely to bleed are those with platelet counts greater than 1.5 million/μL. Polycythemia vera may cause a qualitative defect in platelet function. When possible, surgery should be delayed until the hematocrit and platelet count can be medically reduced. Phlebotomy may help in acute situations. Complication rates as high as 46% have been reported in patients with polycythemia vera undergoing surgery. Spontaneous hemorrhage, thrombosis, a combination of hemorrhage and thrombosis, and infection are the major complications.

Ref.: 28

28. In cirrhotic patients who are actively bleeding, the coagulopathy of end-stage liver disease can be differentiated from DIC most readily by estimation of which of the following factors?

A. Factor II

B. Factor IX

C. Factor VII

D. Factor VIII:C

E. Factor X

ANSWER: D

COMMENTS: Of all of the coagulation factors listed, only factor VIII:C is not produced by hepatocytes. It is produced by reticuloendothelial cells, and its levels are typically increased in the presence of cirrhosis. Reductions in factor VIII:C are observed in patients with DIC because it is consumed along with the other coagulation factors.

Ref.: 15

REFERENCES

1. Williams-Johnson JA, McDonald AH, Strachan GG, Williams EW. Effects of tranexamic acid on death, vascular occlusive events, and blood transfusion in trauma patients with significant haemorrhage (CRASH-2): a randomised, placebo-controlled trial. *West Indian Med J.* 2010;59(6):612–624.
2. Crash-2 Collaborators. The importance of early treatment with tranexamic acid in bleeding trauma patients: an exploratory analysis of the CRASH-2 randomised controlled trial. *Lancet.* 2011;377(9771): 1096–1101.
3. PREPIC Study Group. Eight-year follow-up of patients with permanent vena cava filters in the prevention of pulmonary embolism: the PREPIC (Prévention du Risque d'Embolie Pulmonaire par Interruption Cave) randomized study. *Circulation.* 2005;112(3):416–422.
4. Fairfax LM, Sing RF. Vena cava interruption. *Crit Care Clin.* 2011; 27(4):781–804.
5. Decousus H, Leizorovicz A, Parent F, et al. A clinical trial of vena caval filters in the prevention of pulmonary embolism in patients with proximal deep-vein thrombosis. *N Engl J Med.* 1998;338(7):409–416.
6. Grand'Maison A, Charest AF, Geerts WH. Anticoagulant use in patients with chronic renal impairment. *Am J Cardiovasc Drugs.* 2005;5(5):291–305.
7. Holcomb JB, Del Junco DJ, Fox EE, et al. The prospective, observational, multicenter, major trauma transfusion (PROMMTT) study: comparative effectiveness of a time-varying treatment with competing risks. *JAMA Surg.* 2013;148(2):127–136.
8. Holcomb JB, Tilley BC, Baraniuk S, et al. Transfusion of plasma, platelets, and red blood cells in a 1: 1: 1 vs a 1: 1: 2 ratio and mortality

in patients with severe trauma: the PROPPR randomized clinical trial. *JAMA*. 2015;313(5):471–482.
9. Marino PL. *Marino's the ICU Book*. 4th ed. Philadelphia, PA: Lippincott Williams & Wilkins; 2013.
10. Hébert PC, Wells G, Blajchman MA, et al. A multicenter, randomized, controlled clinical trial of transfusion requirements in critical care. *N Engl J Med*. 1999;340(6):409–417.
11. Salman S. Uremic bleeding: pathophysiology, diagnosis, and management. *Hosp Physician*. 2001;76:45–50.
12. Warkentin TE, Levine MN, Hirsh J, et al. Heparin-induced thrombocytopenia in patients treated with low-molecular-weight heparin or unfractionated heparin. *N Engl J Medicine*. 1995;332(20):1330–1336.
13. Gando S. Disseminated intravascular coagulation. In: Gonzalez E, Moore HB, Moore EE, eds. *Trauma Induced Coagulopathy*. Switzerland: Springer International; 2016:195–217.
14. Emmerich J, Rosendaal FR, Cattaneo M, et al. Combined effect of factor V Leiden and prothrombin 20210A on the risk of venous thromboembolism. *Thromb Haemost*. 2001;86(3):809–816.
15. Colman RW, ed. *Hemostasis and Thrombosis: Basic Principles and Clinical Practice*. Philadelphia, PA: Lippincott Williams & Wilkins; 2006.
16. Rogers FB, Cipolle MD, Velmahos G, Rozycki G, Luchette FA. Practice management guidelines for the prevention of venous thromboembolism in trauma patients: the EAST practice management guidelines work group. *J Trauma*. 2002;53(1):142–164.
17. Schulman S, Kearon C, Kakkar AK, et al. Extended use of dabigatran, warfarin, or placebo in venous thromboembolism. *N Engl J Med*. 2013;368(8):709–718.
18. Schmitz EMH, Boonen K, van den Heuvel DJA, et al. Determination of dabigatran, rivaroxaban and apixaban by ultra-performance liquid chromatography–tandem mass spectrometry (UPLC-MS/MS) and coagulation assays for therapy monitoring of novel direct oral anticoagulants. *J Thromb Haemost*. 2014;12(10):1636–1646.
19. Ives C, Inaba K, Branco BC, et al. Hyperfibrinolysis elicited via thromboelastography predicts mortality in trauma. *J Am Coll Surg*. 2012;215(4):496–502.
20. Knudson MM, Cohen MJ, Reidy R, et al. Trauma, transfusions, and use of recombinant factor VIIa: a multicenter case registry report of 380 patients from the Western Trauma Association. *J Am Coll Surg*. 2011;212(1):87–95.
21. Morrison CA, Carrick MM, Norman MA, et al. Hypotensive resuscitation strategy reduces transfusion requirements and severe postoperative coagulopathy in trauma patients with hemorrhagic shock: preliminary results of a randomized controlled trial. *J Trauma*. 2011;70(3):652–663.
22. Cole HA, Ohba T, Nyman JS, et al. Fibrin accumulation secondary to loss of plasmin-mediated fibrinolysis drives inflammatory osteoporosis in mice. *Arthritis Rheumatol*. 2014;66(8):2222–2233.
23. Rutherford EJ, Brecher ME, Fakhry SM, et al. Hematologic principles in surgery. In: Townsend CM, Beauchamp RD, Evers BM, et al., eds. *Sabiston Textbook of Surgery: The Biological Basis of Modern Surgical Practice*. 18th ed. Philadelphia: Elsevier; 2008.
24. Hunt BJ. Bleeding and coagulopathies in critical care. *N Engl J Med*. 2014;370(9):847–859.
25. Gonzalez EA, Jastrow KM, Holcomb JB, et al. Hemostasis, surgical bleeding and transfusion. In: Brunicardi FC, Andersen DK, Billiar TR, et al., eds. *Schwartz's Principles of Surgery*. 9th ed. New York: McGraw-Hill; 2010.
26. Srivastava A, Brewer AK, Mauser-Bunschoten EP, et al. Guidelines for the management of hemophilia. *Haemophilia*. 2013;19(1):e1–e47.
27. Taylor J. Von Willebrand disease. In: *Hemostasis and Thrombosis*. Switzerland: Springer International Publishing; 2015:23–26.
28. Sethi S, Kumari K. Anesthetic management of a patient with polycythemia vera for nephrectomy. *IJAR*. 2015;3(7):147–149.

CHAPTER 4

NUTRITION, METABOLISM, AND FLUID AND ELECTROLYTES

A. Fluids and Electrolytes

Chetan Aher, M.D., and Ami Shah, M.D.

1. Which one of the following clinical scenarios is associated with hypercalcemia?

A. Fluid resuscitation from shock

B. Rapid infusion of blood products

C. Improper administration of phosphates

D. Malignancy

E. Acute pancreatitis

ANSWER: D

COMMENTS: Infusion of large volumes of **isotonic fluid** can cause a modest reduction in serum calcium levels. The concomitant decrease in magnesium also impairs vitamin D activity and makes correction of the hypocalcemia more difficult. Administration of a **citrate load** during rapid transfusion of blood products can lead to severe hypocalcemia, hypotension, and cardiac failure. In this setting, calcium should be replaced at a dose of 0.2 g/500 mL of blood transfused. Most patients receiving blood transfusions do not require calcium supplementation. **Acute pancreatitis** causes precipitation of calcium salts in the abdomen and may contribute to hypocalcemia. Other common causes include necrotizing fasciitis, renal failure, gastrointestinal fistula, and hypoparathyroidism. In general, calcium replacement should be monitored by measuring the concentration of ionized calcium.

Ref.: 1

2. A 30-year-old, 70-kg woman has symptomatic hyponatremia. Her serum sodium level is 120 mEq/L (normal level, 140 mEq/L). Her sodium deficit is:

A. 500 mEq/L

B. 600 mEq/L

C. 700 mEq/L

D. 800 mEq/L

E. 400 mEq/L

ANSWER: C

COMMENTS: Correction of changes in concentration depends, in part, on whether the patient is symptomatic. If symptomatic **hypernatremia** or **hyponatremia** is present, attention is focused on prompt correction of the abnormal concentration to the point that the symptoms are relieved. Attention is then shifted to correction of the associated abnormality in volume. The sodium deficiency in such patients is estimated by multiplying the sodium deficit (normal sodium concentration minus observed sodium concentration) by total body water in liters (60% of body weight in males and 50% of body weight in females). For the patient in question, the calculation is as follows: total body water = 70 kg × 0.5 = 35 L. Sodium deficit = (140 − 120 mEq/L) × 35 L = 700 mEq sodium chloride.

Initially, half the calculated amount of sodium is infused as 3% sodium chloride. The infusion is given slowly because rapid infusion can cause symptomatic hypovolemia. Rapid correction of hyponatremia can be associated with irreversible central nervous system injury (central pontine and extrapontine myelinolysis). Once the symptoms are alleviated, the patient should be reassessed before beginning the additional infusion of sodium. In patients with profound hyponatremia, a correction of no more than 12 mEq/L/24 h should be achieved. If the original problem was associated with a volume deficit, the remainder of the resuscitation can be accomplished with isotonic fluids (sodium chloride in the presence of alkalosis and sodium lactate in the presence of acidosis). Care must be taken when treating hyponatremia associated with volume excess. In this setting, after the symptoms are alleviated with a small volume of hypertonic saline solution, water restriction is the treatment of choice. Infusion of hypertonic saline solution in this setting has the potential to further expand the extracellular intravascular volume and is contraindicated in patients with severely compromised cardiac reserve. In such a case, peritoneal dialysis or hemodialysis may be preferred for removing excess water.

Ref.: 1

3. Which of the following disturbances is associated with tumor lysis syndrome?

A. Hypocalcemia

B. Hypouricemia

C. Hypokalemia

D. Hypomagnesemia

E. Hypophosphatemia

ANSWER: A

COMMENTS: *Tumor lysis syndrome* is a constellation of electrolyte abnormalities that results from massive tumor cell necrosis secondary to antineoplastic therapy. **Hypocalcemia**, **hyperphosphatemia**, **hyperuricemia**, and **hyperkalemia** may occur. Hypocalcemia results from the release of intracellular stores of phosphate, which binds with ionized serum calcium to form calcium phosphate salts. Chemotherapy directed against solid tumors, especially **lymphomas**, is most commonly associated with tumor lysis syndrome. **Acute renal failure** can occur and prevent spontaneous correction of the electrolyte abnormalities. Hypermagnesemia is not associated with tumor lysis syndrome.

Ref.: 1

4. An elderly patient with adult-onset diabetes mellitus is admitted to the hospital with severe pneumonia. The patient would not be expected to develop:
   A. Hypokalemia
   B. Hyperkalemia
   C. Nonketotic hyperosmolar coma
   D. Hypophosphatemia
   E. Hyponatremia

ANSWER: B

COMMENTS: Elderly patients with adult-onset diabetes mellitus are at risk for the development of **nonketotic hyperosmolar coma** during sepsis. As a result of the development of a nonketotic hyperglycemic hyperosmolar state, hypokalemia and hyperglycemia may also occur. Treatment of these patients should include a reduction in the glucose load provided and the administration of isotonic fluids. Patients may also benefit from the administration of insulin. Systemic bacterial sepsis is also often accompanied by a drop in the serum sodium concentration, possibly because of interstitial or intracellular sequestration. It is treated by withholding free water, restoring extracellular fluid (ECF) volume, and treating the source of sepsis.

Ref.: 1

5. An asymptomatic patient is found to have a serum calcium level of 13.5 mg/dL. Which of the following medications should be avoided?
   A. Bisphosphonates
   B. Thiazide diuretics
   C. Mithramycin
   D. Calcitonin
   E. Corticosteroids

ANSWER: B

COMMENTS: Hypercalcemia can affect the gastrointestinal, renal, musculoskeletal, and central nervous systems. Early symptoms include fatigability, lassitude, weakness, anorexia, nausea, and vomiting. Central nervous symptoms can progress to stupor and coma. Other symptoms include headaches and the three Ps: pain, polydipsia, and polyuria. The critical serum calcium level for hypercalcemia is 16 to 20 mg/mL. Prompt treatment must be instituted at this level, or the symptoms may progress to death. Two major causes of hypercalcemia are **hyperparathyroidism** and **metastatic disease**. Metastatic breast cancer in patients receiving estrogen therapy is the most common cause of hypercalcemia associated with metastases.

Oral or intravenous **phosphates** are useful for reducing hypercalcemia by inhibiting bone resorption and forming calcium phosphate complexes that are deposited in the soft tissues. Intravenous phosphorus, however, has been associated with the acute development of hypocalcemia, hypotension, and renal failure. For this reason, it should be given slowly over a period of 8 to 12 h once daily for no more than 2 to 3 days. Intravenous **sodium sulfate** is effective but no more so than saline diuresis. **Bisphosphonates** reduce serum calcium levels by suppressing the function of osteoclasts and thus reducing the bone resorption of calcium. In some malignant conditions, such as breast cancer, bisphosphonates may be administered prophylactically to prevent hypercalcemia. **Mithramycin** lowers serum calcium levels within 24 to 48 h by inhibiting bone resorption. A single dose may normalize serum calcium levels for several weeks.

Calcitonin is produced by the parafollicular cells of the thyroid gland and functions by inducing renal excretion of calcium and suppressing osteoclast bone resorption. Calcitonin can produce a moderate decrease in serum sodium levels, but the effect is lost with repeated administration. Because **corticosteroids** decrease resorption of calcium from bone and reduce intestinal absorption, they are useful for treating hypercalcemic patients with sarcoidosis, myeloma, lymphoma, or leukemia. Their effects, however, may not be apparent for 1 to 2 weeks. **Chelating agents**, such as ethylenediaminetetraacetic acid (EDTA), are not indicated since they can result in metastatic calcification, acute renal failure, and hypocalcemia. **Thiazide diuretics** are contraindicated because they are calcium sparing (and are often implicated as a cause of iatrogenic hypercalcemia). Acute hypercalcemic crisis from hyperparathyroidism is treated by stabilizing the patient and performing a parathyroidectomy.

Ref.: 1

6. Which of the following statements regarding the distribution, composition, and osmolarity of body fluid compartments is true?
   A. A majority of intracellular water resides in adipose tissue.
   B. The principal intracellular anions are proteins and phosphates.
   C. Sodium determines the effective osmotic pressure between the interstitial and intravascular (plasma) fluid compartments.
   D. Calcium greatly determines the effective osmotic pressure between the intracellular fluid (ICF) and ECF compartments.
   E. The principal intracellular cation is calcium.

ANSWER: B

COMMENTS: The ICF compartment (accounting for 40% of total body weight) is contained mostly within skeletal muscles. The principal intracellular cations are potassium and magnesium, whereas the principal **intracellular anions** are proteins and phosphates. In the ECF compartment (20% of total body weight), which is subdivided into the interstitial (extravascular) and the intravascular (plasma) fluid compartments, the principal cation is sodium, whereas the principal anions are chloride and bicarbonate. The interstitial compartment has a rapidly equilibrating functional component and a slowly equilibrating, relatively nonfunctional component consisting of fluid within connective tissue and cerebrospinal and joint fluid (termed **transcellular water**). Intravascular fluid (plasma) has a higher concentration of nondiffusible organic proteins than interstitial fluids. These plasma proteins act as multivalent anions. As a result, the concentration of inorganic anions is lower, but the total concentration of cations is higher in the intravascular fluid than in the interstitial fluid. This relationship is explained in the **Gibbs–Donnan equilibrium equation**: the product of the concentrations of any pair of diffusible cations and anions on one side of a semipermeable membrane equals the product of the same pair on the other side.

In each body compartment the concentration of osmotically active particles is 290 to 310 mOsm. Although total osmotic pressure represents the sum of osmotically active particles in the fluid compartment, the effective osmotic pressure depends on osmotically active particles that do not freely pass through the semipermeable membranes of the body. The nonpermeable proteins in plasma are responsible for the effective osmotic pressure between plasma and the interstitial fluid compartment (the colloid osmotic pressure). The effective osmotic pressure between the ECF and ICF compartments is due mainly to sodium, the major extracellular cation, which does not freely cross the cell membrane. Because water moves freely between the compartments, the **effective oncotic pressure** within the various body fluid compartments is considered to be equal after fluid equilibration. An increase in the effective oncotic pressure of the ECF compartment (such as an increase in sodium concentration) causes movement of water from the intracellular space to the extracellular space until the osmotic pressure equalizes. Conversely, loss of sodium (hyponatremia) from the extracellular space results in movement of water into the intracellular space. Thus the ICF contributes to correcting the changes in concentration and composition in the ECF. Isotonic ECF losses (losses in volume without change in concentration) generally do not cause transfer of water from the intracellular space as long as the osmolarity remains unchanged. Isotonic volume losses result in changes in ECF volume.

Ref.: 1

7. Which of the following conditions is associated with hypernatremia?

A. Adrenal insufficiency

B. Tumor lysis syndrome

C. Marked hyperglycemia

D. Stevens–Johnson syndrome

E. Excessive loop diuretic administration

ANSWER: D

COMMENTS: Dermatologic conditions such as second-degree burns and exfoliative dermatitis can substantially increase transcutaneous water loss and thereby result in the rapid onset of dehydration and hypernatremia. Tumor lysis syndrome, a condition involving cell breakdown and release of their intracellular contents after some chemotherapies, typically develops in patients treated with vinca alkaloid chemotherapy; it causes hyperkalemia, hyperphosphatemia, hyperuricemia, and ultimately, renal failure. Tumor lysis syndrome does not cause hypernatremia. Adrenal insufficiency, hyperglycemia, and loop diuretics all cause hyponatremia.

Ref.: 1

8. Which of the following humoral factors increases arterial vasodilation while not decreasing protein permeability in the capillary membranes?

A. Bradykinin

B. Nitric oxide (NO)

C. Atrial natriuretic factor

D. Histamine

E. Platelet-activating factor

ANSWER: B

COMMENTS: The **protein permeability** characteristics of capillary membranes are quantified by a numeric value termed the **reflection coefficient**. This value ranges from 0 to 1 and is conceptualized as the fraction of plasma protein that "reflects" back from the capillary wall when water crosses. The higher the coefficient, the more impermeable the capillary is to protein. Therefore the oncotic pressure of the plasma volume declines as the reflection coefficient decreases. Certain intravascular factors can reduce the reflection coefficient and increase arterial vasodilation. Bradykinin, atrial natriuretic factor, histamine, and platelet-activating factor increase microvascular membrane permeability while causing arterial vasodilation. NO, although it causes arterial vasodilation, does not increase microvascular membrane permeability. Membrane permeability causes a shift of fluid and plasma proteins into the interstitium and thereby decreases the intravascular compartment. The protein-rich edema in the interstitium can adversely affect the ability to combat infection.

Ref.: 1

9. A 55-year-old female with a small bowel obstruction is found to have a serum potassium level of 2.8 mmol/L. Her hypokalemia is refractory to aggressive repletion. Which of the following is true?

A. The patient will likely suffer from flaccid paralysis and respiratory compromise until her potassium level is increased to at least 3.0 mmol/L.

B. An electrocardiogram will likely show peaked T waves.

C. Intravenous potassium repletion with a rate of 80 mEq/h should improve her condition.

D. Hypomagnesemia could contribute to her problem.

E. Hypokalemia results in hypopolarization of the resting potential of the cell.

ANSWER: D

COMMENTS: Potassium is the main intracellular ion. Patients with a potassium concentration lower than 3.5 mmol/L have hypokalemia, which results in hyperpolarization of the resting potential of the cell and interferes with neuromuscular function. In severe cases where the serum potassium falls below 2.0 mmol/L, flaccid paralysis with respiratory compromise can occur.

In the setting of hypokalemia, an electrocardiogram may show depressed T waves and U waves. Cardiac arrhythmia, particularly atrial tachycardia with or without a block; atrioventricular dissociation; ventricular tachycardia; and ventricular fibrillation can all result from hypokalemia. Patients on digoxin are at increased risk for hypokalemia-associated arrhythmia. Fatal arrhythmia can occur with IV potassium repletion over 40 mEq/h.

Magnesium levels should be monitored in the setting of hypokalemia as magnesium is an important cofactor for the uptake and maintenance of potassium levels. Supplemental magnesium also reduces the risk of cardiac arrhythmia.

Ref.: 1

10. A 70-kg man is nil per os and receiving maintenance intravenous fluids in the form of 5% dextrose in 0.45% saline after gastrointestinal surgery. Which of the following is true regarding his fluid and electrolyte requirements?

A. His daily water need is 4000 mL.

B. His sodium requirement is 1 g/day.

C. His potassium requirement is 50 mEq/day.

D. Average urine volume is 3000 mL.

E. If he were febrile, his average increase in insensible loss would be 250 mL/day for each degree of fever.

ANSWER: E

COMMENTS: The average individual has an intake of 2000 to 2500 mL of water per day—1500 mL is ingested orally, and the remainder is acquired in solid food. Daily losses include 250 mL in stool, 800 to 1500 mL in urine, and approximately 600 mL as insensible loss. To excrete the products of normal daily catabolism, an individual must produce at least 500 to 800 mL of urine. In healthy individuals, 75% of insensible loss occurs through the skin and 25% through the lungs. Insensible loss from the skin occurs as loss of water vapor through the skin and not by evaporation of water secreted by the sweat glands. In febrile patients, insensible loss through the skin may increase to 250 mL/day for each degree of fever. Losses from sweating can be as high as 4 L/h. In a patient with a tracheostomy who is being ventilated with unhumidified air, insensible loss from the lungs may increase to 1500 mL/day. Average sodium needs are 2 to 4 g/day. Maintenance of potassium requires 100 mEq/day.

Ref.: 1, 2

11. Which of the following statements regarding hypervolemia in postoperative patients is true?

A. Hypervolemia can be produced by the administration of isotonic salt solutions in amounts that exceed the loss of volume.

B. Acute overexpansion of the ECF space is typically not well tolerated in healthy individuals.

C. Excess administration of normal saline can result in metabolic derangement, most commonly hyperchloremic metabolic alkalosis.

D. The most reliable sign of volume excess is peripheral edema.

E. Daily weight measurement in the postoperative period does not help determine fluid status.

ANSWER: A

COMMENTS: The earliest sign of **volume excess** during the postoperative period is weight gain. Normally, during this period the patient is in a catabolic state and is expected to lose weight (1/4 to 1/2 lb/day). Circulatory and pulmonary signs of overload appear late and usually represent massive overload. Peripheral edema does not necessarily indicate excess volume. In a patient with edema but without additional evidence of volume overload, other causes of peripheral edema should be considered. The most common cause of excess volume in a surgical patient is the administration of isotonic salt solutions in amounts that exceed the loss of volume. In a healthy individual, such overload is usually well tolerated. However, if the excess fluid is administered for several days, the ability of the kidneys to secrete sodium may be exceeded, thus resulting in hypernatremia. In the case of excess normal saline administration, hyperchloremic metabolic acidosis may occur.

Ref.: 1, 2

12. With regard to potassium, which of the following statements is true?

A. Normal dietary intake of potassium is 150 to 200 mEq/day.

B. In patients with normal renal function, most ingested potassium remains in the extracellular space.

C. More than 90% of the potassium in the body is located in the extracellular compartment.

D. Critical hyperkalemia (>6 mEq/L) is rarely encountered if renal function is normal.

E. Administration of sodium bicarbonate shifts potassium from the ICF to the ECF.

ANSWER: D

COMMENTS: The average daily dietary intake of potassium is 50 to 100 mEq. In patients with normal renal function and serum potassium levels, most ingested potassium is excreted in urine. More than 90% of the body's potassium stores are within the intracellular compartment at a concentration of 150 mEq/L. Although the total extracellular potassium concentration is just 50 to 70 mEq (4.5 mEq/L), this concentration is critical for cardiac and neuromuscular function. Significant quantities of intracellular potassium are released in response to severe injury, surgical stress, acidosis, and a catabolic state. However, dangerous hyperkalemia (>6 mEq/L) is rarely encountered if renal function is normal. The administration of bicarbonate shifts potassium from the ECF across the cell membrane into the ICF.

Ref.: 1, 2

13. Which of the following electrocardiographic (ECG) findings is associated with hyperkalemia?

A. Inverted T waves

B. Shortened PR interval

C. Peaked P waves

D. Narrowing of the QRS complex

E. T waves higher than R waves in more than one lead

ANSWER: E

COMMENTS: Hyperkalemia occurs when the serum potassium level exceeds 5 mmol/L. As potassium increases, changes in the resting membrane potential of cells impair depolarization and repolarization and lead to cardiac arrhythmias. The signs of hyperkalemia are generally limited to cardiovascular and gastrointestinal symptoms. Gastrointestinal symptoms include nausea, vomiting, intermittent intestinal colic, and diarrhea. ECG changes can be the first manifestation of hyperkalemia and include peaked T waves and a prolonged PR interval, which are characteristic early findings. These ECG changes may be seen with potassium concentrations greater than 6 mEq/L. Symmetrically peaked T waves indicate dangerous hyperkalemia, particularly if the T waves are higher than the R wave in more than one lead. At higher potassium concentrations (7 mmol/L), loss of P waves, slurring, or widening of the QRS complexes occurs. As $[K^+]$ exceeds 8 mmol/L, sudden lethal arrhythmias, such as asystole, ventricular fibrillation, or a wide pulseless idioventricular rhythm, ensue.

Ref.: 1, 2

14. With regard to postoperative hyponatremia, which of the following statements is true?

A. It does not occur when water is used to replace sodium-containing fluids because intracellular reserves often replace these losses.

B. In patients with head injury, hyponatremia despite adequate salt administration is usually caused by occult renal dysfunction.

C. In oliguric patients, cellular catabolism with resultant metabolic acidosis increases cellular release of water and can contribute to hyponatremia.

D. Hyperglycemia is not a cause of hyponatremia.

E. Patients with salt-wasting nephropathy usually have abnormal blood urea nitrogen and creatinine values.

ANSWER: C

COMMENTS: Abnormalities in sodium concentration do not usually occur during the postoperative period if the functional ECF volume has been adequately replaced during the operation. The sodium concentration generally remains normal because the kidneys retain the ability to excrete moderate excesses of water and solute administered during the early postoperative period. Hyponatremia does occur when water is given to replace lost sodium-containing fluids or when the amount of water given consistently exceeds the amount of water lost. In patients with head injury, hyponatremia may develop despite adequate salt administration because of excessive secretion of antidiuretic hormone (ADH) with resultant increased water retention.

Patients with preexisting renal disease and loss of concentrating ability may excrete urine with a high salt concentration. This **salt-wasting** phenomenon is commonly encountered in elderly patients and is often not anticipated because the blood urea nitrogen and creatinine levels are within normal limits. When there is doubt, determination of the urine sodium concentration can help clarify the diagnosis. Oliguria reduces the daily water requirement and can lead to hyponatremia if not anticipated. Cellular catabolism in patients without adequate caloric intake can lead to gain of significant quantities of water released from the tissues. Hyperglycemia may produce a depressed serum sodium level by exerting an osmotic force in the extracellular compartment and thus diluting serum sodium levels.

Ref.: 1, 2

15. Which of the following statements regarding changes in volume status of the ECF compartment is true?

A. Hyponatremia is diagnostic of excess ECF volume.

B. Hypernatremia is diagnostic of depletion of ECF volume.

C. Excess extracellular volume is usually iatrogenic or due to renal or cardiac failure.

D. Central nervous system symptoms appear after tissue signs with acute volume loss.

E. The concentration of serum sodium is directly related to extracellular volume.

ANSWER: C

COMMENTS: The serum concentration of sodium is not necessarily related to the volume status of the ECF compartment. **Volume deficit** or excess can exist with high, low, or normal serum sodium concentrations. Volume deficit is the most frequent volume disorder encountered during surgery. Its most common cause is loss of isotonic fluid (i.e., fluid having the same composition as ECF), for example, through hemorrhage, vomiting, diarrhea, fistulas, or third spacing. With acute volume loss, central nervous system symptoms (e.g., sleepiness and apathy progressing to coma) and cardiovascular signs (e.g., orthostasis, hypotension, tachycardia, and coolness in the extremities) appear first, along with decreasing urine output. Tissue signs (e.g., decreased turgor, softness of the tongue with longitudinal wrinkling, and atonicity of muscles) usually do not appear during the first 24 h. In response to hypovolemia, body temperature may be slightly decreased. It is therefore important to also monitor the body temperature of hypovolemic patients. Signs and symptoms of sepsis may be depressed in volume-depleted patients. The abdominal pain, fever, and leukocytosis associated with peritonitis may be absent until ECF volume is restored.

Volume overload is generally either iatrogenic or the result of renal insufficiency or heart failure. Both plasma and the interstitial fluid spaces are involved. The signs are those of circulatory overload and include distended veins, bounding pulses, functional murmurs, edema, and basilar rales. These signs may be present in young, healthy patients, but these patients can compensate for moderate to severe volume excess without overt failure or pulmonary edema development. In elderly patients, however, congestive heart failure (CHF) with pulmonary edema may develop quite rapidly.

Ref.: 1, 2

16. With regard to hypokalemia, which of the following statements is true?

A. It is less common than hyperkalemia in surgical patients.

B. Respiratory acidosis is associated with increased renal potassium loss.

C. Hypokalemia can cause increased deep tendon reflexes.

D. Flattened T waves and a prolonged QT interval are associated with hypokalemia.

E. Intravenous potassium administration should not exceed 10 to 20 mEq/h.

ANSWER: D

COMMENTS: Hypokalemia is more common than hyperkalemia in surgical patients. Hypokalemia can result from increased renal excretion, prolonged administration of potassium-free fluids, hyperalimentation with inadequate potassium replacement, or gastrointestinal losses. Respiratory and metabolic **alkalosis** results in increased renal potassium loss because potassium is preferentially excreted in an attempt to preserve hydrogen ions. Loss of gastrointestinal **secretions** can also be a significant cause of potassium depletion. This problem is compounded if potassium-free fluids are used for volume replacement. Signs of hypokalemia, including **paralytic ileus**, diminished or absent **tendon reflexes**, weakness, and even flaccid **paralysis**, are related to decreased muscle contractility. ECG changes include **flattened** or **inverted T waves**, U waves, and **prolongation of the QT interval**. The best treatment of hypokalemia is prevention. Gastrointestinal losses should be treated by the administration of fluids containing enough potassium to replace the daily obligatory loss (20 mEq/day), as well as the additional losses in gastrointestinal drainage. As a rule, no more than 40 to 60 mEq of potassium should be added to each liter of intravenous fluid, and the rate of potassium administration should never exceed 40 to 60 mEq/h.

Ref.: 1, 2

17. With regard to abnormalities in serum sodium concentration, which of the following statements is true?

A. Changes in serum sodium concentration usually produce changes in the status of ECF volume.

B. The chloride ion is the main determinant of the osmolarity of the ECF space.

C. Extracellular hyponatremia leads to depletion of intracellular water.

D. Dry, sticky mucous membranes are characteristic of hyponatremia.

E. Preservation of normal ECF has higher precedence than maintenance of normal osmolality.

ANSWER: A

COMMENTS: Although extracellular volume may change without a change in serum sodium concentration (as occurs after isotonic volume losses), changes in serum sodium concentration usually produce changes in ECF volume because the serum sodium concentration is the main determinant of the osmolarity of the ECF space. Alterations in its concentration produce concomitant shifts in water volume. Signs and symptoms of hypernatremia and hyponatremia are not generally present unless the changes are severe or the alteration in sodium concentration occurs rapidly.

Hyponatremia is caused by excessive intake of hypotonic fluids or salt loss that exceeds water loss. With hyponatremia, decreased extracellular osmolarity causes a shift of water into the intracellular compartment. When such a shift occurs, central nervous system symptoms caused by increased intracranial pressure develop, and tissue signs of excess water are noted. Central nervous system symptoms include muscle twitching, hyperactive tendon reflexes, and, when the hyponatremia is severe, convulsions and hypertension. Tissue signs include salivation, lacrimation, watery diarrhea, and "fingerprinting" of the skin. When hyponatremia develops rapidly, signs and symptoms may appear at sodium concentrations of less than 130 mEq/L. Acute dilution of osmolality can occur if patients with an ECF deficit are given sodium-free water. The hyponatremia is exacerbated in hypovolemic patients because of secretion of ADH as a result of the hypothalamic–pituitary response to both elevated ECF osmolality and a reduction in ECF volume. The normal response of the hypothalamic–pituitary axis to hyponatremia is suppression of ADH release, and as the dilute urine is excreted, there is a corrective increase in serum [Na^+]. A moderate or severely hyponatremic patient should have undetectable blood levels of ADH. Preservation of normal ECF has higher precedence than maintenance of normal osmolality. In symptomatic patients, administration of hypertonic (3%) solutions of sodium may be indicated to correct the problem in those with severe hyponatremia who are at risk for seizures. In less severe cases, restriction of free water and judicious infusion of normal saline solution are usually sufficient. In patients with acute hyponatremia and [Na^+] less than 120 mEq/L, the rate of infusion of sodium-containing solutions should not increase serum [Na^+] more rapidly than 0.25 mEq/L/h.

Chronic hyponatremia develops slowly, and patients may have sodium levels as low as 120 mEq/L before becoming symptomatic. Severe hyponatremia may be associated with the onset of irreversible oliguric renal failure. Patients with a closed head injury are sensitive to even mild hyponatremia because of increased intracellular water, which exacerbates the increased intracranial pressure associated with the head injury. The **syndrome of inappropriate release of antidiuretic hormone** (SIADH) and chronic renal failure are frequent causes of hyponatremia. The diagnosis of SIADH can be made only in euvolemic patients who have a serum osmolality of less than 270 mmol/kg H_2O along with inappropriately concentrated urine.

Hypernatremia is the result of excessive free water loss or salt intake. Central nervous system signs and symptoms associated with hypernatremia include restlessness, weakness, delirium, and maniacal behavior. The tissue signs are characteristic and include dryness and stickiness of mucous membranes, decreased salivation and tear production, and redness and swelling of the tongue. Body temperature is usually elevated, occasionally to a lethal level. An acute onset of hypernatremia increases ECF osmolality and contracts the size of the ICF compartment. Patients have moderate hypernatremia if their serum [Na^+] is 146 to 159 mEq/L. Water loss is the most common explanation for acute hypernatremia. Neurologic damage as a result of contraction of brain cell volume is the primary risk associated with hypernatremia. Patients with **diabetes insipidus** or **nephrogenic diabetes insipidus** have a failure to synthesize and release ADH or a failure of the renal tubular cells to respond to ADH, respectively, thus leading to hypernatremia. Treatment of patients with hypernatremia secondary to dehydration involves the administration of water. Hypernatremic patients are frequently hypovolemic, and these patients are treated by the intravenous infusion of isotonic saline solution until the volume deficit has been restored. A rapid decline in ECF osmolality in a severely hypernatremic patient can lead to cerebral injury as a result of cellular swelling. [Na^+] should be lowered at a rate not to exceed 8 mEq/day (Table 4.1). Patients with central diabetes insipidus are treated with desmopressin [1-desamino-8-D-arginine vasopressin (DDAVP)]. **Desmopressin** is a synthetic analogue of ADH.

Ref.: 1, 2

TABLE 4.1 Given a Patient with Hypernatremia (Serum [Na^+] = 160 mEq/L), the Estimated Change in [Na^+] after Infusion of 1 L

$$\frac{\text{Change in }[Na^+]}{L} = \frac{\text{Infusate }[Na^+] - \text{Serum }[Na^+]}{TBW+1}$$

Infusate	Woman Aged 70 Years 50 kg × 0.45 = 22.5 L TBW	Man Aged 20 Years 80 kg × 0.60 = 48.0 L TBW
D_5W	$\frac{0-160}{22.5+1} = -6.8$	$\frac{0-160}{48+1} = -3.3$
D_5 0.2% NaCl	$\frac{34-160}{22.5+1} = -5.4$	$\frac{34-160}{48+1} = -2.6$
D_5 0.45% NaCl	$\frac{77-160}{22.5+1} = -3.5$	$\frac{77-160}{48+1} = -1.7$

D_5W, 5% dextrose in water; TBW, total body water.

18. A 45-year-old alcoholic man is found to have hypomagnesemia. Which of the following statements about magnesium is true?

A. The distribution of nonosseous magnesium is similar to that of sodium.

B. Calcium deficiency cannot be adequately corrected until the hypomagnesemia is addressed.

C. Magnesium depletion is characterized by depression of the neuromuscular and central nervous systems.

D. Magnesium supplementation should be stopped as soon as the serum level has normalized.

E. The treatment of choice for magnesium deficiency is oral magnesium phosphate.

ANSWER: B

COMMENTS: The body contains 2000 mEq of **magnesium**, half of which is contained in bone. Most of the remaining magnesium is **intracellular** (a distribution similar to that of potassium). Plasma levels range between 1.5 and 2.5 mEq/L. Normal dietary intake is 240 mg/day, most of which is excreted in feces. The kidneys excrete some magnesium but can help conserve magnesium when a deficiency is present. **Hypomagnesemia** (like calcium deficiency) is characterized by **neuromuscular** and **central nervous system hyperactivity**. Hypomagnesemia can occur with starvation, malabsorption, protracted loss of gastrointestinal fluid, and prolonged parenteral therapy without proper magnesium supplementation.

An accompanying **calcium deficiency**, cannot be successfully treated until the hypomagnesemia is corrected.

Magnesium deficiency is treated with parenteral administration of magnesium sulfate or magnesium chloride. The extracellular magnesium concentration can be restored rapidly, but therapy must be continued for 1 to 2 weeks to replenish the intracellular component. To avoid magnesium deficiency, patients managed with hyperalimentation should receive 12 to 24 mEq of magnesium daily. Oral supplementation and intramuscular injection are alternative routes for replacement but are not preferred. **Magnesium toxicity** is rare except in the setting of renal insufficiency. Immediate treatment is infusion of **calcium chloride** or **calcium gluconate**; if the symptoms persist, dialysis may be required.

Ref.: 1, 2

19. Which of the following clinical situations can be associated with hypovolemic hyponatremia?

A. CHF

B. SIADH

C. Cirrhosis

D. Hyperglycemia

E. Gastrointestinal losses

ANSWER: E

COMMENTS: Hyponatremia in a surgical patient can be classified into hypervolemic, euvolemic, and hypovolemic categories, which can then be further subclassified according to tonicity (hypertonic, >290 mOsm; isotonic, 280 to 290 mOsm; and hypotonic, <280 mOsm). For simplicity and rapid clinical evaluation, volume status can be used to direct treatment. **Hypervolemic hyponatremia** may be caused by increased intake of water, postoperative secretion of ADH, and high ECF volume states such as cirrhosis and CHF. Hyponatremia can develop in patients with edema and ascites secondary to CHF, nephrotic syndrome, or cirrhosis despite having an expanded overall volume of extracellular water. These patients have an excess of sodium but an even greater proportional increase in water volume. Their pathophysiologic condition entails an overall contracted intravascular volume, which stimulates the release of vasopressin from the hypothalamus centrally. Peripherally, renal hypoperfusion contributes to water retention. Fluid restriction is crucial to the treatment of this type of hyponatremia. In patients with severe hyponatremia, small volumes of hypertonic saline solution may be administered. Diuresis may be used but is generally unsuccessful. Hemodialysis may be performed in extreme circumstances of fluid excess. **Euvolemic hyponatremia** may be caused by hyperglycemia, hyperlipidemia, or hyperproteinemia (termed **pseudohyponatremia** because of relative hyperosmolar protein, lipid, or glucose-rich plasma drawing fluid from the interstitial space and diluting plasma sodium), SIADH, water intoxication, and diuretics. SIADH is characterized by functional reabsorption of free water and subsequent dilution of plasma sodium. **Hypovolemic hyponatremia** may be caused by decreased overall sodium intake, gastrointestinal losses, renal losses associated with the use of diuretics (especially thiazide diuretics), and primary renal disease.

Conversely, hypernatremia can also be subdivided into volume states. Hypervolemic hypernatremia may be caused by iatrogenic sodium administration or mineralocorticoid excess (e.g., aldosteronism, Cushing disease, congenital adrenal hyperplasia). Euvolemic hypernatremia may be associated with renal (renal disease, diuretics, or diabetes insipidus) or nonrenal free water loss through the skin or gastrointestinal tract. Hypovolemic hypernatremia can likewise be subdivided into nonrenal and renal water loss.

Ref.: 1, 2

20. With regard to intraoperative management of fluids, which of the following statements is true?

A. In a healthy person, up to 500 mL of blood loss may be well tolerated without the need for blood replacement.

B. During an operation, functional ECF volume is directly related to the volume lost to suction.

C. Functional ECF losses should be replaced with plasma.

D. Administration of albumin plays an important role in the replacement of functional ECF volume loss.

E. Operative blood loss is usually overestimated by the surgeon.

ANSWER: A

COMMENTS: It is now believed that the routine use of albumin to replace blood and **ECF losses** intraoperatively is not indicated and may be potentially harmful. Maintenance of cardiac and pulmonary function by replacing blood with blood products and ECF with "mimic" solutions can be achieved without the addition of albumin. In general, it is believed that blood should be replaced as it is lost. However, it is usually unnecessary to replace blood loss of less than 500 mL. Operative blood loss is usually underestimated by the surgeon by 15%–40% in comparison to the isotopically measured loss, a factor that may contribute to the detection of anemia during the immediate postoperative period.

Ref.: 1, 2

21. Which of the following statements regarding total body water is true?

A. In males, approximately 40% of total body weight is water.

B. The percentage of total body weight that is water is higher in females than in males.

C. Obese individuals have a greater proportion of water (relative to body weight) than lean individuals.

D. The percentage of total body water decreases with age.

E. The majority of body water is contained within the interstitial fluid compartments.

ANSWER: D

COMMENTS: Approximately 50%–75% of body weight is water. In males, 60% (±15%) of body weight is water, and in females, 50% (±15%) of body weight is water. Age and lean body mass also contribute to differences in the percentage of total body weight that is water. Since fat contains little water, lean individuals have a greater proportion of **body water** than obese individuals of the same weight. Because females have more subcutaneous fat in relation to lean mass than males, they have less body water. Total body water decreases with age as a result of decreasing lean muscle mass. Infants have an unusually high ratio of total body water to body weight: up to 75%–80%. By 1 year of age, however, the percentage of body water approaches that of adults.

Body water is divided into three functional compartments: the **ICF compartment** (40% of body weight) and the **ECF compartment** (20% of body weight), which is further subdivided into the interstitial (15% of body weight) and intravascular (5% of body weight) fluid compartments.

Ref.: 1–3

22. A 62-year-old female takes 40 mg of furosemide twice daily for hypertension and CHF. Which of the following is true?

A. Loop diuretics act on the distal convoluted tubule in the nephron.

B. Magnesium is affected by loop diuretics.

C. Fatigue and muscle weakness are not side effects of her medication.

D. Loop diuretics decrease venous capacitance.

E. Loop diuretics are agonists to the sodium-potassium-chloride cotransporter.

ANSWER: B

COMMENTS: Loop diuretics, such as furosemide, are potent inhibitors of the sodium-potassium-chloride cotransporter. They act by competing for the chloride-binding site at the thick ascending limb of the loop of Henle. The effect is inhibition of sodium reabsorption, resulting in diuresis. Magnesium, potassium, and calcium will likewise be excreted, with the net increase in urine output. Hypomagnesemia can result in fatigue, muscle weakness, numbness, or even convulsions. Therefore it is important to monitor serum levels to prevent depletion while a patient is being treated with a loop diuretic.

Loop diuretics are commonly used for pulmonary edema because of their potency. In addition to inhibition of sodium absorption, they increase blood flow to the kidneys by stimulating vasodilatory prostaglandins and increase venous capacitance, which can quickly relieve pulmonary edema, even before diuresis and natriuresis have occurred. These three mechanisms help decrease ECF volume. Loop diuretics, such as furosemide or bumetanide, are extensively protein bound and must reach their intratubular site of action through active proximal tubular secretion.

Ref.: 1, 3

23. With regard to distributional shifts during an operation, which of the following statements is true?

A. The surface area of the peritoneum is not large enough to account for significant third-space loss.

B. Approximately 1 to 1.5 L/h of fluid is needed during an operation.

C. Blood is replaced as it is lost, without modification of the basal operative fluid replacement rate.

D. Sequestered ECF is predominantly hypotonic.

E. A major stimulus to ECF expansion is peripheral vasoconstriction.

ANSWER: C

COMMENTS: The **functional ECF volume** decreases during major abdominal operations largely because of sequestration of fluid in the operative site as a consequence of (1) extensive dissection, (2) fluid collection within the lumen and wall of the small bowel, and (3) accumulation of fluid in the peritoneal cavity. The surface area of the peritoneum is 1.8 m^2. When irritated, it can account for a functional loss of several liters of fluid that is not readily apparent. It is generally agreed that this lost volume should be replaced during the course of an operation with an isotonic saline solution as a "mimic" of sequestered ECF. Although there is no set formula for intraoperative fluid therapy, useful guidelines for replacement include the following. (1) Blood is replaced as it is lost, regardless of additional fluid therapy, provided that the patient meets the criteria for transfusion: hemoglobin concentration less than 7 g/dL. (2) Lost ECF should be replaced during the operative procedure if there is a delay in replacement until after the operation; fluid management is then complicated by adrenal and hypophyseal compensatory mechanisms that respond to operative trauma during the immediate postoperative period.

Ref.: 1–3

24. With regard to perioperative fluid management, which of the following statements is correct?

A. Insensible loss is approximately 600 mL/day.

B. Intraoperative insensible losses from an open abdomen are less than 250 mL/h.

C. About 200 to 300 mL of fluid is needed to excrete the catabolic end products of metabolism.

D. Lost urine should be replaced milliliter for milliliter.

E. Hypermetabolism and hyperventilation are not important factors in postoperative fluid loss or management.

ANSWER: A

COMMENTS: Postoperative fluid management requires assessment of the patient's volume status and evaluation for possible disorders in concentration or composition. All measured and insensible losses should be treated by replacement with appropriate fluids. In patients with normal renal function, the amount of potassium given is 40 mEq/day for replacement of renal excretion. An additional 20 mEq should be given for each liter of gastrointestinal loss. Insensible water loss is usually constant in the range of 600 mL/day. It can be increased to 1500 mL/day by hypermetabolism, hyperventilation, or fever. Insensible loss is replaced with 5% dextrose in water. Insensible loss may be offset by an insensible gain of water from excessive catabolism in postoperative patients who require prolonged intravenous fluid therapy. Approximately 800 to 1000 mL/day of fluid is needed to excrete the catabolic end products of metabolism. Because the kidneys are able to conserve sodium in a healthy individual, this amount can be replaced with 5% dextrose in water. A small amount of salt is usually added, however, to relieve the kidneys of the stress of sodium resorption. If there is a question regarding urinary sodium loss, measurement of urinary sodium levels helps determine the type of fluid that can best be used. Urine volume should not be replaced milliliter for milliliter because high output may represent diuresis of the fluids given during surgery or the diuresis that takes place to eliminate excessive fluid administration. Sensible or measurable losses such as those from the gastrointestinal tract are usually isotonic and should therefore be treated by replacement in equal volumes with isotonic salt solutions. The type of salt solution selected depends on determination of the patient's serum sodium, potassium, and chloride levels. In general, replacement fluids are administered at a steady rate over a period of 18 to 24 h as losses are incurred.

Ref.: 1–3

25. Which of the following has no effect on the development of hypernatremia?

A. Excessive sweating

B. Hyperlipidemia

C. Lactulose

D. Glycosuria

E. Inadequate maintenance fluids

ANSWER: B

COMMENTS: Hypernatremia is less common than hyponatremia in postoperative patients and is a reflection of elevated serum osmolality and hypertonicity. It is indicative of a deficiency of free water relative to the sodium concentration. Decreased intake of water, increased loss of water, and increased intake of sodium are the main mechanisms responsible for the development of hypernatremia. Loss of the thirst mechanism and an inability to access free water are mechanisms by which hypernatremia secondary to decreased intake of water can develop. Excessive sweating and large evaporative losses are mechanisms of loss of free water. Agents such as lactulose and sorbitol and carbohydrate malabsorption can cause osmotic diarrhea and result in relative losses of hypotonic fluid. Similarly, hyperglycemia causing glycosuria or diuresis in a catabolic patient excreting excess urea can also cause an osmotic diuresis. Both hyperlipidemia and hyperproteinemia are responsible for an entity known as pseudohyponatremia, which occurs when excess lipids or proteins displace water and create a falsely measured hyponatremia.

Ref.: 3

26. With regard to diabetes insipidus, which of the following statements is true?

A. Diabetes insipidus causes hypervolemic hyponatremia.

B. Central diabetes insipidus cannot be corrected by the administration of desmopressin.

C. Treatment of diabetes insipidus requires correction of hypernatremia at a rate faster than 12 mEq/day.

D. Alcohol intoxication can mimic diabetes insipidus.

E. Lithium administration could induce central diabetes insipidus.

ANSWER: D

COMMENTS: Diabetes insipidus is one of the causes of hypovolemic hypernatremia and is marked by a continual production of dilute urine of less than 200 mOsm/kg H_2O in the context of serum osmolarity of ECF greater than 300 Osm/L. Patients can have either central (lack of production of ADH by the hypothalamus) or nephrogenic (lack of response of the distal tubule of the nephron to ADH) diabetes insipidus. Alcohol causes suppression of vasopressin release and can mimic central diabetes insipidus. Treatment of hypernatremia consists of slow correction of sodium by the administration of free water. Whenever hypernatremia develops, a relative free water deficit exists and must be replaced. The water deficit can be approximated by using the following formula: water deficit = total body water × (1 − 140 ÷ serum sodium). Usually, the rate of correction of hypernatremia should not exceed 12 mEq/L/day. The aim should be to correct approximately half the deficit over the first 24 h. Too rapid correction of hypernatremia may lead to cerebral edema and seizures.

Desmopressin is a synthetic analogue of ADH that can be used to mimic arginine vasopressin (AVP) and to differentiate between central and nephrogenic diabetes insipidus. It is the agent of choice for treating patients with central diabetes insipidus because the drug increases water movement out of the collecting duct but does not have the vasoconstrictive effects of ADH. **Central diabetes insipidus** will respond to desmopressin, whereas nephrogenic diabetes insipidus will not. Unlike vasopressin, desmopressin is only renally active and does not have the vasoactive side effects. Lithium and amphotericin B can induce nephrogenic, not central, diabetes insipidus.

Ref.: 1, 3

27. A postoperative patient has a serum sodium concentration of 125 mEq/L and a blood glucose level of 500 mg/dL (normal level, 100 mg/dL). What would the patient's serum sodium concentration be (assuming normal renal function and appropriate intraoperative fluid therapy) if blood glucose levels were normal?

A. 120 mEq/L

B. 122 mEq/L

C. 137 mEq/L

D. 142 mEq/L

E. 147 mEq/L

ANSWER: C

COMMENTS: Serum osmolality is described as the amount of solutes per unit of water. It can be measured with an osmometer, or it can be calculated. It is reported as milliosmoles per liter. Calculation of serum osmolality is performed with the following equation:

$$P_{osm} = 2 \times \text{Na (mEq/L)} + \text{Glucose (mg \%)}/18 + \text{BUN (mg \%)}/2.9$$

The serum concentrations of sodium, urea, and glucose are required, whereas that of chloride is not required for the calculation. Simply doubling the serum sodium concentration provides an adequate estimate of serum osmolality.

As a general rule, each 100-mg/dL rise in the blood glucose level above normal is equivalent to a 1.6- to 3.0-mEq/L fall in the apparent serum sodium concentration. For example, if the patient has a blood glucose level of 500 mg/dL, or 400 mg/dL above normal, this is equivalent to a 12-mEq/L change in the serum sodium level. If this patient has a measured sodium concentration of 125 mEq/L, the sodium concentration is actually 137 mEq/L once the excess extracellular water has been eliminated.

Ref.: 1–3

28. Which one of the following is least useful in the immediate treatment of hyperkalemia?

A. Calcium salts

B. Sodium bicarbonate

C. Potassium-binding resins

D. Glucose and insulin

E. Hemodialysis

ANSWER: C

COMMENTS: The most dreaded complication of **hyperkalemia** is the development of a lethal arrhythmia. Immediate management includes ECG monitoring and cessation of all potassium supplementation and potassium-sparing drugs. **Calcium** is administered intravenously to stabilize the membrane potential and decrease myocardial excitability. It acts in less than 5 min, and the effects last for 30 to 60 min. **Sodium bicarbonate** drives potassium into cells, thereby transiently reducing serum potassium levels. Its actions last 15 to 30 min. **Insulin and glucose** also facilitate entry of potassium into cells, with an almost immediate onset of action. In cases of severe hyperkalemia, **hemodialysis** is the definitive and most rapid method of decreasing extracellular potassium. **Potassium-binding resins**, such as sodium polystyrene sulfonate (Kayexalate), begin lowering serum potassium within 1 to 2 h and last 4 to 6 h. Rectal administration of these binding resins is more effective than oral formulations. However, enemas with sodium polystyrene sulfonate combined with sorbitol have been associated with colon necrosis and perforation. Kaliuresis through the administration of diuretics such as acetazolamide is also effective in reducing serum potassium levels.

Ref.: 1–3

29. Which one of the following is not associated with hypocalcemia?

A. Shortening of the QT interval

B. Painful muscle spasms

C. Perioral or fingertip tingling

D. Seizures in children

E. Prolongation of the QT interval

ANSWER: A

COMMENTS: The symptoms of **hypocalcemia** are generally seen at serum levels of less than 8 mg/dL. Symptoms include numbness and tingling in the circumoral area and in the tips of the fingers and toes. Signs include hyperactive deep tendon reflexes, positive **Chvostek sign**, positive **Trousseau sign**, muscle and abdominal cramps, tetany with carpal pedal spasm, or convulsions. The ECG may show prolongation of the QT interval. Calcium is found in three forms in the body: **protein bound** (≈50%, mostly to albumin); diffusible calcium combined with anions such as bicarbonate, phosphate, and acetate (5%); and **ionized** (≈45%). Patients with severe alkalosis may have symptoms of hypocalcemia despite normal serum calcium levels because the ionized calcium is markedly decreased. Conversely, hypocalcemia without signs or symptoms may be present in patients with hypoproteinemia and a normal ionized fraction. Acute symptoms can be relieved by the intravenous administration of calcium gluconate or calcium chloride. Patients requiring prolonged replacement can be treated with oral calcium, often given with vitamin D.

Ref.: 1–3

30. Which one of the following clinical signs or symptoms is associated with serum sodium concentrations below 125 mEq/L?

A. Restlessness

B. Hallucinations

C. Tachycardia

D. Hyperventilation

E. Hyperthermia

ANSWER: B

COMMENTS: In most patients with **symptomatic hyponatremia**, the serum sodium concentration decreases below 125 mEq/L. When the concentration falls below 125 mEq/L, clinical signs and symptoms may occur, including headache, nausea, lethargy, hallucinations, seizures, bradycardia, hypoventilation, and occasionally coma. Hypothermia, not hyperthermia, occurs.

Ref.: 2, 3

31. Which one of the following is not a stimulus for ECF expansion?

A. Hemorrhage leading to a reduction in blood volume

B. Increased capillary permeability after major surgery

C. Peripheral arterial vasoconstriction

D. Negative interstitial fluid hydrostatic pressure

E. Colloid oncotic pressure

ANSWER: C

COMMENTS: Approximately 85% of the ECF that is within the vascular compartment resides in the venous circulation. Therefore the remaining 15% resides within the arterial system. The vascular compartment, otherwise known as **plasma fluid**, constitutes approximately one-third of the ECF. **Interstitial fluid** (i.e., fluid between the cells) makes up approximately two-thirds of the ECF. The **ECF** constitutes one-third of total body water, whereas the ICF represents two-thirds. Expansion of ECF is primarily driven by three mechanisms, all of which have the final common stimulus of reduction of intravascular volume. The first mechanism, hemorrhage, is directly responsible for the reduction in blood volume. Through various pathways, this drop in volume signals the retention and sequestration of fluid in the intravascular space. Increased capillary permeability, the second mechanism, occurs following major surgery and is due to the loss of endothelial integrity. This loss of integrity is mediated by several humoral factors that act on the endothelium. The end result of the loss of endothelial integrity is extravasation of protein-rich fluid into the interstitium, with a consequent increase in the interstitial fluid space. This constitutes the third mechanism of ECF expansion. Serum albumin is a major determinant of **colloid oncotic pressure**, and hypoalbuminemia could lead to transudation of fluid from the vascular to the interstitial compartment. This concept is expressed mathematically by the **Starling equation**: $Q_f = K_f \times (P_v - P_t) - \delta \times (\text{COP} - \text{TOP})$, where Q_f is fluid flux, K_f is the capillary filtration coefficient, P_v is vascular hydrostatic pressure, P_t is interstitial hydrostatic pressure, δ is a reflection coefficient (which defines the effectiveness of the membrane in preventing flow of solutes), COP is colloid osmotic pressure, and TOP is tissue osmotic pressure.

Ref.: 3

32. A 70-year-old man with sepsis has a pH of 7.18. Which of the following statements is true regarding his metabolic acidosis?

A. Tissue hypoxia leads to increased oxidative metabolism.

B. Acute compensation for metabolic acidosis is primarily renal.

C. Metabolic acidosis results from the loss of bicarbonate or the gain of fixed acids.

D. The most common cause of excess acid is prolonged nasogastric suction.

E. Restoration of blood pressure with vasopressors corrects the metabolic acidosis associated with circulatory failure.

ANSWER: C

COMMENTS: **Metabolic acidosis** results from the retention or gain of fixed acids (e.g., through diabetic acidosis or lactic acidosis) or the loss of bicarbonate (e.g., through diarrhea, small bowel fistula, or renal tubular dysfunction). Initial compensation is **respiratory** (by hyperventilation). **Renal compensation** is slower and occurs through the same means as the renal compensation for respiratory acidosis: excretion of acid salts and retention of bicarbonate. This compensation depends on normal renal function. When kidney damage interferes with the ability to excrete acid and resorb bicarbonate, metabolic acidosis may rapidly progress to profound levels. The most common cause of metabolic acidosis in surgical patients is **circulatory failure**, with tissue hypoxia and anaerobic metabolism, leading to the accumulation of lactic acid. Resuscitation with vasopressors or infusion of bicarbonate does not correct the underlying problem. Replacement of volume with a balanced electrolyte solution, blood, or both results in restoration of the circulation, hepatic clearance of lactate, consumption of the formed bicarbonate, and clearance of carbonic acid by the lung. Excessive use of **bicarbonate** can cause metabolic alkalosis, which, in combination with other sequelae such as hypothermia and low levels of 2,3-diphosphoglycerate (from banked blood), shifts the oxygen–hemoglobin distribution curve to the left and thereby compromises oxygen delivery.

Ref.: 1, 4

33. A 70-kg man with pyloric obstruction secondary to ulcer disease is admitted to the hospital for resuscitation after 1 week of prolonged vomiting. What metabolic disturbance is expected?

A. Hypokalemic, hyperchloremic metabolic acidosis

B. Hyperkalemic, hypochloremic metabolic alkalosis

C. Hyperkalemic, hyperchloremic metabolic acidosis

D. Hypokalemic, hypochloremic metabolic alkalosis

E. None of the above

ANSWER: D

COMMENTS: A common problem seen in patients with persistent emesis is **hypokalemic, hypochloremic metabolic alkalosis**. To compensate for the alkalosis associated with the loss of chloride- and hydrogen ion–rich fluid from the stomach, bicarbonate excretion in urine is increased. The bicarbonate is usually excreted as a sodium salt. However, in an attempt to conserve intravascular volume, aldosterone-mediated sodium absorption occurs and leads to potassium and hydrogen excretion. This compounds the alkalosis and results in a paradoxical aciduria. Management includes resuscitation with isotonic saline solutions and aggressive replacement of lost potassium.

Ref.: 1, 4

REFERENCES

1. Mullins RJ. Shock, electrolytes, and fluid. In: Townsend CM, Beauchamp RD, Evers BM, et al., eds. *Sabiston Textbook of Surgery: The Biological Basis of Modern Surgical Practice*. 18th ed. Philadelphia: WB Saunders; 2008.
2. Shires GT. Fluid and electrolyte management of the surgical patient. In: Brunicardi FC, Andersen DK, Billiar TR, et al., eds. *Schwartz's Principles of Surgery*. 9th ed. New York: McGraw-Hill; 2010.
3. Fenves AZ, Rao A, Emmett M. Fluids and electrolytes. In: O'Leary JP, ed. *The Physiologic Basis of Surgery*. 4th ed. Philadelphia: Lippincott Williams & Wilkins; 2008.
4. Jan BV, Lowry SF. Systemic response to injury and metabolic support. In: Brunicardi FC, Andersen DK, Billiar TR, et al., eds. *Schwartz's Principles of Surgery*. 9th ed. New York: McGraw-Hill; 2010.

B. Endocrine and Metabolic Response to Stress

Vidya A. Fleetwood, M.D., and Shabirhusain S. Abadin, M.D.

1. A 27-year-old male presents with perforated appendicitis. He is in severe discomfort and shows signs of activating his sympathoadrenal axis. All of the following activate the sympathoadrenal and hypothalamic–pituitary axes during stress or injury except:

A. Pain

B. Hypovolemia

C. Acidosis

D. Hypercapnia

E. Acetylcholine

ANSWER: E

COMMENTS: In response to **stress** or injury, neural afferent signals converge on the brain to activate the sympathetic nervous system and hypothalamic stimulation. Catecholamines are released from the sympathetic nervous system and result in increases in blood pressure, heart rate, cardiac output, and minute ventilation. Hypothalamic release of corticotropin-releasing hormone leads to release of corticotropin from the pituitary gland, which in turn induces the adrenal cortex to synthesize and release cortisol. These responses are designed to compensate for lost circulatory volume, maintain organ perfusion, and provide the energy substrates needed for organ function. Pain is a potent activator of these pathways. Hypovolemia simulates baroreceptors in the aorta and carotid bodies, which stimulates these pathways. Chemoreceptors in the carotid bodies and aorta are activated by hypoxemia, acidosis, and hypercapnia. These receptors also trigger the hypothalamic-pituitary-adrenal axis. Cytokines can likewise affect these pathways, though in a less direct manner since they do not have direct neural input into these axes. Acetylcholine has antiinflammatory effects and is not a part of the afferent response to injury.

Ref.: 1

2. The patient above exhibits signs of a systemic inflammatory response. All of the following are a part of the systemic inflammatory response syndrome (SIRS) except:

A. Temperature of 36°C or lower

B. Pulse rate lower than 56 beats/min

C. Respiratory rate of 20 breaths/min or higher

D. White blood cell count of 12,000/μL or greater

E. 10% or greater band forms on complete blood count (CBC) with differential

ANSWER: B

COMMENTS: The clinical spectrum of **SIRS** includes two or more of the following criteria:

- Temperature of 38°C or higher or 36°C or lower
- Pulse rate of 90 beats/min or greater
- Respiratory rate of 20 breaths/min or greater or a Pa_{CO_2} of 32 mmHg or lower
- White blood cell count of 12,000/μL or greater or 4000/μL or lower or 10% or more band forms on the CBC with differential

SIRS is a sterile response. Sepsis includes an identifiable source of infection in addition to SIRS.

Ref.: 2

3. A patient with pheochromocytoma shows signs of an amino acid deficiency, with coarse hair, dry skin and nails, and constipation. Which of the amino acids is critical to the synthesis of catecholamines?

A. Tyrosine

B. Phenylalanine

C. Glutamate

D. Aspartic acid

E. Methionine

ANSWER: A

COMMENTS: Tyrosine from the diet or from conversion of phenylalanine is the prime substrate for the synthesis of catecholamines. Tyrosine is hydroxylated to form dihydroxyphenylalanine (dopa), which undergoes decarboxylation to form dopamine. Dopamine is then hydroxylated to form norepinephrine. Norepinephrine is subsequently methylated in the adrenal medulla to form epinephrine. In patients with pheochromocytoma, tyrosine can be used up and the patient can become tyrosine deficient, exhibiting the symptoms above.

Ref.: 1

4. The patient above undergoes an open adrenalectomy and has an early postoperative fever, indicating inflammation due to cytokine release. All of the following are secreted as a part of the endocrine response to stress except:

A. Corticotropin

B. Antidiuretic hormone (ADH)

C. Growth hormone

D. Thyroid hormone

E. None of the above

ANSWER: E

COMMENTS: **Trauma** induces the release of **hormones**, which directly affect the metabolism of carbohydrates, fats, and proteins. Corticotropin is released from the pituitary gland and stimulates the release of cortisol, which stimulates hepatic gluconeogenesis and increases the release of amino acids from skeletal muscles. Release of ADH from the posterior pituitary gland in response to a decreased effective circulating plasma volume leads to increased peripheral vasoconstriction, increased water reabsorption, increased hepatic gluconeogenesis, and glycogenolysis. Growth hormone is released from the anterior pituitary and increases amino acid uptake and hepatic protein synthesis. Thyroid hormone release increases after injury in response to the release of thyroid-stimulating hormone (TSH) from the anterior pituitary. It induces glycolysis and gluconeogenesis and increases the metabolic rate and heat production.

Ref.: 1

5. A patient presents with an aldosteronoma and clinical evidence of suppression of the renin–angiotensin system. Which of the following is true of the system?

A. It is activated by an increase in the renal tubular sodium concentration.

B. Angiotensinogen is found in the renal medulla.

C. Angiotensin-converting enzyme in the liver converts angiotensin I to angiotensin II.

D. Angiotensin II stimulates the release of aldosterone.

E. Angiotensin II decreases splanchnic vasoconstriction.

ANSWER: D

COMMENTS: The **renin–angiotensin system** is activated by decreases in renal arterial blood flow and renal tubular sodium concentration, as well as increased β-adrenergic stimulation. Renin is secreted from the juxtaglomerular cells of the renal afferent arteriole. It converts angiotensinogen in the liver to angiotensin I. Angiotensin-converting enzyme produced by the lung converts angiotensin I to angiotensin II. Angiotensin II simulates the release of aldosterone, increases peripheral and splanchnic vasoconstriction, and decreases the renal excretion of salt and water.

Ref.: 1

6. A 35-year-old woman presents to you after running her first marathon with complaints of muscle aches. Which of the following is not an action of cortisol in this metabolically stressed patient?

A. It stimulates release of insulin by the pancreas.

B. It induces insulin resistance in muscles and adipose tissue.

C. It stimulates release of lactate from skeletal muscle.

D. It induces release of glycerol from adipose tissue.

E. It leads to immunosuppression.

ANSWER: A

COMMENTS: Cortisol is the major glucocorticoid released during **physiologic stress**. After injury, cortisol levels are elevated in proportion to the degree of stress to the patient. Metabolically, cortisol potentiates the actions of glucagon and epinephrine, which is manifested as hyperglycemia. It also stimulates enzymatic activities favoring hepatic gluconeogenesis. In skeletal muscle, cortisol induces protein degradation and release of lactate; lactate serves as a substrate for hepatic gluconeogenesis. It also potentiates the release of free fatty acids, triglycerides, and glycerol from adipose tissue to provide additional energy sources. In a stressed patient, cortisol induces insulin resistance in muscles and adipose tissue. All these actions are directed at increasing blood glucose levels in the stressed system. Answer A is therefore incorrect because insulin causes a decrease in blood glucose levels. Additionally, glucocorticoids cause depressed cell-mediated immune responses (decreased killer T-cell and natural killer cell function, as well as T-cell generation) and delayed hypersensitivity responses.

Ref.: 2

7. The patient above is found to have marked rhabdomyolysis. Which of the following are effects of epinephrine in response to injury in this patient?

A. It enhances the adherence of leukocytes to vascular endothelial membranes.

B. It stimulates the release of aldosterone.

C. It inhibits the secretion of thyroid hormones.

D. It increases glucagon secretion.

E. It decreases lipolysis in adipose tissue.

ANSWER: D

COMMENTS: The **catecholamines** norepinephrine and epinephrine are increased up to fourfold in plasma immediately after injury. In the liver, epinephrine promotes glycogenolysis, gluconeogenesis, lipolysis, and ketogenesis. It decreases insulin release and increases glucagon secretion. Epinephrine increases lipolysis in adipose tissue and induces insulin resistance in skeletal muscle. The overall effect of these actions is stress-induced hyperglycemia. Catecholamines also increase the secretion of thyroid and parathyroid hormones as a part of the stress response. Epinephrine induces leukocyte demargination from vascular endothelial membranes, which is manifested as leukocytosis.

Ref.: 2

8. Which of the following substances has been shown to be useful as a measurable marker of the response to injury?

A. Tumor necrosis factor-α (TNF-α)

B. Interleukin-2 (IL-2)

C. IL-6

D. IL-10

E. C-reactive protein (CRP)

ANSWER: E

COMMENTS: Cytokines released as a part of the **stress response** have a myriad of effects that both drive and inhibit the inflammatory process. TNF-α is among the earliest detectable cytokines after injury. It is secreted by macrophages, Kupffer cells, neutrophils, natural killer cells, T lymphocytes, mast cells, and endothelial cells, among others. It has a half-life of less than 20 min. TNF-α induces significant shock and catabolism. IL-2 is secreted by T lymphocytes and has a half-life of less than 10 min. It promotes lymphocyte proliferation, immunoglobulin production, and gut barrier integrity. It also regulates lymphocyte apoptosis. IL-6 is released by macrophages, B lymphocytes, neutrophils, basophils, mast cells, and endothelial cells. It has a long half-life and prolongs the survival of activated neutrophils. It is a potent inducer of acute-phase proteins in the liver. IL-10 is secreted by B and T lymphocytes, macrophages, basophils, and mast cells. It is an antiinflammatory cytokine and has been shown to reduce mortality in animal models of sepsis and acute respiratory distress syndrome (ARDS). CRP is useful as a marker of the response to injury because it reflects the degree of inflammation fairly accurately. CRP levels are not subject to diurnal variations and do not change with feeding. Consequently, it is used as a biomarker of inflammation and response to treatment.

Ref.: 2

9. After a gunshot wound to the lower extremity requiring operative exploration and repair of the popliteal artery, a patient has pain, pallor, and coldness of his leg. You suspect reperfusion injury causing compartment syndrome. Which of the following is true regarding reactive oxygen metabolites?

A. Reactive oxygen metabolites are synthesized and stored within leukocytes before being released in response to injury.

B. Reactive oxygen metabolites cause injury by oxidation of unsaturated fatty acids within cell membranes.

C. Cells secreting reactive oxygen metabolites are immune to damage after the release of these metabolites.

D. In ischemic tissue, the mechanisms for the production of reactive oxygen metabolites are downregulated.

E. Reactive oxygen metabolites are quenched by inhibitory cytokines.

ANSWER: B

COMMENTS: Reactive oxygen metabolites are short-lived, highly reactive molecules that cause tissue injury by oxidation of fatty acids within cell membranes. They are produced during anaerobic glucose oxidation, with the resulting production of superoxide anion from the reduction of oxygen. Superoxide anion is further metabolized to hydrogen peroxide and hydroxyl radicals. Cells are not immune to injury from the reactive oxygen metabolites that they release, but they are usually protected from damage by oxygen scavengers such as glutathione and catalases, not inhibitory cytokines. In ischemic tissues, the mechanisms for the production of oxygen metabolites are actually activated, but because of the lack of oxygen supply, the production of reactive oxygen metabolites is kept to a minimum. Once blood flow is restored, oxygen is redelivered, thereby allowing large quantities of reactive oxygen metabolites to be produced, which in turn leads to reperfusion injury. This is the inciting insult in compartment syndrome after the repair of vessels.

Ref.: 2

10. A patient presents with an acute gastrointestinal bleed and receives multiple transfusions of packed red blood cells. The following day, hypoxemia and bilateral infiltrates are observed on his chest x-ray. Which of the following statements about eicosanoids is true?

A. Their synthesis is dependent on the enzymatic activation of phospholipase A_2.

B. They originate from lymphocytes around the site of injury.

C. They are stored within inflammatory cells and released on tissue injury.

D. The production of leukotrienes is dependent on the enzymatic activation of cyclooxygenase.

E. The production of prostaglandins is dependent on the enzymatic activation of lipoxygenase.

ANSWER: A

COMMENTS: Eicosanoids are a class of mediators that includes **prostaglandins**, thromboxanes, leukotrienes, hydroxyeicosatetraenoic acids, and lipoxins. They are secreted by all nucleated cells except for lymphocytes. Phospholipids are converted by phospholipase A_2 into arachidonic acid. Arachidonic acid is then metabolized by cyclooxygenase to yield cyclic endoperoxides and eventually prostaglandins and thromboxanes. Alternatively, arachidonic acid is metabolized by lipoxygenase to yield hydroperoxyeicosatetraenoic acid and, eventually, hydroxyeicosatetraenoic acid and leukotrienes. Eicosanoids are not stored within cells but are synthesized and released in response to hypoxia or direct tissue injury. Other substances such as endotoxin, norepinephrine, vasopressin, angiotensin II, bradykinin, serotonin, acetylcholine, cytokines, and histamine can also induce the production and release of eicosanoids. Eicosanoids have a variety of deleterious effects, including acute lung injury, pancreatitis, and renal failure. They are extremely potent in promoting capillary leakage, leukocyte adherence, neutrophil activation, bronchoconstriction, and vasoconstriction.

Ref.: 2

11. In the patient above, you suspect transfusion-induced acute lung injury and intubate. The next day he has severe diffuse edema. Which of the following is true regarding the kallikrein–kinin system?

A. Bradykinins are potent vasoconstrictors produced in ischemic tissues.

B. Bradykinins are stored in macrophages and released in response to tissue injury.

C. Bradykinin release and elevation are proportional to the magnitude of injury.

D. Bradykinin antagonists have been shown to improve survival in septic trauma patients.

E. Bradykinin release is actually decreased in sepsis.

ANSWER: C

COMMENTS: Bradykinins are vasodilators produced by kininogen degradation by the protease kallikrein. **Kallikrein** circulates in blood and tissues in an inactive form until it is activated by Hageman factor, trypsin, plasmin, factor XI, kaolin, and collagen. Bradykinins increase capillary permeability, which leads to tissue edema. They also increase renal vasodilation, thereby leading to a reduction in renal perfusion pressure, which in turn activates the renin–angiotensin system and culminates in retention of sodium and water. Bradykinins are released during hypoxia and ischemia and after hemorrhage, sepsis, and endotoxemia. Elevations in bradykinins are proportional to the magnitude of the injury present. Studies in which bradykinin antagonists have been used to reduce the effects of sepsis show no improvement in survival.

Ref.: 2

12. Which of the following is true with regard to the complement cascade in the setting of injury, as in acute lung injury in the patient above?

A. Complement deactivates granulocyte activation.

B. Complement induces the release of TNF-α and IL-1.

C. Complement induces the relaxation of endothelial smooth muscle.

D. The complement components C3b and C5b are strong anaphylatoxins.

E. The complement cascade is inhibited by hemorrhage.

ANSWER: B

COMMENTS: Ischemia and endothelial injuries lead to the activation of **complement**, a series of plasma proteins involved in the inflammatory response. Complement is activated with the release of biologically active anaphylatoxins C3a and C5a during hemorrhage. These components cause granulocyte activation and aggregation, increased vascular permeability, smooth muscle contraction, and release of histamine and arachidonic acid metabolites. They also promote the release of TNF-α and IL-1, both major cytokines in the inflammatory response. Although the activation of complement can lead to the destruction and lysis of invading organisms, overactivation may result in tissue destruction and damage, as seen in ARDS.

Ref.: 3

13. A patient presents to the emergency room after a pitchfork puncture wound the day before, concerned about infection. Which of the following is true with regard to the inflammatory response?

A. Clot at the site of injury is the primary chemoattractant for neutrophils and monocytes.

B. Migration of neutrophils to the site of injury is inhibited by the release of serotonin.

C. Mast cells appear at the site of injury after migrating to the injury via chemoattractants such as cytokines.

D. Surgical or traumatic injury is associated with upregulation of cell-mediated immunity via type 1 helper T (T_H1) cells and downregulation of antibody-mediated immunity via type 2 helper T (T_H2) cells.

E. Eosinophils involved in the inflammatory response are inactivated by the complement anaphylatoxins C3a and C5a.

ANSWER: A

COMMENTS: Formation of clot at the site of injury serves as the primary **chemoattractant** for Band monocytes during the **inflammatory** response of the body to injury. Migration of neutrophils along with platelets through the vascular endothelium occurs within hours of injury and is facilitated by serotonin, platelet-activating factor, and prostaglandin E_2. **Mast cells** are preexistent in tissues and are therefore the first to be involved in the inflammatory response. They release histamine, cytokines, eicosanoids, proteases, and TNF-α, which results in local vasodilation, capillary leakage, and recruitment of other inflammatory cells to the area. In severe injuries, there is a reduction in cell-mediated immunity and T_H1 cytokine production and a shift toward antibody-mediated immunity through the action of T_H2 cells. A T_H1 response is favored in lesser injuries, with intact cell-mediated opsonizing capability and antibody immunity against microbial infections and with the activation of monocytes, B lymphocytes, and cytotoxic T lymphocytes. A shift to the T_H2 response is associated with more severe injuries and includes activation of eosinophils, mast cells, and B-lymphocyte antibody production. Eosinophils involved in the inflammatory response are activated by IL-3, granulocyte–macrophage colony-stimulating factor (GM-CSF), IL-5, platelet-activating factor, and the complement anaphylatoxins C3a and C5a.

Ref.: 2

14. In acute wounds as in the patient above, the initial recruitment of neutrophils to endothelial surfaces is mediated primarily by:

A. Immunoglobulins

B. Integrins

C. Selectins

D. All of the above

E. None of the above

ANSWER: C

COMMENTS: In endothelial injury, the initial recruitment of inflammatory leukocytes, specifically **neutrophils**, to the endothelial surfaces is mediated by adhesion molecules known as **selectins**, which are found on cell surfaces. Neutrophil rolling in the first 20 min after injury is mediated by P-selectin, which is stored within endothelial cells. After 20 min, P-selectin is degraded and L-selectin becomes the primary mediator of leukocyte rolling. Firm adhesion and transmigration of neutrophils through the endothelium and into the site of injury are mediated by integrins and the immunoglobulin family of **adhesion molecules**, including intercellular adhesion molecule (ICAM), vascular cell adhesion molecule (VCAM), and platelet–endothelial cell adhesion molecule (PECAM).

Ref.: 2

15. Which of the following regarding macrophages/monocytes is true?

A. Macrophages and monocytes become hyperresponsive to *continued* injury/insult after trauma.

B. Functional impairment in macrophage/monocyte capability may persist for a week and is overcome with the development and growth of newer, more immature monocytes.

C. Macrophages present peptides in association with major histocompatibility complex (MHC) class II molecules to prime $CD8^+$ cytotoxic T lymphocytes.

D. Human leukocyte antigen (HLA)/MHC II expression on monocytes increases after a major injury.

E. Macrophages present peptides in association with MHC class I molecules to prime $CD4^+$ helper T lymphocytes.

ANSWER: B

COMMENTS: After the initial short-lived hyperactivation involving the release of TNF and IL-1, **macrophages** and **monocytes** actually become hyporesponsive. Deactivation of these cells results in a type of immunologic paralysis. With stress, these cells release prostaglandin E_2, which has immunosuppressive effects. It inhibits T-cell mitogenesis, along with IL-1 and TNF-α production. This functional impairment in the patient's innate cellular immunity lasts for up to 7 days, until newly recruited monocytes are produced to bolster the immune response. Additional mediators such as transforming growth factor-β (TGF-β), IL-10, and IL-4 are also secreted after stress or trauma and inhibit the capability of macrophages and monocytes to present antigen to T cells, thereby contributing to impairment in antigen-specific immunity as well. The overall decrease in the adaptive immune response has been found to be associated with decreased resistance to infection. The functional impairment in macrophage/monocyte capability may persist for up to 7 days and is overcome with the development and growth of newer, more immature monocytes, which may lack the abilities of their predecessor monocytes. HLA-DR/MHC II expression on monocytes decreases after a major injury, with prolonged depression being associated with an increased infection rate. Macrophages present peptides in association with MHC class I molecules to prime $CD8^+$ cytotoxic T lymphocytes and peptides in association with MHC class II to prime $CD4^+$ helper T lymphocytes.

Ref.: 4

16. A patient with a history of alcohol abuse presents with profound hepatic failure after a Tylenol overdose. She is hypotensive, and you suspect delayed degradation of nitric oxide (NO) from her failing liver. Which of the following is true regarding NO?

A. NO is inhibited by acetylcholine stimulation.

B. NO is expressed constitutively.

C. NO can induce platelet adhesion and thus lead to microthrombosis.

D. NO has a half-life of 5 min.

E. NO is formed from the oxidation of L-alanine.

ANSWER: B

COMMENTS: NO is derived from the endothelial surfaces in response to acetylcholine stimulation, hypoxia, endotoxins, and cellular injury. It is expressed constitutively at low levels and helps maintain normal vascular smooth muscle relaxation. It reduces platelet adhesion and aggregation, thus making thrombosis of small vessels less likely. It is diffusible, with a half-life measured in seconds. NO is formed from the oxidation of L-arginine via the enzyme NO synthase. In liver failure, NO is not broken down efficiently, leading to hypotension.

Ref.: 2

17. A patient presents with complaints of weight loss and is found to have colon cancer. Which of the following regarding TNF-α is true?

A. It is predominantly a local mediator that induces the classic inflammatory febrile response to injury by stimulating local prostaglandin activity in the anterior hypothalamus.

B. It is effective in promoting the maturation/recruitment of functional leukocytes needed for a normal cytokine response and delays apoptosis of macrophages and neutrophils, which may contribute to organ injury.

C. It has both a proinflammatory and antiinflammatory roles; is a mediator of the hepatic acute-phase response to injury; induces neutrophil activation but also delays disposal of neutrophils; and can attenuate TNF-α and IL-1 activity, thereby curbing the inflammatory response.

D. It is an inducer of muscle catabolism and cachexia during stress by shunting available amino acids to the hepatic circulation as fuel substrates; it also activates coagulation and promotes the expression/release of adhesion molecules, prostaglandin E_2, platelet-activating factor, glucocorticoids, and eicosanoids.

E. It promotes T-cell proliferation, production of immunoglobulins, and gut barrier integrity.

ANSWER: D

COMMENTS: Cytokines are the most potent mediators of the inflammatory response. On a local level, they promote wound healing and proliferation of microorganisms. In excess levels, as sometimes occurs during the response to injury, they may induce hemodynamic instability, which can lead to organ failure or death. There is considerable overlap regarding the effects of cytokines with regard to promoting or attenuating the inflammatory response. Choice A describes IL-1. Choice B describes GM-CSF. Choice C describes IL-6. Choice D describes TNF-α. Choice E describes IL-2. TNF-α is thought to be responsible for the cachexia observed in cancer patients.

Ref.: 2

18. Which of the following is considered an antiinflammatory cytokine?

A. IL-1

B. IL-4

C. IL-6

D. IL-8

E. Interferon-γ (IFN-γ)

ANSWER: B

COMMENTS: The alterations in the hemodynamic, metabolic, and immune responses evident in stressed patients are orchestrated by endogenous polypeptides known as **cytokines**. They are produced by immune cells in direct response to injury, with levels correlating with the degree of tissue damage. Despite considerable overlap in bioactivity among cytokines, they are commonly classified by their predominant effect as proinflammatory or antiinflammatory. Those commonly considered proinflammatory include IL-1, IL-6, IL-8, and IFN-γ. Those usually considered antiinflammatory include IL-4, IL-10, IL-13, and TGF-β.

Ref.: 4

19. Which of the following is true with regard to TNF-α and IL-1?

A. Levels of soluble molecules that antagonize the effects of TNF-α and IL-1 have been shown to be predictive of organ failure.

B. Secretion of TNF-α and IL-1 is conducive to a hypocoagulable state during an acute injury.

C. Secretion of TNF-α and IL-1 in response to injury leads to the downregulation of the synthesis of NO and subsequent vasoconstriction.

D. TNF-α and IL-1 have a long half-life, which makes them effective markers for determining the magnitude and severity of the inflammatory response.

E. TNF-α and IL-1 have no natural antagonists; rather, their systemic effects diminish because of natural cytokine degradation.

ANSWER: A

COMMENTS: TNF-α and **IL-1** are overproduced in patients after posttraumatic inflammation. They induce increased synthesis of NO; activation of the **cyclooxygenase** and **lipoxygenase** pathways, which leads to the formation of thromboxanes and prostaglandins; and production of platelet-activating factor, intracellular adhesion molecules, and selectins, which is conducive to hypercoagulability. TNF-α and IL-1 have a short half-life, thus making them unreliable predictors of the severity of injury in the clinical setting. Soluble molecules that antagonize their effects are more stable and have been found to be predictive of lethal outcome and end-organ failure. IL-1 receptor antagonist (IL-1Ra) binds to the IL-1 receptor and blocks IL-1 activity. Soluble TNF receptors I and II (sTNF-RI and sTNF-RII) bind biologically active TNF and antagonize its effects.

Ref.: 4

20. All of the following with regard to IL-6 are true except:

A. IL-6 is a sensitive marker for the degree of tissue injury.

B. IL-6 induces the synthesis of CRP.

C. IL-6 secretion is inhibited by TNF-α and IL-1.

D. IL-6 levels peak early after injury.

E. IL-6 has antiinflammatory effects.

ANSWER: C

COMMENTS: IL-6 is a very sensitive marker for the degree of tissue injury. It is secreted by monocytes, macrophages, neutrophils, T and B cells, endothelial cells, smooth muscle cells, and fibroblasts. IL-6 expression is induced by bradykinin, TGF-β, platelet-derived growth factor, TNF-α, and IL-1, among others. IL-6 levels peak early after injury, with levels found to be predictive of risk for and mortality from organ failure after trauma. IL-6 induces the synthesis of acute-phase proteins such as fibrinogen, complement factors, α_1-antitrypsin, and CRP. CRP itself is a marker for states with increased inflammation and, in addition, is predictive of adverse outcomes following a secondary surgery. IL-6 also has some antiinflammatory effects, including inhibition of proteases and reduction of TNF-α and IL-1 synthesis; furthermore, it can cause the release of immunosuppressive glucocorticoids.

Ref.: 4

21. All of the following with regard to IL-8 are true except:

A. IL-8 levels after injury have been shown to correlate with the onset of multiorgan failure.

B. IL-8 exerts important inhibitory effects on polymorphonuclear cells.

C. IL-8 is associated with ARDS.

D. Local hypoxia induces the production of IL-8 from macrophages.

E. IL-8 does not produce the hemodynamic instability characteristic of TNF-α and IL-1.

ANSWER: B

COMMENTS: Like IL-6, **IL-8** levels peak within the first 24 h of injury. Prolonged elevation of IL-8 is predictive of the onset of multiorgan failure and even mortality. IL-8 is secreted by monocytes, macrophages, neutrophils, and endothelial cells. It is a potent chemoattractant for polymorphonuclear cells, particularly in the lung, where it is thought to have a role in initiating ARDS. Local hypoxia is thought to play a role in stimulating IL-8 production by pulmonary macrophages. Circulating polymorphonuclear cells migrate in response to IL-8 production, thereby leading to massive infiltration into the lungs, which in turn can progress to full-blown ARDS. Interestingly, IL-8 does not produce the hemodynamic instability characteristic of TNF-α and IL-1.

Ref.: 4

22. Which of the following with regard to IL-10 is true?

A. IL-10 is a strong proinflammatory cytokine.

B. IL-10 is secreted primarily by platelets in response to injury.

C. IL-10 inhibits some proinflammatory cytokines such as IL-1.

D. IL-10 has a short half-life and is therefore not a useful marker for assessing the severity of injury.

E. IL-10 secretion is inhibited by the stress of surgical procedures.

ANSWER: C

COMMENTS: IL-10 originates from T cells and monocytes. It has strong antiinflammatory properties and is capable of inhibiting the synthesis of proinflammatory cytokines such as IL-1 and TNF-α. It also induces a reduction in class II MHC molecules on monocytes, thereby leading to the downregulation of the immune response. IL-10 levels in trauma patients have been shown to reflect the severity of injury and are predictive of patients in whom sepsis or multiorgan dysfunction syndrome will develop. Release of IL-10 is increased in direct proportion to tissue damage, thus suggesting that more invasive surgical procedures augment the release of IL-10.

Ref.: 4

23. A patient in your intensive care unit (ICU) has hyperglycemia at 250 mg/dL 17 h after coronary artery bypass grafting. All of the following regarding insulin therapy are true except:

A. Hyperglycemia increases the morbidity of critically ill patients in the surgical ICU setting without significantly affecting mortality rates.

B. Maintaining blood glucose levels of 80 to 110 mg/dL is beneficial in surgical ICU patients.

C. Hyperglycemia impairs macrophage ability.

D. Insulin has antiinflammatory effects.

E. Hyperglycemia promotes coagulation.

ANSWER: A

COMMENTS: Prospective, randomized data from Van den Berge and colleagues have shown that hyperglycemia increases mortality rates in critically ill surgical ICU patients. Hyperglycemia promotes oxidative stress, coagulation, and phagocyte dysfunction. Advanced glycation end products resulting from hyperglycemia are themselves proinflammatory. Insulin has anabolic, antiinflammatory, and antiapoptotic effects. For all these reasons, **insulin therapy** for **tight blood glucose control** has been shown to improve outcomes in ICU patients. However, maintaining very strict glucose control (80 to 110 mg/dL) has been shown to worsen outcomes and increase mortality, and a higher threshold is recommended.

Ref.: 4

24. The above patient remains intubated and is without enteral feeding for 3 days. Which of the following is the main energy source during critical illness/injury?

A. Skeletal muscle

B. Liver

C. Adipose tissue

D. Kidney

E. Gut

ANSWER: C

COMMENTS: Lipids are nonprotein, noncarbohydrate fuel sources that minimize **protein breakdown** in injured patients. In response to catecholamines released during stress, triglyceride lipase induces fat mobilization/lipolysis from adipose stores. Glycerol is released and provides a substrate for hepatic gluconeogenesis. Fatty acids are released and processed into ketone bodies by the liver to provide an additional fuel source. Free fatty acids can also serve as a direct source of energy for such tissues as cardiac, kidney, liver, and muscle cells.

Ref.: 2

25. When attempting to wean from the ventilator on postoperative day 6, you notice the above patient has persistent hypercapnea and suspect overfeeding. Which of the following is correct with respect to the respiratory quotient (RQ)?

A. RQ = 1: greater oxidation of protein for fuel

B. RQ > 1: overfeeding/greater carbohydrate oxidation

C. RQ = 0.7: greater oxidation of carbohydrate for fuel

D. RQ = 0.85: greater oxidation of fatty acid for fuel

E. RQ < 1: excess breakdown of proteins for fuel

ANSWER: B

COMMENTS: The **RQ** is a unitless number used for the calculation of basal metabolic rate when estimated from carbon dioxide production. It is calculated from the ratio of CO_2 produced and O_2 consumed. The RQ in patients who are in metabolic balance usually ranges from 1.0 (the value expected for pure carbohydrate oxidation) to 0.7 (the value expected for pure fat oxidation). A mixed diet of fat and carbohydrate results in an average value between these numbers. The RQ may rise above 1.0 in an organism oxidizing carbohydrate to produce fat, as in overfeeding. In summary,

RQ = 1: greater oxidation of carbohydrate for fuel
RQ > 1: overfeeding/greater carbohydrate oxidation
RQ = 0.7: greater oxidation of fatty acid for fuel
RQ = 0.85: oxidation of equal amounts of fatty acids and glucose

Ref.: 2

REFERENCES

1. Zukerbraun BS, Harbrecht BG. The physiologic response to injury. In: Peitzman AB, Rhoes M, Schwab CW, et al., eds. *The Trauma Manual: Trauma & Acute Care Surgery*. 3rd ed. New York: Lippincott Williams & Wilkins; 2008.
2. Jan BV, Lowry SF. Systemic response to injury and metabolic support. In: Brunicardi FC, Andersen DK, Billiar TR, et al., eds. *Schwartz's Principles of Surgery*. 9th ed. New York: McGraw-Hill; 2010.
3. Phelan HA, Esatman AL, Frotan A, Gonzales RP. Shock and hypoperfusion states. In: O'Leary JP, Tabuenca A, Capote LR, eds. *The Physiologic Basis of Surgery*. 4th ed. New York: Lippincott Williams & Wilkins; 2008.
4. Faist E, Trentzsch H. The immune response. In: Feliciano DV, Mattox KL, Moore EE, eds. *Trauma*. 6th ed. New York: McGraw-Hill Medical; 2007.

C. Nutrition

Vidya A. Fleetwood, M.D., and Shabirhusain S. Abadin, M.D.

1. For an adult patient consuming a normal diet, which of the following is the most calorically dense energy source?

A. Fat
B. Alcohol
C. Protein
D. Carbohydrate
E. Water

ANSWER: A

COMMENTS: Fat stores can equal 160,000 kcal, with higher stores present in obese individuals. Lean body mass proteins can supply 30,000 kcal of the body's energy stores. Energy in the diet can be provided by carbohydrates (4 kcal/g), fats (9 kcal/g), proteins (4 kcal/g), and alcohol (7 kcal/g).

Ref.: 1

2. A 53-year-old diabetic patient undergoes small bowel resection for volvulus. He now has a prolonged postoperative ileus and has had only 0.45% normal saline for 5 days. In order to limit protein catabolism, how much glucose should be administered in his total parenteral nutrition (TPN)?

A. 1 L of 5% dextrose in water (D_5W)
B. 2 L of D_5W
C. 3 L of D_5W
D. 4 L of D_5W
E. 5 L of D_5W

ANSWER: B

COMMENTS: Blood glucose levels are regulated by hormones in response to carbohydrate intake. Insulin secretion increases with intake of glucose, and glucagon secretion declines, thus allowing an increased uptake of glucose by liver, muscle, and adipose tissue. Conversely, glucagon mobilizes liver glycogen via the cyclic adenosine monophosphate (cAMP) protein kinase system when blood glucose levels decrease because of decreased intake. Glucose tolerance is determined by the rate at which mechanisms of glucose removal can operate. Administration of 100 g of glucose (or 1 mg/kg/min) has a protein-sparing effect that suppresses the use of nitrogen (from amino acids) for gluconeogenesis. D_5W, or 5% dextrose per liter of water, contains 50 g of dextrose per liter.

Ref.: 1

3. A patient with a history of a trauma laparotomy presents with a small bowel obstruction. A nasogastric tube is placed that aspirates greater than 4L of fluid per day. The gastrointestinal tract can secrete and reabsorb how much water in the form of gastric juices per day (in a 70-kg adult male)?

A. 1 to 2 L/day
B. 4 to 5 L/day
C. 6 to 7 L/day
D. 8 to 10 L/day
E. 50 L/day

ANSWER: D

COMMENTS: The end products of protein, carbohydrate, and fat oxidation include water, with 1 g of carbohydrate yielding 0.6 mL of water, 1 g of protein yielding 0.42 mL, and 1 g of fat yielding 1.07 mL. In addition, the gastrointestinal tract may secrete and reabsorb as much as 8 to 10 L/day of water as digestive juices in the following estimated amounts: saliva, 1500 mL; gastric juice, 2500 mL; bile, 500 mL; pancreatic juices, 700 mL; intestinal juices, 3000 mL; and water intake, 2000 mL.

Ref.: 2

4. In the above patient, the decreased insulin–glucagon ratio seen during simple starvation allows:

A. Increased lipogenesis
B. Increased lipolysis
C. Increased protein synthesis
D. Increased glycogen production
E. Decreased lipolysis

ANSWER: B

COMMENTS: During **starvation**, the insulin–glucagon ratio is decreased, which allows activation of lipolysis and suppression of lipogenesis. Lipolysis breaks down fat to free fatty acids, which are used as alternative fuels by many tissues that prefer fat as a fuel source (i.e., kidney, cardiac muscle, and skeletal muscle). The liver oxidizes fatty acids to acetyl CoA, which is then converted to ketones. As **ketone** (acetoacetate and β-hydroxybutyrate) levels rise, they can cross the blood–brain barrier to supply fuel, but some glucose is still required. The use of fatty acids as a primary fuel source allows the sparing of body proteins for gluconeogenesis. This sparing effect is important for maintenance of immune functions and liver and respiratory muscle function. A respiratory quotient (RQ, Vco_2/Vo_2) of 0.6 to 0.7 during simple starvation reflects the fact that fat is the body's primary fuel source during simple starvation.

Ref.: 3

5. During simple starvation, gluconeogenesis is important for:

A. Glycogen storage
B. Lipogenesis to continue to allow adequate fat storage
C. Protein synthesis to progress to allow muscle health
D. Tissues that use only glucose for fuel, such as the brain and blood, and are dependent on this process
E. None of the above

ANSWER: D

COMMENTS: Simple starvation results when nutrient intake does not meet energy requirements. Energy expenditure characteristically decreases to help match energy intake, and metabolic responses occur to preserve the muscle mass. In early fasting, glycogenolysis is the first energy source, followed by gluconeogenesis to maintain a glucose supply to obligate glucose users such as the brain, blood, renal medulla, and bone marrow. Gluconeogenesis requires alanine, glycerol, and lactate; therefore the focus of other organ systems in early fasting is to provide these substrates to the liver.

Initially, during early fasting, the glycogen derived from glycogenolysis supplies glucose for obligatory glucose-using tissues. Lipogenesis is curtailed. The Cori cycle is then activated, which allows glucose to be converted back to lactate through glycolysis in the peripheral tissues. Skeletal muscle releases alanine via the alanine cycle. Through these reactions, alanine and lactate are created for gluconeogenesis.

Ref.: 3

6. Which amino acid is released in large amounts to be used by the liver during simple starvation?

A. Valine

B. Serine

C. Glutamine

D. Cysteine

E. Homocysteine

ANSWER: C

COMMENTS: Protein metabolism adapts to starvation as follows: (1) the synthesis of protein decreases because energy sources for production are not available, (2) protein catabolism is reduced as other fuels become the primary sources of energy for many tissues, and (3) decreased ureagenesis and urinary nitrogen loss reflect protein sparing (in the initial stages of starvation, the rate of urea nitrogen loss is greater than 10 g/day, with a decline to less than 7 g/day after weeks of starvation). Alanine, glutamine, and glycine are released in large amounts to be used by the liver and kidney for net glucose formation.

Ref.: 3

7. A 24-year-old male is made nil per os (NPO) after midnight for lipoma removal the next day. His case is delayed until early evening, and he enters simple starvation. In this patient, glucagon mobilizes which of the following?

A. Glycogen from muscle tissue

B. Liver glycogen

C. Insulin to improve the cellular uptake of glucose

D. Glucose to the liver for storage

E. None of the above

ANSWER: A

COMMENTS: Carbohydrates can be classified as complex (polysaccharides) or simple (mono- and disaccharides). Carbohydrate digestion starts in the mouth with salivary amylase, which hydrolyzes polysaccharide bonds, and continues with pancreatic amylase and the enzymes sucrase, lactase, maltase, and isomaltase from intestinal epithelial cells to yield monosaccharides.

Glucose, a monosaccharide, is the preferred fuel in humans, with all the metabolism beginning or ending with this hexose. Glucose is transported to the liver via the portal circulation and goes on to form pyruvate, glycogen, or fat in adipose tissue.

Glycogen is the stored form of carbohydrates and is present in the liver and the skeletal muscle; the liver glycogen is for general use and can be mobilized at any time using the enzyme **glucose-6-phosphatase**, whereas muscles lack this enzyme and therefore conserve their glycogen for exclusive muscle use.

In times of fasting, glucagon activates the enzyme **glycogen phosphorylase** to facilitate **glycogenolysis**. Glucagon also inhibits glycogen synthase, preventing the formation of new glycogen. Glycogenolysis can provide glucose supplies for 12 to 24 h of fasting.

Ref.: 3, 9

8. A patient presents with lymphoma and a left pleural effusion; upon drainage, the fluid is noted to be chylous. In which of the following is he likely to be deficient?

A. Short-chain fatty acids

B. Medium-chain fatty acids

C. Long-chain fatty acids

D. Calcium

E. Vitamin B_{12}

ANSWER: C

COMMENTS: Fat absorption is through the small intestine and the lymphatics.

Medium- and **short-chain free fatty acids** enter the enterocyte through simple diffusion and are transported from there into the portal system. **Triacylglycerides** (TAGs), cholesterol, and lipids are broken down by pancreatic lipase, cholesterol esterase, phospholipase, and bile salts to form **micelles** and free fatty acids in the intestine. Micelles contain bile salts, **long-chain fatty acids**, and cholesterol. The micelles then fuse with the enterocyte membrane and from there undergo breakdown in the enterocyte.

TAGs are then resynthesized and form **chylomicrons** with phospholipids and cholesterol. These, along with long-chain fatty acids, enter the lymphatics to empty into the thoracic duct.

Chylothorax and other lymphatic or thoracic duct disruptions can result in a profound deficiency of TAGs and long-chain fatty acids.

Ref.: 3, 9

9. A patient presents with a 55% total body surface area (TBSA) burn. Early enteral feeds are started per protocol, and the burn unit director considers glutamine supplementation. Glutamine is an amino acid that:

A. Is categorized as an essential amino acid

B. Is found only in muscle tissue

C. Has been shown to be conditionally essential during stress

D. Maintains stable levels in plasma during stress

E. Can be eliminated from the diet during times of stress

ANSWER: C

COMMENTS: Body proteins are made up of 20 different amino acids, each of which has a different metabolic rate and function in the body. There are three categories of amino acids: (1) essential amino acids, which cannot be synthesized by the body; (2) nonessential amino acids, which can be synthesized de novo in the body; and (3) conditionally essential amino acids, which consist of nonessential amino acids that are considered essential during stress or trauma if their use exceeds the body's capacity for synthesis and an outside source is required.

Glutamine, the most abundant amino acid in the body, is a conditionally essential amino acid; it accounts for 50% of the amino acids in muscle, and its concentrations can fall during times of stress because of the body's inability to meet increases in body requirements for the amino acid. Glutamine is the major amino acid for intestinal mucosa, and some evidence shows improved outcomes in burn patients with glutamine supplementation. Other conditionally essential amino acids include arginine and tyrosine.

Ref.: 4, 19

10. Which amino acids are classified as essential, can be metabolized outside the liver, and are a local source of energy for muscle?

A. Leucine, isoleucine, and valine
B. Alanine, arginine, and lysine
C. Ethionine, glutamine, and lysine
D. Phenylalanine, tyrosine, and histidine
E. None of the above

ANSWER: A

COMMENTS: Essential amino acids are those that cannot be synthesized and must be obtained in the diet. The essential amino acids are valine, leucine, isoleucine, methionine, lysine, threonine, phenylalanine, and tryptophan. Of these, valine, leucine, and isoleucine are branched-chain amino acids; this makes them less susceptible to first-pass metabolism and less amenable to breakdown in the liver. They are easily broken down by muscle and therefore provide an energy source to skeletal muscle. The breakdown products of these amino acids are alanine and glutamine.

Ref.: 5

11. A 65-year-old woman with recently diagnosed nonobstructing colon cancer presents to schedule a right hemicolectomy. She has read about nutrition and healing after her surgery and asks how she can optimize her protein intake. What are the dietary protein recommendations for a 60-kg woman with intact protein stores?

A. 0.7 to 0.8 g/kg/day (42 to 48 g/day)
B. 0.9 to 1.0 g/kg/day (54 to 60 g/day)
C. 1.2 to 1.5 g/kg/day (72 to 90 g/day)
D. 2 to 4 g/kg/day (120 to 240 g/day)
E. 5 to 6 g/kg/day (300 to 360 g/day)

ANSWER: A

COMMENTS: The dietary protein requirement for adults is 0.8 g/kg/day; that is, approximately 20% of the calories consumed should be in the form of protein. One gram of nitrogen equals 6.24 g of protein. In patients undergoing acute stress such as that of surgery, protein intake should rise to 1.2 to 1.5 g/kg/day; in patients with severe stress, such as burns or large nonhealing wounds, protein requirements may rise to 2 to 4 g/kg/day. For burn patients, protein requirements may be calculated by the following formula:

$$\text{Protein} = 1.5 \text{ g/kg/day} + (3 \text{ g} \times \% \text{ TBSA burn})$$

Ref.: 6

12. A patient presents with a perforated Meckel's diverticulum and undergoes terminal ileal resection with reanastomosis. He subsequently develops poor reabsorption of bile acids. What is the primary substrate for the formation of bile acids?

A. Cholesterol
B. Triglycerol
C. Triglycerides
D. Phospholipids
E. Insulin

ANSWER: A

COMMENTS: Three main forms of fat are found in the body: glycerides, phospholipids, and sterols. **Glycerides**, principally triglycerides and triglycerol (fatty acid and glycerol), are the storage forms of fat and are the most abundant forms in food; they account for approximately 95%–98% of ingested fat and the fat in tissues. Triglycerides store calories, protect organs, and act as insulators. **Phospholipids** are ingested in small amounts and are main constituents of cell membranes and myelin sheaths; they are the substrates for prostaglandins, leukotrienes, and thromboxanes. **Sterols** consist primarily of cholesterol. **Cholesterol** is the substrate for the formation of bile acids (the primary bile acids are cholate and chenodeoxycholate) and steroid hormones (aldosterone, progesterone, estrogen, and androgens).

Ref.: 7

13. A 26-year-old patient presents with abdominal pain, weight loss, and steatorrhea. He is found to have severe terminal ileal involvement and structuring. In which of the following vitamins is he least likely to be deficient?

A. Vitamin A
B. Vitamin D
C. Vitamin E
D. Vitamin C
E. Vitamin K

ANSWER: D

COMMENTS: Vitamins can be either water soluble (vitamin C and B vitamins—thiamin, niacin, riboflavin, folate, vitamin B_6, vitamin B_{12}, biotin, and pantothenic acid) or fat soluble (vitamins A, D, E, and K). Patients with steatorrhea, as seen in those with an absent or damaged terminal ileum or those with pancreatitis, can present with deficiencies of the fat-soluble vitamins.

The following are the classic signs of vitamin deficiency:

Vitamin A—dermatitis, night blindness, and poor wound healing
Vitamin D—bone demineralization and osteopenia
Vitamin E—increased platelet aggregation and decreased red blood cell survival
Vitamin K—bruising and hemorrhage

Ref.: 8, 9

14. Which of the following is not a component of the Harris–Benedict equation?

A. Weight
B. Height
C. Age
D. Gender
E. % Lean body mass

ANSWER: E

COMMENTS: The Harris–Benedict equation can be used to predict the basal metabolic rate of a given patient at rest. The equation factors in weight, height, age, and gender form an estimation of caloric needs. It is not an infallible estimate but is commonly used as baseline estimation.

In general, a patient's diet should be broken into 20% protein, 30% fat, and 50% carbohydrates. Protein needs may increase in the postsurgical state or when significant wound healing is necessary, as in burns. Trauma, surgery, sepsis, pregnancy, lactation, and fever can increase basal metabolic needs significantly.

Ref.: 9

15. A 75-year-old female presents with ductal carcinoma in situ for simple mastectomy. She has marked muscle wasting on examination and admits to a poor diet. Which of the following values is most predictive of postoperative mortality?

A. Serum sodium

B. Serum albumin

C. Serum protein

D. Serum creatinine

E. Serum glucose

ANSWER: B

COMMENTS: Nutritional assessment of surgical patients involves evaluation for preexisting malnutrition, comorbidities, risk factors for malabsorption, and substance dependency. A number of laboratory tests may be performed based on the patient's individual risk factors. Multiple test values and anthropomorphic measurements have been used to evaluate the risk of nonhealing and complications after surgery; however, only serum **albumin** has been found to correlate directly with morbidity and mortality. Preoperative albumin levels less than 3 g/dL are associated with an increased risk of developing serious complications within 30 days of surgery, including sepsis, acute renal failure, coma, failure to wean from ventilation, cardiac arrest, pneumonia, and wound infection. A serum albumin level greater than 4.5 carries a <1% risk of mortality, less than 3 carries a 9% risk, and less than 2 carries a 30% risk.

Ref.: 9, 11

16. A 55-year-old woman presents with pneumoperitoneum and is found to have a perforated gastric ulcer with gross intraabdominal spillage. Subsequently, she has sepsis and a prolonged intubation, and tube feeds are started. Which of the following visceral proteins is the best indicator of her immediate nutritional status?

A. Prealbumin

B. Albumin

C. Transferrin

D. Total protein

E. Serum globulin

ANSWER: A

COMMENTS: In patients with a prolonged lack of nutrition, serum markers of nutrition are a helpful way of assessing the adequacy of nutritional supplementation. Serum total protein levels are nonspecific and can be elevated by viral or autoimmune disease processes. Levels of serum albumin, which has a half-life of 18 to 21 days, are helpful in the outpatient setting to assess general nutrition but are poorly reflective of short-term changes while hospitalized. Serum transferrin is commonly used but has a half-life of 8 to 10 days, again reflecting too long a time period to provide day-by-day assessments. Serum prealbumin has a half-life of 10 h to 2 days, depending on which isotype is used, and is commonly obtained to assess the response to supplementation.

Of note, all of these markers are hepatic acute-phase reactants and can decrease in times of stress; therefore the trend is more significant than the absolute value.

Ref.: 9, 10

17. A patient presents to the trauma bay after a house fire with a 65% TBSA burn. He is intubated and remains in the burn unit for 5 days, after which he enters the hypermetabolic flow phase of stress metabolism. Hyperglycemia during stress hypermetabolism can be attributed to:

A. Increased insulin resistance

B. Increased glycogen storage

C. Decreased lipolysis

D. Increased glycogenesis

E. Increased insulin uptake

ANSWER: A

COMMENTS: In contrast to simple starvation, activation of **stress hypermetabolism** occurs following surgery, trauma, or sepsis to provide energy and substrates for tissue repair and to activate immune function and the inflammatory response. In the initial period, known as the **ebb phase**, a decline in oxygen consumption is seen, along with poor circulation, fluid imbalance, and cellular shock lasting 24 to 36 h. As the body adapts (**flow or plateau phase**), enhanced cellular activity and increased hormonal stimulation take place and lead to an elevated metabolic rate, body temperature, and nitrogen loss. This phase can last days, weeks, or months.

Both phases are characterized by hyperglycemia. In the ebb phase, patients manifest impaired glucose tolerance. In the flow phase, patients display frank insulin resistance.

In the hypermetabolic phase, glycogen storage is attenuated and lipogenolysis is increased in an effort to keep up with the grossly increased metabolic demands of wound healing.

Ref.: 12

18. In the patient above, stress hypermetabolism is characterized by:

A. Decreased body temperature

B. Hypoglycemia and glycogenesis

C. Fluid imbalance and increased resting metabolic rate

D. Decreased gluconeogenesis and proteolysis

E. Decreased urinary protein retention

ANSWER: C

COMMENTS: The earliest stages of hypermetabolism are characterized by increases in gluconeogenesis, resting energy expenditure (REE), proteolysis, ureagenesis, and urinary nitrogen loss. Clinical signs include tachypnea, increased body temperature, and tachycardia, with laboratory results showing increased leukocytosis, hyperlactatemia, azotemia, and hyperglycemia. Liver production of glucose during stress is increased through gluconeogenesis and glycogenolysis (Cori cycle), which are stimulated by endocrine (hormonal) changes: increased cortisol, increased glucagon, increased catecholamines, and decreased insulin. Overall use of protein as an oxidative fuel source by the liver is increased, and typically, there is increased turnover of branched-chain amino acids.

Ref.: 12

19. A 59-year-old woman remains intubated due to sepsis after perforated diverticulitis. She has failed multiple trials of extubation due to hypercapnia, which you suspect to be due to overfeeding. Which of the following RQs is characteristic of overfeeding?

A. 0.75

B. 0.85

C. 0.90

D. 1.0

E. 1.05

ANSWER: E

COMMENTS: Calculation of the RQ allows the clinician to alter the nutrient content of feedings to optimize the macronutrient intake. The RQ is the ratio of CO_2 expired (Vco_2) to the amount of O_2 inspired (Vo_2): $RQ = Vco_2/Vo_2$.

The RQ is reflective of the type of energy expenditure. CO_2 is produced when carbohydrates are converted to fat; therefore an elevated RQ (1.0) indicates pure carbohydrate metabolism, and an RQ of >1.0 indicates conversion of carbohydrates into fat and therefore overfeeding.

An RQ of 0.7 is consistent with pure fat metabolism (starvation), 0.8 with pure protein metabolism, and 0.83 with a balanced metabolism. A high RQ, by definition, causes hypercapnia and can lead to difficulty to wean from the ventilator.

Ref.: 9, 13

20. A 35-year-old man is admitted to the intensive care unit (ICU) following a diagnosis of acute pancreatitis. After initial resuscitation, the patient's condition improves and enteral tube feedings are started through a postpyloric tube. Initial intolerance to a tube feeding regimen requires the clinician to:

A. Immediately start TPN

B. Add water to the feeding regimen to dilute the feedings for better tolerance

C. Slow the tube feeding regimen and progress to the goal rate less aggressively

D. Immediately change the tube feeding formula

E. Increase the tube feeding rate per hour

ANSWER: C

COMMENTS: Enteral feedings have been shown to decrease septic complications and are theorized to prevent intestinal bacterial translocation. Complications can be metabolic (e.g., overhydration or underhydration) or gastrointestinal (e.g., diarrhea, nausea, vomiting, delayed gastric emptying, constipation, or abdominal distention). **Diarrhea** has been estimated to occur in 2.3% of the enteral population and in 34%–41% of critically ill patients. Diarrhea may be related to (1) factors associated with the patient's underlying illness or (2) factors related to the tube feeding formula, including too rapid an infusion rate, too rapid initiation or progression, lactose intolerance, microbe contamination, lack of fiber, the osmolality of the formula, or a high fat content in the formula. The diarrhea may be controlled by (1) antimotility agents, (2) changing to continuous feeding, or (3) slowing the rate of tube feeding until tolerance is established, before initiation of medication to control the problem.

Ref.: 14

21. A 67-year-old woman with a history of atrial fibrillation is admitted to the emergency department with complaints of abdominal pain out of proportion to the physical findings. She is found to have superior mesenteric arterial occlusion and undergoes on-table thrombectomy and stenting with small bowel resection. The remaining proximal jejunum measures 100 cm. What is the minimum amount of small intestine required for absorption of nutrients before considering the use of enteral feedings?

A. 20 cm of small intestine

B. 50 cm of small intestine

C. 100 cm of small intestine

D. 120 cm of small intestine

E. 250 cm of small intestine

ANSWER: C

COMMENTS: The functional capacity of the gut must be considered before prescribing enteral nutrition therapy. There must be at least 100 cm of the small intestine for absorption of nutrients with an intact ileocecal valve, or 150 cm with an incompetent ileocecal valve. Relative contraindications for the use of the gastrointestinal tract include gastroparesis, intestinal obstruction, and paralytic ileus. More absolute contraindications include high-output enteric fistula, short bowel syndrome, severe malabsorption, and hemodynamic instability.

Ref.: 9, 14

22. Due to multiple takebacks for "second-look" procedures and attempts at extubation, the patient in the question above remains without enteral nutrition for 8 days. Which type of formula might be appropriate for a patient who has been NPO for more than 1 week and has a partially functioning gastrointestinal tract?

A. Elemental formula

B. Concentrated formula

C. Specialty formula

D. Modular formula

E. Superconcentrated formula

ANSWER: A

COMMENTS: Tube feeding formulas are divided into six types: standard, concentrated, high nitrogen, elemental, fiber containing or blenderized, and special. They differ by nutritional content and texture. **Standard** formulas contain 50%–60% of calories being derived from carbohydrates, 10%–15% from protein, and 25%–40% from fat. They are appropriate for patients with no major enteral restrictions who have been NPO for less than 1 week. **Concentrated** formulas have similar nutritional content but decreased water content, making them suitable for patients with fluid restrictions or those receiving bolus feedings. **Elemental** formulas contain hydrolyzed macronutrients, requiring less energy and mucosal interface to digest; they are appropriate for those who have had a prolonged NPO status or those with tube feed intolerance. **High-nitrogen-protein** formulas provide more than 15% of calories from proteins and are appropriate for those with high protein needs. **Fiber-containing** and blenderized formulas contain increased fiber to decrease diarrhea. Special formulas have special formulations for special patient populations, such as those with renal failure or hepatic failure.

Ref.: 15

23. Which of the following is one of the most common food allergies that must be considered when deciding on a tube feeding formula?

A. Rice allergy

B. Soy allergy

C. Nut allergy

D. Corn syrup allergy

E. Citrus fruit allergy

ANSWER: C

COMMENTS: Food allergy considerations are important when selecting an enteral formula. Nuts, fruits, and milk are the most common food allergy triggers for 20% of the population of allergy sufferers. Gluten tolerance should also be a consideration. Some enteral products contain lactose, which causes bloating, cramping, and diarrhea in some patients. Because of electrolyte imbalances or the need for varied macronutrient content, some patients have needs that cannot be met by the available commercial products. Enteral feeding modules can be used to create a patient-specific formula (**modular formula**) that addresses the carbohydrate, protein, and fat requirements.

Ref.: 16

24. How many calories are provided in one 500-mL bottle of 20% intravenous fat solution?

A. 150 kcal

B. 550 kcal

C. 800 kcal

D. 1000 kcal

E. 4000 kcal

ANSWER: D

COMMENTS: Fat solutions are available in 10%, 20%, and 30% solutions, which provide 1.1, 2.0, and 3.0 kcal/mL of energy, respectively. In this question, 500 mL of a 20% infusion provides 1000 kcal.

Ref.: 17

25. A 65-year-old man is admitted to the hospital because of profuse diarrhea after small bowel resection for an ischemic bowel that resulted in short bowel syndrome. The patient is resuscitated and TPN started. What is the maximum infusion rate for lipids when using TPN?

A. 0.5 g/kg/day

B. 1.5 g/kg/day

C. 2.5 g/kg/day

D. 3.0 g/kg/day

E. 4.0 g/kg/day

ANSWER: C

COMMENTS: A patient whose nutritional needs cannot be met via the oral or enteral route requires **TPN**, the basic goal of which is to meet nutritional needs and maintain or improve metabolic balance safely. Crystalline protein and synthetic amino acids are the **protein** sources for TPN solutions. Commercially available **dextrose** solutions typically contain 15%–35% dextrose. The monohydrate form of dextrose is used for TPN and provides 3.4 kcal/g on oxidation. Carbohydrates should be administered at a rate no greater than 5 mg/kg/min via TPN, which is the maximum oxidation rate of glucose. Fat solutions are considered isotonic and can be administered peripherally or centrally without concern about thrombosis. **Fat solutions** are available in 10%, 20%, and 30% solutions, which provide 1.1, 2.0, and 3.0 kcal/mL, respectively. Monitoring clearance by checking triglyceride levels is key to ensuring tolerance to lipid infusions. Fat should be administered at a rate no faster than 2.5 g/kg/day. Lipid solutions should be administered cautiously to patients with acute respiratory distress syndrome (ARDS), severe liver disease, or increased metabolic stress because fat may exacerbate these conditions. Patients with hypertriglyceridemia (>250 mg/dL), lipid nephrosis, egg allergy, or acute pancreatitis associated with hyperlipidemia should not be given fat emulsions.

Ref.: 17, 18

26. A patient with multiple small bowel resections for Crohn's disease presents with an acute flare. Due to his preexisting short length of bowel and current profuse diarrhea, he is suspected of having functionally a short gut syndrome and is started on TPN. Refeeding syndrome is characterized by which of the following electrolyte abnormalities?

A. Hyponatremia, hypokalemia, and hypercalcemia

B. Hyperphosphatemia, hypokalemia, and hypocalcemia

C. Hypokalemia, hypomagnesemia, and hypophosphatemia

D. Hypocalcemia, hyponatremia, and hypomagnesemia

E. Hyperkalemia, hypernatremia, and hypercalcemia

ANSWER: C

COMMENTS: Refeeding syndrome is a profound metabolic disturbance that can occur in patients who are in severe malnutrition prior to starting TPN. Initiation of TPN can result in markedly decreased serum potassium, magnesium, and phosphorus; this is due to the effects of glucose administration in the previously starved patient. Refeeding can be prevented by evaluating and repleting serum levels of these electrolytes prior to starting TPN.

Ref.: 18

27. After 4 days of TPN, the patient above develops blood glucose levels greater than 300 mg/dL. Hyperglycemia in a surgical patient receiving TPN may best be managed by:

A. Oral hypoglycemics

B. Decreasing the dextrose load and doubling the amount of fat

C. Adding regular insulin to the TPN

D. Discontinuing TPN for 2 weeks and then trying to start TPN again

E. Increasing the concentration of protein and carbohydrate calories and decreasing that of lipids

ANSWER: C

COMMENTS: A number of **metabolic complications** may result from TPN. Excess glucose can (1) increase blood glucose levels and induce hyperosmolar nonketotic coma; (2) lead to dehydration; (3) lead to lipogenesis with subsequent hepatic abnormalities (e.g., fatty liver); and (4) increase CO_2 production, which may compromise respiratory function. Because rebound hypoglycemia can occur with discontinuation of TPN, weaning to 50 mL/h before complete discontinuation is important. Treatment of **hyperglycemia** in TPN patients typically consists of the addition of regular (not long-acting) insulin to the parenteral solution along with stringent monitoring of glucose levels.

Ref.: 18

28. A 40-year-old man undergoes gastric bypass surgery for morbid obesity. This patient should:

A. Eat only high-protein foods

B. Begin a feeding regimen with small amounts of regular foods

C. Begin with small amounts of water

D. Eat high-calorie foods six times a day

E. Eat only small amounts of high-fat foods

ANSWER: C

COMMENTS: Bariatric surgery has emerged as a viable weight-loss method for patients with medically significant obesity and morbidly obese patients who are unable to achieve or sustain weight loss. Nutritional issues are complex in this population. Patients are expected to lose 50%–60% of their presurgery weight. Therefore numerous postoperative nutritional complications are common. Malnutrition, vitamin and mineral deficiencies, failure of weight loss, dehydration, anemia, and dumping syndrome may occur. Oral feeding resumes on postoperative day 1 with small volumes of water. A 3-day progression from clear liquids to pureed foods is recommended, with small-volume feedings of 30 to 60 mL at each feeding. The diet eventually returns to regular foods given in small, frequent meals, along with the following general instructions: (1) stop eating when full; (2) chew food well, to a pulp-like consistency; (3) avoid high-calorie liquids, especially those with ice cream; and (4) make mealtimes last 30 min. Because of bypass of 90% of the stomach, entire duodenum, and a small portion of the jejunum, supplemental nutrient recommendations are necessary. B_6, B_{12}, folate, and calcium deficiencies are common, and these nutrients are usually prescribed as supplements.

Ref.: 20

29. Which of the following is true when considering the nutritional status of a geriatric patient?

A. Muscle wasting can be a pathologic process that is mistaken for normal aging.

B. Liver function does not affect the selection of nutrition regimens.

C. Enteral nutrition is not an option because of slowed gut function.

D. Body mass index (BMI) is the best anthropometric measurement for determining the nutritional status in an elderly patient.

E. Laboratory tests cannot be used to evaluate the nutritional status.

ANSWER: A

COMMENTS: Determining the most appropriate nutrition support interventions in **elderly** surgical patients can be difficult because of the aging process. Use of the BMI and anthropometrics often results in inaccurate measurements because of age-related changes. Many pathologic processes mistaken for normal aging are related to nutrition or affect the nutritional status (anthropometrics and biochemical and hematologic aspects) and can include muscle wasting, weight loss, undernutrition, problems with balance and endurance, declining cognition, and depression. Multiple age-related changes in the renal, liver, cardiovascular, and muscular systems can affect the overall health and nutrition regimens for surgical patients. Enteral nutrition may be an option for an elderly patient with poor nutritional intake before surgery. Commonly, enteral nutrition has been used in patients with dementia, cancer, dysphagia secondary to stroke, and other neurologic problems. Conditions for which the benefits of enteral support have been demonstrated in the elderly are short-term use in those with stroke and cancer when significant decreases in body mass can probably be prevented, the patient is a candidate for physical therapy, or recovery is probable.

Ref.: 21

REFERENCES

1. Blundell JE, Stubbs J. Diet composition and control of food intake in humans. In: Bray GA, Bouchard C, eds. *Handbook of Obesity: Etiology and Pathophysiology*. New York, NY: Marcel Dekker; 2004.
2. Barrett KE, Barman SM, Boitano S, Heddwen B. Regulation of gastrointestinal function. In: Ganong WF, ed. *Review of Medical Physiology*. 22nd ed. New York, NY: McGraw Hill Lange Medical; 2005.
3. Berg JM, Tymoczko JL, Stryer L, eds. *Biochemistry*. New York, NY: WH Freeman; 2002.
4. Saito H, Furukawa S, Matsuda T. Glutamine as an immunoenhancing nutrient. *JPEN J Parenter Enteral Nutr*. 1999;23(suppl 5):S59–S61.
5. Reeds PJ. Dispensable and indispensable amino acids for humans. *J Nutr*. 2000;130:S1835–S1840.
6. Ettinger S. Macronutrients: carbohydrates, protein, and lipids. In: Mahan JK, Escott-Stumps S, eds. *Krause's Food, Nutrition, and Diet Therapy*. 10th ed. Philadelphia, PA: WB Saunders; 2000.
7. Barrett KE, Barman SM, Boitano S, Heddwen B. Digestion and absorption. In: Ganaong WF, ed. *Review of Medical Physiology*. 22nd ed. New York, NY: McGraw Hill Lange Medical; 2005.
8. Food and Nutrition Board, Institute of Medicine. *Dietary Reference Intakes for Vitamin C, Vitamin E, Selenium, and Carotenoids*. Washington, DC: National Academy Press; 2004.
9. Rhee P, Joseph B. Shock, electrolytes, and fluid. In: Townshend CM, Beauchamp RD, Evers BM, Mattox KL, eds. *Sabiston Textbook of Surgery: The Biological Basis of Modern Surgical Practice*. 19th ed. New York, NY: Saunders; 2012.
10. Fuhrman MP, Charney P, Mueller CM. Hepatic proteins and nutritional assessment. *J Am Diet Assoc*. 2004;104:1258–1264.
11. Gibbs J, Cull W, Henderson W, et al. Preoperative serum albumin level as a predictor of operative mortality and morbidity: results from the National VA Surgical Risk Study. *Arch Surg*. 1999;134:36–42.
12. Chioléro R, Revelly J, Tappy L. Energy metabolism in sepsis and injury. *Nutrition*. 1997;13(suppl 9):S45–S51.
13. Holdy KE. Monitoring energy metabolism with indirect calorimetry: instruments, interpretation, and clinical application. *Nutr Clin Pract*. 2004;19:447–454.
14. ASPEN Board of Directors and the Clinical Guideline Task Force. Guidelines for the use of parenteral and enteral nutrition in adult and pediatric patients. *JPEN J Parenter Enteral Nutr*. 2002;26(suppl 1):SA1–SA138.
15. Parrish CR. Enteral formula selection: a review of selected product categories. *Pract Gastroenterol*. 2005;29:44.
16. Malone A. Enteral formula selection. In: Charney P, Malone A, eds. *ADA Pocket 17. Guide to Enteral Nutrition*. vol. 63. Chicago, IL: American Dietetic Association; 2006.
17. Sacks GS, Mayhew S, Johnson D. Parenteral nutrition implementation and management. In: Merritt R, De Legge M, Holcombe B, et al., eds. *The A.S.P.E.N. Nutrition Support Practice Manual*. 2nd ed. Silver Spring, MD: American Society for Parenteral and Enteral Nutrition; 2005.
18. Matarese LE. Metabolic complications of parenteral nutrition therapy. In: Gottschlich MM, Furhman MP, Hammond KA, et al., eds. *The Science and Practice of Nutrition Support: A Case-Based Care Curriculum*. Dubuque, IA: Kendall/Hunt; 2001.
19. Mundi MS, Shah M, Hurt RT. When is it appropriate to use glutamine in critical illness? *Nutr Clin Pract*. 2016;1(4):445–450.
20. Shikovra S. Techniques and procedures: surgical treatment for severe obesity: the state of the art for the new millennium. *Nutr Clin Pract*. 2000;15:13–22.
21. Mitchell-Eady C. Nutritional assessment of the elderly. In: Chernoff R, ed. *Geriatric Nutrition: The Health Professional's Handbook*. Sudbury, MA: Jones & Bartlett; 2006.

CHAPTER 5

SURGICAL INFECTION AND TRANSMISSIBLE DISEASES AND SURGEONS

A. Surgical Infection

Jill Smolevitz, M.D.

1. On the eighth day after an exploratory laparotomy and bowel resection complicated by intraabdominal hypertension, a 65-year-old female who remains intubated in the intensive care unit (ICU) develops a fever of 102°F. An infectious workup reveals a new right lower lobe consolidation. When initiating antibiotic therapy for presumed ventilator-associated pneumonia (VAP), which of the following does not treat *Pseudomonas aeruginosa*?

A. Cefepime

B. Unasyn (ampicillin/sulbactam)

C. Ticarcillin

D. Aztreonam

E. Ciprofloxacin

ANSWER: B

COMMENTS: *P. aeruginosa* is a gram-negative bacillus commonly implicated in VAP. Antipseudomonal antibiotics should be initiated empirically in any patient with VAP prior to isolation of the organism on culture due to the high mortality associated with pseudomonal infection. Antipseudomonal penicillins include ticarcillin and piperacillin. Third- and fourth-generation cephalosporins, such as ceftazidime and cefepime, are effective against *P. aeruginosa* and have a relatively narrow range of activity, making them preferred agents in susceptible isolates. Monobactams (like aztreonam) and carbapenems (meropenem, imipenem) are effective, but have a very broad spectrum of activity, and should be deescalated once susceptibilities are available. Fluoroquinolones are also effective. The polymyxin colistin is also effective, but has an extensive toxicity profile, and should be used cautiously with multiresistant organisms.

Ref.: 1

2. A 67-year-old male remains in the hospital 1 week after undergoing a pancreaticoduodenectomy. He has two intraabdominal closed-suction drains in place, as well as a left internal jugular triple lumen catheter; his Foley catheter was removed on the third postoperative day. On the seventh postoperative day, he becomes febrile to 101.5°F, and a fever workup reveals a growth of *Enterococcus* in two of two peripheral blood cultures. Which of the following is true regarding the diagnosis of a central line–associated bloodstream infection (CLABSI)?

A. It is preferential to begin empiric antimicrobial therapy prior to obtaining cultures.

B. Catheter-site exudate, if present, should not be cultured when there is concern for a line-related bloodstream infection.

C. The subcutaneous portion of the central venous catheter should be cultured, rather than the tip.

D. Paired blood samples (one from the catheter and one from a peripheral vein, or alternatively from greater than two lumens of the same central venous catheter) growing the same organism at levels that meet catheter-related bloodstream infection criteria are required to diagnose a CLABSI.

E. Growth of greater than 10 colony-forming units (cfu) by semiquantitative (roll-plate) culture confirms catheter colonization.

ANSWER: D

COMMENTS: See Question 3.

Ref.: See Question 3

3. Which of the following is true regarding the treatment of catheter-related bloodstream infections?

A. All catheters in cases of confirmed CLABSI should be removed; it is never appropriate to attempt to salvage the infected catheter.

B. Empiric coverage of *Candida* should be initiated in bone marrow or solid organ transplant patients with presumed CLABSI.

C. Empiric antibiotic therapy should include methicillin-resistant *Staphylococcus aureus* (MRSA) coverage as well as gram-negative rod (GNR) coverage, regardless of the severity of illness.

D. Duration of antibiotic therapy in CLABSIs is timed from the day when empiric antibiotics were initiated.

E. The location of a temporary central venous catheter (subclavian versus internal jugular versus femoral) has no influence on the empiric antibiotic agents that should be used.

ANSWER: B

COMMENTS: Central venous catheters are commonly used in many settings in modern health care, but their use is associated with the risk of bloodstream infections, known as CLABSIs. These infections are known to increase morbidity, mortality, and health care costs.

To diagnose a CLABSI, growth of greater than 15 cfu by semiquantitative (roll-plate) culture from at least two samples is required; these two samples may be obtained from the catheter and a peripheral vein or, alternatively, from at least two lumens from the same central venous catheter. The diagnosis of CLABSI is best defined by a colony count threefold greater than that obtained from a peripheral vein. Skin and catheter hubs should be prepared with alcohol, tincture of iodine, or alcohol-based chlorhexidine (>0.5%) with adequate drying time, prior to obtaining cultures; cultures should be obtained by trained phlebotomists if possible.

Management of CLABSI varies based on the organism cultured and the severity of illness, but for all CLABSIs, the duration of antimicrobial therapy is determined on the first day of obtaining negative blood cultures. Preferably, adequate cultures are obtained prior to the initiation of antibiotic therapy. Empiric therapy in uncomplicated cases [i.e., cases without evidence of severe sepsis, endocarditis or osteomyelitis (OM), or without evidence of infection of the catheter tunnel or adjacent abscess] should begin with antibiotics that cover gram-positive cocci. Vancomycin or daptomycin for empiric therapy should be reserved for areas with a high prevalence of MRSA. Empiric GNR coverage should be added in cases of severe sepsis, neutropenia, in patients with known colonization with a GNR organism, or in patients with femoral catheters. Empiric coverage for *Candida*, either with an echinocandin or a fluconazole, should be initiated in patients with severe sepsis plus prolonged broad-spectrum antibiotic use, total parenteral nutrition, hematologic malignancy or receipt of solid organ or bone marrow transplants, or known *Candida* colonization. In most circumstances, the infected catheter should be removed; however, there are certain instances in which salvage of the catheter may be attempted. Antibiotic locks (antibiotic solutions that are instilled into the catheter itself) can be used in conjunction with systemic antimicrobial therapy, particularly in patients in whom catheters are difficult to remove or replace (i.e., tunneled hemodialysis catheters or ports for parenteral nutrition in short gut syndrome). If patients have persistent positive blood cultures after salvage attempt, the catheter should be removed.

Ref.: 2

4. A 78-year-old man with a history of urinary retention and a chronic indwelling urinary catheter is admitted to the hospital from his nursing home with a new-onset altered mental status, and a catheter-associated urinary tract infection (CAUTI) is suspected. Which of the following is true regarding CAUTIs?

A. A 7-day antibiotic treatment is adequate for patients whose symptoms respond promptly to treatment.

B. A CAUTI can be sufficiently diagnosed by the presence of greater than 10^5 cfu/mL of at least one bacterial species in a urine specimen.

C. Urine specimens being sent for culture can be obtained from the catheter bag.

D. Pyuria is a specific indicator for urinary tract infections (UTIs).

E. *Proteus mirabilis* is the most common organism cultured in CAUTIs.

ANSWER: A

COMMENTS: CAUTIs are the most common health care–associated infection worldwide, and the most important factor leading to nosocomial UTIs is urinary catheterization. The best prevention for CAUTIs is avoiding catheterization. There are a limited number of circumstances in which catheterization is appropriate, such as when monitoring urine output in critically ill patients, in patients with acute urinary retention or obstruction, in certain surgical procedures, or to facilitate healing of wounds or pressure ulcers in some patients with urinary incontinence. A CAUTI is diagnosed by the presence of greater than 10^3 cfu/mL of at least one bacterial species in a catheter urine specimen or a midstream-voided urine specimen in addition to clinical signs and symptoms suggestive of infection. Signs and symptoms of a UTI include new-onset fever, rigors, altered mental status, lethargy, malaise, flank pain, costovertebral angle tenderness, hematuria, suprapubic or pelvic discomfort, dysuria, urinary frequency, and urinary urgency. For these symptoms to be attributed to a catheter, the patient must have a current indwelling urinary catheter or have had one within the 48 h preceding his or her symptoms. Without these symptoms, an infection cannot be diagnosed. Catheter-associated asymptomatic bacteriuria is more likely, and this is diagnosed by the presence of greater than 10^5 cfu/mL of at least one bacterial species in a urine specimen. Catheters predispose to bacteriuria and UTIs in a variety of ways, but formation of a biofilm along the catheter itself is the most important predisposing factor. Pyuria is not specific for UTIs; it can be seen in a variety of other renal pathologies and should not be used as a diagnostic criterion for UTI. Urine culture specimens are best collected by removing the catheter, if possible, to obtain a voided midstream specimen, from the tubing or catheter itself in a catheter that has been in place for less than 2 weeks, or by removing any catheter that has been in place for greater than 2 weeks and obtaining a specimen from the new catheter. The duration of antibiotic therapy should be 7 days for patients whose symptoms respond promptly to antibiotics and 10 to 14 days for those whose symptoms respond slowly. *Escherichia coli* is the most common causative organism in CAUTIs, although *Proteus* is commonly cultured in patients with chronic indwelling catheters.

Ref.: 3, 4

5. A 57-year-old Asian American female presents to her hepatologist's office for monitoring of her known chronic hepatitis B infection. Which of the following sets of test results is consistent with chronic active hepatitis B infection?

A. Hepatitis B surface antigen (HBsAg)+ less than 6 months, hepatitis B surface antibody (HBsAb)–, immunoglobulin M (IgM) anti-HBc+, elevated aspartate transaminase (AST), and alanine transaminase (ALT)

B. HBsAg+ greater than 6 months, HBsAb–, HBcAb+, hepatitis B virus (HBV) DNA > 20,000 IU/mL, mildly elevated AST and ALT

C. HBsAg+ greater than 6 months, hepatitis B e antigen (HBeAg)–, HBV DNA < 2000 IU/mL, normal AST and ALT

D. HBsAg–, HBsAb+, HBcAb+, normal AST and ALT

E. HBsAg–, HBsAb+, HBcAb–, normal AST and ALT

ANSWER: B

COMMENTS: Answer A is acute hepatitis B infection; chronic infection requires HBsAg positivity for at least 6 months. A patient with chronic active infection (answer B) exhibits normal to mildly elevated liver enzymes and HBsAg positivity but negative HBsAb since the infection has not been cleared; HBcAb will be positive with chronic infection, and HBeAg may be positive as well if there is a continued high level of viral replication; this is usually accompanied by a high level of HBV DNA. This is different from an inactive carrier state (answer C); these patients have persistent HBV infection of the liver without significant hepatic necrosis or inflammation, so their liver enzymes are not significantly elevated; there is a low level of viral replication, which correlates with negative HBeAg. Patients who have cleared HBV infection have evidence of HBsAb and HBcAb positivity (answer D). Answer E reflects successful vaccination, with only HBsAb positivity on serologic testing.

Ref.: 5

6. Match the antibiotic and its classical toxicity profile.

A. Vancomycin	a. Tendinopathy
B. Aminoglycosides	b. Red man syndrome
C. Isoniazid (INH)	c. Phototoxicity
D. Fluoroquinolones	d. Hepatitis
E. Tetracycline	e. Ototoxicity

ANSWER: A-b, B-e, C-d, D-a, E-c

COMMENTS: Vancomycin is known to cause red man syndrome, a syndrome composed of flushing of the face, neck, and chest. It is better described as a hypersensitivity reaction, rather than a true allergy, because the effect is partly mediated by the speed with which it is transfused. Aminoglycosides can cause ototoxicity (cochlear and vestibular), which is dose dependent. The effects may begin to be seen even after cessation of the drug; aminoglycoside ototoxicity may be irreversible. INH can cause severe, sometimes fulminant, hepatitis that is largely indistinguishable from acute viral hepatitis. The mechanism of toxicity is not clear, but is thought to be related to direct toxicity of the drug or its metabolites, and is more likely to occur when other hepatitis risk factors are present, such as concurrent alcohol consumption, use of other drugs that utilize the cytochrome P450 system for metabolism, previous INH intolerance, or prior or concurrent liver disease. Fluoroquinolone-induced tendinopathy is rare, but it has been documented with almost all drugs in this class. Tetracyclines cause cutaneous phototoxicity, so patients taking tetracyclines are cautioned to avoid sun exposure.

Ref.: 6

7. Which of the following is not a Surgical Care Improvement Project (SCIP) measure for infection prevention in surgical patients?

A. The optimal timing for administration of prophylactic antibiotics is within 1 h of surgical incision.

B. Prophylactic antibiotics should be discontinued within 24 h of the end of surgery; in cardiac surgery, this is lengthened to 48 h.

C. Clippers are preferred to razors for preoperative hair removal, if necessary.

D. Goal blood glucose in the first 48 h following surgery is less than 160 mg/dL.

E. Patients should remain normothermic within the first hour following surgery.

ANSWER: D

COMMENTS: The SCIP summarizes specific tactics aimed at prevention of surgical site infections (SSIs). Of the answer choices listed above, only D is inaccurate; optimal blood glucose within the first 48 h of surgery is less than 200 mg/dL. Hyperglycemia impairs the host immune function and is known to increase the risk of infection in both diabetic and nondiabetic patients. Moderate hyperglycemia (i.e., blood glucose > 200 mg/dL) in the first 24 h following surgery increases the risk of SSIs by a factor of four. Tight blood glucose control has been a matter of debate in recent years, with some arguing that very strict blood glucose control (i.e., less than 110 mg/dL) results in significantly decreased rates of infection. However, postoperative hypoglycemia is associated with increased mortality, so glycemic goals have been relaxed.

The remaining answer choices are correct. Prophylactic antibiotics should be given within 1 h of incision, though 2 h is appropriate for fluoroquinolones and vancomycin, due to the prolonged infusion times for these drugs. They should be discontinued within 24 h of the end of surgery in all cases aside from the cardiac surgery, where 48 h of prophylactic antibiotic therapy is appropriate. Razors should never be used to remove hair prior to procedures due to the increased risk for small breaks in the skin, which might introduce infection; clippers should be used preoperatively. Normothermia, defined as any temperature between 96.8°F and 100.4°F, should be maintained intraoperatively and for at least the first hour following surgery.

Ref.: 6

8. Match the surgical procedure with the most appropriate preoperative prophylactic antibiotic.

A. Elective laparoscopic cholecystectomy	a. Ertapenem
B. Femoral to popliteal arterial bypass with graft	b. Clindamycin
C. Cystoscopy with ureteral stent placement	c. None
D. Right hemicolectomy	d. Cefazolin
E. Parotidectomy	e. Ciprofloxacin

ANSWER: A-c, B-d, C-e, D-a, E-b

COMMENTS: Prophylactic antibiotics administered preoperatively should be targeted to the organisms most likely to be encountered in the operative field. Broad-spectrum antibiotics do not have greater efficacy at preventing SSIs than more narrow-spectrum, targeted choices. The choice of prophylactic antibiotic therapy for intraabdominal surgeries varies widely depending on the exact location within the gastrointestinal tract that is being manipulated. Low-risk biliary tract procedures (e.g., elective laparoscopic cholecystectomy) do not require surgical site infection prophylaxis; however, patients undergoing open or complicated procedures involving the biliary tract should receive antibiotics covering enteric GNRs, *Enterococcus*, and *Clostridia*. Comparatively, colorectal surgery requires broad coverage of enteric GNRs, anaerobes, and *Enterococcus*, which may be accomplished with ertapenem, a carbapenem antibiotic. Cystoscopy with manipulation, such as the placement of ureteral stents, necessitates coverage of enteric GNRs and *Enterococcus*; compared with colorectal surgery, anaerobic coverage is not necessary. Vascular SSIs are most commonly caused by skin flora, such as *Staphylococcus* and *Streptococcus* species, so a first-generation cephalosporin, such as cefazolin, is adequate. In clean-contaminated head and neck cases (i.e., any surgical procedure involving the oropharyngeal mucosa), prophylactic antibiotics should cover both aerobic and anaerobic oral flora (such as *Streptococcus*, *Bacteroides*, and *Peptostreptococcus*).

Ref.: 6, 7

9. A 68-year-old female has been admitted to the emergency room with recurrent *Clostridium difficile* colitis. Her first episode of *C. difficile* colitis was 3 months prior after receiving clindamycin for a mild episode of cellulitis. Two months ago, she had a second episode, treated again with full symptom resolution. On examination, her vital signs are normal and her abdomen is benign, with only mildly tender to deep palpation in the right lower quadrant. Laboratory results are notable for a leukocytosis of 13.4,000 cells per MCL with 86% neutrophils, mild hypokalemia, and positive *C. difficile* stool antigen. An abdominal film shows a colon of normal caliber. What is the most appropriate treatment for this patient?
   A. Oral metronidazole 500 mg every 8 h for 10 to 14 days
   B. Intravenous (IV) metronidazole 500 mg every 8 h for 10 to 14 days
   C. Oral vancomycin 125 mg every 6 h for 10 to 14 days
   D. Oral vancomycin, in a tapered and pulsed fashion over approximately 5 to 7 weeks
   E. IV vancomycin 125 mg every 6 h for 10 to 14 days

ANSWER: D

COMMENTS: See Question 11.

Ref.: See Question 11

10. The patient in the question above is admitted and started on antibiotics, but her condition continues to deteriorate clinically over the next 2 days despite appropriate antibiotic therapy, probiotics, and supportive treatment. Her white blood cell (WBC) count continues to rise to 17.8 and creatinine increases to 1.5 from baseline of 0.8. She has a low-grade fever and marginal urine output, and her abdomen becomes distended, tympanic, and tender. An abdominal obstructive series shows dilation of the entire colon to 10 cm in diameter without evidence of pneumoperitoneum. Which of the following is not an acceptable course of action in treating severe *C. difficile* colitis?
   A. Transitioning from pulsed to standard scheduled oral vancomycin 125 mg every 6 h with the addition of IV metronidazole 500 mg every 8 h
   B. Transitioning from pulsed to standard scheduled oral vancomycin 125 mg every 6 h with the addition of oral fidaxomicin 200 mg every 12 h
   C. Subtotal colectomy
   D. Diverting loop ileostomy with colonic lavage
   E. Metronidazole enemas

ANSWER: E

COMMENTS: See Question 11.

Ref.: See Question 11

11. Which of the following is true regarding the pathophysiology of *C. difficile* infection?
   A. Antimicrobial agents with activity against *C. difficile* are equally as likely to result in *C. difficile* colitis as those without activity against *C. difficile.*
   B. A patient's inability to produce antibody to toxin A is a significant predictor of recurrent *C. difficile* infection.
   C. Advanced age is not considered a risk factor for development of clinical *C. difficile* infection.
   D. Studies have suggested that gastric acid suppression [i.e., use of proton pump inhibitors (PPIs) or H_2 blockers] may be protective against the development of *C. difficile* infection.
   E. Alcohol-based hand sanitizers are effective in removing *C. difficile* spores after contact with an infected patient.

ANSWER: B

COMMENTS (Questions 9–11)**:** Recurrent *C. difficile* colitis is a growing health problem in the United States. Treatment of an initial episode can be accomplished with oral or IV metronidazole (500 mg every 8 h for 10 to 14 days) or oral vancomycin (125 mg every 6 h for 10 to 14 days). IV vancomycin is never acceptable as a treatment for *C. difficile* colitis. More severe initial infections should be treated with vancomycin rather than metronidazole. For a patient's first relapse, if there is no evidence of systemic toxicity, treatment with the initial antibiotic regimen may be appropriate. Second relapses and beyond, however, require oral vancomycin in a tapered and pulsed fashion (see the following chart). Alternatively, fidaxomicin, a macrolytic antibiotic that is bactericidal against *C. difficile*, can be used. With both drugs, probiotics may be added, though their efficacy is still unclear. Fecal microbiota transplant has also been shown to be a cost-effective solution for recurrent *C. difficile* colitis.

For patients developing evidence of systemic toxicity from *C. difficile* colitis, more aggressive therapy is required. Depending on the patient's clinical stability, multiple avenues of treatment are available. Scheduled oral vancomycin or fidaxomicin can be given, with or without IV metronidazole; IV metronidazole may have enhanced efficacy in patients with evidence of bowel dysmotility. The duration of antibiotics in severe *C. difficile* colitis is generally at least 17 to 24 days (1 week beyond standard treatment). Intracolonic vancomycin administration (i.e., vancomycin enema) is also an acceptable treatment method; metronidazole enema is not an accepted treatment, which makes answer E incorrect. Vancomycin enemas are particularly useful in patients who have conditions preventing oral vancomycin from reaching the colon (i.e., end ileostomies, severe ileus, colonic dysmotility, etc.). Patients who are severely ill with toxic megacolon, perforation, uncontrolled sepsis, or multiorgan failure should be considered operative candidates. The two most accepted surgical procedures are subtotal colectomy and diverting loop ileostomy with colonic lavage followed by antegrade vancomycin enemas.

The pathogenesis of *C. difficile* infection rests largely on the disruption of normal colonic flora by other antibiotics. Those with inherent activity against *C. difficile* (i.e., those who have a robust antibody response to toxin A) are less likely to become clinically infected. One study reported that patients who did not develop antibodies to toxin A during their initial infection were 48 times as likely to develop a recurrent infection. Advanced age (>65 years) is predictive of both initial and recurrent infection. Additional patient-specific risk factors for infection include gastric acid suppression (either via PPIs or H_2 blockers), recent gastrointestinal surgery, chemotherapy, stem cell transplant, and obesity. The three classes of antibiotics cited most frequently as causative agents are clindamycin, cephalosporins, and fluoroquinolones, and these agents are generally administered weeks to several months prior to the development of *C. difficile* infection. Concomitant use of multiple antibiotics and prolonged courses of antibiotics have also been found to be risk factors for infection; however, not all patients who are exposed to *C. difficile* and receive antibiotics develop an infection.

Infection control policies are paramount to controlling the nosocomial spread of *C. difficile* infection; patients with active infections should be placed on contact precautions, and all health care workers (HCWs) who encounter the patient should wash their hands with soap and water since *C. difficile* spores are resistant to alcohol-based hand sanitizers.

Tapered and Pulsed Vancomycin Dosing for Recurrent *C. difficile* Infection

Tapered dosing: 125 mg four times daily for 10 to 14 days, followed by 125 mg twice daily for 7 days, and then 125 mg daily for 7 days

Pulse dosing (after completion of the taper): 125 mg every 2 to 3 days for 2 to 8 weeks

Ref.: 8–11

12. Which of the following is true regarding postoperative fever?

A. Urinalysis, urine culture, and chest x-ray must be obtained as part of a complete fever workup in postoperative patients within 72 h of operation.

B. In a febrile postoperative patient, wound cultures should be obtained regardless of the appearance of the wound.

C. Wound infections in the first 24 to 48 h are uncommon but, if present, are worrisome for group A streptococcal or clostridial infection.

D. Fevers persisting for greater than 96 h postoperatively are expected in cases of diffuse intraabdominal infection, such as feculent peritonitis from diverticulitis, even with appropriate surgical management.

E. All of the above.

ANSWER: C

COMMENTS: Fever is a common postsurgical finding, but not all fevers require evaluation. In the first 72 h after surgery, fever is more likely related to postoperative inflammatory responses in the host, rather than infection, when the patient is otherwise asymptomatic or without an indwelling urinary catheter. While fever is expected in postoperative patients with evidence of diffuse infection preoperatively (such as large abscesses, purulent or feculent peritonitis, or necrotizing soft tissue infection), fevers that are persistent for greater than 96 h after appropriate surgical management, or recurrent fevers after 96 h, are concerning for recurrent or incompletely cleared infection. Fevers presenting greater than 96 h postoperatively are more likely to be due to infection. Surgical wounds should only be cultured if there are signs or symptoms suggestive of wound infection (i.e., purulence, tenderness, and erythema). SSIs are most commonly due to the native flora of the organ that was operated upon, but within the first 24 to 48 h of surgery, wound infections are more likely to be due to group A *Streptococcus* (GAS) or *Clostridia*, which are significantly more virulent organisms. Deep venous thrombosis, pulmonary embolism, and superficial thrombophlebitis are other possible etiologies that should be considered in the evaluation of a febrile postoperative patient.

Ref.: 12

13. A 25-year-old male remains nasotracheally intubated in the ICU while undergoing repeated debridements for Ludwig's angina. His infection appears to be adequately drained, although he still has persistent facial swelling. Sinusitis is expected. Which of the following is true regarding sinusitis in critically ill patients?

A. The most important risk factor for sinusitis in critically ill patients is a history of MRSA of the nares.

B. Few sinus infections are polymicrobial; often, only one organism is isolated in culture.

C. The most commonly isolated organism in sinusitis cultures is coagulase-negative *S. aureus.*

D. Computed tomography (CT) scan of the sinuses is the most sensitive diagnostic imaging modality for sinusitis.

E. Incidence of acute sinusitis in nasotracheally intubated patients is approximately 75% after 1 week.

ANSWER: D

COMMENTS: Sinusitis is an infrequent but potentially life-threatening cause of fever in critically ill patients. When the ostia of the sinuses become obstructed (e.g., from nasotracheal intubation, nasogastric tube placement, or maxillofacial trauma), bacterial overgrowth can occur, and when drainage is impaired, infection results; approximately one-third of patients who are nasotracheally intubated develop sinusitis within 1 week. The diagnosis is suggested by clinical findings, including cough, purulent nasal discharge, tooth pain, fever, wheezing, or throat or tooth pain. Normal nasopharyngeal organisms are the most common causes, and infections are often polymicrobial. GNRs are present in approximately two-third of cases of acute sinusitis in critically ill patients; gram-positive rods are isolated in approximately one-third of cases, and fungi are found in 5%–10%. A CT scan of the sinuses is the most sensitive imaging modality for diagnosing sinusitis, although plain films can be obtained as well. Plain films are less sensitive than CT scan, but the accuracy of plain films in diagnosis can be augmented if combined with the findings of nasal endoscopy, when performed by a skilled endoscopist. Needle aspiration of the sinuses to obtain fluid for cultures provides a definitive diagnosis, but a biopsy may be required to rule out invasive fungal sinusitis in immunocompromised patients.

Ref.: 12

14. A 24-year-old male presents to the emergency department after sustaining a puncture wound to his left foot 60 min prior to presentation. On examination, he has a small metal nail protruding from the plantar aspect of his left foot, with moderate surrounding erythema and a small amount of bleeding, but no significant purulence. He is unsure of his tetanus vaccination status. How should the issue of potential tetanus infection be addressed in this patient?

A. Local wound care only

B. Local wound care, IV metronidazole or penicillin for 7 to 10 days

C. Local wound care, IV metronidazole or penicillin for 7 to 10 days, tetanus toxoid

D. Local wound care, IV metronidazole or penicillin for 7 to 10 days, tetanus toxoid, tetanus immunoglobulin

E. No treatment

ANSWER: D

COMMENTS: See Question 15.

Ref.: See Question 15

15. Which of the following is true regarding tetanus infection?

A. Tetanus is caused by tetanus toxin, which is produced by *C. tetani*, an aerobic gram-positive bacillus.

B. Tetanus infection has purely motor neuron effects.

C. Tetanus-prone wounds include contaminated wounds (i.e., soil, saliva, and stool), crush wounds, or burn wounds.

D. Tetanus immunoglobulin is indicated in any patient with an unknown tetanus vaccination history.

E. None of the above.

ANSWER: C

COMMENTS: Tetanus toxin, produced by *C. tetani*, an anaerobic gram-positive bacillus, causes disinhibition of lower motor neurons; it is taken up via lower motor neurons and transported proximally to the spinal cord and brainstem and then into inhibitory neurons, causing a functional denervation of motor neurons. This can result in lockjaw; muscle rigidity; and spasm of respiratory, laryngeal, and abdominal muscles, causing respiratory failure. Autonomic dysfunction can also be seen with tetanus, manifesting as labile blood pressure and heart rate. Tetanus-prone wounds include contaminated wounds (i.e., soil, saliva, and stool), crush wounds, or burn wounds. Treatment of tetanus-prone wounds includes local wound care (i.e., debridement and irrigation) and antibiotic therapy targeted against *C. tetani.* Depending on the completeness of a patient's tetanus vaccination, additional therapy is required, based on the following tables:

Tetanus-Prone Wounds

Previous Tetanus Toxoid Administration	Tetanus Toxoid	Tetanus Immunoglobulin
Less than three doses	Yes	Yes
Three or more doses	No; yes, if the last dose was prior to more than 5 years	No

Clean Wounds

Previous Tetanus Toxoid Administration	Tetanus Toxoid	Tetanus Immunoglobulin
Less than three doses	Yes	No
Three or more doses	No; yes, if the last dose was prior to more than 10 years	No

Tetanus immunoglobulin serves to bind tetanus toxin in the bloodstream to minimize absorption into motor neurons. Muscle spasm and rigidity should be treated if present.

Ref.: 13

16. A 62-year-old man with a history of chronic pancreatitis from alcohol abuse presents to the emergency department with complaints of fevers and abdominal pain. On examination, he is febrile to 100.8°F. He is jaundiced and has right upper quadrant tenderness. His liver enzymes are elevated with a new leukocytosis. A CT scan of the abdomen demonstrates cirrhotic liver morphology, calcifications along the pancreas, and a rim-enhancing hypoechoic liver lesion. Which of the following is true regarding the diagnosis of a pyogenic liver abscess (PLA)?

A. Most PLAs are found in the left hepatic lobe.

B. The most common etiology of PLAs is seeding from another intraabdominal infection via the portal vein.

C. Most PLAs are polymicrobial, and in the United States, *E. coli* is the most commonly isolated organism.

D. Percutaneous drainage is recommended for all PLAs if the drainage is technically feasible.

E. The classic triad of fever, right upper quadrant pain, and malaise is present in many patients with PLAs.

ANSWER: C

COMMENTS: PLAs are relatively uncommon and have vague presenting symptoms. The classic triad of fever, right upper quadrant pain, and malaise is present in only about one-third of patients. PLAs have multiple causes including biliary tract disease causing obstruction, seeding from another intraabdominal infection via the portal vein, hepatic artery seeding or bacteremia, direct extension from an adjacent infection (such as cholecystitis and perinephric abscess), or trauma; a small percentage of cases are cryptogenic. Biliary tract disease is now the most common etiology of PLAs and includes cases of choledocholithiasis, biliary stricture, congenital anomalies of the biliary tree such as choledochal cysts, and obstructing tumors like cholangiocarcinoma or pancreatic adenocarcinoma. Most infections are polymicrobial, and *E. coli* is the most frequently isolated organism in the United States, followed by *Klebsiella pneumoniae*. PLAs occur most frequently in the right lobe of the liver, given its greater portal venous flow. Treatment involves broad-spectrum antibiotics (though particularly targeted against enteric GNRs and anaerobes) with percutaneous drainage for patients who do not improve with 2 to 3 days of appropriate antimicrobial therapy, abscesses greater than 5 cm in diameter, or abscesses at risk of rupture. Surgical intervention is generally reserved for ruptured abscesses, failed response to percutaneous drainage, uncorrected primary pathology (e.g., biliary stricture), or multiloculated abscesses not amenable to percutaneous drainage.

Ref.: 14

17. A 47-year-old man has been admitted to the burn ICU for 4 days after sustaining a 30% total body surface area (TBSA) burn, involving the neck, chest, bilateral upper extremities, and lower extremities, when he begins to clinically decompensate. Which of the following is suggestive or diagnostic of a burn wound sepsis?

A. Conversion of a partial-thickness burn to a full-thickness burn

B. Fevers greater than 100.4°F

C. Burn wound culture swab growing greater than 10^5 organisms per gram of tissue swabbed

D. Inability to tolerate enteral tube feeds for greater than 24 h

E. Failure to improve with broad-spectrum antibiotic administration

ANSWER: A

COMMENTS: Burn wound infections remain a major cause of morbidity and mortality in burn patients, especially in those with greater than 20% TBSA burns. Burn wounds have a greater propensity for infection than the healthy tissue since the wound lacks a barrier to environmental organisms, and devascularized burn tissue provides a protein-rich medium in which bacteria can thrive; in addition, burns cause significant systemic responses that inhibit a patient's normal host defense and healing mechanisms. Most burns are colonized with bacteria early after injury but do not cause systemic symptoms. Topical antimicrobials help to reduce the rate of conversion into invasive wound infections; however, invasive infections do result in systemic symptoms and must be treated. Diagnosis of a burn wound infection requires positive histopathology: the burn must be biopsied, with the growth of $>10^5$ organisms per gram of burn wound tissue. Burn wound infections often manifest with physical changes in the appearance of the burn, such as conversion to a greater degree of burn and surrounding cellulitis. Because most burn patients exhibit the signs of a systemic inflammatory response syndrome (SIRS), the American Burn Association has developed criteria for specifically diagnosing burn wound sepsis:

- At least one of the following:
  - Culture-positive infection (i.e., blood, urine, wound)
  - Pathologic tissue source identified ($>10^5$ bacteria per gram of tissue on quantitative biopsy)
  - Clinical improvement with antimicrobial therapy
- At least three of the following:
  - Temperature greater than 102.2°F or less than 97.7°F
  - Progressive tachycardia
  - Progressive tachypnea
  - Thrombocytopenia that occurs greater than 3 days after initial resuscitation
  - Refractory hypotension
  - Leukocytosis > 12,000 or <4000 WBCs/cells MCL
  - Hyperglycemia
  - Inability to tolerate enteral feedings for >24 h

Ref.: 15

18. Which of the following is not a classical clinical manifestation of GAS infection?

A. Necrotizing soft tissue infection

B. Acute rheumatic fever

C. Toxic shock syndrome

D. Pharyngitis

E. Meningitis

ANSWER: E

COMMENTS: GAS, or group A *S. pyogenes*, is an aerobic gram-positive coccus that is responsible for a wide range of clinical illnesses, accounting for greater than 600 million infections globally each year. The infections caused by GAS vary in clinical severity, from mild cellulitis to life-threatening toxic shock syndrome, as demonstrated by the answer choices above. GAS is also responsible for a variety of postinfectious immune-mediated diseases, such as acute rheumatic fever or poststreptococcal glomerulonephritis. All the answer choices above can be classically attributed to GAS infection except for meningitis, which is more commonly caused by group B *Streptococcus*, particularly in newborns.

GAS, which colonizes epithelial surfaces, is almost universally sensitive to penicillin. Its main virulence factor is the M protein, which is a surface antigen and virulence factor encoded by the *emm* gene, of which there are over 200 types. Different *emm* types are associated with different types of infection; some are known to cause cutaneous infection, while others cause invasive infection. The prevalence of different *emm* types is also socioeconomically distinct, with certain *emm* types being seen in more industrialized areas compared with other types being prevalent in more rural communities. Geography plays a role as well, with variability in the prevalence of *emm* types based on region.

Ref.: 16, 17

19. A 45-year-old man who underwent a splenectomy for immune thrombocytopenic purpura develops a fever. Which of the following is true regarding postsplenectomy sepsis?

A. A fever without other localizing symptoms of infection (such as cough and diarrhea) is usually not worrisome in postsplenectomy patients.

B. Postsplenectomy sepsis is almost never seen in patients who complete the appropriate vaccinations.

C. The most common organism implicated in postsplenectomy sepsis is *Haemophilus influenzae.*

D. Initiation of empiric antibiotics should be delayed until cultures are obtained.

E. Ceftriaxone and vancomycin are an appropriate empiric antibiotic regimen in an asplenic patient with fever.

ANSWER: E

COMMENTS: See Question 20.

Ref.: See Question 20

20. Which of the following statements regarding the risk for postsplenectomy sepsis is true?

A. The indication for splenectomy has no bearing on a patient's risk for developing postsplenectomy sepsis.

B. Adult splenectomy patients have a greater likelihood of developing postsplenectomy sepsis than do children or newborns who require a splenectomy.

C. The risk for postsplenectomy sepsis is highest in the first year after splenectomy, but asplenic patients' increased risk for developing sepsis persists for approximately 10 years following splenectomy.

D. The risk of sepsis is increased in splenectomy patients due to impaired cellular immunity.

E. None of the above.

ANSWER: C

COMMENTS: Asplenic patients (those who have either undergone splenectomy or are functionally asplenic, such as in sickle cell disease) are at an increased risk for a fulminant and potentially rapidly fatal overwhelming bloodstream infection caused by encapsulated organisms. This is due to impaired bacterial clearance, especially of encapsulated organisms (i.e., *S. pneumoniae*, *Neisseria meningitidis*, and *H. influenzae*), and impaired humoral (not cellular) immunity. The risk of developing postsplenectomy sepsis varies based on the indications for splenectomy, the age at which the patient underwent splenectomy (or became functionally asplenic), and the time interval since splenectomy (or functional asplenia). In terms of indication for splenectomy, patients who have undergone splenectomy for trauma are at the lowest risk; those who have undergone splenectomy for hereditary spherocytosis or immune thrombocytopenic purpura are at intermediate risk; and the greatest risk patients are those who are functionally asplenic due to α-thalassemia, sickle cell disease, or portal hypertension. Children (especially those under the age of 5 years) are at a greater risk for developing sepsis than are adults, but this may also be confounded by the indications for splenectomy or functional asplenia in this age group. Overall, the risk for postsplenectomy sepsis is greatest in the first year following splenectomy, but patients who have undergone splenectomy are at an increased risk for sepsis for approximately 10 years following surgery.

Since the year 2000, when universal vaccination with the heptavalent pneumococcal conjugate vaccine (PCV7) in children began, the rates of invasive pneumococcal infection have dropped significantly, and the rates have continued to fall with the development of the 13-valent vaccine (PCV13) in 2010. Patients who undergo splenectomy or are functionally asplenic should receive vaccinations for the encapsulated organisms prior to splenectomy if it is elective or prior to discharge if performed urgently.

Treatment of postsplenectomy sepsis should be rapid. A fever in any postsplenectomy patient should prompt initiation of antimicrobial therapy as it may be the only sign of an impending fulminant infection. Postsplenectomy patients, even those who have undergone vaccination for *S. pneumoniae*, *N. meningitidis*, and *H. influenzae*, should be counseled to seek medical attention with any febrile episode. The most common causative organism is *S. pneumoniae*, so ceftriaxone, which is also active against *H. influenzae* and *N. meningitidis*, is appropriate. Vancomycin should be administered as well due to concerns for penicillin-resistant pneumococcus and β-lactamase–producing *H. influenzae*. Antibiotics should be administered immediately and should not be delayed to obtain cultures.

Ref.: 18

21. A patient with a recurrent duodenal ulcer is referred for surgical consultation. He has been having abdominal pain for the last 2 years. Fifteen months ago, upper endoscopy showed a duodenal ulcer. The patient was treated with ranitidine, and his condition improved, but the symptoms recurred. Upper endoscopy confirmed a recurrent ulcer, and the result of a *Campylobacter*-like organism (CLO) test was positive. The patient was treated with a combination of two antibiotics and a PPI for 2 weeks. Which of the following tests best assesses eradication of *Helicobacter pylori* after completion of treatment?

A. Urea breath test

B. CLO test

C. Biopsy and culture

D. Serum antibody [by enzyme-linked immunosorbent assay (ELISA)]

E. Stool antibody test

ANSWER: A

COMMENTS: Surgery for the treatment of peptic ulcers is indicated only in the following circumstances: intractable hemorrhage, perforation, and obstruction. The patient does not have any of these conditions. Furthermore, *H. pylori* infection, the most important pathophysiologic factor in the development of duodenal ulcer, was never adequately treated. Treatment options for *H. pylori* infection are numerous, but they must always include an H_2 blocker or a PPI plus at least two antibiotics. The antibiotics most commonly used are amoxicillin, clarithromycin, and metronidazole. Bismuth-containing regimens have also been used. Depending on the combination used, the length of treatment varies from 2 to 4 weeks.

Methods of detecting *H. pylori* can be divided into two categories: invasive and noninvasive. Biopsy and the CLO test require endoscopy, but all the other tests do not. Like the CLO test, the urea breath test takes advantage of the ability of *H. pylori* to split urea. However, the urea breath test only requires the patient to "blow," whereas the CLO test is conducted on a piece of tissue. The serologic test for *H. pylori* antibody is useful but of limited value in determining the success of the therapy. There is no stool "antibody" test for *H. pylori*, but a stool antigen test is available and is as sensitive as the urea breath test.

Since there is no need for repeated endoscopy in this patient, the clinician must consider the relative merits of the noninvasive methods. Because antibody test results may remain positive after treatment, the best choice is the urea breath test, which helps determine the presence of live *H. pylori*.

Ref.: 19

22. Which of the following statements regarding anaerobic bacterial infections is true?

A. Anaerobic bacteria are normal inhabitants of the skin and mucous membranes.

B. *Bacteroides* spp. are the most common isolates in intraabdominal anaerobic infections.

C. If appropriate cultures are obtained, anaerobes are found in more than 75% of intraabdominal abscesses.

D. Proper treatment of anaerobic infections consists of surgical drainage, debridement of necrotic tissue, and appropriate antibiotic therapy.

E. All of the above.

ANSWER: E

COMMENTS: Anaerobic bacteria are normal inhabitants of the skin, mucous membranes, and gastrointestinal tract. In fact, anaerobic bacteria outnumber aerobic organisms by more than 10:1 in the oral cavity and by more than 1000:1 in the colon. Therefore it is not surprising that anaerobes are cultured from up to 90% of intraabdominal abscesses. The most common pathogens in this group are *Bacteroides* spp. *Bacteroides fragilis* is an important copathogen in the pathogenesis of intraabdominal abscesses. As with most serious infections, proper treatment involves appropriate drainage of abscesses and debridement of devitalized tissue when present, as well as appropriate antibiotic therapy. Antibiotics with excellent broad-spectrum anaerobic activity include the carbapenems (imipenem, meropenem, and ertapenem), â-lactam/â-lactamase combinations (ampicillin/sulbactam, ticarcillin/clavulanate, and piperacillin/tazobactam), and metronidazole. Although the second-generation cephalosporins (i.e., cefoxitin and cefotetan) and clindamycin also provide anaerobic coverage, over the past decade an increase in resistance of *Bacteroides* organisms to these agents has been observed. For example, as many as 30% of *B. fragilis* isolates are resistant to clindamycin.

Ref.: 20

23. Which of the following clinical situations or laboratory results requires systemic antifungal therapy?

A. A single positive blood culture result obtained from an indwelling intravascular catheter

B. *Candida* identified from a drain

C. Oral candidiasis

D. *Candida* isolated from a drain culture in a patient who recently underwent surgery for colonic perforation

E. Mucocutaneous candidiasis

ANSWER: A

COMMENTS: Candidemia is associated with significant morbidity (e.g., endocarditis, septic arthritis, and ophthalmitis) and mortality (approximately 40%). Management of candidemia, particularly in patients with intravascular devices, remains controversial. Although the bloodstream in some patients—usually those who are immunocompetent—spontaneously clears after removal of the intravascular device, other patients—particularly those who are immunosuppressed—have disseminated disease and require systemic antifungal therapy. There are no accurate diagnostic tests or methods for selecting high-risk patients to determine those who require systemic antifungal therapy. Therefore all patients with at least one positive blood culture result for *Candida* should be treated with an antifungal agent. All nonsurgically implanted lines should be removed, and if continued central venous access is required, a new line should be placed at a new site (not exchanged over a guidewire). Some would attempt to sterilize the bloodstream without the removal of tunneled catheters or subcutaneous ports. However, in patients with persistent candidemia or septic shock, these devices should also be removed. Amphotericin B and fluconazole appear to have similar efficacy in the treatment of candidemia. Voriconazole and caspofungin are new antifungal agents that are also effective against *Candida.* These agents may be particularly useful for non-*albicans* species such as *Candida krusei* or *Candida glabrata*, which are less susceptible to fluconazole. All patients with candidemia should be evaluated for manifestations of disseminated disease, such as ocular involvement or OM. *Candida* identified from a surgical drain most likely represents colonization and does not require systemic antifungal therapy. Mucocutaneous candidiasis can be treated with local nystatin or clotrimazole.

Ref.: 20

24. A 10-year-old boy who recently emigrated from Mexico has had a 2-day illness characterized by fever, odynophagia, dysphagia, and drooling at the mouth. Physical examination reveals the child to be in a toxic condition with a temperature of 102°F (38.9°C), tachycardia, and tachypnea. There is mild tenderness in the submandibular area and few palpable lymph nodes. The suspected diagnosis is epiglottitis, which is confirmed with a CT scan of the neck. Blood culture results are positive. What kind of organism will probably be seen on Gram stain?

A. Gram-positive cocci in pairs and chains
B. Gram-positive cocci in clusters
C. Slender GNRs
D. Gram-negative coccobacilli
E. Spirochetes

ANSWER: D

COMMENTS: The patient has acute epiglottitis, most likely attributable to *H. influenzae* type B, which is recovered from the blood in up to 100% of cases. Classically, the patient is a 2- to 4-year-old boy with a short history of fever, irritability, dysphonia, and dysphagia, which can occur at any time of the year. The widespread use of *H. influenzae* type B vaccine in developed countries has led to a marked decline in invasive disease with this organism. However, the disease is still common in developing countries. *Haemophilus* species are gram-negative coccobacilli. Treatment includes early intubation, with plans for a cricothyroidotomy or a tracheotomy if intubation fails, and an antibiotic such as ceftriaxone or ampicillin/sulbactam.

Ref.: 20

25. Which of the following previously healthy patients scheduled for an operation should undergo human immunodeficiency virus (HIV) antibody testing?

A. A 35-year-old man seen for removal of a lipoma in the anterior triangle of the neck. A routine preoperative complete blood count reveals a WBC count of 4500 cells/mL with a normal differential, hemoglobin level of 13 g/dL, and platelet count of 81,000/mL
B. A 40-year-old man seen for repair of an inguinal hernia. Physical examination reveals white, adherent, nonremovable plaques on the lateral aspect of his tongue
C. A 28-year-old woman seen for the removal of a breast lump in whom a painful vesicular rash along the T8-10 dermatomes develops on the right side
D. A 20-year-old man undergoing nephrectomy for living related-donor transplantation
E. All of the above

ANSWER: E

COMMENTS: Several risk groups have been identified in whom HIV testing is indicated, including persons with sexually transmitted diseases and persons in high-risk categories, such as injected drug users, homosexual and bisexual men, hemophiliacs, patients with active tuberculosis (TB), and pregnant women. Donors of blood or organs should be tested. Certain clinical or laboratory findings should also prompt HIV testing. Such findings include idiopathic thrombocytopenia, oral hairy leukoplakia, reactivation varicella-zoster virus infection involving more than one dermatome, unexplained oral candidiasis, persistent vulvovaginal candidiasis, and herpes simplex virus infection resistant to treatment.

Ref.: 20

26. Which of the following is true regarding the management of hepatic echinococcal disease?

A. Preoperative endoscopic retrograde cholangiopancreatography can be both diagnostic and therapeutic for cyst–biliary communication.
B. Percutaneous drainage of hydatid cysts is contraindicated due to the risk for anaphylaxis.
C. Surgical excision of hydatid cysts need not be preceded by antiparasitic chemotherapy.
D. CT scan is the most sensitive imaging modality to identify communication between hydatid cysts and the biliary tree.
E. Praziquantel is the preferred antiparasitic agent in hydatid cyst disease.

ANSWER: A

COMMENTS: Hydatid cyst disease is caused by *Echinococcus*, with *E. multilocularis* and *E. granulosus* being the most common species causing infection in humans. The definitive hosts of these parasites are dogs, and the intermediate hosts are most commonly sheep or goats; humans are incidental hosts.

Albendazole is the preferred antiparasitic therapy for *Echinococcus*. Mebendazole is also an option, although it has less in vitro activity than albendazole. Benzimidazole agents interfere with parasite glucose absorption.

The goals of drainage procedures, either surgical or percutaneous, for hepatic echinococcal cysts are inactivation of the parasites and evacuation and obliteration of the cyst cavity; surgical procedures also include the removal of the germinal layer of the cyst cavity. Radical surgical procedures, such as pericystectomy, partial hepatectomy, or lobectomy, are preferred over less invasive surgical techniques. PAIR (puncture, aspiration of the cyst, injection of a scolicidal solution such as hypertonic saline, and reaspiration of cyst contents) is generally the preferred percutaneous drainage procedure. Any drainage procedure should be preceded by the use of a benzimidazole (i.e., albendazole or mebendazole) to sterilize the cyst contents and reduce the risk of anaphylaxis and echinococcal dissemination.

Cystobiliary communication is likely relatively common in hepatic echinococcal disease, but the majority of cases are not clinically apparent. Magnetic resonance cholangiopancreatography has a sensitivity of 92% in diagnosing intrabiliary rupture, whereas CT scan has only 75% sensitivity. Endoscopic retrograde cholangiopancreatography (ERCP) is also very sensitive (86%–100%) and can be used for therapeutic intervention. ERCP with sphincterotomy effectively treats cholangitis related to cystobiliary communication, and some studies have shown that it can decrease the rate of postoperative biliary fistula formation.

Ref.: 21, 22

27. A diabetic patient has recently been discharged from the hospital after intracranial bleeding. He is readmitted for aspiration pneumonia. His condition deteriorates rapidly, with hypotension and multiorgan dysfunction. Which of the following treatments is contraindicated?

A. Volume resuscitation

B. Antibiotics

C. Activated protein C

D. Intensive insulin therapy for hyperglycemia

E. Low-dose hydrocortisone

ANSWER: C

COMMENTS: Severe sepsis is characterized by multiorgan dysfunction with or without shock and is due to a generalized inflammatory and procoagulant response to infection. Efforts to improve the outcome with anticytokine therapy along with antibiotics and supportive care have until recently not been associated with improved survival. Recently, a randomized, double-blind, placebo-controlled multicenter trial evaluating recombinant activated protein C has demonstrated a survival benefit in patients with severe sepsis. However, activated protein C treatment was associated with an increased risk for bleeding and is contraindicated in patients with recent hemorrhagic stroke. Fluid resuscitation and antibiotics are mainstays in the treatment of sepsis. Intensive insulin therapy that maintains serum glucose levels at 80 to 110 mg/dL reduces morbidity and mortality in critically ill patients. The mechanism is unknown, but it is possible that correcting hyperglycemia may improve neutrophil function. The use of corticosteroids for sepsis remains controversial. High doses of corticosteroids may in fact worsen outcomes by increasing the frequency of secondary infections. However, low doses of corticosteroids may be beneficial in septic patients who may have "relative" adrenal insufficiency despite elevated levels of circulating cortisol. Although the issue is controversial, the use of low-dose hydrocortisone is not contraindicated in this patient.

Ref.: 23

28. Endocarditis prophylaxis is recommended for which of the following patients?

A. A patient with mitral valve prolapse but without murmur who is undergoing lithotripsy for renal calculi

B. A patient with a history of rheumatic fever and normal cardiac valves who is undergoing prostatic biopsy

C. A patient with a prosthetic aortic valve who is undergoing pulmonary resection

D. A patient with severe hypertrophic cardiomyopathy who is undergoing endoscopic retrograde cholangiography for biliary obstruction

E. A patient previously treated for streptococcal endocarditis who is undergoing colonoscopy

ANSWER: C

COMMENTS: Antibiotic prophylaxis for endocarditis is recommended for patients with certain cardiac conditions who are undergoing any dental procedure that involves the gingival tissues or periapical region of a tooth and for any procedure involving perforation of the oral mucosa. In addition, patients undergoing procedures on the respiratory tract or those with skin or soft tissue infections should also receive prophylaxis. The cardiac conditions associated with the highest risk for adverse outcomes from infective endocarditis for which prophylaxis is indicated prior to the previously listed procedures include prosthetic heart valves, history of infective endocarditis, congenital heart disease (CHD) limited to unrepaired cyanotic CHD, repaired CHD with prosthetic material or devices during the first 6 months after the procedure, repaired CHD with residual defects at the site or adjacent to the site of a prosthesis, and cardiac transplantation recipients with cardiac valvulopathy. Prophylaxis against viridans group streptococci with a penicillin, cephalosporin, or clindamycin is recommended. Routine prophylaxis in patients undergoing gastrointestinal or genitourinary procedures is no longer recommended.

Ref.: 24

29. A patient is infected with HIV. His last $CD4^+$ T-lymphocyte count was 50 cells/mm^3, and his viral load was 100,000 copies/mL. He comes to the hospital with a sudden onset of right hemiparesis. He has been afebrile. A CT scan and magnetic resonance imaging (MRI) of the brain show multiple ring-enhancing lesions in the left cerebral hemisphere. The *Toxoplasma* IgG antibody test result is positive. He has received pyrimethamine and sulfadiazine for 12 days. Neurologically, the patient is stable. Which of the following is the next best step?

A. Repeat MRI of the brain.

B. Continue the same antibiotic therapy for an additional 10 days and reassess.

C. Switch treatment to pyrimethamine with the addition of clindamycin and reassess whether the patient improves clinically in 10 to 14 days.

D. Add corticosteroids to the treatment regimen.

E. Perform a positron emission tomography (PET) or single-photon emission computed tomography (SPECT) scan.

ANSWER: A

COMMENTS: Up to 90% of HIV-infected patients with advanced disease (<100 $CD4^+$ cells/mm^3), multiple ring-enhancing lesions, and a positive *Toxoplasma* IgG antibody have cerebral toxoplasmosis. Empiric treatment with pyrimethamine, sulfadiazine, and folinic acid is recommended. Most patients with central nervous system (CNS) toxoplasmosis respond rapidly to this therapy, with nearly 90% of patients demonstrating neurologic improvement at 2 weeks. Radiographic improvement occurs at a slower pace, with approximately 50% improvement on repeated MRI of the brain occurring within 3 weeks of initiating treatment. For patients who do not improve by 2 weeks, a brain biopsy is indicated. Although lymphoma is the most likely alternative diagnosis in patients with acquired immunodeficiency syndrome (AIDS) and CNS lesions, up to 25% of brain biopsy specimens reveal toxoplasmosis. Thallium-201 (SPECT) or PET scans may provide useful information in that a "cold" lesion revealed by SPECT or hypometabolic lesions seen on PET scanning are consistent with infection. However, false-positive and false-negative results can occur with these functional imaging studies. The addition of corticosteroids may be useful in the treatment of increased intracranial pressure. However, this antiinflammatory effect may make interpretation of clinical and radiographic responses difficult.

Ref.: 25

30. Match each agent in the left-hand column with one or more mechanisms of antimicrobial action in the right-hand column.

A. Carbapenems	a. Impairment of bacterial DNA synthesis
B. Aminoglycosides	b. Inhibition of cell wall synthesis
C. Quinolones	c. Disruption of ribosomal protein synthesis
D. Cephalosporins	d. Disruption of cell wall cation homeostasis
E. Vancomycin	e. Disruption of the cytoplasmic membrane

ANSWER: A-a; B-c, d; C-a; D-b; E-b

COMMENTS: All the antimicrobial agents listed above are bactericidal agents (i.e., their associated mechanisms of action result in bacterial death). Bacteriostatic agents (e.g., tetracyclines, chloramphenicol, erythromycin, clindamycin, and linezolid) act by preventing bacterial growth but do not result in bacterial death. They work primarily through inhibition of ribosomal protein synthesis. Both carbapenems and cephalosporins are â-lactam antibiotics and hence have a similar mode of activity. Enzymes located within the bacterial cytoplasmic membrane are responsible for peptide cross-linkage. These enzymes are called penicillin-binding proteins (PBPs) and are the site at which â-lactam drugs bind. Such binding interferes with bacterial cell wall synthesis and eventually results in cell lysis. Gram-negative bacteria contain a variable number of various PBPs. Each â-lactam antibiotic has different affinities for the different PBPs. Vancomycin is a glycopeptide that also inhibits bacterial cell wall synthesis and assembly. Vancomycin complexes to cell wall precursors and prevents elongation and cross-linkage, thereby making the cell susceptible to lysis. This antibacterial activity is limited to gram-positive organisms. Aminoglycosides bind irreversibly to the 30S bacterial ribosome and interfere with protein synthesis. For this activity to take place, they must penetrate the cell wall, which occurs optimally under aerobic conditions. Unlike other antibiotics that inhibit protein synthesis, aminoglycosides are bactericidal. This feature is due to their disruptive effect on calcium and magnesium homeostasis within the cell wall. Quinolones inhibit topoisomerase II (DNA gyrase) and topoisomerase IV, which impairs DNA synthesis in bacteria. Appreciation of the mechanism of action of antimicrobials may have a bearing on the selection of alternative therapies when bacterial resistance to the drug of choice develops.

Ref.: 26

31. Which of the following statements regarding diabetic foot infections is false?

A. Acute diabetic foot infections are often caused by gram-positive organisms.

B. Chronic diabetic foot infections are polymicrobial.

C. To diagnose an infection in a patient with a chronic wound, a foul odor and redness must be present.

D. MRSA infections are associated with a worse outcome.

E. Impaired host defenses allow low-virulence colonizers such as coagulase-negative staphylococci and *Corynebacterium* spp. to become pathogens.

ANSWER: C

COMMENTS: See Question 32.

Ref.: See Question 32

32. Which of the following regarding the treatment of diabetic foot infections is true?

A. Acute diabetic foot infections are caused by monomicrobial gram-negative aerobes.

B. The use of antibiotics for an uninfected chronic wound facilitates wound closure and prevents future infection.

C. Sharp debridement of necrotic or unhealthy tissue prolongs wound healing and removes a potential reservoir for bacteria.

D. Avoiding direct pressure on the wound facilitates healing.

E. The administration of granulocyte-stimulating factors (GSFs) results in faster resolution of the infection.

ANSWER: D

COMMENTS: Diabetic patients have a higher risk for foot infections because of factors such as vascular insufficiency, decreased sensation, hyperglycemia, and impairment of the immune system, particularly neutrophil dysfunction. Deep tissue biopsy of the infected foot is the preferred method of culture. Acute diabetic foot infections are often caused by monomicrobial aerobic gram-positive cocci (*S. aureus* and â-hemolytic streptococci, especially group B), whereas patients with chronic wounds and those who have recently received antibiotic therapy generally have polymicrobial gram-positive and gram-negative aerobes and anaerobes within their wound, including enterococci, *Enterobacter*, obligate anaerobes, and *P. aeruginosa*. Initial therapy is usually empiric and based on the severity of infection and available microbiology data (culture results or Gram stain). A majority of mild infections can be treated with orally dosed antimicrobials directed against aerobic gram-positive cocci. In patients with more severe infections or extensive chronic infections, parenteral broad-spectrum antibiotics with activity against gram-positive cocci (including MRSA) and gram-negative and obligate anaerobic organisms are warranted. The diagnosis of infection in patients with chronic wounds includes the presence of purulent secretions (pus) and two or more of the following: redness, warmth, swelling or induration, and pain or tenderness. MRSA infections are associated with worse outcomes, and impaired host defenses allow low-virulence colonizers such as coagulase-negative staphylococci and *Corynebacterium* spp. to become pathogens. In addition to antibiotics, early incision and drainage of abscesses with debridement of devitalized tissue, immobilization, and supportive care are important in the total management of a diabetic foot. In the presence of significant vascular insufficiency, revascularization of the distal end of the lower extremity may improve healing and prevent amputation. Radioactive studies using technetium-99 (bone scan) or gallium citrate or indium-labeled leukocyte scans have poor specificity and should not be performed routinely. MRI has become the imaging study of choice for diagnosing OM.

Continued use of antimicrobials is not warranted for the entire time that the wound is open or for the management of clinically uninfected ulceration either to enhance wound healing or as prophylaxis against infection. Local wound care with sharp debridement of necrotic or unhealthy tissue promotes wound healing and removes a potential reservoir of pathogens. Avoiding direct pressure on the wound and providing off-loading devices facilitate wound healing. Administration of granulocyte colony-stimulating factors does not accelerate the resolution of infection but may significantly reduce the need for operative procedures.

Ref.: 27

33. Match each clinical characteristic or agent in the left-hand column with the correct infecting organism or organisms in the right-hand column. More than one answer may apply.

A. Fibrosing mediastinitis	a. *Candida albicans*
B. Amphotericin	b. *Nocardia asteroides*
C. Intertrigo	c. *Actinomyces israelii*
D. Brain abscess	d. *Cryptococcus neoformans*
E. Pelvic mass	e. *Histoplasma capsulatum*

ANSWER: A-e; B-a, d, e; C-a; D-b; E-c

COMMENTS: Amphotericin B remains an important agent for the treatment of systemic mycotic infections, including candidiasis, mucormycosis, cryptococcosis, histoplasmosis, coccidioidomycosis, sporotrichosis, and aspergillosis. Amphotericin B is a fungicidal agent. Binding of amphotericin B to ergosterol in the fungal cell membrane alters permeability, with leakage of intracellular ions and macromolecules, leading to cell death. Adverse events such as infusion reactions and nephrotoxicity are common with the conventional (deoxycholate) form of the drug. New lipid formulations of amphotericin B have been developed and are associated with a reduction in toxicity without sacrificing efficacy. Newer triazoles (voriconazole and posaconazole) and echinocandins (caspofungin, micafungin, and anidulafungin) are emerging as alternative broad-spectrum antifungal agents. Histoplasmosis is predominantly a pulmonary infection caused by *Histoplasma capsulatum*, a dimorphic fungus endemic to the Mississippi and Ohio River valleys and along the Appalachian Mountains. Histoplasmosis has been associated with massive enlargement of the mediastinal lymph nodes secondary to granulomatous inflammation. During the healing process, fibrotic tissue can cause postobstructive pneumonia or constriction of the esophagus or superior vena cava and result in dysphagia or superior vena cava syndrome (or both). Actinomycosis is caused by a group of gram-positive higher-order bacteria that are part of the normal flora found in the oral cavity, gastrointestinal tract, and female genital tract. Typically, infections with *Actinomyces* spp. often occur after disruption of mucosal surfaces and lead to oral and cervical disease, pneumonia with empyema, and intraabdominal or pelvic abscesses. Placement of intrauterine devices has been associated with pelvic abscess secondary to this organism. Sinus tract formation is common as these organisms extend, unrestricted, through tissue planes. High-dose penicillin and surgical drainage are generally required for cure. *Nocardia* spp., other higher-order bacteria, are found in soil, organic matter, and water. Human infection occurs after inhalation or skin inoculation. Chronic pneumonia can occur, usually in immunocompromised patients. Skin lesions and brain abscesses are common with a disseminated infection.

Prolonged treatment with sulfonamides in combination with other antibiotics is required for cure. *C. neoformans* causes meningitis and pulmonary disease. Infection is common in the setting of immunodeficiency, such as organ transplantation and AIDS, but it may also occur in immunocompetent hosts. *C. albicans* is a common inhabitant of the mucous membranes and gastrointestinal tract. Intertrigo is one form of cutaneous candidiasis that occurs in skinfolds where a warm moist environment exists. Vesiculopustules develop, enlarge, rupture, and cause maceration and fissuring. Obese and diabetic patients are at risk for the development of candidal intertrigo. Local care, including nystatin powder, is usually effective.

Ref.: 20, 28

34. Which of the following statements is correct regarding spontaneous bacterial peritonitis (SBP; primary peritonitis) in a cirrhotic patient?

A. Infection is usually polymicrobial.
B. Ascitic fluid culture results are always positive.
C. The most likely pathogenic mechanism is translocation from the gut.
D. Twenty-one days of antibiotic treatment may be adequate.
E. Infection-related mortality has declined to less than 10%.

ANSWER: E

COMMENTS: SBP is a monomicrobial infection, with enteric GNRs accounting for 60%–70% of the episodes of SBP. *E. coli* is the most frequently recovered pathogen, followed by *K. pneumoniae*. Streptococcal species, including pneumococci and enterococci, are also important pathogens. Ascitic fluid culture results are negative in many cases, but inoculation of blood culture bottles at the bedside yields bacterial growth in approximately 80% of cases. SBP most likely develops from the combination of prolonged bacteremia secondary to abnormal host defense, intrahepatic shunting, and impaired bactericidal activity of ascetic fluid. Transmural migration of gut flora and transfallopian spread of vaginal bacteria to the peritoneal space may also occur. Initial antimicrobial treatment should include coverage against aerobic gram-negative organisms. A third-generation cephalosporin, such as cefotaxime or ceftriaxone, is a reasonable choice. The duration of antibiotic treatment is unclear; 2 weeks has been suggested, but shorter courses (5 days) may have similar efficacy. Although the in-hospital mortality rate approaches 40%, infection-related mortality has declined significantly (10%). Unfortunately, the probability of recurrence is 70% at 1 year, with 1- and 2-year survival rates being 30% and 20%, respectively.

Ref.: 29, 30

35. Which of the following patients with cirrhosis benefit from prophylactic antibiotic therapy to decrease the risk for SBP?

A. Patients awaiting liver transplantation
B. Patients hospitalized with acute gastrointestinal bleeding
C. Patients with ascitic fluid protein levels of greater than 1 g/100 mL
D. Patients who have recovered from a previous episode of SBP
E. Patients with ascitic fluid protein levels of less than 1 g/100 mL

ANSWER: C

COMMENTS: Randomized trials have demonstrated that secondary prophylaxis with oral norfloxacin, 400 mg/day, or trimethoprim/sulfamethoxazole, one double-strength tablet five times per week decreases the risk for recurrent SBP from 68% to 20%. However, overall mortality in these patients remains unchanged compared with those not receiving secondary prophylaxis. Another observation is that long-term quinolone use has been associated with the development of infection with quinolone-resistant bacteria. In approximately 30%–40% of patients with cirrhosis hospitalized for acute gastrointestinal bleeding, infection develops during the hospitalization. Norfloxacin (400 mg a day for 7 days) decreases the incidence of infective episodes involving gram-negative bacteria. The risk for SBP increases tenfold in patients with an ascitic fluid protein concentration of less than 1 g/100 mL fluid. Norfloxacin, 400 mg/day, during hospitalization decreases the incidence of SBP in these patients as well. Patients hospitalized while awaiting liver transplantation are probably at risk for SBP and may therefore benefit from antibiotic prophylaxis. Active infection is a contraindication to liver transplantation.

Ref.: 30

36. Which of the following statements regarding secondary peritonitis is false?

A. It usually occurs because of perforation of an intraabdominal viscus.

B. Carbapenems, aminoglycosides, and fourth-generation cephalosporins have equal efficacy in treatment studies.

C. Increased age, cancer, cirrhosis, and systemic illness are factors that increase the mortality rate.

D. Sequestration of bacteria within fibrin clots leads to intraabdominal abscess formation.

E. The most common organism cultured from the abdomen is *E. coli.*

ANSWER: B

COMMENTS: Secondary peritonitis usually occurs because of perforation of an intraabdominal viscus such as perforated peptic ulcer, appendix, or diverticulum or penetrating gastrointestinal trauma. The infection is polymicrobial, with facultative aerobes and anaerobes acting synergistically. One study revealed an average of 2.5 anaerobes and 2 facultative aerobes identified per case of secondary peritonitis. *E. coli* is the most common isolate in culture. *Bacteroides* spp. are the most frequent anaerobes cultured from abdominal infections. About 10^{12} bacteria reside in the colon per gram of feces, with 90% of these bacteria being anaerobic organisms. Any process that impairs immunologic function or is associated with general debilitation increases mortality. Age, cancer, hepatic cirrhosis, and the presence of a systemic illness have been shown to increase mortality. One of the defense mechanisms of the peritoneal cavity is the production of fibrin to sequester bacteria for limiting systemic spread. Such sequestration leads to the formation of intraabdominal abscesses, which generally require drainage for cure. Treatment of secondary peritonitis requires surgical intervention for removal of the source of infection and systemic antibiotics for eradication of residual bacteria. Antibiotics selected should include agents with broad-spectrum coverage for facultative aerobes, gram-negative bacilli, and anaerobes. Carbapenems are a good empiric choice for treatment. Aminoglycosides and fourth-generation cephalosporins lack anaerobic activity.

Ref.: 20, 31

37. Which of the following statements regarding cytomegalovirus (CMV) infection and solid organ transplantation is false?

A. Symptomatic infection occurs 2 to 6 months after transplantation.

B. Patients being treated for acute rejection are at an increased risk for the development of symptomatic CMV infection.

C. Transmission can occur through the donor organ.

D. Reactivation of latent infection is associated with the greatest risk for the development of severe disease.

E. CMV infection may be associated with premature atherosclerosis in cardiac transplant patients.

ANSWER: D

COMMENTS: CMV is the most important pathogen affecting recipients of solid organ transplants. Symptomatic CMV disease may develop in as many as 50% of allograft recipients, usually 2 to 6 months after transplantation. CMV-seronegative recipients who are primarily infected are at the greatest risk for the development of severe CMV disease. Primary infection can occur through the donor organ, unscreened blood products, or intimate contact with a viral shedder. Reactivation of latent infection is less likely to cause severe disease. Patients receiving muromonab-CD3 (OKT3)/antilymphocyte globulin (ALG) therapy for acute rejection also appear to be at risk for the development of CMV disease. In addition to clinical disease directly attributable to CMV infection, CMV has indirect immunomodulatory activity. Symptomatic CMV infections are associated with an increased incidence of bacterial infections and opportunistic infections such as aspergillosis and *Pneumocystis carinii* pneumonia. In heart transplant patients, acute rejection and accelerated atherosclerosis are associated with CMV infection. Ganciclovir is the most commonly used agent for the prevention of CMV infection and disease; however, there is growing concern regarding the emergence of ganciclovir resistance.

Ref.: 32, 33

38. A 28-year-old man who sustained closed-head trauma in a motor vehicle accident a month earlier comes to the emergency department with a 3-day history of progressive headache, fever, and confusion. His wife reports the recent onset of clear drainage from his left naris. Physical examination reveals a temperature of 102°F (38.9°C), a stiff neck, and no rash. Which of the following statements concerning the patient is true?

A. He most likely has bacterial meningitis secondary to *S. aureus.*

B. Antiretroviral prophylaxis has been beneficial in preventing bacterial meningitis after head trauma.

C. Empiric antibiotics should include an extended-spectrum cephalosporin and vancomycin.

D. Corticosteroid administration with antibiotics is not indicated.

E. He requires immediate surgical intervention for repair of cerebrospinal fluid leakage.

ANSWER: C

COMMENTS: The patient probably sustained a basilar skull fracture and a dural rent, with subsequent development of a dural fistula from the subarachnoid space and nasal cavity or paranasal sinuses. Cerebrospinal fluid rhinorrhea may occur and can easily be diagnosed by detecting the presence of $â_2$-transferrin in nasal secretions. In patients with known basilar skull fracture, cerebrospinal fluid rhinorrhea develops in approximately 10% of the cases. Of these patients, bacterial meningitis develops in up to 30%. *S. pneumoniae* is the most common pathogen (65% of cases). Other organisms, such as *H. influenzae*, *N. meningitidis*, and *S. aureus*, account for the remaining cases. Empiric treatment should include an extended-spectrum cephalosporin (ceftriaxone, cefotaxime, or cefepime) and vancomycin since the incidence of â-lactam–resistant pneumococci is increasing. Prophylactic antibiotics have no proven benefit and may predispose to meningitis from antibiotic-resistant gram-negative bacteria. A recent prospective study demonstrated a survival advantage in patients with pneumococcal meningitis who received corticosteroids before or at the time of antibiotic administration. Spontaneous closure of the dural fistula is less likely in patients with a delayed manifestation of cerebrospinal fluid leakage with meningitis, and surgical repair is indicated. Diagnostic studies to identify the site of the fistula and treatment of any CNS infection should be completed before surgical intervention.

Ref.: 34, 35

39. Which of the following statements regarding hepatitis C virus (HCV) infection is false?

A. The prevalence of HCV infection in HCWs is similar to that in the general population.

B. Chronic HCV infection occurs in 75%–85% of patients after acute infection.

C. Hepatic failure because of chronic HCV infection is the most common indication for liver transplantation.

D. Pegylated interferon plus ribavirin is an effective therapy for most patients with chronic HCV infection.

E. Factors associated with the development of cirrhosis include male gender, alcohol use, and coinfection with HIV.

ANSWER: D

COMMENTS: Persons with acute HCV infection are typically asymptomatic (60%–70%) or have a mild clinical illness. Fulminant hepatitis is rare. Chronic HCV infection develops in approximately 75%–80% of persons with acute HCV infection. Cirrhosis develops in 10%–20% of chronically infected individuals, usually after more than 20 years of infection. Liver failure from chronic HCV infection has become the leading indication for liver transplantation. Increased alcohol use, male gender, HIV coinfection, and HCV genotype 1 are associated with more severe liver disease. Hepatocellular carcinoma can be a late complication in 1%–2% of patients with cirrhosis. Antiviral therapy is recommended for individuals at an increased risk for progressive liver disease, as demonstrated by persistently elevated serum transaminase levels, detectable HCV RNA levels, and moderate inflammation in liver biopsy specimens.

The prevalence of HCV infection is highest in injected drug users and patients undergoing hemodialysis. Overall, nearly 2% of the U.S. population has persistent HCV infection. Although transmission of HCV to HCWs occurs after approximately 3% of needlestick exposures involving HCV-infected patients, the prevalence of HCV infection in HCWs, including surgeons, is like the general population.

Ref.: 20, 36

40. Which statement about *Mycobacterium tuberculosis* treatment and prophylaxis is true?

A. Two-drug treatment with INH and rifampin (RIF) for 9 months is standard therapy for active pulmonary TB.

B. Treatment failure can be due to drug resistance or nonadherence.

C. HIV-infected individuals require prolonged therapy for active TB.

D. INH prophylaxis for latent TB is given for at least 12 months.

E. INH prophylaxis should not be given to individuals with recent conversion from purified protein derivative (PPD)-negative to PPD-positive status.

ANSWER: B

COMMENTS: Recent Centers for Disease Control and Prevention (CDC) guidelines recommend that all patients with active pulmonary TB receive four-drug therapy consisting of INH, RIF, pyrazinamide, and ethambutol for the initial 2 months of treatment. For patients with drug-susceptible TB and negative sputum test results after 2 months of therapy, treatment can be completed with 4 months of INH and RIF. Extrapulmonary disease requires 6 to 9 months of treatment, except for meningitis, which is treated for 1 year. HIV-infected individuals are treated similar to non–HIV-infected patients with TB. However, significant drug–drug interactions may occur with antiretroviral agents and TB drugs and may alter therapeutic decisions. Treatment failures are generally due to nonadherence by patients to multidrug regimens. Currently, local health departments have directly observed therapy programs to improve compliance with and completion of anti-TB medication regimens. Another cause of treatment failure is infection with multidrug-resistant strains of *M. tuberculosis*. Conditions associated with a higher rate of resistance include TB in those known to have a higher prevalence of drug resistance, such as Asians or Hispanics and previously treated individuals; the persistence of culture-positive sputum after 2 months of therapy; and known exposure to drug-resistant TB.

Certain individuals are at considerable risk for the development of active TB once infected (latent TB). TB skin testing (Mantoux/PPD) is useful for identifying latent TB in high-risk individuals. Three cut points have been recommended for defining a positive tuberculin reaction: greater than 5 mm, greater than 10 mm, and greater than 15 mm of induration. Persons considered at highest risk (>5 mm of induration) include individuals with HIV infection, recent contacts with TB patients, and organ transplant patients. Individuals also at risk (>10-mm induration) include injectable drug users, residents of nursing homes and prisons, hospital employees, and recent immigrants from countries with a high prevalence of TB. These individuals, who are at a considerable risk for the development of active TB once infected, should receive 9 months of INH therapy.

Ref.: 37

41. Which of the following is true regarding the bacteriology of vascular graft infections?

A. *S. epidermidis* is the most commonly isolated organism.

B. Fungal graft infections are uncommon, but when they do occur, they are most common in immunocompromised patients.

C. Gram-negative organisms are implicated most frequently in thoracic aortic and carotid artery graft infections.

D. Gram-negative infections are often less virulent and have fewer major complications than do gram-positive infections.

E. None of the above.

ANSWER: B

COMMENTS: See Question 42.

Ref.: See Question 42

42. Which of the following clinical scenarios raises concern for vascular graft infection?

A. New-onset gastrointestinal bleeding in a patient with a history of abdominal aortic endograft placement

B. The presence of a draining sinus tract 3 cm distal to a forearm arteriovenous graft for hemodialysis

C. A slowly growing pulsatile mass in the groin of a patient with a history of an aortofemoral bypass graft

D. CT scan demonstrating the presence of a fluid collection adjacent to an abdominal aortic graft

E. All of the above

ANSWER: E

COMMENTS: Vascular graft infections can manifest in a variety of ways, and surgeons must maintain a high index of suspicion for graft infection. There are multiple mechanisms by which vascular grafts can become infected: perioperative contamination (including from lymphatic disruption), seeding from bacteremia, contiguous spread from an adjacent infectious process, and erosion of the graft into the gastrointestinal or genitourinary tracts. Grafts are more prone to infection than natural tissue since bacteria adhere to graft material and form a biofilm that resists the body's natural immunologic defenses. The most likely organisms in vascular graft infections are gram-positive cocci such as *S. aureus* (the most common pathogen) and *S. epidermidis*, but the incidence of GNR infections is significantly increased in abdominal aortic, aortofemoral, and infrainguinal vascular graft infections. Gram-negative infections are more virulent than gram-positive infections, because gram-negative organisms produce proteases, elastases, and other destructive enzymes, which can cause anastomotic disruption and vessel rupture. In the vast majority of cases of vascular graft infection, the prosthetic material must be excised for complete eradication of the infection.

Ref.: 38

43. Suspicion of OM in a diabetic foot ulcer should be raised in all of the following except:

A. A deep ulcer that overlies a bony prominence

B. An ulcer that does not heal after 2 weeks of appropriate therapy

C. A patient with a swollen foot and a history of foot ulceration

D. Unexplained high WBC count or inflammatory markers in a patient with a diabetic foot ulcer

E. Evidence of cortical erosion and periosteal reaction on plain radiography

ANSWER: B

COMMENTS: See Question 44.

Ref.: See Question 44

44. Which of the following is true regarding OM in a diabetic foot?

A. A nuclear medicine-tagged WBC scan is the best way to diagnose OM.

B. The only reported successful treatment of OM includes resection of the infected bone.

C. A presumptive diagnosis of OM cannot be made even if bone destruction is seen on plain film underneath an ulcer.

D. A bone biopsy is often difficult to perform and invasive and should be avoided.

E. Selected patients may benefit from implanted antibiotics, hyperbaric oxygen therapy, or revascularization.

ANSWER: E

COMMENTS: OM impairs healing of the wound and acts as a nidus for recurrent infection. It should be suspected in any deep or extensive ulcer, in one that overlies a bony prominence, and in an ulcer that does not heal after 6 weeks of appropriate therapy. In addition, concern for OM is raised in a patient with a swollen foot and a history of foot ulceration, the presence of a "sausage toe" (red, swollen digit), unexplained high WBC count, or inflammatory markers. Bone destruction underneath an ulcer seen on radiographs or probing of an ulcer down to bone is OM until proved otherwise. MRI is the most useful available imaging modality to diagnose OM, as well as to characterize any underlying soft tissue infection. The "gold standard" for diagnosis of OM remains isolation of bacteria from a bone sample with concomitant histologic findings of inflammatory cells and osteonecrosis.

When treating a diabetic foot infection, if there are no hard signs to indicate the presence of OM and plain radiographs do not demonstrate any evidence of bone pathology, the patient should be treated for about 2 weeks for the soft tissue infection. If there is a persistent concern for OM, plain films should be repeated in 2 to 4 weeks to look for evidence of cortical erosion, periosteal reaction, or mixed radiolucency and sclerosis. Radioisotope scans are more sensitive than plain radiographs for diagnosis but are expensive and can be time consuming. If findings on plain films are only consistent with but not characteristic of OM, the clinician should consider the following: (1) additional imaging studies—MRI is preferred but nuclear medicine scans with leukocyte or immunoglobulin techniques would be the second choice; (2) empiric treatment for an additional 2 to 4 weeks with repeated radiographs to look for progression of bone changes; and (3) bone biopsy (operative or percutaneous fluoroscopic or CT guidance), especially if the etiologic pathogen or susceptibilities need to be established. Some physicians would perform biopsies for midfoot or hindfoot lesions because these are more difficult to treat and lead to higher-level amputations.

Traditionally, resection of a bone with chronic OM was necessary for cure; however, some nonrandomized case series report clinical success in 65%–80% of patients treated nonoperatively with prolonged (3 to 6 months) antibiotic therapy. When treatment of OM fails, the clinician should consider whether the original diagnosis was correct; whether there is any remaining necrotic or infected bone or surgical hardware that needs to be removed; and whether the antimicrobials selected were appropriate, achieved an effective concentration within the bone, and were used for a sufficient duration. Selected patients may benefit from implanted antibiotics, hyperbaric oxygen therapy, revascularization, long-term or intermittent antibiotic administration, or amputation.

Ref.: 27

45. Which of the following regarding hospital-acquired pneumonia (HAP), VAP, and health care–associated pneumonia (HCAP) is false?

A. They are the most common nosocomial infections.

B. They are usually caused by aerobic gram-negative bacilli.

C. They are rarely due to viral or fungal pathogens in immunocompetent patients.

D. Infection resulting from aspiration is usually due to anaerobes.
E. Gram-positive coccal isolates are more common patients with head trauma.

ANSWER: A

COMMENTS: See Question 46.

Ref.: See Question 46

46. Which of the following are risk factors for HAP, VAP, or HCAP caused by multidrug-resistant pathogens?

A. Hospitalization for 5 or more days
B. Antimicrobial therapy or hospitalization in the preceding 90 days
C. Home wound care
D. Immunosuppressive disease or therapy
E. All of the above

ANSWER: E

COMMENTS: HAP, HCAP, and VAP are the second most common nosocomial infections after UTI. They result in significant morbidity and mortality. They are due to a wide spectrum of bacterial pathogens and are often polymicrobial, especially in patients with acute respiratory distress syndrome. They are rarely due to viral or fungal agents in immunocompetent patients. Isolation of *Candida* from endotracheal aspirates of immunocompetent patients usually represents colonization.

Common pathogens include aerobic gram-negative bacilli, including *P. aeruginosa*, *E. coli*, *K. pneumoniae*, and *Acinetobacter* spp. There has been an emergence of pneumonia associated with gram-positive cocci (*S. aureus*, particularly MRSA), and it is more commonly seen in diabetics, patients with head trauma, and those hospitalized in the ICU. Infection with anaerobic organisms may follow aspiration in nonintubated patients but is rare in VAP.

Early-onset HAP or VAP occurring within the first 4 days of hospitalization carries a better prognosis than do late-onset infections (5 days or more), which are more likely to be due to multidrug-resistant bacterial pathogens and result in increased morbidity and mortality. Additional risk factors for multidrug-resistant bacterial pathogens such as *Pseudomonas, Acinetobacter* spp., MRSA, and *K. pneumoniae* include antimicrobial therapy or hospitalization in the preceding 90 days, a high frequency of antibiotic resistance in the community or in the specific hospital unit, and immunosuppressive disease or therapy. Risk factors for multidrug-resistant pathogens in patients with HCAP include residence in a nursing home or long-term care facility, home infusion therapy, chronic dialysis within 30 days, home wound care, and a family member with a multidrug-resistant pathogen.

P. aeruginosa is the most common gram-negative bacterial pathogen that causes multidrug-resistant HAP/VAP, with some isolates being susceptible only to polymyxin B. Most MRSA infections are treated successfully with linezolid, although MRSA isolates resistant to linezolid are emerging.

Early administration of a broad-spectrum antibiotic in adequate doses and deescalation of the initial antibiotic therapy based on cultures and clinical response are essential. Failure to adequately treat the infection because of delayed initiation of appropriate therapy has been associated with increased mortality. Guidelines have been established by the American Thoracic Society and the Infectious Disease Society of America for empiric therapy in immunocompetent adults with bacterial causes of HAP, VAP, or HCAP; treatment should include either ceftriaxone, a fluoroquinolone, ampicillin/sulbactam, or ertapenem if there is no suspicion of a multidrug-resistant pathogen.

Ref.: 39

47. Which of the following antimicrobial agents is considered safe in pregnancy?

A. Ganciclovir
B. Albendazole
C. Ketoconazole
D. Streptomycin
E. Erythromycin

ANSWER: E

COMMENTS: Multiple antimicrobial agents are contraindicated in pregnancy. Of the answer choices listed above, erythromycin is the only agent considered safe. Most penicillins and cephalosporins are safe as well. Ganciclovir, ketoconazole, and albendazole are teratogenic in the first trimester. Streptomycin has been shown to cause ototoxicity in fetuses.

Ref.: 40

REFERENCES

1. Kanj S, Kanafani Z. Current concepts in antimicrobial therapy against resistant gram-negative organisms: extended-spectrum beta-lactamase-producing Enterobacteriaceae, carbapenem-resistant Enterobacteriaceae, and multidrug-resistant *Pseudomonas aeruginosa*. *Mayo Clin Proc*. 2011;86(3):250–259.
2. Mermel LA, Allon M, Bouza E, et al. Clinical practice guidelines for the diagnosis and management of intravascular catheter-related infection: 2009 update by the Infectious Diseases Society of America. *Clin Infect Dis*. 2009;49(1):1–45.
3. Nicolle LE. Catheter associated urinary tract infections. *Antimicrob Resist Infect Control*. 2014;3(1):1.
4. Hooton TM, Bradley SF, Cardenas DD, et al. Diagnosis, prevention, and treatment of catheter-associated urinary tract infection in adults: 2009 International Clinical Practice Guidelines from the Infectious Diseases Society of America. *Clin Infect Dis*. 2010;50(5):625–663.
5. Lok ASF, McMahon BJ. Chronic hepatitis B. In: Rodes J. Benhamou JP, Blei AT, et al. eds. *Hepatology*. 2007;45(2):507–539.
6. Barie PS. Surgical infections and antibiotic use. In: *Sabiston Textbook of Surgery*. 19th ed. Saunders, Philadelphia; 2012:240–280.
7. Bandyk DF. Vascular surgical site infection: risk factors and preventative measures. *Semin Vasc Surg*. 2008;21(3):119–123.
8. Bakken JS, Borody T, Brandt LJ, et al. Treating *Clostridium difficile* infection with fecal microbiota transplantation. *Clin Gastroenterol Hepatol*. 2011;9(12):1044–1049.
9. Louie TJ, Miller MA, Mullane KM, et al. Fidaxomicin versus vancomycin for *Clostridium difficile* infection. *N Engl J Med*. 2011;364(5):422–431.
10. Owens RC, Donskey CJ, Gaynes RP, Loo VG, Muto CA. Antimicrobial-associated risk factors for *Clostridium difficile* infection. *Clin Infect Dis*. 2008;46(1):S19–S31.
11. Bartlett JG. Narrative review: the new epidemic of *Clostridium difficile*–associated enteric disease. *Ann Intern Med*. 2006;145(10):758–764.
12. O'Grady NP, Barie PS, Bartlett JG, et al. Guidelines for evaluation of new fever in critically ill adult patients: 2008 update from the American College of Critical Care Medicine and the Infectious Diseases Society of America. *Crit Care Med*. 2008;36(4):1330–1349.
13. Hassel B. Tetanus: pathophysiology, treatment, and the possibility of using botulinum toxin against tetanus-induced rigidity and spasms. *Toxins*. 2013;5(1):73–83.
14. Longworth S, Han J. Pyogenic liver abscess. *Clin Liver Dis*. 2015;6(2):51–54.
15. Greenhalgh DG, Saffle JR, Holmes JH, et al. American Burn Association consensus conference to define sepsis and infection in burns. *J Burn Care Res*. 2007;28(6):776–790.

16. Nasser W, Beres WB, Olsen RJ, et al. Evolutionary pathway to increased virulence and epidemic group A *Streptococcus* disease derived from 3,615 genome sequences. *Proc Natl Acad Sci.* 2014;111(17):E1768–E1776.
17. Walker MJ, Barnett TC, McArthur JD, et al. Disease manifestations and pathogenic mechanisms of group A *Streptococcus*. *Clin Microb Rev.* 2014;27(2):264–301.
18. Rubin LG, Schaffner W. Care of the asplenic patient. *N Engl J Med.* 2014;371(4):349–356.
19. Suerbaum S, Michetti P. *Helicobacter pylori* infection. *N Engl J Med.* 2002;347:1175–1186.
20. Mandell GL, Bennett JE, Dolin R. *Principles and Practice of Infectious Diseases*. 5th ed. Philadelphia: Churchill Livingstone; 2000.
21. Smego RA, Sebanego P. Treatment options for hepatic cystic echinococcosis. *Int J Infect Dis*. 2005;9(2):69–76.
22. Ramia JM, Figueras J, De la Plaza R, Garcia-Parreño J. Cysto-biliary communication in liver hydatidosis. *Langenbeck Arch Surg*. 2012;397: 881–887.
23. Bernard GR, Vincent JL, Laterre PF, et al. Efficacy and safety of recombinant human activated protein C for severe sepsis. *N Engl J Med.* 2001;344:699–709.
24. Wilson W, Taubert KA, Gewitz M, et al. Prevention of infective endocarditis: guidelines from the American Heart Association. *J Am Dent Assoc*. 2007;138:739–745.
25. Dolin R, Masur H, Saag MS. *AIDS Therapy*. 2nd ed. Philadelphia: Churchill Livingstone; 2003.
26. Katzung BG. *Basic and Clinical Pharmacology*. 8th ed. New York: McGraw-Hill; 2001.
27. Lipsky BA, Berendt AR, Deery HG, et al. Diagnosis and treatment of diabetic foot infections. *Clin Infect Dis*. 2004;39:885–910.
28. Garrett Jr HE, Roper CL. Surgical intervention in histoplasmosis. *Ann Thorac Surg*. 1986;42:711–722.
29. Bhuva M, Ganger D, Jenssen D. Spontaneous bacterial peritonitis: an update on evaluation, management, and prevention. *Am J Med.* 1994;97:169–175.
30. Such J, Runyon BA. Spontaneous bacterial peritonitis. *Clin Infect Dis*. 1998;27:669–674.
31. Anaya DA, Dellinger EP. Surgical infections and choice antibiotics. In: Townsend CM, Beauchamp RD, Evers BM, et al, eds. *Sabiston Textbook of Surgery: The Biological Basis of Modern Surgical Practice*. 18th ed. Philadelphia: WB Saunders; 2008.
32. Simon DM, Levin S. Infectious complications of solid organ transplantations. *Infect Dis Clin North Am*. 2001;15:521–549.
33. Razonable RR. *Infections in solid organ transplant recipients*. Conference Report: Highlights from the 40th Annual Meeting of Infectious Diseases Society of America; October 24–27, 2002.
34. de Gans J, van de Beek D. European Dexamethasone in Adulthood Bacterial Meningitis Study Investigators. Dexamethasone in adults with bacterial meningitis. *N Engl J Med.* 2002;347:1549–1556.
35. Chawdhury MH, Tunkel AR. Antibacterial agents in infections of the central nervous system. *Infect Dis Clin North Am*. 2000;14: 391–408.
36. Centers for Disease Control and Prevention. Recommendations for prevention and control of hepatitis C virus infection and HCV-related chronic disease. *MMWR Recomm Rep*. 1998;47(RR-19):1–39.
37. American Thoracic Society. CDC, Infectious Diseases Society of America. Treatment of tuberculosis. *MMWR Recomm Rep*. 2003;52 (RR-11):1–77.
38. Back M. Local complications: graft infection. In: Cronenwett JL, Johnston KW, eds. *Rutherford's Vascular Surgery*. 8th ed. Philadelphia: Elsevier Health Sciences; 2014:654–672.
39. American Thoracic Society. Infectious Diseases Society of America. Guidelines for the management of adults with hospital-acquired, ventilator-associated, and healthcare-associated pneumonia. *Am J Respir Crit Care Med.* 2005;171:388–416.
40. Weller T, Jamieson C. Antibiotics in pregnancy. In: Rubin P, Ramsay M, eds. *Prescribing in Pregnancy*. Malden, MA: Blackwell Publishing; 2008:36–55.

B. Transmissible Diseases and Surgeons

Michael Tran, M.D.

1. A patient with a known history of tuberculosis (TB) is scheduled for bronchoscopy. Which of the following statements is correct?

    A. The endoscopy staff should wear a powered air-purifying respirator (PAPR) during bronchoscopy.

    B. The endoscopy staff should take prophylactic isoniazid (INH) for 3 days after the procedure.

    C. Bronchoscopy should be performed with the patient under general anesthesia and the use of endotracheal intubation.

    D. Bronchoscopy should be deferred if the patient's tuberculin skin test result is positive.

    E. Bronchoscopy is contraindicated until the result of the purified protein derivative (PPD) test is available.

ANSWER: A

COMMENTS: Health care providers are at an increased risk for exposure to **TB** during cough-inducing or aerosolizing procedures, such as bronchoscopy, endotracheal intubation, or suctioning. Respiratory protection requires the use of a particulate filter respirator or a PAPR. The latter device provides filtered air to a hood that is worn. Use of a PAPR may be recommended when prolonged exposure is possible, such as during bronchoscopy. The risk for infection depends on the concentration of droplet nuclei and the duration of exposure. The diagnosis of pulmonary TB is made presumptively on the basis of the tuberculin skin test and chest radiograph results and confirmed by acid-fast bacilli (AFB) smear and culture results. Bronchoscopy is indicated for the diagnosis of patients with undiagnosed pulmonary infection and for the exclusion of cancer, regardless of the skin test results.

Ref.: 1

2. Which of the following is not considered a standard precaution for reducing the spread of transmissible diseases?

    A. Hand washing before contact with a patient

    B. Hand washing after glove removal

    C. Wearing gloves during contact with a patient

    D. Negative pressure airflow

    E. Eye protection

ANSWER: D

COMMENTS: Standard, or universal, precautions are designed to prevent the spread of transmissible disease by contact with blood, body fluids, or any other potentially infected material. These precautions apply to *all* patients *all* the time. Hand washing is fundamental and should be performed before and between each contact with a patient and after glove removal. Gloves are worn when contacting a potentially contaminated area. Surgical masks and eye protection are required if mucous membrane or eye exposure is possible. Gowns are a part of standard precautions when more extensive blood or fluid exposure may occur. Specific engineering controls for airflow and processing of air are integral to preventing the spread of certain airborne pathogens and as such are not a component of basic standard precautions. Specific procedures for infection control are mandated by federal regulatory agencies. Surgeons and all health care workers (HCWs) must be familiar with the specific infection control policies and procedures established at their places of work.

Ref.: 1

3. A 60-year-old woman with a history of multiple soft tissue abscesses has a recurrent abscess on her right thigh. This patient had a recent hospitalization for exacerbation of congestive heart failure, during which she was in the hospital for 5 days. Because of her history of previous methicillin-resistant *Staphylococcus aureus* (MRSA) abscesses, vancomycin therapy is started. On morning rounds, all of the following precautions should be taken except:

    A. Washing hands before examining the patient

    B. Wearing gloves while examining the patient

    C. Wearing a mask while examining the patient

    D. Wearing a gown while examining the patient

    E. Washing hands after examining the patient

ANSWER: C

COMMENTS: Contact precautions are indicated in this patient and include washing one's hands both before and after leaving the patient's room and donning both a gown and gloves while in the patient's room. Wearing a mask is not indicated for patients who are on contact precautions.

Ref.: 1

4. A 68-year-old woman is admitted to the hospital for neurosurgery after being found comatose at home. The patient lives alone, but her neighbor states that she has been "acting strangely" for the last several weeks. No additional history is available. Magnetic resonance imaging of the brain reveals evidence of focal cerebritis and enlarged ventricles along with enhancement of the basilar meninges. A chest radiograph shows upper lobe consolidation. Results of a rapid human immunodeficiency virus (HIV) test are positive. The patient is taken to the operating room for placement of a ventricular drain. Which type of isolation would be needed for this patient in the postoperative period?

    A. Standard and airborne precautions

    B. Airborne precautions

    C. Droplet precautions

    D. Contact precautions

    E. Reverse isolation

ANSWER: A

COMMENTS: This **HIV**-infected patient has evidence of meningitis, cerebritis, and upper lobe pneumonia. The unifying diagnosis is pulmonary and cerebral **TB**. This patient requires airborne precautions.

A variety of infection control measures are implemented to decrease the risk for transmission of microorganisms in hospitals. Standard precautions are used for the care of all patients. Hand washing between patient contact and the use of barrier protection, such as gloves, gowns, and masks, to minimize exposure to potentially infectious body fluids (e.g., blood, feces, and wound drainage) are important components of standard precautions and all infection control programs.

In addition to standard precautions, **airborne precautions** are used for patients with known or suspected illness transmitted via small airborne droplets (≤5 μm). TB, measles, smallpox, and varicella (chickenpox) are examples of diseases requiring airborne precautions. Because these organisms can be dispersed widely by air currents and may remain suspended in the air for long periods, special air handling and ventilation are necessary. Patients requiring airborne precautions are placed in "negative pressure" rooms, and all persons entering the room require an N95 mask.

In addition to standard precautions, **droplet precautions** are used for patients with suspected or proven invasive disease caused by *Haemophilus influenzae* or *Neisseria meningitidis* (e.g., pneumonia, meningitis, or sepsis) or other respiratory illnesses such as diphtheria, pertussis, pneumonic plague, influenza, mumps, and rubella. The droplets produced by these illnesses are usually generated by coughing but are larger than the droplets described earlier (>5 μm), travel only short distances (<3 ft), and do not remain suspended in air. Patients require a private room, and persons entering the room require a surgical mask.

In addition to standard precautions, contact precautions apply to specific patients infected or colonized with epidemiologically important organisms that spread by direct contact with a patient or contact with items in the patient's environment. These organisms may demonstrate antibiotic resistance and include MRSA, vancomycin-resistant *S. aureus*, vancomycin-resistant enterococci (VRE), and multidrug-resistant gram-negative bacilli. Enteric pathogens such as *Clostridium difficile* and skin infections such as impetigo (group A streptococci), herpes simplex, and scabies also require contact precautions.

Ref.: 2

5. Which of the following statements regarding MRSA is true?

A. The treatment of choice is clindamycin.

B. MRSA can only be found in the health care setting.

C. MRSA is more virulent than methicillin-sensitive *S. aureus*.

D. Treatment of surgical patients with intranasal mupirocin decreases wound infection rates with MRSA.

E. Hospitalized patients colonized with MRSA require contact isolation.

ANSWER: E

COMMENTS: Staphylococci are the most common cause of nosocomial infections in surgical patients. Recent reports suggest that carriage of MRSA in the community has increased, and more infections with this organism are being seen in persons without health care–associated risks.

At the beginning of the antibiotic era, *S. aureus* was susceptible to penicillins. Resistance developed to penicillin via β-lactamase production, and new antibiotics were discovered, including the penicillinase-resistant penicillins (methicillin, oxacillin, nafcillin, etc.). MRSA is by definition resistant to methicillin. Methicillin is not used in clinical practice because it induces interstitial nephritis, but it is still used in the laboratory to differentiate methicillin-susceptible *S. aureus* (MSSA) from MRSA. Vancomycin or linezolid can be used to treat MRSA. *S. aureus* strains with intermediate susceptibility to vancomycin and vancomycin-resistant *S. aureus* have been reported in the United States.

Although some studies suggest that mortality after MRSA infection is higher than that after MSSA infection, the increased death rate is most likely due to comorbid conditions and not due to differences in virulence between MSSA and MRSA. Hospitalized patients colonized with MRSA require contact isolation to avoid the spread of the bacteria to other patients. A recent prospective, randomized, placebo-controlled study showed that intranasal mupirocin did not significantly reduce *S. aureus* surgical site infections.

Ref.: 3–5

6. Which of the following statements regarding hand hygiene is true?

A. The use of soap and water for hand washing is required before and after each contact with a patient.

B. HCWs should clean their hands with an antiseptic-containing agent before and after each contact with a patient.

C. Adherence to hand hygiene guidelines by HCWs is high.

D. Application of alcohol-based products to the palmer surface of the hands and fingers is adequate for hand washing.

E. VRE and MRSA are rarely seen on the hands of HCWs.

ANSWER: B

COMMENTS: Hand washing by HCWs may be the single most effective measure for preventing nosocomial infection. The spread of bacteria, particularly antibiotic-resistant organisms such as MRSA and VRE, from contaminated HCWs to patients is well documented. Despite recommendations to wash hands before and after all contact with patients, adherence to such policies by HCWs has been poor. Although hand washing with soap and water is required when hands are visibly soiled with blood, alcohol-based products may be used instead of soap and water as long as the hands are not visibly soiled. Alcohol-based products are superior to antimicrobial soaps for standard hand decontamination. Alcohol-based hand rubs have the broadest spectrum of antimicrobial activity among the available hand hygiene products, and their use results in a rapid reduction in microbial skin counts. The ability to make these rubs available at the entrance to patients' rooms, at the bedside, or in pocket-sized containers to be carried by HCWs may improve compliance with hand hygiene policies. Alcohol-based hand rubs must be applied to all surfaces of the hands and fingers, and the hands and fingers should be rubbed together until they are dry. The Centers for Disease Control (CDC) has recently published guidelines for hand hygiene in health care settings that include recommendations for hand-washing antisepsis, hand hygiene techniques, and surgical hand antisepsis.

Ref.: 6

7. A surgical resident performs endotracheal intubation of a patient. The patient is unknown to the resident, and the resident had not worn a mask during intubation. Subsequently, the resident is informed that the patient has active TB. The resident has had previous negative PPD tests. The appropriate measure for the resident is:

A. No intervention is necessary.

B. The resident should have a PPD test performed, and prophylactic INH started regardless of the result.

C. The resident should have a PPD test performed, and prophylactic INH started only if the result is positive and the resident does not have symptoms of active infection.

D. The resident should have a PPD test performed, and INH started only if the result is positive and symptoms develop in the resident.

E. The resident does not need a PPD test but should have chest radiography performed.

ANSWER: C

COMMENTS: Exposure to ***Mycobacterium tuberculosis*** is determined by skin testing. If there is any concern for exposure to an active disease, especially in a high-risk situation such as intubation in which the resident is directly exposed to respiratory secretions, the patient should have a PPD test performed. If the PPD results are positive, the resident should begin treatment with INH. A chest radiograph should not be performed in place of the PPD test. If symptoms develop, a chest radiograph is warranted. Infection develops in less than 10% of exposed individuals. Skin testing is performed at least annually in HCWs. The majority of PPD-positive individuals have old exposures. However, when the PPD test results are positive, a chest radiograph and sputum for AFB smear and culture are obtained. **INH prophylaxis** is indicated for persons younger than 35 years with positive skin test results and those older than 35 years with high-risk conditions (i.e., HIV infection, injected drug use, contact with a known TB source, from a medically underserved population, foreign born, or those with abnormal chest radiograph results). The duration of prophylaxis is 6 to 12 months. Active pulmonary TB is diagnosed by sputum AFB smear or culture analysis (or both). The standard treatment of active disease involves a multidrug regimen with INH, rifampin (RIF), and other drugs (pyrazinamide, ethambutol, or streptomycin) for months. Surgical therapy (usually resection) is occasionally necessary for patients who fail medical therapy or for those in whom persistent problems develop, such as a residual lung cavity or destruction, bronchiectasis, or hemoptysis.

Ref.: 7

8. A 60-year-old immigrant from China is admitted to the hospital with fevers and a cough productive of bloody sputum. A chest radiograph demonstrates a right upper lobe infiltrate. The patient's TB exposure is unknown. Which of the following precautions is appropriate?

A. No precautions are necessary.

B. The patient should be admitted to a shared room but be required to wear a mask.

C. The patient should be admitted to a private room but does not need a mask during transport.

D. The patient should be admitted to a private room and should wear a mask during transport.

E. The patient should be admitted to a negative pressure private room and wear a mask during transport.

ANSWER: E

COMMENTS: Airborne precautions are necessary to reduce the exposure of staff and other patients to individuals with suspected pulmonary or laryngeal **TB**. Early recognition of patients at risk for TB is critical, including patients with possible symptoms of TB and those at a higher risk for active disease. Typical symptoms include persistent cough, bloody sputum, fever, night sweats, and weight loss. A chest radiograph may show a cavitary lesion or upper lobe infiltrate. Individuals at a higher risk include the homeless, elderly, known contacts of TB cases, injected drug users, foreign-born individuals, and patients with HIV infection, renal failure, malignancy, or immunosuppression. The largest growing proportion of new TB cases is in the HIV-infected and immunosuppressed population. Persons with suspected TB must have their face covered with a surgical mask during transport and should be admitted to a private negative airflow room equipped with engineering controls specifically designed to reduce airborne exposure. Precautions must be implemented promptly for any suspected case and should not be delayed to wait for confirmation by AFB culture results, which may take weeks. Staff entering the patient's room must wear special particulate filter respirators (fit testing required) or equivalent respirator systems. Use of appropriate respiratory equipment for the protection of HCWs is mandated by the Occupational Safety and Health Administration (OSHA) and the National Institute of Occupational Safety and Health (NIOSH).

Ref.: 7

9. The operating surgeon is stuck with a needle while performing elective repair of an inguinal hernia. The patient is known to be HIV negative, but his hepatitis C virus (HCV) status is unknown. The patient has a known history of intravenous drug abuse. In addition, the operating surgeon is hepatitis B immune because of previous vaccination. Which one of the following measures is appropriate?

A. Prophylactic antiviral treatment

B. Administration of HCV vaccine and immunoglobulin if the surgeon is HCV antibody negative

C. Baseline testing of the surgeon and patient for HCV and follow-up testing of the surgeon at 4 to 6 months

D. No testing for the surgeon is indicated if the patient tests negative for HCV

E. Prophylactic administration of HCV immunoglobulin in addition to baseline testing of both the surgeon and patient and follow-up testing of the surgeon in 4 to 6 months

ANSWER: C

COMMENTS: Anytime that someone is inadvertently stuck with a needle from a patient with unknown **HCV status**, both the patient and the person stuck should undergo baseline testing for HCV. In addition, the person stuck should have follow-up testing at 4 to 6 months. There is no treatment that has proven efficacy in reducing the risk for seroconversion with HCV; therefore no prophylaxis for HCV infection is currently indicated.

Ref.: 7, 9

10. A surgical resident is placing a central venous catheter in a patient who is HIV positive and is stuck with the needle. Which of the following regarding postexposure prophylaxis is true?

A. No prophylaxis is necessary; however, the surgical resident should have a baseline HIV test performed and follow-up tests in 3 and 6 months.

B. The resident should have a baseline HIV test performed and follow-up testing in 3 and 6 months and, in addition, begin combined triple antiretroviral therapy.

C. The resident should have a baseline HIV test performed and follow-up testing in 3 and 6 months and, in addition, begin single antiretroviral therapy.

D. The resident should have a baseline HIV test performed and follow-up testing in 3 and 6 months and, in addition, begin therapy with two antiretroviral drugs.

E. The resident should begin combined triple antiretroviral therapy and have an HIV test performed in 6 months.

ANSWER: B

COMMENTS: Most occupationally **acquired HIV infection** has been documented in nurses or laboratory technicians. Postexposure drug prophylaxis should be initiated as soon as possible, ideally within 2 h. In cases where the status of the source is unknown, standard **serologic testing** (enzyme immunoassay and Western blot) is indicated, but the results may take several days. A rapid HIV test can now give results within 1 h. However, serologic test results may be negative in infected individuals for 3 to 12 weeks following the acquisition of the virus. The decision to start postexposure drug prophylaxis must therefore consider any known risk factors that the source may have, regardless of the serologic results. **Postexposure prophylaxis** consists of multidrug therapy with a combination of nucleoside and protease inhibitors. Adverse side effects are frequent and sometimes severe. Recommendations for postexposure prophylaxis continue to evolve. The most effective method of reducing the risk for transmission of HIV to a person stuck with a needle from a known HIV-positive patient is to begin combined triple antiretroviral therapy. The first dose should be given after exposure as soon as possible. Besides a baseline HIV test, this person should undergo an additional follow-up testing at both 3 and 6 months.

Ref.: 7, 9

11. A nonimmune surgical resident is stuck by a contaminated needle from a hepatitis B surface antigen (HBsAg)-positive source. Which of the following is the correct initial treatment?

A. None because the patient does not have active hepatitis B virus (HBV) infection and is immune to HBV

B. Interferon

C. Vaccination against HBV

D. Hepatitis B immune globulin (HBIG)

E. Vaccination against HBV and administration of HBIG

ANSWER: E

COMMENTS: The best method of preventing **occupational HBV infection** is to vaccinate all HCWs at risk if they do not have natural immunity from previous infection. When exposure occurs, the affected area should be immediately and thoroughly washed with soap and water. The source is tested for HBV, HCV, and HIV. If the source tests positive for HBV, nonimmune individuals are given HBIG for passive prophylaxis and are vaccinated. If a previously vaccinated individual incurs a needle injury, titers should be checked and a dose of vaccine given if titers are not detected. Interferon is not used for prophylaxis following acute exposure but may be useful for some patients with chronic HBV or HCV infection.

Ref.: 8

12. Which of the following is an important risk factor for transmission of HIV to the surgeon after a percutaneous injury?

A. The source patient has advanced HIV infection with a CD4+ T-cell count less than 50 cells/mm3.

B. The surgeon sustains a deep puncture injury.

C. Blood was visible on the sharp object causing the injury.

D. The injury was caused by a device that had entered a blood vessel of the source patient before injury.

E. All of the above.

ANSWER: E

COMMENTS: See Question 13.

13. What is the approximate probability of transmission of HCV to an HCW through a needlestick injury from an infected source?

A. 0.3%

B. 3%

C. 15%

D. 30%

E. 50%

ANSWER: B

COMMENTS: The risk for **transmission of HIV** after percutaneous exposure to HIV-infected blood is about 0.3%. This risk is influenced by several factors, including depth of the injury and the presence of undiluted blood on the device causing the injury. Exposure to blood from patients in the terminal stages of acquired immune deficiency syndrome (AIDS), which probably reflects high titers of circulating virus, also increases the risk to HCWs. Although no prospective study demonstrating benefit from postexposure prophylaxis with antiretroviral agents has been completed, a retrospective case-control study suggests that in those who receive zidovudine prophylaxis after exposure, the odds of HIV infection were reduced significantly (by approximately 80%). Postexposure prophylaxis, which now includes at least two antiretroviral agents, should be started immediately (within 72 h) in HCWs with high-risk injuries.

HCWs are at risk for contracting transmissible viral disease when stuck by needles with contaminated blood or by exposure of mucosal membranes to blood or other body fluids. The risk for documented seroconversion is approximately 3%–10% for HCV. The risk for HBV infection after needlestick injury is 5%–30%. The risk for HCV infection following mucous membrane or other cutaneous exposure has not been defined. The risk for HIV infection with mucous membrane exposure is about 0.1%. When exposure occurs, the infected area should be washed thoroughly with soap and water. The source should be tested for infection with HBV, HCV, and HIV. The risk of contracting HIV infection is greatest with hollow needles, with deep intramuscular injury, or when the exposure involves a greater amount of virus (i.e., from a larger amount of blood or a source with late-stage HIV infection).

Ref.: 8, 9, 11

14. A surgical resident is stuck with an HCV-contaminated hollow-bore needle. Which of the following tests should be done initially?

A. Detection of HCV RNA

B. Detection of HCV surface antigen

C. Detection of HCV antibodies by enzyme immunoassay

D. Measurement of viral load

E. Detection of HCV core antigen

ANSWER: C

COMMENTS: The initial screening test for HCV is an antibody immunoassay. The person stuck with the contaminated needle should have baseline testing performed. Since it can take up to 6 months for a person to seroconvert, called the window period, people who have been stuck with a contaminated needle not only require baseline testing but will also need follow-up testing in 6 months.

Ref.: 9

15. Which of the following blood tests confirms HCV infection?

A. Detection of HCV RNA

B. Detection of HCV surface antigen

C. Detection of HCV antibodies by enzyme immunoassay

D. Detection of HCV antibodies and alanine aminotransferase levels of 500 to 1000 u/L

E. Measurement of HCV viral load

ANSWER: A

COMMENTS: The **screening test for HCV** is an immunoassay for anti-HCV antibodies. Although the results are positive in 90% of patients infected with HCV, the predictive value of the test is limited when the prevalence of infection is low. In addition, anti-HCV antibodies may not be detectable for up to 18 weeks following exposure. Their presence does not differentiate the state of infection. Qualitative reverse transcriptase polymerase chain reaction (RT–PCR) for detection of HCV RNA is confirmatory. Infection may also be confirmed by recombinant immunoblot assay for HCV antibody.

Ref.: 9

16. A 36-year-old man with HIV infection and a CD4+ count less than 500 cells/mm^3 has an incarcerated ventral hernia. In addition to standard precautions, which one of the following is recommended?

A. Avoidance of prosthetic mesh

B. Broader preoperative prophylactic antibiotic coverage than for a patient who is HIV negative

C. Prophylactic trimethoprim/sulfamethoxazole in addition to standard preoperative antibiotics

D. Disposable surgical instruments

E. None of the above

ANSWER: E

COMMENTS: Beyond the universal precautions that are used for all patients, there are no specific recommendations regarding the preoperative or intraoperative management of patients with HIV infection. Operative treatment should be performed according to the surgical condition and antiretroviral drug therapy administered according to the status of the HIV disease. Prophylactic antibiotics or prosthetic materials are used for the same indications in HIV-infected individuals as in non–HIV-infected individuals. Trimethoprim/sulfamethoxazole is used for the prophylaxis of *Pneumocystis carinii* pneumonia in patients with clinical AIDS but has nothing to do with surgical prophylaxis. Standard surgical instruments and sterilization techniques are appropriate. The use of disposable instruments is often convenient and simple when performing minor procedures outside the main operating room.

Ref.: 9

17. What is the prevalence of HCV infection in the United States?

A. 0.2%

B. 2%

C. 5%

D. 10%

E. 20%

ANSWER: B

COMMENTS: The prevalence of HCV in the United States is approximately four times greater than that of HIV infection. The rate in HCWs, including general, orthopedic, and oral surgeons, is no higher. As would be expected, some populations have a much higher prevalence, including hemophiliacs (60%–90%), injectable drug users (60%–90%), and chronic hemodialysis patients (up to 60%).

Ref.: 9, 10

18. During an emergency appendectomy, a surgical resident sustains an injury from a contaminated hollow-bore needle with spontaneous bleeding. Which one of the following blood-borne organisms is most likely to be transmitted, assuming that the patient was infected with all of them?

A. HIV

B. HBV

C. HCV

D. *Plasmodium* spp. (malaria)

E. *Treponema pallidum* (syphilis)

ANSWER: B

COMMENTS: All the organisms mentioned in the list are potentially transmissible through the exposure described. After significant exposure to **blood-borne pathogens**, the risk is about 30% for acquiring hepatitis B, 3% for hepatitis C, and 0.3% for HIV disease. Malaria and syphilis may be acquired through blood transfusion, and acquisition through a needlestick is theoretically possible. Because of the high risk associated with hepatitis B exposure, it is recommended that all HCWs be vaccinated against HBV. In the event that a nonimmune HCW is exposed to HBV, it is recommended that the HCW receive HBIG within 7 days of the exposure and also start a vaccination series. Postexposure prophylaxis with antiretroviral drugs may be indicated after exposure to HIV-infected blood. There is no postexposure prophylaxis available against HCV.

Ref.: 12

19. A surgical resident sustains a needlestick injury with a hollow-bore needle contaminated with the blood of a patient who is hepatitis B antigen positive. The resident completed a series of three hepatitis B vaccines 1 year ago, but his antibody response was not checked. Which of the following statements best describes the management of this case?

A. Observation only is indicated since the source does not have active HBV infection.

B. The resident needs a booster of hepatitis B vaccine.

C. The resident should receive HBIG immediately.

D. The resident should receive HBIG and a hepatitis B vaccine booster immediately.

E. The resident needs to be tested for anti–hepatitis B antibody immediately. If the test result is negative, proceed as in option D.

ANSWER: E

COMMENTS: HCWs who sustain injuries from needles contaminated with blood containing **HBV** have a risk for the development of serologic evidence of HBV infection as high as 62%. The source patient is hepatitis B antigen positive, which is an indication of active HBV infection. The resident has been vaccinated against HBV, but his immune status is unknown and should be determined. If the resident is anti–hepatitis B antibody positive, no intervention is necessary. However, if the resident is anti–hepatitis B antibody negative, HBIG (which can be given up to 7 days after the exposure) and a hepatitis B vaccine booster should be administered. If the resident was never vaccinated, HBIG should be administered immediately and the hepatitis B vaccination series begun.

Ref.: 13

20. Which of the following precautions regarding care for patients with *C. difficile* is true?

A. Only gloves are required when examining the patient.

B. Stethoscopes do not need to be cleaned after use.

C. The patient should be placed in a private room.

D. All visitors should wear gloves, a gown, and a mask.

E. Alcohol-based hand sanitizers are adequate to clean hands after exiting a patient's room.

ANSWER: C

COMMENTS: *C. difficile* is spread by direct contact, and thus contact precautions must be followed. Appropriate precautions include donning a gown and gloves and washing hands both before entering and after leaving the patient's room. Alcohol-based hand sanitizers do not kill *C. difficile*, and thus hand washing with soap and water, particularly after leaving a patient's room, is required. There is no indication for anyone to wear a mask in this patient's room. In addition, the patient should be placed in a private room. It is also ideal to have a disposable stethoscope dedicated to that patient to avoid spreading *C. difficile*. If not available, the stethoscope must be cleaned thoroughly after use.

Ref.: 1, 14

21. Which of the following clinical conditions is identified by the presence of antibodies in the serum against HBsAg (anti-HBs) in the absence of hepatitis B core antigen (anti-HBc) and HBsAg?

A. The patient is susceptible to HBV infection.

B. The patient is immune because of HBV vaccination.

C. The patient has an active acute infection with HBV.

D. The patient has chronic active hepatitis with HBV.

E. The patient has recovered from an HBV infection with subsequent natural immunity.

ANSWER: B

COMMENTS: Testing for HBsAg will be positive in both patients who have been immunized against HBV and those who were previously infected. To distinguish the two clinical situations, one must use other tests. HBsAg positivity indicates an active infection, either acute or chronic. Anti-HBc–positive results indicate that a person either currently has an active infection or has been infected with HBV in the past. If both are negative in the setting of positive anti-HBs, the person has been vaccinated but never infected with HBV.

Ref.: 8, 14

22. Which of the following markers is the most clinically useful for monitoring the course of a person infected with HIV?

A. Viral load

B. CD4+ T-cell count

C. Serum neopterin

D. Serum oligoclonal immunoglobulins

E. Serum p24 antigen level

ANSWER: B

COMMENTS: The **CD4+ T-cell count**, although somewhat imperfect, is the most useful determination for monitoring the course of an HIV infection. The normal CD4+ count is greater than 600 cells/mm^3, with most counts ranging from 800 to 1200 cells/mm^3. Symptomatic disease usually begins when the CD4+ count falls below 300 to 400 cells/mm^3. Opportunistic infections begin to occur when the CD4+ cell count is less than 200 cells/mm^3. The time course of this decline in CD4+ T-cell count is prolonged and may take more than 10 years. Direct quantification of viral load with plasma viremia shows increasing viral titers as the disease progresses. β_2-Microglobulin is shed into the serum in HIV-infected patients and reflects increased lymphocyte turnover. **Neopterin** is produced by macrophages stimulated by interferon. Although both are found in increasing amounts as HIV infection progresses, neither of these two determinations is specific for HIV infection, and they are generally used in a research setting. Determination of p24 antigen is specific for HIV but not very sensitive.

Ref.: 7, 15

23. The chance of an HIV-infected individual transmitting infection best correlates with which of the following?

A. CD4+ T-cell count

B. Viral load

C. Absolute lymphocyte count less than 1000 cells/mm^3

D. Active opportunistic infection

E. Whether the patient is currently receiving antiretroviral therapy

ANSWER: B

COMMENTS: Blood measurements of **viral load** reflect the risk for transmission of HIV by any route: parenteral, sexual, or perinatal. The risk of acquiring HIV infection through occupational exposure also correlates with the viral load in the source. Both viral load and the CD4+ count reflect the stage of the disease as patients with late viral infection have low CD4+ levels and high viral counts. Opportunistic infections are also more prevalent as CD4+ counts fall and immunodeficiency worsens. **Clinical AIDS** is defined in patients with positive HIV serologic findings when CD4+ counts are less than 200 cells/mm^3 or when one of a number of defined associated conditions exists. The list of these

AIDS-defining conditions includes specific opportunistic infections, neoplasms, and degenerative conditions.

Ref.: 7, 9, 16

24. A 28-year-old woman with AIDS has right upper quadrant pain and is found to have acute cholecystitis on ultrasound examination. Which of the following is the appropriate therapy?

A. The patient should begin antibiotic therapy but should undergo no surgical intervention because of her immune status.

B. The patient should begin antibiotic therapy and have a percutaneous cholecystostomy tube placed.

C. The patient should begin antibiotic therapy and undergo open cholecystectomy.

D. The patient should begin antibiotic therapy and undergo laparoscopic cholecystectomy.

E. None of the above.

ANSWER: D

COMMENTS: AIDS and **HIV** infection are not contraindications to **laparoscopy**. These patients should be managed according to routine general surgery principles. A patient with AIDS and acute cholecystitis should be treated with appropriate antibiotics and laparoscopic cholecystectomy unless the patient is not stable enough or has other comorbid conditions that make surgery too dangerous.

Ref.: 17

25. The operative mortality rate after laparotomy in patients with AIDS has most closely been associated with which of the following?

A. Total lymphocyte count less than 1000 cells/mm^3

B. CD4+ T-cell count less than 500/mm^3

C. Active opportunistic infection

D. Duration of HIV infection

E. Emergency surgery

ANSWER: E

COMMENTS: Prognostic factors in AIDS patients undergoing abdominal operations have not been extensively analyzed. The cumulative operative mortality rate after major abdominal procedures is approximately 20%. Most deaths are related to the patient's underlying disease and not to specific operative complications. Emergency operations have been associated with higher mortality rates than elective procedures, particularly in patients with intestinal perforations because of opportunistic infections such as cytomegalovirus (CMV). However, there is no convincing evidence that patients with HIV infection without AIDS-defining criteria have an inordinate risk for death or complications after abdominal surgery.

Ref.: 18

26. Laparotomy is performed on a 26-year-old, HIV-positive man who has been hospitalized with abdominal pain, intractable diarrhea, and a perforated viscus. He has a 2-cm cecal perforation, and the colon is dilated throughout. Select the most appropriate therapy.

A. Primary repair of the perforation with placement of a drain

B. Primary repair of the perforation with a diverting ileostomy

C. Ileocecal resection with primary anastomosis

D. Ileocecal resection with primary anastomosis and a diverting ileostomy

E. Abdominal colectomy with ileostomy and a Hartmann procedure

ANSWER: E

COMMENTS: Infection of the gastrointestinal tract with CMV is one of the most common causes of **intestinal perforation in HIV-infected patients** and is an AIDS-defining condition. The diagnosis is based on the demonstration of intranuclear inclusion bodies on a biopsy specimen. Initial treatment consists of antiviral agents and support. Surgery is indicated for perforation, bleeding, or obstruction as a result of stricture formation. CMV perforations are most frequently ileocolic in location. They can involve the small intestines, stomach, or duodenum. Operative management of colon perforations is resection without anastomosis. Determination of the extent of resection has various considerations, but since the entire colon is typically involved, total abdominal colectomy is often advisable. Such patients are often desperately ill, and appropriate and timely surgical intervention and aggressive support are necessary for their survival.

Ref.: 14, 19

27. A 32-year-old, HIV-positive injectable drug user is admitted following a seizure. Examination reveals a pronator drift. A computed tomography (CT) scan of the head with intravenous contrast material shows two ring-enhancing lesions. Which of the following statements is true?

A. Primary central nervous system (CNS) lymphoma is the most likely diagnosis.

B. Biopsy should be performed for all enhancing lesions in HIV-infected patients.

C. Toxoplasmosis is the most likely diagnosis.

D. Pyrimethamine is an effective agent for primary prophylaxis of this condition but is not very effective for its treatment.

E. The neurologic symptoms are unrelated to AIDS.

ANSWER: B

COMMENTS: Ten percent of AIDS patients experience a neurologic symptom as the first sign of their illness, and one or more neurologic deficits eventually develop in 40% of AIDS patients. Major **HIV-related CNS** diseases include HIV encephalopathy, meningitis, myelopathy, opportunistic infections [progressive multifocal leukoencephalopathy (PML) caused by papovavirus, CMV, herpes, *Toxoplasma gondii*, and *Cryptococcus neoformans*], neoplasms (primary CNS lymphoma), and cerebrovascular complications. *T. gondii*, the protozoan that causes toxoplasmosis, accounts for 50%–70% of focal brain lesions in these patients and is the most common cause of focal enhancing lesions on CT. Ten percent to 25% of focal lesions are **CNS lymphomas**. Primary CNS lymphoma is a rare intracranial tumor in the general population, in whom it accounts for only 1.5% of primary brain tumors. However, it is significantly more common in HIV-infected patients, even when compared with other immunosuppressed populations. Current management recommendations for HIV-infected patients with focal brain lesions include 2 to 3 weeks of empiric treatment of toxoplasmosis, followed by biopsy if the radiologic or clinical condition deteriorates.

Ref.: 7, 15, 20

28. Which of the following is true regarding current CDC recommendations for influenza vaccinations and HCWs?

A. HCWs have greater than 99% vaccination coverage.

B. The most common reason reported for not getting vaccinated is that HCWs do not need the vaccine.

C. Influenza vaccines are made with only killed viruses.

D. With rare exceptions, people aged 6 months and older are recommended to receive the vaccine.

E. HCWs are legally mandated by the CDC to receive the annual vaccine.

ANSWER: D

COMMENTS: By occupation, early season flu vaccination coverage was highest among pharmacists (86.7%), nurse practitioners/physician assistants (85.8%), physicians (82.2%), nurses (81.4%), and other clinical professionals (72.0%). Flu vaccination coverage was the lowest among administrative and nonclinical support staff (59.1%) and assistants or aides (46.6%). By work setting, early season flu vaccination coverage was the highest among health care personnel working in hospitals (78.7%). Flu vaccination coverage was the lowest among health care personnel working in long-term care facilities (54.4%). Early season flu vaccination coverage was higher among health care personnel whose employers required (85.8%) or recommended (68.4%) that they be vaccinated, compared with those whose employer did not have a policy or recommendation regarding flu vaccination (43.4%).

Among unvaccinated health care personnel, the most common reasons were that they felt the vaccinations did not work or were unneeded. The seasonal flu vaccine protects against the influenza viruses that research indicates will be most common during the upcoming season.

The findings of a recent CDC review of related published literature indicate that influenza vaccination of health care personnel can enhance patient safety. These recommendations may be considered by state and other federal agencies when making or enforcing laws; however, the CDC does not issue any requirements. There are no legally mandated vaccinations for adults, except for persons entering military service. The CDC does recommend certain immunizations for adults, depending on age, occupation, and other circumstances, but these immunizations are not required by law.

Everyone 6 months of age and older should get a flu vaccine every season according to recommendations from the CDC's Advisory Committee on Immunization Practices (ACIP) dated February 24, 2010. Flu vaccines DO NOT cause the flu. They are made with either killed or weakened viruses.

Ref.: 21

29. Which of following is correct regarding influenza vaccines?

A. The nasal spray influenza vaccine protects against four types of influenza viruses.

B. The live attenuated influenza vaccine can cause flu in rare cases.

C. The nasal spray influenza vaccine is approved for use in individuals aged 6 months and older.

D. Trivalent vaccines protect against one type of influenza A viruses and two types of influenza B viruses.

E. HCWs may receive the nasal spray vaccine even when caring for posttransplant patients.

ANSWER: A

COMMENTS: The seasonal flu vaccine protects against the influenza viruses that research indicates will be most common during the upcoming season. Trivalent vaccines are made to protect against three flu viruses: two influenza A (H1N1 and H3N2) viruses and an influenza B virus. Quadrivalent vaccines protect against four viruses: the same viruses as the trivalent vaccine as well as an additional B virus. All nasal spray flu vaccines are quadrivalent. The nasal spray is approved for use in people aged 2 through 49 years. Flu vaccines do not cause the flu. Flu vaccines are made with either inactivated or live attenuated viruses.

Health care providers should not get the nasal spray vaccine if they are providing medical care for immunocompromised patients such as patients in bone marrow transplant units. The flu shot is preferred for vaccinating HCWs who are in close contact with severely immunocompromised patients. These HCWs may still get nasal spray vaccine, but they must avoid contact with such patients for 7 days after getting vaccinated.

Ref.: 21–23

30. Indications for antiviral treatment of influenza include which of the following?

A. Individuals aged less than 2 years or older than 65 years

B. HCWs

C. Postoperative patients

D. Patients with hypertension

E. Women who are less than 4 weeks postpartum

ANSWER: A

COMMENTS: Antiviral treatment with a neuraminidase inhibitor is recommended for all persons with suspected or confirmed influenza who are at a higher risk for influenza complications due to age or underlying medical conditions. These include children aged less than 2 years; adults aged 65 years and above; persons with chronic pulmonary (including asthma), cardiovascular (except hypertension alone), renal, hepatic, hematologic (including sickle cell disease), and metabolic disorders (including diabetes mellitus) or neurologic and neurodevelopment conditions [including disorders of the brain, spinal cord, peripheral nerve, and muscle such as cerebral palsy, epilepsy (seizure disorders), stroke, intellectual disability (mental retardation), moderate-to-severe developmental delay, muscular dystrophy, or spinal cord injury]; immunosuppressed patients; women who are pregnant or postpartum (within 2 weeks after delivery); persons aged less than 19 years who are receiving long-term aspirin therapy; American Indians/Alaska Natives; persons who are morbidly obese [i.e., with a body mass index (BMI) of 40 or greater]; and residents of nursing homes and other chronic-care facilities.

Ref.: 24

31. Regarding antiviral treatments for influenza, which of the following is correct?

A. Amantadine is the preferred primary antiviral agent.

B. Influenza is 100% susceptible to oseltamivir.

C. Antiviral treatment reduces the duration of symptoms by 3 days.

D. Antiviral treatment should be initiated within 48 h of illness onset for benefit to occur.

E. None of the above.

ANSWER: D

COMMENTS: Oseltamivir or zanamivir are the primary antiviral agents recommended for the prevention and treatment of influenza. Most influenza A and B virus strains are susceptible to oseltamivir and zanamivir. Sporadic oseltamivir-resistant 2009 H1N1 virus infections have been identified; 98.2% of the 2009 H1N1 viruses tested for surveillance were susceptible to oseltamivir, and 100% of them were susceptible to zanamivir. Resistance to adamantanes remains high among influenza A viruses currently circulating. Therefore amantadine and rimantadine are not recommended for antiviral treatment or chemoprophylaxis of currently circulating influenza A virus strains.

Zanamivir or oseltamivir can reduce the duration of uncomplicated influenza A and B illnesses by approximately 1 day when administered within 48 h of illness onset compared with placebo. Minimal or no benefit was reported in healthy children and adults when antiviral treatment was initiated more than 2 days after onset of uncomplicated influenza.

Ref.: 24, 25

32. Which of the following is true regarding treatment of hepatitis C?

A. Sofosbuvir has an equivalent sustained virologic response (SVR) to that of pegylated interferon and ribavirin.

B. Pegylated interferon must be used with sofosbuvir for the treatment of all genotypes of HCV.

C. Sofosbuvir can be used in combination with other drugs to treat four genotypes of HCV.

D. Simeprevir can be used in all genotypes of HCV.

E. None of the above.

ANSWER: C

COMMENTS: Sofosbuvir and simeprevir are two medications approved by the U.S. Food and Drug Administration (FDA) in 2013 for the treatment of chronic hepatitis C. SVR is used as a marker for cure and is defined as undetectable HCV RNA 24 weeks after the completion of antiviral therapy. Clinical trials demonstrated that sofosbuvir and simeprevir can help achieve SVR in 80%–95% of patients after 12 to 24 weeks of treatment. Previously, the mainstay of treatment of HCV was pegylated interferon and ribavirin, which helped achieve an SVR of 50%–80%.

Sofosbuvir is a nucleotide analogue inhibitor of the HCV NS5B polymerase enzyme, which plays an important role in HCV replication. The drug is approved for two chronic hepatitis C indications: interferon-free therapy for chronic HCV infection and combination therapy with pegylated interferon and ribavirin for treatment-naïve adults with HCV genotype 1 and 4 infections or combination therapy with ribavirin for adults with HCV genotypes 2 and 3 infection. Simeprevir is a protease inhibitor that blocks a specific protein needed by the HCV to replicate. It is used in combination with pegylated interferon-alfa and ribavirin for genotype 1 infections only.

Ref.: 26

33. Which of the following is incorrect regarding personal protective equipment (PPE) when caring for a patient with confirmed Ebola virus disease (EVD)?

A. Single-use (disposable) boot covers that extend to mid-calf are recommended.

B. A disposable gown or coveralls are recommended for body protection.

C. An apron is recommended in addition to a disposable gown.

D. Double gloving is required.

E. Droplet protection with only a standard surgical mask is required.

ANSWER: E

COMMENTS: For Ebola precautions, there are multiple PPE recommendations. For the body, a single-use (disposable) impermeable gown extending to at least mid-calf or single-use (disposable) impermeable coverall is worn. A single-use (disposable) apron that covers the torso to the level of the mid-calf should be used over the gown or coveralls if patients with Ebola are vomiting or have diarrhea and should be used routinely if the facility is using a coverall that has an exposed, unprotected zipper in the front. An apron provides additional protection, reducing the contamination of gowns or coveralls by body fluids and providing a way to quickly remove a soiled outer layer during patient care. Respiratory protection is provided with either a PAPR or an N95 respirator. Two pairs of single-use (disposable) examination gloves with extended cuffs should be worn so that a heavily soiled outer glove can be safely removed and replaced during care. At a minimum, outer gloves should have extended cuffs. Double gloving also allows potentially contaminated outer gloves to be removed during doffing to avoid self-contamination. Single-use (disposable) boot covers that extend to at least mid-calf are also recommended. In addition, single-use (disposable) ankle-high shoe covers ("surgical booties") worn over boot covers may be considered to facilitate the doffing process, reducing contamination of the floor in the doffing area, thereby reducing contamination of underlying shoes.

Ref.: 27

34. A patient presents with suspected Ebola virus disease (EVD). Which of the following regarding EVD is true?

A. Symptoms typically present 1 to 3 days after exposure.

B. One of the early signs and symptoms of EVD is mucosal bleeding.

C. On presentation, signs and symptoms are relatively specific to EVD.

D. Ebola can be transmitted by exposure of mucous membranes to bodily fluids.

E. Fatality is commonly due to uncontrollable hemorrhage.

ANSWER: D

COMMENTS: Initial signs and symptoms for EVD are nonspecific and include constitutional symptoms of subjective fever, chills, myalgias, and malaise. Thus these nonspecific symptoms may be confused for other common diseases such as pneumonia or influenza. These symptoms typically occur 8 to12 days after exposure. Gastrointestinal symptoms such as abdominal pain, diarrhea, nausea, and emesis can develop after 5 days. Other symptoms such as chest pain, shortness of breath, headache, or confusion may also develop. Patients often have conjunctival injection. Seizures may occur, and cerebral edema has been reported.

Patients may develop a diffuse erythematous maculopapular rash by day 5 to 7 (usually involving the neck, trunk, and arms) that can desquamate. Bleeding is not present in all cases; however, petechiae, ecchymosis/bruising, or oozing from venipuncture sites and mucosal hemorrhage can be seen.

Ebola virus enters the patient through mucous membranes, breaks in the skin, or parenterally. Ebola virus appears to trigger a release of proinflammatory cytokines with subsequent vascular leak and impairment of clotting. This ultimately results in multiorgan failure, septic shock, and death.

Ref.: 28

35. Which of the following is true regarding guidelines for surgical protocol for possible or confirmed Ebola cases?

A. Leg covering is not needed provided shoe covers are worn.

B. A fluid-resistant or N95 mask does not need to be worn.

C. Extralong surgical gloves are not needed as long as operation room (OR) staff are double gloved.

D. Scalpels instead of electrocautery should be used to limit the production of smoke and potentially aerosolized Ebola virus.

E. Elective surgical procedures should not be performed.

ANSWER: E

COMMENTS: As experience with Ebola is evolving quickly, it is imperative that guidelines are provided to aid surgeons and OR staff with the care of patients who may have confirmed or suspected Ebola infection. Elective surgical procedures should not be performed in cases of suspected or confirmed Ebola. For patients with probable or early confirmed Ebola, emergency surgery can be considered. However, patients with severe active EVD would likely not tolerate or survive an operation.

Recommended PPE includes Association for the Advancement of Medical Instrumentation (AAMI) Level 4 Impervious Surgical Gowns and leg coverings that have full plastic film coating over the fabric and not just over the foot area. Face protection is strongly recommended with the use of a surgical helmet; if it is not available, a long full plastic face shield to come down over the neck is recommended. Fluid-resistant surgical masks or N95 masks should be worn. Double gloves should be worn. The outer layer of gloves should be extralong surgical gloves to provide better protection of the forearms.

General technical considerations are to limit the amount of sharps used and use of instruments over fingers to handle sharps. Use of blunt electrocautery over scalpels is recommended.

Ref.: 29

36. Which of the following is true regarding the risk of *C. difficile* infection (CDI)?

A. Admission to a room previously occupied by a patient with a CDI increases the risk of CDI.

B. Previous exposure to antibiotics does not increase the risk of CDI.

C. Proton pump inhibitors (PPIs) do not increase the risk of CDI.

D. Rates of CDI are decreasing.

E. None of the above.

ANSWER: A

COMMENTS: Two of the biggest risk factors for CDI are previous exposure to antibiotics, particular broad-spectrum antibiotics, and exposure to the organism. Exposure to the organism is often in a health care facility setting. Other factors that increase the risk of CDI include older age, gastrointestinal surgery, nasogastric tube feeding, reduced gastric acid, use of PPIs, and concurrent disease, including inflammatory bowel disease. In a recent study, it was found that in the group of patients that stayed in a room that had a prior occupant **without** a CDI, 4.6% of the patients developed a CDI. In patients that stayed in a room that had a prior occupant **with** a CDI, 11.0% of the patients developed a CDI. From 2000 to 2005, the incidence of CDI in adults increased from 5.5/10,000 to 11.2/10,000.

Ref.: 30, 31

37. One of your patients who recently has been on antibiotics has been having abdominal pain and diarrhea. You suspect the possibility of CDI. Which of the following regarding testing for *C. difficile* is true?

A. Solid stool or diarrhea sample should be sent for concern of *C. difficile.*

B. Repeated testing should be performed when the first test is negative.

C. Resolution of symptoms can be seen with the absence of toxin A and B.

D. PCR testing is superior to toxin A and B enzyme immunoassay.

E. None of the above.

ANSWER: D

COMMENTS: Only stool from patients with diarrhea should be tested for *C. difficile*. Because *C. difficile* carriage is increased in patients on antimicrobial therapy, only diarrheal stools warrant testing. Several studies have shown that repeat testing after a negative test is positive in <5% of specimens and it increases the likelihood of false positives. There is no evidence that repeat testing can enhance the sensitivity or negative predictive values. It is recommended that nucleic acid amplification tests for *C. difficile* toxin genes such as PCR are superior to toxins A and B enzyme immunoassay as a standard diagnostic test for CDI. Studies have shown that both toxin A and B enzyme immunoassay may remain positive for as long as 30 days in patients who have resolution of symptoms.

Ref.: 31

REFERENCES

1. Centers for Disease Control and Prevention. Healthcare-associated infections (HAIs). Available at: www.cdc.gov/hai.
2. Garner JS. Guidelines for isolation precautions in hospitals. The Hospital Infection Control Practices Advisory Committee. *Infect Control Hosp Epidemiol*. 1996;17:53–80.
3. Perl TM, Cullen JJ, Wenzel RP, et al. Intranasal mupirocin to prevent postoperative *Staphylococcus aureus* infections. *N Engl J Med*. 2002;346:1871–1877.
4. Salgado CD, Farr BM, Calfee DP. Community-acquired methicillin-resistant *Staphylococcus aureus*: a meta-analysis of prevalence and risk factors. *Clin Infect Dis*. 2003;36:131–139.
5. Centers for Disease Control and Prevention. Vancomycin-resistant *Staphylococcus aureus*—Pennsylvania, 2002. *MMWR Morb Mortal Wkly Rep*. 2002;51:902.
6. Boyce JM, Pittet D. Healthcare Infection Control Practices Advisory Committee, HICPAC/SHEA/APIC/IDSA Hand Hygiene Task Force. Guidelines for hand hygiene in healthcare settings: recommendations of the Healthcare Infection Control Practices Advisory Committee and the HICPAC/SHEA/APIC/IDSA Hand Task Force. Society for Healthcare Epidemiology of America Association for Professionals in Infection Control/Infectious Diseases Society of America. *MMWR Recomm Rep*. 2002;51(RR-16):1–45.
7. Preventing Surgical Site Infections: A Surgeon's Perspective. Centers for Disease Control and Prevention. Available at: wwwnc.cdc.gov/eid/article/7/2/70-0220_article.htm.
8. Dellinger EP. Surgical infections. In: Mulholland MW, Lillemoe KD, Doherty GM, eds. *Greenfield's Surgery: Scientific Principles and Practice*. 4th ed. Philadelphia: Lippincott Williams & Wilkins; 2006.

9. Bartlett JG. Occupational exposure to HIV and other blood-borne pathogens. In: Cameron JL, ed. *Current Surgical Therapy*. 9th ed. Philadelphia: CV Mosby; 2008.
10. Centers for Disease Control and Prevention. Recommendations for prevention and control of hepatitis C (HCV) virus and HCV-related chronic disease. *MMWR Recomm Rep*. 1998;47(RR-19):1–39.
11. Dolin R, Masur H, Saag MS. *AIDS Therapy*. 2nd ed. Philadelphia: Churchill Livingstone; 2003.
12. Mandell GL, Bennett JE, Dolin R. *Principles and Practice of Infectious Diseases*. 5th ed. Philadelphia: Churchill Livingstone; 2000.
13. U.S. Public Health Service. Updated U.S. Public Health Service guidelines for the management of occupational exposures to HBV, HCV, and HIV and recommendations for postexposure prophylaxis. *MMWR Recomm Rep*. 2001;50(RR-11):1–52.
14. Anaya DA, Dellinger EP. Surgical infections and choice antibiotics. In: Townsend CM, Beauchamp RD, Evers BM, et al., eds. *Sabiston Textbook of Surgery: The Biological Basis of Modern Surgical Practice*. 18th ed. Philadelphia: WB Saunders; 2008.
15. Centers for Disease Control and Prevention. Public Health Service guidelines for the management of health care worker exposures to HIV and recommendations for postexposure prophylaxis. *MMWR Recomm Rep*. 1998;47(RR-7):1–33.
16. Centers for Disease Control and Prevention. Revised classification system for HIV infection and expanded surveillance case definition for AIDS among adolescents and adults. *MMWR Recomm Rep*. 1992;41(RR-17):1–19.
17. HIV InSite website by the University of California San Francisco, Section of Surgery in Patients with HIV. Available at: http://hivinsite.ucsf.edu.
18. Deziel DJ, Hyser MJ, Doolas A, Bines SD, Blaauw BB, Kessler HA. Major abdominal operations in acquired immunodeficiency syndrome. *Am Surg*. 1990;56:445–450.
19. Beck DE, Wexner SD. *Fundamentals of Anorectal Surgery*. New York: McGraw-Hill; 1992.
20. HIV InSite website by the University of California San Francisco, Section of Toxoplasmosis and HIV. Available at: http://hivinsite.ucsf.edu.
21. Centers for Disease Control and Prevention. Influenza vaccination information for health care workers. Available at: http://www.cdc.gov/flu/healthcareworkers.htm.
22. Centers for Disease Control and Prevention. Flu vaccine safety information. Available at: http://www.cdc.gov/flu/protect/vaccine/general.htm.
23. Centers for Disease Control and Prevention. Making Better Influenza Virus Vaccines. Available at: wwwnc.cdc.gov/eid/article/12/1/05-1043_article.
24. Centers for Disease Control and Prevention. Use of antivirals: background and guidance on the use of influenza antiviral agents. Available at: http://www.cdc.gov/flu/professionals/antivirals/antiviral-use-influenza.htm.
25. Centers for Disease Control and Prevention. Antiviral drug resistance among influenza viruses: guidance on the use of influenza antiviral agents. Available at: http://www.cdc.gov/flu/professionals/antivirals/antiviral-drug-resistance.htm.
26. Centers for Disease Control and Prevention. Hepatitis C FAQs for health professionals: management and treatment. Available at: http://www.cdc.gov/hepatitis/hcv/hcvfaq.htm#section4.
27. Centers for Disease Control and Prevention. Guidance on personal protective equipment (PPE) to be used by healthcare workers during management of patients with confirmed Ebola or persons under investigation (PUIs) for Ebola who are clinically unstable or have bleeding, vomiting, or diarrhea in U.S. hospitals, including procedures for donning and doffing PPE. Available at: http://www.cdc.gov/vhf/ebola/healthcare-us/ppe/guidance.html.
28. Centers for Disease Control and Prevention. Ebola virus disease (EVD) information for clinicians in U.S. healthcare settings. Available at: http://www.cdc.gov/vhf/ebola/healthcare-us/preparing/clinicians.html.
29. Wren SM, Kushner AL. Surgical protocol for possible or confirmed Ebola cases. Available at: https://www.facs.org/surgeons/ebola/surgical-protocol.
30. Shaughnessy MK, Micielli RL, DePestel DD, et al. Evaluation of hospital room assignment and acquisition of *Clostridium difficile* infection. *Infect Control Hosp Epidemiol*. 2011;32(3):201–206.
31. Surawicz CM, Brandt LJ, Binion DG, et al. Guidelines for diagnosis, treatment, and prevention of *Clostridium difficile* infections. *Am J Gastroenterol*. 2013;108(4):478–498.

CHAPTER 6

TRANSPLANTATION AND IMMUNOLOGY

Edie Chan, M.D., and Shannon Zielsdorf, M.D.

1. Which of the following statements regarding rejection of solid organ transplants is true?

A. Hyperacute rejection begins in the operating room with reperfusion of the transplanted organ.

B. Liver transplants are especially susceptible to hyperacute rejection.

C. Most immunosuppressive medications are used to prevent chronic rejection.

D. The major cause of graft failure is acute rejection.

E. Chronic rejection is characterized histologically by lymphocyte infiltration.

ANSWER: A

COMMENTS: There are three types of **solid organ rejection** that are based on the timing of the rejection: hyperacute rejection, acute rejection, and chronic rejection. The immunologic mechanism varies among these types of rejection. **Hyperacute rejection** occurs immediately and is the result of preformed antibodies binding to the allograft on reperfusion of the organ. Hyperacute rejection is due to ABO incompatibility or a high titer of antidonor human leukocyte antigen (HLA)-I antibodies in the recipient. For kidney, heart, pancreas, and lung transplants, current protocols include preoperative testing for ABO incompatibility or HLA antibodies (or both). For reasons not completely elucidated, liver transplants are resistant to this process. Liver transplants are performed without HLA matching and can be performed without ABO typing, although the ABO type is usually matched.

Acute rejection occurs days to weeks following transplantation. Since acute rejection is initiated by T-cell immunity, most medications for preventing and treating it are directed toward T-cell suppression. Microscopically, acute rejection is characterized by a lymphocytic infiltrate, with plasma cells and eosinophils being seen on tissue biopsy specimens.

Chronic rejection occurs months to years after transplantation and is the major cause of graft failure and mortality with all organ transplants. There is loss of normal histologic structure, fibrosis, and atherosclerosis, with intergraft expression of certain cytokines. Chronic rejection is the final common pathway of various insults, including repeated bouts of acute rejection, drug toxicity, chronic mechanical obstruction, recurrent infections, noncompliance with immunosuppressive medications, and pretransplant organ issues such as ischemia time and older organ donors. There is no defined therapy for chronic rejection, but it is believed that a better understanding of cytokine-mediated atherosclerosis would help in the development of treatments and prevention of chronic rejection.

Ref.: 1

2. A 30-year-old woman with lupus receives a kidney transplant. Two hours later, she is anuric. Vital statistics of the kidney include cold ischemia time of 10 h, a 60-year-old donor, a negative crossmatch, and panel-reactive antibody (PRA) of 80%. Select the best next step of management.

A. Immediate angiogram to evaluate for (and treat) an arterial occlusion

B. Immediate sonographic studies to verify vessel patency

C. Immediate reexploration

D. Immediate administration of high-dose steroids to empirically treat rejection

E. Magnetic resonance angiography to determine vessel patency

ANSWER: B

COMMENTS: The most common cause of delayed graft function following kidney transplantation is **acute tubular necrosis** (ATN). However, ATN is usually characterized by urine production in the range of 10 to 30 mL/h, which generally declines to 0 to 5 mL/h over the first 24 h. Although surgical complications such as vascular thrombosis and ureteral obstruction are rare, they must be excluded in patients who have anuria immediately after kidney transplantation. The initial test of choice is a **Doppler ultrasound** to verify vessel patency, exclude the presence of a fluid collection secondary to a hematoma or urinoma that may be impinging on the graft, and rule out arterial or venous obstruction from kinking of one or both vessels. If no flow is seen in either the renal artery or vein, reexploration is indicated. Ultrasound is a quick, reliable, and noninvasive test to evaluate vessels and detect hydronephrosis and fluid collections; it should be performed before returning to the operating room.

Ref.: 2

3. A 30-year-old type 1 brittle diabetic patient with diabetic nephropathy receives a simultaneous pancreas and kidney (SPK) transplant. Which of the follow statements is true?

A. Elevation of plasma glucose levels in the early postoperative period are indicative of pancreas rejection.

B. Bladder drainage is preferred because it is associated with fewer complications.

C. Most surgeons prefer enteric drainage because the incidence of complications attributed to bladder drainage, such as acidosis and urinary tract infections, is decreased.

D. Most surgeons prefer bladder drainage because avoiding contamination with enteric contents reduces the incidence of infections.

E. The preferred enteric drainage of the pancreatic allograft is the cecum.

ANSWER: C

COMMENTS: Rejection of the pancreas is almost completely reliant on monitoring for renal allograft rejection and dysfunction because: (1) pancreas allograft rejection has no reliable early marker and (2) discordant rejection of allografts is rare in SPK transplantation. The exocrine pancreas is affected by acute rejection first. In contrast, beta cells have considerable function reserve because the islets of Langerhans are scattered sparsely throughout the exocrine pancreas. Therefore in long-term post-transplant patients, elevated glucose is a late sign of rejection because it takes time for dysfunction of the majority of the islets to cause hyperglycemia. Elevation of glucose in the immediate postoperative period can be a sign of vascular compromise.

Enteric drainage of pancreas transplants has a lower leak rate than those drained into the bladder. However, a leak from an enteric anastomosis is more likely to result in graft loss. An enteric leak also threatens the patient's life given the potential catastrophic course of intraabdominal sepsis in an immunocompromised patient. Long-term complications of **bladder drainage** include recurrent urinary tract infections and metabolic acidosis from the loss of bicarbonate into the bladder. For these reasons, bladder drainage is commonly converted to enteric drainage. The preferred site for enteric drainage is the small bowel.

Ref.: 3, 4

4. Which of the following is true regarding allocation of liver allografts for transplantation?

A. Allocation of cadaveric liver allografts is dependent on model for end-stage liver disease (MELD), length of time on the waitlist, ABO compatibility, HLA compatibility, and PRA results.

B. Allocation of cadaveric liver allografts for patients with hepatocellular carcinoma (HCC) requires the recipient to be on the waitlist for at least 6 months.

C. Allocation of cadaveric liver allografts for status 1A or 1B candidates is immediately assigned a MELD score of 40, which is the highest score possible on the waitlist.

D. Cadaveric renal or liver allografts with hepatitis C virus (HCV) are routinely allocated to both HCV-positive and HCV-negative recipients.

E. The time-to-transplant on the waitlist has decreased since using the MELD score for cadaveric liver allograft allocation; however, there has been no significant change in the mortality rate while on the waitlist.

ANSWER: B

COMMENTS: Within a designated geographical region or "donor service area," allocation of cadaveric liver allografts is dependent first on ABO compatibility and MELD score and then on the length of time on the waitlist (if MELD scores are equal for two candidates). The MELD score, which is based on total bilirubin level, serum creatinine level, and international normalized ratio, was initially developed to estimate the 3-month mortality risk in cirrhotic patients after transjugular intrahepatic portosystemic shunt (TIPS) placement and later validated for predicting 3-month transplant waiting list mortality. Since MELD was initiated for organ allocation in February 2002, its use has resulted in a shorter time to transplant. Thus it also resulted in significantly fewer dropouts and deaths while on the transplant list. Of note, MELD allocation does not apply to status 1A or 1B candidates.

Patients with HCC who have **stage T2 lesions** are given a MELD score of 28 after 6 months on the liver transplant waitlist. The MELD score exception for HCC was previously 22 and given immediately upon listing. However, this caused preferential organ allocation to HCC patients and higher dropout rates for non-HCC candidates. Delaying the score assignment—which was initiated in October 2015—should address this disparity. Furthermore, after the exception score assignment, HCC patients are given extra MELD points for each additional 3-month period on the waitlist; the score exception for HCC is capped at 34.

HCV-positive liver allografts without severe inflammation or fibrosis can be used for HCV-positive recipients. The literature has shown that there are no differences in HCV recurrence, graft survival, or patient survival in HCV-positive recipients receiving an HCV-positive allograft compared with those receiving an HCV-negative allograft. The use of HCV-positive liver allografts for HCV-negative recipients should be reserved for cases of extreme necessity. However, the availability of the new efficacious and tolerable direct-acting antivirals (DAAs) may change HCV-positive allograft allocation in the future and expand the organ donor pool for HCV-negative candidates as well.

Ref.: 5–8

5. With respect to de novo postrenal transplant diabetes mellitus, which of the following statements is true?

A. It is more common in African-American recipients.

B. Most patients inevitably require long-term insulin therapy.

C. Risk factors include advanced age and previous history of hyperlipidemia.

D. It has become less common since the introduction of tacrolimus.

E. Its incidence does not correlate with steroid dosage.

ANSWER: A

COMMENTS: New-onset diabetes after transplantation (NODAT) occurs at rates of 9.1%, 16%, and 24% at 12, 24, and 36 months after transplantation, respectively. Steroids, cyclosporine, and tacrolimus are diabetogenic. There is a direct relationship between steroid dosage and the incidence of NODAT. **Tacrolimus**-based immunosuppressive therapy was associated with a 15% incidence of NODAT. Rates are dose dependent and fall with decreased levels of tacrolimus. **Cyclosporine**-based immunosuppressive therapy resulted in only a 9% incidence of NODAT. Risk factors include age, obesity, family history of diabetes, and African-American race. The potential mechanisms include decreased insulin secretion, increased insulin resistance, and a toxic effect of tacrolimus and cyclosporine on pancreatic beta cells. In only 25% of patients with NODAT does persistent hyperglycemia develop, and 50% of patients in this group ultimately require insulin replacement therapy.

Ref.: 9

6. Regarding liver transplantation for patients chronically infected with HCV, which of the following statements is true?

A. Posttransplant reinfection with HCV occurs in approximately 50% of patients.
B. Posttransplant treatment of HCV is a contraindication due to the extensive drug interactions between DAAs and immunosuppressive agents.
C. Posttransplant reinfection with HCV causes cirrhosis in approximately 80% of patients at 5 years after liver transplantation.
D. The clinical course of HCV after reinfection is less virulent than that of the original infection.
E. Allograft failure secondary to recurrence of HCV infection is currently the most common cause of death and retransplantation in recipients with HCV infection.

ANSWER: E

COMMENTS: The most common indication for liver transplantation worldwide is **HCV infection**. Most patients with chronic HCV who develop cirrhosis have had the infection for more than 20 years. After liver transplantation, these patients uniformly become reinfected within a matter of days. Cirrhosis develops much earlier in the transplanted allograft, with approximately 5% to over 20% of patients exhibiting cirrhosis on biopsy at 5 years following transplantation.

DAAs, such as sofosbuvir, simeprevir, and daclatasvir, have revolutionized the treatment of HCV infection. Specifically, the treatment of liver transplant candidates and recipients can now be safely and effectively done. Several factors must be taken into account when determining a treatment regimen for these patients, such as genotype, liver and renal function, concurrent use of immunosuppressive agents, and timing of treatment (if occurring in the posttransplant period). Recent studies on HCV patients receiving DAA(s) with ribavirin following liver transplantation showed promising sustained virologic responses (SVRs) in both treatment-naïve and treatment-experienced patients. In this setting, the magnitude of long-term benefits of DAAs, which are both efficacious and well tolerated, is yet to be determined. However, as of now, the most common cause of death and retransplantation in recipients with HCV infection is recurrence of hepatitis C.

Ref.: 10, 11

7. Which of the following statements regarding interleukins (ILs) is true?
A. All ILs upregulate the immune system.
B. IL-8 is a neutrophil chemotactic factor.
C. ILs are only produced by leukocytes.
D. IL-10 produces fever and inflammation.
E. Prednisone upregulates the effect of IL-1.

ANSWER: B

COMMENTS: *ILs* are a group of cytokines that function in various ways to upregulate and downregulate the immune system. IL-3 functions as a hematopoietic growth factor. IL-4, IL-6, and IL-10 are the ILs that have known inhibitory functions. Specifically, IL-4 inhibits the secretion of cytokines by macrophages, IL-6 inhibits tumor necrosis factor (TNF), and IL-10 inhibits monocyte/macrophage function and counteracts the inflammatory cytokines. IL-4, IL-6, and IL-10 also have other stimulatory functions.

ILs are produced by a variety of cells, including macrophages and monocytes, T and B lymphocytes, mast cells, stromal cells of the thymus and bone marrow, fibroblasts, epithelial cells, and endothelial cells. Most of the ILs stimulate a particular variety of leukocytes. IL-8 attracts neutrophils to the site of inflammation by movement through the vascular endothelium. IL-1 is responsible for fever and inflammation and also leads to the proliferation of T and B cells. *Glucocorticoid* administration inhibits the synthesis of IL-1 (among others), thus downregulating the inflammatory and immune response.

Ref.: 12–14

8. Which of the following statements is true regarding liver transplantation in the pediatric population?
A. HCC is the most common malignancy in children, leading to transplantation.
B. Portoenterostomy for biliary atresia is inferior to liver transplant in infants; therefore if transplantation is an option, it is the optimal treatment.
C. Inborn errors of metabolism with or without injury to the liver can be an indication for liver transplantation.
D. Polycystic kidney and liver disease is the most common indication for liver transplantation in children.
E. The two main grafts used for pediatric liver transplantation are an allograft from a pediatric donor of similar size or an adult donor's right lobe.

ANSWER: C

COMMENTS: Urea cycle defects, Crigler-Najjar syndrome, homozygous familial hypercholesterolemia, and primary hyperoxaluria are examples of **metabolic disorders** that do not injure the liver but have been treated with liver transplantation. The principal goal of treatment is correcting the metabolic error. Crigler-Najjar syndrome is the prototype for this decision-making process. The severe deficiency of bilirubin uridine diphosphate–glucuronyl transferase results in the systemic accumulation of bilirubin; this leads to neurologic injury. It can be treated for some time with phototherapy and bilirubin-binding agents. Nevertheless, medical management inevitably fails, and these patients require a liver transplant prior to their teenage years.

Biliary atresia is the most common specific indication for liver transplantation in children: 41% of pediatric transplants overall and 65% of transplants in children under the age of 1 year. The general strategy for treating biliary atresia is maximizing overall outcome. Successful portoenterostomy prolongs survival out of infancy, and it does not jeopardize the patient at the time of transplantation in the future. Moreover, survival statistics following a portoenterostomy reveal that this approach is as good as early transplantation.

Hepatoblastoma is the most common malignancy in children, leading to transplantation. The most important principle of hepatoblastoma treatment is complete removal. Therefore hepatic resection is also an option, if size and anatomic location allow it.

Organ size is of utmost importance in pediatric transplantation given that the majority of children reach end-stage disease before 2 years of age. Unfortunately, most pediatric liver donors are too large for the typical pediatric recipient, causing excessively long waiting times and high pretransplant mortality among small children. Over the past 10 years, there has been a substantial expansion in the availability of donor grafts for pediatric liver transplantation due to surgical innovations, from both living and deceased donors. Left lateral lobe grafts are generally used when the donor-to-recipient weight ratio exceeds 4, and left lobe grafts are used when the ratio is between 2 and 4. Right lobe grafts have been used in teenagers as in adult-to-adult procedures.

Ref.: 15

9. A 40-year-old man who underwent kidney transplant 1 year ago is seen in the office with an enlarged groin lymph node. Labs show an elevated *Epstein-Barr virus* (EBV), and an excisional lymph node biopsy reveals B-cell **posttransplant lymphoproliferative disorder (PTLD.)** He is given acyclovir, and his immunosuppression is decreased; however, this treatment fails. What is the next best step?

A. Change immunosuppressive agents.

B. Add radiation therapy to positive lymph node basins.

C. Add rituximab.

D. Perform transplant nephrectomy.

E. Add cyclophosphamide, hydroxydaunomycin (doxorubicin,) oncovin (vincristine), and prednisone (CHOP).

ANSWER: C

COMMENTS: Posttransplant lymphoproliferative disorder represents a spectrum of diseases related to EBV infection, including infectious mononucleosis, benign proliferation of B cells, and lymphoma. In a transplant recipient, clones of EBV-transformed B cells are generated as a result of infection with EBV from the donor or personal contact. Because of impaired immunity, transplant recipients are unable to control the clonal expansion of EBV-infected B cells. Risk factors for the development of PTLD include young age; use of antilymphocytic globulin or polyclonal antibodies as induction agents, such as OKT3 and antithymocytoglolubin; EBV seronegativity prior to transplant with primary infection after transplant; and cytomegalovirus (CMV)-negative recipients who receive an organ from a CMV-positive donor.

Patients with elevated serum levels of EBV are usually treated by decreasing the dosage of immunosuppressive agents and by administering either acyclovir or ganciclovir. When PTLD is unresponsive to initial reduction of immunosuppression, patients can be treated with the anti–B-cell (anti-CD20) antibody rituximab (Rituxan). For high-risk CD20-positive PTLD, those refractory to rituximab, or T-cell PTLD, the treatment of choice is cytotoxic chemotherapy such as CHOP (cyclophosphamide, hydroxydaunorubicin [doxorubicin], oncovin [vincristine], and prednisone).

In specific (and rare) situations, local radiation therapy is considered in conjunction with the aforementioned treatment to control localized PTLD. Finally, transplant nephrectomy is atypical and reserved as a last resort for PTLD.

Ref.: 16

10. Liver transplantation may be contraindicated for which of the following?

A. A 42-year-old patient with cirrhosis and prior alcohol use 7 months ago

B. A 60-year-old patient with a single, 5-cm-diameter HCC

C. A 55-year-old patient with liver failure and uncorrected pulmonary hypertension

D. A 37-year-old patient with liver failure and hepatopulmonary syndrome

E. A 52-year-old patient with liver failure and portal vein thrombosis

ANSWER: C

COMMENTS: Patients with alcoholic liver disease who are abstinent for more than 6 months and have good psychosocial support are considered good candidates for liver transplantation because of the low risk for alcohol recidivism. As a group, their long-term survival rate may be one of the highest because they are often not subject to viral hepatitis and other progressive diseases that may recur in the transplanted liver. Alcohol use is frequently encountered in patients who are evaluated for other diseases, and they too should be abstinent for a certain defined period. Patients also receive additional points for HCC and hepatopulmonary syndrome.

The ideal deceased donor liver allocation scheme for **HCC** should result in minimum patient dropout from the waiting list due to progression of HCC, minimize disease recurrence after transplantation, and be comparable to other patients in terms of pretransplant and posttransplant survival. The Milan criteria have been extensively studied to meet these standards and are the tumor inclusion standards used in most Western countries for allocation of deceased donor organs. The Milan criteria are a single tumor of 5-cm diameter or up to three tumors up to 3 cm in diameter. Furthermore, some tumors beyond the criteria may be downstaged to within Milan criteria (by various interventional radiology procedures) with the ultimate goal of transplantation.

Hypoxemia from **severe pulmonary hypertension** is an absolute contraindication to transplantation. Pulmonary hypertension is defined as a mean pulmonary artery pressure greater than 25 mmHg with normal pulmonary capillary wedge pressure. The overall prevalence of pulmonary hypertension in the general population is 0.13%, although in patients with portal hypertension, it is significantly higher at 0.73%. For patients with liver failure, pulmonary hypertension can be classified as mild (mean pulmonary pressure of 25 to 35 mmHg), moderate (mean pulmonary pressure of 35 to 45 mmHg), or severe (mean pulmonary pressure > 45 mmHg.) Pulmonary artery pressure higher than 50 mmHg despite therapy correlates with a nearly 100% mortality rate. Patients with untreated severe pulmonary hypertension who undergo liver transplantation are at very high risk for cardiac death from right ventricular failure immediately following reperfusion. Fortunately, for moderate and severe pulmonary hypertension, treatment with the prostacyclin epoprostenol by constant infusion can reduce pulmonary pressure to a range at which liver transplantation can be successful. Bosentan, a nonselective endothelin receptor antagonist, can also be used. While liver transplantation may be contraindicated in patients with severe pulmonary hypertension unresponsive to medical treatment, for patients who do respond, they can be gradually weaned from the prostacyclin after transplantation, and pulmonary pressure will remain normal.

Hepatopulmonary syndrome is essentially the opposite of pulmonary hypertension. Pulmonary capillaries serving unoxygenated areas of the lung respond to the liver disease by dilating, which impedes oxygen diffusion and increases intrapulmonary shunting. As a result, patients require increasing amounts of supplemental oxygen. However, transplantation is curative, and the shunt fraction is reduced to normal often within a few days, although complete resolution may take up to 15 months. Transplantation before development of severe hypoxemia ($PaO_2 < 50$ mmHg) may improve outcomes and result in less need for postoperative ventilator support.

Portal venous thrombosis was previously a contraindication for liver transplant given early experiences with worse outcomes, including intraoperative deaths related to issues with the portal vein. However, as transplantation experience improved and key operative technique included extensive dissection to the confluence of the splenic and superior mesenteric vein (SMV), survival and portal vein patency also improved. Preoperative evaluation of the vascular anatomy is paramount. Diagnostic imaging is usually ultrasonography with Doppler or computed tomography (CT); however, it can also include magnetic resonance imaging (MRI) or portal venography. The armamentarium of treatments includes portal thromboendovenectomy, a vein jump graft to the SMV, or vein grafting to alternative inflow such as the coronary vein.

Ref.: 17–19

11. After orthotopic liver transplantation (OLT) 10 years earlier for HCV cirrhosis, a 50-year-old man is hospitalized for fluid overload and is found to have a worsening renal function. If this is due to toxicity of an immunosuppressive agent, which of the following medications has the patient likely been taking?

A. Sirolimus (Rapamune)

B. Tacrolimus (Prograf)

C. Mycophenolate (Cellcept, Myfortic)

D. Prednisone

E. Azathioprine (Imuran)

ANSWER: B

COMMENTS: All immunosuppressive agents have toxicities, but using various combinations of the agents at lower dosages can minimize these toxicities. Both **tacrolimus** and **cyclosporine** are calcineurin inhibitors and cause renal vasoconstriction, which can lead to acute nephrotoxicity by reducing renal blood flow. They can also cause chronic nephrotoxicity from hyaline thickening in the afferent arterioles, interstitial fibrosis, tubular atrophy, and glomerulosclerosis. Calcineurin inhibitor nephrotoxicity is common: up to 20% of liver recipients experience chronic renal failure by 5 years posttransplant. In addition, both tacrolimus and cyclosporine can cause neurotoxicity, such as headaches, tremors, confusion, agitation, seizures, or coma. Lastly, in addition to nephrotoxicity and neurotoxicity, tacrolimus has been associated with an increase in posttransplant diabetes and further potentiates the hyperglycemic effects of steroids.

Sirolimus binds to the same immunophilin as tacrolimus. However, this complex inhibits the serine/threonine protein kinase, mammalian target of rapamycin (mTOR), instead of calcineurin. It is not nephrotoxic, although it can cause proteinuria. Common toxicities of sirolimus are hyperlipidemia as well as cytopenias. Additionally, an increased risk of hernias has been reported due to its impact on fibrogenesis and interference with wound healing.

Mycophenolate inhibits purine synthesis, which is essential for the proliferative responses of T and B cells to mitogens. This impacts both cellular immunity and antibody production. It can cause gastrointestinal side effects, such as diarrhea, flatulence, bloating, and abdominal pain. **Azathioprine** is a prodrug that is converted into the active form of 6-mercaptopurine and thus prevents purine synthesis as well. Myelosuppression is the most common side effect, with more than 50% of recipients experiencing significant cytopenias. It can also cause gastrointestinal disturbances, although not nearly as often as mycophenolate.

Ref.: 20

12. Which of the following statements regarding T cells is true?

A. T cells complete development in the thymus and then migrate to the bone marrow.

B. The various types of T cells can be identified by the binding of specific monoclonal antibodies to antigens on the cell surface.

C. Helper T cells can be activated to produce antibodies.

D. Cytotoxic T cells can destroy target cells by recognizing foreign antigens at the target cell nucleus.

E. Cell-mediated immunity can be transferred passively in serum.

ANSWER: B

COMMENTS: T lymphocytes mature in the thymus, whereas B lymphocytes mature in the fetal liver and the bone marrow. The thymus, liver, and bone marrow are referred to as the primary lymphoid organs. **T lymphocytes** subsequently migrate to the secondary lymphoid organs: the spleen, lymph nodes, and dispersed lymphoid tissues found in the bronchus, urogenital tract, and gut (i.e., Peyer patches). The T lymphocytes circulate through the bloodstream from these points in search of nonself antigens.

Lymphocytes that differentiate into T cells and B cells express various clusters of antigens on their membranes. All T cells express the cell surface antigen–specific receptor designated CD3, whereas B cells express the cell surface antigen–specific receptors CD19 and CD20. **$CD3^+$ T cells** can be distinguished and subdivided further by the expression of additional differentiation antigens on the T-cell surface (T-cell receptors), such as cytotoxic T cells (CD3/CD8), suppressor T cells (CD3/CD8), helper/inducer T cells (CD3/CD4), and delayed-type hypersensitivity T cells (CD3/CD4). **Cytotoxic T cells** are capable of destroying a target cell by recognizing a foreign or "modified-self" antigen and class I major histocompatibility complex (MHC) molecules on the target-cell surface. **Helper T cells** consist of T_H1 and T_H2 cells. They appear to work together in a regulatory circuit, with each having a negative effect on the other. T_H1 cells are proinflammatory and release interferon gamma (IFN-α). T_H2 cells release ILs to promote B-cell differentiation and maturation. **Delayed-type hypersensitivity T cells** bring macrophages and other inflammatory cells to areas in which delayed-type hypersensitivity reactions occur through the production of various chemokines.

Ref.: 12, 13

13. Which of the following patients should be considered for the TIPS procedure?

A. A 45-year-old woman with portal hypertension causing bleeding esophageal varices; MELD score 14; she needed a blood transfusion and two endoscopies for variceal bleeding in the past 6 months.

B. A 52-year-old with alcohol-related cirrhosis; MELD score 20; his liver disease is complicated by poorly controlled hepatic encephalopathy and ascites requiring paracentesis every other week.

C. A 60-year-old woman with portal hypertension causing ascites; MELD score 15; she is on the maximum dose of diuretics and still requires paracentesis every other week.

D. A 39-year-old woman with cirrhosis due to autoimmune hepatitis; MELD score 16; her liver disease is complicated by recurrent hospitalizations for pleural effusion causing dyspnea for which she was started on a trial of diuretics.

E. A 65-year-old man with HCV-related cirrhosis; MELD score 40; he is currently intubated in the intensive care unit (ICU) for hemorrhagic shock secondary to bleeding esophageal varices.

ANSWER: C

COMMENTS: Due to TIPS, there has been a dramatic shift away from open surgical portosystemic shunts for the treatment of refractory portal hypertension. TIPS is especially useful in those awaiting transplant because it acts as a bridge to liver transplantation without distorting the extrahepatic vascular anatomy or tissue planes. Multiple studies concluded that TIPS did not significantly affect the course of a transplant operation. There was no difference in operative times, transfusion requirements, or short-term survival.

The indications for TIPS are refractory variceal bleeding, ascites, hepatic hydrothorax, and Budd–Chiari syndrome. Most important, conservative management of the aforementioned sequelae of portal hypertension must first fail prior to considering TIPS as treatment, which is why A and D are incorrect. The use of early TIPS (within 72 h of control of variceal bleeding) in patients at high risk for rebleeding, such as those with a MELD score > 18 or a transfusion requirement of >4 units of red blood cells within a 24-h period, is associated with a reduced rate of treatment failure and mortality compared with continued medical and endoscopic therapy. Furthermore, when bleeding cannot be controlled after two trials of endoscopic intervention within a 24-h period, TIPS is the usual salvage treatment.

The relative contraindications for TIPS are refractory hepatic encephalopathy and high MELD, which is why B and E are incorrect. TIPS may worsen liver function by depriving the liver of portal venous blood, thereby increasing the risk of hepatic encephalopathy as well as liver decompensation. Patients with a MELD score ≤ 14 have an excellent survival rate after TIPS. However, patients with a MELD score > 24 have a 30-day mortality rate that approaches 30%. TIPS placement in patients with intermediate MELD scores of 15 to 24 should be determined on a case-by-case basis, depending on the patient and physician's judgment as well as the likelihood of liver transplantation in the near future.

Interestingly, the MELD score has been used for organ allocation on the transplant waiting list since 2002. However, it was originally studied and validated for predicting survival in cirrhotic patients after the TIPS procedure.

Ref.: 21

14. Which of the following is true regarding organ preservation for liver transplantation?

A. University of Wisconsin (UW) solution contains phosphate, which replenishes the depleted intracellular levels caused by degradation of adenosine triphosphate (ATP) during cold ischemia time.

B. Hypothermic machine perfusion (HMP) has become the gold standard treatment for liver allografts from donation after cardiac death (DCD).

C. UW solution contains lactobionic acid, which counteracts oxygen free radical production during reperfusion.

D. It is better to perform the back-table liver dissection after packaging and travel time as opposed to immediately after organ procurement.

E. Glutathione was added to UW solution in order to buffer the intracellular acidosis created during cold ischemia time.

ANSWER: D

COMMENTS: **UW solution** was allowed for clinical use in the United States in 1987. Aside from the introduction of immunosuppressants like cyclosporine, the development of preservation solutions like UW is one of the most influential factors in the evolution of liver transplantation. Organ sharing across long distances was made possible because the liver grafts could be preserved for more than 15 h.

The electrolyte composition mimics the intracellular environment—high potassium and low sodium—in order to limit transmembranous fluid and electrolyte shifts. Instead of glucose, this solution contains raffinose and **lactobionic acid**, which are osmotic membrane-impermeable agents. They offset transmembranous water movement to prevent cellular edema. UW solution contains a **phosphate buffer** to prevent the intracellular acidosis caused by anaerobic glycolysis during cold ischemia. **Adenosine** in UW solution acts as a substrate for the resynthesis of ATP after reperfusion. The antioxidant **glutathione** and **allopurinol** were added to neutralize and block the production of oxygen radicals generated during reperfusion, respectively.

Hypothermia is induced during liver procurement by infusing the arterial inflow with chilled UW solution and applying ice slush around the organ in the operative field. Most enzymes decrease in activity at a low temperature, and therefore oxygen metabolism is significantly reduced at core liver temperatures of 0°C to 4°C. There is evidence that low temperatures below 4°C are guaranteed for nearly 1 h when the back-table preparation is performed after organ transportation in the icebox. Furthermore, experimental data revealed reduced ischemia–reperfusion injury and better early graft function following cold storage at 0°C compared with 5°C. These two findings highlight the advantage of performing the back-table liver dissection after proper organ packaging and transportation.

HMP with or without oxygenation provides protection by the deactivation of mitochondrial respiration and decreased production of reactive oxygen species. HMP uses lower perfusion pressures, low flow rates, and modified colloid solutions instead of blood. Only a few clinical trials have been performed; however, they have revealed promising results: lower rates of early allograft dysfunction (5% versus 25% in matched cold storage group) as well as significantly reduced expression of proinflammatory cytokines and ICAM-1. These encouraging results show a great potential for HMP, especially in DCD and extended-criteria donor liver allografts, in order to continue expanding the donor pool. However, as of yet, it is not the gold standard for organ preservation of any kind.

Ref.: 22

15. Which of the following statements regarding TNF is true?

A. TNF-α is produced only by monocytes and macrophages.

B. Release of TNF is stimulated by exotoxins.

C. TNF enhances the anticoagulant activity of endothelial surfaces.

D. TNF is responsible for the cachexia associated with metastatic disease.

E. Glucocorticoids have essentially no effect on TNF-α expression.

ANSWER: D

COMMENTS: **TNF** is so named because of its ability to cause hemorrhagic necrosis in methylcholanthrene-induced sarcomas in mice. **TNF-α** is produced primarily by monocytes and macrophages but also by neutrophils and natural killer (NK) cells. It stimulates the activity of neutrophils, induces endothelial cells to produce IL-1, and induces synovial cells and fibroblasts to produce prostaglandin E2 and collagenase. TNF-α enhances the procoagulant activity of endothelial surfaces, increases vascular permeability, degranulates neutrophils, and stimulates the release of superoxides and arachidonic acid metabolites. In gram-negative shock, **endotoxin** stimulates the release of TNF-α, which leads to hypotension, disseminated intravascular coagulation, and even death. TNF stimulates catabolism in muscle and fat cells, thereby leading to an increase in anaerobic glycolysis, protein breakdown, and lipolysis. It is largely responsible for the **cachexia** associated with metastatic disease. It is produced in lesser quantities when **glucocorticoids** are present because they downregulate the signaling pathway that transcribes the TNF gene.

Ref.: 13, 14

16. Which statement is true regarding the pancreas allograft of an SPK transplantation?

A. Despite the increased risk of hemorrhage, some institutions use heparin for anticoagulation after SPK to prevent the increased risk of allograft vascular thrombosis.

B. Early hemorrhage after SPK is often from rupture of a pseudoaneurysm due to direct erosion by leaking pancreatic exocrine enzymes.

C. Thrombosis is the most common indication for repeat laparotomy after SPK.

D. Allograft pancreatitis is easily distinguishable from acute rejection based on specific CT scan findings and the magnitude in elevation of lipase and amylase levels.

E. Acute rejection is the most common cause of early pancreas allograft failure after SPK.

ANSWER: A

COMMENTS: The blood flow to the pancreas is much lower than that to the kidney. This physiology as well as donor-specific and recipient-specific risk factors increases the incidence of allograft venous or arterial thrombosis. Venous thrombosis is twice as common as arterial thrombosis. Either of them is by far the most common cause of early graft loss after SPK, at approximately 5%. Given this risk, some transplant centers routinely use heparin for anticoagulation in the immediate postoperative period, although this is not the gold standard.

Early hemorrhage after SPK is the most common indication for repeat laparotomy. It is often due to vascular anastomoses or thrombus-sealing small vessels coming into contact with proteolytic and fibrinolytic exocrine secretions that leak from the pancreas surface. Unlike allograft thrombosis, early bleeding has little impact on the ultimate outcome. Late hemorrhage after SPK is uncommon. It is associated with the rupture of a pseudoaneurysm or vascular anastomosis that has been eroded by direct contact with leaking pancreatic exocrine enzymes.

Allograft pancreatitis can result from cold storage and ischemia–reperfusion injury. It can also occur from reflux into the pancreatic duct, which is more common with bladder drainage. Reflux can also occur during the transplantation itself: after pancreatic reperfusion but prior to the duodenal drainage anastomosis, excessive distention of the stapled duodenum with pancreatic fluid can result in postoperative pancreatitis. Unfortunately, both allograft pancreatitis and acute rejection present with the same symptoms, similar lab results, and an edematous pancreas seen on CT scan.

Ref.: 4

17. A 60-year-old woman with end-stage renal disease (ESRD) on dialysis is blood type O, has a recent PRA result of 15%, and has now been offered a blood type O cadaveric renal transplant. The crossmatch on this potential donor is positive. Which of the following statements is true?

A. A positive crossmatch indicates a higher likelihood that this patient will inevitably suffer graft loss from chronic cellular rejection.

B. A positive crossmatch is an absolute contraindication to cadaveric renal transplantation.

C. Additional immunotherapy can prevent hyperacute rejection and should be given to this patient in the perioperative period.

D. This patient's low PRA result typically predicts a higher likelihood of donor-specific antibodies.

E. This patient's sister is blood type A and wishes to be a living related kidney donor for her. This is a valid option because ABO incompatibility is no longer an absolute contraindication to kidney transplantation.

ANSWER: E

COMMENTS: Hyperacute rejection of a transplanted kidney generally occurs within minutes of reperfusion and is due to the presence of preformed immunoglobulin G (IgG) antibodies in the recipient's serum. These antibodies attach to major histocompatibility antigens (HLA-A, HLA-B, and HLA-DR) on the donor vascular endothelium. The test for donor-specific antibodies is called a **crossmatch** and is performed on all potential donors just before transplantation.

A positive crossmatch result is a relative contraindication to cadaveric renal transplantation. With cadaveric kidneys, there is insufficient time for preoperative plasmapheresis and intravenous immunoglobulin until a negative crossmatch is obtained. This increases the risk of immunologic graft loss. However, patients undergoing living related renal transplantation with a positive crossmatch result can be treated to remove the antibody (through one or both of the aforementioned treatments). Agents such as rituxamab (anti-CD20) can also be used to decrease antibody production. Plasmapheresis, intravenous immunoglobulin, and rituximab infusion combined with modern immunosuppression have allowed kidney transplantation from an **ABO-incompatible donor** to be performed with an acceptable success rate.

Potential recipients of ABO-compatible renal allografts develop donor-specific HLA antibodies of the IgG class from antigen exposure because of transfusions, pregnancy, or previous transplants. The presence of donor-specific antibodies can be predicted by periodically testing the reactivity of the recipient's serum to a panel of common A, B, and DR antigens and expressing the result as a percentage. This test is referred to as the **PRA**. The higher the PRA result at the time of transplantation, the more likely a patient is to have an episode of antibody-mediated rejection.

Ref.: 23, 24

18. A 62-year-old woman comes to the emergency department complaining of nausea and vomiting. She underwent OLT for alcoholic cirrhosis 5 weeks earlier. Her white blood cell count is 1.0 cell/mL. Which of the following is the most likely cause of her clinical symptoms?

A. Wound infection

B. CMV

C. Pneumonia

D. Bowel obstruction

E. Rejection

ANSWER: B

COMMENTS: CMV has the highest incidence of infection in seronegative recipients who receive seropositive organs. To decrease, but not eliminate, the risk of this infection, an extended period of prophylaxis with acyclovir or gancyclovir is usually given to all recipients. Early CMV disease occurs most commonly between 3 and 8 weeks after transplantation. Late CMV disease can also occur, and the risk of this increases with treatments for rejection with agents such as antithymocyte globulin. CMV infection is usually an acute, systemic infection that can result in gastritis, hepatitis, pneumonitis, retinitis, and bone marrow suppression. CMV infection rarely involves only one organ and seldom causes chronic nephropathy. The mainstay of therapy is **ganciclovir**.

Ref.: 25

19. A 58-year-old man with HCV cirrhosis undergoes an OLT and receives induction immunosuppression with rabbit antithymocyte globulin (rTAG). Regarding rTAG, which of the following statements is true?

A. It competitively binds IL-2 receptors without activating it, thereby blocking IL-2 stimulation of T cells.

B. The cytokine release syndrome associated with rTAG administration cannot be prevented; however, it resolves within a short period of time.

C. Serum sickness is a common side effect whose occurrence peaks approximately 48 h after the first administration of rTAG.

D. It causes a depletion of lymphocytes that lasts for 2 to 6 months.

E. It is effective against both T cells and B cells.

ANSWER: E

COMMENTS: rTAG is an antilymphocyte globulin commonly used for induction therapy. It has polyclonal antibodies against T-cell antigens (CD2, CD3, CD4, CD8, CD11a, CD25, CD44, and CD45) and B-cell antigens (CD19, CD20, CD21, and CD40) as well as antibodies against HLA-DR and HLA class I. Because they are depleting antibodies, the effects last for an extended period of time. Clinical trials have shown it to be an effective drug for preventing acute rejection after transplantation.

When the antibodies bind the T-cell receptor, they actually activate the T cell prior to its destruction. This releases cytokines that induce a systemic inflammatory response syndrome (SIRS), causing fever, rigors, hypotension, and, possibly, severe pulmonary edema. This reaction is usually mitigated by premedication with an antihistamine (diphenhydramine), an antipyretic (acetaminophen), and corticosteroids (hydrocortisone). Serum sickness is another reaction that can develop from rTAG, usually more than 7 days after the initial dose. It is due to a reaction to the proteins in the antibodies derived from nonhuman animal sources. It manifests as high fever, polyarthralgias, jaw pain, rash, or renal dysfunction. Treatment is high-dose steroids with the addition of plasmapheresis in steroid-resistant cases. Fortunately, it only occurs in up to 6% of liver recipients. More common side effects are leukopenia and thrombocytopenia.

Basiliximab (Simulect) is a mouse–human chimeric anti-CD25 monoclonal antibody that blocks stimulation of T cells by competitively binding to the IL-2 receptor without activating it. Due to its chimeric nature, it has a remarkably low incidence of side effects. **Alemtuzumab (Campath)** is a humanized monoclonal antibody against CD52 that is expressed on 95% of peripheral T and B cells as well as monocytes and macrophages. Use of this drug leads to depletion of B cells for approximately 2 to 6 months, while T cells recover only about 50% from baseline after 36 months. Interestingly, worse patient and graft survivals have been reported when alemtuzumab was used in HCV-positive patients. Therefore it should be avoided in this patient population.

Ref.: 12, 20

20. A 35-year-old man with a body mass index of 22 underwent kidney transplantation 6 weeks earlier for focal segmental glomerulosclerosis. He has a sense of fullness in his pelvis and increased urinary frequency. On physical examination, the ipsilateral lower extremity is painless but noticeably swollen. Ultrasound of the lower extremities is negative for deep venous thrombosis. An ultrasound of the transplanted kidney shows normal flow and heterogeneous fluid collection adjacent to the bladder. What is the best initial management of this problem?

A. Percutaneous drainage

B. Percutaneous drainage with sclerosis

C. Reexploration of the surgical site

D. Observation

E. Laparoscopic internal marsupialization

ANSWER: A

COMMENTS: Lymphoceles develop after kidney transplantation in up to 50% of recipients usually as a result of inadequate ligation of the iliac lymphatics. They do not require intervention if asymptomatic. However, if they compress the kidney, ureter, or bladder, an intervention is necessary. Initial treatment usually involves percutaneous drainage. If the lymphocele recurs, most surgeons would place a percutaneous external drain under ultrasound or CT guidance. **Percutaneous drainage with sclerosing agents** such as povidone-iodine can be used, but such treatment can have a directly toxic effect on the transplanted kidney. If the lymphocele reaccumulates and becomes symptomatic after removal of the external drain, **internal drainage** by marsupialization is indicated. The marsupialization involves fenestrating the peritoneum to drain the lymphocele into the peritoneal cavity. This can be done as an open procedure or laparoscopically with ultrasound guidance.

Ref.: 2

21. Which of the following statements regarding the immune response is true?

A. The primary immune response is more intense and rapid than the secondary immune response.

B. A cell-mediated immune response consists primarily of T lymphocytes.

C. T lymphocytes are the precursors of plasma cells, which produce antibodies.

D. The immune response has three phases, the first being the establishment of memory.

E. Immunoglobulins (IgG versus IgE versus IgM) are all identical except at the variable region.

ANSWER: B

COMMENTS: The **immune response** is characterized by a series of reactions triggered by an immunogen. Immunogens include substances recognized as foreign, or "nonself" (such as virus, bacteria, and histoincompatible tissues), as well as substances that are "altered-self" or "modified-self" (such as most tumor antigens). All immune responses, whether primary or secondary, are characterized by three phases: (1) **cognitive phase** (recognition of nonself antigen), (2) **activation phase** (proliferation of immunocompetent cells or lymphocytes), and (3) **effector phase** (development of immunologic memory). The primary immune response is the result of the first exposure to a specific antigen. The secondary response results from a second (or subsequent) exposure to the same antigen. It is more rapid and more intense than the primary response and is a result of the phenomenon of immunologic memory.

There are two basic types of immune responses: cell-mediated (or cellular immunity), which is mediated primarily by T lymphocytes, and humoral immune response, which is mediated primarily by B lymphocytes. **T lymphocytes** mature in the thymus from multipotent cells derived from the bone marrow.

B lymphocytes differentiate into antibody-producing plasma cells after activation. They develop in the fetal liver and the bone marrow. B lymphocytes are precursors of plasma cells and can be identified by specific antigen-binding sites on their surface. **Plasma cells** ultimately produce the antibodies (or immunoglobulins) that are found in serum and that may be transferred passively in serum. Within a subgroup of **immunoglobulins**, IgG versus another IgG, the variable portions consist of both the light and heavy chains. However, the number of chains is constant: an **IgG** has two heavy chains and two light chains joined by disulfide bonds that create a dimeric structure, whereas the **IgM** structure is made of multiple chains that create a pentamer.

Ref.: 12, 13

22. A 32-year-old woman is seen in the emergency department with an acute onset of confusion. Her laboratory work reveals markedly elevated transaminase levels, hyperbilirubinemia, and coagulopathy. Which of the following is not a potential indication for transplantation in a patient with fulminant hepatic failure?

A. Progressive jaundice over the past 2 weeks

B. Overdose of acetaminophen

C. Acute infection with hepatitis A virus (HAV)

D. Prothrombin time greater than 100 s

E. Acute fatty liver of pregnancy

ANSWER: A

COMMENTS: Fulminant hepatic failure can be caused by a multitude of injuries to the liver, including but not limited to acetaminophen toxicity and infection with HAV, hepatitis B virus (HBV), EBV, parvovirus, CMV, varicella-zoster virus (VZV), and herpes simplex virus. Other causes include *Bacillus cereus* infection; drug-induced liver injury by isoniazid, anabolic steroids, antiretroviral drugs, and other illicit drugs such as ecstasy; and pregnancy-related disorders (such as acute fatty liver of pregnancy and the syndrome of hemolysis, elevated liver enzymes, and low platelet count [HELLP]).

Though not standardized, most centers follow the criteria established by the **King's College Hospital** in London. The criteria in patients with acetaminophen overdose are persistent acidosis (pH < 7.30) *or* prothrombin time longer than 100 s *plus* serum creatinine levels greater than 300 μmol/L (>3.4 mg/dL) *and* grade 3 or 4 encephalopathy. In nonacetaminophen causes of fulminant hepatic failure, the criteria are a prothrombin time longer than 100 s irrespective of encephalopathy *or* any three of the following: cryptogenic hepatitis or other drug toxicity, age less than 10 years or more than 40 years, jaundice, duration of encephalopathy less than 7 days, prothrombin time longer than 50 s, or serum bilirubin level greater than 300 μmol/L (17.5 mg/dL). By definition, jaundice progressing over more than a 7-day period would exclude a diagnosis of fulminant hepatic failure even though the encephalopathy may be acute in onset.

Ref.: 26, 27

23. Mr. Smith is a 58-year-old man with chronic HBV cirrhosis who presents for OLT. His labs on the day of the transplant show absence of HBV DNA, presence of e antigen, and MELD score 29. Regarding his risk of recurrent HBV, which of the following statements in true?

A. Lamivudine is the preferred prophylaxis in this patient.

B. This patient's lab results have no bearing on his risk for recurrence.

C. This patient has a higher risk of recurrence than patients with fulminant HBV infection.

D. Hepatitis B immunoglobulin (HBIg) has no role in the posttransplant period.

E. This patient only has an indication for posttransplant prophylaxis.

ANSWER: C

COMMENTS: The major advances in prophylaxis and treatment of **HBV recurrence** after OLT have improved the overall survival rates: previously between 40% and 60%, now it is as high as 80% and 90% at 5 years. The optimal prophylaxis in patients with viral replication before OLT (such as the patient in this question given the presence of e antigen) is using an antiviral with a high genetic barrier to the development of resistance, such as entecavir or tenofovir, or the use of combinations of antivirals. Therefore using lamivudine or adefovir as single agents is ill advised given the high risk for resistance. Of note, however, in patients without viral replication before OLT, there is no evidence that preoperative antiviral therapy is useful.

Posttransplant therapy typically includes a combination of antivirals and HBIg. This combination approach reduces the HBV recurrence rate to 0%–10% at 1 to 2 years after OLT. HBIg likely acts by binding to and neutralizing circulating virions and by inhibiting cell-to-cell infection. However, the exact mechanism of action is not completely understood.

Patients with replicative disease at the time of transplant—those who test positive for e antigen or for HBV DNA—have an increased risk for recurrent infection. Alternatively, patients with fulminant hepatic failure secondary to HBV infection or those with hepatitis D coinfection have the lowest risk for the development of recurrent infection.

Ref.: 28

24. In a uremic diabetic patient who undergoes SPK transplantation, which of the following statements regarding the secondary complications of diabetes and pancreatic transplantation is true?

A. Diabetic retinopathy is irreversible; however, there is generally no further progression after pancreatic transplantation.

B. Recurrence of diabetic nephropathy in renal allografts is inevitable.

C. Diabetic neuropathy is irreversible; however, there is generally no further progression after pancreatic transplantation.

D. Advanced diabetic neuropathy is improved with pancreatic transplantation; however, overall survival rates in this patient population are unchanged.

E. Diabetic gastropathy is reversed by 3 years after transplantation.

ANSWER: A

COMMENTS: Diabetic retinopathy has not been shown to reverse with successful transplantation. Furthermore, stabilization of retinopathy takes 3 years after transplantation. During this time, this patient population should have a close ophthalmic follow-up, and if any indication for laser treatment for proliferative retinopathy develops, he or she should undergo the treatment. Interestingly, the early improvement in vision that is reported by patients is likely due to resolution of macular edema. This can be a result of either euglycemia from the pancreatic transplant or improved fluid balance from the simultaneous kidney transplant—or, most likely, a combination of both processes.

With normoglycemia after pancreatic transplantation, **diabetic nephropathy** can not only be halted but associated histologic changes can also be reversed. This reversal is seen in patients with normoglycemia for at least 5 years.

The combination of diabetes and severe neuropathy leads to a lower survival rate. Improvement in long-term glucose control results in improved neural function and subsequently improved survival rates. Patients with **neuropathy** have improvement in both motor and sensory indices following successful pancreatic transplantation, but it takes many months for this benefit to become evident. **Diabetic gastropathy** stabilizes but is not reversed by pancreatic transplantation.

Ref.: 3, 4

25. Which of the following statements is true regarding the deceased kidney allocation scheme (KAS)?

A. Wait time for point accrual in the KAS begins at the time of official referral to a transplant center.

B. Cadaveric renal allografts are allocated nationwide, as opposed to locally, if the donor organ matches all six HLA antigens of a recipient.

C. Previous living kidney donor status assigns the most points within the KAS and therefore the highest priority in order to allocate the next ABO-compatible allograft to that waitlist candidate.

D. Transplant candidates with panelreactive antibodies (PRA) results of 98%–100% are given no preferential treatment in the KAS. Unfortunately, this translates to a very low likelihood of undergoing transplantation.

E. The KAS takes into account details of the recipient only; the donor profile is reviewed by the surgeon on an individual, but not standardized, basis.

ANSWER: B

COMMENTS: A new **KAS** went into effect in December 2014 that focused on "longevity matching," which preferentially allocates the best quality of allografts to the transplant candidate with the longest predictive survival. Deceased allografts are given a **kidney donor profile index (KDPI)** based on 10 factors, such as donor age, specific medical history, cause of death, and most recent laboratory values. Waitlist candidates are assigned a score as well, the **expected posttransplant survival (EPTS)**. This is essentially a risk stratification of the recipient that takes into account four factors: age, dialysis duration, prior solid organ transplant, and diabetes status. The overall aim is to have patients with the top 20th percentile of EPTS receive organs with the top 20th percentile KDPI score. Furthermore, the KAS is based on a point system, within which a significant number of points given are based on the level of sensitization (or PRAs). After the KDPI and EPTS classes are established, **HLA sensitization** is given first preference. In fact, high PRAs (100%, 99%, and 98%) are allocated at the national, regional, and local levels, respectively.

Next preference is zero HLA mismatch. HLA antigens are inherited on chromosome 6, and although multiple HLA antigens have been identified, kidney recipients and donors undergo tissue typing for only three antigens: HLA-A, HLA-B, and HLA-DR. Since these antigens are inherited from each parent, usually as a codominant allele, offspring have two HLA-A antigens, two HLA-B antigens, and two HLA-DR antigens. **HLA matching** for all six antigens has resulted in improved long-term outcome in patients undergoing both living related and cadaveric renal transplantation. As a result, cadaveric organs that match for all six antigens are allocated nationwide.

Prior living donors get the next preference. In addition, in order to benefit candidates with limited resources who might be late to get on the transplant list, points accrued for wait time are given per year since the date of initiation of dialysis or the date of listing with GFR < 20 mL/min, whichever occurred first.

Ref.: 29

26. Six months after renal transplantation, a 56-year-old woman is admitted to the hospital with high fever, an elevated serum creatinine level, disseminated vesicular skin lesions, and bilateral pulmonary infiltrates. Which of the following statements is most accurate?

A. This is most likely due to primary VZV infection.

B. Superinfection with bacterial pneumonia is rare.

C. The gold standard of treatment for disseminated disease includes corticosteroids.

D. The immunosuppressive drug regimen should be maintained given the transplant was performed less than 1 year ago.

E. The initial treatment is varicella-zoster immune globulin.

ANSWER: A

COMMENTS: The incidence of **herpes zoster (shingles)** is 7.9% in renal transplant recipients, and it usually occurs during the first 9 months after transplantation as a result of high levels of immunosuppression. **Disseminated VZV**, usually due to **primary VZV infection**, is rare but can be associated with pneumonia, encephalitis, disseminated intravascular coagulation, and graft dysfunction.

Initially, intravenous—followed by oral—acyclovir usually prevents systemic dissemination and leads to rapid healing of the skin lesions. The levels of immunosuppressive agents should be drastically reduced to prevent death. Furthermore, if a seronegative transplant patient is inadvertently exposed to a person with shingles or VZV infection, varicella-zoster immune globulin should be given for prophylaxis.

Airborne and contact isolation is necessary to prevent the spread of infection to other patients. **Bronchoscopic examination** should be considered to rule out superinfection with bacterial, fungal, or other opportunistic organisms, especially if the patient does not respond to intravenous antivirals.

Ref.: 25

27. Which of the following statements is true regarding the immunosuppressive agent tacrolimus?

A. It inhibits T cells by inhibiting de novo purine synthesis.

B. It is better to use in posttransplant liver patients who have baseline chronic kidney disease.

C. It is not a maintenance immunosuppressive agent; rather, it is used for induction and refractory acute rejection.

D. It reduces the synthesis of IL-2 and IFN-γ as well as inhibits secretion of IL-1 from macrophages.

E. It is associated with significantly fewer episodes of acute steroid-resistant or refractory rejection.

ANSWER: E

COMMENTS: Tacrolimus was first isolated from *Streptomyces tsukubaensis*. It is approximately 100 times more potent than cyclosporine. Large number of studies have demonstrated that tacrolimus was associated with significantly fewer episodes of acute steroid-resistant or refractory rejection. It first binds to the immunophilin FK506–binding protein, which then binds to calcineurin to form a larger complex. **Calcineurin** is a calcium-dependent protein that plays a crucial role in the activation of transcription of the IL-2 gene within T cells. Inhibition prevents further phosphorylation and stops the second messenger cycle, thereby halting T-cell activation and proliferation. It can be nephrotoxic; therefore its use in liver recipients with significant chronic kidney disease should be determined on a case-by-case basis. It is not used for induction or refractory acute rejection. **Steroids**, such as prednisone, decrease the synthesis of IL-2 and IFN-γ. They also inhibit the secretion of IL-1 from macrophages.

Ref.: 12, 20

28. Which of the following statements regarding interferons is true?

A. IFN-γ is produced by macrophages.

B. Interferon production is inhibited by infection.

C. Interferons have a direct antiproliferative effect on T_H2 cells.

D. Cytokine production by macrophages is inhibited by interferons.

E. Pegylated interferon-α (PEG–IFN-α) is a highly effective and easily tolerated treatment option for HCV liver disease.

ANSWER: C

COMMENTS: Interferons are glycoproteins produced by a variety of cells in response to viral infection or other stimulants. Interferons block viruses in two ways: through signaling pathways and by inhibition of the translation machinery (protein synthesis). The three major classifications of interferons are based on their cells of origin: **interferon-α**, produced mainly by macrophages; **interferon-β**, produced by epithelial cells, fibroblasts, and macrophages; and **interferon-γ**, produced by T lymphocytes and NK cells. Interferons have a direct antiproliferative effect on cells but can also induce differentiation. Interferons decrease the activity of T_H2 cells but promote the differentiation of immature CD4+ cells into committed T_H1 cells. This explains their usefulness as anticancer agents, although some anticancer effects may also result from stimulation of the cytotoxic activity of macrophages, NK cells, and cytotoxic T cells. Interferons stimulate a variety of cells to release other mediators and cytokines.

Dual therapy with PEG–IFN-α and ribavirin was the gold standard treatment for patients infected with HCV. The reported SVR rate after 24 or 48 weeks of treatment was only 42%–84%, depending on the specific genotype. In addition, PEG–IFN-α has many side effects that make patients intolerant or even ineligible for treatment. However, interferon-based therapy is becoming second line since the emergence of new oral DAA medications such as sofosbuvir. Multiple randomized controlled trials have shown that sofosbuvir and ribavirin regimens have higher SVR and greater tolerability with even shorter treatment periods, such as 12-week courses.

Ref.: 13, 14, 30, 31

29. Which of the following statements regarding liver ischemia–reperfusion injury is true?

A. Cold ischemia is more deleterious to sinusoidal endothelial cells (SECs) than to hepatocytes.

B. Warm ischemia time between 90 and 120 min is typically well tolerated.

C. Activated proteases, like calpain, are responsible for the increased intracellular calcium concentration seen during cold ischemia time.

D. The significant increase in superoxide radical production is seen mostly during cold ischemia time.

E. During warm ischemia time, the supply of ATP decreases, while the demand remains the same.

ANSWER: A

COMMENTS: The period of time between flushing the allograft with cold preservation solution during procurement and packaging it with ice for transport until eventually transferring it into the recipient operative field is deemed the **cold ischemia time**. There are multiple mechanisms during cold ischemia that cause a depletion of ATP and instigate cellular death. First, aerobic metabolism changes to anaerobic, which decreases the amount of ATP production by 19-fold. Second, intracellular acidosis develops due to the end product of anaerobic glycolysis, which inevitably inhibits key glycolytic enzymes and blocks further anaerobic energy production. Intracellular acidosis and depletion of ATP activate many pathways that lead to increased intracellular calcium, cellular membrane permeability, and cell death. Third, increased intracellular calcium concentrations activate important proteases such as calpain (a nonlysosomal cysteine protease) and matrix metalloproteinases (MMPs). These proteases interrupt the protective endothelial layer of glycoproteins, which expose and activate SEC surfaces. These exposed and activated surfaces are the prerequisite for platelet and leukocyte adhesion, which are the beginning of a sterile inflammatory immune response after reperfusion. This mechanism may explain why SECs are significantly more affected than hepatocytes by cold ischemia time. Finally, hypoxanthine is a degradation product of ATP and inevitably forms **superoxide radicals** when further degraded in the presence of oxygen. Ischemia promotes the conversion of specific oxidases to increase this reaction; however, it is quite slow during cold preservation given the short supply of molecular oxygen. Upon organ reperfusion, this mechanism drastically increases superoxide radical production, which is highly toxic to liver cells via cell membrane damage by lipid peroxidation.

The period between bringing the allograft into the operative field for the recipient vascular anastomoses and actually finishing the anastomoses to reperfuse the organ is deemed the **warm ischemia time**. The liver core temperature progressively increases to 12°C, 17°C, and 20°C after 30, 40, and 50 min, respectively. During this time, the higher temperature results in a higher energy demand; however, it further depletes ATP because it is still under anoxic conditions. Because hepatocytes have high energy demands at 20°C, warm ischemia time is more deleterious to them as opposed to SECs. Very long periods (>90 min) of rewarming alone have the potential to result in organ failure.

Ref.: 22

30. Which of the following statements regarding T-cell activation is true?

A. Antigen recognition is not specific, which allows clonal expansion and differentiation.

B. Antigen expression requires the T cells to be MHC compatible with the antigen-presenting cells.

C. T cells produce IL-1 in response to antigen presentation.

D. Plasma cells are responsible for the synthesis of IL-2.

E. T cells recognize soluble antigens.

ANSWER: B

COMMENTS: When an antigen enters a lymph node or the spleen, it may first be phagocytized by a macrophage, which processes the antigen and expresses it on the cell surface for presentation to B and T cells. Macrophages that do this are called antigen-presenting cells (APCs). Other APC**s** include dendritic cells (a macrophage-like cell found in the skin, lymph nodes, and other tissues) and a subset of B lymphocytes. Recognition of the antigen is highly specific and accomplished only by T lymphocyte clones that have a receptor specific to that antigen. T cells also require interaction with the MHC of the APC; they do not directly recognize unbound circulating antigens. When the antigen is presented to the T cells, *macrophages* produce IL-1 while T cells produce IL-2 and increase the expression of IL-2 receptors on the surface. This activation by IL-2 causes T cells to proliferate.

Ref.: 12, 13

31. A 26-year-old man is found to be brain-dead after a gunshot wound to the head. His family consents to organ donation. Which of the following is a contraindication to organ donation?

A. Positive hepatitis B core antibody

B. Active hepatitis C

C. History of basal cell carcinoma 5 years ago

D. Donor liver biopsy with 10% steatosis

E. Creutzfeldt–Jakob disease

ANSWER: E

COMMENTS: There are both absolute and relative contraindications to **organ donation. Absolute contraindications** include transmissible agents that may cause death or severe disease in the recipient. These include Creutzfeldt–Jakob disease and other prion diseases such as kuru. Other contraindications include disseminated or invasive viral infections, mycobacterial infections, fungal infections, or systemic bacterial infections such as methicillin-resistant *Staphylococcus aureus* (MRSA). Interestingly, human immunodeficiency virus (HIV) is no longer an absolute contraindication to organ donation due to the bill, the HIV Organ Policy Equity Act, which was passed by the U.S. Senate in 2013. The first liver transplantation (and the first U.S. kidney transplantation) from an HIV-positive donor to HIV-positive recipients occurred at Johns Hopkins Hospital in March 2016.

Active malignancy is an absolute contraindication to donation. Low-grade skin cancers such as basal cell carcinoma do not exclude a donor. Five-year disease-free survival in the donor from any cancer is considered cured by United Network for Organ Sharing (UNOS). However, the type and biological behavior of the tumor should be considered. Late recurrence is seen with breast and lung cancer, and therefore additional caution is warranted even beyond the 5-year disease-free interval.

Relative contraindications include age of the donor, hepatic steatosis, damaged organs, infection, and viral infection. Age more than 60 years places a donated organ in the extended-criteria category. Steatosis greater than 60% has an unacceptably high risk for primary nonfunction and is contraindicated. However, livers with steatosis of less than 30% have not been shown to have higher rates of nonfunction or lower graft survival rates than nonfatty livers.

Liver transplantation from hepatitis B core antibody–positive donors results in a 22%–100% seroconversion rate in hepatitis B core antibody-negative recipients. HBV-positive livers can be transplanted with concurrent postoperative treatment with HBIg and lamivudine. The ideal recipient for a hepatitis B core antibody–positive donor is a patient who already has hepatitis B and would undergo treatment after transplantation regardless of donor status. Likewise, donors with hepatitis C should donate to hepatitis C–positive recipients. Historically, the disease was transmitted universally; recipients with hepatitis C inevitably reinfected the new liver even if it was hepatitis C negative. However, the new DAAs for hepatitis C may change this; it is yet to be determined.

Ref.: 32, 33

32. The incidence of primary nonfunction of a liver allograft following transplantation ranges from 2% to 10%. Immediately after the liver transplantation procedure, which of the following is associated with this clinical syndrome?

A. Metabolic alkalosis

B. Hyperkalemia

C. Hypertensive crisis

D. Low-output heart failure

E. Excessive bile output (if a T-tube biliary drainage catheter is in place)

ANSWER: B

COMMENTS: Primary nonfunction of a liver allograft is a poorly understood clinical syndrome associated with markedly abnormal function of the allograft, manifesting with severe coagulopathy, acidosis, hyperkalemia, poor mental status, continued hyperdynamic cardiac function with high cardiac output, low systemic vascular resistance with liver failure, poor bile output, and usually renal failure. Recipients with normally functioning grafts have marked metabolic alkalosis secondary to metabolism of the citrate component of bicarbonate (from banked blood given during the transplant procedure) by the liver graft during the immediate posttransplant period. Within the first 24 h of liver transplantation, patients with normally functioning grafts return to normal cardiac hemodynamics.

The most specific pretransplant predictor of primary nonfunction is the amount of **macrosteatosis** (extracellular fat globules) in the liver allograft. Studies have shown that when greater than 30% of the cross-sectional area of a liver biopsy specimen exhibits macrosteatosis, the incidence of primary dysfunction may reach 13%. Other possible predictors of primary nonfunction include high levels of vasopressor support in the donor and longer cold ischemia time. Although a variety of strategies have been used in attempts to ameliorate this syndrome, the only treatment is prompt retransplantation.

Ref.: 34

33. Which of the following statements is true?

A. Infection with CMV following kidney transplantation is the strongest predictor of poor long-term survival.

B. The incidence of symptomatic CMV infection is declining secondary to the use of screening tests.

C. Patients at highest risk for the development of CMV infection are those who test seropositive for CMV IgG.

D. CMV infection is more likely than infection with polyomavirus (BK) to cause chronic allograft nephropathy.

E. CMV infection can be indistinguishable from acute EBV infection.

ANSWER: B

COMMENTS: With the development of the effective antiviral agent ganciclovir, acute rejection—not CMV infection—is now the strongest predictor of poor allograft survival. The incidence of CMV infection is declining probably because of very effective tests for viral load in the serum, such as CMV pp65 antigen and CMV DNA testing, as well as early prophylaxis. Patients who are at the highest risk for CMV are those who test seronegative for CMV IgG and receive an allograft from a donor seropositive for CMV IgG. CMV infection is usually an acute, systemic infection that can result in gastritis, hepatitis, pneumonitis, retinitis, and bone marrow suppression. CMV infection rarely involves only one *organ* and seldom causes chronic nephropathy.

Infection with **polyomavirus** is usually isolated to the kidney and the urinary system. BK virus can cause nephropathy in the transplanted kidney. Active infection is associated with progressive loss of graft function, a condition also known as polyomavirus-associated nephropathy. Acute infection with **EBV** generally causes inflammation of the gastrointestinal tract in the form of gastritis, enteritis, or colitis and is thus clinically similar to CMV infection. The two can easily be distinguished by checking serum viral loads with quantitative CMV DNA and EBV DNA testing. In addition, biopsy specimens from inflamed gastrointestinal mucosa can be specifically stained for each virus.

Ref.: 35

34. Which of the following would exclude a patient with HCC from becoming a transplant candidate?

A. A single 1-cm lesion in the liver with microvascular invasion

B. Two lesions, each less than 2 cm

C. A solitary 1-cm HCC lesion in the lung

D. A single 4.8-cm HCC lesion in segment VIII

E. Portal vein thrombus

ANSWER: C

COMMENTS: OLT is an excellent option for stage I and stage II HCC. It has an advantage over resection because of the multifactorial nature of **HCC**. In addition, resection is often not feasible because approximately 80%–90% of patients with HCC also have cirrhosis. OLT allows excision of the tumor and removal of the underlying disease, which should decrease the likelihood of recurrence. OLT can be considered for any stage I or stage II tumor. This limits OLT to patients without distant metastases and to those with negative lymph nodes and either T1 or T2 disease. T1 disease is a solitary tumor without vascular invasion (regardless of size). T2 disease is a solitary tumor with vascular invasion or a combination of tumors all less than 5 cm in size. These groupings were developed on the basis of the way in which these tumors behave.

Conventionally, OLT is an option for tumors that fall within the Milan criteria. The Milan criteria are a solitary tumor less than 5 cm in diameter or multiple tumors up to three in number, all smaller than 3 cm. However, there have been multiple studies that showed the same survival rate with extended criteria, such as the University of California San Francisco (UCSF) criteria and the Dallas criteria. If expanded tumor inclusion criteria are used, pretransplant ablation therapy is recommended in order to achieve good posttransplant outcomes.

Distant metastasis is an absolute contraindication to transplantation. Portal vein thrombosis is a relative contraindication to transplantation. If it is due to HCC, it is a contraindication. If it is from bland portal vein thrombi, then OLT is still an option. Unfortunately, differentiating the two is a diagnostic challenge.

Ref.: 17, 36

REFERENCES

1. Markmann JF, Yeh HA, Naji A, et al. Transplantation of abdominal organs. In: Townsend Jr CM, Beauchamp RD, Evers BM, Mattox KL, eds. *Sabiston Textbook of Surgery: The Biological Basis of Modern Surgical Practice*. 18th ed. Philadelphia: WB Saunders; 2008.
2. Allen RD. Vascular complication after kidney transplantation. In: Morris PJ, Knechtle SJ, eds. *Kidney Transplantation: Principles and Practice*. 6th ed. Philadelphia: WB Saunders; 2008.
3. Gruessner AC, Gruessner RWG. Pancreas and kidney transplantation for diabetic nephropathy. In: Morris PJ, Knechtle SJ, eds. *Kidney Transplantation: Principles and Practice*. 7th ed. Philadelphia: PA. Elsevier Saunders; 2014[Chapter 36].
4. Akyol M. Pancreas transplantation. In: Forsythe JL, ed. *Transplantation: Companion to Specialist Surgical Practice*. 5th ed. Philadelphia: WB Saunders; 2014.
5. Kamath PS, Kim WR. The model for end-stage liver disease (MELD). *Hepatology*. 2007;45(3):797–805.
6. U.S. Department of Health and Human Services. Organ Procurement and Transplantation Network. Revised Liver Policy Regarding HCC Exception Scores. HRSA. Available at: https://optn.transplant.hrsa.gov/news/revised-liver-policy-regarding-hcc-exception-scores/. Accessed October 6, 2015.
7. Khwaja K, Pomfret EA. The current allocation system (MELD). In: Busuttil RW, Klintmalm GK, eds. *Transplantation of the Liver*. 3rd ed. Philadelphia: WB Saunders; 2015.
8. Busuttil RW, DiNorcia J, Kaldas FM. Positive viral serologic results in extended criteria donors. In: Busuttil RW, Klintmalm GK, eds. *Transplantation of the Liver*. 3rd ed. Philadelphia: WB Saunders; 2015.
9. Kasiske BE, Israni AJ. Cardiovascular Complications after renal transplantation. In: Morris PJ, Knechtle SJ, eds. *Kidney Transplantation: Principles and Practice*. 6th ed. Philadelphia: WB Saunders; 2008.
10. Davis GL. Recurrent hepatitis C after transplantation. In: Busuttil RW, Klintmalm GK, eds. *Transplantation of the Liver*. 3rd ed. Philadelphia: WB Saunders; 2015.
11. Cholongitas E, Pipili C, Papatheodoridis G. Interferon-free regimens for the treatment of hepatitis C virus in liver transplant candidates or recipients. *World J Gastroenterol*. 2015;21(32):9526–9533.
12. Grainger DK, Ildstad ST. Transplantation immunology and immunosuppression. In: Townsend Jr CM, Beauchamp RD, Evers BM, Mattox KL, eds. *Sabiston Textbook of Surgery: The Biological Basis of Modern Surgical Practice*. 18th ed. Philadelphia: WB Saunders; 2008.
13. Bromberg JS, Magee JC. Transplant immunology. In: Mulholland MW, Lillemoe KD, Doherty GM, et al., eds. *Greenfield's Surgery: Scientific Principles and Practice*. 4th ed. Philadelphia: Lippincott Williams & Wilkins; 2006.
14. Alarcon LH, Fink MP. Mediators of the inflammatory response. In: Townsend Jr CM, Beauchamp RD, Evers BM, Mattox KL, eds. *Sabiston Textbook of Surgery: The Biological Basis of Modern Surgical Practice*. 18th ed. Philadelphia: WB Saunders; 2008.

15. Lin HC, Alonso EM, Superina RA, et al. General criteria for transplantation in children. In: Busuttil RW, Klintmalm GK, eds. *Transplantation of the Liver*. 3rd ed. Philadelphia: WB Saunders; 2015.
16. Gallego-Orozco JF, Campsen J. Posttransplant lymphoproliferative disorder in transplant-related malignancies. In: Busuttil RW, Klintmalm GK, eds. *Transplantation of the Liver*. 3rd ed. Philadelphia: WB Saunders; 2015.
17. Khungar V, Fox AN, Brown RS. Current indications, contraindications, delisting criteria, and timing for transplantation. In: Busuttil RW, Klintmalm GK, eds. *Transplantation of the Liver*. 3rd ed. Philadelphia: WB Saunders; 2015.
18. Steadman RH, Ramsay MA. Portopulmonary hypertension and hepatopulmonary syndrome. In: Busuttil RW, Klintmalm GK, eds. *Transplantation of the Liver*. 3rd ed. Philadelphia: WB Saunders; 2015.
19. Schnickel GT, Busuttil RW. Diagnosis and operative strategy in portal vein thrombosis and other venous anomalies. In: Busuttil RW, Klintmalm GK, eds. *Transplantation of the Liver*. 3rd ed. Philadelphia: WB Saunders; 2015.
20. McKenna GJ, Klintmalm GB. Induction and maintenance of immunosuppresion. In: Busuttil RW, Klintmalm GK, eds. *Transplantation of the Liver*. 3rd ed. Philadelphia: WB Saunders; 2015.
21. Shah VH, Kamath PS. Portal hypertension and variceal bleeding. In: Feldman M, Friedman LS, Brandt LJ, eds. *Sleisenger and Fordtran's Gastrointestinal and Liver Disease*. 10th ed. Philadelphia: WB Saunders; 2016.
22. Petrowsky H, Clavien PA. Principles of liver preservation. In: Busuttil RW, Klintmalm GK, eds. *Transplantation of the Liver*. 3rd ed. Philadelphia: WB Saunders; 2015.
23. Fuggle SV, Taylor CJ. Histocompatibility in renal transplantation. In: Morris PJ, Knechtle SJ, eds. *Kidney Transplantation: Principles and Practice*. 6th ed. Philadelphia: WB Saunders; 2008.
24. Stegall MD, Gloor JM. Transplantation in the sensitized recipient and across ABO blood groups. In: Morris PJ, Knechtle SJ, eds. *Kidney Transplantation: Principles and Practice*. 6th ed. Philadelphia: WB Saunders; 2008.
25. Holt CD, Winston DJ. Viral infections after transplantation. In: Busuttil RW, Klintmalm GK, eds. *Transplantation of the Liver*. 3rd ed. Philadelphia: WB Saunders; 2015.
26. Durazo FA, Ton MJ. Unusual indications for transplantation. In: Busuttil RW, Klintmalm GK, eds. *Transplantation of the Liver*. 3rd ed. Philadelphia: WB Saunders; 2015.
27. O'Grady J. Transplantation for fulminant hepatic failure. In: Busuttil RW, Klintmalm GK, eds. *Transplantation of the Liver*. 3rd ed. Philadelphia: WB Saunders; 2015.
28. Roche B, Samuel D. Transplantation for hepatitis A and B. In: Busuttil RW, Klintmalm GK, eds. *Transplantation of the Liver*. 3rd ed. Philadelphia: WB Saunders; 2015.
29. Chopra B, Sureshkumar KK. Changing organ allocation policy for kidney transplantation in the United States. *World J Transplant*. 2015;5(2):38–43.
30. Gonzalez SA, Davis GL. Antiviral therapy in natural history of hepatitis C. In: Busuttil RW, Klintmalm GK, eds. *Transplantation of the Liver*. 3rd ed. Philadelphia: WB Saunders; 2015.
31. World Health Organization. Guidelines for the screening, care, and treatment of persons with hepatitis C infection. Available at: http://www.who.int/hiv/pub/hepatitis/hepatitis-c-guidelines/en/. Accessed April 2014.
32. Burroughs SG, Burnett SK, Ghobrial RM. Donor selection and management. In: Busuttil RW, Klintmalm GK, eds. *Transplantation of the Liver*. 3rd ed. Philadelphia: WB Saunders; 2015.
33. Sifferlin A. First transplant from HIV-positive donor performed in U.S. *Time Magazine*. 30 March 2016. Available at: http://time.com/4276422/first-transplant-from-hiv-positive-donor-performed-in-u-s/.
34. Petrowsky H, Busuttil RW. Graft failure. In: Busuttil RW, Klintmalm GK, eds. *Transplantation of the Liver*. 3rd ed. Philadelphia: WB Saunders; 2015.
35. Fishman JA, Davis JO. Infection in renal transplant recipients. In: Morris PJ, Knechtle SJ, eds. *Kidney Transplantation: Principles and Practice*. 6th ed. Philadelphia: WB Saunders; 2008.
36. Onaca N, Stone MJ, Fulmer JM, Klintmalm GB. Transplantation for primary hepatic malignancy. In: Busuttil RW, Klintmalm GK, eds. *Transplantation of the Liver*. 3rd ed. Philadelphia: WB Saunders; 2015.

CHAPTER 7

PERIOPERATIVE CARE AND ANESTHESIA

Behnoosh Shayegan, M.D., and David M. Rothenberg, M.D.

A. Perioperative Care

1. Maintaining perioperative serum glucose levels between 80 and 110 mg/dL in diabetic patients undergoing cardiac surgery may:

A. Have no effect on postoperative complications

B. Increase the incidence of deep sternal wound infections

C. Increase the incidence of hypoglycemia

D. Promote osmotic diuresis

E. Decrease in-hospital mortality

ANSWER: C

COMMENTS: Diabetes mellitus impairs wound healing due to the effects of hyperglycemia and macrovascular and microvascular disease–induced tissue hypoperfusion. Hyperglycemia is a known risk factor for postoperative deep sternal wound infection because it alters the normal physiologic response to infection. It is associated with impaired phagocytosis, lymphocyte dysfunction, immunoglobulin inactivation, activation of the complement component C3, and impaired deposition of collagen in wounds. In this regard, a tight control of blood glucose levels during the postoperative period may improve wound healing and reduce the incidence of postoperative sternal wound infections. Sternal wound infection rates approach those found in nondiabetic patients when blood glucose levels are maintained less than 180 to 200 mg%. Correction of the blood glucose levels to normal may restore both neutrophil chemotaxis and phagocytosis and may increase $CD4^+$ cell counts, often found to be depressed in patients with poorly controlled diabetes. Although studies support the postoperative benefit of tight glucose control, it is difficult to discern the beneficial effects of lowering serum glucose versus those of insulin itself, as insulin plays the role of an antiinflammatory and antioxidant hormone. In a 2012 Cochrane Database analysis, tight glucose control was not associated with a significant reduction in hospital mortality, but there was an increased risk of hypoglycemia, which could, if not monitored properly, negate the beneficial effects of normoglycemia.

Ref.: 1–3

2. In addition to determining blood glucose levels, the perioperative management of a patient with diet-controlled diabetes mellitus should include which of the following considerations?

A. Determination of glycosylated hemoglobin (HbA1c) level before surgery

B. Subcutaneous administration of regular insulin for glucose levels above 140 mg%

C. Metformin initiated 3 days prior to surgery

D. Intravenous (IV) insulin therapy 1 h prior to surgery

E. Oral liquid carbohydrate initiated 3 h prior to surgery

ANSWER: A

COMMENTS: Patients with diet-controlled diabetes mellitus do not require any special preoperative measures other than monitoring serum glucose. Initiating insulin and/or oral hypoglycemic drugs is not necessary, and they may cause hypoglycemia. Oral hypoglycemic agents stimulate insulin secretion (sulfonylurea) or decrease intestinal absorption (metformin). Patients should withhold these the morning of surgery to prevent perioperative hypoglycemia, and, in particular, metformin should not be administered as it has been associated with drug-induced lactic acidosis. Increasing carbohydrate consumption will cause hyperglycemia and may place the patient at risk of osmotic diuresis, electrolyte imbalance, and possible infection. HbA1c accounts for 4%–7% of the total hemoglobin. Poor control of diabetes mellitus will result in higher HbA1c levels. Data suggest that patients undergoing elective surgery should have their procedure postponed until HbA1c levels are less than 9%.

Ref.: 4, 5

3. When evaluating a patient with known or suspected adrenal insufficiency, which of the following statements is false?

A. Glucocorticoid therapy should be adjusted in response to the anticipated surgical stress.

B. Signs and symptoms of acute adrenal insufficiency may mimic those of septic shock.

C. Hypernatremia, hypokalemia, and hypoglycemia commonly occur.

D. Sudden development of hypotension requires hydrocortisone 50 to 100 mg IV.

E. Dexamethasone does not interfere with the corticotropin stimulation test.

ANSWER: C

COMMENTS: Adrenal insufficiency may be classified as primary or secondary. The main causes of secondary insufficiency include exogenous glucocorticoids, operative correction of endogenous hyperadrenalism, and abnormalities of the hypothalamus or pituitary gland. The hypothalamus secretes corticotropin-releasing factor, which stimulates the anterior pituitary to release adrenocorticotropic hormone (ACTH). ACTH stimulates the adrenal production of cortisol. Cortisol activates a negative feedback mechanism that affects both the hypothalamus and the anterior pituitary. Acute or relative adrenal insufficiency is a rare condition that may be manifested clinically as septic shock. It is associated with hypotension, nausea, vomiting, abdominal pain, weakness, and dizziness. Hyponatremia and hyperkalemia are often manifested due to the loss of mineralocorticoid and glucocorticoid secretion. The diagnosis should be considered in any patient with a history of tuberculosis or any patient undergoing long-term glucocorticoid therapy. While diagnostic studies are being considered, suspected adrenal insufficiency should be treated with 50 to 100 mg of hydrocortisone or its equivalent. Dexamethasone may also be used and has the benefit of not interfering with the ACTH stimulation test, but it lacks the mineralocorticoid effect of hydrocortisone. Laboratory studies should include determinations of serum cortisol, electrolytes, blood urea nitrogen, and creatinine levels, as well as a complete blood count (CBC). If blood pressure fails to return to normal within 2 h of administration of the hydrocortisone, other diagnoses should be considered. If adrenal insufficiency is supported by the patient's response to hydrocortisone and a serum cortisol level of less than 20 mg/dL, an ACTH stimulation test may be used to confirm the diagnosis, but it is often unnecessary. A normal response includes a baseline cortisol level greater than 20 mg/dL and an elevation of the cortisol level of at least 7 mg/dL following an ACTH bolus. A patient who demonstrates a normal response to ACTH stimulation (i.e., a cortisol level > 600 mg/L at 30 min) does not require additional glucocorticoid therapy. An abnormal response to ACTH stimulation indicates that either the hypothalamic-pituitary-adrenal (HPA) axis is not intact or the adrenal gland is insufficient or both. In patients for whom surgical intervention results in the need for perioperative glucocorticoid therapy, the ACTH stimulation test can be used to determine when the function of the HPA axis normalizes.

Ref.: 6

4. A patient with a history of glucocorticoid-dependent rheumatoid arthritis is scheduled for colon resection. Which of the following statements is false?

A. Intraoperative hypoperfusion should be treated with hydrocortisone 100 mg IV.

B. The patient is at an increased risk of infection.

C. The patient may benefit from concomitantly administered epidural analgesia.

D. An ACTH stimulation test may be indicated prior to elective reversal of the colostomy.

E. Etomidate may be safely administered for anesthesia induction and maintenance.

ANSWER: E

COMMENTS: Long-term corticosteroid (CS) therapy will likely suppress the HPA and, in turn, may lead to acute adrenal insufficiency during periods of stress. If acute adrenal insufficiency is present, the patient should improve following hydrocortisone administration. Patients maintained on CSs are at an increased risk of postoperative infection, impaired wound healing, increased skin friability, and gastrointestinal bleeding. Epidural anesthesia reduces the perioperative stress response in patients at risk of adrenal insufficiency. The ACTH stimulation test assesses the integrity of the HPA axis. Although a negative test result indicates that perioperative CSs are not necessary, a positive result indicates that CS replacement therapy may be helpful, but it does not predict the clinical response to surgical stress. There is considerable variation in cortisol secretion among individuals undergoing surgery. However, cortisol secretion rates greater than 200 mg/day on the first postoperative day are rare. Patients who have received more than 80 mg/day of hydrocortisone or its equivalent for longer than 3 weeks may be considered to be at risk of the HPA-axis suppression. They require perioperative stress therapy with 50 to 100 mg of hydrocortisone, followed by 100 to 150 mg in three divided doses. Tapering to preoperative maintenance doses may be accomplished in 2 to 3 days depending on the patient's hemodynamic status. The anesthetic induction drug etomidate is a sedative-hypnotic that inhibits the 11β-hydroxylase enzyme that converts 11β-deoxycortisol into cortisol and predictably reduces cortisol synthesis for up to 48 h after a single intubating dose and is contraindicated in patients chronically treated with CSs. This agent is often used by paramedical personnel to intubate the trachea for respiratory failure in the field and should be suspected as a contributory factor in patients with persistent hemodynamic compromise in the setting of failed resuscitation.

Ref.: 7, 8

5. Which of the following statements concerning perioperative management of patients with pheochromocytoma is false?

A. α-Adrenergic blockade with phenoxybenzamine may require 2 to 4 weeks of therapy.

B. β-blockade is useful as a primary antihypertensive agent.

C. Clinical criteria confirm adequate α-adrenergic blockade.

D. Intraoperative hypotension following resection of the tumor is best treated with vasopressin and/or methylene blue.

E. Sevoflurane is the preferred anesthetic agent vs. desflurane.

ANSWER: B

COMMENTS: Preoperative management of patients with pheochromocytoma requires control of hypertension and effective arterial blood volume. α-Adrenergic blockade is imperative in preventing intraoperative hypertensive crises and improving the ability to restore intravascular volume following tumor excision. Phenoxybenzamine is the drug most commonly used for α-adrenergic blockade. Therapy may be required for 2 to 4 weeks and is considered effective when symptoms have disappeared, blood pressure < 160/90 mmHg, orthostatic hypotension is resolved, no ST-segment changes are noted on electrocardiogram (ECG), and there are no more than five premature ventricular contractions per minute. If a patient's symptoms have not resolved or if the pulse is higher than 100 beats/min, β-adrenergic blockade therapy is added. β-Adrenergic blockers should not be used for tachycardia until α-adrenergic blockade has been established, or a hypertensive crisis can occur. Other classes of medications have been investigated, including α_1-antagonists and calcium channel blockers. Calcium channel blockade may be particularly effective in patients with coronary vasospasm. Once the catecholamine-secreting tumor is removed, persistent vasodilation may result in hypovolemia, thereby increasing the need for aggressive IV fluid therapy. In this regard, invasive central venous or pulmonary artery catheter monitoring and transesophageal echocardiography are often necessary. Intraoperative hypertension is treated with sodium nitroprusside, nicardipine, nitroglycerin, fenoldopam, and/or magnesium, which is a potent catecholamine receptor–release inhibitor. Cardiac arrhythmias are best treated with short-acting β-blockers such as esmolol. Vasopressin is most effective to treat perioperative hypotension; however, methylene blue has been shown to be useful for more severe vasoplegic states. Desflurane is best avoided as it is associated with an increase in sympathetic stimulation.

Ref.: 9, 10

6. A 33-year-old woman is scheduled for elective cholecystectomy. Preoperative evaluation shows the presence of moderate hypothyroidism. Select the next most appropriate action:

A. Proceed with surgery with the knowledge that minor perioperative complications could develop.

B. Postpone surgery until a euthyroid state is achieved.

C. Proceed with surgery while beginning treatment with levothyroxine.

D. Proceed with surgery while beginning treatment with thioamides.

E. Proceed with surgery if severe clinical symptoms are not present.

ANSWER: B

COMMENTS: Mild to moderate hypothyroidism is a diagnosis that applies to patients who are not in myxedema coma and do not exhibit severe clinical symptoms. Systolic and diastolic myocardial function is impaired in patients with chronic hypothyroidism, with congestive heart failure occasionally occurring in hypothyroid patients in the absence of underlying heart disease. Hypothyroidism causes a decrease in cardiac output by reducing the heart rate and contractility. Patients with hypothyroidism are predisposed to pericardial effusion and may have a higher incidence of atherosclerotic heart disease. Hypoventilation may be present because of respiratory muscle weakness and impaired pulmonary response to hypoxia and hypercapnia. These patients have decreased gut motility, constipation, and hyponatremia because of a reduction in the clearance of free water. Hypothyroidism is also associated with a decrease in red blood cell mass, which causes normochromic normocytic anemia. Although elective procedures may be performed on these patients safely, they are at an increased risk for hypotension and congestive heart failure, along with postoperative gastrointestinal and neuropsychiatric complications. Elective operations should be postponed in these patients, but urgent or emergency ones can be performed, provided that thyroid replacement is begun with levothyroxine. Thioamides are used for the treatment of hyperthyroidism.

Ref.: 11

7. Which of the following drugs is not recommended for the perioperative management of thyroid storm?

A. Propranolol

B. Propylthiouracil

C. Iodine solution

D. Aspirin

E. Acetaminophen

ANSWER: D

COMMENTS: Like patients with hypothyroidism, patients with hyperthyroidism should also not undergo elective surgery until clinical euthyroidism has been achieved. β-Blockers (propranolol) will control the symptoms of increased adrenergic tone, whereas thioamides (propylthiouracil) will block the synthesis of a new hormone. Iodine solution (iopanoic acid) has been used both to decrease the vascularity of the gland and to block the release of thyroid hormone. Acetaminophen is preferred over aspirin to treat hyperpyrexia because aspirin may increase serum levels of free thyroxine (T4) and triiodothyronine (T3) by interfering with protein binding. In emergency situations, hydration; cooling blankets; and a combination of CS, β-blockade, and iopanoic acid therapy can restore patients to an acceptable state of euthyroidism even if this treatment does not normalize thyroid-stimulating hormone levels. It may be difficult to differentiate thyroid storm from malignant hyperthermia. A medical history, clinical symptoms, and routine laboratory tests are necessary. A clinical score to assess the likelihood of thyroid storm has been suggested, and this involves the use of seven clinical variables: body temperature, heart rate, central nervous system (CNS) symptoms, gastrointestinal symptoms, congestive heart failure, atrial fibrillation, and jaundice. Total scores exceeding 45 were indicative of thyroid storm.

Ref.: 12–14

8. Which of the following statements is true regarding the use of epidural anesthesia/analgesia (EA) in patients with severe chronic obstructive pulmonary disease (COPD) who are undergoing abdominal surgery when compared with the use of perioperative opiates?

A. The use of EA is associated with a decrease in postoperative pneumonia.

B. The use of EA facilitates postoperative ambulation and feeding.

C. The use of EA is associated with a decrease in ventilator dependency.

D. The use of EA is associated with unplanned postoperative tracheal intubation.

E. All of the above.

ANSWER: E

COMMENTS: In patients with COPD, the concomitant use of EA may decrease perioperative morbidity and, as shown in some studies, mortality. Although procedures involving the lower part of the abdomen can frequently be performed solely with epidural and/or spinal anesthesia, upper abdominal operations usually require supraumbilical incisions, which necessitate higher sensory levels of anesthesia. Patients with severe COPD may not tolerate high levels of anesthesia due to decreased expiratory reserve volume, ineffective cough, and inability to clear secretions. General anesthesia with mechanical ventilation may allow better control of ventilation and therefore oxygenation in these patients. Studies have been inconclusive regarding whether EA results in a decreased incidence of postoperative pulmonary complications in non-COPD patients. Generally, it is believed that the risk for postoperative pulmonary complications is independent of the choice of intraoperative anesthesia. However, perioperative EA may decrease the risk for complications after upper abdominal and thoracic surgery.

Ref.: 15, 16

9. Which of the following regarding pulmonary function tests (PFTs) is true?

A. Functional residual capacity (FRC) is the lung volume after forced expiration.

B. FRC is not altered by atelectasis.

C. Forced vital capacity (FVC) is the lung volume after maximal expiration and inhalation.

D. Minute ventilation is FVC × respiratory rate.

E. Positive end-expiratory pressure (PEEP) does not improve FRC.

ANSWER: C

COMMENTS: Tidal volume (TV) is the volume of gas exchanged during normal breathing and is ~6 to 8 mL/kg. Inspiratory volume is the additional gas that can be inspired above normal TV. Expiratory reserve volume is the additional gas that can be forcefully exhaled after expiration of normal TV. Residual volume is the lung volume remaining after maximal expiration. Lung capacities are composed of two or more lung volumes. Vital capacity (~60 mL/kg) is the total volume of gas that can be expired after full inhalation to residual volume. Inspiratory capacity is the maximum amount of air that can be inspired. Total lung capacity is the maximum amount of air that can fill the lungs. FRC is the amount of air that is remaining in the lungs after a normal expiration (see Fig. 7.1). General anesthesia, tobacco use, COPD, acute respiratory distress syndrome (ARDS), obesity, and trauma all decrease FRC and promote atelectasis. PEEP improves FRC by recruiting and reexpanding alveoli.

Figure 7.1:

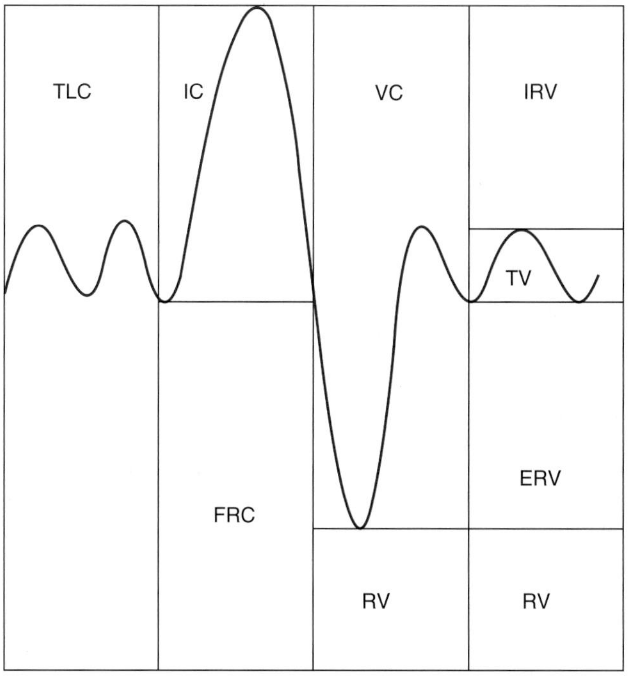

Fig. 7.1 Diagram of normal lung volumes and capacities. Lung capacities are composed of two or more volumes. *ERV*, expiratory reserve volume; *FRC*, functional residual capacity; *IC*, inspiratory capacity; *IRV*, inspiratory reserve volume; *RV*, residual volume; *TV*, tidal volume; *TLC*, total lung capacity; *VC*, vital capacity.

Ref.: 17–19

10. Regarding preoperative PFTs, which of the following statements is/are false?

A. PFTs help predict postoperative pulmonary complications in patients undergoing abdominal operations.

B. PFTs conducted before and after bronchodilator therapy are useful in determining optimal management.

C. The history and physical examination are more useful than PFTs in predicting postoperative pulmonary complications.

D. Patients with an FRC less than 50% of FVC should undergo ventilation-perfusion testing before pneumonectomy.

E. All of the above.

ANSWER: A

COMMENTS: Routine use of preoperative PFTs in all patients with preexisting pulmonary disease is controversial. PFTs have a positive predictive value for postoperative pulmonary complications in patients undergoing lung resection. However, the routine use of PFTs for abdominal operations often does not predict postoperative pulmonary complications. Instead, PFTs can be used as tools to provide optimal preoperative management and assist in the postoperative care of patients (i.e., patients with reactive airway disease whose PFTs improve with bronchodilator therapy). Clinical factors such as smoking, wheezing, and increased sputum production on the preoperative workup are more predictive of potential postoperative complications. Patients with an FRC less than 50% of FVC who are scheduled for lung resection should undergo ventilation-perfusion studies to determine their predicted postoperative pulmonary function.

Ref.: 20

11. A 25-year-old asthmatic patient is scheduled for elective inguinal hernia repair. In the holding area, he exhibits bilateral wheezing on auscultation. Which of the following would be the best initial approach to perioperative management for this patient's surgery?

A. Perform a field block with local anesthesia and sedate with IV ketamine and propofol.

B. Administer albuterol nebulizer treatment preoperatively and proceed with general anesthesia sevoflurane via a laryngeal mask airway (LMA).

C. Postpone surgery for 4 to 6 weeks.

D. Perform surgery with spinal anesthesia.

E. Administer hydrocortisone 100 mg IV and proceed with general anesthesia with desflurane administered via an endotracheal tube.

ANSWER: C

COMMENTS: Although inguinal hernia repair is a minor risk surgical procedure, unexpected complications may occur that could worsen bronchospasm in a patient with active asthma. A single treatment is unlikely to be adequate therapy, and resolution often requires 4 to 6 weeks of treatment in order for bronchial reactivity to resolve. The use of spinal or local anesthesia with or without sedation does not ensure that the patient will not require a general anesthetic, particularly if the spinal block or sedation is inadequate. Indeed, a high-sensory/motor-level spinal anesthetic may lead to significant parasympathetic tone and worsen bronchospasm. Elective surgery in this setting should be postponed.

Ref.: 21, 22

12. An 85-year-old with severe COPD is scheduled for elective cholecystectomy. The risk for postoperative pulmonary complications can be minimized in this patient by all of the following except:
    A. Cessation of smoking for at least 8 weeks
    B. Prophylactic antibiotics for patients with productive yellowish sputum
    C. Perioperative incentive spirometry
    D. Laparoscopic technique
    E. Inspiratory-to-expiratory ratio of 1:1 during mechanical ventilation

ANSWER: E

COMMENTS: Patients with COPD are at an increased risk for postoperative pulmonary complications. The risk can be reduced if effective measures are taken in the perioperative period. Patients should be instructed to stop smoking. However, frequently, there is insufficient time to achieve the beneficial effects of this maneuver. It may require at least 8 weeks of cessation before any decrease in postoperative pulmonary complications may be realized. Cessation for as little as 24 h will improve carbon monoxide levels, but secretions may still be problematic, as mucociliary function often requires a longer time to return to normal. Increased sputum production or a change in the color of sputum is an indication that an underlying infection could exist. If a pulmonary infection is present, antibiotic therapy should be instituted and the patient treated for the appropriate amount of time before undergoing surgery. Incentive spirometry may help prevent postoperative pulmonary complications, along with deep breathing, coughing, and chest physical therapy. The cholecystectomy should be done laparoscopically, if possible, to avoid a painful upper abdominal incision and to preserve better diaphragmatic function. COPD patients need a prolonged expiratory phase during mechanical ventilation to prevent auto-PEEP by exhalation time and minimize increases in airway pressure.

Ref.: 23

13. A 45-year-old male 5′10″ in height with a body mass index (BMI) 44 kg/m^2 and a history of continuous positive airway pressure (CPAP)-dependent obstructive sleep apnea is likely to present with each of the following preoperative test abnormalities except:
    A. ECG: P Pulmonale
    B. PFTs: Vital capacity, 2.5 cm^3
    C. CBC: Hemoglobin, 16.5 gm%
    D. Electrolytes: HCO_3^-, 30 mEq/L
    E. Chest x-ray (CXR): Flattened diaphragms

ANSWER: E

COMMENTS: Morbidly obese patients (BMI > 40 kg/m^2) have an increased incidence of obstructive sleep apnea. Obstructive sleep apnea may lead to chronic arterial hypoxemia and hypercapnia, which in turn may cause polycythemia, pulmonary hypertension, and right heart failure. Perioperative findings may include ECG changes of right atrial or ventricular strain (peaked P waves), elevated hemoglobin and serum bicarbonate, and diminished vital capacity. CXR findings are more consistent with restrictive lung disease and would likely show diminished, and not hyperexpanded, lung volumes.

Ref.: 24

14. A 67-year-old obese patient with a history of diabetes mellitus and hypertension undergoes revision of a right total hip arthroplasty. Which of the following reasons would place this patient at an increased risk for developing postoperative deep-vein thrombosis (DVT)?
    A. Venous stasis
    B. Polycythemia
    C. Decreased ambulation
    D. Length of surgery
    E. Associated ischemic heart disease

ANSWER: E

COMMENTS: Obese patients are at a much higher risk than nonobese patients for developing DVT. Venous stasis increases the risk for DVT. Increased abdominal weight leads to decreased venous return secondary to compression of the inferior vena cava. Polycythemia, common in obese patients with sleep apnea, leads to decreased vascular flow. If an obese patient has difficulty walking preoperatively, it is likely that postoperative mobilization will be poor, leading to an increased risk for DVT. Prolonged operations result in longer periods of venous stasis during the operation. Preventive therapy should be instituted before induction of anesthesia by administering regular heparin or low-molecular-weight heparin along with intermittent sequential venous compression stockings. It is important to institute early ambulation in this patient population. Neuraxial anesthesia may also decrease the incidence of DVT in patients undergoing total hip arthroplasty.

Ref.: 25

15. A morbidly obese patient with a history of obstructive sleep apnea presents for coronary artery bypass graft surgery. Which of the following statements is true regarding general anesthesia and airway management in this patient?
    A. Large neck circumference makes intubation difficult but does not compromise mask ventilation.
    B. The diagnosis of obstructive sleep apnea should not alter management.
    C. Hypoxemia following induction of anesthesia and during intubation is likely due to diminished FRC.
    D. Awake intubation is not contraindicated.
    E. LMA management is preferred because of decreased airway trauma.

ANSWER: D

COMMENTS: Management of a morbidly obese patient's airway can be difficult. The approach to endotracheal intubation must take into consideration a number of factors. These patients often have short, thick necks; large tongues; limited mouth and neck mobility; and increased thoracic and abdominal pressure. For these reasons, both ventilation and intubation can be difficult. Patients with obstructive sleep apnea frequently have redundant soft tissue in the airway, which may make visualization of the vocal cords extremely difficult. In fact, obese patients with sleep apnea and abnormalities on airway examination should be considered for awake intubation. In experienced hands, awake fiberoptic intubation with the prior topical application of local anesthetic and proper sedation is ideal and is not contraindicated even for patients with coronary artery disease. If general anesthesia is induced and difficulty with intubation and ventilation ensues, obese patients can rapidly become hypoxemic. This is due to both an increased rate of oxygen consumption and decreased FRC. Oxygenation with 100% O_2 before induction of anesthesia may decrease the rate of desaturation, but it does not eliminate this risk and may promote atelectasis by causing denitrogenation. This may be overcome after endotracheal intubation by performing an alveolar recruitment maneuver and increasing the level of PEEP. LMA airway management is contraindicated in these patients because of the increased risk for aspiration and the need for higher airway pressures.

Ref.: 26

16. Atrial fibrillation with a heart rate of 110 beats/min develops in a 65-year-old male 3 days following a coronary arterial bypass graft operation. Blood pressure is 100/74 mmHg, and laboratory test values are normal. Which of the following is true?

A. The patient is not at an increased risk for stroke.

B. The duration and cost of the patient's hospital stay will be increased.

C. Cardioversion is indicated.

D. Initiate anticoagulant therapy with heparin within 6 h.

E. All of the above.

ANSWER: B

COMMENTS: Atrial fibrillation may occur in 20%–50% of patients undergoing open heart surgery and increases the patient's risk of stroke due to clots forming in the atrial appendage. Perioperative atrial fibrillation may be related to autonomic nervous system changes associated with an inflammatory response. Although it may seem logical that rhythm conversion would be more advantageous than rate control, this is not true. Controlling the ventricular response rate either pharmacologically or by ablation of the atrioventricular node and implantation of a pacemaker allows the use of less toxic medications, which results in fewer adverse drug reactions and hospitalizations. Statistics show that the duration of the hospital stay will increase by an average of 1 to 2 days, and the median cost will increase significantly. The duration of atrial fibrillation is crucial to determining therapy. This patient has atrial fibrillation with a rapid ventricular response. Treating this patient with β-blockers such as metoprolol or calcium channel blockers, such as diltiazem, would be appropriate. Calcium channel blockers are especially advantageous in patients who cannot tolerate β-blockade. Digoxin may also be used; however, it may be ineffective in high-adrenergic states such as those present postoperatively. Amiodarone is also an appropriate and effective therapy. Cardioversion is not indicated as an initial management step in this patient since there is no hemodynamic instability. Moreover, the majority of the patients in whom atrial fibrillation develops revert to sinus rhythm with medical management.

The risk for thromboembolism in patients who do not convert to sinus rhythm is markedly increased after 48 h. Therefore anticoagulation should be strongly considered in patients with an indeterminate duration of atrial fibrillation, even in the immediate postoperative period. A reasonable treatment plan consists of IV heparin, titrated to maintain a partial thromboplastin time of two to three times normal and subsequent administration of warfarin to maintain an international normalized ratio between 2.0 and 3.0. The addition of anticoagulation therapy considerably decreases the risk of stroke.

Ref.: 27, 28

17. A 65-year-old man with a long-standing history of hypertension and a smoking history of 25 pack/year is scheduled for elective laparoscopic hernia repair. His blood pressure is 150/90 mmHg. The ECG shows nonspecific ST-segment changes. Appropriate interventions would include which of the following?

A. Canceling the procedure

B. Obtaining a more detailed history regarding the level of exercise and daily activity

C. Requesting a cardiac consultation

D. Perioperative administration of a β-blocker and changing the operation to open hernia repair with local anesthesia

E. None of the above

ANSWER: B

COMMENTS: Current recommendations regarding preoperative cardiac evaluation for noncardiac surgery are based on the theory that random testing and screening for cardiac disease in the absence of clinical findings or changes in a patient's history are not cost effective and do not appear to reduce perioperative cardiovascular morbidity and mortality. The approach to the patient needs to consider both the surgical risk factors for a cardiac complication and the patient's cardiac risk factors.

High-risk predictors of cardiac complications include recent myocardial infarction (MI); unstable angina; decompensated heart failure; severe valvular heart disease, in particular aortic stenosis; and high-grade arrhythmias. Advanced age, poor exercise tolerance, chronic kidney disease, cerebrovascular disease, and insulin-dependent diabetes are also considered to increase the perioperative risk of cardiac morbidity and mortality. High-risk surgical procedures include any emergency procedure; acute trauma (e.g., hip fracture); procedures involving the heart, aorta, or other major vasculature; and prolonged procedures entailing large blood loss and fluid shifts.

If the patient's history and exercise tolerance have been stable and routine laboratory studies such as ECGs are unchanged, elective procedures of low to intermediate risk can proceed without additional intervention. However, when the history and physical findings suggest progression of coronary artery disease, the urgency of surgery must be considered, and further evaluation may be in order. Cardiac consultation should be used to answer specific questions regarding disease status and to assist in optimizing medical therapy and not simply to request "clearance." Anesthesiologists strongly believe that "clearance" is a part of their process since they are responsible for the patient's well-being during the procedure. Appropriate use of consultation services may include further testing when indicated by changes in a patient's history or findings on physical examination. As a general rule, if nothing in the history or physical examination indicates a need for intervention, the operation may proceed.

Although available data indicates that appropriate β-blockade therapy may reduce the incidence of preoperative morbidity and mortality, there is no evidence that one type of anesthetic technique is superior to another for myocardial protection. The approach should involve optimizing the patient's condition and making reasonable predictions of risk rather than attempting alternative measures in the hope of reducing the likelihood of complications.

Ref.: 29

18. A patient is scheduled for a colon resection for diverticulitis. His history is significant for asthma, hypertension, and insulin-dependent diabetes. He had two drug-eluting coronary stents placed 12 months ago. He is currently symptom free and exercises three times per week to six metabolic equivalents (METs). Preoperative testing should include which of the following?

A. Transesophageal echocardiogram

B. Troponin C level

C. Adenosine-stress test

D. Coronary angiography

E. None of the above

ANSWER: E

COMMENTS: In the absence of a change in a patient's clinical history, symptoms, or physical findings, only routine testing appropriate for age and gender needs to be conducted. In patients with good functional capacity (METs ≥ 4) without symptoms, no further testing is warranted. Patients who have undergone coronary artery bypass grafting within 5 years or had normal findings during an interventional cardiac workup within 2 years also do not need further testing unless dictated by changes in the history or findings on physical examination. When indicated, exercise stress testing is the preferred test. Routine treadmill testing provides much useful information, including the patient's functional capacity, areas of myocardium in which ischemia may occur, and a heart rate at which ischemia may occur. For patients who cannot exercise on a treadmill, chemical stress testing is the next preferred method of assessing ventricular function. Adenosine, however, should not be administered to patients with asthma as it may precipitate bronchospasm. Angiography is generally reserved for patients with known cardiac disease, recent MI, unstable angina, or severe stenotic valvular disease. In such patients, an acute intervention, such as angioplasty with stenting or balloon valvuloplasty, may be indicated before noncardiac surgery.

Ref.: 29

19. In patients with intermediate predictors of cardiac risk who are scheduled for high-risk surgical procedures, which of the following interventions can reduce perioperative mortality?

A. Intraoperative ST-segment analysis

B. Preoperative administration of β-blockade therapy

C. Intraoperative transesophageal echocardiography monitoring

D. Prophylactic administration of IV nitroglycerin

E. Regional anesthesia in conjunction with general anesthesia

ANSWER: B

COMMENTS: It is unclear whether certain anesthetic techniques or intraoperative monitoring methods can reliably reduce perioperative mortality. Continuous ST-segment monitoring is a noninvasive, safe, readily available, and inexpensive component of routine intraoperative monitoring. Although it has proven useful in the early detection of myocardial ischemia, it has not been shown to favorably affect the overall incidence of perioperative MI or death. Regional anesthesia "seems safer" than general anesthesia; however, few randomized, controlled studies have supported this belief. Transesophageal echocardiography is safe and provides pertinent information regarding volume status, contractility, and regional wall-motion abnormalities. However, it requires an experienced operator and may not always be obtainable, particularly during procedures involving the thorax and upper part of the abdomen. Perioperative nitroglycerin administration has been used to optimize cardiac perfusion in high-risk patients because it causes dilation of epicardial vessels and effectively treats angina, yet it does not reduce mortality.

Preoperative β-blockade therapy rapidly became a common practice when initial data showed a reduction in perioperative and long-term complications related to myocardial morbidity and mortality from MI. It seems to work by reducing myocardial oxygen demand and stabilizing intravascular plaques and thrombi. Unfortunately, the PeriOperative Ischemia Evaluation (POISE) trial suggested that although β-blockers reduced cardiac risk, they were associated with an increased risk of stroke and mortality from noncardiac complications. Additional studies have confirmed improved cardiac outcome but with the significant drawbacks of bradycardia, hypotension, and increased stroke risk. Controversy exists regarding the timing of initiating and type of β-blockade. Current guidelines state that β-blocking medications should be continued in patients who have been receiving them on a chronic basis. In patients at an intermediate or high risk [revised risk cardiac index (RCRI) ≥ 3 risk factors], β-blocking therapy may be started 2 to 7 days prior to elective surgery, but not on the same day. However, it should not be added in patients at an increased risk of stroke or congestive heart failure. Selective β-blockade with bisoprolol has been associated with fewer postoperative strokes than that with either atenolol or metoprolol. Calcium channel blockers and α_2-agonists have not been shown to have the same effect as β-blockade.

Ref.: 29–32

20. A 65-year-old male undergoes repair of an infrarenal abdominal aortic aneurysm. Evidence-based strategies for intraoperative renal protection prior to aortic cross-clamp placement include administration of which of the following?

A. Fenoldopam

B. Isotonic saline

C. Mannitol

D. Furosemide

E. Low-dose dopamine

ANSWER: B

COMMENTS: None of these drugs has been shown to consistently offer renal protection during the surgical repair of an abdominal aortic aneurysm, although all have theoretical benefits. Fenoldopam preserves medullary blood flow and decreases systemic vascular resistance and, hence, mean arterial blood pressure. Mannitol causes an osmotic diuresis and, in theory, prevents microtubular obstruction from cellular debris and is an oxygen free-radical scavenger. It is the most commonly administered agent for renal protection prior to aortic cross-clamping, but scientific data are lacking. Loop diuretics, such as furosemide, reduce the metabolism of tubular cells and should enable patients to better tolerate ischemia. The so-called low-dose dopamine has been shown to have no benefit as serum levels do not correlate with dosage. Therapeutic measures with proven efficacy for renal protection prior to aortic cross-clamping include volume resuscitation and maximizing cardiac output. Other modalities such as *N*-acetylcysteine or bicarbonate infusions have shown no evidence of perioperative renal protection.

Ref.: 33

21. Regarding urinary retention after ambulatory surgery, which of the following statements is false?

A. It is most frequently associated with herniorrhaphy and anorectal procedures.

B. It is greater with spinal anesthesia than general anesthesia.

C. It can frequently be asymptomatic.

D. Ambulatory surgery patients may be discharged prior to voiding.

E. It can be caused by excessive administration of IV fluids.

ANSWER: B

COMMENTS: Patients at risk for postoperative urinary retention include those with a previous history of retention and those undergoing procedures such as herniorrhaphy and anorectal operations. Both spinal anesthesia and general anesthesia are predisposing factors, especially when the latter is associated with the use of anticholinergic drugs or high-dose opiates. Although bladder overdistention is a significant factor contributing to postoperative urinary retention, many patients are asymptomatic, with bladder volumes exceeding 600 mL. Although low-risk patients may be discharged safely without the requirement to void, consideration should be given to catheterization of high-risk patients before discharge. Patients at high risk for postoperative urinary retention should have ready access to a medical facility and be instructed to return to a medical facility if still unable to void 8 to 12 h after discharge from an ambulatory surgical facility. Judicious use of IV fluids may reduce the incidence of postoperative urinary retention in patients at high risk.

Ref.: 34

22. Initial treatment of a postdural puncture headache (PDPH) after spinal anesthesia for a total knee arthroplasty includes all of the following except:

A. Epidural blood patch

B. Increasing oral fluid intake

C. Bed rest

D. Oral analgesics

E. IV caffeine

ANSWER: A

COMMENTS: PDPH results from decreased intracranial pressure (ICP) secondary to leakage of cerebrospinal fluid from the dural defect created by the spinal needle. The incidence of PDPH can be decreased primarily by reducing the needle size and, to a lesser extent, by using needles of improved design (pencil point vs. cutting). Increased oral fluid intake, remaining recumbent, and the use of oral analgesics may reduce cephalgia as well as other symptoms, such as visual disturbances, auditory disturbances, and nausea. While the recumbent position may offer symptomatic relief, it is not an option for patients who must be ambulatory to prevent DVT formation and to benefit from physical therapy, as is the case following total knee arthroplasty. Caffeine may also be helpful in reducing symptoms. An epidural blood patch is a more aggressive approach that is typically reserved for severe, persistent symptoms or for those who cannot remain supine. Epidural injection of 10 to 20 mL of autologous blood collected from a fresh venipuncture is associated with successful relief of severe, persistent PDPH symptoms in 90% of patients.

Ref.: 35

23. Which statement about postoperative nausea and vomiting (PONV) after ambulatory surgery is false?

A. It is associated with opiate use.

B. It occurs less frequently following anesthetic induction or maintenance with propofol.

C. Antiemetic therapy should be administered to all patients before ambulatory surgery.

D. It is increased in adults who are not required to ingest oral fluids before discharge.

E. Wound hematoma is not a risk factor for PONV.

ANSWER: C

COMMENTS: PONV is one of the most prevalent factors leading to delay in discharge from ambulatory surgical centers or unanticipated hospitalization after outpatient procedures. Both pain and the treatment of pain with opiates are associated with an increased risk for PONV. Multimodal analgesia with the use of nonopiate drugs, such as ketorolac or acetaminophen; adjuvant methods of analgesia, such as wound infiltration with local anesthetics; peripheral nerve blocks; or regional anesthesia may reduce opiate use and associated PONV. Use of propofol for anesthesia induction is known to reduce the incidence of PONV. Although the effect is lessened after long surgical procedures, a continuous infusion or repeated dose prior to emergence from anesthesia may increase its antiemetic efficacy. Because of the cost and side effects of antiemetic drugs, prophylaxis for all patients undergoing ambulatory surgery is not recommended. However, prophylaxis for patients at a high risk for PONV may be cost effective by reducing the length of the postoperative stay and improving patient satisfaction. Risk factors for PONV include female gender, history of PONV or motion sickness, nonsmoking status, and postoperative opiate use. Although oral fluid intake before discharge does not increase the risk for PONV in adult patients, eliminating oral fluid intake as a discharge criterion does not reduce the risk for PONV. Therefore patients should be allowed to decide to accept or decline oral fluids as they desire before discharge.

Ref.: 36

24. Patients with liver dysfunction may be at an increased risk for surgery. Which of the following statements about this is false?

A. Laparoscopic surgery can be safely performed in patients with acute hepatitis A.

B. Sevoflurane reduces hepatic arterial blood flow less than halothane.

C. Hypercapnia increases portal blood flow.

D. Fentanyl elimination is not appreciably altered in patients with cirrhosis.

E. Patients with Child class B cirrhosis undergoing cardiac surgery have a high mortality rate.

ANSWER: A

COMMENTS: Routine laboratory screening of otherwise healthy surgical candidates for unsuspected liver disease should not be performed. However, a carefully taken history to identify risk factors for liver disease permits adequate initial evaluation. Celiotomy leads to a greater reduction in hepatic arterial blood flow than extraabdominal or laparoscopic operations. Halothane is now rarely, if ever, used, but it is the inhalational agent that has the greatest effect on decreasing the hepatic blood flow. Hypercapnia should be avoided since it triggers sympathetic splanchnic stimulation and leads to decreased portal flow. Fentanyl, sufentanil, or remifentanil are the opiates of choice as the metabolism of morphine may be prolonged in patients with liver disease.

The Child-Turcotte-Pugh and the Model for End-Stage Liver Disease (MELD) classifications are the most useful predictors of mortality and morbidity in patients with cirrhosis. MELD scores of less than 10, 10 to 14, and higher than 14 correspond to classes A, B, and C, respectively. Postoperatively, bilirubin levels and prothrombin times should be monitored closely. Cardiac surgery is associated with a high mortality rate in patients with cirrhosis, particularly classes B and C, because of the higher risk for infection and bleeding. Surgery, in general, should be avoided in patients with acute hepatitis of any etiology due to the increase in postoperative liver failure and death.

Ref.: 37

25. A 66-year-old male undergoes laparotomy for perforated diverticulosis. In the intensive care unit (ICU), the patient remains on mechanical ventilation with $FiO_2 = 0.5$ and intravenous (IV) norepinephrine 5 μg/min. The arterial blood gas (ABG) analysis reveals the following: pH, 7.29; $PaCO_2$, 38 mmHg; PaO_2, 72 mmHg; HCO_3^-, 18 mEq/L.
The acid–base disturbance is best described as:

A. Respiratory acidosis
B. Metabolic acidosis and respiratory alkalosis
C. Respiratory acidosis and metabolic alkalosis
D. Metabolic acidosis and respiratory acidosis
E. None of the above

ANSWER: D

COMMENTS: This patient is clearly acidemic (pH < 7.40) and has a metabolic acidosis evident by his bicarbonate level being <24 mEq/L. This is likely secondary to hyperlactatemia from sepsis. In this setting, an appropriate respiratory compensation would be to hyperventilate (or have the mechanical ventilation adjusted to increase minute ventilation) so that the $PaCO_2$ would be approximately 33 to 34 mmHg. This is based on the formula for compensation for metabolic acidosis: ΔHCO_3^- (1.2) = $\Delta PaCO_2$. In this regard, the serum bicarbonate change is 6 mEq/L (from normal of 24 mEq/L), with an appropriate decrease in $PaCO_2$ being 7 mmHg or to 33 mmHg. The patient's $PaCO_2$ of 38 mmHg is inappropriately elevated, signifying a secondary respiratory acidosis even though the absolute value of $PaCO_2$ is < 40 mmHg.

Ref.: 38

26. A 33-year-old, 70-kg female undergoes a 4-h colon resection under general anesthesia. Intraoperative blood loss is 300 mL, and the patient received 3.5 L of 0.9% saline. In the postanesthesia care unit (PACU), the patient is breathing 2 L oxygen by nasal cannula and receiving IV morphine for analgesia. Vital signs are stable. Laboratory data reveal the following: Na^+, 141 mEq/L; Cl^-, 115 mEq/L; HCO_3^-, 18 mEq/L; K^+, 3.9 mEq/L; ABGs: pH, 7.34; $PaCO_2$, 33 mmHg; PaO_2, 92 mmHg.
The most likely etiology of the patient's laboratory findings is:

A. Metabolic acidosis secondary to hyperlactatemia
B. Respiratory alkalosis secondary to pain
C. Respiratory acidosis secondary to residual anesthesia
D. Metabolic acidosis secondary to hyperchloremia
E. Respiratory acidosis secondary to morphine

ANSWER: D

COMMENTS: Saline resuscitation is associated with developing hyperchloremia, which in turn can cause not only a slight dilution of the serum bicarbonate but also an actual renal loss of bicarbonate due to a disproportionate proximal and distal tubule reabsorption of chloride and excretion of bicarbonate. In this regard, 0.9% saline is unphysiologic and should best be used to manage patients with chloride deficiency, as is often seen in patients who have severe vomiting or nasogastric suctioning. In order to avoid perioperative hyperchloremic acidosis, a physiologic isotonic solution should be used, such as Plasma-Lyte or Normosol. Ringer's lactate is also unphysiologic as the ratio of sodium to chloride (130 mEq/L:109 mEq/L) makes it a relatively hyperchloremic solution.

Ref.: 39

27. An 80-year-old, fully oriented female requires urgent surgery for a small bowel obstruction. She has a preexisting do not resuscitate (DNR) order based on quality-of-life issues. Prior to surgery, what is the best means to address the DNR order?

A. Recommend to the patient to discontinue the order and reinstate after surgery.
B. Automatically rescind as surgery takes precedence over the order.
C. Automatically maintain the order for surgery.
D. Discuss with patient's daughter and abide by the daughter's wishes.
E. Cancel the surgery, if the patient desires to maintain the order for the procedure.

ANSWER: A

COMMENTS: The DNR order applies in two clinical situations, medical futility and quality of life. Physicians determine futility, and patients determine the quality of life. In the purest sense of the order, it only implies that acute resuscitation [e.g., cardiopulmonary resuscitation (CPR) and advanced cardiac life support (ACLS)] will not be attempted should the patient suffer a cardiac arrest. It does not mean withholding any other lifesaving support (e.g., vasopressors, IV fluids, and mechanical ventilation). In the preoperative phase of care, both the American Society of Anesthesiologists and the American College of Surgeons recommend a period of "required reconsideration." This means a discussion should take place with the patient, if competent (or an established surrogate or durable power of attorney, if not competent), with the recommendation to rescind the order for the duration of the procedure and anesthetic and reinstate it when the patient is either in an ICU or in the surgical ward. In this way, the surgery, which may improve the quality of life, can be performed without "tying the hands" of the anesthesiologist. Patients have the right to maintain the DNR order, but all parties, including the surgeons and the anesthesia team, must agree to operate under those conditions.

Ref.: 40–42

28. A 45-year-old male presents for emergency splenectomy following a motor vehicle collision. The patient states that he is a Jehovah's Witness (JW) and would rather die than take a blood transfusion. The patient's starting hemoglobin is 8.5 gm%. Which of the following is the most appropriate management in the case of this patient?

A. Request a consent order to transfuse, if necessary.

B. Administer fresh frozen plasma as a red cell substitute.

C. Honor the patient's wishes and do not transfuse blood, even if massive hemorrhage ensues.

D. Obtain consent from his spouse to transfuse once anesthesia has been initiated.

E. None of the above.

ANSWER: C

COMMENTS: JWs are members of a fundamental Christian sect that believes in the literal translation of the Bible as it pertains to ingestion of blood: *God decreed that Noah and his offspring "must not eat the blood, because the life is in the blood"* (Genesis 9). The JW name was adopted in 1931 as the group evolved from its origins in the Bible Student movement, founded in the late 1870s by Charles Taze Russell. Originally, only eating meat containing blood was prohibited; this was a common interpretation of the Bible. The proscription of blood transfusions did not become mandatory until around 1950 through the efforts of a series of progressively more rigid leaders. Currently, the Watchtower Society, which issues rules for JW members, prohibits transfusion of both donated and autologous whole blood and blood products including red cells, white cells, platelets, and plasma. The use of fractions such as albumin, immunoglobulins, and hemophiliac preparations is open to interpretation and may be up to the individual.

Management of patients who are JWs may be challenging and result in ethical and emotional conflicts for the physician. Guidelines have emerged based on the religious rights of the individual and on case law. Specifically, competent adult patients have the right to refuse blood products, even if it results in their death. However, each adult patient should have his or her wishes discussed privately so as to avoid the semblance of external coercion. In many cases, individuals will consent to transfusion, if it is clearly lifesaving, in spite of their membership in the JW church. However, they usually do not want their friends or even their family to know because of the social stigma that it carries within their community.

Parents may refuse transfusions for their children; however, this may be overridden by a court order. Remarkably, many, although not all, parents express relief when the decision is taken out of their hands. Court orders may also be sought for patients who are deemed incompetent at the time of their consent. Fresh frozen plasma might be acceptable for an individual JW patient, but it is not useful in the management of massive hemorrhage without red cell therapy. Waiting until anesthesia is induced to ask the spouse for permission is unethical and would represent coercion. Clearly, these issues must be discussed in private with each JW patient or parent, whenever possible, and documented.

Ref.: 43

29. A 78-year-old male with a history of hypertension develops acute delirium while recovering in the ICU 2 days following a pancreatectomy for pancreatic cancer.
Vital signs: BP, 150/100 mmHg; HR, 110 bpm; RR, 20 beats per min; T, 36ºC; SaO_2, 99%
Neurologic examination: no focal defects
Lab data: Na^+, 130 mEq/L; Glucose, 140 mg%
ABGs: pH, 7.46; $PaCO_2$, 32 mmHg; PaO_2, 98 mmHg
Medications: morphine, scopolamine patch, metoprolol, and furosemide
Which of the following is the next best step in this patient's management?

A. Administer lorazepam.

B. Continue scopolamine.

C. Initiate free water restriction.

D. Continue morphine.

E. Initiate dexmedetomidine.

ANSWER: E

COMMENTS: Postoperative delirium is a common occurrence in critically ill patients and, if severe, may lead to significant morbidity and mortality. Risk factors include advanced age, sleep deprivation, preexisting cognitive impairment, environmental disruptions (e.g., excessive noise or light), and medications, especially benzodiazepine, anticholinergics, and opiates. Ensuring a quiet environment by discontinuing unnecessary alarms, avoiding unnecessary patient awakenings, and discontinuing known offending drugs is the mainstay of therapy. In addition, it has been shown that the α_2-agonist dexmedetomidine imparts excellent anxiolysis and analgesia without disrupting normal sleep physiology. In addition, it will decrease the heart rate and blood pressure in a similar fashion as clonidine.

Ref.: 44–46

30. Which of the following statements in regard to delaying elective noncardiac surgery is true?

A. Elective noncardiac surgery should be delayed for at least 1 week after coronary artery balloon angioplasty without stent placement.

B. Elective noncardiac surgery should be delayed at least 3 months after placement of a bare-metal stent for MI.

C. Risk of stent thrombosis or ischemia after percutaneous coronary intervention (PCI) for MI is minimal, and surgery should not be postponed.

D. Elective noncardiac surgery should ideally be postponed 1 year after drug-eluting stent placement.

E. All of the above.

ANSWER: D

COMMENTS: Patients who have suffered an acute MI are commonly treated with PCI with stenting. Because of the risk of stent thrombosis and acute death, they are typically treated with dual antiplatelet therapy (DAPT) after stent placement for 6 to 12 months. This usually consists of aspirin 75 to 100 mg daily plus clopidogrel 75 mg daily. Elective noncardiac surgery is often required in this patient population. The timing of elective surgery after PCI involving angioplasty, with or without stenting, depends on the temporally related risks of vessel thrombosis, restenosis, and bleeding related to the antiplatelet therapy used. Cessation of DAPT prior to the recommended duration of use, as well as the prothrombotic and proinflammatory state associated with surgery, contributes to an increased risk of adverse perioperative cardiovascular events and death.

If feasible, surgery should be postponed for at least 30 days after the placement of a bare-metal stent and 1 year after the placement of a drug-eluting stent. If surgery is more time sensitive and the risk of delaying surgery outweighs the risks of ischemia and stent thrombosis, 6 months is acceptable.

After balloon angioplasty alone, patients should be treated with DAPT, and elective noncardiac surgery should be scheduled at least 14 days post PCI.

In patients with an increased risk of bleeding, aspirin should be continued alone. In patients in whom bleeding can be catastrophic, such as those undergoing neurosurgical procedures, suspending both antiplatelet agents may be reasonable.

Ref.: 47, 48

REFERENCES

1. Buchleitner AM, Martinez-Alonso M, Hernandez M, Solal MD. Perioperative glycaemic control for diabetic patients undergoing surgery. *Cochrane Database Syst Rev*. 2012;9:CD007315.
2. Sato H, Carvalho G, Sato T, Lattermann R, Matsukawa T, Schricker T. The association of perioperative glycemic control, intraoperative insulin sensitivity, and outcomes after cardiac surgery. *J Clin Endocrinol Metab*. 2010;95:4338–4344.
3. Wiener RS, Wiener DC, Larson RJ. Benefits and risks of tight glucose control in critically ill adults: a meta-analysis. *JAMA*. 2008;300: 933–944.
4. Halkos ME, Puskas JD, Lattouf OM, et al. Elevated preoperative hemoglobin A1c is predictive of adverse events after coronary artery bypass surgery. *J Thorac Cardiovasc Surg*. 2008;136:631–640.
5. Stryker LS, Abdel MP, Morrey ME, Morrow MM, Kor DJ, Morrey BF. Elevated postoperative blood glucose and preoperative hemoglobin A1c are associated with increased wound complications following total joint arthroplasty. *J Bone Joint Surg Am*. 2013;95:808–814.
6. Yong SL, Coulthard P, Wrzosek A. Supplemental perioperative steroids for surgical patients with adrenal insufficiency. *Cochrane Database Syst Rev*. 2012;12:CD005367.
7. Bornstein SR. Predisposing factors for adrenal insufficiency. *N Engl J Med*. 2009;360:2328–2339.
8. Vinclair M, Broux C, Faure P, et al. Duration of adrenal inhibition following a single dose of etomidate in critically ill patients. *Intensive Care Med*. 2008;34:714–719.
9. Kinney MA, Narr BJ, Warner MA. Perioperative management of pheochromocytoma. *J Cardiothorac Vasc Anesth*. 2002;16:359–369.
10. Ramakrishna H. Pheochromocytoma resection: current concepts in anesthetic management. *J Anaesthesiol Clin Pharmacol*. 2015;31: 317–323.
11. Stathoatos N, Wartofsky L. Perioperative management of patients with hypothyroidism. *Endocrinol Metab Clin North Am*. 2003;32:503–518.
12. Chiha M, Samarasinghe S, Kabaker AS. Thryoid storm: an updated review. *J Intensive Care Med*. 2015;30:131–140.
13. Bahn Chair RS, Burch HB, Cooper DS, et al. Hyperthyroidism and other causes of thyrotoxicosis: management guidelines of the American Thyroid Association and American Association of Clinical Endocrinologists. *Thyroid*. 2011;21:593–646.
14. Burch HB, Wartofsky L. Life-threatening thyrotoxicosis. Thyrotoxic storm. *Endocrinol Clin North Am*. 1993;22:263–277.
15. Hausman Jr MS, Jewell ES, Engoren M. Regional versus general anesthesia in surgical patients with chronic obstructive pulmonary disease: Does avoiding general anesthesia reduce the risk of postoperative complications? *Anesth Analg*. 2015;120:1405–1412.
16. Pöpping DM, Elia N, Van Aken HK, et al. Impact of epidural analgesia on mortality and morbidity after surgery: systematic review and meta-analysis of randomized controlled trials. *Ann Surg*. 2014;259: 1056–1067.
17. Salome CM, King GG, Berend N. Physiology of obesity and effects on lung function. *J Appl Physiol*. 2010;108:206–211.
18. Reinius H, Jonsson L, Gustafsson S, et al. Prevention of atelectasis in morbidly obese patients during general anesthesia and paralysis: a computerized tomography study. *Anesthesiology*. 2009;111:979–987.
19. Kavanagh BP, Hedenstierna G. Respiratory physiology and pathophysiology. In: *Miller's Anesthesia*. 8th ed. Philadelphia: Elsevier Churchill Livingstone; 2015:444–472.
20. Smetana GW, Lawrence VA, Cornell JE. Preoperative pulmonary risk stratification for noncardiothoracic surgery: systematic review for the American College of Physicians. *Ann Intern Med*. 2006;144: 581–595.
21. Woods BD, Sladen RN. Perioperative considerations for the patient with asthma and bronchospasm. *Br J Anaesth*. 2009;103(suppl 1):i57–i65.
22. Warner DO, Warner MA, Barnes RD, et al. Perioperative respiratory complications in patients with asthma. *Anesthesiology*. 1996;85: 460–467.
23. Qaseem A, Snow V, Fitterman N, et al. Risk assessment for and strategies to reduce perioperative pulmonary complications for patients undergoing noncardiothoracic surgery: a guideline from the American College of Physicians. *Ann Intern Med*. 2006;144:575–580.
24. Poirier P, Giles TD, Bray GA, et al. Obesity and cardiovascular disease: pathophysiology, evaluation, and effect of weight loss. An update of the 1997 American Heart Association scientific statement on obesity and heart disease from the obesity committee of the council on nutrition, physical activity and metabolism. *Circulation*. 2006;113: 898–918.
25. Mantilla CB, Horlocker TT, Schroeder DR, Berry DJ, Brown DL. Risk factors for clinically relevant pulmonary embolism and deep venous thrombosis in patients undergoing primary hip or knee arthroplasty. *Anesthesiology*. 2003;99:552–560.
26. American Society of Anesthesiologists Task Force on Perioperative Management of Patients with Obstructive Sleep Apnea. Practice guidelines for the perioperative management of patients with obstructive sleep apnea: an updated report by the American Society of Anesthesiologists Task Force on Perioperative Management of Patients with Obstructive Sleep Apnea. *Anesthesiology*. 2014;120:268–286.
27. Fuster V, Ryden LE, Cannom DS, et al. 2011 ACCF/AHA/HRS focused updates incorporated into the ACC/AHA/ESC 2006 guidelines for the management of patients with atrial fibrillation: a report of the American College of Cardiology Foundation/American Heart Association Task Force on Practice Guidelines. *J Am Coll Cardiol*. 2011;57:e101–e198.
28. Hillis LD, Smith PK, Anderson JL, et al. 2011 ACCF/AHA guideline for coronary bypass surgery: a report of the American College of Cardiology Foundation/American Heart Association Task Force on Practice Guidelines developed in collaboration with the American Association of Thoracic Surgery, Society of Cardiovascular Anesthesiologists, and Society of Thoracic Surgeons. *J Am Coll Cardiol*. 2011;58:e123–e210.
29. Devereaux PJ, Sessler DI. Cardiac complications in patients undergoing major noncardiac surgery. *N Engl J Med*. 2015;373:2258–2269.
30. Ng JLW, Chan MTV, Gelb AW. Perioperative stroke in noncardiac, nonneurosurgical surgery. *Anesthesiology*. 2011;115:879–890.
31. Ashes C, Judelman S, Wijeysundera DN, et al. Selective β1-antagonism with bisoprolol is associated with fewer postoperative strokes than atenolol or metoprolol: a single-center cohort study of 44,092 consecutive patients. *Anesthesiology*. 2013;119:777–787.
32. Davis C, Tait G, Carroll J, Wijeysundera DN, Beattie WS. The Revised Cardiac Risk Index in the new millennium: a single centre prospective cohort re-evaluation of the original variables in 9,519 consecutive patients. *Can J Anaesth*. 2013;60:855–863.
33. Josephs SA, Thakar CV. Perioperative risk assessment, prevention, and treatment of acute kidney injury. *Int Anesthesiol Clin*. 2009;47:89–105.
34. Baldini G, Bagry H, Aprikian A, Carli F. Postoperative urinary retention: anesthetic and perioperative considerations. *Anesthesiology*. 2009;110:1139–1157.
35. Basurto Ona X, Martínez García L, Solà I, BonfillCosp X. Drug therapy for treating post-dural puncture headache. *Cochrane Database Syst Rev*. 2011 Aug 10;(8):CD007887.
36. Gan TJ, Diemunsch P, Habib AS, et al. Consensus guidelines for the management of postoperative nausea and vomiting. *Anesth Analg*. 2014;118:85–113.
37. Rothenberg DM, O'Connor CJ, Tuman KJ. Anesthesia and the hepatobiliary system. In: *Miller RD, ed. Miller's Anesthesia*. 8th ed. Philadelphia: Elsevier Churchill Livingstone; 2015:2244–2261.
38. Cocoma SM, Rothenberg DM. Acute acid-base disorders. In: *Roberts, PR, Todd SR, eds. Comprehensive Critical Care*. Adult. Mount Prospect, IL: Society of Critical Care; 2012:623–639.
39. Moritz ML, Ayus JC. Maintenance intravenous fluids in acutely ill patients. *N Engl J Med*. 2016;374:290–291.
40. Speicher PJ, Lagoo-Deenadayalan SA, Galanos AN, Pappas TN, Scarborough JE. Expectations and outcomes in geriatric patients with do-not-resuscitate orders undergoing emergency surgical management of bowel obstruction. *JAMA Surg*. 2013;148:23–28.
41. Rothenberg DM. What are the ethical issues with perioperative DNR orders? In: *Thompson DR, Kaufman D, eds. Critical Care Ethics: A Practice Guide*. 3rd ed. Mount Prospect, IL; 2014:215–219. L: Society of Critical Care.

42. Rothenberg DM. Informed refusal—DNR orders in the patient undergoing anesthesia and surgery and at the end-of-life. In: *Van Norman GA, Jackson S, Rosenbaum SH, Palmer SK, eds. Clinical Ethics in Anesthesiology: A Case-based Textbook*. Cambridge, UK: Cambridge University Press; 2011:13–18.
43. West JM. Informed refusal—the Jehovah's Witness patient. In: *Van Norman GA, Jackson S, Rosenbaum SH, Palmer SK, eds. Clinical Ethics in Anesthesiology: A Case-based Textbook*. Cambridge, UK: Cambridge University Press; 2011:19–26.
44. Pisani MA, Kong SY, Kasl SV, Murphy TE, Araujo KL, Van Ness PH. Days of delirium are associated with 1-year mortality in an older intensive care unit population. *Am J Respir Crit Care Med*. 2009;180:1092–1097.
45. Vasilevskis EE, Ely EW, Speroff T, Pun BT, Boehm L, Dittus RS. Reducing iatrogenic risks: ICU-acquired delirium and weakness–crossing the quality chasm. *Chest*. 2010;138:1224–1233.
46. Pandharipande PP, Sanders RD, Girard TD, et al. Effect of dexmedetomidine versus lorazepam on outcome in patients with sepsis: an a priori-designed analysis of the MENDS randomized controlled trial. *Crit Care*. 2010;14:R38.
47. Stefanini GG, Holmes DR. Drug-eluting coronary-artery stents. *N Engl J Med*. 2013;368:254–265.
48. Cutlip D, Windecker S, Cohn SL. Noncardiac surgery after percutaneous coronary intervention. In: Saperia GM, ed. *UpToDate*. UpToDate. Waltham, MA. UpToDate; 2016.

B. Anesthesia

Behnoosh Shayegan, M.D., and David M. Rothenberg, M.D.

1. Which of the following precautions should be taken to decrease the risk of fire during a tracheostomy?

A. Decrease FiO_2 from 0.5 to 0.4.

B. Avoid air/oxygen gas mixture and instead utilize nitrous oxide/oxygen.

C. Utilize a polyvinyl chloride endotracheal tube.

D. Allow adequate time for flammable skin prepping solutions to dry.

E. All of the above.

ANSWER: D

COMMENTS: Airway fires occur most often during laser airway surgery but can take place in any oxygen-rich environment where igniting stimuli may exist. A fire requires the three components known as the "fire triad," which includes an oxidizer, ignition source, and fuel. Any combustible material, including polyvinyl chloride tubing, surgical drapes, and human tissue, can ignite. If an airway fire occurs, both the surgeon and the anesthesiologist should take the following steps simultaneously:

- Remove the tracheal tube.
- Stop the flow of all airway gases.
- Remove all flammable and burning materials from the airway.
- Pour saline or water into the patient's airway.

Mask ventilation should be performed until the trachea can be safely reintubated. Consider bronchoscopy to determine the extent of the airway damage and to remove any foreign bodies that may be present. If severe, it may be necessary to leave the trachea intubated while administering oxygen.

Prevention of airway fire is crucial. If possible, nitrous oxide should be avoided, and the lowest, safest FiO_2 level should be used. Ignition sources, such as electrocautery, should be used as far as possible from oxide-rich environments. All flammable skin prepping solutions should be given adequate time to dry. Laser-safe endotracheal tubes should be used for airway laser procedures.

Ref.: 1, 2

2. Effective management of gastric acid aspiration includes which of the following?

A. Suctioning and controlled ventilation with positive end-expiratory pressure (PEEP)

B. Tracheal intubation and saline lavage of the lungs

C. Prophylactic antibiotic therapy

D. Prophylactic steroid therapy

E. Diuresis

ANSWER: A

COMMENTS: Gastric aspiration may be fatal, with the severity of the injury determined by the volume and pH of the gastric fluid aspirated. Fluid with a pH < 2.5 and a volume > 0.4 mL/kg (approximately 30 mL for an adult) is associated with a greater degree of pulmonary damage. Most cases of aspiration are considered acute chemical pneumonitis rather than infection. Therefore initial management with antibiotics is not warranted. Initial treatment should begin with intubation, suctioning of aspirated fluid, testing the pH of the fluid (if readily available), and positive pressure ventilation with PEEP. The level of PEEP is determined by the ability to adequately oxygenate (goal $PaO_2 > 60$ mmHg), ideally with the $FiO_2 < 0.6$. Saline lavage is not indicated as it has been suggested to aggravate the injury. Prophylactic steroid therapy has not been shown to be beneficial and therefore is not indicated. With the initiation of positive pressure ventilation and loss of fluid into the damaged lung parenchyma, patients are often intravascularly depleted. Thus empiric diuretic therapy is not appropriate.

Ref.: 3–5

3. A 30-year-old man with no past medical history undergoes emergency hernia repair. He has a 10-pack-per-year smoking history. What is his American Society of Anesthesiologists (ASA) physical status classification?

A. ASA class I

B. ASA class IIE

C. ASA class III

D. ASA class V

E. None of the above

ANSWER: B

COMMENTS: The ASA physical status class risk stratification system is based on the patient's comorbid conditions and is a rudimentary aid in predicting preoperative risks. The addition of "E" denotes an emergent surgery.

ASA Physical Status Classification

Classification	Definition	Examples
ASA I	Healthy patient	Healthy
ASA II	Patient with mild systemic disease	Smoker, pregnancy, obesity (body mass index [BMI] < 40), well-controlled hypertension (HTN) or diabetes mellitus (DM), mild asthma
ASA III	Patient with severe systemic disease	Poorly controlled HTN or DM, chronic obstructive pulmonary disease (COPD), morbid obesity
ASA IV	Patient with severe systemic disease that is a constant threat to life	Myocardial infarction (MI), cerebrovascular accident (CVA), sepsis, end-stage renal disease (ESRD)
ASA V	Moribund patient	Ruptured abdominal aortic aneurysm (AAA), trauma
ASA VI	Brain dead patient, organ donor	

Ref.: 6, 7

4. Which of the following regarding the inflammatory response following tissue injury is true?

A. Injury leads to platelet-inhibition factor release from endothelium.

B. There is an antiinflammatory response that leads to a return to homeostasis-accompanied suppression of the innate immune system.

C. Macrophages play an important role in wound healing.

D. The degree of inflammation is not proportional to injury severity.

E. All of the above.

ANSWER: C

COMMENTS: The degree of the systemic inflammatory response following trauma is proportional to tissue injury severity and is an independent predictor of subsequent organ dysfunction. Macrophages play a dominant role in wound healing by releasing growth factors and cytokines. Injury leads to platelet activating factor release from the endothelium along with tissue factor (factor III) release necessary for initiation of thrombin formation. The clinical features of the injury-mediated systemic inflammatory response, characterized by increased body temperature, heart rate, respirations, and white blood cell count, are similar to those observed with infection.

Ref.: 8, 9

5. Intubation of an obtunded patient with a closed head injury, who is breathing spontaneously, is best accomplished by which of the following?

A. Topical lidocaine application to the nares, spontaneous ventilation, and "blind" nasal intubation

B. Induction with etomidate, muscle relaxation with succinylcholine, and oral tracheal intubation

C. Placing a laryngeal mask airway

D. Awake tracheostomy with local anesthesia

E. Awake rigid laryngoscopy

ANSWER: B

COMMENTS: Securing an airway in the trauma patient can be challenging. Concurrent cervical injury and instability should be suspected in a patient with a head injury. Airway management should be done while maintaining in-line axial cervical stabilization. The ideal method to secure the airway in a trauma patient with increases in intracranial pressure (ICP) would be via etomidate, which can decrease cerebral blood flow and the cerebral metabolic rate, therefore decreasing ICP. Etomidate also preserves blood pressure and heart rate in the trauma patient. Succinylcholine causes a small, transient increase in ICP (approximately 4 mmHg), but these increases are offset by the ICP-reducing effect of etomidate and hyperventilation. In addition, the muscle paralysis induced by succinylcholine prevents coughing, which may increase ICP by 50 to 70 mmHg, allowing for rapid-sequence induction and intubation in a trauma patient who is presumed to be an aspiration risk. Nasal intubation carries the risk of damage to the cribriform plate when preexisting fractures are present, and epistaxis can cause airway compromise in an obtunded patient. Tracheostomy should be performed whenever airway distortion prevents prompt intubation by other methods. In some situations, tracheostomy is the appropriate initial approach to securing the airway. Placing a laryngeal mask airway would only be a temporizing measure for those situations where ventilation failed during the course of airway management.

Ref.: 10–12

6. Succinylcholine should be avoided in patients with which of the following?

A. Recent burns (2 h) of 40% of the body surface area

B. Chronic kidney disease (K^+ of 4.4 mEq/L)

C. Acute spinal cord injury (complete T4) 8 h ago

D. Age < 2 years

E. Burns to 40% of the body surface area 5 days ago

ANSWER: E

COMMENTS: Succinylcholine is a depolarizing muscle relaxant, which causes paralysis by depolarizing the motor end plate via repeated generation of action potentials. This results in an efflux of potassium ions and a transient rise in extracellular potassium levels. This increase is approximately 0.5 to 1 mEq/L in patients without neurologic deficits or severe muscular injury. Since the number of motor end plates is markedly increased (i.e., sensitization) 3 to 5 days after neurologic or muscular injury, administration of depolarizing muscle relaxants, such as succinylcholine, at this time can cause large increases in extracellular potassium and cardiac arrest. Therefore succinylcholine should be used only in the acute setting (immediately after injury) for patients with burns or spinal cord injury in whom such sensitization is not observed within the first 1 to 2 days of injury. Although routine succinylcholine use in children is not common practice, due to the associated risks of bradycardia, hyperkalemia in undiagnosed muscular dystrophies, and malignant hyperthermia (MH), its use is not contraindicated. The presence of chronic kidney disease does not preclude the use of succinylcholine if serum potassium levels are within the normal range.

Ref.: 13, 14

7. Which of the following is the most common cause of intraoperative hypothermia 2 h after induction of anesthesia?

A. Redistribution

B. Conduction

C. Evaporation

D. Convection

E. Radiation

ANSWER: E

COMMENTS: Two main mechanisms of heat loss in the operating room are through impaired thermoregulation from anesthesia and low ambient temperature of the operating room. Redistribution of body heat from the core to the periphery is the most common cause of hypothermia in the first hour after induction of anesthesia. After that, heat is lost to the environment through four main mechanisms:

Radiation—Heat loss into the surrounding atmosphere
Convection—Heat loss through contact with colder air currents
Evaporation—Heat loss from the change of liquid to vapor
Conduction—Heat loss through direct contact with a cold surface

The main source of heat loss after the first hour of surgery is radiation.

Maintaining normothermia intraoperatively is crucial since hypothermia suppresses phagocytic activity, thereby reducing oxidative bacterial killing by neutrophils and leading to wound infection. As a result of hypothermia, reflexive peripheral vasoconstriction occurs, which causes decreased blood flow to the surgical wound, decreased oxygen delivery, and increased surgical site infections.

The two most efficacious methods for preventing hypothermia in the operating room are prewarming and forced-air systems.

Other measures to increase temperature include heating IV fluids and airway gases.

Ref.: 15–17

8. Which of the following is true regarding MH?

A. Unusually low end-tidal carbon dioxide ($EtCO_2$) may be an early sign of MH.

B. MH may be triggered by nitrous oxide.

C. MH may be triggered by succinylcholine.

D. Increased core temperature is an early sign of MH.

E. There is no family correlation with MH.

ANSWER: C

COMMENTS: MH is a rare, potentially fatal condition. MH is transmitted genetically as an autosomal dominant trait with variable penetrance. It is thought that an abnormal gene causes a defect in the calcium channels in the sarcoplasmic reticulum of skeletal muscle cells. Administration of a triggering agent causes an uncontrolled release of calcium from the sarcoplasmic reticulum, which results in a hypermetabolic response in the skeletal muscle. MH should be suspected in a patient with a suspicious family history. Genetic testing is possible, but testing of a skeletal muscle biopsy is more common. Elevated serum creatinine phosphokinase levels may be seen in MH-susceptible patients, but this test is not useful for screening because of its poor specificity.

A fulminant episode is characterized by muscle rigidity, fever, tachycardia, respiratory and metabolic acidosis, severe hypermetabolism, arrhythmias, and eventual cardiovascular collapse. MH can occur minutes to several hours after the administration of triggering agents, such as succinylcholine or potent (halogenated) inhaled agents. Nitrous oxide is not a trigger for MH. The earliest, most sensitive, and most specific sign of MH is an unexplained rise in $EtCO_2$ levels despite increases in minute ventilation, followed by tachycardia, frequently with multifocal premature ventricular contractions. Increases in temperature are a relatively late finding.

Treatment involves cessation of the triggering anesthetics, administration of dantrolene (a skeletal muscle relaxant), forced cooling of the patient, increasing isotonic saline IV fluids to minimize renal dysfunction from myoglobinuria and widespread rhabdomyolysis, and monitoring of blood gas and potassium levels. Early recognition and rapid treatment are critical for survival. Avoidance of triggering agents in patients suspected of MH susceptibility is the safest and easiest method of treatment.

Ref.: 18, 19

9. Which of the following statements regarding the toxicity of local anesthetics is false?

A. Neurologic symptoms almost always precede those of cardiac toxicity.

B. The site of injection is an important determinant of toxicity.

C. The addition of a 1:100,000 epinephrine solution allows the administration of higher doses of local anesthetics.

D. The relative toxicity of local anesthetics, in decreasing order, is bupivacaine, ropivacaine, and lidocaine.

E. Pregnancy has no effect on local anesthetic toxicity.

ANSWER: E

COMMENTS: Local anesthetics can be classified into amides or esters. Systemic toxicity from local anesthetics primarily involves the central nervous system (CNS) and the cardiovascular system. Local anesthetics cross the blood–brain barrier; therefore CNS toxicity usually occurs at doses well below those that result in cardiovascular toxicity. Manifestations of CNS toxicity include confusion, dizziness, tinnitus, somnolence, and seizures. Cardiovascular toxicity is due to direct blocking effects on both cardiac and vascular smooth muscle and is generally manifested as cardiovascular collapse. Ventricular arrhythmias and asystole are the most common findings on the electrocardiogram (ECG). Lipophilicity is the predominant determinant of local anesthetic toxicity. More lipophilic drugs, such as bupivacaine and ropivacaine, are considered to have a higher toxicity profile than less lipophilic drugs, such as lidocaine.

Systemic absorption of local anesthetics is highly dependent on the vascularity of the injection site and the presence or absence of epinephrine. Epinephrine causes vasoconstriction and allows a higher maximum dose of local anesthetic to be safely administered without toxicity. Absorption of local anesthetics occurs most rapidly, with the highest serum levels from the highly vascular intercostal space, and is slowest with the lowest serum levels from infiltration of local subcutaneous tissue.

Pregnancy reduces not only the toxic threshold but also the dose of local anesthetic needed for therapeutic purposes. The enlargement of the epidural veins seen with progressive enlargement of the uterus decreases the size of the epidural space and the volume of cerebrospinal fluid in the subarachnoid space. The decreased volume of these spaces facilitates the spread of local anesthetic. Biochemical changes of pregnancy, particularly progesterone, play a role in toxicity and spread of local anesthetics. Progesterone itself has potent sedative effects.

Ref.: 20–22

10. Which of the following statements regarding propofol is false?

A. Induction and sedation doses for children are higher than those for adults.

B. Pain from propofol injection is prevented by prior midazolam treatment.

C. Propofol does not suppress the respiratory system.

D. The incidence of postoperative nausea and vomiting (PONV) is decreased with propofol-based anesthesia.

E. Propofol does not have analgesic properties.

ANSWER: C

COMMENTS: Propofol is a nonbenzodiazepine, nonbarbiturate, short-acting intravenous anesthetic with hypnotic properties. Stemming from its chemical structure as a substituted derivative of phenol, it is insoluble in water and is formulated as a 1% emulsion similar to parenteral lipid formulations. Propofol can be administered safely in most patients with egg allergy if there is no history of anaphylaxis. Induction doses are higher for children and adolescents than for adults and should be reduced for elderly patients, hypovolemic patients, and those with poor cardiac reserve. Propofol produces profound dose-dependent respiratory depression that frequently leads to apnea in patients premedicated with other sedatives. It also causes pain on injection; hypotension; and decreased systemic vascular resistance, oxygen consumption, and ICP. After single-bolus administration, propofol is rapidly redistributed (within 2 to 8 min) and rapidly hydrolyzed by the plasma. Emergence from anesthesia occurs rapidly after discontinuation of propofol, thus making it particularly suitable for short procedures and longer sedation, as in the intensive care unit (ICU). Propofol has antiemetic properties and, when administered as part of a total intravenous anesthetic, may cause less PONV than inhalational anesthetics.

Ref.: 23, 24

11. Which of the following statements regarding midazolam is true?

A. Midazolam's effects can be reversed with naloxone.

B. Midazolam does not cause respiratory depression.

C. Midazolam only causes anterograde amnesia.

D. Midazolam has no active metabolites.

E. Midazolam is minimally metabolized.

ANSWER: C

COMMENTS: Midazolam is a short-acting benzodiazepine used for its anxiolytic, anterograde amnestic, sedative, hypnotic, and anticonvulsant properties. It does not cause retrograde amnesia. Midazolam differs from other benzodiazepines in both structure and solubility. An imidazole side ring imparts stability and ease of rapid hepatic metabolism, and a water-soluble structure allows painless injection. Two active metabolites of midazolam exist and accumulate when continuous infusions are used. Like other benzodiazepines, midazolam produces dose-dependent respiratory depression (often synergistically when administered with other sedatives or opiates). All benzodiazepines should be used cautiously in elderly patients and in those with hepatic dysfunction as the half-life of these drugs is significantly increased.

Ref.: 23

12. Which of the following statements regarding neuromuscular blockade by nondepolarizing agents is false?

A. The effects are prolonged by aminoglycosides.

B. Vagolytic side effects occur with *cis*-atracurium.

C. Nondepolarizing agents may trigger MH.

D. Vecuronium undergoes primarily hepatic metabolism.

E. Train-of-four monitoring effectively predicts the degree of blockade.

ANSWER: C

COMMENTS: Nondepolarizing muscle relaxants currently in clinical use include vecuronium, *cis*-atracurium, and rocuronium. Nondepolarizing muscle relaxants interfere with transmission at the neuromuscular junction by competing with acetylcholine for available receptor sites. These effects may be reversed by anticholinesterases, which prolong the half-life of acetylcholine to overcome the competitive inhibition of the muscle relaxant. The effect of nondepolarizing agents can be prolonged by aminoglycosides, clindamycin, tetracycline, and other antibiotics; hypothermia; hypercapnia; and magnesium. Vagolytic activity is common with rocuronium but not with other agents. Except for *cis*-atracurium (which is metabolized by Hofmann elimination), the metabolism of nondepolarizing agents occurs in the liver, with varying amounts of biliary or renal metabolism and excretion. Train-of-four monitoring involves the administration of stimuli percutaneously to a peripheral nerve four times over a 1-s period and noting the distal muscular response. If fewer than two of the stimuli result in muscle contraction, more than 95% of the receptors may be blocked.

Ref.: 13, 25, 26

13. Which of the following statements regarding flumazenil is true?

A. It is a benzodiazepine antagonist that acts by competitive inhibition.

B. It has been used successfully to reverse the clinical effects of opiate overdose.

C. It is indicated for patients with suspected tricyclic antidepressant overdoses.

D. It reverses the respiratory depressant actions but not the sedative effects of benzodiazepines.

E. It does not improve hepatic encephalopathy.

ANSWER: A

COMMENTS: Flumazenil is a benzodiazepine-specific antagonist that competitively inhibits the activity of benzodiazepines at the benzodiazepine–receptor complex. Flumazenil does not antagonize the CNS effects of gamma-aminobutyric acid (GAB) Aergic-acting drugs (ethanol, barbiturates, or general anesthetics), nor does it antagonize the effects of opiates. Flumazenil antagonizes the sedation, impaired recall, psychomotor impairment, and ventilatory depression produced by all benzodiazepines. Use of flumazenil is contraindicated in patients treated with benzodiazepines for status epilepticus or tricyclic antidepressant overdose due to lowering of the seizure threshold. Case reports have demonstrated a remarkable improvement in the encephalopathic changes associated with liver failure. Flumazenil should not be used as the only agent for treating hepatic encephalopathy, but it may be helpful in patients resistant to conventional medical therapy.

Ref.: 23, 27

14. Which one of the following regarding inhaled anesthetics is false?

A. The minimum alveolar concentration (MAC) of an inhaled anesthetic is the alveolar concentration where 50% of patients do not move with an incision.

B. Nitrous oxide can expand air-filled spaces.

C. The speed of induction of an inhaled anesthetic is determined by its blood:gas solubility.

D. All volatile inhaled anesthetics can be triggers for MH.

E. The MAC does not change with age.

ANSWER: E

COMMENTS: Inhaled anesthetics produce anesthesia by enhancing inhibitory channels and blunting excitatory channels in the brain. The MAC of inhaled anesthetic is the alveolar concentration where 50% of patients do not move with incisional stimuli. It is determined by and dependent on many factors:

Factors That Increase MAC	Factors That Decrease MAC
• Infants < 1 year	• Age
• Hypernatremia	• Hyponatremia
• Hyperthermia	• Hypothermia
• Chronic Alcohol Abuse	• Acute Alcohol Intoxication
	• Anemia
	• Hypercarbia
	• Hypoxia
	• Metabolic Acidosis
	• Pregnancy

All inhaled anesthetics are considered volatile agents except nitrous oxide. They all cause a decrease in systemic vascular resistance, arterial blood pressure, and myocardial function. They also blunt the normal respiratory response to hypoxia and hypercarbia and relax airway smooth muscles. Although inhaled anesthetics produce an increase in cerebral blood flow, they cause a decrease in cerebral metabolic rate. Volatile anesthetics are potent triggers for MH, along with succinylcholine.

The blood:gas solubility of inhaled anesthetics determines the speed of induction. The more soluble a gas is, the slower its speed of induction.

Ref.: 28–30

15. With regard to pulse oximetry studies, which of the following is true?

A. Pulse oximetric analysis is unaffected by tissue perfusion.

B. Methemoglobinemia results in a displayed arterial oxygen saturation of approximately 85%.

C. Oxygen saturation measurements may be artificially decreased in the presence of carboxyhemoglobin.

D. A standard pulse oximeter measures light absorption at four wavelengths.

E. Ambient light will not affect oximetric readings.

ANSWER: B

COMMENTS: The use of pulse oximetry studies has led to a marked improvement in the care and safety of patients in the operating room, postanesthesia care unit, and ICU. The concept of oximetry is based on Beer's law, which relates the concentration of a solute in suspension (in this case, hemoglobin) to the intensity of light transmitted through the solution. Pulse oximetric analysis measures the oxygen saturation only of pulsatile blood using two wavelengths of light (red and infrared). The ratio of the pulse-added absorbencies of these two wavelengths is determined by the arterial oxygen saturation. Pulse oximetry may be difficult to perform in patients who are suffering from any type of shock or tissue hypoperfusion. Because both oxyhemoglobin and carboxyhemoglobin absorb red light similarly, the pulse oximeter reads the sum of the two hemoglobins and produces an artificially elevated reading of oxygen saturation. Direct measurement of saturation from an arterial blood gas sample is required to confirm the presence of carbon monoxide. Methemoglobinemia, a disorder that may occur with nitroglycerin toxicity, inhaled nitric oxide therapy, or topical tetracaine or benzocaine local anesthetics, results in a displayed oxygen saturation of approximately 85%. Methemoglobin does not absorb red light in the same manner as oxyhemoglobin or deoxyhemoglobin. The absorbance of red and infrared light by methemoglobin is nearly equal and results in a displayed saturation of approximately 85%. Because ambient light can affect pulse oximeter readings, it is occasionally necessary to cover the probe to avoid artifactual readings.

Ref.: 31, 32

16. While transporting an intubated patient from the operating room to the ICU, the pressure gauge on the size E compressed gas cylinder containing O_2 reads 1100 psi. How long can O_2 be delivered at a flow rate of 5 L/min?

A. 10 min

B. 5 min

C. 60 min

D. 125 min

E. 220 min

ANSWER: C

COMMENTS: A full E cylinder reading 2200 psi contains approximately 625 L of O_2. Boyle's law states that for a fixed mass of gas at constant temperature, the product of pressure and volume is constant. Boyle's law allows estimation of the volume of gas remaining in a closed container by measuring the pressure within the container. When the pressure gauge reads 1100 psi, the volume of gas in the cylinder is half that of a full cylinder (or about 625 L ÷ 2 = 312.5 L). At a flow rate of 5 L/min, the cylinder in question will last approximately 1 h. This information is important when portable sources of oxygen are being used during transport and diagnostic procedures remote from the OR.

Ref.: 33

17. After administration of epidural anesthesia to the T3 dermatome in a patient with severe COPD undergoing open cholecystectomy, which of the following is least likely to occur?

A. Increased heart rate

B. Decreased venous return

C. Decreased alveolar ventilation

D. Systemic hypotension

E. Decreased heart rate

ANSWER: A

COMMENTS: On average, after administration of epidural anesthesia, central neuraxial blockade at any dermatome level leads to sympathetic blockade two spinal segments higher than and motor blockade two spinal segments lower than the site of administration. At the T3 dermatome level, blockade of the cardiac accelerator nerves (T1–4) and unopposed vagal activity results in relative bradycardia despite hypotension caused by the reduction in venous return secondary to vasodilation. In addition, motor nerve blockade of intercostal muscle function reduces alveolar ventilation and may precipitate respiratory compromise in a patient with underlying pulmonary disease, particularly if a significant fraction of intercostal muscle function is impaired.

Ref.: 34, 35

18. Which of the following is least likely to occur in conjunction with a surgically induced stress response?

A. Increased secretion of thyroid-stimulating hormone

B. Hypercoagulability

C. Suppression of the immune response

D. Increased secretion of adrenocorticotropic hormone (ACTH)

E. Increased metabolic rate

ANSWER: A

COMMENTS: Current evidence suggests that many adverse perioperative events can be attributed to the effects of the stress response. Somatic or visceral pain can trigger the systemic release of catecholamines and neuroendocrine hormones. Hormones released in response to stress include growth hormone, ACTH, vasopressin, prolactin, cortisol, glucagon, and renin-angiotensin-aldosterone. In contrast, secretion of thyroid-stimulating hormone is decreased by the stress response. The overall systemic effects of the stress response lead to increased metabolic activity, a hypercoagulable state, and a less effective immune response to infectious agents.

Ref.: 36, 37

19. All of the following cause a right shift of the oxygen–hemoglobin dissociation curve except:

A. Fever

B. Metabolic acidosis

C. Increased 2,3-DG production

D. Respiratory acidosis

E. Fetal hemoglobin (HbF)

ANSWER: E

COMMENTS: The oxygen–hemoglobin dissociation curve plots the relationship between the proportion of saturated hemoglobin (SaO_2) and the partial pressure of oxygen (pO_2). The P50 is the oxygen tension at which 50% of the hemoglobin is saturated and is normally 26.7 mmHg. A rightward shift of the curve increases the P50 and thereby lowers the hemoglobin's affinity for oxygen (increased release to tissues). A leftward shift decreases the P50 and increases hemoglobin's affinity for oxygen, thereby reducing its availability to tissues. Increases in temperature, 2,3-BPG, and pCO_2 and decreases in pH all cause a right shift. HbF causes a left shift in the curve.

Ref.: 38, 39

20. A 44-year-old patient undergoing laparoscopic hepatic resection has a sudden decrease in $EtCO_2$ and becomes tachycardic and hypotensive. Which of the following is the most likely cause?

A. Venous air embolism (VAE)

B. MH

C. Excessive depth of anesthesia

D. Disconnection from breathing circuit

E. Decreased depth of anesthesia

ANSWER: A

COMMENTS: Air embolism is a potentially life-threatening event, which occurs when air enters the venous system from an operative field that is above the level of the heart and where venous sinusoids do not collapse under the influence of atmospheric pressure. It is most common in neurosurgical procedures in the sitting position but may also occur during laparoscopic surgeries on solid structures (e.g., liver, uterus, and hip). The two main factors that influence mortality are the volume of gas entering the venous system and the rate at which it accumulates. The clinical presentation of VAE includes cardiovascular, pulmonary, and neurologic changes. Tachyarrhythmias, as well as ST-segment changes, are common. Hypotension results as a decrease in cardiac output. Decreased $EtCO_2$, desaturation, and hypoxia may also be seen with VAE. Detection of VAE includes transesophageal echocardiogram (most sensitive) and precordial Doppler. Management includes discontinuing insufflation, flooding the field with saline, increasing FiO_2, and hemodynamic support. MH leads to an increase in $EtCO_2$, and excessive depth of anesthesia causes a gradual decline in blood pressure and $EtCO_2$; disconnection causes complete loss of $EtCO_2$ without changes in blood pressure or heart rate, and light anesthesia causes tachycardia and hypertension.

Ref.: 40–42

REFERENCES

1. Modest VM, Alfille PH. Anesthesia for laser surgery. In: *Miller's Anesthesia*. 8th ed. Elsevier Churchill Livingstone; 2015:2598–2611.
2. American Society of Anesthesiologist. Practice advisory for the prevention and management of operating room fire. *Anesthesiology*. 2008;2008(108):786–801.
3. Practice Guidelines for Preoperative Fasting and the Use of Pharmacologic Agents to Reduce the Risk of Pulmonary Aspiration. Application to Healthy Patients Undergoing Elective Procedures: an updated report by the American Society of Anesthesiologists Committee on Standards and Practice Parameters. *Anesthesiology*. 2011;114:495–511.
4. Lanspa MJ, Jones BE, Brown SM, Dean NC. Mortality, morbidity, and disease severity of patients with aspiration pneumonia. *J Hosp Med*. 2013;8:83–90.
5. Marik PE. Aspiration pneumonitis and aspiration pneumonia. *N Engl J Med*. 2001;344:665–671.
6. Wijeysundera DN, Sweitzer B-J. Preoperative evaluation. In: *Miller's Anesthesia*. 8th ed. Elsevier Churchill Livingstone; 2015:1085–1155.
7. Skaga NO, Eken T, Sovik S, et al. Pre-injury ASA physical status classification is an independent predictor of mortality after trauma. *J Trauma Injury Infect Crit Care*. 2007;63:972–978.
8. Lenz A, Franklin GA, Cheadle WG. Systemic inflammation after trauma. *Injury*. 2007;38:1336–1345.
9. Marik PE, Flemmer M. The immune response to surgery and trauma: implications for treatment. *J Trauma Acute Care Surg*. 2012;73:801–808.
10. Mccunn M, Grissom TE, Dutton RP. Anesthesia for trauma. In: *Miller's Anesthesia*. 8th ed. Elsevier Churchill Livingstone; 2015:2423–2459.
11. Baird CRW, Hay AW, McKeown DW, Ray DC. Rapid sequence induction in the emergency department: induction drug and outcome of patients admitted to the intensive care unit. *Emerg Med J*. 2009;26:576–579.
12. Perkins ZB, Wittenberg MD, Nevin D, Lockey DJ, O'Brien B. The relationship between head injury severity and hemodynamic response to tracheal intubation. *J Trauma Acute Care Surg*. 2013;74:1074–1080.
13. Martyn JJA. Neuromuscular physiology and pharmacology. In: *Miller's Anesthesia*. 8th ed. Elsevier Churchill Livingstone; 2015:423–443.
14. Meakin GH. Neuromuscular blocking drugs in infants and children. *Contin Educ Anaesth Criti Care Pain*. 2007;7:143–147.
15. Sessler DI. Temperature regulation and monitoring. In: *Miller's Anesthesia*. 8th ed. Elsevier Churchill Livingstone; 2015:1622–1646.
16. Seamon MJ, Wobb J, Gaughan JP, et al. The effects of intraoperative hypothermia on surgical site infection: an analysis of 524 trauma laparotomies. *Ann Surg*. 2012;225:789–795.
17. Beltramini AM, Salata RA, Ray AJ. Thermoregulation and risk of surgical site infection. *Infect Control Hosp Epidemiol*. 2011;32:603–610.
18. Zhou J, Bose D, Allen PD, Pessah IN. Malignant hyperthermia and muscle-related disorders. In: *Miller's Anesthesia*. 8th ed. Elsevier Churchill Livingstone; 2015:1287–1314.
19. Litman RS, Rosenberg H. Malignant hyperthermia-associated diseases: state of the art uncertainty. *Anesth Analg*. 2009;109:1004–1005.
20. Berde CB, Strichartz GR. Local anesthetics. In: *Miller's Anesthesia*. 8th ed. Elsevier Churchill Livingstone; 2015:1028–1054.
21. Zink W, Graf BM. The toxicity of local anesthetics: the place of ropivacaine and levobupivacaine. *Curr Opin Anaesthesiol*. 2008;21:645–650.
22. Bourne E, Wright C, Royse C. A review of local anesthetic cardiotoxicity and treatment with lipid emulsion. *Local Reg Anesth*. 2010;3:11–19.
23. Vuyk J, Sitsen E, Reekers M. Intravenous anesthetics. In: *Miller's Anesthesia*. 8th ed. Elsevier Churchill Livingstone; 2015:821–863.
24. Vasileiou I, Xanthos T, Koudouna E, et al. Propofol: a review of its non-anaesthetic effects. *Eur J Pharmacol*. 2009;605:1–8.
25. Murphy GS, Brull SJ. Residual Neuromuscular block: lessons unlearned. Part I: Definitions, incidence, and adverse physiological effects of residual neuromuscular block. *Anesth Analg*. 2010;111:120–128.
26. Brull SJ, Murphy GS. Residual neuromuscular block: lessons unlearned. Part II: Methods to reduce the risk of residual weakness. *Anesth Analg*. 2010;111:129–140.

27. Marraffa JM, Cohen V, Howland MA. Antidotes for toxicological emergencies: a practical review. *Am J Health Syst Pharm*. 2012;69: 199–212.
28. Perouansky M, Pearce RA, Hemmings HC. Inhaled anesthetics. In: *Miller's Anesthesia*. 8th ed. Elsevier Churchill Livingstone; 2015: 614–637.
29. Forman SA, Ishizawa Y. Inhaled anesthetic pharmacokinetics. In: *Miller's Anesthesia*. 8th ed. Elsevier Churchill Livingstone; 2015: 638–669.
30. Eger EI. Characteristics of anesthetic agents used for induction and maintenance of general anesthesia. *Am J Health Syst Pharm*. 2004;61 (suppl 4):S3–10.
31. Chitilian HV, Kaczka DW. Vidal Melo MF. Respiratory monitoring. In: *Miller's Anesthesia*. 8th ed. Elsevier Churchill Livingstone; 2015: 1541–1579.
32. Ortega R, Hansen CJ, Elterman K, Woo A. Pulse oximetry. *N Engl J Med*. 2011;364. e33.
33. De Ruyter ML. Medical gas supply. In: *Faust's Anesthesiology Review*. 4th ed. Elsevier Inc; 2015.
34. Brull R, MacFarlane AJR, Chan VWS. Spinal, epidural and caudal anesthesia. In: *Miller's Anesthesia*. 8th ed. Elsevier Churchill Livingstone; 2015:1684–1720.
35. Freise H, Van Aken HK. Risks and benefits of thoracic epidural anaesthesia. *Brit J Anaesth*. 2011;107:859–868.
36. Finnerty CC, Mabvuure NT, Ali A, et al. The surgically induced stress response. *J Parenter Enteral Nutr*. 2013;37:21S–29S.
37. Huiku M, Uutela K, van Gils, et al. Assessment of surgical stress during general anaesthesia. *Brit J Anaesth*. 2007;98:447–455.
38. Hall JE. Transport of oxygen and carbon dioxide in blood and tissue fluids. In: *Guyton and Hall Textbook of Medical Physiology*. 13th ed. Elsevier Inc; 2016:527–537.
39. Dash RK, Bassingthwaighte JB. Erratum to: Blood HbO_2 and $HbCO_2$ dissociation curves at varied O_2, CO_2, pH, 2,3-DPG and temperature levels. *Ann Biomed Eng*. 2010;38:1683–1701.
40. Kim CS, Kim JY, Kwon J, et al. Venous air embolism during total laparoscopic hysterectomy: comparison to total abdominal hysterectomy. *Anesthesiology*. 2009;111:50–54.
41. Park EY, Kwon J, Kim KJ. Carbon dioxide embolism during laparoscopic surgery. *Yonsei Med J*. 2012;53:459–466.
42. Jayaraman S, Khakhar A, Yang H, et al. The association between central venous pressure, pneumoperitoneum, and venous carbon dioxide embolism in laparoscopic hepatectomy. *Surg Endosc*. 2009;23:2369–2373.

CHAPTER 8

FUNDAMENTALS OF SURGICAL TECHNOLOGY

A. Principles of Minimally Invasive Surgery

Philip Omotosho, M.D., and Jonathan A. Myers, M.D.

1. Which of the following is not a characteristic of carbon dioxide (CO_2) as an insufflation gas?

A. Rapidly absorbed
B. Relatively inexpensive
C. Negligible physiologic consequences
D. Low risk of gas embolism
E. Readily available

ANSWER: C

COMMENTS: CO_2 is the most commonly used insufflation gas in laparoscopic surgery. The main reasons are its ready availability and relatively inexpensive cost. However, the gas does not support combustion and is rapidly eliminated. CO_2 pneumoperitoneum is associated with significant physiologic changes in major organ systems, including cardiopulmonary and renal effects, as well as changes in intracranial pressure and mesenteric blood flow.

Ref.: 1

2. Which of the following hemodynamic parameters decreases during laparoscopy with CO_2 pneumoperitoneum?

A. Mean arterial pressure
B. Pulmonary vascular resistance
C. Systemic vascular resistance
D. Heart rate
E. Peripheral blood flow

ANSWER: E

COMMENTS: CO_2 pneumoperitoneum produces consistent cardiopulmonary effects, but the magnitude of these effects depends on several factors, including the anesthetic agent, underlying cardiopulmonary status, and metabolic factors. CO_2 pneumoperitoneum causes diminished venous return in the cardiovascular system, which produces decreased preload, stroke volume, and cardiac output. In addition, direct myocardial depression due to CO_2 pneumoperitoneum reduces stroke volume and cardiac output. These changes produce a compensatory increase in heart rate and systemic and pulmonary vascular resistance. Increased intraabdominal pressure on the aorta, vena cava, and splanchnic vasculature along with the compensatory release of renin and vasopressin produces increased systemic vascular resistance and decreased peripheral blood flow.

Ref.: 1

3. Which of the following conditions represents a contraindication to advanced laparoscopic operations?

A. Pregnancy
B. Morbid obesity
C. Contraindication to general anesthesia
D. Previous laparotomy
E. Cirrhosis

ANSWER: C

COMMENTS: The indications for laparoscopic surgery are generally the same as those for open surgery, but several factors may complicate or increase the difficulty associated with laparoscopic surgery. High-risk [American Society of Anesthesiologists (ASA) class IV] patients are not ideal candidates for laparoscopic surgery because of the prerequisite for establishing pneumoperitoneum. Gas-less laparoscopy with regional anesthesia has been used in the past to avoid the use of gas insufflation. Yet high-risk patients may not tolerate the increased intraabdominal pressure required for adequate visualization. Morbid obesity, previous abdominal surgery, and pregnancy are no longer considered contraindications to laparoscopy. However, these patients with these conditions might be at an increased risk for the development of complications of surgery and anesthesia, so adequate preoperative preparation is essential. Morbidly obese patients may be difficult to intubate and might require large doses of muscle relaxants. Proper positioning is paramount to prevent nerve injuries. Selecting an appropriate access point for establishing pneumoperitoneum is important in those who have previously undergone laparotomy. Ultrasound imaging of the abdominal wall (visceral sliding technique) and selection of the left upper quadrant as a point of entry (Palmer's point) are useful techniques. These considerations are important in pregnant patients to maintain adequate fetal blood flow and prevent uterine injury. Although it increases the likelihood of complications, early cirrhosis with preserved hepatic synthetic function is no longer considered an absolute contraindication to laparoscopy.

Ref.: 1

4. Which of the following does not routinely increase during laparoscopic surgery?

A. Airway pressure

B. Pulmonary capillary wedge pressure

C. Vital capacity

D. Diaphragmatic excursion

E. Intrathoracic pressure

ANSWER: C

COMMENTS: Unlike the indirect cardiac effects, almost all respiratory changes during laparoscopic surgery are directly attributable to the mechanical effects of increased intraabdominal pressure. This produces increased diaphragmatic excursion, which in turn causes increased airway pressure and decreased vital capacity, functional reserve capacity, and thoracic compliance. The combination of these factors typically requires a 15% increase in minute ventilation for compensation, even in healthy subjects.

Ref.: 1

5. Which of the following is not a recommended technique for initial trocar placement during laparoscopic surgery?

A. Veress needle insufflation followed by blind trocar placement

B. Open placement of a Hasson cannula without pneumoperitoneum

C. Optical trocar placement

D. Blind trocar placement without pneumoperitoneum

E. All of the above

ANSWER: D

COMMENTS: Initial intraperitoneal access for laparoscopic surgery may be obtained with a number of open or closed approaches. One standard closed method involves inserting a Veress needle to achieve insufflation, most commonly at the umbilicus or in the left upper quadrant, followed by blind trocar placement. Another closed technique involves using an optical trocar to visualize the abdominal wall layers during insertion. Open access techniques use a direct cut-down, and the fascia and peritoneum are opened under direct visual inspection. A blunt Hasson trocar is then placed and secured before peritoneal insufflation. Blind trocar placement alone is not a recommended technique for abdominal access. With appropriate training and good surgical judgment, all of the remaining methods listed can be used safely.

Ref.: 2

6. Which of the following insufflation gases should not be used with radiofrequency (RF) electrosurgery ("electrocautery")?

A. CO_2

B. Nitrous oxide

C. Argon

D. Helium

E. None of the above

ANSWER: B

COMMENTS: CO_2 is the most commonly used gas for peritoneal insufflation, but alternative gases are available. Nitrous oxide has been used for procedures performed under local anesthesia because it does not cause the acid–base disturbances associated with CO_2 pneumoperitoneum and may cause less postoperative pain. However, it supports combustion, and its use is not recommended in procedures that require RF electrosurgery. Use of inert gases, such as helium and argon, also prevents acid–base problems; however, these agents are rarely used because they are expensive and have low solubility, which may increase the risk for gas embolism. In addition, argon may cause significant cardiac depression.

Ref.: 2

7. Select the most appropriate site for initial trocar placement in a patient undergoing laparoscopic Nissen fundoplication with a previous midline scar from the xiphoid to the pubis:

A. Umbilical

B. Suprapubic

C. Left upper quadrant

D. Left lower quadrant

E. Right upper quadrant

ANSWER: C

COMMENTS: The most appropriate site for the placement of the initial trocar for a laparoscopic operation depends on several factors, including the procedure to be performed; the size and shape of the patient; the location of previous incisions; and the presence of organomegaly, hernias, or masses. Frequently, the umbilicus is the site of choice, but alternatively, nonmidline sites may be used in patients with previous abdominal surgery. The area of previous incisions should be avoided, and the chosen site should be lateral to the rectus muscle to avoid the major abdominal wall vessels. Laparoscopic Nissen fundoplication often requires a trocar in the left subcostal position, thus making this an ideal choice for this patient.

Ref.: 2

8. Thirty minutes into a laparoscopic procedure, visualization becomes inadequate to proceed. The insufflation monitor shows an intraabdominal pressure of 20 mmHg and no flow of CO_2. What is the most likely explanation?

A. An empty CO_2 canister

B. CO_2 leak from the abdominal wall

C. Inadequate muscle relaxation

D. Improper insufflator settings

E. Dislodged insufflation tubing

ANSWER: C

COMMENTS: When visualization inexplicably deteriorates during a laparoscopic procedure, the cause is most often an inadvertent loss of the pneumoperitoneum that has been maintaining the operative exposure. This may occur for several reasons, but in this case, the intraabdominal pressure is high with no gas flow in the presence of decreased pneumoperitoneum. This scenario is most commonly caused by abdominal muscle contraction because of inadequate paralysis, but occlusion of the insufflation tubing could produce similar findings. Peritoneal gas leaks via trocar sites or through a trocar may produce impaired visualization, but this will be manifested as low pressure and a high gas flow rate.

Ref.: 2

9. Shortly following CO_2 insufflation, the heart rate of an otherwise healthy 50-year-old woman undergoing laparoscopic cholecystectomy decreases to 40 beats/min. What is the most likely cause of her bradycardia?

A. Gas embolism

B. Unrecognized hemorrhage

C. CO_2 pneumoperitoneum

D. Anesthetic drugs

E. Capnothorax

ANSWER: C

COMMENTS: Cardiac arrhythmias are not uncommon during laparoscopic surgery and occur in up to 25% of patients. The most frequent insufflation-associated arrhythmia is sinus bradycardia, although tachycardia and premature ventricular contractions may also occur. Bradycardia has been attributed to the vasovagal effect of stretching the peritoneum during insufflation; therefore gradual insufflation at a low flow rate is advisable to avoid this complication.

Ref.: 2

10. During laparoscopic paraesophageal hernia repair, the patient's end-tidal CO_2 increases to 48 mmHg and the airway pressure rises. Blood pressure and heart rate are stable. What is the most appropriate next step?

A. Place a chest tube for capnothorax.

B. Increase minute ventilation.

C. Convert to an open operation.

D. Immediately desufflate the abdomen.

E. Proceed with the intervention.

ANSWER: B

COMMENTS: CO_2 diffuses across the peritoneum into the venous circulation where it is carried to the lungs for alveolar elimination. Hypercapnia may result, and an increase in expired CO_2 is typical. The mechanical effects of pneumoperitoneum increase diaphragmatic excursion and airway pressure and can be anticipated in any laparoscopic procedure. A 15% increase in minute ventilation is usually required to compensate for these effects, even in healthy patients. Some patients with a severe cardiopulmonary impairment may present with severe hypercapnia that cannot be controlled in this manner and may require conversion to an open procedure. Immediate release of the pneumoperitoneum should be the surgeon's first maneuver when acute hemodynamic instability develops during the course of a laparoscopic procedure.

Ref.: 2

11. Which of the following is true regarding infection, tumor growth, and laparoscopic surgery?

A. Immunosuppression is increased in comparison with an open surgery.

B. The acute-phase proteins interleukin-6 (IL-6) and C-reactive protein are elevated after laparotomy.

C. The catecholamine response after laparoscopy is reduced in comparison to laparotomy.

D. Current studies demonstrate increased port site metastasis after a laparoscopic colectomy.

E. Survival is improved after a laparoscopic colon resection.

ANSWER: C

COMMENTS: Reversible immunosuppression occurs after both open and laparoscopic procedures. Several acute-phase proteins, such as IL-6 and C-reactive protein, which correlate with the physiologic stress response, are reduced after laparotomy. However, the magnitude of immunosuppression is considerably lower after laparoscopy. This is supported in studies that demonstrate significantly more depressed cell-mediated immunity in patients undergoing laparotomy than in those undergoing laparoscopy. A decreased stress response to laparoscopic surgery is also supported by a reduced catecholamine response to laparoscopic versus open cholecystectomy.

Regarding tumor growth and spread of neoplasms, early studies demonstrated the existence of port site metastasis after a laparoscopic colon surgery. Theories for this include aerosolization of neoplastic cells in the peritoneum, direct implantation of cells during removal of specimens, and local trauma from the procedure, resulting in hematogenous spread. However, the Clinical Outcomes of Surgical Therapy (COST) study, published in 2003, demonstrated that "in experienced hands, laparoscopic and open colectomy were equivalent techniques with no oncologic disadvantage to patients."

Ref.: 3, 4

12. Following insertion of a Veress needle, what is the initial maneuver to confirm intraperitoneal placement?

A. Saline drop test

B. Aspiration of the needle

C. Flushing the needle

D. Measuring insufflation pressure

E. Starting high-flow insufflation

ANSWER: B

COMMENTS: When using the Veress needle technique, free entry of the needle into the peritoneal cavity must be confirmed before beginning insufflation. Usually, two audible clicks are heard as the needle traverses the fascia and peritoneum. Following suspected entry, the needle is aspirated to ensure that no blood, urine, or intestinal contents are returned. Subsequently, a saline drop test is confirmatory of intraperitoneal needle placement when saline in the needle hub flows freely through the needle. Insufflation should be initiated only after the confirmation of needle position. Low insufflation pressure should also be confirmed at this time.

Ref.: 5

13. Which of the following is not a potential advantage of robotic-assisted laparoscopy compared with standard laparoscopy?

A. Improved ergonomics

B. Reduced operative times

C. Increased manual dexterity

D. Reduced fatigue of assistants

E. Elimination of tremor

ANSWER: B

COMMENTS: The introduction of laparoscopy represented a revolution in the care of patients undergoing abdominal surgical procedures by reducing surgical invasiveness. This major advantage is proven and well documented. However, laparoscopic approaches often increased procedure complexity and added significant learning curves, both for surgeons experienced in open technique and for new trainees. In addition, certain difficulties became apparent with increasing utilization of laparoscopy: rigidity and limited fine movement of long instruments, amplification of natural tremor, ergonomic challenges associated with positioning and available instrumentation, and fatigue. Robotic systems have been developed to address some of these limitations and potentially further increase the adoption of laparoscopy. These systems allow automated camera function and retraction and limit the demands on assistants while allowing the surgeon to maintain a comfortable sitting position during operation. In addition, robotic arms provide seven degrees of freedom and mimic the mobility of the human wrist. However, most robotic-assisted procedures have been shown to take longer than the standard laparoscopic or open variants for a variety of reasons, including the time required for robot setup. Moreover, the robotic arms are not attached to the operating table, and changes in patient positioning often require removal of the arms and replacement after repositioning. Currently, these systems are also limited by their large size and associated higher cost.

Ref.: 6, 7

14. In the United States, recommendations for human natural-orifice transluminal endoscopic surgery (NOTES) procedures from the Natural Orifice Surgery Consortium for Assessment and Research (NOSCAR) include which of the following?

A. Informed consent

B. Institutional Review Board (IRB)-approved research protocol

C. Use of laparoscopy to confirm hemostasis and security of luminal closure

D. Inclusion of cases in a national NOTES registry

E. All of the above

ANSWER: E

COMMENTS: Since 2005, rapid development of NOTES has occurred primarily in acute animal survival models, but diagnostic transgastric peritoneoscopy and transgastric and transvaginal cholecystectomy have been successfully performed in human patients. NOSCAR was developed to guide the research, development, and clinical application of these technologies. Because these procedures all remain experimental at present, NOTES must be performed in the United States under an IRB-approved protocol with laparoscopic confirmation of hemostasis and secure luminal closure. NOSCAR has also requested that all cases be recorded in a national registry to facilitate data collection regarding their safety and efficacy.

Ref.: 8

REFERENCES

1. Jamal MK, Scott-Connor CH. Patient selection and practical considerations in laparoscopic surgery. In: Soper NJ, Swanstrom LL, Eubanks WS, eds. *Mastery of Endoscopic and Laparoscopic Surgery*. 3rd ed. Philadelphia: Lippincott Williams & Wilkins; 2009.
2. Fingerhut A, Millat B, Borie F. Prevention of complications in laparoscopic surgery. In: Soper NJ, Swanstrom LL, Eubanks WS, eds. *Mastery of Endoscopic and Laparoscopic Surgery*. 2nd ed. Philadelphia: Lippincott Williams & Wilkins; 2005.
3. Are C, Raman S, Talamini M. Physiologic consequences of laparoscopic surgery. In: Soper NJ, Swanstrom LL, Eubanks WS, eds. *Mastery of Endoscopic and Laparoscopic Surgery*. 2nd ed. Philadelphia: Lippincott Williams & Wilkins; 2005.
4. Nagle D. Laparoscopic colon surgery. In: Cameron JL, ed. *Current Surgical Therapy*. 9th ed. Philadelphia: CV Mosby; 2008.
5. Kaban GK, Czerniach DR, Novitsky YW, et al. Special access techniques in laparoscopic surgery. In: Soper NJ, Swanstrom LL, Eubanks WS, eds. *Mastery of Endoscopic and Laparoscopic Surgery*. 2nd ed. Philadelphia: Lippincott Williams & Wilkins; 2005.
6. Gould JC, Melvin WS. Surgical robotics. In: Soper NJ, Swanstrom LL, Eubanks WS, eds. *Mastery of Endoscopic and Laparoscopic Surgery*. 3rd ed. Philadelphia: Lippincott Williams & Wilkins; 2009.
7. Higgins RM, Frelich MJ, Bosler ME, Gould JC. Cost analysis of robotic versus laparoscopic general surgery procedures. *Surg Endosc*. 2017;31:185–192.
8. Swanstrom LL, Soper NJ. New developments in surgical endoscopy: natural orifice transluminal endoscopic surgery. In: Soper NJ, Swanstrom LL, Eubanks WS, eds. *Mastery of Endoscopic and Laparoscopic Surgery*. 3rd ed. Philadelphia: Lippincott Williams & Wilkins; 2009.

B. Principles of Surgical Endoscopy

Donnamarie Packer, M.D., Benjamin R. Veenstra, M.D., and Edward F. Hollinger, M.D., Ph.D.

1. A major disadvantage of a flexible fiberoptic endoscope is:

A. Loops in the scope
B. Image quality
C. Size of the scope
D. Fragility of the fibers
E. Inadequate scope length

ANSWER: D

COMMENTS: Initial endoscopy technology utilized fiberoptic light transmission. Two bundles of fine glass fibers are packed together. Light from an emitting source is transferred through one bundle while the image is reflected back to the viewing optic. The image clarity is dependent on the orientation and fibers remaining intact. A reflective layer envelopes the fibers allowing light to bounce back and forth within the fiber, prohibiting minimal light loss. However, if any fibers fracture, light transmission is compromised and the image develops dark spots affecting the image quality. Fiber fragility affects long-term device functionality. Newer endoscope technology utilizes a charge-coupled device (CCD) chip–based camera at the tip of the endoscope relaying a digital image to a video processor. Photocell receptor density on the CCD chip determines the image resolution and allows for higher image quality with smaller scope diameters.

***Ref.:** 1*

2. Endoscopy equipment requires thorough cleaning after each use; however, sterilization is not attained. Many cleaning methods exist, but the advantage of disinfecting equipment with glutaraldehyde as opposed to ethylene oxide gas is which of the following?

A. Removes gross contaminants
B. Does not require an overnight cycle
C. Less toxic
D. Less corrosive on equipment
E. Does not require gross contaminant removal

ANSWER: B

COMMENTS: Endoscopes are a valuable tool diagnostically and therapeutically. However, cases of infection associated with their use have been documented, although low. To prevent the spread of infection, all endoscopes must undergo high-level disinfection after each use. Gross contamination must be mechanically removed with thorough cleaning to allow a high level of disinfection. The major cause of infection transmission is inadequate cleaning and failure to follow recommended cleaning procedures. The endoscope is immersed in a disinfectant, and all channels are perfused. Glutaraldehyde is a commonly used and U.S. Food and Drug Administration-approved disinfectant with a 12-min use time. Ethylene oxide gas is available for endoscope sterilization but requires 12-h processing and aeration.

***Ref.:** 2*

3. A 68-year-old male with a history of a cardiac murmur is being scheduled for a screening colonoscopy. Which of the follow is true regarding antibiotic prophylaxis for endocarditis prevention?

A. Prophylactic antibiotics are indicated in a patient with a prosthetic mitral valve with planned colonoscopy.
B. Prophylactic antibiotics are indicated in instances of mitral regurgitation with planned colonoscopy polypectomy.
C. Prophylactic antibiotics are indicated in a patient with a prosthetic mitral valve with planned esophagogastroduodenoscopy (EGD).
D. Prophylactic antibiotics are indicated in a patient with a prosthetic mitral valve with planned sclerotherapy of esophageal varices.
E. Not indicated in any of the above scenarios.

ANSWER: D

COMMENTS: The risk for bacterial endocarditis after endoscopic procedures is very low. The mean frequency of bacteremia during upper endoscopy and colonoscopy is 4.5%. Bacteremia occurs briefly but rarely leads to clinically significant complications. The highest risk for bacteremia is seen with esophageal stricture dilation and sclerotherapy of esophageal varices. Cardiac lesions at the highest risk for infective endocarditis are prosthetic cardiac valves, history of prior bacterial endocarditis, surgical systemic-pulmonary shunts, and complex congenital heart disease. Prophylactic antibiotic coverage should be provided in cases with high risk for cardiac lesions and for procedures that have a high frequency of bacteremia.

***Ref.:** 3, 4*

4. A 50-year-old male presents with complaint of melena for 1 month with associated fatigue and weight loss. Which of the following is true regarding common bowel preparations available?

A. Ideal preparations allow fluid and electrolyte balance shifts.
B. Iso-osmotic preparations contain polyethylene glycol.
C. During active colitis, bowel preparations do not cause mucosal changes that may alter pathologic diagnosis.
D. Hyperosmotic preparations are safe in renal failure patients.
E. Iso-osmotic preparations are osmotic balance absorbable electrolyte solutions.

ANSWER: B

COMMENTS: Colonoscopies require proper preparation to allow for thorough evaluation of the colonic mucosa. Ideal preparations reliably empty the colon of all fecal material, do not affect the histology of the mucosa, require short ingestion time, and do not lead to fluid or electrolyte balance shifts. Two common categories of preparations include iso-osmotic preparations containing polyethylene glycol and hyperosmotic preparations containing sodium phosphate. Iso-osmotic preparations are useful because they do not cause a significant change in weight, electrolytes, hematocrit, or histologic appearance of the mucosa. In addition, iso-osmotic preparations are safely used in patients with electrolyte imbalances, liver disease, congestive heart failure, and renal failure.

Ref.: 5

5. A commonly available over-the-counter bowel preparation is magnesium citrate. Which of the following is true regarding hyperosmotic preparations?

A. They cause limited fluid influx into the lumen of the bowel.

B. They are safe to use in renal failure.

C. They lead to cholecystokinin release to stimulate fluid secretion and promote intestinal motility.

D. Oral phosphates given in large doses for bowel preparation can lead to hypophosphatemia and hypercalcemia.

E. They require large volume ingestion to obtain results.

ANSWER: C

COMMENTS: Hyperosmotic preparations draw fluid into the lumen of the bowel to encourage evacuation; smaller volume ingestion is therefore required and is better tolerated by the patient. However, they can lead to dehydration if the patients do not replenish their losses. In addition, magnesium citrate, a hyperosmotic preparation, utilizes cholecystokinin release to stimulate fluid secretion and intestinal motility. Lastly, sodium phosphate preparations have been studied and found to alter serum electrolytes and extracellular fluid, leading to hyperphosphatemia and hypokalemia. Relative contraindications for hyperosmotic preparations include renal failure, congestive heart failure, and ascites.

Ref.: 6

6. A 35-year-old female presenting with newly diagnosed choledocholithiasis is being prepared for endoscopic retrograde cholangiopancreatography (ERCP) under general anesthesia. Which screening tests should be done?

A. Basic metabolic panel (BMP)

B. Partial prothrombin time (PTT)/prothrombin time (PT)/ international normalized ratio (INR)

C. Pregnancy

D. Type and screen

E. All of the above

ANSWER: C

COMMENTS: Assessing a patient for risks associated with anesthesia is an important physician skill. Prior to endoscopy, the surgeon should review the patient's history of medical illness, medications, previous endoscopies, allergies, and bleeding tendencies. Screening tests are not routinely indicated prior to conscious sedation endoscopy unless the patient's medical history or physical examination warrants them. The American Society for Gastrointestinal Endoscopy recommends the following for routine testing. Coagulation studies and routine cross-matching for bleeding abnormalities in patients with clinical risk factors. Hemoglobin and electrolytes are not indicated without a history of anemia. An electrocardiogram (ECG) should be performed if there is a history of arrhythmia. As for potentially fertile women, routine pregnancy test is indicated prior to general anesthesia and if fluoroscopy is planned, however it is not indicated for conscious sedation.

Ref.: 7

7. According to the American Society of Anesthesiology (ASA) task force, what is the primary cause of morbidity in patients undergoing endoscopy?

A. Airway obstruction

B. Perforation of gastrointestinal (GI) tract

C. Hypotension

D. Bleeding

E. Pharyngeal trauma

ANSWER: A

COMMENTS: Practice guidelines for sedation and analgesia for nonanesthesiologists set forth by the ASA task force recommend that all patients undergoing moderate sedation should be monitored with pulse oximetry, exhaled CO_2 monitoring, and blood pressure and heart rate at 5-min intervals. For deep sedation with propofol, end-tidal CO_2 capnography and continuous ECG should be routinely performed. According to the ASA task force, primary causes of morbidity during endoscopy stem from medication and induce hypoventilation and airway obstruction. In addition, pulse oximetry alone is insufficient to monitor hypoventilation since it does not provide data on ventilation, and capnography should be utilized.

Ref.: 8, 9

8. A 78-year-old male underwent EGD for evaluation of dysphagia. Endoscope insertion was difficult, and postprocedure, the surgeon is concerned about perforation. Which of the following is an early sign of possible perforation?

A. Chest wall rigidity

B. Hypotension

C. Hypoxia

D. Neck stiffness

E. Cervical crepitus

ANSWER: E

COMMENTS: The most common complications arising from upper GI endoscopy include cardiopulmonary complications related to sedation and analgesia, oxygen desaturations, and perforation of the upper GI tract (0.03%). Risk for perforation can be decreased by visualizing the lumen during scope advancement at all times and avoiding excessive force. If perforation is suspected, an upper GI study with water-soluble contrast should be performed. Concerning signs of perforation are dependent upon the location of perforation and include cervical crepitus, substernal chest pain, and abdominal pain or rigidity.

Ref.: 10

9. Routine upper endoscopy usually requires the patients to be on their left side. Under what circumstance would you need to position the patients on their right side for an upper endoscopy procedure?

A. Barrett's esophagus

B. Acute upper GI bleed

C. Unable to intubate the pylorus

D. Unable to navigate past an esophageal stricture

E. Esophageal varix banding

ANSWER: B

COMMENTS: Standard upper endoscopy positioning recommends the patient lay on his or her left side with head slightly elevated and positioned near the endoscopy tower. However, during an acute upper GI bleed, blood will pool in the fundus of the stomach while positioned with the left side down and may preclude a lesion from being visualized. Rolling the patient to a right-side down position will empty the fundus of blood and clot and allow for a complete examination.

Ref.: 11

10. On reaching the duodenal bulb, what technical scope manipulations will allow maneuvering of the sharp turn of the superior angle of the duodenum?

A. Dial down, dial right, rotate shaft clockwise

B. Dial up, dial left, rotate shaft counterclockwise

C. Dial up, dial right, rotate shaft clockwise

D. Dial up, dial right, rotate shaft counterclockwise

E. Dial down, dial left, rotate shaft clockwise

ANSWER: C

COMMENTS: Several technical maneuvers are documented to help aid visualization during upper endoscopy. Duodenal intubation and retroflexion of the gastroesophageal (GE) junction continue to be two technical skills required to complete a thorough upper endoscopy. On passing the pylorus, the duodenal bulb should come into view. Advancement then leads to the sharp turn of the superior angle of the duodenum. To maneuver this angle, one simultaneously dials up, right and twists the shaft clockwise (right-hand maneuver). To visualize the GE junction, withdraw the endoscope into the antrum and deflect the tip of the endoscope all the way up while rotating counterclockwise and withdrawing the scope pulling into the proximal body and cardia.

Ref.: 12

11. A 45-year-old male whose uncle died of colon cancer schedules an appointment to discuss his need for screening colonoscopy. When should he have his first screening colonoscopy, and what should be the frequency of his endoscopic follow-up?

A. Immediately and then every 5 years

B. Immediately and then every 10 years

C. Starting at age 50 and then every 10 years

D. Starting at age 50 and then every 5 years

E. Starting 10 years prior to the age his uncle was diagnosed and then every 5 years

ANSWER: C

COMMENTS: Colorectal cancer is the third most common type of cancer and the second leading cause of cancer-related death in the United States. Convincing evidence exists that screening for colorectal cancer with fecal occult blood testing, sigmoidoscopy, or colonoscopy detects early-stage cancer and adenomatous polyps and reduces mortality. Current recommendations include initiation of screening at 50 years of age with repeat screening every 10 years if initial colonoscopy is normal. For patients with a first-degree relative with colorectal cancer or adenomas prior to age 60, screening should be initiated at 40 years of age or 10 years prior to the youngest-affected relative, with a repeat every 5 years. For patients with a first-degree relative with colorectal cancer or adenomas after age 60, screening should be initiated at age 40, with a repeat every 10 years.

Ref.: 13

12. A 25-year-old female with newly diagnosed familial adenomatous polyposis (FAP) returns to the surgical office to discuss continued care and treatment. Which of the following is true about the endoscopic care of FAP?

A. Individuals at risk or affected by FAP need an annual screening colonoscopy or flexible sigmoidoscopy beginning at 25 years of age.

B. In addition to colon cancer, FAP patients must also undergo annual computed tomography (CT) enterography for small bowel carcinoma screening.

C. Postsurgical surveillance should include lower endoscopy of rectum or ileal pouch every 3 years.

D. Stomach endoscopic screening includes random fundic gland polyp sampling and requires surgical resection for low-grade dysplasia.

E. Gastric and duodenal screening should start at 25 to 30 years of age and be repeated routinely depending on the Spigelman stage of polyposis.

ANSWER: E

COMMENTS: FAP is an inherited condition with a mutation in the adenomatous polyposis coli gene (*APC*) leading to nearly 100% risk for future colon cancer. Individuals at risk or with classic FAP symptoms should undergo colorectal cancer screening by means of annual colonoscopy, beginning at puberty. In addition to colorectal cancer, FAP patients are at an increased risk for gastric and duodenal tumors. FAP screening should include regularly scheduled upper endoscopy every 6 months to 4 years, depending on the Spigelman stage of duodenal polyposis. Random sampling of gastric fundic gland polyps should be included in FAP screening upper endoscopy. Gastric or duodenal resections should be reserved for high-grade dysplasia only. Preventative colectomy with ileorectal anastomosis is a single-stage procedure with slightly less morbidity than the ileal pouch–anal anastomosis (IPAA) surgery, but some rectal cancer risk remains, and yearly proctoscopy is essential. Even after total proctocolectomy and IPAA, adenomas and cancers may occur in the anal transition zone and in the pouch itself; lifelong endoscopic surveillance is required.

Ref.: 13

13. On insertion of the colonoscope, the rectum of a 68-year-old female with a history of a hysterectomy was easily traversed. The rectosigmoid junction was then encountered, and advancement was difficult. Which of the following is a useful technique to pass the rectosigmoid junction?

A. Partially withdraw and "jiggle" the scope.

B. Torque tip around the junction to keep the sigmoid loop short.

C. Advance scope making a large loop and reduce the loop after entering descending colon.

D. Apply external pressure to sigmoid to hold down the loop and prevent further scope looping.

E. All of the above.

ANSWER: E

COMMENTS: The rectosigmoid junction can be difficult to traverse for novice endoscopists. This is particularly evident in patients with a history of pelvic operations. Removal of pelvic organs allows the colon to fall more deeply into the pelvis, increasing angulation. In addition, adhesions may lead to tethering, making angulations more acute. Occasionally, the sigmoid may stretch into a large loop with scope advancement. When this occurs, meaningful advancement ceases. Techniques that may be helpful include partially withdrawing and "jiggling" the scope, accepting the large loop and attempting to reduce the loop once the rectosigmoid junction has been hooked by the tip of the scope, or applying external pressure to the sigmoid to hold down the sigmoid and prevent looping.

Ref.: 14, 15

14. Relative segments of the colon are identifiable by their endoscopic appearance. Which of the following is true?

A. The splenic flexure is readily identifiable by a slight bluish discoloration.

B. The sigmoid and descending colon are much larger in diameter and distend more easily.

C. A triangle appearance of the transverse colon makes it easily identifiable.

D. On passing the hepatic flexure, the diameter decreases as the ascending colon is entered.

E. Cecal confirmation requires only transillumination in the right lower quadrant.

ANSWER: C

COMMENTS: Several identifiable features of each segment of the colon are notable. The rectal segment is easily distended with three valves that require minimal scope torque to traverse. The sigmoid can be difficult to pass depending on the patient's prior surgical history, especially in prior pelvic operations. Endoscopically, the sigmoid diameter is smaller, and the muscular walls are identifiable by rhythmic contractions around the scope. The splenic flexure appears as a sharp, slit-like turn at the proximal descending colon. In addition, a transmitted cardiac pulsation may be noted. The transverse colon is marked by a triangular appearance. In many cases, a combination of advancement and suctioning is needed to cross the transverse colon. The hepatic flexure often has a bluish hint due to its close approximation to the liver. The ascending colon is notable for its large diameter and easy distensibility. Lastly, the cecal position is confirmed by the crow's foot appearance created by the tenia coalescence and identification of the appendiceal orifice.

Ref.: 15

15. A 58-year-old male arriving for his routine screening colonoscopy admits that he had difficulty completing all of the prescribed bowel preparation. As the colonoscopy is started, significant stool burden is identified. Which of the following is correct?

A. Continue procedure.

B. Irrigate with silicone particle-based antifoam.

C. Insufflate to expose.

D. Aggressively irrigate stool from mucosa.

E. Abandon and reschedule.

ANSWER: E

COMMENTS: If solid or copious stool is encountered, the procedure should be abandoned and rescheduled after discussing with the patient the need for adequate preparation. If stool is predominately liquid, the substance may be aspirated to permit thorough examination. Stool suctioning is best done by positioning the liquid at the bottom of the screen where the suction channel is located. Flushing saline through the suction channel may be needed if debris blocks the lumen. The U.S. Multi-Society Task Force on Colorectal Cancer defines an adequate preparation as one that allows confidence that lesions greater than 5 mm generally are not obscured by residual colonic contents. The Boston Bowel Prep Scale allows for accurate scoring of the degree of preparation, and scores of 0 to 1 have statistically significant miss rates compared with scores of 2 to 3.

Ref.: 16, 17

16. A 48-year-old female with a family history of colorectal cancer underwent screening colonoscopy. During colonoscopy, a large, yellowish nonobstructing lesion was identified within the sigmoid (Fig. 8-B.1). Which of the following is correct?

A. Documentation by photo as characteristics are not concerning

B. Excision by piecemeal polypectomy

C. Cold biopsy alone is sufficient

D. Excision by snare polypectomy

E. Excision by saline mucosal elevation

ANSWER: A

COMMENTS: Colonic lipomas are the second most common benign tumors after adenomatous polyps. Lipomas of the GI tract appear on imaging as well-demarcated spherical or ovoid masses with homogeneous fat density. On endoscopy, these lesions appear as yellowish submucosal lesions covered by normal mucosa. If nonobstructing, they do not need to be biopsied or resected. Endoscopists can palpate using closed biopsy forceps to assess for a soft and spongy consistency looking for indentation (pillow sign). Endoscopic ultrasound shows a uniformly hyperechoic mass arising from the submucosal layer. No intervention is needed for smaller or asymptomatic lipomas.

Ref.: 18

17. A 78-year-old male on postoperative day 3 after an emergent abdominal aortic aneurysm repair experiences hematochezia, abdominal distention, and worsening clinical status. Emergent endoscopy is planned to assess for ischemia. What can be done to minimize the risk for insertion trauma?

A. Complete colonoscopy quickly to limit the amount of insufflation.

B. Use carbon dioxide for insufflation.

C. Use higher insufflation pressures to allow for thorough mucosal evaluation.

D. Position the patient on his back.

E. Rigid proctoscope alone is sufficient to assess for colonic ischemia.

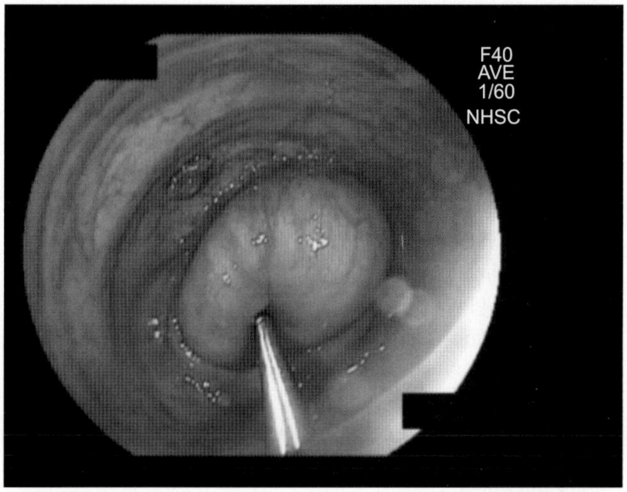

Fig. 8-B.1 *(With permission from: Hsu-Heng Yen. Colonoic lipoma.* Video Journal and Encyclopedia of GI Endoscopy *1(3):661–662.)*

ANSWER: B

COMMENTS: When clinical concern for colonic ischemia exists, a colonoscopy is indicated to assess the extent of ischemia. Mild ischemia or resolving ischemia may appear similar to colitis. Severe ischemia is evidenced by white, green, or black discoloration of the mucosa. If the mucosa appears black, ischemia is likely full thickness and surgical intervention is required. Ischemia is likely to occur at vascular watershed regions of the superior and inferior mesenteric artery (splenic flexure) or the superior rectal and middle rectal arteries (rectosigmoid junction). When performing a colonoscopy in the setting of colonic ischemia, the surgeon should proceed with caution to prevent perforation. Specifically, limited insufflation and gentle scope manipulation may reduce the risk for perforation, and use of CO_2 insufflation is beneficial as it is absorbed quickly.

Ref.: 19, 20

18. A 28-year-old female presents with symptoms consistent with choledocholithiasis, and an ERCP is planned. Which of the following has been used to successfully reduce the risk for pancreatitis with ERCP?

A. Allopurinol

B. Balloon dilation instead of sphincterotomy

C. Selective bile duct cannulation prior to contrast injection

D. Somatostatin

E. Rectal acetaminophen

ANSWER: C

COMMENTS: Post-ERCP pancreatitis remains the most common complication after the procedure, with an incidence of 3%–5%. Post-ERCP pancreatitis is defined as increased abdominal pain associated with three times the normal serum amylase. Much research has gone into the medical and procedural prevention of this complication. Freeman et al. analyzed patient risk factors and found that balloon sphincter dilation, difficult papillary cannulation, pancreatic sphincterotomy, and multiple pancreatic duct injections were independent risk factors for post-ERCP pancreatitis. Techniques used to decrease pancreatitis include selective common bile duct cannulation with guidewire prior to contrast injection, pancreatic duct stenting for difficult papillary cannulations, and limiting contrast injection in the pancreatic duct. Current research for medical prevention of post-ERCP pancreatitis reveals that rectal administration of nonsteroidal antiinflammatory medication reduces the incidence of pancreatitis.

Ref.: 21, 22

19. During an ERCP for retained stone after laparoscopic cholecystectomy, a ballooned sphincteroplasty was performed for stone extraction. Bleeding was noted at the site of sphincteroplasty during the procedure. Which of the following is the most efficacious technique utilized for hemostasis?

A. Band ligation

B. Endoscopic clips

C. Argon plasma coagulation

D. Balloon tamponade

E. Epinephrine injection

ANSWER: D

COMMENTS: Bleeding is a known complication after endoscopic biliary sphincterotomy. The incidence of postsphincterotomy bleeding varies from 1% to 10% and can occur immediately or several days after the initial sphincterotomy. Approach to hemostasis depends on the severity. Many cases are managed endoscopically by epinephrine injection and thermal or mechanical methods. In a small percentage of patients, endoscopic hemostasis is unsuccessful and angiographic embolization is required. In the above question, the most efficient initial hemostasis method would be balloon tamponade because the endoscopic balloon would still be in place. Inflation of the balloon within the sphincteroplasty site or adjacent to it with manual pressure will often stop or slow bleeding and allow time for the preparation of other hemostatic devices if needed.

Ref.: 23

20. During an EGD for acute upper GI bleeding, active bleeding from a visible vessel was identified. Vessels up to what size are typically controlled by coaptive thermal techniques?

A. 1 mm

B. 1.5 mm

C. 2 mm

D. 2.5 mm

E. 3 mm

ANSWER: C

COMMENTS: Coaptive thermal techniques utilize a probe passed via the endoscope that can apply pressure to tamponade and simultaneously apply thermal coagulation. Bipolar and heater probe devices are most commonly used. Monopolar cautery is also available but has a higher full-thickness injury rate. Important variables in achieving hemostasis include probe size, force of application, power setting, and duration of energy delivery. Vessels up to 2 mm are well controlled by coaptive techniques.

Ref.: 23

21. During an EGD for acute upper GI bleeding, active bleeding from a shallow gastric ulcer was identified. Hemostasis was achieved by epinephrine injection. Several factors have been identified that are associated with the risk for rebleeding. Which of the following is NOT a risk factor for rebleeding?

A. Ulcer size

B. Pigmented dark adherent clot

C. Visible vessel

D. Anemia

E. Age > 40 years

ANSWER: E

COMMENTS: Upper GI bleeding is not without significant morbidity, and initial endoscopic treatment is useful in hemodynamically stable patients. However, rebleeding after endoscopic evaluation does occur. Important factors associated with the risk for rebleeding include active bleeding on endoscopy with visible vessels (the highest rebleeding risk), pigmentation of clots signifying maturation, ulcers > 2 cm, age > 60 years, significant comorbidities, patient presenting in shock, coagulopathy, and anemia. Actively bleeding ulcers and those with a visible vessel warrant endoscopic therapy. In cases of rebleeding, repeat endoscopy can be attempted and has been shown to reduce the need for surgery without increasing mortality and is associated with a few complications.

Ref.: 24

22. A 68-year-old male with significant dysphagia after a stroke underwent percutaneous gastrostomy tube placement for use during his rehabilitation. Which of the following is NOT a contraindication to percutaneous endoscopic gastrostomy (PEG) tube placement?

A. Ascites

B. Gastric dysmotility

C. Diffuse gastric cancer

D. Combative, neurologically altered patients

E. Head and neck cancer

ANSWER: E

COMMENTS: PEG tube placement is a useful method to obtain enteral nutrition access in an increasing patient population. Indications include any patient with a functional GI tract who is unable to take oral nutrition independently or needs gastric decompression. However, PEG tubes are contraindicated in a patient with ascites, gastric dysmotility, documented reflux and aspiration, or diffuse gastric cancer or in a combative, neurologically impaired patient who may dislodge access prior to tract maturation. Patients struggling with ascites are likely to suffer chronic persistent drainage around the PEG and are at risk for bacterial or fungal peritonitis due to seeding of the ascites. Gastric dysmotility and documented reflux with aspiration will only be worse when feeding the stomach via PEG tube and are indications for a percutaneous gastrojejunostomy tube. In head and neck cancer, seeding of the gastric tract has been documented, but it is very rare and can be reduced even further with the use of the "push technique" instead of the pull technique of PEG placement.

Ref.: 25

23. Multiple techniques of PEG tube placement have been described. Which of the following describes the safe tract technique?

A. Insufflation of the stomach with palpation of the gastric wall visible endoscopically

B. Insufflation of the stomach and transillumination of the anterior abdominal wall through the gastric wall with the endoscope light source

C. Visualization of needle entering gastric lumen endoscopically

D. Continuous aspiration with saline-filled syringe observing for air or enteric contents prior to endoscopic visualization of needle in gastric lumen

E. Combined endoscopic and laparoscopic PEG insertion allowing confirmation of only gastric penetration by PEG tube

ANSWER: D

COMMENTS: The safe tract technique is recommended for all patients undergoing PEG tube placement to prevent inadvertent colonic placement. Using a saline-filled syringe and continuous suction, a needle is passed through the anterior abdominal wall while observing gastric lumen endoscopically. If air or enteric contents are noted in the syringe prior to visualization of the needle within the gastric lumen, the suspicion of inadvertent bowel placement should be made and the needle should be removed and a new location chosen. In addition to the safe tract technique, position and placement choice by easy palpation transmission and light transillumination can be utilized by the endoscopist.

Ref.: 26

REFERENCES

1. American Society for Gastrointestinal Endoscopy. Report on emerging technology. *Gastrointest Endosc*. 2011;74:1–6.
2. Guideline for disinfection and sterilization in healthcare facilities. Available at: https://www.cdc.gov/hicpac/pdf/guidelines/Disinfection_Nov_2008.
3. Nelson DB. Infectious disease complications of GI endoscopy: part I, endogenous infections. *Gastrointest Endosc*. 2003;57(4):546–556.
4. Hirota WK, Petersen K, Baron TH, et al. Guidelines for antibiotic prophylaxis for GI endoscopy. *Gastrointest Endosc*. 2003; 58:475–482.
5. Siegel JD, Palma JA. Medical treatment of constipation. *Clin Colon Rectal Surg*. 2005;18(2):76–80.
6. Hsu CW, Imperiale TF. Meta-analysis and cost comparison of polyethylene glycol lavage versus sodium phosphate for colonoscopy preparation. *Gastrointest Endosc*. 1998;48:282.
7. American Society for Gastrointestinal Endoscopy. Position statement on routine laboratory testing before endoscopic procedures. *Gastrointest Endosc*. 2008;68:827–838.
8. American Society of Anesthesiologists Task Force on Sedation and Analgesia by Non Anesthesiologists. Practice guidelines for sedation and analgesia by nonanesthesiologists. *Anesthesiology*. 2002; 96(4):1004–1017.
9. Schauer PR, Schwesinger WH, Page CP, Stewart RM, Levine BA, Sirinek KR. Complications of surgical endoscopy. A decade of experience from a surgical residency training program. *Surg Endosc*. 1997; 11(1):8–11.
10. Ponsky JL. *Complications of Endoscopic and Laparoscopic Surgery, Prevention and Management*. Philadelphia: Lippincott-Raven; 1997:292.
11. Society of American Gastrointestinal and Endoscopic Surgeons. Fundamentals of endoscopic surgery: upper gastrointestinal endoscopy. Available at: www.fesdidactic.org.

12. Lee SH, Park KU. Technical skills and training of upper gastrointestinal endoscopy for new beginners. *World J Gastroenterol.* 2015;21(3): 759–785.
13. Anthony T, Simmang C, Hyman N, et al. Standard Practice Task Force, American Society of Colorectal Surgeons. Practice parameters for the surveillance and follow-up of patients with colorectal cancer. *Dis Colon Rectum.* 2004;47:807–817.
14. Clancy C, Burke JP, Chang KH. The effect of hysterectomy on colonoscopy completion: a systematic review and meta-analysis. *Dis Colon Rectum.* 2014;57(11):1317–1323.
15. Cotton PB, Williams CB. *Practical Gastrointestinal Endoscopy. The Fundamentals.* 5th ed. Malden, MA: Blackwell Publishing Ltd; 2003.
16. Clark BT, Protiva P, Nagar A. Quantification of adequate bowel preparation for screening or surveillance colonoscopy in men. *Gastroenterology.* 2016;150(2):396–405.
17. American Society for Gastrointestinal Endoscopy. Guideline: Bowel preparation before colonoscopy. *Gastrointest Endosc.* 2015;81 (4):781–793.
18. Jiang L, Jiang LS, Li FY, et al. Giant submucosal lipoma located in the descending colon: a case report and review of the literature. *World J Gastroenterol.* 2007;13:5664–5667.
19. Sajid MS, Caswell J, Bhatti MI. Carbon dioxide insufflation vs conventional air insufflation for colonoscopy: a systematic review and meta-analysis of published randomized controlled trials. *Colorectal Dis.* 2015;17(2):111–123.
20. Fitzgeral JF, Hernandez LO. Ischemic colitis. *Clin Colon Rectal Surg.* 2015;28(2):93–98.
21. Freeman ML, DiSario JA, Nelson DB. Risk factors for post-ERCP pancreatitis: a prospective, multicenter study. *Gastrointest Endosc.* 2001;54:425–434.
22. Li X, Tao LP, Wang CH. Effectiveness of nonsteroidal anti-inflammatory drugs in prevention of post ERCP pancreatitis: a meta-analysis. *World J Gastroenterol.* 2014;20(34):123–129.
23. Ferreira LE, Baron TH. Post-sphincterotomy bleeding: who, what, when, and how. *Am J Gastroenterol.* 2007;102(12):2850–2858.
24. Lau JY, Sung JJ, Lam YH. Endoscopic retreatment compared with surgery in patients with recurrent bleeding after initial endoscopic control of bleeding ulcers. *N Engl J Med.* 1999;340(10):751–756.
25. Azar AR, Kurtz A, Farkas DT. Percutaneous endoscopic gastrostomy: indications, technique, complications and management. *World J Gastroenterol.* 2014;20(24):7739–7751.
26. Foutch PG, Talber GA, Waring JP. Percutaneous endoscopic gastrostomy in patients with prior abdominal surgery: virtues of the safe tract. *Am J Gastroenterol.* 1988;83(2):147–150.

C. Principles of Ultrasound

MacKenzie D. Landin, M.D., Benjamin R. Veenstra, M.D., and Edward F. Hollinger, M.D., Ph.D.

1. Which of the following most accurately represents the average speed at which ultrasound waves move through the human body?

A. 350 m/s

B. 2000 m/s

C. 500 cm/s

D. 1540 m/s

E. 800 m/s

ANSWER: D

COMMENTS: Sound moves through biologic tissue at a speed that is dependent on tissue density. Sound moves more slowly through less dense matter, such as air (330 m/s), and more quickly through high-density material, such as bone (4050 m/s). The average **speed of sound** through human tissue is 1540 m/s. Specific examples of propagation speeds through tissue are 1459 m/s for fat, 1520 m/s for the brain, 1550 m/s for the liver, 1560 m/s for kidneys, and 1580 m/s for muscle. Because most soft tissues have similar density and therefore sound passes through them at a similar speed, ultrasound machines are designed on the assumption that the speed of sound through soft tissues is 1540 m/s.

Ref.: 1

2. Concerning acoustic impedance, which of the following statements is true?

A. It can be amplified by increasing the gain on the ultrasound equipment.

B. It is influenced by the density of the tissue and the velocity of the sound wave.

C. It permits the operator to distinguish between two structures even if their densities are the same.

D. It is calculated by multiplying the amplitude of the waves by the density of the tissue.

E. The greater the difference in impedance between two tissues, the lesser the energy reflected to the transducer.

ANSWER: B

COMMENTS: Diagnostic ultrasonography is centered on the analysis of sound waves that have been reflected back to the ultrasound transducer. Impedance is the acoustic resistance to sound traveling in a medium. **Acoustic impedance** is dependent on the speed of sound in the tissue and the density of the tissue. It can be calculated as acoustic impedance = density × velocity. Sound wave properties are not the only parameters that shape ultrasound physics. The medium (tissue) carrying the sound is a major contributor to events. The compressibility of a material determines, in part, the way that sound is carried along within that material. Because sound forms compressions and rarefactions, the ability of the tissue to be compressed and stretched determines just how well sound can be propagated through the tissue. Hard tissues (e.g., bone) are difficult to compress and thus *impede* the formation of compressions and rarefactions when they carry sound waves. As a result, hard materials have high acoustic impedance when compared with softer tissues (e.g., muscle), which have low acoustic impedance. Therefore the ease with which sound is transmitted through a substance is termed *impedance*. The interface between two adjacent tissues serves as a major source for reflecting sound waves back to the transducer. When two adjacent tissues have different impedance values, the sound wave reflects back to the transducer. The greater the difference in impedance between the two tissues, the lesser the energy transferred to the next tissue and the more the energy reflected back. Fortunately, differences in impedance between most soft tissues are small. These small differences are enough to cause reflection of the sound waves to provide the information for generating an image; at the same time, the differences are small enough to allow enough amplitude for the passage of some sound waves past the tissue interface into deeper tissues. These differences in impedance are sufficient to make ultrasound a workable diagnostic modality. Increasing the gain on the machine does not affect any of these parameters.

Ref.: 1, 5

3. Which of the following statements regarding transducers is false?

A. Higher-frequency transducers have poor penetration and good resolution.

B. The higher the frequency, the shorter the wavelength.

C. Longer wavelengths result in deeper penetration.

D. Axial resolution is independent of frequency.

E. The piezoelectric effect is defined as the "conversion of electrical to mechanical energy."

ANSWER: D

COMMENTS: Ultrasound transducers contain crystals. When a sound wave mechanically deforms one of the crystals, voltage is produced. The corollary is also true: when a crystal has voltage applied to it, it deforms and a sound wave is generated. This is described as the piezoelectric effect and has practical applications to the field of ultrasonography. The crystals used in ultrasound machines initially act as speakers that send out and receive sound waves. The returning sound that is reflected back causes the crystals to vibrate and generate voltage.

High-frequency transducers provide high-resolution images at the expense of tissue penetration. In ultrasonography, three types of resolutions exist: axial resolution, lateral resolution, and temporal resolution. **Axial resolution** is the ability to distinguish one object from another object below it. It is dependent on frequency. By definition, a higher frequency means a shorter wavelength. Because the depth of penetration is dependent on the wavelength, a higher frequency results in less tissue penetration. **Lateral resolution** is the ability to differentiate between two objects that are next to each other. It is independent of the frequency and is dependent on the width of the beam. **Temporal resolution** is the perception of real-time movement and is dependent on the frame rate.

Ref.: 1, 5

4. Which of the following descriptors regarding echogenicity is not true?
   A. Hyperechoic tissues are brighter than the surrounding tissue.
   B. Hypoechoic tissues are less bright than the surrounding tissue.
   C. Isoechoic tissues are similar in appearance to the surrounding tissue.
   D. Anechoic tissues appear as black sonographic images.
   E. Simple cysts are hyperechoic.

ANSWER: E

COMMENTS: Echogenicity refers to the appearance of a specific tissue or structure on the ultrasound image relative to its ability to reflect the ultrasound wave. A region in a sonographic picture in which echoes are brighter than those in nearby structures is referred to as hyperechoic. In contrast, hypoechoic areas appear darker than surrounding areas. Isoechoic areas appear similar to surrounding structures, and anechoic areas appear dark or black, without echoes, on a sonographic image. Simple cysts appear as anechoic images with posterior enhancement.

Ref.: 1, 5

5. Which of the following is not characteristic of the sonographic appearance of a malignant thyroid nodule?
   A. Hypoechoic in comparison with the surrounding tissue
   B. Peripheral calcifications
   C. Irregular margins
   D. Absence of cystic areas
   E. Heterogeneity

ANSWER: B

COMMENTS: Head and neck cancers comprise 1.5%–2% of all malignancies. There are 22 to 55 new cases per million people annually. Ultrasound has proven useful in the evaluation of **thyroid carcinoma**. Suspicious ultrasound findings that are concerning for malignancy include irregular borders, indistinct contours, microcalcifications smaller than 2 mm without acoustic shadowing, posterior shadowing behind lesions, hypervascular lesions, and regional lymphadenopathy. When microcalcifications are present (psammoma bodies), they are located in the interior of the lesion, not at the periphery. In addition, cystic thyroid masses are usually benign.

Ref.: 2

6. Which of the following statements regarding focused abdominal sonography for trauma (FAST) is true?
   A. It can reliably evaluate the retroperitoneum.
   B. It can quickly detect the presence of pericardial fluid or a pleural effusion.
   C. It is useful in detecting a cardiac contusion.
   D. It is considered a replacement for computed tomography (CT).
   E. It can reliably detect diaphragmatic injuries.

ANSWER: B

COMMENTS: FAST has become a vital component in the initial evaluation of trauma patients. Currently, the primary focus of the FAST examination is to detect fluid presumed to be blood, but as time progresses, more advanced applications will undoubtedly arise. The examination is completed quickly during a primary survey (of an unstable patient) or a secondary survey (of a stable patient) and focuses on detecting fluid in the pericardial space and dependent portions of the abdomen. The examination is divided into three parts: cardiac, abdominal, and thoracic. The cardiac examination consists of a sagittal view in the subxiphoid region. The abdominal examination focuses on longitudinal views of the left and right upper quadrants and a transverse view of the pelvis. The thoracic portion is an upward scan from the upper abdominal quadrants and can detect pleural effusions or pneumothorax. Despite the usefulness of the FAST examination, it does have limitations. The FAST examination can quickly evaluate for the presence of both pericardial fluid and pleural effusion. However, it does not evaluate the retroperitoneum and does not detect a cardiac contusion. CT still has many practical applications in trauma patients and has not been fully replaced by the FAST examination. Transabdominal ultrasound has several advantages over CT, including cost, portability, safety, and speed of the examination. However, ultrasound examinations are operator dependent. The quality of the images, or lack thereof, depends on the technical expertise of the person operating the ultrasound machine.

Ref.: 3

7. Which of the following is not a sonographic characteristic of an inflamed gallbladder?
   A. Gallbladder distention
   B. Pericholecystic fluid
   C. Wall thickness of 2 mm
   D. Sonographic Murphy's sign
   E. Gallstones

ANSWER: C

COMMENTS: The sonographic diagnosis of **cholelithiasis** is generally indicated by the presence of a mobile, hyperechoic, intraluminal object (i.e., gallstone) with posterior shadowing. If these three criteria are not met, the diagnosis is less certain. In the presence of cholecystitis, a sonogram may display the following: gallbladder distention, pericholecystic fluid, a sonographic Murphy's sign, and gallstones. Gallbladder wall thickness is considered abnormal if it is greater than 3 mm.

Ref.: 4, 5

8. Regarding vascular arterial ultrasound imaging, which of the following statements is true?
   A. In Doppler ultrasound of blood flow, the reflected wave returning to the transducer has the same frequency as the transmitted wave.
   B. For Doppler ultrasound, the transducer should be held at a 90-degree angle to the body.
   C. Arterial stenosis leads to decreased flow velocity.
   D. Carotid artery duplex ultrasound scanning allows assessment of arterial plaque morphology, as well as estimation of the degree of carotid artery stenosis caused by the plaque.
   E. In dialysis access patients, duplex ultrasonography does not generally assess arterial inflow for arteriovenous (AV) fistulas or grafts accurately.

ANSWER: D

COMMENTS: Doppler ultrasound relies on the fact that the sound wave that has been reflected back to the transducer from a moving object has a different frequency than does the transmitted wave. The change in frequency is known as the Doppler shift, named after the Austrian physicist Christian Doppler who described it in 1842. If the transducer is held at a 90-degree angle while performing Doppler ultrasonography, regardless of the actual velocity in a blood vessel, the ultrasound machine will read zero velocity. This is because the theoretical velocity is calculated by the equation $V = \Delta fc/2f \cos\theta$ (where V is velocity, c is the speed of sound in soft tissue, Δf is the change in frequency of reflected versus transmitted sound waves, f is the frequency of transmitted sound, and $\cos\theta$ is the angle between the ultrasound wave and the direction of motion of the target). Because the cosine of 90 degrees is zero, the theoretical velocity would be zero if the transducer is held at a 90-degree angle to the target. The ideal angle of insonation is 60 degrees. Analysis of the Doppler shift is used to determine the speed and direction of blood flow. Unless the arterial stenosis is so severe that blood flow is slowed almost to zero, the velocity increases in arterial stenosis. As its name implies, duplex ultrasonography uses two diagnostic modalities: (1) high-resolution gray-scale B-mode imaging (anatomic information) and (2) Doppler spectral analysis of blood flow patterns (physiologic information). The B-mode imaging allows visualization of plaque location, composition, and morphology. Soft plaques and plaques with an irregular intimal surface (ulceration) may be relatively unstable and pose more risk for cerebral thromboembolic events and stroke compared with dense fibrous plaques with a smooth intimal lining. Doppler spectral measurement of flow velocities allows accurate assessment of the degree of carotid artery stenosis. As with other ultrasound diagnostic modalities, the accuracy and reliability of vascular ultrasound imaging are dependent on the skill and experience of the operator. Ultrasound imaging is very useful in patients requiring hemodialysis access. Vein mapping can be performed preoperatively to determine the best vessels to support an AV fistula and postoperatively to assess fistula maturation. It can also be used to assess the arterial inflow for a fistula or graft. Ultrasound of new AV grafts may be limited by air trapped in the wall of the prosthetic graft.

Ref.: 1, 5

9. Which of the following statements best describes the use of breast ultrasound imaging?

A. It should be used instead of breast biopsy.

B. It can be used to distinguish between cystic and solid masses.

C. It is considered an initial screening test to evaluate the entire breast.

D. It can be used to define microcalcifications.

E. It should not be used in lieu of stereotactically guided biopsies even if the lesion is detected ultrasonographically.

ANSWER: B

COMMENTS: As the technology of breast ultrasonography has continued to improve, its application has increased. Although breast ultrasound can aid in the performance of breast biopsy and other interventional modalities, ultrasound images cannot replace the information that biopsy provides. **Breast ultrasound** is used in the workup of a palpable breast mass to aid in the differentiation of a cystic from a solid mass. A simple cyst in the breast appears anechoic in comparison to the surrounding breast tissue. Breast ultrasound is performed early in the workup of breast lesions, but it is not generally used as a screening tool. It is difficult to adequately characterize (and often to even visualize) microcalcifications with breast ultrasound. If suspicious calcifications are seen on mammography, stereotactic biopsy should be performed for a thorough evaluation. Ultrasound-guided biopsy should be used preferentially whenever the lesion has been defined sonographically.

Ref.: 5

10. Which of the following statements regarding attenuation is false?

A. It is dependent on the absorption of sound waves.

B. It is dependent on the scattering of sound waves.

C. It is dependent on the reflection of sound waves.

D. It is dependent on the refraction of sound waves.

E. None of the above.

ANSWER: D

COMMENTS: Attenuation is a combination of the **absorption, scattering**, and **reflection** of sound waves. Ultrasound waves are absorbed as they move through tissue. The denser the tissue, the greater the absorption of sound. Absorption occurs because the sound energy is converted to heat. The less dense the tissue, the more easily the pulse passes through the tissue (also known as through-transmission) and is not absorbed. When sound waves encounter tissues of greater density, they can be scattered off the edge of the tissue (e.g., bone) in different directions. They can also be reflected back toward the transducer when the sound pulse meets an interface between two tissues of different densities and consequentially two different acoustic impedances. The sound pulses can also be refracted. Refraction is a change in the direction of sound when sound encounters an interface between two tissues. The frequency of sound remains constant; therefore the wavelength must change to accommodate the difference in the speed of sound in two different tissues. As the wavelength changes, the sound wave is redirected.

Ref.: 1, 5

11. What is the *least* desirable angle to determine the Doppler frequency shift?

A. Zero degrees

B. 35 degrees

C. 45 degrees

D. 60 degrees

E. 90 degrees

ANSWER: E

COMMENTS: The Doppler principle explains why an ambulance has a higher pitch when driving toward a person and a lower pitch when driving away. When an ambulance approaches an observer, the sound is compressed as the distance shortens between the ambulance siren and the observer. The wavelength of the sound is compressed, and the frequency is higher. As the ambulance drives away, the sound spreads out over the distance between the siren and the observer and the wavelength stretches resulting in decreased frequency. The Doppler principle can also help to determine the speed of a moving object. The ultrasound transducer generates a sound pulse that is transmitted through tissues to the vessel of interest. The frequency of the generated sound is known. The pulse is reflected back to the transducer off the moving target (the red blood cells within the vessel). The frequency of the reflection can be calculated. The goal is to determine the speed of the moving target.

The Doppler equation is as follows: $f_o - f_r = [2f_oV)/c]\cos\theta$

f_o = frequency of original sound pulse

f_r = frequency of reflected sound pulse

V = velocity of target of interest

c = speed of sound in tissue

θ = angle between the direction of the moving target and the reflected sound pulse

At a Doppler angle of 90 degrees, when the sound is perpendicular to the direction of blood flow, the cos 90 = 0, and there will be no Doppler frequency shift. When the sound is parallel to the direction of blood flow, i.e., the Doppler angle is 0, cos 0 = 1 and the Doppler shift will be the largest. With this idea in mind, the calculated velocity can change based upon the Doppler shift.

Ref.: 5

12. Which of the following statements regarding acoustic shadowing is false?

A. It is the result of the reflection of sound waves.

B. It is the result of the refraction of sound waves.

C. It is the result of the absorption of sound waves.

D. Gases cause high acoustic shadowing.

E. None of the above.

ANSWER: B

COMMENTS: Acoustic shadowing is the result of both the **reflection** and **absorption** of part of the sound wave as it is transmitted through tissue. The concept of refraction does not play a role in acoustic shadowing. Gases cause high acoustic shadowing. When sound pulses reach a gas–tissue interface, a large amount of the sound pulse is reflected, and it interacts with the interface in front of the gas, in turn, causing secondary reflections that eventually reflect back to the transducer. This series of reflections produces a "dirty" appearance. As stones are denser tissues, they absorb more than they reflect. When sound waves reflect off stones, there is less sound energy available to generate secondary reflections and as such the shadow is more "clean."

Ref.: 1, 5

13. Posterior enhancement is most significant for which structure?

A. Bone

B. Fat

C. Cyst

D. Muscle

E. Stone

ANSWER: C

COMMENTS: As sound passes through tissue, it is attenuated either by absorption, scattering, or reflection. The higher the tissue density, the greater the attenuation. When sound moves through a fluid, the attenuation is less and more of the sound energy passes through, a principle called through-transmission. If there is a solid tissue behind the fluid-filled structure, when the sound pulse meets the solid tissue, it will be reflected back to the transducer. This reflection produces a picture where the cyst is darker than the bright solid tissue. If there is a solid–solid interface, the pulses reflected back would produce an image with less bright structures. However, solid tissues that attenuate sound less than the solid tissues surrounding them will also have increased through-transmission and will have posterior enhancement.

Ref.: 5

14. In which of the following scenarios would one most likely expect mirror image artifact?

A. Ultrasound for FAST examination

B. Ultrasound of the gallbladder in the evaluation of cholecystitis

C. Ultrasound of the renal pelvis in the evaluation of stone disease

D. Ultrasound of the bladder

E. None of the above

ANSWER: D

COMMENTS: A **mirror image** is produced by the reflection of an ultrasound wave over a highly reflective surface. A typical mirror is a surface that is in between two tissues of different acoustic impedances. Images are exactly replicated when the mirror is flat, whereas an image is distorted when the surface of the mirror is curved. Gas can act as a mirror as it reflects sound, instead of light, and it reflects almost all of the sound transmitted to it. The lungs, which are gas containing, can act as a mirror, and the diaphragm, liver, or other structures like the kidneys can be seen as mirror images. Imagine a patient with metastatic colon cancer, and there is a concern for metastatic lesions to the liver. If an ultrasound is used to examine the liver, the ultrasound wave generated by the transducer passes through the abdomen, and one part of the wave reaches a liver metastasis, while another continues to the diaphragm, and a mirror image of a metastasis can be seen across the diaphragm in the position of the lung. When the bladder is viewed on ultrasound, if there is gas in the rectum, the wave will be reflected off the bladder and off the gas-filled rectum, producing a mirror image; in this case it would appear as a large cyst posterior to the bladder.

Ref.: 5

15. Which of the following findings is consistent with perforated acute appendicitis?

A. External diameter > 4 cm

B. Compressible cecum

C. Asymmetric appendiceal thickening

D. Fluid within the lumen of the appendix

E. Appendicolith

ANSWER: C

COMMENTS: Acute appendicitis can be diagnosed in some patients on ultrasound, most often children, due to their size and the superficial nature of the appendix in this age group. Ultrasound findings of appendicitis include a noncompressible appendix with an external diameter > 6 cm. These findings have a negative predictive value of 98%. Appendicoliths are present in only one-third of patients. Lymphadenopathy is seen in one-half of all patients. If free fluid, asymmetric appendiceal thickening, or mesenteric inflammation and ileus are seen, this is concerning for appendiceal perforation.

Ref.: 4, 5

16. Which of the following statements regarding ultrasound of the small bowel is false?

A. The most prominent layers of the small bowel are the submucosa (bright) and muscularis propria (dark).

B. Normal small bowel wall thickness is less than 3 mm.

C. Doppler ultrasound can be used to demonstrate normal bowel wall vascularity.

D. Normal small bowel loops are compliant, easily displaced, and demonstrate slow peristalsis.

E. Exaggerated or decreased peristalsis as well as increased bowel wall thickening is a sign of abnormal small bowel.

ANSWER: C

COMMENTS: Doppler ultrasound does not show normal bowel wall vascularity. The layers of the bowel wall are as follows: superficial mucosa (bright), deep mucosa including lamina propria (gray), submucosa (bright), muscularis propria (dark), and serosa (bright). The serosa/superficial mucosa appears bright because there is fluid within the bowel itself or ascites between bowel loops. Due to the thickness of each layer as well as the contrast between layers, the submucosa and muscularis propria are the easiest to identify in poor conditions. Blood supply to the small bowel originates from the mesentery, but it delivers supply through branches and small collaterals. Therefore the vascular supply is not easily seen on color Doppler. Abnormal small bowel can be identified by changes in bowel wall thickness, irregularities of the lumen, abnormal peristalsis, blood flow (exaggerated in areas of inflammation), or mesentery (lymphadenopathy/matting).

Ref.: 4, 5

17. When performing sonography of the pediatric abdomen, all of the following are true except:

A. In a child with malrotation, the superior mesenteric artery (SMA) will be on the right and the superior mesenteric vein (SMV) will be on the left on a transverse view of the abdomen.

B. If the patient has intussusception, you will see target sign on a longitudinal view.

C. Splenic torsion will show a high position of the spleen.

D. Constipation can be diagnosed on ultrasound.

E. Commonly used for diagnosis of pyloric stenosis.

ANSWER: C

COMMENTS: Ultrasonography of the pediatric abdomen has aided in diagnosing acute illness and preventing exposure of children to radiation from CT. While ultrasound has many uses, it is limited by the patient's body habitus, normal anatomic variants (retrocecal appendix), and the technician's skill. Diseases like malrotation, intussusception, and pyloric stenosis can be diagnosed with ultrasound. Patients with malrotation may have evidence of small bowel obstruction (dilated loops of bowel), evidence of ischemia (free fluid in the abdomen, decreased flow on the Doppler mode), or even change in orientation of the SMV and superior mesenteric week. In normal development, the abdominal contents exit the developing abdomen at 10 weeks and rotate 270 degrees counterclockwise before returning to the abdomen. This stretches the mesentery, ensuring that the terminal ileum is in the right lower quadrant. In malrotation, the abdominal contents never rotate and therefore the mesentery is short and the bowel can volvulize. The SMA will be to the right of the SMV on ultrasound imaging.

In a child with intussusception, the bowel has telescoped on itself and appears as a "target" with the rings being folds of bowel on itself. These children may have intermittent abdominal pain and bleeding and can be treated with air-contrast enema.

When a child has splenic torsion, the spleen usually rotates and rests inferiorly within the left lower quadrant. There will be an absence of flow within the vessels on ultrasound.

If a child has a significant stool burden, in the case of a patient with constipation, the stool can be visualized on ultrasound within the lumen of the bowel. There will be no through-transmission of the ultrasound waves. Ultrasound remains a key tool in the diagnosis of pyloric stenosis.

Ref.: 6

18. During laparoscopic cholecystectomy, the so-called "Mickey Mouse" view of the hepatoduodenal ligament can be obtained with laparoscopic ultrasound to help delineate important anatomy. Which of the following lists all of the structures seen when the proper view is obtained?

A. Portal vein, common hepatic duct, and inferior vena cava (IVC)

B. Portal vein, common hepatic duct, and hepatic artery

C. Portal vein, common hepatic duct, and cystic artery

D. Portal vein, common bile duct, and hepatic artery

E. Portal vein, common bile duct, and cystic artery

ANSWER: D

COMMENTS: Intraoperative ultrasound during laparoscopic cholecystectomy is a useful tool for the general surgeon. This skill can be employed when there is a concern for choledocholithiasis, bile duct injury, ambiguous anatomy, or when there is an unsuspected finding during the case, like a mass. Typically, the ultrasound probe is placed through a 5-mm port, and a longitudinal view of the biliary tree and gallbladder is obtained. A color Doppler can be applied to discern the portal vein and hepatic artery from the common bile duct. Flow is depicted as blue if it is away from the transducer and red if it is toward the transducer. When a transverse view is applied, the "Mickey Mouse" view can be obtained. The portal vein represents the face, the right ear is the common bile duct, and the left ear is the hepatic artery. The ultrasound is limited in obese patients as fat causes acoustic impedance. Also, if a patient has pancreatic calcifications, these can mimic the appearance of distal common bile duct stones.

Ref.: 7

REFERENCES

1. Machi J, Staren ED. *Ultrasound for Surgeons*. 2nd ed. Philadelphia: Lippincott Williams & Wilkins; 2005.
2. Kharachenko VP, Kotlyarov PM, Mogutov MS, et al. *Ultrasound Diagnostics of Thyroid Diseases*. New York: Springer; 2010.
3. Mclean A. *Critical Care Ultrasound Manual*. Philadelphia: Elsevier; 2012.
4. Maconi G. *Ultrasound of the Gastrointestinal Tract*. New York: Springer; 2006.
5. Hertzberg B, Middleton W. *Ultrasound: The Requisites*. 3rd ed. Philadelphia: Elsevier; 2016.
6. Babcock DS. Sonography of the acute abdomen in the pediatric patient. *J Ultrasound Med*. 2002;21(8):887–899.
7. Lalla M, Arregui ME. Laparoscopic ultrasound of the biliary tree. In: Soper NJ, Scott-Conner CE, eds. *The SAGES Manual: Volume 1. Basic Laparoscopy and Endoscopy*. 3rd ed. New York: Springer; 2012.

D. Principles of Surgical Energy Use

MacKenzie D. Landin, M.D., Benjamin R. Veenstra, M.D., and Edward F. Hollinger, M.D., Ph.D.

1. Current can be diverted from the targeted tissue of interest by all of the following except:

A. Insulation failure
B. Direct coupling
C. Antenna coupling
D. Capacitative coupling
E. Facilitative coupling

ANSWER: E

COMMENTS: All of the above answer choices can result in diversion of current from target tissue except facilitative coupling. Insulation failure occurs when there is a break in the insulation of the device. These breaks are often small and not visible. The smaller the violation of the insulated layer, the greater the density of current to the nontarget tissue. Direct coupling occurs when a conductive element conducts current to an element outside the intended circuit. An example of this situation is when a monopolar device is activated adjacent to a retractor and the current arcs from the monopolar device to the retractor, causing thermal injury to the tissue that is being retracted. Antenna coupling is energy from the activated device. Then, the energy is released and captured (or coupled) by another parallel device and transferred to tissue outside the targeted field. This can occur during a laparoscopic case when the cord for the monopolar device and the camera cord are parallel to one another, or bundled. When the monopolar device is activated, the camera cord absorbs the energy and transfers it to the tissue adjacent to the camera. Antenna coupling is prevented by not bundling cords together, which does not allow the cords to run parallel to each other. Capacitative coupling occurs when electrical energy is stored within a device. A capacitor is two conductors separated by an insulator. If a cord from a monopolar device is wrapped around a clamp, the clamp can become a capacitor. After the monopolar device is activated, the clamp can store the energy and damage the tissue it is attached to. Facilitative coupling is not a described entity.

Ref.: 1, 2

2. All of the following are true regarding the use of argon gas in argon devices with the exception of:

A. Known risk of gas emboli
B. Known risk of pneumatosis
C. Known risk of intraabdominal hypertension
D. Known risk of arrhythmia
E. Noncontact fulguration of the tissues

ANSWER: E

COMMENTS: Argon gas is an ionizable, inert, and noncombustible gas. Argon gas is used to transfer electrical current from a surgical device to the tissue of interest. Argon devices are monopolar and cause fulguration of tissue without requiring contact. There are risks associated with these devices. Argon can be absorbed by the patient and can cause arrhythmias. If the argon is absorbed into the vasculature, it can result in a gas embolus significant enough to cause hypotension, jugular venous distension, and the classic murmur from an air–liquid interface, the "mill-will" murmur. If a patient develops an argon gas embolus, the patient should be treated with 100% oxygen and placed in the left lateral decubitus position to prevent air from escaping the right ventricle. From this position, the gas can then be aspirated through central venous access. If the argon device comes into contact with the mucosa of the colon or small bowel, pneumatosis can result from argon deposition into the submucosa. As this monopolar device uses a gas as its medium for energy transfer, the peritoneal cavity must be continuously ventilated during laparoscopic cases to prevent intraabdominal hypertension.

Ref.: 1, 3

3. Using the "pure cut" function on a monopolar instrument results in tissue:

A. Desiccation
B. Vaporization
C. Fulguration
D. Ablation
E. Coagulation

ANSWER: B

COMMENTS: The cut function of a monopolar instrument vaporizes tissue. Electrical energy is converted to kinetic energy, which causes an increase in the intracellular temperature to greater than 100°C (thermal energy). The rise in temperature results in the contents of the cells being converted from a liquid to a gas state, generating steam. The cell rapidly expands and ruptures due to the increase in the intracellular volume, releasing steam. The explosive force is speculated to cause acoustic vibrations that contribute to the cutting effect. The coagulation function of the monopolar instrument causes the contents of the cell to be heated to a temperature between 45°C and 100°C. There is a loss of intracellular water, causing desiccation, and proteins are denatured. Fulguration is a type of superficial protein coagulation created by the establishment of an array of current arcs in the gap between the electrode and the underlying tissue. Fulguration requires the use of modulated high-voltage waveforms, typically produced by the "coagulation" output of the electrosurgical generator and a "no-touch" technique. Tissue temperatures become higher than with either vaporization or "white coagulation," typically exceeding 200°C and resulting in organic molecular breakdown and carbonization. Fulguration is most effective for superficial coagulation and desiccation of superficial, capillary, and small arteriolar bleeding ("ooze"). Ablation is applying energy to the tissue to temperatures consistent with coagulation and avoiding carbonization and vaporization.

Ref.: 2–4

4. Monopolar instruments have:

A. Only a dispersive electrode

B. Only an active electrode

C. Two active and one dispersive electrode

D. Both an active and a dispersive electrode, with a *separate* "grounding pad"

E. Both an active and a dispersive electrode, in which the "grounding pad" *is* the dispersive electrode

ANSWER: E

COMMENTS: Monopolar instruments have an active electrode and a dispersive electrode. The active electrode is attached to the device and used within the surgical field. The active electrode has a specific size and shape, usually small, to focus current to the targeted tissue to avoid thermal injury to tissues not of interest. The current flows from the active electrode through the tissues to the dispersive electrode; thus the patient is included in the circuit. The term "grounding pad" has traditionally been used as a synonym for the dispersive electrode, but this is no longer being used. Bipolar instruments are designed to have both electrodes located within the device. The target tissue is gripped between the two blades and is desiccated and coagulated by the device. The current that is generated by the device heats the tissue to 60°C to 90°C and is delivered in a continuous low-voltage waveform.

Ref.: 2–4

5. Which of the following is most ideal when sealing a vessel?

A. Continuous low-voltage waveforms

B. Continuous high-voltage waveforms

C. Intermittent low-voltage waveforms

D. Intermittent high-voltage waveforms

E. Intermittent alternating voltage waveforms

ANSWER: A

COMMENTS: Use of a continuous low-voltage waveform is the most effective means of sealing a blood vessel. Continuous low-voltage wavelengths apply a consistent amount of energy, which causes desiccation and protein denaturation without vaporization. The low-voltage wavelength causes more even coagulation compared with a high-voltage wavelength. High-voltage wavelengths heat superficial tissue, increasing the impedance and preventing appropriate transmission of energy to deep layers. The most effective method of sealing a vessel is to compress it with forceps. This prevents the flow of blood within the lumen from removing thermal energy as well as bringing together the walls of the lumen, which facilitates the seal being formed.

Ref.: 3

6. Choose the best placement for the location of the dispersive electrode:

A. Over the hip of a patient with a history of a hip replacement

B. Over the hip of a patient without a history of hip replacement

C. Over the lateral thigh

D. Over the anterior thigh in a patient with a history of skin graft at this site

E. Over the wrist

ANSWER: C

COMMENTS: The dispersive electrode works by diverting the current and absorbing it over a large surface area. The larger the surface area, the smaller the thermal change, and thus the smaller the risk of a patient sustaining a burn injury. In order to absorb the current evenly, the dispersive electrode should never be placed over bony prominences, metal implants, scar tissue, hair-bearing areas, pressure points, limbs with circulatory compromise, or sites of skin injury. The dispersive electrode should also NEVER be cut to size. If there is partial detachment of the grounding pad, the current or density of the current can increase, and the dispersive electrode can become active and cause a burn.

Ref.: 3

7. With regard to bipolar and monopolar devices:

A. Both use direct current (DC).

B. Both use alternating current (AC).

C. Bipolar uses AC, while monopolar uses DC.

D. Bipolar uses DC, while monopolar uses AC.

E. Neither requires an electrosurgical unit (ESU).

ANSWER: B

COMMENTS: DC, when applied to a cell, causes positive ions (K^+, Na^+) to move toward the negative electrode and negative ions (Cl^-, HCO_3^-) to move to the positive electrode. A common power source of DC electricity is the battery. This is not used with electrosurgery and thus plays no role in the function of monopolar or bipolar devices. When the current alternates (when the polarity switches), the ions move past one another toward the oppositely charged electrodes. As they oscillate, friction is generated, and this form of mechanical energy is converted to thermal energy, causing an increase in intracellular temperature. A common power source of AC electricity is the standard wall outlet. This principle is the basis for electrosurgery and thus for both the monopolar and bipolar devices. These both require an ESU.

Ref.: 2, 3

8. Which of the following regarding ultrasonic energy devices is true?

A. They use DC.

B. They use AC.

C. They require a dispersive electrode.

D. They generate smoke, similar to electrosurgical devices.

E. Thermal spread is equivalent to electrosurgical devices.

ANSWER: B

COMMENTS: Ultrasonic devices also use the principle of AC, but in a different way than the standard monopolar or bipolar device. A standard outlet delivers AC, and the electrical energy is converted to mechanical energy by the device. The handpiece contains crystals that, when stress is applied, generate electric energy. Likewise, when the crystals are placed in an electric field, they exhibit stress. This is called the piezoelectric effect. The handpiece has jaws that oscillate and cut through the tissue and generate heat. Ultrasonic devices are unique in that the energy supplied is transferred directly to the tissue and therefore no current travels through the patient. If no current is traveling through the patient, then there is no need for a dispersive electrode and no concern for electromagnetic interference. Ultrasonic shears do not generate smoke. Although thermal spread is still a factor with ultrasonic devices, the amount is considered less than that of traditional electrosurgical devices, generally 1 to 3 mm.

Ref.: 2, 3

9. Which of the following regarding the pediatric population and electrosurgery is true?

A. In neonates, the dispersive electrodes should be placed over the abdomen.

B. It is permissible to use monopolar devices on infants less than 1 lb.

C. Smaller anatomy requires smaller instruments and therefore less chance of thermal injury.

D. Infant tissue is a good conductor of current.

E. It is acceptable to cut an adult dispersive electrode to size on a neonate in an emergency situation.

ANSWER: D

COMMENTS: Children are a special population to be cognizant of when using electrosurgical devices. General principles for adults do not always apply to children. When placing dispersive electrodes on children, it is important to remember that the dispersive electrode should NEVER be cut to size. The electrode should be placed on the back, thigh, or torso of an infant. Electrodes should be placed between the scapulae of a neonate. For infants less than 1 lb, it is not recommended to use monopolar devices. Children have greater body surface area to volume, but less total body surface area overall, and can be hurt if devices are overlapped. Children also have greater total body water content than adults. Current flows better in tissue with higher water content as there is less impedance. Therefore infant tissue, which has a high water content, is a good conductor of current. As the size of the surgical field decreases, the size of the instruments also decreases. Small instruments concentrate the current, and therefore there is a higher density of current delivered by the electrosurgical device. If this device is not used carefully, injury can occur.

Ref.: 2, 3

10. What is the first step to take if there is an intraoperative fire?

A. Remove all burning drapes from the patient

B. Turn off insufflation gas

C. Turn off all anesthetic gases

D. Extinguish the fire

E. Initiate Code Red Alert per hospital protocol

ANSWER: C

COMMENTS: Intraoperative fires are rare but serious events. The best way to prevent an operating room fire is to understand the use and maintenance of energy devices. If an intraoperative fire were to occur, the first step is to discontinue all anesthetic gas use and remove the patient from the ventilator circuit. If there is any airway fire, the endotracheal tube should be removed and the patient should be supported with room air. Second, any burning materials should be removed from the patient, and finally, the fire should be extinguished.

Ref.: 3

11. Electromagnetic interference is a concern for patients with pacemakers when using energy devices. Of the following, which device would not generate any electromagnetic interference?

A. Monopolar electrosurgical device

B. Monopolar endoscopic device

C. Radiofrequency ablation (RFA)

D. Ultrasonic device

E. Bipolar electrosurgical device

ANSWER: D

COMMENTS: While bipolar is favored over monopolar devices in patients with a pacemaker, it is ultrasonic devices that do not generate any electromagnetic interference. If other devices must be used in patients with implantable devices, there are several methods one can employ to minimize risk. Implantable devices include not only pacemakers but also defibrillators, deep brain stimulators, spinal cord stimulators, and cochlear implants. Ideally, monopolar devices should only be used in cut mode for short periods. The dispersive electrode should be placed as close to the active electrode as possible. The patient's pacemaker should be reprogrammed to an asynchronous mode to avoid pacemaker inhibition. However, patients who are at risk of ventricular tachycardia or ventricular fibrillation should be discussed prior to reprogramming their device.

Ref.: 3, 4

12. A 65-year-old male with metastatic colon cancer to his liver presents to the hepatology clinic to discuss treatment options. Due to his comorbidities and significant disease burden, he is suggested to undergo RFA of his liver lesions. Which of the following are possible pitfalls regarding the use of RFA?

A. Incomplete ablation of the tumor

B. Uneven delivery of energy

C. Damage to surrounding tissues

D. All of the above

E. None of the above

ANSWER: D

COMMENTS: RFA is a type of electrosurgical tool that causes ablation of tissue by heating the cell to high temperatures, causing vaporization and carbonization. The current is delivered in an alternating fashion, agitating ions. When the ions are agitated, their friction generates heat, and the thermal energy causes coagulation. RFA can be performed for several reasons. Some of those reasons include palliation or if a tumor is unresectable due to location or tumor burden, if the patient is a poor surgical candidate, or if the patient is being considered for transplantation. RFA can require up to four dispersive electrodes. Burns can be sustained around the dispersive electrodes if there are too few or if they are placed inappropriately. There can be incomplete ablation of the tumor, and benign tissue can be damaged by RFA. If there are blood vessels within the target field, they can distort the delivery of energy or absorb some of the energy, affecting the overall efficacy of treatment of the target.

Ref.: 3, 5

13. All of the following are true for RFA as opposed to microwave ablation, except for which of the following?

A. Requires a dispersive electrode

B. Uses alternating low-voltage current

C. Uses dielectric tissue heating, which is not affected by tissue impedance

D. Heat is transferred by conduction as opposed to radiation

E. None of the above

ANSWER: C

COMMENTS: RFA and microwave ablation are both methods of tissue destruction. RFA involves an electrode that is placed within the target tissue. The electrode receives high-frequency, alternating, low-voltage current, causing the tissue ions to oscillate, generate friction, and raise the intracellular temperature. The amount of water content is critical in that if the tissue becomes desiccated, heat cannot be generated appropriately. Also, resistance affects the ablation process, meaning if the tissue gets heated to too high of a temperature, the charred tissue will prevent appropriate treatment of additional target tissue. An example of this is the burnt crust of the bread with a doughy center. In RFA, tissue heating is affected by tissue impedance. RFA also utilizes several dispersive electrodes.

Microwave ablation uses electromagnetic waves rather than electrical current. An ablation antenna is placed within the target tissue. Microwave energy is applied to the antenna and "broadcasted" from the antenna in a spherical pattern through the tissue. Dipole molecules within the target field align themselves. The field itself rapidly alternates polarity, causing the dipole molecules to rapidly alternate orientation. The field changes so quickly that the molecules lag behind, causing resistive heating. As there is no current flow within the field, there is no need for a dispersive electrode. The heating is uniform. There is energy loss in microwave ablation with impedance mismatch. When the waves move from one tissue to another, they encounter differences in impedance. If the difference is small, only minimal waves are reflected. If the difference in impedance is large, the amount of waves reflected back will also be large. Any reflected waves can cause heating.

Ref.: 3, 5

14. After successful treatment by RFA, which of the following is the most appropriate recommendation for follow-up?

A. Ultrasound examination 1 week postoperatively and then at 3-month intervals

B. Magnetic resonance imaging (MRI) 2 weeks after surgery and then at 6-month intervals

C. MRI every 3 months after surgery

D. Computed tomography (CT) 1 week postoperatively and then at 3-month intervals

E. Positron emission tomography (PET)-CT every 3 months after surgery.

ANSWER: D

COMMENTS: Although intraoperative ultrasound is used to facilitate proper placement of the RFA probe and for intraoperative monitoring, it is not sensitive for distinguishing the difference between treated tissue and tumor recurrence. CT or MRI best visualizes the adequacy of ablation following treatment. The appropriate follow-up imaging schedule is either CT or MRI 1 week postoperatively, followed by repeated studies at 3-month intervals thereafter. Tumor marker studies are usually done at 3-month intervals as well. After RFA, peritumoral hyperemia is seen on cross-sectional imaging as rim enhancement around the ablation zone, which is indistinguishable from tumor enhancement. Persistent rim enhancement, months after the treatment, is diagnostic of recurrent (or residual) disease. PET may also help diagnose recurrence, but findings in the treated area or areas in the perioperative period are usually nonspecific.

Ref.: 6

REFERENCES

1. Voyles CR. *Prevention and Management of Laparoendoscopic Surgical Complications*; Society of Laparoendoscopic Surgeons, Miami, FL, 2006.
2. Alkatout I, Schollmeyer T, Hawaldar NA, Sharma N, Mettler L. Principles and safety measure of electrosurgery in laparoscopy. *J Soc Laparoendoscopic Surg*. 2012;16:130–139.
3. Feldman LS, Fuchshuber PR, Jones DB. *The SAGES Manual on the Fundamentals of Surgical Energy Use*. New York: Springer; 2012.
4. Sobolewski CJ. Electrosurgery: the newest surgical devices. *Contemporary OB/GYN*. 2013. http://contemporaryobgyn.modernmedicine.com/contemporary-obgyn/content/tags/aesculap/electrosurgery-newest-energy-based-devices.
5. Brace CL. Radiofrequency and microwave ablation of the liver, lung, kidney and bone: organ-specific ablation. *Curr Probl Diagn Radiol*. 2009;38(3):135–143.
6. Billhook AJ. Colorectal cancer metastatic to the liver: radiofrequency ablation. In: Cameron JL, ed. *Current Surgical Therapy*. 9th ed. St. Louis: CV Mosby; 2007.

SECTION II

ACUTE AND CRITICAL CARE

CHAPTER 9

CRITICAL CARE

A. Acute Care Surgery

Nicole Siparsky, M.D., and Alfred Guirguis, D.O., M.P.H.

1. An 18-year-old man has a 12-h history of vague, periumbilical abdominal pain, anorexia, and nonbilious vomiting. The pain is localized to the right lower quadrant. On examination, he is found to have tenderness over McBurney's point. Which of the following best explains the localization of pain in the right lower quadrant of the abdomen?

A. Inflammation of the visceral peritoneum's visceral nerve fibers

B. Inflammation of the visceral peritoneum's somatic nerve fibers

C. Inflammation of the parietal peritoneum's parietal nerve fibers

D. Inflammation of the parietal peritoneum's somatic nerve fibers

E. Distention of the appendiceal lumen

ANSWER: D

COMMENTS: Typically, early in the course of appendicitis, distention of the appendiceal lumen triggers the visceral nerves that course to the superior mesenteric artery ganglia and produces vague pain that is perceived in the periumbilical region. As appendiceal inflammation progresses and involves the parietal peritoneum, somatic pain fibers are triggered. These are thinly myelinated, fast-conducting fibers that course to the spinal nerve roots T7 to L2. Movement of the inflamed parietal peritoneum will trigger these fibers and is the cause of "rebound tenderness." Muscle rigidity is an involuntary spasm of the abdominal muscles in response to peritoneal inflammation.

Ref.: 1, 2

2. A 65-year-old man presents to the emergency room with epigastric pain of several days' duration. He has not eaten in 3 days. He has felt dizzy since the morning of admission. Two weeks ago, his rheumatologist prescribed 800 mg of ibuprofen every 6 h for joint pain. He is alert, oriented, and well appearing in the triage bay. Which of the following findings does NOT suggest shock in this patient with abdominal pain?

A. Diaphoresis

B. Pallor

C. Altered mental status

D. Heart rate 110 beats/min

E. Systolic blood pressure 100 mmHg

ANSWER: E

COMMENTS: Initial evaluation of patients with acute abdominal pain should include assessment for signs of shock. Shock is a clinical syndrome defined by inadequate organ perfusion. Symptoms of shock include alteration in mentation, cool and clammy skin, and oliguria. In cases of bleeding, shock can be classified by the volume of blood lost and the severity of alteration of mental status, pulse, blood pressure, and urine output. Patients with class I or class II blood loss typically have a normal blood pressure. However, the definition of "low blood pressure" is controversial. In general, most providers assume a cautious position when they observe a systolic blood pressure less than 100 mmHg, especially in communities in which hypertension is common.

Immediate intravenous access and resuscitation should be initiated. In this case, the patient's recent history of ulcerogenic medication (ibuprofen, a nonsteroidal antiinflammatory drug) and epigastric pain is suggestive of a peptic ulcer. Further evaluation is needed to ascertain the source of his dizziness. He is likely to be dehydrated. He may also be bleeding, although he has not passed blood yet.

Class	Pulse	Blood Pressure	Mental Status	Urine Output	Blood Loss
I	<100	Normal	Anxious	>30 mL/h	<15%
II	>100	Normal	Anxious	20–30 mL/h	15%–30%
III	>120	Decreased	Confused	5–15 mL/h	30%–40%
IV	>140	Decreased	Lethargic	Nil	>40%

Ref.: 3, 4

3. Which of the following statements is true regarding normal peritoneal fluid?

A. The abdominal cavity contains 150 to 200 mL of fluid.

B. The abdominal cavity contains fluid that is isotonic to blood.

C. The protein content of peritoneal fluid is 3 g/dL.

D. Mesothelial cells absorb solutes via gradient-driven passive osmosis.

E. Inflammation of the peritoneum increases its permeability.

ANSWER: E

4. Which of the following statements about bacterial contamination of the peritoneal cavity is false?
   A. Bacterial contamination of the peritoneum triggers degranulation of mesothelial cells, which initiates the systemic inflammatory response.
   B. Once the systemic response is initiated, the endothelial cells increase their permeability to complement, opsonins, and fibrin.
   C. Serum levels of catecholamines decrease in response to mast cell degranulation.
   D. Ninety percent of the bacteria are cleared by phagocytosis and the reticular endothelial system.
   E. Bacteria in the peritoneum may enter the systemic circulation through subdiaphragmatic lymphatics.

ANSWER: C

COMMENTS QUESTIONS 3, 4: Normally, the peritoneum contains 50 to 100 mL of fluid, with solute concentrations being equal to those found in plasma. The protein content is less than that of plasma. Fluid is absorbed by the mesothelial cells lining the peritoneum through endocytosis. Solutes with a molecular weight less than 30 kDa are easily absorbed. Inflammation of the peritoneum increases its permeability. Gravity and the negative pressure created by exhalation under the diaphragm affect the movement of the peritoneal fluid. The right paracolic gutter allows unhindered movement of fluid from the pelvis to the right subdiaphragmatic area, whereas the phrenicocolic ligaments obstruct flow through the left paracolic gutter. The subdiaphragmatic lymphatics play a major role in the absorption of peritoneal fluid and clearance of solutes and bacteria, which progress into the systemic circulation through the thoracic duct. Once circulating, more than 90% of bacteria will be cleared by Kupffer cells and the reticuloendothelial system.

Bacterial contamination of the abdomen triggers mast cells to degranulate, thereby initiating a local and systemic cascade of events. Locally, mesothelial and endothelial cells increase their permeability and allow products of complement, opsonins, and fibrin to enter the peritoneal cavity freely. This increased permeability depletes intravascular volume as fluid shifts into the peritoneal cavity. The systemic inflammatory response syndrome (SIRS) is initiated and consists of an increase in serum levels of catecholamines, glucocorticoids, aldosterone, and vasopressin. The resulting tachycardia and increased renal absorption of sodium and water help to sustain perfusion in the stress state by expanding the intravascular volume and increasing the cardiac output.

Ref.: 5

5. A 55-year-old man comes to the emergency department with a 6-h history of acute, diffuse abdominal pain. On examination, his heart rate is 115 beats per min, his blood pressure is 95/60 mmHg, his respiratory rate is 22 breaths per min, and his oxygen saturation is 93% on a 4-L nasal cannula. He is alert, is answering questions without dyspnea, and has diffuse abdominal rigidity and tenderness. Upright chest x-ray demonstrates extraluminal air under the diaphragm. Initial management should be:
   A. Immediate administration of broad-spectrum intravenous antibiotics
   B. Rapid infusion of 2 L of intravenous crystalloid through a peripheral venous catheter
   C. Rapid infusion of 2 L of intravenous crystalloid through a central venous catheter
   D. Immediate endotracheal intubation for airway control
   E. Rapid transport to Radiology for a stat computed tomography (CT) scan

ANSWER: B

6. Regarding the patient in Question 5, which of the following statements is true?
   A. No further radiologic workup is required.
   B. CT scanning with intravenous contrast is required to confirm the diagnosis.
   C. Bedside sonographic imaging is preferred over CT imaging to confirm the diagnosis.
   D. Diagnostic peritoneal lavage can be performed at the bedside to rule out intestinal perforation.
   E. An abdominal x-ray series is needed to confirm the diagnosis.

ANSWER: A

COMMENTS QUESTIONS 5, 6: The initial evaluation of a patient with abdominal pain should include assessment for signs of hemodynamic instability and shock, including tachycardia, hypotension, pallor, decreased skin turgor, and decreased urine output. Establishing intravenous access and delivering hydration are immediate priorities. For a patient with hypotension, boluses of crystalloid (lactated Ringer's or normal saline solution) should be given through a peripheral intravenous catheter.

Most patients do not require endotracheal intubation and mechanical ventilation in the emergency department. Evidence of impending ventilatory failure, including tachypnea, shallow breathing, lethargy or alteration in mentation, hypercapnia ($Paco_2 > 50$ mmHg), acidosis (pH < 7.35), or a hypoxic shunt refractory to oxygen ($Pao_2 < 60$ mmHg on an Fio_2 of 100%) should prompt consideration for intubation.

Patients with a rigid abdomen and free air revealed by x-ray do not require further radiographic workup. Time would be unnecessarily wasted pursuing CT or sonographic imaging in a patient who needs prompt surgical exploration.

Ref.: 1, 5

7. A 35-year-old woman experiences an acute onset of epigastric and right upper quadrant pain several hours after a large dinner. She has had similar episodes in the past that resolved after a few hours. This episode persists, and she has fever and nonbilious vomiting. What is the most likely source of the abdominal pain?
   A. Perforated ulcer
   B. Acute appendicitis
   C. Bowel obstruction
   D. Cholecystitis
   E. Diverticulitis

ANSWER: D

8. A 60-year-old man with chronic alcoholism awakens at 3:00 a.m. with severe, sharp epigastric pain. Three hours later, he

develops diffuse abdominal pain. What is the most likely source of the abdominal pain?

A. Perforated ulcer
B. Acute appendicitis
C. Bowel obstruction
D. Cholecystitis
E. Diverticulitis

ANSWER: A

9. A 55-year-old man with a 2-day history of abdominal distention, vomiting, crampy abdominal pain, and obstipation is experiencing severe, diffuse abdominal pain. What is the most likely source of the abdominal pain?

A. Perforated ulcer
B. Acute appendicitis
C. Bowel obstruction
D. Cholecystitis
E. Diverticulitis

ANSWER: C

10. A 65-year-old man with a history of chronic constipation has a 3-day history of abdominal distention without a bowel movement. He has fever and abdominal pain in the left lower quadrant. What is the most likely source of the abdominal pain?

A. Perforated ulcer
B. Acute appendicitis
C. Bowel obstruction
D. Cholecystitis
E. Diverticulitis

ANSWER: E

COMMENTS QUESTIONS 7–10: It is important to obtain a thorough history in determining a patient's diagnosis and tailoring the initial workup in the management of an acute abdomen. Differentiating between patients who require immediate intervention and those who can undergo a more gradual workup is also essential to avoid unnecessary delays in treatment.

Biliary colic is a crampy or sharp pain in the epigastrium or right upper quadrant, which occurs after meals. It may be associated with nausea and/or vomiting. It results from gallbladder contraction against a transiently obstructed cystic duct. In such cases, the patient experiences pain until the stone/sludge passes. If the duct obstruction persists, acute inflammation ensues and results in acute cholecystitis, a syndrome of right upper quadrant pain, nausea/vomiting, and fever.

Patients with a perforated ulcer will classically remember the exact moment when the perforation occurred. There may be a prolonged period of mild discomfort in the epigastrium, which precedes the perforation, as well as a period of diminished pain after perforation; however, this is quickly followed by the severe pain of diffuse chemical peritonitis. Risk factors include a previous history of peptic ulcer disease, untreated *Helicobacter pylori* infection, use of ulcerogenic medications (e.g., steroids and nonsteroidal antiinflammatory drugs), alcohol abuse, and conditions associated with ulcers (e.g., head injury, burns).

When vomiting is part of the history, it is important to differentiate between patients with mechanical obstruction of the bowel, bile duct, or pancreatic duct and patients who have a secondary ileus. A patient with acute appendicitis and periumbilical pain may have one or two episodes of nonbilious emesis before localization of pain in the lower right quadrant. The early abdominal pain and vomiting associated with appendicitis may resemble gastroenteritis. However, in appendicitis, pain is the predominant clinical feature and precedes diarrhea and vomiting in most instances. With gastroenteritis, the vomiting is typically more profuse and frequent and may be accompanied by profuse diarrhea as well.

A history of new-onset obstipation, changes in stool patterns, and fever may suggest diverticulitis. If the pain is diffuse, it may herald a free perforation, causing diffuse contamination of the peritoneal cavity. If the pain is localized, it may represent a contained perforation or diverticular abscess. This type of pain typically occurs in the lower left quadrant. In contrast, weight loss, cachexia, a slow decrease in stool caliber, and mild cramping reflect a more gradual process, such as malignancy, which permits elective workup and treatment.

Ref.: 1, 5–7

11. A 65-year-old alcoholic man has been experiencing epigastric and periumbilical pain associated with nonbilious vomiting for one day. He denies melena or hematemesis. In the past, he has had several episodes of similar pain that sometimes radiated to the back. He denies any previous surgery or medical problems. He is afebrile; his blood pressure is 120/80 mmHg, his pulse is 110 beats per min, and his mucous membranes are dry. His abdomen is not distended and does not have any surgical scars. Bowel sounds are present but diminished. His abdomen is soft, and he exhibits voluntary guarding of the epigastrium. His serum amylase level is 550 U/L. A CT scan is performed on admission to the hospital. Which of the following findings requires immediate intervention?

A. Diffuse pancreatitis with patchy areas of necrosis
B. Pancreatic pseudocyst formation measuring 3 cm in diameter without findings of intestinal obstruction
C. Diffuse pancreatitis with splenic vein thrombosis
D. Diffuse pancreatitis with nonbleeding splenic artery pseudoaneurysm formation
E. Diffuse pancreatitis with gallstones

ANSWER: D

COMMENTS: A patient with pancreatitis can have severe abdominal pain and rigidity. Surgery should be avoided except for complications (e.g., infected pancreatic necrosis or symptomatic pseudocyst). Initial management of a patient with acute pancreatitis should include bowel rest, intravenous resuscitation, and monitoring in the intensive care unit (ICU) when appropriate. Causes of pancreatitis should be investigated, including gallstones, hyperlipidemia, and drugs (i.e., thiazides). Alcohol abuse is a common cause of pancreatitis, but the fact that a patient abuses alcohol should not dismiss the necessity for a thorough workup. After stabilization and resuscitation, diagnostic studies are conducted to define the pancreas and biliary tree. Sonographic studies can screen for stones but may not provide a good evaluation of the retroperitoneum because of overlying bowel gas.

CT scanning with intravenous contrast administration will demonstrate pancreatitis, as well as its complications (pancreatic necrosis, pseudocyst, fistula, splenic vein thrombosis, and splenic artery pseudoaneurysm). Splenic artery pseudoaneurysm is an uncommon but dangerous complication; if left untreated, pseudoaneurysm rupture is associated with a high mortality rate. A mesenteric angiogram with embolization is usually successful in managing this unusual complication. Small, asymptomatic, uninfected pseudocysts do not require drainage. Cholecystectomy can be delayed until the patient's condition improves, but it is best performed prior to discharge from the hospital. Pancreatic necrosis is best managed in a step-up approach, with necrosectomy performed in a delayed fashion. Splenic vein thrombosis may result in venous hypertension; approximately half of these patients will develop gastric varices, which may bleed.

Ref.: 8–11

12. A 59-year-old diabetic male with acute lymphoblastic leukemia is hospitalized for chemotherapy. Shortly after his therapy, he develops a fever and lethargy. He becomes hypotensive, tachycardic, and oliguric. Blood cultures are obtained, which grow gram-positive cocci within 24 h. His white blood cell count is 0.02 K/μL. He is transferred to the ICU for septic shock. He receives a large volume of crystalloid infusion for hypotension. He develops anasarca. The following morning, the patient complains of perineal and scrotal pain. On examination, he is noted to have mild induration of the perineum and scrotum, with minimal associated erythema; no crepitus or fluctuance is noted. Which of the following is the most important determinant of mortality in this patient?

A. Inadequate initial debridement
B. Inadequate initial antibiotic therapy
C. Inadequate initial fluid resuscitation
D. Delayed intestinal diversion
E. Delayed nutritional therapy

ANSWER: A

COMMENTS: This patient is suffering from Fournier's gangrene or necrotizing soft tissue infection (NSTI) of the perineum and scrotum. Most NSTIs are polymicrobial. Toxin production contributes to tissue edema and loss of microvascular integrity, while cytokine production results in systemic inflammation. The result of these events is septic shock, microvascular thrombosis, and rapid spread of infection. The treatment is emergent wide surgical debridement of affected tissues.

Patients with NSTI appear ill (anxious, diaphoretic) and may recall a skin break within 48 h of presentation. More than half of the patients will not recall a skin break. Most report pain out of proportion to examination. Erythema and swelling are the most common signs of NSTI, although they occur late in the infection. These are the same findings of nonnecrotizing cellulitis, which explains why NSTI is frequently misdiagnosed. Crepitus and necrosis are present in less than one third of the patients.

Systemic illness, pain out of proportion to examination, pain outside the area of obvious involvement, and immunosuppression (e.g., diabetes, chemotherapy, immunosuppressants, corticosteroids, and advanced age) should raise the provider's index of suspicion for NSTI. Although positive imaging studies support the diagnosis, negative studies do not rule it out, thereby causing unnecessary delays in definitive treatment. Operative exploration may uncover dishwater or murky discharge, tissue necrosis (microscopic or gross), lack of bleeding tissue, and lack of tissue resistance to finger dissection. Wide, sharp dissection to bleeding tissues remains the standard of care. Although often necessary for wound healing, intestinal diversion and nutrition are not immediate priorities.

Ref.: 11

13. A 68-year-old homeless, otherwise healthy-appearing woman with a history of prior abdominal surgeries is admitted to the hospital with a small bowel obstruction. She undergoes unsuccessful nonoperative management for 48 h, followed by laparotomy and lysis of adhesions. On induction of anesthesia, she aspirates and develops rapidly progressive chemical pneumonitis. She is admitted to the ICU for respiratory failure and requires ventilator support. In the postoperative period:

A. Start parenteral nutrition immediately. Wait for bowel sounds and a bowel movement before starting enteral nutrition.
B. Start parenteral nutrition immediately. Wait for a 6-h gastric residual volume of <400 mL before starting enteral nutrition.
C. Continue crystalloid infusion. Wait for a 6-h gastric residual volume of <400 mL before starting enteral nutrition. Start parenteral nutrition after 5 days of bowel rest (which includes the 2 days preceding surgery).
D. Wait for 24 h before starting enteral nutrition, regardless of the 6-h gastric residual volume.
E. Wait for 48 h before starting enteral nutrition, regardless of the 6-h gastric residual volume.

ANSWER: C

14. The patient suffers from an ileus and does not tolerate tube feeding attempts. Parenteral nutrition is started at 25 kcal/kg per day. The following day, the patient suffers a witnessed seizure, and frequent premature ventricular contractions are noted on telemetry. The serum phosphate and magnesium levels are measured and noted to be low. Which of the following is true in patients with prolonged inanition (>7 days) due to postoperative ileus?

A. Patients with malnutrition or a history of substance abuse should start parenteral nutrition at 50 kcal/kg/day.
B. Patients with malnutrition or a history of substance abuse should start parenteral nutrition at 30 kcal/kg/day.
C. Patients with malnutrition or a history of substance abuse should start parenteral nutrition at 10 kcal/kg/day.
D. Patients with malnutrition or a history of substance abuse should not receive parenteral nutrition.
E. Patients with prolonged inanition should not receive parenteral nutrition.

ANSWER: C

COMMENT: Following abdominal surgery, ileus is a common finding. However, the resolution of ileus is not well associated with the presence of bowel sounds or subjective flatus. Most patients will experience a return of bowel function before these findings are noted.

If it is possible, the gut should be fed. Patients who are unable to eat (e.g., intubated) may still receive tube feeding through a nasogastric tube. Gastric residual monitoring every 6 h is a safe way to identify patients who are intolerant of feeding due to ileus or gastric dysmotility. In the Gastric residual volume during enteral nutrition in ICU patients (REGANE) trial, a prospective, randomized trial of ICU patients, 6-h gastric residual volumes less than 500 mL were not associated with increased complications (e.g., pneumonia, length of stay, ventilator days).

If the patient is unable to receive enteral nutrition due to postoperative ileus, parenteral nutrition should be considered after 5 days of bowel rest. The timing of parenteral nutrition administration is controversial. The risks of parenteral nutrition exceed the benefits for most patients who have been on bowel rest for less than 5 days. Likewise, the benefits clearly outweigh the risks for patients who have been on bowel rest for greater than 14 days. For most patients, parenteral nutrition should be considered after 5 to 7 days of bowel rest. The literature supports the earlier initiation of parenteral nutrition in chronically malnourished patients.

Parenteral nutrition should be avoided if the patient can eat or receive enteral nutritional support or if the anticipated starvation is less than 5 days. Similarly, it should be avoided in sepsis, terminal illness, uncontrolled hyperglycemia, fungemia, bacteremia, and shock. Last, it should be avoided if patients do not accept artificial feeding in their advanced directives.

Patients who suffer from malnutrition [body mass index (BMI) <16, unintentional weight loss >15% over 3 to 6 months, poor intake >10 days] and electrolyte disturbances (hypokalemia, hypophosphatemia, hypomagnesemia) are at risk for refeeding syndrome with parenteral nutrition administration. In such patients, it has been recommended that feeding start below goal at 10 kcal/kg/day. The patient should be closely monitored on telemetry, electrolytes should be checked daily, and electrolyte deficiencies should be corrected.

Ref.: 12–16

15. Which of the following is NOT associated with infusion of normal saline for large-volume intravenous fluid resuscitation?

A. Renovascular constriction

B. Hyperchloremic metabolic acidosis

C. Lactic acidosis

D. Anasarca

E. Decrease in strong ion difference

ANSWER: C

COMMENT: Large-volume normal saline administration for resuscitation of surgical patients can be problematic. Normal saline (0.9% saline) provides a superphysiologic chloride load, which leads to a decrease in the strong ion difference and hyperchloremic metabolic acidosis. Normal saline also causes renovascular constriction. However, it does not cause lactic acidosis. The administration of lactated Ringer's solution to patients with poor liver function results in lactic acidosis.

Ref.: 17, 18

16. A 60-year-old healthy woman presents to the emergency room with right breast pain. She notes that her pet cat slept with her the night before, lying on her chest. She notes the acute onset of diffuse swelling, itching, and redness. Physical exam reveals the patient to be afebrile with a normal blood pressure and heart rate. There is diffuse right breast warmth and tenderness; the nipple appears slightly retracted. No masses or nipple discharge are encountered. The skin is intact. The left breast is normal in appearance and exam. What is the diagnostic test that will correctly diagnose this patient's condition?

A. Ultrasound

B. Magnetic resonance imaging (MRI)

C. Mammogram

D. Shave biopsy of the skin

E. Full-thickness biopsy of the skin

ANSWER: E

COMMENTS: This patient has inflammatory breast cancer (IBC). It is commonly misdiagnosed as cellulitis, mastitis, and breast abscess. Antibiotic therapy is commonly prescribed, without clinical improvement. A high index of suspicion is needed to accurately diagnose this condition early on.

The hallmark of IBC is a dermal lymphatic invasion. A full-thickness skin biopsy should be obtained to confirm the diagnosis. While mammogram and ultrasound are useful in ruling out concurrent malignancy, they are insufficient in confirming the diagnosis. Once the diagnosis is made, staging is performed to determine the treatment.

Ref.: 19

17. A 27-year-old woman presents to the emergency room with right upper quadrant abdominal pain. She is 35 weeks pregnant. Her BMI is 34. She notes that she has experienced nausea and vomiting daily during her pregnancy. She has a temperature of 100.1°F, blood pressure 110/70 mmHg, and heart rate 100 beats per min. An ultrasound is performed, but due to the large fetus, the gallbladder and appendix are not visualized. Which of the following is true about imaging this pregnant patient?

A. Both abdominal MRI and CT scan expose the fetus to a dose of ionizing radiation, which exceeds the maximum safe dose of ionizing radiation during pregnancy.

B. Both abdominal MRI and CT scan expose the fetus to a dose of ionizing radiation, which is below the maximum safe dose of ionizing radiation during pregnancy.

C. Neither abdominal MRI nor CT scan exposes the fetus to a dose of ionizing radiation.

D. MRI exposes the fetus to ionizing radiation.

E. CT scan exposes the fetus to ionizing radiation.

ANSWER: E

COMMENTS: Pregnant women represent a challenging surgical patient population because it can be difficult to distinguish normal symptoms of pregnancy from pathology. Approximately 1% of pregnant patients require surgery each year. Delays in the diagnosis of common conditions, including appendicitis and cholecystitis, contribute to poor maternal and fetal outcomes. For patients in whom imaging is indicated, ultrasound remains a safe, low-cost option. However, ultrasound is uncommonly helpful; the likelihood of visualizing the appendix is low, and it delays definitive diagnosis. CT scan (2.6 cGy), x-ray (0.00007 cGy), and hepatobiliary iminodiacetic acid (HIDA) scan (0.15 cGy) expose the fetus to doses of ionizing radiation that are below the maximum accepted dose for an entire pregnancy (5 cGy). The risk of radiation-induced childhood malignancy is highest during the first 15 weeks of pregnancy, when the organs and nervous system are developing.

For these reasons, many experts advocate MRI as a first-line imaging modality in the pregnant patient. It does not employ ionizing radiation and is felt to be safe for the fetus, although the risk to the fetus is unknown. To date, animal studies have not shown teratogenic effects of electromagnetic radiation. There is a potential risk of increased local generation of heat, which is why it is advised to avoid MRI in the first trimester of pregnancy if possible.

Ref.: 20, 21

18. A 65-year-old obese man undergoes emergent coronary artery bypass grafting (CABG) on cardiopulmonary bypass. He requires large-volume resuscitation due to the long operative time. After surgery, he develops rhabdomyolysis, oliguria, and volume overload. On the morning after surgery, he undergoes endotracheal intubation and mechanical ventilation for respiratory failure due to volume overload. His abdomen becomes distended. An abdominal x-ray reveals a gas pattern consistent with ileus; there is mildly dilated small bowel with a paucity of gas in the colon. A nasogastric tube is placed for intestinal decompression, but his abdomen remains tender, distended, and firm. An ultrasound of the right upper quadrant reveals a normal gallbladder without stones and a normal common bile duct. He grimaces on examination and endorses pain by nodding his head. Bladder pressure is measured to be 22 mmHg. What is the appropriate next step?

A. Heavily sedate and paralyze the patient. Repeat bladder pressure.

B. Heavily sedate the patient. Repeat the bladder pressure the following day.

C. Perform a decompressive laparotomy with a temporary abdominal closure.

D. Perform a decompressive laparoscopy to drain the ascites noted on ultrasound.

E. Obtain a CT scan to rule out acute bowel ischemia.

ANSWER: A

COMMENTS: This patient has developed abdominal compartment syndrome (ACS). During large-volume resuscitation associated with an inflammatory response, capillary leak leads to edema of the abdominal wall and intestine. The abdominal wall becomes less compliant, the intestines swell, and ascites production ensues. The resulting intraabdominal hypertension results in decreased abdominal organ perfusion by occluding capillaries and veins. Oliguria heralds acute renal failure, while hypoventilation signals the onset of respiratory failure.

Capillary leak is observed in many surgical settings, including sepsis, acute respiratory distress syndrome (ARDS), and SIRS and following cardiopulmonary bypass. Cardiopulmonary bypass generates a capillary leak through the activation of the complement and inflammation cascades. Similar systemic manifestations are observed in conditions such as necrotizing pancreatitis and burns, and with large-volume blood transfusion.

To diagnose ACS, bladder pressure should be measured in a supine patient who is placed in a flat position. Pressures less than 20 mmHg are reassuring. However, for pressures exceeding 20 mmHg, the measurement must be repeated in the setting of paralysis, which removes external forces contributing to abdominal hypertension. In the setting of heavy sedation and paralysis, pressures exceeding 20 mmHg warrant further investigation. Typically, to salvage the abdominal organs, permit ventilation, and prevent acute renal failure, a decompressive laparotomy is warranted. This can be performed in the ICU for unstable, critically ill patients. The abdomen is often maintained with a temporary sterile occlusive dressing during this time, until the capillary leak and abdominal hypertension resolve. Laparoscopy is typically not sufficient to decompress the abdomen and can worsen abdominal hypertension.

In some cases, heavy sedation and paralysis are sufficient to decrease the abdominal pressure below 20 mmHg. In such cases, the ACS may be managed nonoperatively, until the abdominal hypertension resolves.

A CT scan is not necessary or useful in the diagnosis of ACS.

Ref.: 22–24

19. An 85-year-old woman is admitted to the ICU with septic shock. She was previously healthy and did not take medications. She receives crystalloid resuscitation and broad-spectrum antibiotic therapy. Her blood cultures grow gram-negative rods. Her lipase is mildly elevated. An ultrasound of the abdomen reveals a common bile duct of 9 mm; there is no wall thickening or pericholecystic fluid. Endoscopic retrograde cholangiopancreatography (ERCP) reveals pus on entry into the common bile duct. A sphincterotomy is performed, and the common bile duct is cleared of sludge and small stones. Following ERCP, her pancreatitis resolves, and within 48 h, she becomes pain free. What is the appropriate next step in this patient's management?

A. Place a percutaneous cholecystostomy tube to prevent cholecystitis.

B. Perform a cholecystectomy prior to discharge.

C. Allow the patient to recover from sepsis, and delay cholecystectomy for 2 weeks.

D. Allow the patient to recover from sepsis. No cholecystectomy is warranted given the patient's resolution of symptoms.

E. Perform an HIDA scan; proceed to cholecystectomy if the gallbladder is not visualized.

ANSWER: B

COMMENTS: This patient suffered from septic shock secondary to cholangitis, which resulted from acute biliary obstruction by gallstones. She also suffered from gallstone pancreatitis. In most cases, patients who suffer from this condition will require cholecystectomy to prevent future complications of gallstone disease, including recurrent cholangitis, liver failure, pancreatitis, and cholecystitis.

In the past, there was much debate regarding the timing of surgery for patients who experience gallstone pancreatitis. However, the literature has produced ample data to support same-stay cholecystectomy, which helps to avoid future complications of gallstones and excessive health care costs arising from readmission for biliary symptoms. In a study of gallstone pancreatitis patients by McCullough, 20% of the patients awaiting surgery were readmitted for biliary symptoms arising from persistent pain, recurrent pancreatitis, and acute cholecystitis. Similarly, a recent study of patients who did not undergo same-stay cholecystectomy reported a readmission rate of 24.9%.

However, as with all procedures, the risks and benefits must be weighed. As the population ages, surgeons will encounter an increasing number of elderly patients. Elderly patients who undergo cholecystectomy experience a higher mortality rate and length of stay than the general population. In a study of 1017 nonagenarians, the overall mortality was 5.6%; the laparoscopic cholecystectomy group experienced a lower mortality rate of 3.8% and a shorter hospital stay (5 days) than their open cholecystectomy counterparts. Similarly, in a review of Medicare patients who underwent laparoscopic cholecystectomy, there were 0.8% deaths (509 patients), which were associated with age more than 84 years, prolonged length of stay, operations performed on day 3 or thereafter in the hospitalization, and chronic diseases. The overall adverse outcome rate was 24%.

Ref.: 25–28

20. A 60-year-old man is admitted to the hospital with painless bright red blood per rectum. He noted the onset 1 h prior to presentation. He is tachycardic and hypotensive. His examination is normal except for bright red blood and clots noted in the rectal vault. A nasogastric lavage reveals normal gastric fluid without blood. He is admitted to the ICU for further evaluation. Which of the following is most likely to ultimately be both diagnostic and therapeutic for this patient?

A. Tagged red blood cell (RBC) scan
B. Upper endoscopy
C. CT scan
D. Mesenteric angiogram
E. Colonoscopy

ANSWER: D

COMMENT: This patient is experiencing hematochezia or fresh blood per rectum. In this case, the patient's nasogastric lavage does not reveal blood, suggesting that a stomach source is unlikely. A duodenal bleed cannot be ruled out, but it is less likely than a colonic bleed, given the fresh appearance of the blood. The patient without prior history is most likely to be having a diverticular bleed from the lower gastrointestinal tract.

Acute gastrointestinal hemorrhage is a common problem. In most cases, the first step in evaluating a patient with a gastrointestinal bleed (GIB) is to determine whether the source is upper (stomach, duodenum) or lower (small intestine, colon, rectum, and anus). Blood is a natural cathartic; typically, when present in the stomach, bleeding will induce hematemesis and/or can be identified by nasogastric tube lavage. Similarly, blood that empties into the intestine stimulates gut emptying. Unless the bleed is very brisk, melena is usually observed. Most patients with hematochezia have either a very brisk GIB or a lower GIB close to the rectum.

The three most common sources of colonic bleed are diverticulosis (30%–40%), ischemia (5%–10%), and anorectal disorders (5%–15%). Approximately 80% of diverticular bleeds stop spontaneously. Less common disorders, such as aortoenteric fistula, radiation proctitis, and Crohn's colitis, are often suggested by the patient's past medical and surgical history.

The imaging selection should be based on the source of bleeding and suspected rate of bleeding. With improved critical care and endoscopy, most patients with GIB can be successfully supported through localizing imaging studies, such that they rarely require undirected emergent surgery. Most upper GIBs can be confirmed (and, in many cases, treated) with upper endoscopy. Most lower GIBs can be localized by tagged RBC scan, which will detect bleeding at a rate of 0.1 mL/min; however, the test may take hours to complete, so it is a suboptimal option for a briskly bleeding patient.

For patients who appear to be bleeding briskly, or in whom resuscitation efforts fail, mesenteric angiography can be performed. CT angiography is inferior to traditional angiography because it exposes the patient to an intravenous dye load with no benefit, whereas traditional mesenteric angiography also permits selective embolization of the bleeding mesenteric vessel. A bleed rate of 1 mL/min is required to visualize the bleed by angiography. Colonoscopy is a useful study but is often limited by the large amount of blood in the colon. If a diverticular bleed is seen, epinephrine injection, cautery, or clips may be helpful.

Surgical intervention for lower GIB can be challenging. The mortality of emergent subtotal colectomy for bleeding approximates 30%. Blind hemicolectomy results in rebleeding in more than 50% of patients, while operations based on tagged RBC scans result in reoperation 30% of the time. For this reason, surgery is typically reserved for endoscopic or angiographic treatment failures.

Ref.: 29, 30

REFERENCES

1. Silen W. *Cope's Early Diagnosis of the Acute Abdomen*. 19th ed. New York, NY: Oxford University Press; 1996.
2. Jaffe B, Berger D. The appendix. In: Brunicardi F, Andersen D, Billiar T, et al., eds. *Schwartz's Principles of Surgery*. 9th ed. New York, NY: McGraw-Hill; 2010.
3. Rhee P. Shock, electrolytes, and fluid. In: Townsend CM, Beauchamp RD, Evers BM, et al., eds. *Sabiston Textbook of Surgery: The Biological Basis of Modern Surgical Practice*. 19th ed. Philadelphia, PA: Elsevier Saunders; 2012:66–119.
4. Cherkas D. Traumatic hemorrhagic shock: advances in fluid management. *Emerg Med Pract*. 2011;13(11):1–19.
5. Postier R, Squires R. Acute abdomen. In: Townsend CM, Beauchamp RD, Evers BM, et al., eds. *Sabiston Textbook of Surgery: The Biological Basis of Modern Surgical Practice*. 18th ed. Philadelphia, PA: WB Saunders; 2008.
6. Martin R, Rossi R. The acute abdomen: an overview and algorithms. *Surg Clin North Am*. 1997;77(6):1227–1243.
7. Duncan C, Riall T. Evidence-based current surgical practice: calculous gallbladder disease. *J Gastrointest Surg*. 2012;16(11):2011–2025.
8. Butler J, Eckert G, Zyromski N, et al. Natural history of pancreatitis-induced splenic vein thrombosis: a systematic review and meta-analysis of its incidence and rate of gastrointestinal bleeding. *HPB (Oxford)*. 2011;13(12):839–845.
9. Gooszen H, Besselik M, van Santvoort H, et al. Surgical treatment of acute pancreatitis. *Langenbecks Arch Surg*. 2013;398(6):799–806.
10. Vujic I. Vascular complications of pancreatitis. *Radiol Clin North Am*. 1989;27(1):81–91.
11. Sarani B, Strong M, Pascual J. Necrotizing fasciitis: current concepts and review of the literature. *JACS*. 2009;208(2):279–288.
12. Braga M, Ljungqvist O, Soeters P, et al. ESPEN guidelines on parenteral nutrition: surgery. *Clin Nutr*. 2009;28(4):378–386.
13. Braunschweig C, Levy P, Sheean P, et al. Enteral compared with parenteral nutrition: a meta-analysis. *Am J Clin Nutr*. 2001;74(4):534–542.
14. Heyland D, MacDonald S, Keefe L, et al. Total parenteral nutrition in the critically ill patient: a meta-analysis. *JAMA*. 1998;280(23):2013–2019.
15. Walmsley R. Refeeding syndrome: screening, incidence, and treatment during parenteral nutrition. *J Gastroenterol Hepatol*. 2013;28(4):113–117.
16. Montejo J, Minambres E, Bordeje L, et al. Gastric residual volume during enteral nutrition in ICU patients: the REGANE study. *Intensive Care Med*. 2010;36(8):1386–1393.
17. Chowdhury A, Cox E, Francis S, et al. A randomized, controlled, double-blind crossover study on the effects of 2-L infusions of 0.9% saline and Plasma-Lyte 148 on renal blood flow velocity and renal cortical tissue perfusion in healthy volunteers. *Ann Surg*. 2012;256(1):18–24.
18. Moritz M, Ayus J. Maintenance intravenous fluids in acutely ill patients. *N Engl J Med*. 2015;373(14):1350–1360.
19. Jaiyesimi A, Buzdar A, Hortobagyi G. Inflammatory breast cancer: a review. *J Clin Oncol*. 1992;10(6):1014–1024.

20. Mikami BE. Surgery in the pregnant patient. In: Townsend Beauchamp, Evers Mattox, eds. *Sabiston Textbook of Surgery: The Biological Basis of Modern Surgical Practice*. 19th ed. Philadelphia, PA: Elsevier Saunders; 2012:2029–2045.
21. Konrad J, Grand D, Lourenco A. MRI: first-line imaging modality for pregnant patients with suspected appendicitis. *Emerg Med Clin North Am*. 2003;21(3):711–735.
22. DeWolf A, Poelaert J, Herck I, et al. Surgical decompression for abdominal compartment syndrome after emergency cardiac surgery. *Ann Thorac Surg*. 2008;85(6):2133–2135.
23. Iberti T, Kelly K, Gentili D, et al. A simple technique to accurately determine intra-abdominal pressure. *Crit Care Med*. 1987;15(12): 1140–1142.
24. Barie ES. The intensive care unit: the next-generation operating room. In: Britt LD, Trunkey DD, Feliciano DV, eds. *Acute Care Surgery: Principles and Practice*. New York: Springer Science+Business Media, LLC; 2012:118.
25. McCullough L, Sutherland F, Preshaw R, et al. Gallstone pancreatitis: does discharge and readmission for cholecystectomy affect outcome? *HPB*. 2003;5(2):96–99.
26. Irojah B. Are they too old for surgery? Safety of elective cholecystectomy in nonagenarians. *JACS*. 2015;221(4):e83.
27. Fry D, Pine M, Locke D, et al. Composite measurement of outcomes in Medicare inpatient laparoscopic cholecystectomy. *JACS*. 2015; 221(1):102–109.
28. Murphy P, Paskar D, Parry N, et al. Implementation of an acute care surgery service facilitates modern clinical practice guidelines for gallstone pancreatitis. *JACS*. 2015;221(5):975–981.
29. Tavakkolizadeh A. Acute gastrointestinal hemorrhage. In: Townsend Beauchamp, Evers Mattox, eds. *Sabiston Textbook of Surgery: the Biological Basis of Modern Surgical Practice*. 19th ed. Philadelphia, PA: Elsevier Saunders; 2012:1160–1181.
30. Cirocchi R, Grassi V, Cavaliere D, et al. New trends in acute management of colonic diverticular bleeding: a systematic review. *Medicine*. 2015;94(44):e1710.

B. Gynecology

Nicole Siparsky, M.D.

1. A 65-year-old woman undergoes a routine abdominal hysterectomy and bilateral salpingo-oophorectomy for uterine prolapse. Intraoperatively, the surgeon notes ascites, a 3-cm adnexal mass, and lesions in the omentum, spleen, and small bowel. A gynecologic oncologist is not available for consultation. A biopsy of an accessible omental lesion is read as adenocarcinoma, most likely of gynecologic origin, on frozen section. What is the most appropriate surgical strategy?
   A. Abdominal hysterectomy and bilateral salpingo-oophorectomy as planned
   B. Abdominal hysterectomy, bilateral salpingo-oophorectomy, omentectomy, small bowel resection, and splenectomy
   C. Abdominal hysterectomy, bilateral salpingo-oophorectomy, pelvic and para-aortic lymph node dissection, omentectomy, splenectomy, and small bowel resection
   D. Terminate the procedure; arrange for palliative care consultation for metastatic adenocarcinoma
   E. Terminate the procedure; arrange gynecologic oncologist consultation for further surgical evaluation

ANSWER: E

COMMENT: At presentation, 75% of women with epithelial ovarian cancer have disease throughout the peritoneal cavity, involving the para-aortic or inguinal lymph nodes (stage III), or tumor that has spread to other distant sites (stage IV). Treatment of invasive epithelial ovarian cancer includes hysterectomy; bilateral salpingo-oophorectomy; omentectomy; peritoneal biopsy of the diaphragm, bilateral paracolic gutters, bilateral pelvis, and cul-de-sac; and lymph node sampling. If the cell type is mucinous, an appendectomy is also performed to rule out a metastasis from the appendix. Optimal debulking/cytoreduction is defined as residual disease no greater than 1 cm in diameter. Studies have consistently shown that surgical treatment by nongynecologic oncologists and low-volume providers contributes to suboptimal surgical management and shorter median survival.

Ref.: 1–5

2. Which of these options is the most common cause of death in patients with ovarian cancer?
   A. Uremia
   B. Anemia
   C. Liver failure
   D. Bowel obstruction
   E. Respiratory failure

ANSWER: D

3. A 40-year-old woman who previously received surgical therapy for ovarian cancer returns to the emergency room with a small bowel obstruction. A computed tomography scan of the abdomen reveals ascites and diffuse metastases involving the omentum, mesentery, liver, and abdominal wall. Which palliative procedure carries the lowest risk of complications?
   A. Enteroenterostomy
   B. Gastroenterostomy
   C. Insertion of a central venous catheter and administration of parenteral nutrition
   D. Percutaneous endoscopic venting gastrostomy
   E. Nasogastric tube decompression

ANSWER: E

COMMENTS QUESTIONS 2, 3: One of the most common problems faced by women with recurrent advanced ovarian cancer is bowel obstruction.

Palliative surgical options for patients suffering from malignant gynecologic bowel obstruction include gastrointestinal bypass, ostomy creation for intestinal diversion, and palliative tube gastrostomy for intestinal decompression. In cases of gastric or small bowel obstruction, gastrostomy tube decompression can be achieved with minimal pain and a brief recovery period when other options are not advisable. However, for patients with high-grade obstruction, external drainage of any kind often results in dehydration and malnutrition.

Rectosigmoid resection is the most common bowel operation performed for these patients (65%), and colostomy is a part of the procedure in 30% of these patients. Small bowel resection is also commonly performed in women treated surgically for recurrence or palliation. In one study, over half of the women who underwent gynecologic surgery for malignancy later underwent surgery for small bowel obstruction. Only 9% of these obstructions were due to adhesions.

Although surgical intervention for obstruction is undertaken in hopes of improving the quality of life, the median survival after surgery is only 10 to 12 weeks for ovarian cancer patients and 2.5 months for other gynecologic malignancies. In most cases, recurrent gynecologic malignancies are incurable. Therefore any palliative procedure should be weighed against this dismal prognosis.

The complication rates for any surgical intervention warrant careful consideration. Even a minimally invasive procedure, such as venting gastrostomy, carries a substantial risk. In one series, 28% of patients experienced complications, and more than half required a revision procedure. However, venting gastrostomy is excellent in palliating symptoms of nausea, vomiting, and distention.

Although it remains highly controversial, parenteral nutrition is being increasingly considered for patients with malignant bowel obstruction or complications of abdominal cancer recurrence and progression. The risks of catheter insertion (pneumothorax), catheter maintenance (infection, thrombosis), and administration of parenteral nutrition (liver disease) are substantial. In some series, nearly half of the patients experienced a complication related to parenteral nutrition.

For many patients, hospice management alone may be preferable to any of these interventions. Many hospice centers can accommodate decompressive nasogastric tubes for patient comfort. Similarly, portable suction devices are available for hospice care in the patient's home.

Ref.: 3, 6–12

4. A 49-year-old G0P0 perimenopausal woman with 1 year of abnormal uterine bleeding was taken to the operating room (OR) for a total abdominal hysterectomy and bilateral salpingo-oophorectomy. Intraoperatively, the uterus was found to have a deeply invasive adenocarcinoma, confirmed by frozen section. What is the most appropriate operative strategy in addition to completing the total abdominal hysterectomy and bilateral salpingo-oophorectomy?

A. Irrigate and close.
B. Perform pelvic washings and pelvic and para-aortic lymph node dissection.
C. Perform pelvic washings, omentectomy, and pelvic lymph node dissection.
D. Perform pelvic and para-aortic lymph node dissection.
E. Perform pelvic washings and omentectomy.

ANSWER: B

COMMENTS: According to the International Federation of Gynecologists and Oncologists (FIGO) Surgical Staging recommendation, optimal staging for endometrial cancer requires total abdominal hysterectomy and bilateral salpingo-oophorectomy along with pelvic washings and pelvic and para-aortic lymph node dissection. Omentectomy is a part of cytoreductive surgery for ovarian carcinoma and pseudomyxoma peritonei, but it is not necessary for endometrial carcinoma. All other options are incomplete.

Ref.: 3

5. Which of the following is FALSE about endometrial cancer?

A. Obesity is a risk factor.
B. Smoking is a risk factor.
C. Diabetes is a risk factor.
D. Stage of invasion is the most important prognostic indicator.
E. Histology is an important prognostic factor.

ANSWER: B

COMMENTS: Patients who have complex hyperplasia with atypia on endometrial biopsies have a 20%–30% chance for the development of or concurrent presence of adenocarcinoma. Risk factors for hyperplasia include obesity, hypertension, diabetes, anovulation, and unopposed estrogen use. Unlike many other cancers, smoking is not an independent risk factor. Stage and histology are the most important prognostic factors for endometrial cancer, especially the presence of extrauterine disease and particularly pelvic and para-aortic lymphadenopathy.

Ref.: 6, 13, 14

6. A 23-year-old woman is undergoing an emergent cesarean section for fetal compromise during labor. Although the baby is successfully delivered, the mother continues to bleed heavily. Operative blood loss is 2 L. She is normothermic, and her total operative time is 3 h. Her hemoglobin level has dropped from 10 to 7 g/dL. Her platelet count is 175,000/mm^3. Brisk bleeding appears to be coming from near the uterine vessels, but no single bleeding vessel can be identified. What intraoperative option would best control the bleeding?

A. Administration of platelets
B. Bilateral ligation of the anterior division of the hypogastric artery
C. Ligation of the internal iliac vein
D. Use of fibrin sealant
E. Bilateral ligation of the anterior and posterior branches of the hypogastric artery

ANSWER: B

7. As the case in Question 6 is concluded, it is noted that she has received eight units of packed red blood cells and a large volume of crystalloid. She continues to bleed diffusely in the pelvis. What is the best next step in the management of this hemorrhage?

A. Ligate the bilateral internal iliac arteries
B. Administer platelets and fresh frozen plasma.
C. Administer prothrombin complex concentrate (PCC).
D. Pack the pelvis, close the abdomen with a temporary dressing, and reoperate in 24 to 48 h.
E. B and D.

ANSWER: E

COMMENTS QUESTIONS 6, 7: The uterine artery originates from the anterior branch of the internal iliac artery. In cases of life-threatening uterine hemorrhage, ligation of the bilateral internal iliac arteries can be lifesaving. However, it can be complicated by buttock/thigh claudication, injury to the nearby external iliac artery and pelvic nerves, and, less commonly, spinal and bladder ischemia. For this reason, selective ligation of the bilateral anterior branches of the internal iliac artery is preferred.

Of note, there is extensive collateral uterine circulation, and bleeding may not be completely controlled with this maneuver. Similarly, bilateral arterial embolization is an alternative method to decrease uterine bleeding but is not 100% effective.

The most widely accepted transfusion strategy hails from the trauma literature. Large-volume blood loss is replaced with a restrictive, balanced approach, incorporating blood products early when patients do not respond to a 2-L crystalloid challenge. The equal transfusion of red blood cells (RBCs), fresh frozen plasma (FFP), and platelets (1:1:1) is thought to facilitate a more balanced transfusion, thereby avoiding dilutional coagulopathy. Similarly, aggressive replacement of clotting factors with PCC is gaining popularity. Once dilutional coagulopathy has set in, application of pelvic pressure with tight packing plus reoperation in 24 to 48 h after full resuscitation has also been shown to be effective.

An additional option is percutaneous embolization of the bilateral hypogastric arteries while the abdomen is packed. Surprisingly, pelvic embolization for postpartum hemorrhage does not seem to adversely impact later menses. In one series, 60% of embolized patients later carried pregnancies to term and delivered healthy babies.

Ref.: 3, 6, 13, 15–17

8. One year after completing pelvic radiation therapy for cervical cancer, a patient began having symptoms of bowel obstruction. Which segment of bowel is most commonly affected?

A. Jejunum

B. Terminal ileum

C. Cecum

D. Sigmoid colon

E. Rectum

ANSWER: B

9. Two years after completing pelvic radiation therapy, a patient developed progressive rectal bleeding and anemia. Radiation proctitis is diagnosed. All of the following are acceptable treatment options except:

A. Proctoscopy and formalin instillation

B. Colonoscopy with rectal biopsies to rule out neoplasia and focal cautery

C. Colonoscopy without biopsies and argon cautery

D. Cortisone enemas

E. Resection of the affected bowel

ANSWER: B

COMMENTS QUESTIONS 8, 9: Radiation therapy is commonly part of the treatment of pelvic malignancy and is very effective. However, early and late complications are common. Late complications include bleeding from radiation-induced vascular ectasias, fibrotic stenosis, and adhesions. The terminal ileum and other segments of bowel may fall into the radiation field or be fixed in the pelvis physiologically from previous surgery.

Hemorrhagic proctitis is managed in a stepwise manner based on the severity of bleeding. Local treatment with steroid or mesalamine enemas, as well as supportive red blood cell transfusion, is first employed. Colonoscopy with focal cautery can also be performed. However, biopsies are avoided because of the risk of fistula formation. Proctoscopy and application of dilute formalin (applied broadly by enema or selectively using soaked cotton-tip application) often work well. In occasional severe cases, resection may be indicated. This is often accompanied by an ostomy.

Ref.: 3, 6, 13

10. Potential sites for ureteral injury during abdominal hysterectomy with bilateral salpingo-oophorectomy include all of the following except:

A. Transection of the round ligaments

B. Transection of the uterine arteries

C. Transection of the cardinal ligaments

D. Transection of the infundibulopelvic ligaments

E. Inadvertent cautery thermal injury

ANSWER: A

COMMENTS: Anatomic knowledge of the course of the ureters in the pelvis is essential for preventing ureteral injury. The ureters travel in the retroperitoneal space in the abdominal and pelvic segments. In the abdomen, they travel in a caudal and medial fashion, from the kidneys to the bladder, along the anterior surface of the psoas muscle. The ureters cross the iliac vessels as they enter the pelvis and travel in the medial leaf of the parietal peritoneum. They course near the ovarian and uterine vessels. Thus they are susceptible to injury during transection of the infundibulopelvic ligaments and uterine arteries. The ureters travel through the cardinal ligaments about 1 to 2 cm lateral to the cervix.

Removal of the cervix during hysterectomy places the ureter at risk for injury. In general, the ureters do not travel near the round ligaments, which are anterior pelvic structures. Therefore this is not a common site for ureteral injury.

Ref.: 8, 14

11. Regarding tubo-ovarian abscesses (TOAs), which of the following is false?

A. Initial outpatient oral antibiotic therapy is considered a suboptimal treatment.

B. Initial therapy should be nonsurgical.

C. TOAs are present in ~50% of patients with pelvic inflammatory disease (PID).

D. Unilateral removal can be used as conservative therapy for women desiring fertility.

E. TOA symptoms may mimic those of acute appendicitis.

ANSWER: C

COMMENTS: TOAs are present in 10% of women with PID. They are more common in women with concurrent bacterial vaginosis or human immunodeficiency virus (HIV) infection. TOAs contain a mixture of anaerobic and facultative or aerobic organisms. Therefore antibiotic therapy should cover a wide range of organisms, including *Neisseria gonorrhoeae* and *Chlamydia trachomatis*. Initial therapy with oral antibiotics does not provide sufficient serum antibiotic levels to treat TOAs. Broad-spectrum intravenous antibiotics should be used as initial therapy. If the patient's symptoms do not improve over a 24- to 48-h period, drainage should be considered. TOAs can be drained laparoscopically or with radiographic guidance. There appears to be no difference in outcome between these approaches. Radiographic-guided placement of a drain is a common approach. The drain is left in place for at least several days while antibiotics are continued. Midline pelvic TOAs may be drained through a posterior colpotomy. Cultures may guide subsequent antibiotic choices.

For patients who are not candidates for conservative procedures, resection of TOAs via laparotomy is commonly done. Unilateral TOAs may be treated with unilateral adnexectomy for patients desiring fertility. Large or recurrent TOAs, involving both ovaries or the uterus, may be treated with hysterectomy and/or bilateral salpingo-oophorectomy. The abdominopelvic cavity should be irrigated extensively. The vaginal cuff should be left open. An intraperitoneal catheter is placed into the resection bed for postoperative drainage.

Ruptured TOAs are surgical emergencies. These patients usually have acute and progressive pelvic pain, may be hemodynamically unstable, and may quickly progress to septic shock. The mortality rate associated with a ruptured TOA is 5%–10%. Delay in diagnosis and treatment results in even higher mortality rates. Therefore patients should undergo prompt surgical treatment via laparotomy soon after they are resuscitated and hemodynamically stabilized.

Ref.: 8, 14

12. A 30-year-old woman in the second trimester of her first pregnancy develops an asymptomatic, reducible umbilical hernia. She hopes to have at least three children. Which of the following is true?

A. Suture repair of a primary umbilical hernia is as effective as mesh repair in women of reproductive age.

B. Mesh repair of the umbilical hernia is superior to suture repair in preventing hernia recurrence in women of reproductive age.

C. Repair of the umbilical hernia should be performed immediately to prevent incarceration.

D. Repair of the umbilical hernia should be delayed until after delivery unless symptoms of incarceration occur.

E. Hernia repair should be deferred until childbearing is completed.

ANSWER: A

COMMENT: Until recently, the impact of pregnancy on umbilical hernia recurrence was not clear. Still, the optimal timing for hernia repair in women of reproductive age remains to be established.

The "watchful waiting" strategy is a popular way of managing hernias in pregnant women. Pregnant women who develop a hernia without incarceration may be observed for the duration of the pregnancy. Hernia repair may be performed in the postpartum period. Hernia repair does not need to be deferred until childbearing is completed. Some centers perform suture repair of umbilical and inguinal hernias at the time of cesarean section with good results.

The theory of increased "mesh strain" with future pregnancies remained largely unexplored until a 2016 nationwide Danish study was published. A cohort of 224 women underwent epigastric/umbilical hernia repair followed by additional pregnancies. With a median follow-up of 3.8 years, 16% developed recurrence after mesh repair while only 10% recurred after suture repair. This suggests that mesh repair did not protect women of reproductive age against hernia recurrence with subsequent pregnancies. This is in contrast to the general belief that hernia repairs with mesh are superior to sutured repairs. This difference is probably due to the generally better condition and fascial strength of pregnant women compared with patients having repairs of umbilical and ventral hernias.

Ref.: 18–20

REFERENCES

1. American College of Obstetricians and Gynecologists. ACOG Committee Opinion: number 280, December 2002. The role of the generalist obstetrician-gynecologist in the early detection of ovarian cancer. *Obstet Gynecol.* 2002;100:1413–1416.
2. McDonald, Modesitt. The incidental postmenopausal adnexal mass. *Clinical Obstet Gynecol.* 2006;49(3):506–516.
3. Townsend Jr C, Beauchamp R, Evers BM, eds. *Sabiston Textbook of Surgery: The Biological Basis of Modern Surgical Practice.* 18th ed. Philadelphia: WB Saunders; 2004.
4. Sanai F, Bzeizi K. Systematic review: tuberculous peritonitis: presenting features, diagnostic strategies and treatment. *Aliment Pharmacol Ther.* 2005;22(8):685–700.
5. Schrag D, Earle C, Xu F, et al. Associations between hospital and surgeon procedure volumes and patient outcomes after ovarian cancer resection. *J Natl Cancer Inst.* 2006;98(3):163–171.
6. Hoskins W. *Principles and Practice of Gynecologic Oncology.* 3rd ed. Philadelphia: Lippincott Williams & Wilkins; 2000.
7. Tamussino K, Lim P, Webb M, Lee RA, Lesnick TG. Gastrointestinal surgery in patients with ovarian cancer. *Gynecol Oncol.* 2001;80(1):79–84.
8. Thompson J, Rock A. *Te Linde's Operative Gynecology.* 9th ed. Philadelphia: Lippincott Williams & Wilkins; 2003.
9. DeEulis T, Yennurajalingam S. Venting gastrostomy at home for symptomatic management of bowel obstruction in advanced/recurrent ovarian malignancy. *J Palliat Med.* 2015;18(8):722–728.
10. Furnes B, Svensen R, Helland H, Ovrebo K. Challenges and outcome of surgery for bowel obstruction in women with gynecologic cancer. *Int J Surg.* 2016;27:158–164.
11. Hoda D, Jatoi A, Burnes J, Loprinzi C, Kelly D. Should patients with advanced, incurable cancers ever be sent home with total parenteral nutrition? A single institution's 20-year experience. *Cancer.* 2005;103(4):863–868.
12. Rath K, Loseth D, Muscarella P, et al. Outcomes following percutaneous upper gastrointestinal decompressive tube placement for malignant bowel obstruction in ovarian cancer. *Gynecol Oncol.* 2013;129(1):103–106.
13. DiSaia P. *Clinical Gynecologic Oncology.* 6th ed. St. Louis: CV Mosby; 2002.
14. Herbst A, Mishell D, Stenchever M. *Comprehensive Gynecology.* 4th ed. St. Louis: Mosby–Year Book; 2001.
15. Fiori O, Deux J, Kambale J, Uzan S, Bougdhene F, Berkane N. Impact of pelvic arterial embolization for intractable postpartum hemorrhage on fertility. *Am J Obstet Gynecol.* 2009;200(4):384.e1–e4.
16. Holcomb J, Tilley B, Baranjuk S, the PROPPR Study Group, et al. Transfusion of plasma, platelets, and red blood cells in a 1:1:1 vs 1:1:2 ratio and mortality in patients with severe trauma: the PROPPR randomized clinical trial. *JAMA.* 2015;313(5):471–482.
17. Napolitano L, Kurek S, Luchette F, the American College of Critical Care Medicine of the Society of Critical Care Medicine; Eastern Association for the Surgery of Trauma Practice Management Workgroup, et al. Clinical practice guideline: red blood cell transfusion in adult trauma and critical care. *Crit Care Med.* 2009;37(12):3124–3157.
18. Buch K, Tabrizian P, Divino C. Management of hernias in pregnancy. *J Am Coll Surg.* 2008;207(4):539–542.
19. Ochsenbein-Kolble N, Demartines N, Ochsenbein-Imhof N, Zimmerman R. Cesarean section and simultaneous hernia repair. *Arch Surg.* 2004;139(8):893–895.
20. Oma E, Jensen K, Jorgensen L. Recurrent umbilical or epigastric hernia during and after pregnancy: a nationwide cohort study. *Surgery.* 2016;159(6):1677–1683.

C. Neurosurgery

Adam P. Smith, M.D., Richard W. Byrne, M.D., and Nicole Siparsky, M.D.

1. Which of the following statements regarding intracranial pressure (ICP) monitoring is false?

A. Ventricular pressure catheters are the standard for ICP monitoring.

B. ICP monitoring should be performed in salvageable patients with a Glasgow Coma Scale (GCS) score of 3 to 8 after resuscitation and abnormal findings on head computed tomography (CT).

C. Risk factors for elevated ICP after head injury include age younger than 40 years, open basal cisterns on CT, and systolic blood pressure higher than 90 mmHg.

D. Normal ICP is 0 to 15 mmHg or 0 to 20 cm H_2O.

E. ICP can be measured with either an intraparenchymal or a ventriculostomy monitor.

ANSWER: C

2. Which statement is true regarding elevated ICP associated with brain herniation?

A. The pupils are always dilated in the setting of brain herniation.

B. After the pupils become fixed and dilated, no functional recovery is possible.

C. Cortical sulci effacement may not be observed in the setting of increased posterior fossa pressure from a cerebellar hematoma.

D. In a patient with a unilateral supratentorial mass and increased ICP, weakness will always be observed on the contralateral side of the body.

E. Compression of the oculomotor nerve during brain herniation causes pupillary constriction.

ANSWER: C

COMMENTS QUESTIONS 1, 2: Increased ICP is typically generated by increasing the volume of water or blood in the cranium. Conditions favoring cerebral edema include hypoosmolarity, hyponatremia, syndrome of inappropriate antidiuretic hormone, rapid fluid shifting (e.g., dialysis), hypoventilation, hypercarbia, brain metastases, reperfusion injury, and intracranial bleeding (with or without mass effect). Liver failure may contribute to acute-onset intracranial hypertension.

ICP monitoring is appropriate in patients with abnormal GCS score of 3 to 8 and abnormal findings on head CT. Selected patients with normal findings on CT and risk factors for intracranial hypertension may also be candidates for ICP monitoring. Risk factors include age > 40 years, systolic blood pressure < 90 mmHg, decerebrate or decorticate posturing, or a suspicious mechanism of injury. CT findings of brain swelling with elevated ICP include slit ventricles, flattening or loss of normal cortical sulci patterns, blurring of normal gray–white junctions, and effacement of the basal cisterns.

Ventricular catheters are an accurate, low-cost, and reliable method to monitor ICP, thus making them preferred over parenchymal, subarachnoid, subdural, or epidural devices. The risks of ICP monitoring include a 1% risk for hemorrhage and 5% risk for infection. Therefore the procedure is not appropriate for all patients with head injury and especially those with coagulopathy or thrombocytopenia. Colonization rates do appear to be related to the type of device, with parenchymal monitors carrying the highest rates.

With a sustained elevation of ICP, the brain will herniate through the dural attachments and bony prominences inside the cranium. Elevated pressure in the supratentorial compartment leads to a downward pressure on the brain. This forces the medial temporal lobe(s), including the uncus, through the incisura, resulting in uncal herniation. In this process, the oculomotor nerve is compressed, resulting in dilation of the pupils.

The overall mortality rate associated with herniation syndromes leading to fixed and dilated pupils has been reported to be as high as 75%. If medical therapy is instituted immediately and the pupils return to normal, a small chance of survival exists, although the likelihood of a favorable outcome is low. If the pupils do not respond to therapy, it is unlikely that the patient will recover to more than a vegetative state.

Some brain herniation syndromes are associated with normal or constricted pupils. Herniation of the frontal lobes into and beneath the falx may not affect the pupils at all. Similarly, pressure from a pontine hemorrhage may disrupt the descending sympathetic fibers and result in pinpoint pupils (myosis) from unopposed parasympathetic tone. Elevated ICP in the posterior fossa may result in coma from brainstem compression, but the supratentorial compartment may appear relatively unaffected on imaging studies.

Ref.: 1–10

3. A healthy young man fell two stories from a hotel balcony, resulting in an isolated cervical spine fracture. In the emergency department he is hypotensive and bradycardic. Which of the following treatments is *contraindicated*?

A. Crystalloid volume challenge

B. Phenylephrine

C. Dopamine

D. Norepinephrine

E. Epinephrine

ANSWER: B

COMMENTS: Neurogenic shock should be suspected in any patient with cervical spine trauma associated with hypotension and bradycardia. Traumatic sympathetic chain disruption is characterized by the sudden loss of sympathetic tone and the predominance of parasympathetic tone. Trauma to the cervical spinal cord may include disruption of adjacent descending sympathetic neurons. Common features of neurogenic shock include hypotension, bradycardia, warm and dry extremities, peripheral vasodilation, venous pooling, and decreased cardiac output.

As smooth muscle in the vasculature relaxes and blood pressure decreases, cardiac drive is also lost and compensatory reflexive tachycardia does not occur. The first-line therapy is similar to that for other forms of shock and involves placing the patient in the Trendelenburg position and beginning fluid resuscitation. However, excessive volume loading should be avoided since it may lead to pulmonary edema without improvement in hypotension.

The administration of vasopressor agents should be considered early in neurogenic shock. An agent with only α-adrenergic properties may result in reflexive bradycardia. Therefore agents with α- and β-adrenergic properties are preferred because they will combat reflexive bradycardia. In the past, dopamine was a popular choice for vasopressor therapy in this situation. Although no formal recommendations exist regarding which vasopressor agent to use, dopamine's popularity is waning because its dose-dependent effects can prove difficult to manage. Dopamine, norepinephrine, and epinephrine are all effective in providing combined α- and β-adrenergic support for a patient in neurogenic shock.

Ref.: 1–3, 11, 12

4. Which of the following is true regarding brain death?

A. A neurosurgeon must perform the brain death examination.

B. Once the patient demonstrates loss of cranial nerve function, brain death can be pronounced.

C. The brain death examination is not affected by ethanol, opiates, or benzodiazepines.

D. The brain death examination can be performed in a hypotensive patient.

E. Confirmation of the brain death examination findings with electroencephalography (EEG) is not required to pronounce brain death.

ANSWER: E

COMMENTS: Brain death is a clinical diagnosis established by physical examination and confirmed with additional testing. Brain death is also a legal definition established in the national Uniform Determination of Death Act as cessation of vital brain function. State laws mandate other details of brain death determination, such as who is qualified to perform the testing (i.e., neurologist or intensivist) or the type of confirmatory testing required. In turn, most institutions have created policies founded in sound medical practice but that also reflect the state's particular laws regarding brain death testing and declaration.

In a study of 30 years of brain death determinations challenged in courts, the standards of brain death determination were felt to be solid. However, the timing, accuracy, and documentation of brain death generated a tremendous amount of conflict among family members, practitioners, and hospitals. Timely assessment and disclosure of the brain death diagnosis to family members proved to be a common key issue.

The cornerstone of brain death determination remains physical examination and apnea testing, which demonstrate (1) coma or unresponsiveness, including no cerebral motor response to pain; (2) absence of all brainstem reflexes, including absence of the pupillary response, oculocephalic reflex, cold caloric testing, corneal reflex, jaw reflex, cough reflex, or gag reflex; and (3) apnea.

Supportive diagnostic testing should provide evidence of central nervous system (CNS) dysfunction that is compatible with the clinical diagnosis of brain death. These should exclude confounding medical conditions, drug intoxication or poisoning, and hypothermia ($T \leq 32°C$).

In most cases, the brain death examination consists of two examinations separated in time, which is often at least 6 h. Because the apnea test can destabilize an already potentially unstable patient, it is generally performed only after the second brain death examination when brain death is highly suspected. Prerequisites for the apnea test are (1) a core temperature greater than 36.5°C, (2) systolic blood pressure higher than 90 mmHg, (3) euvolemia, (4) normal P_{CO_2}, and (5) normal serum electrolyte levels.

After the apnea test, confirmatory tests are optional, including (1) cerebral angiography, CT cerebral angiography, or transcranial Doppler ultrasonography to demonstrate the absence of intracerebral blood flow; (2) EEG to confirm the absence of electrical activity of brain; or (3) technetium-99m hexamethylpropyleneamine oxime brain scan, which shows no uptake of the isotope.

Ref.: 1, 3, 10, 13, 14

5. Which of the following is true regarding the management of elevated ICP?

A. Hemicraniectomy is the first-line therapy for elevated ICP.

B. Hypertonic saline is superior to mannitol for osmotherapy.

C. Prolonged hyperventilation is a benign method for lowering elevated ICP.

D. Maintenance of elevated cerebral perfusion pressure (CPP) may be more important for an improved neurologic outcome at the expense of high ICP.

E. Persistent hyperventilation is an effective method to sustain alkalization and combat acidosis in the brain for long periods.

ANSWER: D

COMMENTS: CPP is calculated by the formula CPP = MAP − ICP, where MAP is the mean arterial pressure and ICP is the intracranial pressure. Therefore as ICP rises to malignant levels, CPP falls. This is problematic in the treatment of elevated ICP because attempts to continue perfusing the brain (elevating CPP) can occur only by elevating blood pressure (MAP). Increasing blood pressure with already elevated ICP leads to a loss of the brain's normal autoregulatory mechanisms, which eventually results in even higher ICP. Much debate exists over whether to focus treatment on CPP or ICP. Early studies indicated that greater than a 20-mmHg elevation in ICP for sustained intervals was associated with poor neurologic outcome. Later studies indicated that CPP less than 60 mmHg was also associated with worse outcome. Recent preliminary studies, however, have shown that aggressive maintenance of CPP at a level higher than 60 mmHg, even with prolonged ICP higher than 50 mmHg for more than 48 h, may still lead to a good neurologic outcome.

The initial steps in controlling elevated ICP include medical therapies such as raising the head of the bed, maintaining the patient's head straight, hyperventilation, and hyperosmolar therapy. Hyperventilation is a quick and easy way to lower ICP in theory, for lowering P_{CO_2} will decrease cerebral blood flow and reverse brain parenchymal and cerebrospinal fluid (CSF) acidosis. However, hyperventilation is not without consequence. Disadvantages include induced vasoconstriction to the point where ischemia develops. The alkalization of CSF is also very short-lived with hyperventilation. In a direct comparison of hyperventilation and no hyperventilation in patients with severe head injury, some studies have shown a statistically significant worse outcome in the hyperventilation group, mainly because of ischemia induced by the prolonged therapy. However, temporary hyperventilation is still a useful tool to lower ICP until other measures can be instituted. The usual hyperosmolar agents used in the setting of traumatic brain injury are mannitol and hypertonic saline. Mannitol has three postulated effects: (1) plasma expansion, which improves cerebral rheology; (2) antioxidant effect, which improves the cerebral reaction to ischemia; and (3) osmotic diuresis, which lowers MAP and then ICP in a slightly delayed fashion. This third mechanism, however, could be detrimental if diuresis decreases MAP to a point of reduced CPP. Regardless, a level III randomized controlled trial showed improved outcome with mannitol therapy. Hypertonic saline, in contrast, reduces ICP while preserving or improving CPP. Although it is questioned whether the reduction in ICP by hypertonic saline is greater than that by mannitol, few studies have directly compared the two, and they are rarely compared in equimolar doses. Additionally, despite hypertonic saline's proved effect on control of ICP, no evidence of improved outcome exists. As a result, there is insufficient evidence to support the use of hypertonic saline over mannitol for osmotherapy in adults.

Hemicraniectomy has an important role in the treatment of elevated ICP; however, it is rarely used as first-line therapy except in some cases of malignant stroke.

Ref.: 2, 3, 6, 15–17

6. Which of the following statements regarding subarachnoid hemorrhage (SAH) is most accurate?

A. Normal findings on CT of the brain exclude the possibility of SAH.
B. Aneurysms occur most frequently on the basilar artery.
C. Surgical or endovascular treatment is recommended for patients who are neurologically intact and have an uncomplicated aneurysmal SAH.
D. The use of hypertension, hypervolemia, hemodilution (triple-H therapy), and calcium channel blockers is contraindicated for the treatment of vasospasm.
E. Aneurysms are the most common cause of SAH.

ANSWER: C

COMMENTS: Trauma is the most common cause of SAH, although aneurysms are the most common "nontraumatic" etiology. In the traumatic setting, patients commonly complain of only mild headache, and the neurologic sequelae are rarely as profound as observed in those with aneurysmal SAH. Sudden severe headache followed by altered consciousness is the usual clinical pattern of a stroke due to aneurysmal rupture causing SAH. Focal neurologic deficits may occur, but they are less common than those seen with strokes due to occlusion of major intracranial arteries. The sequelae vary depending on the size of the hemorrhage and range from headache to death. Although CT is the diagnostic method of choice to confirm SAH, approximately 15%–20% of patients with documented hemorrhage have normal findings on CT within 24 h of the onset of SAH. It is therefore important to perform a lumbar puncture when SAH is suspected and CT is negative for SAH. Maintenance of a high red blood cell count (often >100,000/mm^3) in the first and last tube is indicative of SAH rather than traumatic lumbar puncture. Furthermore, the presence of xanthochromia, yellow discoloration due to bilirubin in the CSF, indicates hemorrhage. However, xanthochromia may not be present if the hemorrhage occurred in the preceding few days. Angiography is helpful to confirm the presence of an aneurysm and is the gold standard for diagnosis. CT angiography and magnetic resonance angiography are also helpful but may miss smaller aneurysms because of their limited resolution. Most intracranial aneurysms arise from the large intracranial arteries of the circle of Willis and at the origin of the vertebrobasilar arteries. The most common sites of aneurysms, in decreasing order of prevalence, are the anterior communicating artery and posterior communicating artery (nearly equal prevalence), middle cerebral artery, and vertebrobasilar system.

Not all aneurysms rupture. Autopsy studies of asymptomatic subjects demonstrate a 4%–5% prevalence of aneurysms. The risk for rupture and need for treatment of aneurysms found incidentally (no SAH) are much-debated topics. Recent studies have used the size and location of incidentally found nonruptured aneurysms to stratify the risk for rupture. Multiple aneurysms are present 20% of the time and tend to be symmetrical in distribution or arise from the same parent artery on opposite sides of the circulation. Aneurysms felt to be congenital in nature and not caused by hypertension, but risk factors, predominantly hypertension, smoking, and alcohol abuse, are believed to induce rupture. The incidence of rupture is highest in patients between the ages of 40 and 60 years. Since the overall risk of rupture is relatively low and there is little predictive information, the necessity for and type of treatment must be discussed with the patient based on the clinician's estimate of the individual's risk for rupture.

After initial rupture, the aneurysm thromboses, but if left untreated, it may rerupture at an incidence of 4% on the first day and 1.5% every subsequent day to a risk of approximately 20% at 2 weeks and about 50% at 6 months. Therefore it is commonly recommended that surgical correction be performed within 48 to 72 h, if possible. Antifibrinolytics, such as ε-aminocaproic acid, have been found to decrease the rate of rebleeding during the time preceding treatment. Current options for definitive treatment involve either craniotomy for clipping or endovascular coiling (with or without stenting) of the aneurysm. Vasospasm, or delayed ischemic neurologic deficit, is a common entity in patients with SAH. Symptomatic vasospasm occurs in approximately 15% of patients with SAH and results in the highest morbidity in patients surviving the initial hemorrhage. It can be aggressively treated after a ruptured aneurysm is secured by either clips or coils. It often occurs in a delayed fashion after the initial hemorrhage (usually after the third day) and is seen most commonly between the sixth and eighth days after hemorrhage and up until 2 weeks. There is no definitive way to predict whether or when vasospasm will occur. A calcium channel blocker (nimodipine) and relative hypertension, hypervolemia, and hemodilution (triple-H therapy) are the medical therapies most commonly recommended for combating vasospasm.

Ref.: 2, 18

7. Which of the following statements regarding subdural hematomas (SDHs) is false?

A. Acute SDHs are generally unilateral and have a poorer prognosis than chronic SDHs.
B. Adequate treatment of an acute SDH usually consists of drainage through bur holes.
C. Chronic SDHs frequently recur.
D. Chronic SDHs should be suspected in elderly patients with progressive changes in mental status, even without a definite history of trauma.
E. SDHs carry a worse prognosis than epidural hematomas.

ANSWER: B

COMMENTS: SDHs are caused by rupture of veins traversing the subdural space or by arterial bleeding from parenchymal lacerations. Their symptoms and treatment depend on the rapidity of hematoma formation. All types of SDHs (acute, subacute, or chronic) have in common the presence of a decreased level of consciousness out of proportion to the observed focal neurologic deficit.

Acute SDHs cause progressive neurologic deficit within 48 h of injury. They usually follow severe head trauma and are unilateral. They often have both arterial and venous sources of bleeding and can progress rapidly. The diagnosis should be considered in any patient with a history of head injury who exhibits deteriorating neurologic status or who is unresponsive with a focal neurologic deficit. The hematomas are solid and easily visualized on CT as a hyperdense collection or sometimes a hypodense collection in the hyperacute setting when there is active bleeding. They can be bilateral, and adjacent intracerebral hematomas are often present. Treatment requires formal craniotomy with removal of solid clot and control of bleeding points.

Subacute SDHs are defined as those more than 48 h but less than 2 weeks old. Patients are usually less severely injured than those with acute SDHs, and marked fluctuation of the level of consciousness or a headache should alert physicians to the diagnosis. With large hematomas, third-nerve palsy with dilation of the pupils is a warning sign that midbrain compression secondary to temporal lobe herniation is occurring. CT may not identify the collection because the hematoma becomes isodense 10 to 12 days after its formation, and bilateral hematomas may be present. Craniotomy is required for hematoma evacuation.

Chronic SDHs most often develop in the elderly, frequently without a clear history of trauma. They can occur months after the initial injury and should be suspected in patients with decreasing or fluctuating mental status out of proportion to the focal neurologic deficit. The hematoma is commonly liquid, and drainage via bur holes is often adequate. However, chronic SDHs frequently recur when associated with subdural membranes, which may then require formal craniotomy to strip the superficial membrane. Subdural-peritoneal shunting may also eventually be necessary. Because of the tremendous mass effect on the brain from an SDH, mortality may be as high as 60% and can approach 90% in patients older than 80 years without surgical treatment.

Ref.: 2–4, 7

8. Which of the following statements regarding peripheral nerve injuries is false?

A. Neurapraxic injury does not require surgical resection of the nerve root involved to eliminate pain.

B. Axonal regeneration progresses at a rate of 1 mm/day after a 10- to 20-day lag period.

C. Denervation atrophy of muscles becomes irreversible after 12 to 15 months.

D. Restoration of sensory loss is not possible after muscle atrophy secondary to denervation is complete.

E. Recovery is influenced by the cause of the injury, the patient's age, the type of nerve injured, and the severity of injury to nearby vessels and bone.

ANSWER: D

COMMENTS: There are several classifications of nerve injuries. The Seddon's classification uses three terms to classify nerve injuries: neurapraxia, axonotmesis, and neurotmesis.

With neurapraxia, anatomic continuity of the nerve is preserved, and there is often incomplete motor paralysis with little muscle atrophy and considerable sparing of sensory and autonomic function. Operative repair is not indicated, and the quality of recovery is excellent.

Axonotmesis is the loss of axonal continuity without interruption of the investing myelin tissue. There is complete motor, sensory, and autonomic paralysis and progressive muscle atrophy. Operative repair is not indicated, and recovery occurs at a rate of about 1 mm/day.

Neurotmesis is a more severe injury, with significant disorganization within the nerve or actual disruption of continuity of the nerve and its investing myelin tissues. It is common with penetrating trauma and less common with compression injury, such as that seen with surgical positioning. Recovery is impossible without operative repair. After disruption, axonal sprouting begins within 10 to 20 days. After operative repair, distal growth occurs at a rate of 1 mm/day after the initial 10- to 20-day lag period. The degree of recovery is a function of the patient's age (with greater recovery in younger patients), type of nerve involved (pure motor or sensory nerves recover better than mixed motor and sensory nerves), level of nerve injury (distal is better), and duration of denervation (shorter tends to be better). Early repair of the severed nerve has the advantage of clearer anatomy and a longer period for regeneration, but late repair also has advantages. If more than 12 to 15 months is required for regenerating axons to reach a denervated muscle, a significant degree of denervation atrophy will have occurred and is irreversible. In contrast, a sensory loss may be recovered after prolonged periods of denervation, and thus a nerve repair can provide protective sensory function in the atrophied distal extremity. With peripheral nerve injury, the site of injury and nerve activity can be detected by electromyography only after 2 to 3 weeks. A rare late consequence of peripheral nerve injury is causalgia, a painful condition causing burning sensations, swelling, and skin changes in the distribution of a partially injured mixed peripheral nerve. It is believed to be caused by "sensitization" of the traumatized nerve with sympathetic hyperactivity. Treatment consists of medications or sympathectomy in intractable cases.

Ref.: 5, 19, 20

9. Spinal cord injuries may lead to several distinct syndromes. Which of the following incorrectly describes the syndrome listed?

A. In anterior spinal artery syndrome, a bilateral loss of motor and pain sensation occurs with preservation of position and vibratory sensation.

B. In posterior spinal artery syndrome, a bilateral loss of position and vibration sensation occurs with preservation of motor and pain sensation.

C. In central cord syndrome, bilateral motor and pain sensation is lost, worse in the lower extremities than in the upper extremities and worse in the proximal ends of extremities than in the distal ends of extremities.

D. In Brown-Sequard syndrome, ipsilateral motor and position sensation is lost along with contralateral pain and temperature sensation.

E. In cauda equina syndrome, a unilateral or bilateral loss of motor and sensory function occurs in the distribution of multiple nerve roots, including bladder areflexia and stool incontinence.

ANSWER: C

COMMENTS: The syndromes of spinal cord injury are named according to the area of injury and have deficits related to the tracts running in that area of the spinal cord. The anterior two thirds of the spinal cord hold the corticospinal tracts and the spinothalamic tract. Injury to this area via compression or infarction of the anterior spinal artery leads to paralysis and loss of pain and temperature sensation below the level of the lesion, with sparing of proprioception, which runs in the dorsal columns. The posterior spinal cord holds the dorsal columns, which are involved in position and vibratory sense and are supplied by the paired posterior spinal arteries. Lesions in this area result in the loss of these modalities below the level of the lesion, with sparing of motor and pain/temperature sensation. The cervical central spinal cord consists of gray matter, crossing fibers of the spinothalamic tract, and motor fibers to the upper extremities. An injury here causes central cord syndrome. Most common in the elderly with preexisting cervical stenosis, injury is caused by neck hyperextension in which hypertrophied paraspinal ligaments compress the already stenosed cervical cord. This leads to weakness and loss of pain sensation in the arms more than in the legs and distally worse than proximally. Central cord syndrome was originally thought to occur as a result of somatotopy of the corticospinal tract and ischemia from cord impingement, but this theory has recently been questioned. Axial hemisection of the spinal cord from penetrating trauma leads to Brown–Sequard syndrome. Deficits associated with this syndrome are loss of ipsilateral motor, position, and vibratory sensations and contralateral pain and temperature sensations because of the crossing fibers of the spinothalamic tracts. The nerve roots of the cauda equina arise from the distal spinal cord at L1–2. Compression of nerve roots of the cauda equina leads to variable loss of all functions of the nerve roots involved, along with radicular pain.

Ref.: 19, 21, 22

10. Which of the following is true regarding pediatric trauma?

A. Spinal cord injury without radiologic abnormality (SCIWORA) is a diagnosis made after neurologic symptoms are present despite normal findings on magnetic resonance imaging (MRI).

B. Because of their inability to speak, the GCS cannot be used in infants.

C. Age younger than 3 years, findings such as nonparietal skull fractures, isolated SDH in the absence of witnessed trauma, retinal hemorrhages, and long-bone fractures at varying stages of healing are most consistent with accidental trauma.

D. Spinal cord injuries are relatively uncommon in young children.

E. Interpretations of pediatric spinal radiographs are similar to those of adults, and pathologic fractures and subluxations are usually easily identified.

ANSWER: D

COMMENTS: SCIWORA is an injury originally described in children in the 1980s before the advent of MRI. Signs of myelopathy were present in pediatric patients after known cervical spine trauma, but plain radiography and CT showed no pathology. Therefore the current definition does not necessarily include the complete absence of imaging abnormalities because abnormal MRI findings may very well be present. The incidence has been reported to be as high as 36% in children with traumatic myelopathy. Because MRI has become a mainstay imaging modality in the evaluation of cervical trauma, children in whom SCIWORA has been diagnosed have been shown to exhibit ligamentous or disk injury, complete spinal cord transection, spinal cord hemorrhage, or, occasionally, normal findings on MRI. SCIWORA most commonly results from hyperflexion or hyperextension movements. Because the adult GCS assessment is not appropriate for the functional level of infants, particularly in its verbal and motor aspects, a modified version known as the pediatric GCS has been developed. It still uses the eye, verbal, and motor components but to an age-appropriate level for infants. Nonaccidental trauma is most common in children younger than 3 years. Nonparietal skull fractures, isolated SDHs without witnessed trauma, retinal hemorrhages, and long-bone fractures at various stages of healing are common inclusion signs for this diagnosis. Injuries to the spinal cord make up less than 5% of all childhood spinal injuries. The spinal ligaments are lax, and the facet joints are oriented more horizontally in children, thus making vertebral body subluxation and ligamentous injury more common than fractures or cord injuries. Because of the incomplete fusion of ossification centers in a pediatric patient's spine, radiolucencies may falsely appear to be fractures and make interpretation of pediatric spine imaging challenging. Such radiolucencies may occur in the anterior arch of C1 and the junction of the dens with the body of C2, a finding representing persistent synchondrosis that may mimic a fracture.

Ref.: 2, 4, 6, 22

REFERENCES

1. Kandel ER, Schwartz JH, eds. *Principles of Neural Sciences, Part II*. London: Edward Arnold; 1981.
2. Greenberg MS. *Handbook of Neurosurgery*. New York: Thieme Medical Publishers; 2001.
3. Narayan RK, Rosner MJ, Pitts LH, et al. *Guidelines for the Management of Severe Head Injury*. Chicago: Brain Trauma Foundation; 1995.
4. Schmidek HH, Sweet WH. *Operative Neurosurgical Techniques*. 3rd ed. Philadelphia: WB Saunders; 1995.
5. Greenfield LJ. *Surgery*. 3rd ed. Philadelphia: Lippincott Williams & Wilkins; 2001.
6. Bullock MR, Povlishock JT. Guidelines for the management of severe traumatic brain injury. Editor's Commentary. *J Neurotrauma*. 2007; 24(Suppl 1):2.
7. Atlas SW. *Magnetic Resonance Imaging of the Brain and Spine*. New York: Raven Press; 1991.
8. Ritter AM, Muizelaar JP, Barnes T, et al. Brain stem blood flow, pupillary response, and outcome in patients with severe head injuries. *Neurosurgery*. 1999;44:941–948.
9. Clusmann H, Schaller C, Schramm J. Fixed and dilated pupils after trauma, stroke, and previous intracranial surgery: Management and outcome. *J Neurol Neurosurg Psychiatry*. 2001;71:175–181.
10. Wahlster S, Wijdicks EF, Patel PV, et al. Brain death declaration: practices and perceptions worldwide. *Neurology*. 2015;84(18): 1870–1879.
11. Consortium for Spinal Cord Medicine. Early acute management in adults with spinal cord injury: a clinical practice guideline for healthcare professionals. *J Spinal Cord Med*. 2008;31(4):403–479.
12. Furlan JC, Fehlings MG. Cardiovascular complications after acute spinal cord injury: pathophysiology, diagnosis, and management. *Neurosurg Focus*. 2008;25(5):E13.
13. Greer DM, Varelas PN, Haque S, Wijdicks EF. Variability of brain death determination guidelines in leading U.S. neurologic institutions. *Neurology*. 2008;70:284–289.
14. Burkle CM, Schipper AM, Wijdicks EF. Brain death and the courts. *Neurology*. 2011;76(9):837–841.

15. Young JS, Blow O, Turrentine F, Claridge JA, Schulman A. Is there an upper limit of intracranial pressure in patients with severe head injury if cerebral perfusion pressure is maintained? *Neurosurg Focus*. 2003;15(6):E2.
16. Muizelaar JP, Marmarou A, Ward JD, et al. Adverse effects of prolonged hyperventilation in patients with severe head injury: a randomized clinical trial. *J Neurosurg*. 1991;75:731–739.
17. Boone MD, Oren-Grinberg A, Robinson TM, Chen CC, Kasper EM. Mannitol or hypertonic saline in the setting of traumatic brain injury: What have we learned? *Surg Neurol Int*. 2015;6:177. [Published online].
18. Ross JS, Masaryk TJ, Modic MT, Ruggieri PM, Haacke EM, Selman WR. Intracranial aneurysms: evaluation of MR angiography. *AJR Am J Roentgenol*. 1990;155:159–165.
19. Schwartz SI, Shires GT, Spencer FC. *Principles of Surgery*. 7th ed. New York: McGraw-Hill; 1999.
20. Sabiston Jr DC. *Textbook of Surgery*. 15th ed. Philadelphia: WB Saunders; 1997.
21. Way LW. *Current Surgical Diagnosis and Treatment*. 10th ed. Norwalk, CT: Appleton & Lange; 1994.
22. Menezes AH, Sonntag VK, Benzel EC, et al. *Principles of Spinal Surgery*. New York: McGraw-Hill; 1991.

D. Urology

Nicole Siparsky, M.D.

1. A 55-year-old belted passenger is admitted to the hospital following a rollover, high-speed motor vehicle crash. He complains of abdominal pain. He has a tender left abdomen with left flank ecchymosis. He voids blood-tinged urine in the trauma bay. Abdominal ultrasound reveals hematoma around the left kidney. Which of the following is true?

A. Renal contusions are best treated by observation until the gross hematuria subsides.

B. Parenchymal lacerations secondary to blunt trauma require surgical repair because of the risk for vascular aneurysm formation and secondary infection.

C. Nonexpanding retroperitoneal hematomas encountered during laparotomy should be explored to rule out a vascular compromise.

D. On exploring a perinephric hematoma, Gerota's fascia is opened to control the vessels.

E. Ultrasound examination of the kidneys is equivalent to computed tomography (CT) scan in the evaluation of renal trauma.

ANSWER: A

COMMENTS: A spectrum of renal injuries may occur following blunt trauma. Renal contusions are the most common renal injury and are managed conservatively with bed rest and observation.

CT provides accurate staging of renal injury: the severity of injury, presence of active bleeding, and vessel involvement, if any. Parenchymal lacerations confined to the renal cortex may also be treated nonoperatively if the patient is stable and there is no active bleeding. Deeper lacerations extending into the calyceal system may require intervention.

When an expanding, pulsatile, or uncontained retroperitoneal hematoma is encountered at laparotomy, it should be explored. The key surgical principle in the approach to an injured kidney is to obtain control of the vascular pedicle first. If Gerota's fascia is incised first, the tamponade effect may be released, and a significant hemorrhage could occur and possibly lead to nephrectomy.

Nonvisualization of the renal artery on CT may be caused by total avulsion of the renal artery and vein, renal artery thrombosis, absence of the kidney, or severe contusion, resulting in major vascular spasm. Traditionally, nonvisualization of the kidneys has been further evaluated with renal angiographic studies.

Ref.: 1, 2

2. A 64-year-old woman with symptoms typical of cholelithiasis undergoes an ultrasound of the abdomen that detects an asymptomatic, solid left renal mass. Which of the following should be the next examination?

A. Excretory urographic studies

B. Renal angiographic studies

C. CT of the abdomen

D. Radionuclide scanning of the urinary tract

E. Renal biopsy

ANSWER: C

COMMENTS: CT of the abdomen is the single most useful examination for the workup of patients suspected of having renal cell carcinoma. In addition to confirming the solid nature of a renal mass, it can demonstrate local extension; venous and caval involvement; and distant metastases to the liver, adrenal gland, and visualized skeleton.

Renal cell carcinoma, which probably arises from the proximal tubular epithelium, is the most common *primary* renal cancer; it accounts for approximately 86% of all primary malignant renal cancers. Of the remainder, 12% are Wilms tumor and 2% are renal sarcoma. The foregoing comments refer to primary renal tumors, but the most common asymptomatic renal masses are metastatic, with the lung being the most frequent primary site.

Treatment and prognosis of renal cell carcinoma are determined by the anatomic extent of the disease. Treatment of local disease focuses on tumor removal by radical nephrectomy. Solid renal masses are rarely subjected to biopsy, and they are diagnosed by pathologic examination of the excised kidney. Surgery alone offers an excellent prognosis in patients with early lesions that are confined within the renal cortex. Percutaneous ablation of renal masses may be appropriate for small masses, defined as less than 3 cm.

Regional lymphadenectomy has not been shown to result in increased survival. Metastases frequently occur by the hematogenous as well as lymphatic route, which may negate any theoretical advantage of even more radical local surgery. The presence of a limited tumor thrombus in the vena cava with right-sided carcinomas may not adversely affect the long-term outcome if the thrombus is removed completely. In the presence of distant metastases, nephrectomy may still be appropriate to control bleeding, pain, or infection.

Immunotherapy may result in remission of the cancer in a small percentage of patients. In select circumstances, patients with isolated metastases have benefited from resection of their metastatic disease.

Ref.: 3

3. Which of the following statements about renal calculi is true?

A. A low-oxalate diet increases urinary excretion of calcium oxalate.

B. A low-calcium diet reduces urinary excretion of calcium oxalate.

C. Ammonium magnesium phosphate (struvite) is more soluble in acidic urine.

D. Uric acid is more soluble in alkaline urine.

E. Most stones <4-mm diameter will not pass without intervention.

ANSWER: D

COMMENTS: Determination of stone composition is important for both recognition of the underlying abnormality and institution of appropriate therapy. Most urinary calculi (up to 75%) are calcium oxalate stones, and approximately one half of these are mixtures of calcium oxalate and phosphate. The serum calcium level should be checked in patients with these stones, and if elevated, parathyroid hormone levels should be determined as well. Calcium phosphate and calcium oxalate stones are not generally altered by variations in urinary pH within the normal range.

Ammonium magnesium phosphate (struvite) stones are next in frequency and are usually associated with infection. They form in alkaline urine, and their solubility is increased in acidic urine. Because urea-splitting organisms form ammonia and alkalinize the urine in the presence of infection, adequate pH manipulation cannot be obtained without control of the infection.

Uric acid stones are typically radiolucent, and their solubility is increased by alkalinization. The solubility of cystine is increased in alkaline urine.

The simple presence of a renal or ureteral calculus alone is not an indication for intervention by invasive techniques. Medical management, including analgesics, antibiotics, and appropriate urinary pH adjustments, often results in the spontaneous passage of stones. Smaller stones (<4 mm), in particular, can be expected to pass 90% of the time. There is no evidence that excessive hydration facilitates the passage of renal or ureteral calculi. Indeed, it may increase pain. α-Antagonist and calcium channel blocker medications have been shown to significantly decrease the time to passage of distal ureteral stones.

Surgical management is indicated when calculi produce persistent obstruction, intractable pain, or a stone associated with impaired renal function. Techniques for stone removal include ureteroscopic manipulation, percutaneous nephrolithotomy, open nephrolithotomy, and extracorporeal shock wave lithotripsy (ESWL).

Ref.: 4, 5

4. Resection of a sigmoid cancer necessitates excision of a segment of the left pelvic ureter to 3 cm distal to the bifurcation of the common iliac artery. Which of the following is the best option for reconstruction of the ureter?
   A. Ileal substitution
   B. Transureteroureterostomy
   C. Nephrectomy
   D. Psoas bladder hitch
   E. Renal autotransplantation

ANSWER: D

COMMENTS: In this situation, simple *in situ* ureteroneocystostomy is not possible. An end-to-side anastomosis of the severed ureter to the opposite ureter (ureteroureterostomy) may be successful but may jeopardize the contralateral ureter. This approach is contraindicated in patients with a history of nephrolithiasis, transitional cell carcinoma, or recurrent pyelonephritis. A broad U-shaped flap (Boari flap) can be rotated off the bladder, fashioned in the shape of a cylinder, and anastomosed to the severed ureter. Another solution is to mobilize the bladder extensively and hitch it to the psoas muscle to permit ureteral implantation (termed *psoas hitch*). With this technique, the bladder can often be brought as high as the common iliac artery. Mobilization of the kidney may provide 2 to 3 cm of ureteral length as well. Autotransplantation or ileal substitution of the ureter is reserved for large mid- or proximal-ureteral injuries. Nephrectomy may be considered for a nonfunctioning kidney with differential function consisting of less than 20% of the total glomerular filtration rate as quantified on a nuclear medicine study; however, every effort should be made to preserve the renal unit.

Ref.: 1

5. Which of the following is not a principle of repair of an intraoperative ureteral injury?
   A. Use of nonabsorbable suture material
   B. Spatulation of the transected ends
   C. Foley catheter drainage
   D. Placement of a drain next to the repair
   E. Ureteral stent

ANSWER: A

COMMENTS: Ureteral injuries are usually iatrogenic and occur during the course of retroperitoneal dissection for various abdominal and pelvic conditions. In cases of transection, repair should be carried out with absorbable suture material and an indwelling intraureteral stent. Nonabsorbable sutures should be avoided because they may serve as a nidus for calculus formation. Extensive ureteral dissection should be avoided to preserve the segmental blood supply. Spatulation reduces the incidence of anastomotic stricture in the severed ureter. Drains should be placed to accommodate an anastomotic leak. When injury involves the pelvic ureteral segment, ureteroneocystostomy may be preferable. Tube nephrostomy serves to divert urine from the repair site. This may facilitate healing at the anastomotic site but is only occasionally employed when primary repair is performed. Foley catheter drainage is important in the immediate postoperative period because an intraureteral stent allows reflux of bladder urine to the anastomosis.

Ref.: 1

6. A 22-year-old man suffers a pelvic fracture during a motor vehicle crash. He is admitted to the hospital for pain control and further evaluation. He complains of inability to void several hours later and is noted to have a distended abdomen. CT scan of the abdomen and pelvis reveals a distended bladder with contrast extravasation from the urethra; there is no free fluid in the abdomen. Which of the following constitutes appropriate initial treatment?
   A. Passage of a transurethral catheter
   B. Suprapubic tube cystostomy
   C. Percutaneous urethrostomy
   D. Retropubic urethrostomy
   E. Bilateral percutaneous nephrostomy tubes

ANSWER: B

COMMENTS: Blunt pelvic trauma is the most common cause of a urethral injury. Urethral disruption may cause the classic triad of blood at the meatus, a palpable bladder, and inability to urinate. Approximately 10% of pelvic fractures in males result in a urethral injury. Disruption usually occurs at or above the membranous portion of the urethra because the anterior prostatic and membranous portions are relatively fixed by the puboprostatic ligaments and the urogenital diaphragm.

A urethral injury should be suspected if blood is noted at the meatus or if the patient is unable to void clear urine. Urethral catheterization should not be attempted under these circumstances. The risk of inserting a catheter is that partial disruption may be converted to complete disruption. Instead, a retrograde urethrogram should be obtained to confirm the suspected diagnosis.

In most cases, the complications of incontinence, stricture, and impotence are minimized by the performance of suprapubic cystostomy and delayed repair of a urethral injury. Percutaneous nephrostomy tubes will not decompress the bladder and therefore leave the patient at risk for bladder rupture. Perineal urethrostomy does not divert the urine proximal to the site of injury and is of no value in such a situation. Immediate retropubic surgical realignment has a place in selected clinical situations, such as major bladder neck laceration, prostatic fragmentation, or severe dislocation of the prostate with severely displaced bone fragments.

The site of bladder rupture with pelvic fracture is usually extraperitoneal because it has been caused by the shearing force of the pelvic fracture. Isolated extraperitoneal bladder rupture is treated with 7 to 10 days of Foley catheter drainage. Blunt injury *without* pelvic fracture is associated with intraperitoneal rupture, particularly if the bladder is full at the time of injury. This perforation is typically at the dome of the bladder. A bladder injury should be suspected in any patient with lower abdominal trauma if there is any hematuria or the patient is unable to void.

Single-view cystography may miss a significant injury. Anterior, posterior, lateral, oblique, and, in particular, postvoid films are necessary. Alternatively, a CT cystogram may be performed by injecting 300 to 400 mL of contrast material through a Foley catheter followed by CT of the pelvis. The usual treatment of intraperitoneal rupture involves a two-layer, watertight closure with absorbable suture and transurethral or suprapubic bladder drainage.

An iatrogenic injury recognized at the time of an operation does not generally require suprapubic cystotomy but does require repair with absorbable suture and urethral catheter drainage for 5 to 7 days. It is also necessary to be vigilant that the Foley catheter does not become obstructed, such as with blood, and cause the bladder to become distended.

Ref.: 6, 7

7. One hour after a prolonged transurethral resection of the prostate (TURP), a 70-year-old man with mild coronary artery disease experiences bradycardia, hypertension, confusion, nausea, and headache. What is the most likely cause?

   A. Hyperkalemia

   B. Hypokalemia

   C. Hypernatremia

   D. Hyponatremia

   E. Anemia

ANSWER: D

COMMENTS: The patient is most likely suffering from transurethral resection (TUR) syndrome, which is caused by excessive absorption of irrigant solution and results in hyponatremia. The usual irrigation fluid is 1.5% glycine, which has an osmolarity of 200 mOsm/L, compared with the normal serum osmolarity of 290 mOsm/L. Excessive systemic absorption of the solution can result in a dilutional hyponatremia, hypoproteinemia, and decreased serum osmotic pressure. Extremely low sodium levels (<110 mEq/L) may result in severe cerebral edema and subsequent seizures. Treatment of TUR syndrome traditionally consists of terminating the procedure as rapidly as possible, administration of furosemide intraoperatively or postoperatively, and instillation of a 0.9% NaCl (and in severe cases, 3% NaCl) solution over a 3- to 6-h period. Newer bipolar resecting equipment allows the use of 0.9% normal saline to fill the bladder, which has dramatically decreased the incidence of TUR syndrome. However, these patients may still suffer from fluid overload as a result of absorption of this isotonic fluid.

Ref.: 8, 9

8. A 14-year-old boy is brought to the emergency department with a 4-h history of acute, severe left scrotal pain. Examination reveals a high-riding left testicle with severe pain on palpation. Urinalysis does not reveal any evidence of red or white blood cells. Which of the following is the treatment of choice at this point?

   A. Heat, scrotal elevation, and antibiotics

   B. Manual attempt at detorsion

   C. Analgesics and reexamination

   D. Doppler examination of testicular blood flow

   E. Surgical exploration

ANSWER: E

COMMENTS: When examining the acutely painful scrotum, one should attempt to differentiate epididymitis from testicular torsion, but it may not be possible. Doubtful cases should be treated as testicular torsion until proved otherwise. Testicular torsion occurs when the tunica vaginalis of the testicle has not adhered to the surrounding scrotal tissues. Because irreversible testicular ischemia occurs within 4 h (and as early as 2 h) when there is complete torsion, prompt surgical exploration is indicated even if the diagnosis is uncertain. Doppler examination may be helpful for assessing testicular blood flow. Nuclear medicine scans are reliable and may be used judiciously. Manual detorsion is not usually successful but may be attempted if the scrotum is not swollen. It may relieve the pain, but exploration is still necessary because residual torsion may still exist. At the time of exploration, the involved testis should be anatomically fixated after detorsion is performed (orchiopexy). The contralateral testis should undergo a similar procedure prophylactically because the same anatomic abnormality is often found in both testes.

Ref.: 7

9. A 32-year-old man arrives at the emergency department with an exquisitely painful and "woody" feeling penile erection of 18-h duration. Which of the following is not a therapeutic option?

   A. Aspiration of blood from the corpora cavernosa

   B. Irrigation of the corpora cavernosa with papaverine

   C. Creation of a communication between the glans penis and a corporal body with a biopsy needle or scalpel blade

   D. Side-to-side anastomosis between the corpus spongiosum and corpus cavernosum

   E. Exchange transfusions

ANSWER: B

COMMENTS: Priapism is a prolonged pathologic penile erection in the absence of sexual stimulation. There are two major types: ischemic ("low flow") and nonischemic ("high flow"). In the ischemic priapism, the patient experiences pain, and blood gas analysis of aspirated corporal blood shows acidosis and hypoxemia. Ischemic priapism requires emergency treatment. Nonischemic priapism is not usually painful and requires only conservative management and reassurance. Most cases of priapism are idiopathic. Some known causes are sickle cell disease, leukemic infiltration of veins draining the penis, and certain medications, such as anticoagulants and antidepressants. Frequently, simple aspiration of blood from the corpus cavernosum can resolve the tumescence. If this fails, irrigation of the corpus with a dilute solution of epinephrine or norepinephrine may work. This has the dual effect of decompressing the corpus and the venous obstruction that goes with it, as well as diminishing arterial flow. Papaverine is used to treat impotence. It increases penile blood flow by directly relaxing vascular smooth muscle. This is clearly contraindicated in priapism. The glans penis is an extension of the corpus spongiosum and is not usually affected by priapism. Shunts between it and the corpus cavernosa created with biopsy needles or scalpel blades or removal of a portion of the glandular corporal septum may provide a path of egress for blood trapped in the penis. If all else fails, formal spongiosum-to-cavernosum shunts may be created. There is a high incidence of impotence after priapism lasting 24 h or longer. When priapism is secondary to sickle cell anemia, exchange transfusions and other medical therapies, including oxygenation, hydration, and alkalinization, may be indicated.

Ref.: 10

10. Which of the following matches a layer of the scrotum with its corresponding fascial layer in the abdominal wall?

A. Cremasteric fascia—Internal oblique muscle

B. Tunica vaginalis—External oblique fascia

C. Dartos fascia—Transversalis fascia

D. External spermatic fascia—Scarpa's fascia

E. Internal spermatic fascia—Peritoneum

ANSWER: A

COMMENTS: As the testes descend in the fetus, the scrotal wall is formed from layers of the abdominal wall. Scarpa's fascia is continuous with the dartos fascia. The external oblique aponeurosis corresponds to the external spermatic fascia and is attached to the external inguinal ring. The internal oblique muscle gives rise to the cremasteric muscle and fascia. The transversalis fascia is continuous with the internal spermatic fascia. The transversus abdominis muscle terminates superior to the triangle of Hesselbach and therefore does not have a scrotal counterpart. The tunica vaginalis is a bilayered scrotal structure that is continuous with the peritoneum. They are connected by the processus vaginalis, which normally closes in infancy. Persistence of the processus vaginalis may result in a hydrocele.

Ref.: 11, 12

11. A 65-year-old woman with a history of hypertension, diabetes, and diverticulosis presents to the primary care physician with symptoms of a recurrent urinary tract infection with dysuria. She noted some bubbles in her urine with recent voids. Which of the following is true regarding this woman's symptoms?

A. Barium enema is the most sensitive imaging test for enterovesical fistula.

B. An oral charcoal test will localize an enterovesical fistula to the small bowel.

C. Pneumaturia is the most common initial sign/symptom of enterovesical fistula.

D. The diagnosis of an enterovesical fistula can be made 90% of the time with cystoscopy.

E. Inflammatory bowel disease is the most common cause of enterovesical fistula.

ANSWER: C

COMMENTS: Enterovesical fistulas are abnormal connections between the bowel and bladder. The sigmoid colon is the most common segment of involved bowel, and sigmoid diverticulitis accounts for 70% of cases. Other causes include Crohn's disease, malignancy, radiation injury, trauma, and iatrogenic injury. At presentation, patients have pneumaturia or air in the urine 50%–80% of the time and fecaluria or urinary tract infection 40% of the time.

CT of the abdomen and pelvis with oral contrast enhancement is the most sensitive imaging modality for detecting an enterovesical fistula. The classic triad of CT scan findings is a thickened bladder wall adjacent to a thickened loop of bowel, air in the bladder in the absence of instrumentation, and colonic diverticula. Barium enema has low sensitivity for the detection of fistulas; however, the first voided specimen after the test may be centrifuged and examined radiographically to increase its diagnostic yield. Oral charcoal administration and subsequent blackening of the urine will make the diagnosis of enterovesical fistula but will not provide anatomic localization. Cystoscopy will frequently reveal changes in the bladder mucosa, but a fistula tract is identified only approximately 35% of the time. A biopsy should be performed for any endoscopically identified fistula tract in the setting of previous malignancy to evaluate for a malignant fistula.

Ref.: 13

REFERENCES

1. McAninch J, Santucci R. Renal and ureteral trauma. In: Wein A, Kavoussi L, Novick A, et al., eds. *Campbell-Walsh Urology*. 9th ed. Philadelphia: WB Saunders; 2007.
2. Heyns C. Renal trauma: indications for imaging and surgical exploration. *BJU Int*. 2004;93(8):1165–1170.
3. Campbell S, Novick A, Bukowski R. Renal tumors. In: Wein A, Kavoussi L, Novick A, et al., eds. *Campbell-Walsh Urology*. 9th ed. Philadelphia: WB Saunders; 2007.
4. Pearle M, Lotan Y. Urinary lithiasis: etiology, epidemiology, and pathogenesis. In: Wein A, Kavoussi L, Novick A, et al., eds. *Campbell-Walsh Urology*. 9th ed. Philadelphia: WB Saunders; 2007.
5. Prezioso D, Strazzullo P, Lotti T, et al. Dietary treatment of urinary risk factors for renal stone formation. A review of CLU working group. *Arch Ital Urol Androl*. 2015;87(2):105–120.
6. Morey A, Rozanski T. Genital and lower urinary tract trauma. In: Wein A, Kavoussi L, Novick A, et al., eds. *Campbell-Walsh Urology*. 9th ed. Philadelphia: WB Saunders; 2007.
7. Olumi A, Richie J. Urologic surgery. In: Townsend C, Beauchamp R, Evers B, et al., eds. *Sabiston Textbook of Surgery: The Biological Basis of Modern Surgical Practice*. 18th ed. Philadelphia: WB Saunders; 2008.
8. Fitzpatrick J. Minimally invasive and endoscopic management of benign prostatic hyperplasia. In: Wein A, Kavoussi L, Novick A, et al., eds. *Campbell-Walsh Urology*. 9th ed. Philadelphia: WB Saunders; 2007.

9. Ho H, Yip S, Lim K, et al. A prospective randomized study comparing monopolar and bipolar transurethral resection of prostate using transurethral resection in saline (TURIS) system. *Eur Urol.* 2007;52(2):517–522.
10. Burnett A. Priapism. In: Wein A, Kavoussi L, Novick A, et al., eds. *Campbell-Walsh Urology*. 9th ed. Philadelphia: WB Saunders; 2007.
11. Brooks J. Anatomy of the lower urinary tract and male genitalia. In: Wein A, Kavoussi L, Novick A, et al., eds. *Campbell-Walsh Urology*. 9th ed. Philadelphia: WB Saunders; 2007.
12. Turnage R, Richardson K, Li B, et al. Abdominal wall, umbilicus, peritoneum, mesenteries, omentum, and retroperitoneum. In: Townsend C, Beauchamp R, Evers B, et al., eds. *Sabiston Textbook of Surgery: The Biological Basis of Modern Surgical Practice*. 18th ed. Philadelphia: WB Saunders; 2008.
13. Rovner E. Urinary tract fistula. In: Wein A, Kavoussi L, Novick A, et al., eds. *Campbell-Walsh Urology*. 9th ed. Philadelphia: WB Saunders; 2007.

CHAPTER 10

SURGICAL CRITICAL CARE

Brett Fair, M.D., and Christopher Knapp, M.D.

1. A 76-year-old man with hypertension, chronic renal insufficiency, and Child class A cirrhosis is admitted to the intensive care unit (ICU) after emergency exploratory laparotomy for ruptured appendicitis. His vital signs are a temperature of 97.3°F, heart rate (HR) of 129 beats/min, blood pressure (BP) of 220/90 mmHg, respiratory rate (RR) of 30 breaths/min, and oxygen saturation (Sao_2) of 90%. The patient is agitated and trying to pull his drains and nasogastric tube. He does not appear to respond to commands. Select the best choice to sedate this patient.

A. Lorazepam, 5 mg intravenously (IV)

B. Four-point restraints while trying to reason with the patient

C. Morphine delivered by patient-controlled anesthesia (PCA) with settings of 1 mg every 6 min and a 30-mg 4-h lockout

D. Diprivan and fentanyl drip

E. Placement of an epidural catheter for analgesia

ANSWER: D

COMMENTS: In the ICU, management of pain can be difficult and is often complicated by an inability to communicate with the patient and by the patient's physiologic instability, comorbid conditions, or delirium. Several methods have been developed to help assess sedation, including the Riker Sedation-Agitation Scale and the Ramsay Scale. This patient has both renal and hepatic dysfunction, which makes lorazepam an incorrect choice. It has a slow onset and intermediate half-life. In this situation, a faster-acting drug is preferable because the patient is obviously agitated. A Diprivan and fentanyl drip is the best answer because Diprivan is a general anesthetic agent with a rapid onset and ultrashort duration of action. Side effects of this medication include a risk for hypotension, high cost, pain on injection, and potential for hypertriglyceridemia. It has no analgesic effect and therefore additional medication is required to control the pain. Fentanyl is a better choice for analgesia because of the patient's renal failure and its rapid onset of action relative to morphine, which can take 5 to 10 min.

The use of four-point restraints without additionally sedating the patient is not a good option. Again, PCA is not a good option for a patient intubated and needing further sedation because of agitation. Moreover, morphine and its active metabolites (morphine-3-glucuronide and morphine-6-glucuronide) can accumulate in patients with renal insufficiency. Finally, placing an epidural catheter in an agitated patient would be difficult and dangerous to the patient and staff.

Ref.: 1–3

2. A 53-year-old man with coronary artery disease, Child class B alcoholic cirrhosis, and chronic renal insufficiency is admitted to the ICU after undergoing exploratory laparotomy and resection of necrotic small bowel from an incarcerated ventral hernia. He is septic and continues to require mechanical ventilation. Arterial blood gas analysis revealed a pH of 7.59, Pco_2 of 20 mmHg, Po_2 of 59 mmHg, HCO_3 of 21 mEq/L, base deficit of −2, and Sao_2 of 88%. The nurse calls because the ventilator alarms continue to go off. The patient is actually breathing at a rate of 43 breaths/min. After adequately sedating him, he is still dyssynchronous with the ventilator. Which paralytic agent is the most appropriate for this patient?

A. Pancuronium

B. Cisatracurium

C. Vecuronium

D. Succinylcholine

E. Rocuronium

ANSWER: B

COMMENTS: The best choice is cisatracurium, a nondepolarizing neuromuscular blocker and one of the most commonly used paralytics in the ICU. It, along with atracurium, is metabolized by plasma ester hydrolysis and Hofmann elimination and is therefore the best choice in this patient with both hepatic and renal dysfunction. Pancuronium is long acting but contraindicated in patients with coronary artery disease because it has a vagolytic effect and induces tachycardia. Vecuronium is intermediate acting (30 min) but is cleared by the kidney and liver. Succinylcholine is a short-acting depolarizing neuromuscular blocker, usually for facilitation of endotracheal intubation. Rocuronium has a rapid onset and intermediate duration thus making it a better choice for short procedures, as opposed to the needs of this patient, who must be sedated for a longer period.

Ref.: 1

3. Which of the following statements concerning radial artery cannulation is true?

A. Aortic systolic pressure is higher than radial systolic pressure.

B. The Allen test is an outdated mode of assessing the collateral flow of the ulnar and radial arteries.

C. The incidence of infection is higher with catheters placed by surgical cutdown.

D. The catheter should be replaced every 3 days.

E. Intermittent flushing to keep the catheter free of clots is desirable.

ANSWER: C

COMMENTS: The incidence of complications after arterial catheterization seems to be operator independent, unlike the case with pulmonary artery (PA) catheterization. Known risk factors include intermittent punctures, age younger than 10 years, prolonged catheterization (>4 days), anticoagulant therapy, and use of a catheter larger than 20 gauge or made of polypropylene rather than Teflon. The radial artery is the site most frequently used for catheterization, provided that the ulnar artery and palmar arterial arch are patent. Therefore the Allen test should be performed before attempting radial artery catheterization. A normal test result consists of a palmar blush within 7 s after the ulnar artery is released. Most patients with arterial thrombosis remain asymptomatic. Symptoms can be minimized by placing lines in arteries with good collateral circulation. Most thrombi (43%) are present at the time of catheter removal and another 30% develop within 24 h. A higher incidence of thrombosis occurs within the first 24 h when surgical cutdown is performed (48% vs. 23% with percutaneous placement), but the incidence of thrombosis at 1 week is the same for both methods of placement. Brachial artery cannulation has a high incidence of embolic occlusion of the distal arteries (5%–41%) and should therefore be avoided. Infection remains the most common complication. Predisposing factors are prolonged catheterization, surgical cutdown, local inflammation, preexisting bacteremia, and failure to change the saline flush fluid, transducer, and flush tubing every 48 h. The need for intermittent arterial catheter replacement is not established and indeed is controversial. The aortic mean arterial pressure (MAP) and diastolic arterial pressure are slightly higher than the radial MAP and diastolic arterial pressure. However, systolic pressure is consistently higher in the radial artery than in the aorta. This discrepancy increases with distal progression, smaller arterial caliber, and age and is explained by the reflection of pressure waves from capillary beds, which results in augmentation of the systolic and reduction of the diastolic values measured.

Ref.: 4

4. A 70-kg, 72-year-old man known to suffer from congestive heart failure (CHF), arthritis, diabetes mellitus, and a first-degree heart block is intubated in the ICU on postoperative day 2 after exploratory laparotomy for perforated sigmoid diverticulitis. His urine output has dropped to 10 mL/h for the last shift, and he is hypotensive despite several fluid boluses. A PA catheter is placed through the right internal jugular vein with some difficulty. As the line is advanced to 50 cm, the patient has a 14-beat run of ventricular tachycardia, which resolves when the catheter is pulled back. It is finally advanced to 62 cm, and the balloon is inflated with 3 cc of air. As the line is being secured, a large amount of blood is noted in the endotracheal tube and the patient becomes hypotensive. Select the best intervention for this patient:

A. Place external pacing wires and administer lidocaine to treat the ventricular tachycardia.

B. Place a double-lumen endotracheal tube and occlude the appropriate bronchus with a Fogarty catheter.

C. Pull the PA catheter back 2 cm with the balloon inflated.

D. Suction the endotracheal tube while deflating the balloon by 2 cc of air.

E. Obtain a chest radiograph to confirm the correct placement of the line.

ANSWER: B

COMMENTS: The indications for PA catheters and their value in patients with sepsis or hemodynamic instability are uncertain, but they may be useful in the management of patients unresponsive to the use of fluids and vasoactive agents. Dysrhythmias occur in 12%–67% of patients undergoing catheterization but are usually self-limited, premature ventricular contractions. Complete heart block can develop in patients with preexisting left bundle branch block. A prophylactic pacing wire should be used in these patients. Prophylactic lidocaine and full inflation of the balloon may prevent ventricular ectopy. Hemoptysis in patients with a PA catheter suggests the diagnosis of perforation or rupture. Mechanisms involved in PA rupture include (1) overinflation of the balloon, (2) incomplete balloon inflation (<75%) with the exposed tip being forced through the wall, and (3) pulmonary hypertension. An "overwedge" pattern suggests eccentric balloon inflation, overdistention, or both. If hemoptysis develops, the catheter should be pulled back, with the balloon deflated. Massive hemoptysis necessitates placement of a double-lumen endotracheal tube and occlusion of the bronchus on the side of the rupture with a Fogarty catheter. Emergency thoracotomy is needed. Looping or knotting of the catheter may occur in the right ventricle during insertion and can be avoided if no more than 10 cm of the catheter are inserted after a ventricular tracing is identified and before a PA tracing appears. Although catheter-related sepsis occurs in only up to 2% of insertions, bacterial colonization takes place in 5%–35% of catheterizations. Infections are more common when the catheter is left in place for more than 72 h or when it is inserted via an antecubital vein.

Ref.: 5, 6

5. A 51-year-old morbidly obese female who has a known history of symptomatic cholelithiasis is admitted to the ICU after presenting to the emergency department (ED) with severe epigastric pain. Her temperature is 100.5°F; HR, 115 beats/min; and BP, 123/84 mmHg. Her laboratory values are significant for a white blood cell (WBC) count of 15,000/mm^3 and a lipase of 1547. A computed tomography (CT) scan shows peripancreatic inflammation with a small fluid collection. What is the next best step in the management of this patient?

A. Central line placement for monitoring of central venous pressure (CVP)

B. Broad-spectrum antibiotics

C. Placement of an enteral feeding tube and initiation of tube feeding

D. Percutaneous drain placement

E. Cholecystectomy

ANSWER: C

COMMENTS: Acute pancreatitis may have a variable presentation dependent on both etiology and severity. If the patient is presenting with signs of shock and organ hypoperfusion, initial interventions must be targeted toward the improvement of oxygen delivery. Additionally, CT is helpful in determining if pancreatic necrosis with or without infection is present. Typically, infected pancreatic necrosis will present with air within the peripancreatic fluid collection, necessitating drainage or debridement. The role of prophylactic antibiotics in severe pancreatitis has been debated without consensus. A small number of randomized trials found benefit with fewer infectious complications when antibiotics are given prophylactically. However, this has not been widely reproducible. Cholecystectomy should be performed prior to the patient's discharge from the hospital, but not in the acute setting. Early enteral feeding, typically beyond the second portion of the duodenum, is preferable over parenteral nutrition and is associated with fewer infectious complications.

Ref.: 7

6. Of the following parameters, which is the best predictor of successful extubation?
   A. Increase in $Paco_2$ of less than 10 mmHg during a spontaneous breathing trial (SBT)
   B. Spontaneous tidal volume (Vt)
   C. 10-s head raise
   D. Rapid shallow breathing index (RSBI)
   E. Minute ventilation

ANSWER: D

COMMENTS: Many measures are utilized in order to determine the appropriateness for a trial of extubation. The RSBI is RR divided by Vt. A value of more than 105 predicts failure of extubation in over 95% of patients, while an RSBI less than 105 predicts success in over 80% of patients. Other factors can be useful in the decision to extubate; however, they are individually not as reliable as the RSBI. The importance of reliable and objective indicators for successful liberation from the ventilator is tied to the avoidance of complications such as ventilator-associated pneumonia (VAP), along with a decreased requirement for sedative medications.

Ref.: 8

7. A 44-year-old male heroin user is intubated in the surgical intensive care unit (SICU) after undergoing debridement of a lower extremity wound. His vital signs are a temperature of 102.3°F, HR of 134 beats/min, and BP of 80/40 mmHg with a MAP of 55 mmHg. A triple lumen catheter is placed, and CVP reads 12 mmHg. Norepinephrine is started, and despite being at the upper limit of the recommended dose, the MAP increases to 62 mmHg. What is the next best step?
   A. Fluid bolus
   B. Echocardiography
   C. Dobutamine
   D. Epinephrine
   E. Vasopressin

ANSWER: D

COMMENTS: This patient remains in septic shock postoperatively from debridement of an infected wound. We can presume the source to be the wound and therefore source control has been obtained. He should remain on broad-spectrum antibiotics and achieve certain parameters as directed by goal-directed therapy. He is intubated, which mandates a goal CVP of 10 to 12 mmHg. If he were extubated, a lower CVP of 8 to 10 mmHg would be appropriate, given the absence of positive pressure ventilation. This indicates he is volume resuscitated or has an adequate preload. If you are concerned about cardiac function, or need an indicator other than CVP to determine the volume status, echocardiography is indicated. However, this patient remains hypotensive despite norepinephrine, and something must be done in the interim. The first vasopressor used in septic shock should be norepinephrine. If a second vasopressor is required, it is now recommended that epinephrine be added to norepinephrine to achieve a MAP greater than 65 mmHg. Vasopressin may be added subsequently, but the dose should not exceed 0.03 units/min.

Ref.: 9

8. Which of the following is an indication to give calcium gluconate in a patient with hyperkalemia?
   A. Serum potassium of 6.2
   B. Electrocardiogram (ECG) changes consistent with hyperkalemia
   C. The patient does not have preexisting renal disease
   D. Both A and B
   E. All of the above

ANSWER: B

COMMENTS: While mild hyperkalemia is well tolerated, severe hyperkalemia results in a predictable progression of cardiac effects. Classically, peaked T waves are the first to appear on ECG, followed by a widened QRS complex, loss of P wave, appearance of "sine" waves, and eventually ventricular fibrillation. Emergent treatment of hyperkalemia focuses first on the antagonization of the depolarizing effect that a high level of potassium has on the cardiac membranes. Calcium should be administered (1) to any patient with a serum potassium level of 6.5 or greater or (2) to any patient with ECG changes consistent with hyperkalemia regardless of the potassium level. Other treatment of acute hyperkalemia includes redistribution of potassium to the intracellular space with insulin or β-agonists (albuterol). Ultimately, the elimination of excess potassium from the body is achieved by administering loop diuretics, sodium bicarbonate, Kayexalate, or hemodialysis.

Ref.: 10

9. You are asked to see a 24-year-old male with no medical problems who sustained a gunshot wound to the right thigh 1 h prior to arrival. He is afebrile with an HR of 136 beats/min and a BP of 90/60 mmHg. He is initially alert and asking for water but becomes confused during your brief interview. He is in which class of hemorrhagic shock?
   A. I
   B. II
   C. III
   D. IV
   E. More information is needed

ANSWER: C

COMMENTS: This patient presents with hemorrhagic shock with altered mental status, tachycardia, and hypotension. Driven to maintain adequate oxygen delivery, early changes in vital signs are representative of the body's attempt to preserve homeostasis after the rapid loss of a significant amount of its circulating volume. Early care is directed toward eliminating ongoing sources of exsanguination, along with restoration of intravascular volume. The degree of derangement is reliably linked to the volume of blood loss and classified according to the following table. This patient's constellation of findings places him within class III shock, and he has an estimated blood loss of 1.5 to 2 L. This estimate may help in guiding volume resuscitation to give an understanding of how much volume has been lost. The choice of fluid replacement has been the subject of much debate and investigation. Generally, for moderate-to-severe shock, resuscitation is carried out with a combination of both crystalloid and colloid solutions. In the acute setting, hemoglobin is an unreliable indicator; rather, therapy should be aimed at restoring adequate intravascular volume and normalized hemodynamics.

Classification of Hemorrhage

	Class			
Parameter	**I**	**II**	**III**	**IV**
Blood loss (mL)	<750	750–1500	1500–2000	>2000
Blood loss (%)	<15%	15–30%	30–40%	>40%
Pulse rate (beats/min)	<100	>100	>120	>140
Blood pressure	Normal	Decreased	Decreased	Decreased
Respiratory rate (breaths/min)	14–20	20–30	30–40	>35
Urine output (mL/hour)	>30	20–30	5–15	Negligible
CNS symptoms	Normal	Anxious	Confused	Lethargic

Ref.: 11

10. A 33-year-old unhelmeted male is brought to the ED after a motorcycle crash. His temperature is 99.4°F, HR is 95 beats/min, BP is 110/65 mmHg, and RR is 10 breaths/min with an Sao_2 of 94% on room air. He makes incomprehensible sounds, withdraws extremities, and opens eyes to painful stimuli. He is intubated in the ED and placed on the ventilator for transfer to the ICU. On head CT, he is found to have small subarachnoid hemorrhage and a nondepressed skull fracture. The remainder of his trauma workup is negative. In addition to head-of-bed elevation and frequent monitoring of neurologic status, which of the following is indicated?

A. IV mannitol bolus

B. Hypertonic saline infusion

C. Craniotomy

D. Hypothermia

E. Insertion of intracranial pressure (ICP) monitor at bedside

ANSWER: E

COMMENTS: Normal ICP ranges from 5 to 15 mmHg. Because of the bony calvarium, any increase in ICP results in an equivalent decrease in cerebral perfusion pressure (CPP), which is the difference between MAP and ICP. Goals for treatment of closed head injuries are to maintain adequate CPP through the use of various maneuvers to lower ICP.

This patient has suffered a severe head injury, as evidenced by his Glasgow coma score (GCS) of 8. He has an abnormal head CT with intracranial hemorrhage and has a significant risk (50%–60%) of elevations of ICP. For all patients with head injury, abnormal CT scan, and GCS less than 9, and ICP monitoring should be considered. One should also consider the placement of a monitor if the patient will be unable to be examined for a prolonged period [i.e., in the operating room (OR)]. There are conflicting data regarding the potential mortality benefit of ICP monitors; however, numerous data published since 2012 indicate improved outcomes when they are placed in these patients. Mannitol and hypertonic saline are indicated for the treatment of elevated ICP, indicated by invasive monitoring or a change in physical examination (unilateral blown pupil). Hypothermia was found in a recent study to have no benefit in patients with traumatic brain injury and elevated ICP.

Ref.: 12–14

11. When comparing early tracheostomy (<10 days after endotracheal intubation) versus late tracheostomy (>10 days after endotracheal intubation), which of the following is true?

A. Incidence of VAP is the same

B. Decreased mortality in those undergoing early tracheostomy at 28 days

C. Shorter ICU length of stay

D. No difference in sedation requirements

E. Improved patient satisfaction

ANSWER: C

COMMENTS: The timing of tracheostomy continues to be a debated topic in both the critical care and trauma literature. The general division between early and late tracheostomy creation is at 10 days after endotracheal intubation. For patients predicted to have prolonged ventilator requirements, the optimal timing of tracheostomy remains uncertain. Early trials suggested a mortality benefit; however, this result has not been reproduced in more recently published data. There does however seem to be a decrease in the incidence of VAP, along with decreased sedation requirements, more ventilator-free days, and shorter ICU length of stay. Trials with longer follow-up are still ongoing; however, there is some evidence that there may be a long-term mortality benefit for early tracheostomy, though more data are needed to establish this conclusion. While pulmonary hygiene and ease of care are improved with tracheostomy, there are no definitive data suggesting improved patient satisfaction with early versus late tracheostomy creation.

Ref.: 15–17

12. A 53-year-old woman with a history of metastatic lung cancer is admitted to the ICU after video-assisted resection of the right middle lobe. Initial vitals are an HR of 104 beats/min, BP of 64/43 mmHg, and RR of 34 breaths/min. After multiple fluid boluses, the patient remains hypotensive, so a PA catheter is placed and secured at 43 cm. The following values were determined: PA pressure, 38/27 mmHg; CVP, 26 mmHg; PA occlusion pressure (PAOP), 27 mmHg; and cardiac index, 2.0 L/min/m^2. Which of the following explains the clinical scenario?

A. CHF from sepsis

B. Malignant pleural effusion

C. Cardiac tamponade

D. Hypovolemia

E. Pneumothorax

ANSWER: C

COMMENTS: There are many potential causes of pericardial tamponade, with lung cancer, renal failure, tuberculosis, breast carcinoma, and lymphoma and leukemia being among the most common. Hemodynamic monitoring with a PA catheter can help determine the diagnosis by showing equalization of right ventricular diastolic pressure, a PA diastolic pressure, and a PAOP within 2 to 3 mmHg of each other, along with the elevated mean right atrial pressure. With small effusions most patients are asymptomatic, but with fluid in excess of 500 mL, patients can experience the onset of dyspnea, cough, chest pain, tachycardia, and jugular venous distention. Pulsus paradoxus, hypotension, cardiogenic shock, and paradoxical movement of the jugular venous pulse are also signs to be noted. This patient has pericardial tamponade and is unlikely to improve with medical management. Pericardial drainage is recommended in all patients with large effusions because of recurrence rates in the 40%–70% range. Administration of a fluid bolus is an appropriate measure but likely to be temporary. For immediate decompression, one can perform bedside pericardiocentesis. Definitive treatment of persistent symptomatic pericardial effusions is surgical pericardiectomy.

Ref.: 18

13. Which of the following treatments of a hypotensive patient is correct?

A. Pericardiocentesis in a 54-year-old man after myocardial infarction (MI) with adequate volume status and hypotension refractory to inotropic agents

B. Cardiac pacing in a 73-year-old woman taking digitalis with atrial fibrillation on the ECG, a ventricular response rate of 40, and an adequate volume status

C. Intraaortic balloon pump (IABP) in a 47-year-old woman with sepsis from pyelonephritis, good volume, and an echocardiogram showing no mechanical defects

D. Inotropic agents in a 68-year-old woman with metastatic breast cancer, distended neck veins, and PA catheter readings showing normalization of right and left heart pressure

E. Clamping of the infrarenal aorta in a patient with a gunshot wound to the chest and low right and left atrial pressure

ANSWER: B

COMMENTS: Cardiogenic shock most commonly occurs as a consequence of acute left ventricular infarction. However, it may also be due to right ventricular infarction, ruptured papillary muscle, ruptured ventricular wall, acute aortic valvular insufficiency, mitral regurgitation, and a ventricular septal defect. However, before assuming that the hypotension is caused by a cardiogenic mechanism, one must be sure that there is adequate blood volume. Therefore a patient who is hypotensive with low right and left atrial pressure should undergo fluid administration as the initial management. If cardiac performance improves with fluid administration alone, cardiogenic shock is probably not present. If adequate filling pressures are attained and the hypotension persists in the absence of mechanical defects, arrhythmia, and sepsis, a primary pump problem probably exists and should be managed with inotropic agents. One form of cardiogenic shock is cardiac tamponade, which is seen in traumatized patients, postoperative cardiac patients, and those suffering from uremia and certain malignancies. Pericardial tamponade has a trend toward equalization of pressures in the right and left sides of the heart. In a patient who is overdigitalized or hypokalemic, a very low ventricular rate in response to atrial fibrillation or flutter may result in hypotension and should be managed with cardiac pacing. If a patient remains in cardiogenic shock despite adequate blood volume, appropriate HR, absence of a mechanical or valvular defect, appropriate administration of inotropic agents, and restoration of pressure and coronary blood flow, support via IABP counterpulsation may be needed. IABP counterpulsation is most beneficial in patients with severe left ventricular dysfunction. It assists in left ventricular systolic unloading by directly reducing stroke work, which in turn reduces myocardial oxygen consumption during the cardiac cycle, and in diastolic augmentation, which raises arterial BP and provides better coronary arterial perfusion during diastole and improved delivery of oxygen to the myocardium. Patients with hemodynamic compromise secondary to right ventricular MI require fluid resuscitation and inotropic support. Any preload reducers must be avoided. Afterload reducers in the presence of hypotension are not warranted.

Ref.: 1

14. The alarm on the cardiac monitor continues to go off on a 73-year-old man with CHF and diabetes mellitus who was recently transferred to the ICU. He appears calm and is sitting up in bed watching a baseball game. His vital signs are an HR of 155 beats/min, BP of 125/84 mmHg, RR of 18 breaths/min, and Sao_2 of 96%. An ECG taken 7 days ago is normal. The most recent one, taken 24 h previously, shows that his previously distinct P waves have been replaced with rapid, polymorphic, irregular P waves that are irregular and occurring at a rate greater than 300/min. The ECG is repeated and confirms the presence of an arrhythmia. At this point, which is the best initial intervention for this patient?

A. Anticoagulation with a heparin drip

B. Cardioversion with paddles and settings at 260 J up to three times

C. Repeat ECG in 48 h

D. Restoration of sinus rhythm by pharmacologic means such as amiodarone or diltiazem

E. Morphine, 4 mg by IV push, to alleviate the pain

ANSWER: D

COMMENTS: The most common sustained dysrhythmia is atrial fibrillation, which has a prevalence of 5% in persons older than 65 years. There are numerous causes that may trigger new-onset atrial fibrillation, including ischemia, MI, hypertension, electrolyte imbalance, pulmonary embolism (PE), and digoxin toxicity. Initially, an ECG should be obtained, and if the arrhythmia is symptomatic, it should be treated aggressively. New-onset atrial fibrillation with a duration of less than 48 h is a clear indication to restore sinus rhythm by either electrical or pharmacologic means. This can be performed with IV calcium channel blockers, amiodarone, or β-blockers, which are usually effective in rapid conversion. Cardioversion should be performed in patients who are hemodynamically instable. Cardioversion in patients with atrial fibrillation for longer than 48 h is contraindicated until they are fully anticoagulated. Acute intervention may not be necessary in patients with a history of well-tolerated arrhythmia.

Ref.: 1, 19

15. A 58-year-old woman is found to have meningococcemia and sepsis. On examination, she is confused, agitated, and in respiratory distress. She is intubated and placed on assist-control (AC) ventilation. A central line is placed and several fluid boluses are given but she is still hemodynamically unstable. A continuous drip of a vasoactive drug is started. After administration, her HR remains at 105 beats/min, MAP rises to 70 from 45 mmHg, cardiac output (CO) drops to 2.8 from 3.3 L/min, and systemic vascular resistance increases to

1150 from 500 dynes·s/cm^5. Based on the changes observed, which drug was most likely administered?

A. Dobutamine

B. Dopamine

C. Phenylephrine

D. Epinephrine

E. Milrinone

ANSWER: C

COMMENTS: Inotropic agents increase cardiac contractility by increasing the concentration and availability of intracellular calcium. Catecholamines act by binding to adrenergic receptors. Each type of receptor controls a particular cardiovascular function (Table 10.1). Epinephrine, norepinephrine, dopamine, and dobutamine are all catecholamines. The α_1-receptor mediates arterial vasoconstriction by causing contraction of the vascular smooth muscle, and the α_2-receptor induces constriction of venous capacitance vessels. The β_1-receptor stimulates myocardial contractility, and the β_2-receptor causes relaxation of bronchial smooth muscle and relaxation of vascular smooth muscle in skeletal muscle beds. The dopamine receptors cause relaxation of the vascular smooth muscle. The dopamine-1 receptor induces relaxation of renal and splanchnic vascular smooth muscle, and the dopamine-2 receptor

TABLE 10.1 Hemodynamic Response Receptors

Drug	Dose (μg/kg/min)	HR	MAP	CO	SVR	α	β₁	β₂
Dopamine	5	↑	↑	↑			+	
	5–20	↑↑	↑↑	↑	↑↑	++	++	
Dobutamine	2–20	↑↑	↑	↑	↓		++	+
Epinephrine	0.01–0.1	↑↑	↑↑	↑	↑↑	++	++	+
Phenylephrine	10–100 (μg/min)		↑↑	↓	↑↑	++		
Norepinephrine	1–20 (μg/min)	↑	↑↑	↑	↑↑	++	+	
Milrinone	0.3–1.5			↑↑	↓			

CO, Cardiac output; *HR*, heart rate; *MAP*, mean arterial pressure; *SVR*, systemic vascular resistance.
↑, increase
↓, decrease
+, positive

inhibits the uptake of norepinephrine at the sympathetic nerve terminal, which results in a prolonged action of norepinephrine at the motor end plate. The effects of dopamine are unpredictable, and the side effects might be significant. Thus its use in the ICU has been ebbing. The response to catecholamines in normal individuals is different from that in critically ill patients. Receptor populations change over short periods, and upregulation and downregulation can occur depending on the disease state. It is important that catecholamines be administered for a predetermined effect. If the effect is not attained with the particular catecholamine chosen, the dose should be adjusted or another agent used.

Ref.: 1

16. You are consulted for a long-term enteral feeding access in a patient with a recent stroke. Despite speech therapy, he is unable to maintain adequate nutrition with by-mouth (PO) intake alone. Which of the following is an absolute contraindication to percutaneous endoscopic gastrostomy (PEG) placement?

A. Active infection

B. Hepatitis with large ascites

C. History of abdominal surgery

D. Peptic ulcer disease

E. Expected survival of less than 6 months

ANSWER: B

COMMENTS: Placement of a PEG tube is a viable and safe option for many critically ill patients or those who are unable to maintain adequate PO intake. There are few contraindications and complications when performed on a properly selected patient population. The technique of PEG placement relies on the principles of transillumination of the entry site with a lighted gastroscope and 1:1 palpation. These steps are critical to ensure the stomach and anterior abdominal wall are sufficiently opposed, and there are no other organs (i.e., transverse colon) that may be injured during tube insertion. Contraindications to PEG include irreversible coagulopathy, hemodynamic instability, oropharyngeal or esophageal mass unable to be passed by a gastroscope, a history of total gastrectomy, massive ascites, or portal hypertension with varices. There are reports of successful PEG placement with small-to-moderate ascites and the concurrent use of paracentesis; however, the complication rate in this population is much higher suggesting the risks of the procedure outweigh the benefits.

Ref.: 20

17. Which of the following conditions is not usually associated with elevated dead space ventilation?

A. 42-year-old female after MI with CHF and a CO of 1.5 L/min

B. 28-year-old woman on post partum [?] day 1 with shortness of breath, a Pa_{O_2} of 60 mmHg, and segmental clots bilaterally in the pulmonary arteries

C. 52-year-old Hispanic immigrant with a long-standing ventricular septal defect and PA pressure of 80/52 mmHg

D. 22-year-old man after multiple gunshot wounds, massive transfusions, and a mean arterial to inspired oxygen ratio (Pa_{O_2}/FiO_2) of 180

E. 62-year-old woman smoker with the following ventilator settings: controlled mandatory ventilation at a rate of 12 breaths/min, FiO_2 of 60%, Vt of 600 mL, and positive end-expiratory pressure (PEEP) of 5 cm H_2O

ANSWER: E

COMMENTS: The most common causes of increased dead space in critically ill patients are decreased CO, PE, pulmonary hypertension, acute respiratory distress syndrome (ARDS), and excessive PEEP, all of which directly cause decreased blood flow to the pulmonary vasculature. In dead space ventilation with a high ventilation/perfusion ($\dot{V}/\dot{Q}$) ratio, there is decreased blood flow to ventilated areas, which primarily affects the elimination of carbon dioxide. In ARDS, some areas of the lung are perfused but not ventilated. Alveoli may be filled with secretions, exudate, blood, or edema, thereby increasing the shunt fraction. Other areas of the lung may be ventilated but not perfused, which accounts for the dead space ventilation. PEEP can cause dead space ventilation by decreasing CO and stenting alveoli open, which causes the surrounding capillaries to collapse and thereby decreases alveolar perfusion. Carbon dioxide production and the dead space–tidal volume ratio (Vds/Vt) determine minute ventilation. The anatomic dead space includes the volume of the airways to the level of the bronchiole (150 mL). Dead space can also include alveoli that are well ventilated but poorly perfused. When combined, the anatomic and alveolar dead space constitutes the physiologic dead space, which is essentially the volume of gas moved during each tidal breath that does not participate in gas exchange.

Ref.: 19, 21

18. A 17-year-old female with asthma is brought to the OR for ruptured ectopic pregnancy. Postoperatively, she is dyspneic and in acute respiratory failure. She is intubated and transferred to the surgical ICU where her ventilator is set to AC mode, RR of 18 breaths/min, FiO_2 of 0.80, Vt of 600 mL, and PEEP of 0 mmHg. She was sedated and paralyzed for the intubation and is not breathing over the ventilator settings. After examining the patient and the flow pattern on the ventilator, changes in the settings are made. A change in which ventilator setting would best limit the intrinsic PEEP?

A. Increase in Vt

B. Decrease in the inspiratory flow rate

C. Increase in PEEP

D. Decrease in RR

E. Change from AC mode to synchronized intermittent mandatory ventilation (SIMV)

ANSWER: D

COMMENTS: Intrinsic PEEP (commonly known as auto-PEEP) is a state at end exhalation in which there is incomplete gas emptying, which can elevate alveolar volume and pressure. It is the threshold pressure needed to be overcome to initiate inspiratory flow. Severe bronchospasm increases the expiratory time needed, and patients in status asthmaticus or severe chronic obstructive pulmonary disease (COPD) are at risk for intrinsic PEEP. If combined with narrowed airways, such as in asthma, and parenchymal noncompliance, the inspiratory work of breathing is increased. Therefore there is an imbalance of respiratory muscle strength and work of breathing leading to respiratory failure.

During mechanical ventilation, when the expiratory time is insufficient to allow full exhalation of a ventilator breath, expiratory flow is still occurring when the next ventilator breath is delivered. To best limit intrinsic PEEP, one can decrease the RR, thereby giving the patient more time to exhale between breaths. In addition, decreasing Vt will allow minimal improvement. One should also limit the inspiratory time to leave more time in the respiratory cycle for exhalation. Avoidance of hyperinflation and overdistention at the expense of minute ventilation, otherwise known as permissive hypercapnia, is an important method of ventilatory management in asthmatics.

Ref.: 22, 23

19. A 65-year-old male who is 7 days out from a three-vessel coronary artery bypass remains intubated for respiratory failure despite normal hemodynamics. He is sedated with propofol and failed an SBT earlier this morning. The nurse asks if you would like to hold his sedation. Which of the following is true with regard to daily sedation awakening trials (SATs)?

A. The risk of self-extubation is too high to justify SAT after failed SBT.

B. SAT performed daily decreases overall sedation requirements for ventilated patients.

C. SAT alone is associated with lower rates of delirium.

D. Daily paired SAT and SBT are associated with fewer ventilator days and decreased ICU length of stay.

E. When part of an ICU protocol, daily SAT is associated with decreased overall mortality.

ANSWER: D

COMMENTS: The concept of daily interruption in sedation has been widely adopted by ICUs despite little convincing evidence of its independent efficacy. A number of studies have demonstrated improved time-to-extubation with combined SAT and SBT versus SBT alone. However, SAT has been shown to be equivalent to no SAT in many more recent trials. In these studies, there was no decrease in time-to-extubation, sedation requirement, and ICU stay or mortality. In line with no change in sedation requirements, there also has been no proven improvement in the incidence of ICU delirium with routine SAT. SAT can be associated with adverse events such as patient removal of the endotracheal tube or other lines; however, when performed in an appropriate setting, there was also no significant increase in these adverse events.

Ref.: 24–26

20. With regard to ventilatory mechanics, which of the following statements is true?

A. The work of breathing at rest consumes 10% of total-body oxygen consumption (Vo_2).

B. COPD is associated with an increase in the work of breathing as a result of increased expiratory work.

C. The work of breathing may increase to 75% of the total-body Vo_2 in postoperative patients.

D. Airway pressure reflects the compliance of only the lungs.

E. Compliance is measured as the change in pressure divided by the change in volume.

ANSWER: B

COMMENTS: For patients with COPD, the work of breathing is increased because of increased expiratory work, not inspiratory work. It can be assessed by preoperative pulmonary function testing and optimized by preoperative chest physical therapy, bronchodilators, and antibiotics if infection is present. The work of breathing at rest consumes 2% of the total-body Vo_2 and can be markedly increased, up to 50% of total Vo_2, in postoperative patients because of increased airway resistance and decreased compliance of the lung, chest wall, and diaphragm. The proper use of volume-cycled ventilators and pressure support (PS) ventilation can take over most of the work of breathing during the postoperative period. Compliance is defined as the change in pressure associated with each milliliter increase in the lung volume. Measuring airway pressure reflects the compliance of the chest wall and diaphragm, as well as that of the lungs. In relaxed patients this is of little importance, but in restless patients, intraesophageal or intrapleural pressure provides a more accurate measure of compliance. In acute respiratory failure, decreased compliance is usually associated with decreased functional residual capacity. Less compliant lungs need ventilatory management that maintains inflation of alveoli by the use of PEEP and recruits closed alveoli by elevating peak inspiratory pressure. However, because positive airway pressure may overdistend already-ventilated alveoli, the peak inspiratory pressure should be kept below 40 cm H_2O.

Ref.: 27, 28

21. A 53-year-old man with chronic kidney disease, severe COPD, and systolic heart failure after MI is in your ICU. He is unable to tolerate the Trendelenburg position during the placement of a central line in the right internal jugular vein. Immediately after placement, he becomes diaphoretic and complains of difficulty in breathing. He then becomes obtunded, tachycardic, and progressively tachypneic. His BP is 80/50 mmHg, and he has bilateral breath sounds by auscultation. Which of the following should be performed immediately?

A. Left lateral decubitus and Trendelenburg position, then aspiration from the central line

B. Heparinization

C. Removal of the central line

D. Fluid bolus

E. Dobutamine

ANSWER: A

COMMENTS: Though uncommon, air embolism is a potentially lethal complication of the central line placement. Providers must be familiar with its presentation and immediate, lifesaving treatment maneuvers. Presentation depends upon the exact volume of air that enters the venous system. The lethal dose for humans has been estimated at 3 to 5 mL/kg/min; however, cardiovascular compromise can be seen with rates less than 1.5 mL/kg per min. The incidence of air embolism with central line placement is reported as between 0.2% and 1%. Physical examination for a significant air embolism will demonstrate hemodynamic instability and, often, hypoxia, along with a "mill-wheel" murmur in the precordium. Immediate intervention is Durant's maneuver—left lateral decubitus and Trendelenburg position in order to entrap air in the apex of the ventricle. Aspiration via central venous catheter may then allow removal of some amount of the air in the system.

Ref.: 29

22. A family meeting is called for a 69-year-old man who was intubated 6 days earlier for pneumonia and respiratory distress. He is now awake, alert, and asking for removal of the tube. His family wants to know when and whether he will be extubated. Which of the following characteristics of this patient meets conventional weaning criteria?

A. Negative inspiratory force of −10 cm H_2O

B. A respiratory frequency/tidal volume (RF/Vt) ratio of 105 or less

C. Correction of underlying pulmonary and nonpulmonary complications

D. Pulse oximetry reading of 92%

E. Vital capacity of 12 to 15 mL/kg and peak inspiratory pressure of less than 25 cm H_2O

ANSWER: A

COMMENTS: Many indices have been proposed to predict weaning outcome and success or failure of extubation. Most surgical patients (90%) are weaned from mechanical ventilation in less than 1 week. Conventional weaning criteria include (1) measurements of oxygenation with a pulse oximeter (best determined by arterial blood gas analysis, with an $Sao_2 > 90\%$ and any FiO_2 usually being adequate for weaning) and (2) measurements of ventilation, such as an RR less than 24 breaths/min, $Paco_2$ less than 50 mmHg, peak inspiratory pressure below 30 cm H_2O, Vt of at least 5 to 8 mL/kg, and a vital capacity double the Vt value. Failure to satisfy these conventional criteria is associated with unsuccessful weaning in as many as 63% of patients. The rapid, shallow breathing test (RF/Vt) is performed by having the patient breathe room air for 1 min. When RF/Vt is 105 or less, successful weaning occurs in 78% of patients, and when RF/Vt is less than 80, the success rate is 95%. Conversely, an RF/Vt value of 105 or higher is accompanied by a failure rate of 95%. Another method often described is the Simple Object Access Protocol (SOAP) assessment: (1) ability to clear secretions, (2) adequate oxygenation (Pao_2/FiO_2 ratio > 200 mmHg, which requires an FiO_2 of 0.4 to 0.5 and PEEP < 8 cm H_2O), (3) ability to protect the airway, and (4) adequate pulmonary function. Clinical judgment and correction of underlying pulmonary and nonpulmonary complications continue to be the best guide to successful weaning. In addition, helpful ventilation scores include an FiO_2 of less than 40%, continuous positive airway pressure (CPAP) of 3 cm H_2O, effective static compliance greater than 50 mL/cm H_2O, dynamic compliance greater than 40 mL/cm H_2O, ventilator minute ventilation of less than 10 L/min, and a triggered ventilatory rate of less than 20 breaths/min. The duration of ventilatory support is not correlated with survival rates at discharge. Forty-one percent of long-term ventilated patients survive. Because muscle atrophy is often present, a progressive ventilatory withdrawal plan designed to restore muscle function should be used. Intermittent mandatory ventilation, PS ventilation, and weaning by T-piece have been used effectively.

Ref.: 30

23. A 29-year-old firefighter is intubated in the ICU after being exposed to smoke. She has thick yellow secretions that require frequent suctioning along with the administration of bronchodilators. On hospital day 5, she has a percutaneous central venous catheter placed through the right internal jugular vein. Several hours later, she undergoes respiratory arrest. Her peak inspiratory pressure has risen from 24 to 41 cm H_2O, and her plateau pressure has stayed at 16 cm H_2O. Choose which of the following is the most likely reason for the respiratory arrest:

A. Tension pneumothorax

B. Flash pulmonary edema

C. Pulmonary embolism (PE)

D. Endotracheal tube obstruction

E. Auto-PEEP with breath stacking

ANSWER: D

COMMENTS: This patient has an obstruction of the endotracheal tube. The key to identifying this problem is recognizing the components of the patient's respiratory pressure as shown in Table 10.2, most importantly the peak inspiratory and plateau pressures. The peak inspiratory pressure is the pressure required to overcome the resistance in the endotracheal tube and airways, as well as the compliance of the airways. The inspiratory plateau pressure is the pressure generated to overcome the elastance of the lung parenchyma, pleural space, and chest wall. This patient had increasing peak inspiratory pressure, so her problem was related to the tube, not the lung itself. Tension pneumothorax and flash pulmonary edema are associated with increases in both peak inspiratory pressure and inspiratory plateau pressure. PE also does not change the inspiratory pressure.

Ref.: 28

24. A 73-year-old woman weighing 60 kg is admitted to the hospital with acute pancreatitis. She is aggressively resuscitated with fluid but becomes hypotensive and has increasing work of breathing and O_2 requirements within the next 12 h. The patient is transferred to the ICU and intubated. A PA catheter is placed, and the wedge pressure is 8 cm H_2O. Arterial blood gas analysis shows values of a pH of 7.36, a Pao_2 of 62, a Pco_2 of 42, a serum bicarbonate of 21, and a base deficit of −2 with Sao_2 of 90%. Which of the following ventilation strategies is most appropriate for this patient?

A. Pressure-control ventilation (PCV) with a pressure of 40 cm H_2O and an inverse ratio ventilation of 3:1

B. SIMV with a Vt of 720 mL and an RR set to keep the pH at 7.4

C. AC ventilation with a Vt of 600 mL and prone positioning

D. AC ventilation with a Vt of 360 mL and an RR to keep the pH above 7.2

E. SIMV with a Vt of 600 and an FiO_2 of 100%

ANSWER: D

COMMENTS: See Question 25.

TABLE 10.2 Patient's Respiratory Pressures

	Day 1	Day 2	Day 3	Day 4	Day 5
FiO_2	0.6	0.6	0.55	0.5	0.5
PEEP	10	10	8	5	5
PIP	25	23	24	32	41
Plateau pressure	17	18	18	17	16
RR	20	19	23	24	27
O_2 Sat	91	89	94	95	93

FiO_2, Fractional concentration of oxygen in inspired gas; *O_2 Sat*, O_2 saturation; *PEEP*, positive end-expiratory pressure; *PIP*, peak inspiratory pressure; *RR*, respiratory rate.

Ref.: 31–33

25. Which one of the following criteria **is** included in the definition of ARDS?

A. Onset within 1 week of a clinical insult

B. Chest radiograph showing pulmonary infiltrate (unilateral or bilateral)

C. Hypoxemia with Pao_2 to FiO_2 ratio < 200 mmHg

D. Normal PA wedge pressure

E. Infectious origin

ANSWER: A

COMMENTS: Because the principal physiologic problem in ARDS is hypoxemia refractory to increasing FiO_2, therapy is centered on the provision of mechanical ventilation to maximize oxygen delivery while minimizing lung injury. PEEP is used to improve oxygenation and lung compliance and should be optimized with the help of pressure–volume curves to facilitate the maintenance of open alveoli and diffusion of oxygen into the pulmonary capillaries. For a given FiO_2, Pao_2 usually increases on the administration of PEEP in patients with ARDS. However, excessive PEEP (>15 cm H_2O) can be hazardous and lead to pneumothorax from barotrauma and decreased venous return to the heart. Overdistention of alveoli can be prevented by keeping the peak inspiratory pressure below 35 cm H_2O. Newer ventilatory methods attempt to enhance alveolar recruitment, maintain alveolar patency throughout the respiratory cycle, maintain an Sao_2 of greater than 90%, avoid dynamic hyperinflation (volutrauma), and reduce the risk for oxygen toxicity. Spontaneous, augmented low-volume ventilation, with PS ventilation being used as a primary ventilatory support mode, directs flow to regions of low ventilation/perfusion. Diuretics in cases of obvious fluid overload and cardiac decompensation and broad-spectrum antibiotics in cases of established pulmonary infection or other sources of sepsis may be useful for patients with ARDS. The consensus conference on ARDS (ARDSnet.org) showed that a volume-restricted ventilation strategy reduced mortality. In this well-accepted study, 861 patients were randomly assigned to either a traditional-volume ventilation strategy (12 mL/kg of ideal body weight with plateau pressures < 50 cm H_2O) or low-Vt ventilation (6 mL/kg with plateau pressures < 30 cm H_2O). The study was halted early because of significantly reduced overall mortality (31.0% vs. 39.1%, P < .0007). Permissive hypercapnia was allowed, and sodium bicarbonate was given to maintain pH higher than 7.2.

The patient developed ARDS, probably because of acute pancreatitis and systemic inflammatory response syndrome (SIRS). Criteria used to define ARDS have been recently revised. The Berlin definition developed in 2013 now stratifies ARDS based upon the degree of hypoxemia. All types of ARDS include an acute onset within 1 week of clinical insult, bilateral pulmonary infiltrates on chest radiographs, and some degree of hypoxemia not fully explained by cardiac failure. There does not have to be an infectious process for a patient to have ARDS, and no longer are patients with cardiac failure excluded from having coexisting ARDS. ARDS and acute lung injury have now been combined and categorized based on the severity of the Pao_2/FiO_2 ratio: mild (200 to 300), moderate (100 to 200), and severe (<100). The lung response can be divided into an exudative phase (24 to 96 h), with leakage of proteinaceous fluid into the pulmonary interstitium and corresponding damage to the alveolar–capillary interface; an early proliferative phase (3 to 10 days), with proliferation of alveolar type II cells, cellular infiltration of the septum, and organization of hyaline membranes; and a late proliferative phase (7 to 10 days), with fibrosis of the alveolar septum, ducts, and hyaline membranes. Frequently, the radiographic changes can lag behind the clinical picture in ARDS considerably.

Ref.: 34

26. A 59-year-old woman with a long-standing history of gastroesophageal reflux disease (GERD) underwent a Nissen fundoplication that was complicated by 2 L of blood loss and hypotension in the OR. Her vital signs are an HR of 103 beats/min, a BP of 100/70 mmHg, an RR of 16 breaths/min, and an Sao_2 of 96%. Her urine output was 15 mL of urine/h over the last 4 h. Laboratory results include a urine osmolality of 600 mOsm/kg, urine sodium concentration of 15 mEq/L, plasma sodium concentration of 140 mEq/L, urine creatinine concentration of 20 mg/dL, and plasma creatinine concentration of 1.5 mg/dL. What is the next step in management?

A. Flushing the Foley catheter with 60 mL of normal saline

B. Hemodialysis

C. Nephrology consultation

D. Decompressive laparotomy for abdominal compartment syndrome (ACS)

E. Administration of a 1000-mL fluid bolus of normal saline as a fluid challenge

ANSWER: E

COMMENTS: Acute renal failure is a serious morbidity for postsurgical patients, with mortality rates greater than 50%. Renal failure can be prerenal, renal, or postrenal. The most common cause in surgical patients is hypovolemia, as is the case in this patient from blood loss in the OR. Some indicators for prerenal causes include urine osmolality greater than 500 mOsm/kg, fractional excretion of sodium (FE_{Na}) of less than 1%, and urine sodium concentration of less than 20 mEq/L, whereas an FE_{Na} greater than 3% and urinary sodium concentration greater than 40 mEq/L are indicative of parenchymal or postrenal causes. Medications, IV contrast material–induced nephropathy, rhabdomyolysis, and transfusion reactions are all options to consider. This patient's FE_{Na} is 0.8%.

Ref.: 35, 36

27. A 46-year-old brittle diabetic and hypertensive woman is brought to the ICU after being found unresponsive in her bed. After undergoing a CT scan of her head, abdomen, and pelvis with IV contrast media, she is transferred to the ICU. The ICU team places a central line, orders an echocardiogram, and places a bladder catheter. Her urine output has been approximately 10 mL/h for the last 4 h. Her FE_{Na} is calculated to be 2.4%. Which of the following is not consistent with acute tubular necrosis (ATN)?

A. Oliguria

B. FE_{Na} greater than 2%

C. Urine osmolality of 200 mOsm/kg

D. Creatinine clearance greater than 125 mL/min

E. Sodium wasting

ANSWER: D

COMMENTS: A creatinine clearance of 125 mL/min represents a normal renal function. ATN is characterized by a rise in plasma creatinine concentration [decrease in creatinine clearance or glomerular filtration rate (GFR)], a urine volume that is reduced (oliguric) or normal, changes in the findings on urinalysis, and a FE_{Na} greater than 1%–2%. Oliguria, or urine output less than 500 mL/24 h, is a frequent but not an absolute feature of ATN. Whether oliguria occurs may depend on the severity of the renal injury or the relative reabsorption of filtrate at the tubular level. Even if a patient's GFR falls to 10 L/day (normal, 180 L/day), a urine output of 1 to 2 L/day would still be normal as long as 8 to 9 L of filtrate was reabsorbed. In cases of well-preserved tubular function, as in prerenal forms of acute kidney injury (ARF), FE_{Na} is low, consistent with the sodium-avid state. As tubular dysfunction progresses, the ability of nephrons to reabsorb sodium is disrupted, and a greater percentage of the filtered sodium is excreted in urine. As a result, FE_{Na} will be greater than 1%–2% because of inappropriate sodium wasting by altered tubular function. Loss of urinary concentrating ability is an early feature of ATN. A urine osmolality of less than 350 mOsm/L is consistent with ATN, whereas an osmolality greater than 500 mOsm/L suggests a prerenal cause of ARF. However, lower values can be seen during prerenal ARF thus limiting the value of this test as a sole indicator of tubular function.

Ref.: 35, 36

28. A 62-year-old man with peripheral vascular disease, diabetes, and bilateral tissue loss in the lower extremities is admitted for angiography of his lower extremities. He has chronic renal failure and his serum creatinine level is 5.0 mg/dL, which has been his baseline for the last 3 years. Which of the following agents is indicated to reduce the risk for IV contrast–induced nephropathy?

A. Calcium channel blocker

B. Aggressive diuresis

C. Saline volume expansion before and after the procedure

D. Acetylcysteine given only after exposure to contrast material

E. Mannitol and saline hydration

ANSWER: C

COMMENTS: In most cases, radiocontrast agents can lead to a reversible form of ARF. The pathogenesis is not well established, but two proposed mechanisms of injury are renal vasoconstriction and direct tubular toxic effects. The risk is minimal in patients with normal renal function, including those with diabetes, and the renal failure is nonoliguric and transient in most cases. Severe renal failure requiring short- or long-term dialysis is rare and most likely to occur in patients whose baseline creatinine level is greater than 4 mg/dL. Risk factors for the development of contrast-induced nephropathy include underlying chronic renal failure with a plasma creatinine level greater than 1.5 mg/dL, diabetic nephropathy with renal insufficiency, CHF, multiple myeloma, and a large volume of contrast material. Saline volume expansion in the precontrast and postcontrast periods is the only preventive measure consistently shown to be of benefit. Hydration with furosemide may increase the risk for contrast-induced nephropathy when compared with saline alone. Furthermore, the use of saline solution and mannitol does not have any benefit over the use of saline alone. Calcium channel blockers given to minimize renal vasoconstriction after exposure to contrast media have not been conclusively shown to prevent renal failure. The role of nonionic contrast agents is not clearly defined. Studies seem to support the use of isosmolar nonionic agents in high-risk patients, especially those with diabetes. There are conflicting data on the role of acetylcysteine and sodium bicarbonate infusions in the prevention of contrast-induced nephropathy, but given its relatively safe side-effect profile and the few series supporting its use, use of both can be justified, particularly in high-risk patients. A rational approach to preventing contrast-induced nephropathy in high-risk patients, such as the patient in question, would include acetylcysteine (600 mg orally twice daily the day before and on the day of exposure to contrast material), saline volume expansion before and after the procedure, and an isosmolar nonionic contrast agent. Several recent meta-analyses have shown that sodium bicarbonate infusion can decrease the damage associated with contrast-induced nephropathy if given both before and after the procedure as well. The former may be more important for patients with renal dysfunction and diabetes.

Ref.: 35, 37

29. Choose the situation that does not require immediate renal replacement therapy.

A. A 27-year-old bipolar patient, after running a half marathon, taking a prescribed lithium dose and found to have ataxia, confusion, and inverted T waves

B. A 68-year-old man after sigmoid colectomy with new-onset seizures and blood urea nitrogen (BUN) of 150 mg/dL

C. A 58-year-old man after a motor vehicle collision with multiple long-bone fractures, BUN of 120 mg/dL, creatinine of 2.8 mg/dL, and diffuse bleeding

D. A 71-year-old woman with diabetes maintained on an insulin drip after total abdominal hysterectomy and bilateral salpingo-oophorectomy with an FE_{Na} of 0.7% and urine output less than 20 mL/h for last 7 h

E. A 45-year-old man with respiratory distress after massive resuscitation for a septic episode, bilateral lung haziness on chest radiography, and coarse crackles who is unresponsive to diuretics

ANSWER: D

COMMENTS: Indications for acute dialysis treatment include (1) persistent hyperkalemia refractory to medical management; (2) pulmonary edema unresponsive to conventional therapy; (3) severe acidemia; (4) symptoms of uremia such as anorexia, nausea, and vomiting; (5) uremic encephalopathy, seizures, asterixis, uremic pericarditis, and uremic bleeding; and (6) overdose with a dialyzable toxin such as lithium or ethylene glycol. Renal replacement therapy is needed in 1%–2% of patients with ARF, and as many as 15% of patients may ultimately require dialysis at some point in their life. It may be indicated for symptomatic fluid overload, sepsis, uremic complications, and severe electrolyte or acid-base disorders. Frequently in the ICU, continuous renal replacement therapy is superior to intermittent hemodialysis or peritoneal dialysis, but in the United States, it is only used in 10%–20% of ICU patients. Proponents of this method over others argue that it allows better hemodynamic stability and prevention of shifts in intracerebral water, minimizes the risk for infection, and provides continuous control of fluid status and acid-base abnormalities. Complications include the need for anticoagulation and a high level of nursing care.

Ref.: 1, 38–40

30. A 68-year-old woman with a history of GERD, cholelithiasis, and coronary artery disease is seen in the ED with nausea, vomiting, and epigastric pain. Laboratory tests showed amylase and lipase values of 259 and 1782 units/L, leukocytosis of 18,300/mm^3, and a prothrombin time (PT) and international normalized ratio (INR) of 47 s and 1.9, respectively. The patient received 6 L of crystalloid solution because of hypotension and required intubation. After 48 h, the hemoglobin has dropped by 2 g. What are the factors that have the strongest correlation with stress-related bleeding in critically ill patients?

A. Mechanical ventilation and hypotension

B. Coagulopathy and renal failure

C. Steroids and sepsis

D. Mechanical ventilation and steroids

E. Mechanical ventilation and coagulopathy

ANSWER: E

COMMENTS: Risk factors for stress-related mucosal lesions are mechanical ventilation longer than 48 h, coagulopathy, significant burns, and head injury. These lesions have been found in 25%–100% of ICU patients within 48 h of admission, but clinically significant bleeding occurs in only 5%–10%. Patients with risk factors should receive prophylaxis until consuming an enteral diet of at least 50% of their caloric intake.

Ref.: 1, 41

31. You are caring for a 55-year-old male who is in the ICU 5 days after multiple blunt traumatic injuries. He was intubated in the OR for the repair of a femur fracture on hospital day 1 and has not yet been extubated. He continues to fail his SBT with RSBI higher than 105. What is the most effective strategy to liberate this patient from the ventilator?

A. PS wean

B. AC ventilation with daily SBT

C. SIMV wean

D. Early tracheostomy before day 10

E. PCV with daily SBT

ANSWER: A

COMMENTS: The most efficient strategy to wean patients from the ventilator has been studied many times and remains somewhat controversial. It is clear that the most effective way to identify those patients who are ready to have a trial of extubation is the daily SBT. However, those who have failed repeated SBTs may require a more targeted and purposeful weaning technique in order to avoid the complications associated with the long-term mechanical ventilation in the ICU setting. Early tracheostomy, when compared to late tracheostomy, does improve ICU length of stay and number of ventilator days; however, it has not shown direct benefit over other modes of weaning mechanical ventilation and will lead to a higher rate of tracheostomy. When compared directly, SIMV weaning is not as effective as PS weaning, and there is some evidence that PS weaning improves diaphragmatic dysfunction over both AC and pressure-control modes. Regardless of strategy, daily SBT and reassessment of readiness for extubation remain appropriate.

Ref.: 42, 43

32. A 37-year-old woman comes to the ED complaining of a severe headache. She undergoes an emergency head CT scan, which shows subarachnoid hemorrhage; an angiogram identifies an arteriovenous malformation, which is subsequently embolized. Four days later, her serum sodium concentration is 122 mEq/L. Which is the most correct statement regarding the syndrome of inappropriate secretion of antidiuretic hormone (SIADH) and cerebral salt wasting (CSW)?

A. SIADH and CSW share the same underlying pathophysiology and cannot be reliably distinguished.

B. SIADH and CSW can be differentiated by measuring urine sodium and serum uric acid concentrations.

C. SIADH and CSW can be differentiated by measuring urine osmolality and sodium concentration.

D. Assessment of extracellular fluid volume will best differentiate between SIADH and CSW.

E. Regardless of the diagnosis, treatment of the hyponatremia is the same.

ANSWER: D

COMMENTS: Hyponatremia is common in the setting of central nervous system disease. Most often it results from inappropriate SIADH. With SIADH, the hyponatremia initially results from ADH-induced water retention. This volume expansion activates natriuretic mechanisms that induce the loss of sodium and water, with the patient typically being restored to a nearly euvolemic state. With chronic SIADH, the loss of sodium (and often potassium) is much more significant than the water retention. CSW is characterized by hyponatremia and loss of extracellular volume from inappropriate sodium wasting in urine. Patients with CSW meet the laboratory criteria for SIADH: hyponatremia, elevated urine osmolality (>100 mOsm/kg), elevated urine sodium concentration (>40 mEq/L), and low serum uric acid concentration. However, they also have clinical evidence of hypovolemia (decreased skin turgor, elevated hematocrit, decreased weight, and hypotension) rather than the nearly euvolemic state seen with SIADH. Furthermore, volume repletion with isotonic saline in patients with CSW will lead to a dilute urine (and eventual correction of the hyponatremia), whereas isotonic saline administration may worsen the hyponatremia of SIADH because the sodium is retained while the water is excreted. SIADH is usually treated by fluid restriction; however, this must be done with caution in patients with SIADH because of the risk of hypotension and cerebral infarction. Isotonic saline may be used but requires careful monitoring of the serum sodium concentration; if a further fall in serum sodium occurs, a switch to hypertonic saline may be necessary. CSW generally responds well to volume repletion with isotonic saline. Salt tablets and mineralocorticoids (such as fludrocortisones) may also be useful as adjunctive measures.

Ref.: 44, 45

33. A patient is admitted to the surgical ICU after a prolonged laparoscopic cholecystectomy, which required conversion to an open procedure. The patient was reintubated for respiratory distress in the recovery area. Upon arrival to the unit, you obtain an arterial blood gas: pH 7.46, $Paco_2$ 23, and Pao_2 85. Which of the following is true?

A. The primary problem is metabolic with respiratory compensation.

B. No changes should be made to the ventilation as the kidneys will compensate for this abnormality.

C. This acid-base disturbance is consistent with septic shock.

D. Minute ventilation should be decreased.

E. PEEP should be increased.

ANSWER: D

COMMENTS: Arterial blood gas is commonly used to adjust ventilation parameters in order to optimize a patient's respiratory function and maintain homeostasis. This patient has a respiratory alkalosis with low $Paco_2$ contributing to increased pH. Pao_2 is in the normal range and will maintain saturation of hemoglobin with oxygen. Adding PEEP will increase the Pao_2 and is unnecessary for this patient. Decreasing the minute ventilation, however, either by changing the RR or Vt, will increase CO_2 retention and thereby decrease the pH. This patient's primary disturbance is respiratory distress, and while the renal system does compensate for prolonged acid-base disturbance, it requires a much longer duration than do our respiratory compensatory mechanisms. Sepsis is generally associated with metabolic or lactic acidosis.

Ref.: 46

34. An 80-kg, 65-year-old woman with severe lupus is admitted to the ICU after exploratory laparotomy for sigmoid diverticulitis (Hinchey type IV). She is given a stoma and brought to the ICU intubated. Her vital signs are a temperature of 97.5°F, HR of 105 beats/min, BP of 70/50 mmHg, and Sao_2 of 96%. In the first hour her urine output is 20 mL; she has received 4 L of crystalloid and one unit of packed red blood cells (PRBCs), and her antibiotics have been redosed. Her CVP is 10 mmHg, but she remains hypotensive. Choose the next intervention that will be most beneficial?

A. Additional 2 L of a normal saline bolus

B. Hydrocortisone, 100 mg IV

C. Administration of furosemide for low urine output

D. Initiation of vasopressor therapy with norepinephrine or dopamine

E. Aggressive rewarming

ANSWER: D

COMMENTS: In a patient in septic shock who is adequately volume resuscitated (shown by a CVP of 10 mmHg) and is unresponsive to fluid challenges, vasopressor therapy should be started. Administration of vasopressors can quickly restore BP; in the Surviving Sepsis Guidelines, norepinephrine administered centrally is the initial vasopressor of choice. Epinephrine, phenylephrine, and vasopressin should not be administered as the initial vasopressor to patients in septic shock. Epinephrine can be used as the first alternative agent in septic shock when BP is poorly responsive to norepinephrine. Dobutamine should be used in patients with myocardial dysfunction as evidenced by elevated cardiac filling pressures and low CO. In general, the rate of fluid administration should be reduced if cardiac filling pressures increase without concurrent hemodynamic improvement.

Ref.: 47

35. Norepinephrine therapy is started in the patient in Question 34. Later, vasopressin, 0.03 units/min, is added, but the patient remains hypotensive with a MAP below 55 mmHg. Her hemoglobin concentration is 9.0 g/dL. After performing an echocardiogram, dobutamine infusion was started at a maximum of 20 mcg/kg/min; pH is 7.21 with a Pco_2 of 34 mmHg. The patient remains hypotensive. What is the next step?

A. Increase the cardiac index to predetermined supranormal levels.

B. Administer hydrocortisone, 100 mg IV.

C. Have a family discussion about withdrawing care.

D. Perform an adrenocorticotropic hormone (ACTH) stimulation test.

E. Switch the ventilatory mode to AC.

ANSWER: B

COMMENTS: Although there is still much debate in the critical care literature about steroids, IV corticosteroids are recommended in patients with septic shock who despite adequate fluid replacement require vasopressor therapy to maintain adequate BP. Random cortisol levels may be helpful in determining a patient's benefit from steroid therapy, although it is not required. Consideration can be made to discontinue corticosteroid therapy in patients with a random cortisol level of greater than 25 mcg/dL. An ACTH stimulation test is not recommended to identify the subset of patients with septic shock who should receive hydrocortisone.

Ref.: 48

36. A 70-kg, 33-year-old woman who had not seen a physician in 10 years arrives at the ED with symptoms of dyspnea, fatigue, weight gain, diplopia, and dysphagia following an urgent laparoscopic cholecystectomy 10 days ago. On examination, she is awake and alert. She is afebrile with an HR of 80 beats/min, BP of 120/70 mmHg, and RR of 29 breaths/min. Her heart sounds are normal and breaths are bilateral and shallow. She has ptosis and significant proximal muscle weakness in all extremities. She is drooling slightly and having difficulty swallowing. Her vital capacity is 500 mL and her laboratory tests are pending. Which of the following treatments is the most appropriate to initiate next?

A. Administration of pyridostigmine
B. Endotracheal intubation
C. Administration of steroids
D. Administration of IV immunoglobulin
E. Administration of levothyroxine

ANSWER: B

COMMENTS: This patient is having a myasthenic crisis, which is a consequence of an autoimmune attack on the acetylcholine receptor complex. There is clinical weakness that is mostly marked after prolonged muscle exertion and should be considered in any patient with respiratory distress and cranial nerve findings. The myasthenic crisis with respiratory failure develops in approximately 20% of patients and necessitates intubation. It can be precipitated by bronchopulmonary infections, sepsis, surgical procedures, tapering of steroid medications, pregnancy, and some drugs. Upper airway muscle weakness can lead to the collapse of the airways and aspiration. Patients with marginal vital capacity (<15 mL/kg), weak cough or voice, and worsening negative inspiratory force should be considered for intubation.

Ref.: 49

37. A 73-year-old male with stage IV colon cancer is intubated in the ICU 5 days after undergoing palliative resection of his primary tumor. He becomes acutely febrile and tachycardic with increased oxygen requirement. His BP drops to 88/50 mmHg. A bedside echocardiogram demonstrates a hyperdynamic left ventricle and right ventricular strain. Which of the following is the optimal treatment for this patient?

A. Surgical embolectomy
B. Systemic tissue plasminogen activator (tPA)
C. Catheter-directed tPA
D. Initiation of therapeutic heparin drip
E. Placement of inferior vena cava (IVC) filter

ANSWER: C

COMMENTS: Therapeutic anticoagulation is the mainstay of treatment for confirmed or suspected PE. The goal range for partial thromboplastin time (PTT) in the treatment of venous thromboembolism is 60 to 90 s, and the drip should be titrated to this value. Massive PE is defined as hypotension with systolic BP < 90 mmHg, while submassive PEs are those with systolic BP > 90 mmHg but with right heart strain or right ventricular dilation on echocardiogram. Thrombolysis is an option for many nonsurgical patients diagnosed with massive or submassive PE. Contraindications to systemic tPA include recent head trauma, ischemic stroke (within 3 weeks), any prior intracranial hemorrhage, or neoplasm. Relative contraindications include age > 75, recent surgery (within 3 to 4 weeks), pregnancy, or remote ischemic stroke. For patients with massive or submassive PE who do not meet criteria for systemic tPA, a more recent consideration is catheter-directed tPA. While more studies are ongoing, early randomized trials of catheter-directed tPA in postsurgical patients have demonstrated improvement in right ventricle (RV) function at 24 h without increase in bleeding complications.

Ref.: 50, 51

38. Which of the following sites for central venous catheter placement is associated with the lowest rate of catheter-associated blood stream infections?

A. Internal jugular vein
B. Subclavian vein
C. Femoral vein
D. Both A and B are equivalent
E. All sites are equivalent if sterile technique is maintained

ANSWER: B

COMMENTS: See Question 39.

Ref.: 52, 53

39. You are attempting to place a central venous catheter in the right internal jugular vein of a hemodialysis patient who is in the ICU after below-knee amputation for a severe diabetic foot infection. Which of the following is true regarding the central line placement?

A. The widespread use of ultrasound has been shown to reduce complication rates regardless of the site.
B. The risk of complication increases after three attempts by the same proceduralist.
C. If ultrasound is used, a chest radiograph is unnecessary prior to attempts on the contralateral side.
D. Routine exchange of catheters reduces infectious complications.
E. Aspiration of dark blood confirms appropriate venous placement.

ANSWER: B

COMMENTS: Nearly 15% of patients who receive central venous catheters will have an associated complication. While there is an obvious risk associated with their placement, many of these complications are related to catheter-associated infection or thrombosis. Experience reduces the likelihood of complications with line placement, and it has been shown that the complication rate after three attempts is nearly six times that of the complication rate after only one attempt by any one proceduralist. Ultrasound does reduce the risk of complication with internal jugular catheter placement but does not reliably improve outcomes with subclavian catheter placement. Regardless of the use of ultrasound guidance, pneumothorax is a potential complication and does not obviate the need for a chest x-ray.

A recent meta-analysis demonstrated 4.5 infections per 1000 femoral venous catheter placements versus only 1.2 infections per 1000 subclavian venous catheter placements. Likewise, subclavian catheters were also demonstrated to be associated with fewer bloodstream infections than internal jugular venous catheters.

Ref.: 52, 53

40. A 66-year-old woman who has been in the ICU for 2 weeks following total hip replacement complicated by massive infection and sepsis is complaining of right calf pain. She gets out of bed to go to physical therapy and develops severe dyspnea, tachycardia, and hypotension. Pulse oximetry reading is 75%. A CT angiogram shows bilateral clots in the pulmonary arteries. With regard to PE, which of the following is true?

A. Early chest radiographic abnormalities are rarely present in patients with PE.

B. A shunt abnormality is present early after the PE and a V/Q abnormality becomes the mechanism for hypoxemia in later stages.

C. Thrombolytic therapy has been shown to reduce mortality rates in comparison to heparin in patients with PE.

D. Heparin should never be given until the diagnosis of PE is absolute.

E. More than 33% of patients with PE have negative lower extremity duplex studies for deep vein thrombosis (DVT).

ANSWER: E

COMMENTS: DVT occurs in 30% of ICU patients and is monitored by governing bodies in the United States; all ICUs should have a prevention protocol. High-risk factors are thoracic or general procedures requiring general anesthesia for longer than 30 min, active malignancy, neurosurgical procedures, coronary artery bypass grafting (CABG), CHF, and respiratory failure, along with the traumatic injury. ICU patients almost always have at least one risk factor and need prophylaxis. Options include pharmacologic treatment with low-molecular-weight heparin (LMWH), unfractionated heparin, or pneumatic compression devices.

In regard to diagnosis, duplex ultrasound has a specificity and sensitivity greater than 95%. Many emboli can be silent, but symptoms of small-to-medium emboli are usually pulmonary (i.e., dyspnea, chest pain, and cough). Tachypnea and tachycardia are present as well. Massive PE often produces cardiovascular findings such as elevated PA pressure and right heart strain. Angiography is the definitive diagnostic technique for this disease, but a helical CT scan of the chest with infusion has shown excellent specificity. Even without pulmonary infarction, radiographic abnormalities appear as diaphragmatic elevation, atelectasis, and effusion. For treatment of DVT, heparin therapy over a period of 5 to 7 days with an overlap with warfarin constitutes the treatment of choice. Warfarin should be continued for 6 to 12 weeks for calf vein and large-vein thrombosis and up to 6 months for PE.

Ref.: 1, 54

41. A 25-year-old male patient with Von Hippel–Lindau (VHL) syndrome is found to have bilateral adrenal masses identified on a CT of the abdomen. His medication list includes both an angiotensin-converting enzyme (ACE) inhibitor and calcium channel blocker for hypertension. As part of his preoperative preparation, what medication(s) should he receive?

A. β-blockade

B. α-blockade

C. α-blockade followed by β-blockade

D. β-blockade followed by α-blockade

E. Hydrocortisone

ANSWER: C

COMMENTS: A rare genetic syndrome, VHL is associated with numerous benign tumors that have potential malignant transformation or other physiologic consequences. Pheochromocytoma is one of these associated lesions and should be suspected in any young patient with the disorder and hypertension. All patients with pheochromocytoma should undergo preoperative α-blockade to negate the activity of the tumor. Typically this is accomplished with twice-daily dosing of phenoxybenzamine or another α-blocking medication. The dose is generally started at a low level and increased until orthostatic hypotension develops. At this point, with the patient sufficiently α-blocked, there is often rebound tachycardia for which a β-blocker is then started. These medications are continued through the perioperative period until the patient has had the pheochromocytoma surgically excised. If the patient is also adrenally insufficient, stress-dose steroid at the time of the operation may be indicated.

Ref.: 55

42. A 56-year-old male with hypertension and diabetes is anticoagulated following an emergent right femoral-popliteal arterial bypass. He has been continually oozing from his fasciotomy sites, and his hemoglobin has drifted down in the past 3 days to a level of 7.8 g/dL. On review of his chart you see that in the preoperative clearance note from cardiology he had a hemoglobin level of 13.0 g/dL and no significant cardiac disease. His family is concerned about how pale he has been during this ICU stay. His vital signs are an HR of 86 beats/min, BP of 128/69 mmHg, and Sao_2 of 96%. What is the appropriate answer regarding a blood transfusion for this patient at this time?

A. Transfuse five units of PRBCs to reach the preoperative hemoglobin level of 13 g/dL.

B. Check complete blood count (CBC) levels daily and hold transfusion until the hemoglobin level is lower than 9 g/dL.

C. Start erythropoietin at 40,000 units daily.

D. Transfuse PRBCs to a level greater than 10 g/dL.

E. Check daily CBC levels and hold transfusion until the hemoglobin level is lower than 7 g/dL.

ANSWER: E

COMMENTS: Anemia is very common in critically ill patients; in the United States, approximately 85% of patients spending more than 1 week in the ICU receive one or more units of PRBCs in their first week. Blood is a scarce and expensive resource and is associated with morbidity, including transfusion reactions, infections, and worse outcomes. Historically, patients received transfusions if their hemoglobin level dropped below 10 g/dL. However, a multicenter prospective randomized clinical trial in 1999 showed that transfusion for a hemoglobin level of less than 7 g/dL had the same 30-day mortality rate as transfusion when the hemoglobin level was less than 10 g/dL (except in patients with the significant cardiac disease). This patient had preoperative cardiac clearance and is not presently showing any signs of hemodynamic instability.

Patients with anemia of critical illness have been shown to have a blunted response to both endogenous and exogenous erythropoietin. A multicenter trial showed a mild increase in hemoglobin, but it is unclear in the literature whether this improves clinical outcomes.

Ref.: 1, 56, 57

43. The routine use of which of the following is associated with a lower rate of VAP in the ICU setting?

A. Ventilator weaning protocol

B. Chlorhexidine oral rinse

C. Daily sedation vacation

D. H_2 blocker

E. Maintaining the head of bed at 30 to 45 degrees

ANSWER: A

COMMENTS: Most of the items are routinely included on "VAP bundles" in ICUs across the country, although not all are aimed at specifically preventing VAP. The use of H_2 blockers and DVT prophylaxis are indicated for nearly all mechanically ventilated patients given their increased risk for stress ulcer and thromboembolic disease; however, they play no role in the reduction of pneumonia or liberation from the ventilator. Chlorhexidine oral rinse and head-of-bed elevation are also standard practice for ventilated patients, and while not often harmful, their efficacy has been unable to be proven or widely replicated in randomized trials. It is widely accepted, however, that an established ventilator weaning protocol does reduce overall days of mechanical ventilation, which in turn results in a decreased rate of VAP. Daily SATs do not have a significant effect on ventilator days, ICU length of stay, or rates of VAP. Other considerations include the role of early tracheostomy as well as newer technologies like endotracheal tubes with the aspiration of subglottic secretions and their potential applications going forward.

Ref.: 58, 59

44. A 47-year-old man with hepatitis C cirrhosis and hepatocellular carcinoma is in the ICU following orthotopic liver transplant. Preoperatively, he developed renal failure secondary to hepatorenal syndrome and remains on dialysis but otherwise is recovering well. On postoperative day 5, his platelet count is noted to be 70,000 per microliter from 150,000 per microliter one day prior. What is the most likely diagnosis?

A. Consumptive coagulopathy

B. Laboratory error

C. Hemodilution

D. Heparin-induced thrombocytopenia

E. Idiopathic thrombocytopenic purpura (ITP)

ANSWER: D

COMMENTS: See Question 45.

Ref.: 56, 57

45. For the patient in Question 44, the diagnosis of heparin-induced thrombocytopenia (HIT) is confirmed. What is the next best step?

A. Argatroban drip

B. Oral anticoagulation with Coumadin

C. Hold all anticoagulation

D. Lepirudin

E. Transition from heparin to Lovenox

ANSWER: A

COMMENTS: Type II HIT has developed in this patient. Type I HIT occurs in 1%–2% of patients and causes transient sequestration of platelets with a drop in the count to less than the normal range or a 50% fall in the platelet count within the normal range. In general, this is of little consequence. Platelet levels normalize in a few days after heparin is discontinued. Type II is more severe, and antiplatelet antibodies develop in 0.1%–0.2% of patients exposed to heparin. It is associated with thrombotic complications in more than 30% of cases and should be suspected in a patient in whom resistance to anticoagulation, thromboembolic events, and a fall in the platelet count greater than 30% or a count of less than 100,000/mm^3 develop. Once HIT is suspected, all sources of heparin, including LMWH, should be discontinued. Warfarin can worsen the prothrombotic state and should not be used before complete anticoagulation is achieved with argatroban or lepirudin, both antithrombin agents.

Lepirudin undergoes renal elimination, which should be noted in situations such as this patient with renal insufficiency. Argatroban is metabolized hepatically and is the best choice in this situation.

Ref.: 56, 57

46. A 60-year-old man with renal failure who has been undergoing dialysis for the past 2 years is admitted for cellulitis surrounding the fistula site on his right upper extremity. Antibiotics are started, and the patient is observed. On hospital day 4, his fistula clots and he is taken to the OR for revision. On the following day, he is febrile, coughing up thick green sputum, and dyspneic despite having undergone dialysis that morning. A chest radiograph shows an infiltrate in his right lower lobe, and laboratory tests show a WBC count of 18,000/mm^3. Which characteristic of nosocomial pneumonia listed below is not correct?

A. Characterized by onset within 24 h of hospital admission

B. Purulent sputum

C. Isolation of the pathogenic organism from blood or the lung

D. Elevated WBC count

E. Infiltrate on chest radiography

ANSWER: A

COMMENTS: Hospital-acquired pneumonia (HAP) is the second most common of all nosocomial infections in the United States. The Centers for Disease Control and Prevention's definition of nosocomial pneumonia is a clinical one that requires pneumonia to occur more than 48 h after hospital admission and excludes any infections that are present or incubating at admission. The other two criteria include appropriate findings on physical examination *or* an infiltrate on chest radiography plus one of the following: purulent sputum, isolation of the pathogenic organism from blood or the lung, identification of a virus from the lower respiratory tract, or serologic or pathologic evidence of recent infection. Many clinical studies have shown that early, appropriate, and adequate antibiotic therapy can reduce the mortality rate from HAP, currently listed as anywhere from 24% to 76%. The American Thoracic Society presumes that early-onset pneumonia is due to *Haemophilus influenzae*, methicillin-susceptible *Staphylococcus aureus*, *Streptococcus pneumoniae*, or anaerobes. Late-onset HAP occurs more than 4 days after admission and is usually caused by gram-negative organisms, especially *Pseudomonas aeruginosa*, *Acinetobacter*, Enterobacteriaceae (*Klebsiella*, *Enterobacter*, *Serratia*), or methicillin-resistant *S. aureus* (MRSA). Broad-spectrum antibiotics should be started early and deescalated, not escalated, when culture sensitivities are known. This patient does not require intubation at this time, and low-volume, lung-protective ventilation is best used for ARDS. Patients with HAP do not need bronchoscopy daily. Chest therapy, elevation of the head of the bed, and ambulation are all methods to improve pulmonary toilet.

Ref.: 60, 61

47. A 27-year-old patient presented with a prolonged ICU course for Fournier's gangrene. Upon admission 5 days ago he had arterial and central lines placed along with a Foley catheter, which has since been removed. He now complains of diffuse body ache, anorexia, and cough with thin, white sputum. He has not had flatus or a bowel movement for 24 h. Chest radiography shows bilateral haziness at the costophrenic angles. Physical examination shows no acute distress, crackles in the lung bases bilaterally, and a swollen right arm. He has some redness around the right side of his neck and chest while his abdomen is soft, distended, and tympanitic but nontender. Vital signs include a temperature of 101.6°F, HR of 100 beats/min, BP of 128/75 mmHg, and Sao_2 of 96%. Lab findings include WBC of 18,500/mm^3, sodium concentration of 140 mEq/L, potassium of 4.3 mEq/L, BUN of 21 mg/dL, creatinine level of 0.8 mg/dL, and liver profile within normal limits. What is the most likely diagnosis?

A. Acalculous cholecystitis

B. HAP

C. Catheter-related bloodstream infection

D. Perforated peptic ulcer

E. Viral respiratory infection

ANSWER: C

COMMENTS: The most likely diagnosis is a catheter-related bloodstream infection. He had a catheter placed on an emergency basis and is now experiencing fevers and malaise, with cellulitis evident in the right side of his neck. His infection can explain the anorexia, ileus, and elevated WBC count. Catheter-related bloodstream infection is seen in approximately 5% of patients with indwelling catheters and should be suspected if any erythema or purulence is identified at the catheter site. The subclavian vein is the preferred site for the reduction of infection, over internal jugular or femoral locations. Once an infection is suspected, blood should be drawn through the line and peripherally for culture, and immediate removal of the catheter is suggested and the tip sent for culture. A catheter–peripheral colony-forming unit (CFU) ratio of 8 signifies line sepsis, and a catheter tip culture with 25 CFUs confirms a catheter-related infection.

Ref.: 61, 62

48. A 45-year-old male is recovering from multiorgan failure after laparotomy for a perforated gastric ulcer. He has been afebrile for 48 h and is not taking any antibiotics. His WBC count is normal and renal failure has resolved. Encephalopathy is improving, and oxygenation is adequate, although attempts to wean him from the ventilator have been unsuccessful. Neurologic examination shows symmetrical quadriparesis with sparing of the face and depressed deep tendon reflexes. Spinal tap is normal. Which of the following statements is true concerning his condition?

A. Nerve biopsy often shows demyelination or inflammation.

B. Failure to wean from the ventilator is due to phrenic nerve involvement.

C. Corticosteroids are the treatment of choice.

D. Serum antibodies against acetylcholine receptors are always present.

E. Plasmapheresis is the initial treatment of choice.

ANSWER: B

COMMENTS: Critical illness polyneuropathy (CPU) is an axonal motor sensory neuropathy that accompanies sepsis with encephalopathy. It is due to primary axonal degeneration and affects motor fibers more than sensory fibers. Frequently, it is manifested as a failure to wean a patient from the ventilator because of phrenic nerve involvement despite clinical improvement. Symmetrical quadriparesis with facial sparing and depressed deep tendon reflexes is characteristic, and electromyography confirms the diagnosis. Spinal fluid is normal, unlike the case in patients with Guillain-Barré syndrome. Facial involvement and detection of antibodies against acetylcholine are characteristic of myasthenia gravis. Nerve biopsy shows axonal degeneration without demyelination or inflammation. Treatment is supportive, and corticosteroids are contraindicated.

Ref.: 63, 64

49. A 63-year-old man is admitted to the ICU following a Hartmann procedure for Hinchey type IV diverticulitis 5 days earlier. The patient is intubated and maintained on AC ventilation, is tachycardic, and is febrile to 101°F. The nurse has noticed an increase in tracheobronchial secretions that are purulent in character. A chest radiograph shows a new infiltrate in the right lung. Which of the following statements is false regarding this patient's condition?

A. The most likely organism involved is methicillin-sensitive *S. aureus*.

B. The frequency of ventilator circuit changes does not influence the incidence of this complication.

C. Kinetic beds and elevation of the head of the patient to 45 degrees decrease its incidence.

D. The risk for development of this complication is highest in the second week.

E. Qualitative cultures or secretions are preferred over quantitative culture techniques.

ANSWER: D

COMMENTS: VAP has significant costs and a mortality of about 25%. The risk of acquiring VAP is highest in the first week (3% per day), thereafter decreasing to 2% per day in the second week and to 1% per day in the third week. VAP is generally categorized as early (<48 h after intubation) or late (occurring after 5 to 7 days of intubation). Early-onset VAP is associated with bacteria that are normally sensitive to antibiotics (*S. aureus, H. influenzae*, and *S. pneumoniae*), whereas late-onset VAP is typically associated with antibiotic-resistant bacteria (MRSA, *P. aeruginosa, Acinetobacter*, and *Enterobacter* species). The major risk factors for VAP include trauma, burns, and stay in neurosurgical units as opposed to medical ICUs. Known risk factors include patients older than 60 years who require prolonged (>48 h) mechanical ventilatory support, aspiration, a nasogastric tube, failure to elevate the head of the bed, and endotracheal cuff pressures of less than 20 cm H_2O. Orotracheal intubation carries a lower incidence of VAP than nasotracheal intubation. Because contamination of ventilator circuits is universal, the ventilator circuit change interval does not affect the incidence of VAP. Heat and moisture exchangers may be associated with a slightly lower incidence of VAP than heated humidifiers. Drainage of subglottic secretions is associated with a decreased incidence of VAP, especially early-onset VAP. Kinetic beds and positioning of patients at 45 degrees from the horizontal are also associated with a decreased incidence. Previous exposure to antibiotics in a prolonged preoperative hospitalization exposes patients to health care–related infections. Selective digestive decontamination has been reported to be associated with a decreased incidence of VAP, yet these therapies should be time limited to prevent the growth of resistant organisms. The suspicion for VAP in this patient with a prolonged period of ventilation and new onset of fever, leukocytosis, and purulent sputum should be high, particularly if the chest radiograph shows a new infiltrate. The diagnosis is best established by quantitative culture of secretions obtained from the lower respiratory tract. The two techniques used include protected specimen brush (PSB) sampling and bronchoalveolar lavage (BAL). A threshold of 1000 CFU/mL for PSB and 10,000 CFU/mL for BAL is currently recommended. The presence of less than 50% neutrophils in BAL fluid has also been used to exclude pneumonia. Even though the effect of these techniques on patient outcome is unclear, they have resulted in a significant reduction in the use of antibiotics.

Ref.: 65

50. A 22-year-old man involved in a motor vehicle accident is found to have a thoracic spine fracture (T6) and paraplegia. The patient is hypotensive with a systolic BP of 70 mmHg, is bradycardic with a pulse of 48 beats/min, and is breathing comfortably. Which of the following would be the most appropriate initial treatment?

A. Isotonic fluid administration

B. Steroid administration within 24 h of the injury

C. Immediate intubation

D. α-Agonist administration

E. Immediate magnetic resonance imaging

ANSWER: A

COMMENTS: Neurogenic shock refers to a condition characterized by hypotension and bradycardia that results from the interruption of the sympathetic nervous system pathways within the spinal cord. Common causes include sensory stimulation, such as severe pain, exposure to unpleasant events or sights, high spinal anesthesia, and traumatic spinal cord injury. Clinical characteristics include a BP that is often low, as in other forms of shock. However, the pulse rate is usually slower than normal, and the skin is flushed, warm, and dry. CO is reduced secondary to decreased blood return to the heart because of the increased capacitance of the arterioles and venules. Since the heart receives sympathetic input, there is a difference between injuries above and below T4. The former depresses cardiac function and decreases venous return. The bradycardia is caused by sympathectomy of the spinal injury above the level of T4 with no capacity for compensatory tachycardia. Treatment of neurogenic shock secondary to spinal cord injury is usually more complicated not only because of more prolonged hypotension but also because of the presence of coincident hypovolemic shock resulting from associated injuries. Such patients often require ventilatory support as a result of decreased spontaneous respiration and loss of the accessory muscles for breathing. Aggressive fluid therapy should be instituted early under continuous cardiovascular monitoring. Persistent hypotension necessitates recognition of possible hemorrhagic shock, and a vasopressor such as ephedrine or phenylephrine may be needed. If the injury is below T4, a pure α-agonist may aggravate the reflex bradycardia. Thus a drug with mixed chronotropic and inotropic effects (e.g., norepinephrine or dopamine) is preferred. A nasogastric tube should be inserted because gastric atony, dilation, and hypersecretion develop in these patients. Treatment of milder forms of neurogenic shock consists of removing the nociceptive stimulus. Neurogenic shock resulting from high spinal anesthesia can usually be treated with a vasopressor such as ephedrine or phenylephrine, each of which increases CO by direct effects on the heart and by increasing peripheral vasoconstriction. Although the administration of steroids remains controversial, their usefulness for blunt spinal cord injury has been suggested when they are given within 8 h of injury and their administration is extended for 48 h.

Ref.: 66, 67

51. Which of the following is associated with the greatest in-hospital mortality?

A. An ICU patient with an increase in the Sequential Organ Failure Assessment (SOFA) score by 2 points in 24 h

B. A patient in the ED with altered mental status and an RR of 25 breaths/min but no hypotension

C. An ICU patient requiring one vasopressor with a serum lactate value of 2 mmol/L

D. A patient on the medical ward who is alert and oriented but hypotensive and tachypneic

E. All represent sepsis with equal in-hospital mortality

ANSWER: C

COMMENTS: In the newest definitions of sepsis and septic shock, the Society of Critical Care Medicine has identified the utility of the SOFA score and its association with in-hospital mortality. The variables include the Pao_2:FiO_2 ratio, platelet count, serum creatinine, and bilirubin. Sepsis may now be indicated by an increase in an individual patient's SOFA score by 2 points, which is associated with a 10% increase in in-hospital mortality. The quick SOFA, or qSOFA, has been advocated for the rapid assessment of patients and consists of three variables: mental status, tachypnea (RR > 22 breaths/min), and hypotension (systolic BP < 100 mmHg). If at least two of these criteria are met, there should be a high index of suspicion for sepsis in these patients and admission to an intensive care setting is appropriate. Lastly, they identified that the combination of hypotension requiring at least one vasopressor along with a serum lactate value of 2 mmol/L or greater in the absence of hypovolemia is associated with a 40% in-hospital mortality rate. These two criteria are now recognized and utilized as the definition of septic shock.

Ref.: 68

52. A 28-year-old male with a history of depression is brought into the ED by a family member who believes the patient is overdosed on acetaminophen. On further questioning the patient admits to ingesting "a few handfuls" of acetaminophen tablets approximately 18 h prior to the arrival to the hospital. On assessment, the patient is awake; however, he is confused. His vital signs are an HR of 105 beats/min, BP 102/77 mmHg, RR 18 breaths/min, and Sao_2 of 99%. Lab values are significant for arterial pH 7.32, INR 3.1, and creatinine 4.2. What is the best first step for management of this patient?

A. Administration of IV *N*-acetylcysteine

B. Stress-dose steroids

C. Aggressive fluid resuscitation with normal saline

D. Activated charcoal

E. Urgent evaluation for liver transplantation

ANSWER: A

COMMENTS: Fulminant hepatic failure is classically defined as the development of severe liver injury with impaired synthetic function (INR $\geq$ 1.5) and new encephalopathy in patients without preexisting liver disease. In the United States, the most common causes of acute liver failure are acetaminophen overdose and viral hepatitis. Acetaminophen toxicity can be difficult to predict, as there are often no early symptoms and the modified Rumack-Matthew nomogram is widely used to predict poisoning severity following acetaminophen overdose. The use of activated charcoal for gastrointestinal decontamination is useful for patients who present within 4 h of acetaminophen ingestion; however, activated charcoal should be used with caution in patients who may not be able to protect their airway. *N*-acetylcysteine is the most effective antidote for acetaminophen toxicity, and initiation of therapy within 8 h of ingestion is associated with greatly decreased morbidity. The King's College Criteria is used to identify patient's with a poor prognosis with acetaminophen-induced fulminant hepatic failure. An arterial pH less than 7.3 or a combination comprising INR greater than 6.5, creatinine greater than 3.4 mg/dL, and grade III/IV encephalopathy are strong predictors of poor prognosis. Patients who continue to deteriorate despite appropriate medical therapy should be considered for liver transplantation.

Ref.: 69, 70

53. A 30-year-old female with a history of nonalcoholic steatohepatitis underwent a spontaneous vaginal delivery complicated by uterine atony and a large-volume bleeding, refractory to fundal massage, medical management, and uterine artery embolization. Hemostasis eventually is achieved after the patient underwent exploratory laparotomy and hysterectomy; however, the patient required rapid transfusion of 15 units of PRBCs during her resuscitation. Postoperatively, the patient is extubated and transferred to the surgical ICU for monitoring. Shortly after arrival, the patient complains of perioral numbness and paresthesias in her feet. What is the most likely cause of the patient's symptoms?

A. Metabolic alkalosis due to alkaline transfusions

B. Overadministration of IV crystalloids

C. Low serum calcium levels in the transfused blood

D. Citrate toxicity

E. Hyperkalemia due to hemolysis of transfused blood

ANSWER: D

COMMENTS: Massive blood transfusion is classically defined as transfusion of 10 units of red blood cells within 24 h; however, many other definitions have been proposed. There are many physiologic alterations associated with massive blood transfusion that require careful monitoring. Large-volume transfusion of red cells can dilute serum coagulation proteins and platelets leading to a prolongation in PT and activated partial thromboplastin time (aPTT). Additionally, transfused blood is anticoagulated with sodium citrate and citric acid. Rapid transfusion of red blood cells can overwhelm a patient's ability to metabolize the excess citrate, which can bind ionized calcium and can lead to clinically significant hypocalcemia. Generally, very rapid transfusion is required to cause significant hypocalcemia; however, those with preexisting liver disease are at a greatly increased risk. Administration of either calcium gluconate or calcium chloride is an acceptable treatment of hypocalcemia following massive transfusion.

Ref.: 71, 72

54. A 67-year-old-male is brought emergently to the OR for the management of freely perforated diverticulitis. During the procedure the patient is unstable, requiring multiple vasopressors as well as large-volume fluid resuscitation. At the completion of the case, the patient was stabilized and transferred to the SICU intubated with nasogastric decompression. The patient is noted to have worsening abdominal distension throughout the night and decreasing urine output despite multiple crystalloid boluses. On examination, the patient has a Richmond Agitation-Sedation Scale score of −1. He has a tense abdomen with a healthy appearing ostomy and an abdominal surgical drain with minimal serosanguinous drainage. His vital signs are a temperature of 37.2°C, HR 98 beats/min, and BP 144/92 mmHg. He is mechanically ventilated, with peak airway pressures of 38 cm H_2O and plateau pressures of 28 cm H_20. Intravesicular pressure is measured to be 22 mmHg. What is the next best step in managing this patient?

A. Increase the patient's sedation

B. Decrease the patient's Vt

C. Administration of a paralytic agent

D. Broadening of antibiotic therapy

E. Emergent return to the OR for reexploration

ANSWER: A

COMMENTS: ACS is defined as an end-organ dysfunction in the setting of intraabdominal hypertension. Intraabdominal hypertension refers to sustained intraabdominal pressures $\geq$ 12 mmHg. Clinically, there is no defined intraabdominal pressure for ACS as end-organ dysfunction can occur at a variety of pressures between different patients; however, intraabdominal pressures $\geq$ 25 mmHg are frequently associated with ACS. Bladder pressures are widely used as a surrogate measurement for intraabdominal pressure. ACS can occur in a variety of clinical settings, including trauma, burns (>30% of the total body surface area), liver transplantation, and postsurgical patients. Additionally, large-volume resuscitation has been associated with increased occurrence of ACS. The diagnosis of ACS is generally made with the triad of a tense abdomen, decreased urine output despite fluid resuscitation, and increased airway pressures, all in the setting of abdominal hypertension. For patients with progressive renal dysfunction or worsening shock, the definitive management of ACS is a decompressive laparotomy. In patients where there is a concern for the impending development of ACS, supportive care measures can be made to decrease intraabdominal pressures. Nasogastric and rectal decompression, deep sedation, chemical paralysis, limited fluid administration, and ventilator support to reduce airway pressures may be used. In the above scenario, the patient is minimally sedated and may have improved intraabdominal pressures with increased sedative dosing.

Ref.: 73, 74

REFERENCES

1. Adams CA, Biffl WL, Cioffi WG. Surgical critical care. In: Townsend CM, Beauchamp RD, Evers BM, et al., eds. *Sabiston Textbook of Surgery: The Biological Basis of Modern Surgical Practice*. 17th ed. Philadelphia: WB Saunders; 2008.
2. Winters B. Analgesia and sedation in critical care medicine. In: Cameron JL, ed. *Current Surgical Therapy*. 9th ed. Philadelphia: CV Mosby; 2008.
3. Milbrandt EB, Ely EW. Agitation and delirium. In: Fink MP, Abraham E, Vincent JL, et al., eds. *Textbook of Critical Care*. 5th ed. Philadelphia: WB Saunders; 2005.
4. Moran SE, Pei KY, Yu M. Hemodynamic monitoring: arterial and pulmonary artery catheters. In: Gabrielli A, Layon AJ, Yu M, eds. *Civetta, Taylor & Kirby's Critical Care*. 4th ed. Philadelphia: Lippincott Williams & Wilkins; 2009.
5. Rhodes A, Grounds RM, Bennett ED. Hemodynamic monitoring. In: Fink MP, Abraham E, Vincent JL, et al., eds. *Textbook of Critical Care*. 5th ed. Philadelphia: WB Saunders; 2005.
6. Gaspardone A, De Luca L. ST elevation myocardial infarction (STEMI) contemporary management strategies. In: Gabrielli A, Layon AJ, Yu M, eds. *Civetta, Taylor & Kirby's Critical Care*. 4th ed. Philadelphia: Lippincott Williams & Wilkins; 2009.
7. Nathens AB, Curtis JR, Beale RJ, et al. Management of the critically ill patient with severe acute pancreatitis. *Crit Care Med*. 2004;32(12):2524–2536.
8. Yang KL, Tobin MJ. A prospective study of indexes predicting the outcome of trials of weaning from mechanical ventilation. *N Engl J Med*. 1991;324(21):1145–1450.
9. Dellinger RP, Levy MM, Rhodes A, et al. Surviving sepsis campaign: international guidelines for management of severe sepsis and septic shock. *Crit Care Med*. 2013;41:580–637.
10. Weisberg L. Management of severe hyperkalemia. *Crit Care Med*. 2008;36(12):3246–3252.
11. Gutierrez G, Reines HD, Wulf-Gutierrez ME. Clinical review: hemorrhagic shock. *Crit Care*. 2004;8(5):373–381.
12. Mendelson A, Gillis C, Henderson WR, Ronco JJ, Dhingra V, Griesdale DE. Intracranial pressure monitors in traumatic brain injury: a systematic review. *Can J Neurol Sci*. 2012;39(5):571–576.
13. Yuan Q, Wu X, Sun Y, et al. Impact of intracranial pressure monitoring on mortality in patients with traumatic brain injury: a systematic review and meta-analysis. *J Neurosurg*. 2015;122(3):574–587.
14. Andrews P, Sinclair HL, Rodriguez A, et al. Hypothermia for intracranial hypertension after traumatic brain injury. *N Engl J Med*. 2015;373:2403–2412.
15. Siempos II , Ntaidou TK, Filippidis FT, Choi AM. Effect of early versus late or no tracheostomy on mortality and pneumonia of critically ill patients receiving mechanical ventilation: a systematic review and meta-analysis. *Lancet Respir Med*. 2015;3(2):150–158.
16. Gomes Silva B, Andriolo RB, Saconato H, Atallah AN, Valente O. Early versus late tracheostomy for critically ill patients. *Cochrane Database Syst Rev*. 2012;(3):CD007271.
17. Hosokawa K, Nishimura M, Egi M, Vincent JL. Timing of tracheotomy in ICU patients: a systematic review of randomized controlled trials. *Crit Care*. 2015;19:424.
18. Schmalfuss CM. Pericardial disease. In: Gabrielli A, Layon AJ, Yu M, eds. *Civetta, Taylor & Kirby's Critical Care*. 4th ed. Philadelphia: Lippincott Williams & Wilkins; 2009.
19. Marini JJ, Dries DJ, Perry JF. The lung structure and function. In: Gabrielli A, Layon AJ, Yu M, eds. *Civetta, Taylor & Kirby's Critical Care*. 4th ed. Philadelphia: Lippincott Williams & Wilkins; 2009.
20. Rahnemai-Azar A, Rahnemaiazar AA, Naghshizadian R, et al. Percutaneous endoscopic gastrostomy: indications, technique, complications and management. *World J Gastroenterol*. 2014;20(24):7739–7751.
21. Laghi F. Weaning from mechanical ventilation. In: Gabrielli A, Layon AJ, Yu M, eds. *Civetta, Taylor & Kirby's Critical Care*. 4th ed. Philadelphia: Lippincott Williams & Wilkins; 2009.
22. Corbridge TC, Corbridge SJ. Severe asthma exacerbation. In: Fink MP, Abraham E, Vincent JL, et al., eds. *Textbook of Critical Care*. 5th ed. Philadelphia: WB Saunders; 2005.
23. Katsaounou PA, Vassilakopoulos T. Severe asthma exacerbation. In: Gabrielli A, Layon AJ, Yu M, eds. *Civetta, Taylor & Kirby's Critical Care*. 4th ed. Philadelphia: Lippincott Williams & Wilkins; 2009.
24. Mehta S, Burry L, Cook D, et al. Daily sedation interruption in mechanically ventilated critically ill patients cared for with a sedation protocol: a randomized controlled trial. *JAMA*. 2012;308(19):1985–1992.
25. Burry L, Rose L, McCullagh IJ, Fergusson DA, Ferguson ND, Mehta S. Daily sedation interruption versus no daily sedation interruption for critically ill adult patients requiring invasive mechanical ventilation. *Cochrane Database Syst Rev*. 2014;(7):CD00917.
26. Girard T, Kress JP, Fuchs BD, et al. Efficacy and safety of a paired sedation and ventilator weaning protocol for mechanically ventilated patients in intensive care (Awakening and Breathing Controlled Trial): a randomized controlled trial. *Lancet*. 2008;371(9607):126–134.
27. Caples SM, Hubmayr RD. Respiratory system mechanics and respiratory muscle function. In: Fink MP, Abraham E, Vincent JL, et al., eds. *Textbook of Critical Care*. 5th ed. Philadelphia: WB Saunders; 2005.
28. Marino PL. *Principles of Mechanical Ventilation: The ICU Book*. 2nd ed. Philadelphia: Lippincott Williams & Wilkins; 1998.
29. Gordy S, Rowell S. Vascular air embolism. *Int J Crit Illn Inj Sci*. 2013;3(1):73–76.
30. Rajan T, Hill NS. Noninvasive positive-pressure ventilation. In: Fink MP, Abraham E, Vincent JL, et al., eds. *Textbook of Critical Care*. 5th ed. Philadelphia: WB Saunders; 2005.
31. Ware LB, Bernard GR. Acute lung injury and acute respiratory distress syndrome. In: Fink MP, Abraham E, Vincent JL, et al., eds. *Textbook of Critical Care*. 5th ed. Philadelphia: WB Saunders; 2005.
32. Marino PL. *Acute Respiratory Distress Syndrome: The ICU Book*. 2nd ed. Philadelphia: Lippincott Williams & Wilkins; 1998.
33. Ventilation with lower tidal volumes as compared with traditional volumes for acute lung injury and the acute respiratory distress syndrome. The Acute Respiratory Distress Syndrome Network. *N Engl J Med*. 2000;342:1301–1308.
34. Fanelli V, Vlachou A, Ghannadian S, Simonetti U, Slutsky AS, Zhang H. Acute respiratory distress syndrome: new definition, current and future therapeutic options. *J Thorac Dis*. 2013;5(3):326–334.
35. Bagshaw SM, Bellomo R. Acute renal failure. In: Gabrielli A, Layon AJ, Yu M, eds. *Civetta, Taylor & Kirby's Critical Care*. 4th ed. Philadelphia: Lippincott Williams & Wilkins; 2009.
36. Kulaylat MN, Dayton MT. Surgical complications. In: Townsend CM, Beauchamp RD, Evers BM, et al., eds. *Sabiston Textbook of Surgery: The Biological Basis of Modern Surgical Practice*. 18th ed. Philadelphia: WB Elsevier; 2008.
37. Barrett BJ. Contrast dye-induced nephropathy. In: Fink MP, Abraham E, Vincent JL, et al., eds. *Textbook of Critical Care*. 5th ed. Philadelphia: WB Saunders; 2005.
38. Mullins RJ. Acute renal failure. In: Cameron JL, ed. *Current Surgical Therapy*. 9th ed. Philadelphia: CV Mosby; 2008.
39. Bellomo R, D'Intini V. Renal replacement therapy in the ICU. In: Fink MP, Abraham E, Vincent JL, et al., eds. *Textbook of Critical Care*. 5th ed. Philadelphia: WB Saunders; 2005.
40. Balogun RA, Okusa MD. Lithium. In: Fink MP, Abraham E, Vincent JL, et al., eds. *Textbook of Critical Care*. 5th ed. Philadelphia: WB Saunders; 2005.
41. Mendez-Tellez PA, Dorman T. Postoperative respiratory failure. In: Cameron JL, ed. *Current Surgical Therapy*. 9th ed. Philadelphia: CV Mosby; 2008.
42. Boles J-M, Bion J, Connors A, et al. Weaning from mechanical ventilation. *European Resp J*. 2007;29(5):1033–1056.
43. McConville J, Kress J. Weaning patients from the ventilator. *N Engl J Med*. 2012;367:2233–2239.
44. Berl T, Taylor J. Disorders of water balance. In: Fink MP, Abraham E, Vincent JL, et al., eds. *Textbook of Critical Care*. 5th ed. Philadelphia: WB Saunders; 2005.
45. Huston JM, Eachempati SR, Barie PS. Preoperative and postoperative care. In: Cameron JL, ed. *Current Surgical Therapy*. 9th ed. Philadelphia: CV Mosby; 2008.
46. Breen P. Arterial blood gas and pH analysis. Clinical approach and interpretation. *Anesthesiol Clin North Am*. 2001;19(4):885–906.
47. Dellinger RP, Levy MM, Carlet JM, et al. Surviving sepsis campaign: international guidelines for management of severe sepsis and septic shock. *Intensive Care Med*. 2008;34:17–60.
48. Annane D, Sebille V, Charpentier C, et al. Effect of treatment with low doses of hydrocortisone and fludrocortisones on mortality in patients with septic shock. *JAMA*. 2002;288:862–871.
49. Juel VC, Bleck TP. Neuromuscular disorders in the ICU. In: Fink MP, Abraham E, Vincent JL, et al., eds. *Textbook of Critical Care*. 5th ed. Philadelphia: WB Saunders; 2005.
50. Kucher N, Boekstegers P, Müller OJ, et al. Randomized, controlled trial of ultrasound-assisted catheter-directed thrombolysis for acute intermediate-risk pulmonary embolism. *Circulation*. 2014;129(4):479–486.

51. Jaff M, McMurthy MS, Archer SL, et al. Management of massive and submassive pulmonary embolism, iliofemoral deep vein thrombosis, and chronic thromboembolic pulmonary hypertension: a scientific statement from the American Heart Association. *Circulation*. 2011;123(16):1788–1830.
52. Marik PE, Flemmer M, Harrison W. The risk of catheter-related bloodstream infection with femoral venous catheters as compared to subclavian and internal jugular venous catheters: a systematic review of the literature and meta-analysis. *Crit Care Med*. 2012;40(8):2479–2485.
53. Hind D, Calvert N, McWilliams R, et al. Ultrasonic locating devices for central venous cannulation: meta-analysis. *BMJ*. 2003;327(7411):361.
54. Banner MJ. Bedside assessment and monitoring of pulmonary function and power of breathing in the critically ill. In: Gabrielli A, Layon AJ, Yu M, eds. *Civetta, Taylor & Kirby's Critical Care*. 4th ed. Philadelphia: Lippincott Williams & Wilkins; 2009.
55. The Washington manual of Surgery. In: Klingensmith ME, Chen LE, Glasgow SC, et al., eds. Chapter 21 *Endocrine Surgery*. 5th ed. Philadelphia: Lippincott, Williams & Wilkins; 2008, p 358–359.
56. Pineo GF, Hull RD. Pulmonary embolism. In: Fink MP, Abraham E, Vincent JL, et al., eds. *Textbook of Critical Care*. 5th ed. Philadelphia: WB Saunders; 2005.
57. Hallal A, Schulman C, Cohn S. Anemia of critical illness. In: Fink MP, Abraham E, Vincent JL, et al., eds. *Textbook of Critical Care*. 5th ed. Philadelphia: WB Saunders; 2005.
58. Wip C, Napolitano L. Bundles to prevent ventilator-associated pneumonia: How valuable are they? *Curr Opin Infect Dis*. 2009;22(2): 159–166.
59. Maselli DJ, Restrepo MI. Strategies in the prevention of ventilator-associated pneumonia. *Ther Adv Respir Dis*. 2010;5(2):131–141.
60. Fagon JY, Chastre J. Nosocomial pneumonia. In: Fink MP, Abraham E, Vincent JL, et al., eds. *Textbook of Critical Care*. 5th ed. Philadelphia: WB Saunders; 2005.
61. Bohnen JMA. Antibiotics for critically ill patients. In: Cameron JL, ed. *Current Surgical Therapy*. 9th ed. Philadelphia: CV Mosby; 2008.
62. Seger D. Poisoning: overview of approaches for evaluation and treatment. In: Fink MP, Abraham E, Vincent JL, et al., eds. *Textbook of Critical Care*. 5th ed. Philadelphia: WB Saunders; 2005.
63. Leijten FS, de Weerd AW. Critical illness polyneuropathy: a review of the literature, definition and pathophysiology. *Clin Neurol Neurosurg*. 1994;96:10–19.
64. Valenstein E, Musulin M. Neuromuscular disorders. In: Gabrielli A, Layon AJ, Yu M, eds. *Civetta, Taylor & Kirby's Critical Care*. 4th ed. Philadelphia: Lippincott Williams & Wilkins; 2009.
65. Leroy OY, Alfandari S. Respiratory infections in the ICU. In: Gabrielli A, Layon AJ, Yu M, eds. *Civetta, Taylor & Kirby's Critical Care*. 4th ed. Philadelphia: Lippincott Williams & Wilkins; 2009.
66. Vitarbo EA, Levi ADO. Spinal cord injury. In: Fink MP, Abraham E, Vincent JL, et al., eds. *Textbook of Critical Care*. 5th ed. Philadelphia: WB Saunders; 2005.
67. Muehlschlegel S, Greer DM. Neurogenic shock. In: Gabrielli A, Layon AJ, Yu M, eds. *Civetta, Taylor & Kirby's Critical Care*. 4th ed. Philadelphia: Lippincott Williams & Wilkins; 2009.
68. Singer M, Deutschman CS, Seymour CW, et al. The third international consensus definitions for sepsis and septic shock. *JAMA*. 2016;315(8): 801–810.
69. Rumack BH, Matthew H. Acetaminophen poisoning and toxicity. *Pediatrics*. 1975;55(6):871–876.
70. Keays R, Harrison PM, Wendon JA, et al. Intravenous acetylcysteine in paracetamol induced fulminant hepatic failure: a prospective controlled trial. *BMJ*. 1991;303(6809):1026–1029.
71. Howland W, Schweizer O, Carlon GC, Goldiner PL. The cardiovascular effects of low levels of ionized calcium during massive transfusion. *Surv Anesthesiol*. 1978;22(4):384.
72. Collins JA. Problems associated with the massive transfusion of stored blood. *Surgery*. 1974;75(2):274–295.
73. Kirkpatrick AW, Roberts DJ, De Waele J, et al. Intra-abdominal hypertension and the abdominal compartment syndrome: updated consensus definitions and clinical practice guidelines from the World Society of the Abdominal Compartment Syndrome. *Intensive Care Med*. 2013;39(7):1190–1206.
74. O'Mara MS, Slater H, Goldfarb IW, Caushaj PF. A prospective, randomized evaluation of intra-abdominal pressures with crystalloid and colloid resuscitation in burn patients. *J Trauma*. 2005;58(5): 1011–1018.

CHAPTER 11

TRAUMA

Purvi P. Patel, M.D.

1. The primary survey is best described by which sequence of steps?

A. Airway, Blood pressure, Pulses, Breath sounds, Extremities

B. Airway, Breathing, Circulation, Disrobe, Extremities

C. Airway, Breathing, Circulation, Disability, Exposure

D. Access, Blood pressure, Chest compressions, Disability, Endotracheal intubation

E. Airway intubation, Bilateral chest tube placement, Central line placement

ANSWER: C

COMMENTS: The Advanced Trauma Life Support (ATLS) Program of the American College of Surgeons has put forth a general framework on how to approach and manage an injured patient. To streamline care, the A, B, C, D, E, and F sequence has been endorsed, which represents Airway, Breathing, Circulation, Disability, Exposure, and Focused Assessment with Sonography for Trauma (FAST). This comprises the primary survey with the goal of identifying life-threatening injuries and supporting oxygenation, ventilation, and perfusion. A team leader confirms that each system is intact and then moves to the next step with continued reassessment and interventions as needed. Common interventions include endotracheal intubation or cricothyroidotomy, placement of chest tubes and central venous catheters (CVCs), and, rarely, an emergency department (ED) thoracotomy. This is followed by a secondary survey that allows for a head-to-toe examination and a brief medical history.

Ref.: 1, 2

2. A middle-aged male is found lying on the ground in an alley and is brought into the trauma bay for additional evaluation. His vital signs are stable. The only sign of trauma is a large scalp laceration. The patient is confused with a Glasgow Coma Scale (GCS) score of 7. The decision is made to intubate the patient. What is the correct order for rapid-sequence intubation in trauma?

A. In-line cervical immobilization, preoxygenation, cricoid pressure, induction, paralysis, intubate, confirm placement with CO_2 detector

B. In-line cervical immobilization, preoxygenation, cricoid pressure, paralysis, induction, intubate, confirm placement with CO_2 detector

C. In-line cervical immobilization, preoxygenation, cricoid pressure, induction, intubate, confirm placement with CO_2 detector, paralysis

D. Tilt head back in sniffing position, preoxygenation, cricoid pressure, induction, paralysis, intubate, confirm placement with CO_2 detector

E. Tilt head back in sniffing position, preoxygenation, cricoid pressure, paralysis, induction, intubate, confirm placement with CO_2 detector

ANSWER: A

COMMENTS: The most commonly used method for securing a trauma patient's airway is orotracheal intubation. Rapid-sequence intubation consists of preoxygenating the patient for 3 min with bag-valve-mask ventilation while maintaining in-line cervical stabilization, applying cricoid pressure to limit aspiration, administering an induction agent followed by a paralytic, performing laryngoscopy, and then placing an endotracheal tube. In-line cervical stabilization should be maintained with the help of an assistant, not a rigid cervical spine collar. Common medications used include etomidate, ketamine, and succinylcholine. Etomidate is an induction agent that has a quick onset of action and is indicated for patients with a suspected brain injury or open globe because it does not cause an increase in intracranial pressure (ICP). However, it can cause adrenal insufficiency in rare cases. Ketamine is a dissociative anesthetic that can cause tachycardia and hypertension as common side effects. Succinylcholine should be avoided in patients with burns or a spinal cord injury because it can cause a rise in the serum potassium concentration and can lead to severe hyperkalemia. Confirmation of tube placement should be completed with a carbon dioxide detector and chest x-ray.

Ref.: 3, 4

3. A 72-year-old female presents after being ejected during a high-speed motor vehicle crash. Her heart rate (HR) is 155 beats/min, and blood pressure is 60/35 mmHg. Emergency medical technicians (EMT) were not able to obtain intravenous (IV) access. What is the best access for this patient so that fluid resuscitation can be initiated?

A. Saphenous vein cut down

B. Ultrasound-guided left internal jugular vein triple-lumen catheter

C. Right subclavian triple-lumen catheter using landmarks

D. Intraosseous (IO) access at the humerus

E. IO access at the tibia

ANSWER: D

COMMENTS: When traditional vascular access methods have not been successful, IO access can provide a means to give resuscitative fluids, medications, blood, and contrast. The IO route has been demonstrated to have a significantly higher first-attempt success rate and can be completed in a much quicker fashion and with fewer complications. Even experienced providers have difficulty placing a CVC using landmarks. CVC in trauma has about a 50% success on the first pass and requires an average of 8 min to place. In contrast, IO placement is over 90% successful and takes approximately 1 min to place. Ultrasound guidance has been shown to improve central line placement. However, it is not always practical in an emergency setting because it may not be readily available, takes time to set up, and space around a patient is limited. Many sites have been utilized for IO access. Although IO use is limited to the anterior tibia in the pediatric population, cadaver studies in adults showed the best flow rates with minimal placement or dislodgement issues in the sternum followed by the humerus. The humerus is now the preferred position.

Ref.: 5, 6

4. A 17-year-old female presents after a motor vehicle crash and is in hemorrhagic shock. A massive transfusion protocol is triggered. What is the optimal ratio in damage control resuscitation?

A. 2 plasma:1 platelet:1 red blood cell

B. 1 plasma:1 platelet:1 red blood cell

C. 1 plasma:1 platelet:3 red blood cells

D. 2 plasma:1 cryoprecipitate:1 red blood cell

E. 1 plasma:1 cryoprecipitate:1 red blood cell

ANSWER: B

COMMENTS: Approximately 1%–3% of trauma patients require a massive transfusion. The US Department of Defense's Prospective Observational Multicenter Major Trauma Transfusion (PROMMITT) study demonstrated that early transfusion with higher plasma-to-platelet ratios was associated with decreased mortality. The Pragmatic, Randomized Optimal Platelets and Plasma Ratios (PROPPR) trial demonstrated the optimal ratio of 1 plasma:1 platelet:1 red blood cell versus 1 plasma:1 platelet:2 red blood cells was associated with more patients achieving hemostasis with fewer hemorrhage-related deaths without increased complications. The overall 24-h and 30-day mortality was equal between groups. Both these studies support the early use of balanced transfusion therapy in an exsanguinating injured patient.

Ref.: 7, 8

5. A 77-year-old male with a history of atrial fibrillation on dabigatran, a direct thrombin inhibitor, presents after a fall from a ladder. His HR is 130 beats/min and irregular, blood pressure is 82/44 mmHg, and FAST is positive, with fluid in the right upper quadrant (RUQ) and pelvis. Prior to proceeding to the operating room, what is the best reversal agent for this patient's anticoagulation?

A. Fresh-frozen plasma

B. Prothrombin complex concentrates

C. Protamine sulfate

D. Idarucizumab

E. Platelets

ANSWER: D

COMMENTS: As the population grows older and more novel anticoagulants are prescribed, trauma surgeons need to know how to manage and reverse these medications acutely in a bleeding patient. Warfarin, a vitamin K antagonist, has traditionally been managed with fresh-frozen plasma and vitamin K injections. Recombinant factor VII has also been used to treat these patients and cirrhotics with an elevated international normalized ratio (INR). However, there is an increased prothrombotic risk potential with this therapy. Newer therapies include either 3- or 4-factor prothrombin complex concentrates (PCCs) that contain variable amounts of factors II, VII, IX, and X and proteins C and S and rapidly reverse the effects of warfarin within 30 min. Heparin and low-molecular-weight heparin (LMWH) are reversed with variable dosing of protamine sulfate. The effects of platelet inhibitors including aspirin and clopidogrel can be minimized with desmopressin and platelet transfusions. Novel agents including direct thrombin or factor Xa inhibitors can be managed with activated charcoal and PCC. A monoclonal antibody, idarucizumab, specifically adheres to the thrombin-binding site of dabigatran, rendering it inactive within a minute of dosing.

Ref.: 9, 10

6. A 75-year-old morbidly obese male presents after a motorcycle crash. The primary survey demonstrates an intact airway, diminished breath sounds from the left chest, GCS of 10, and limited movement of upper extremities. His HR is 122 beats/min, and blood pressure is 80/44 mmHg. A left chest tube is placed with 1 L of bloody output. The patient has 2 L of saline infused. His HR decreases to 116 beats/min, and blood pressure is 86/48 mmHg. FAST was indeterminate. What is the next best step to evaluate for intraabdominal hemorrhage?

A. Serial abdominal examinations

B. Diagnostic peritoneal tap

C. Computed tomography (CT)

D. Exploratory laparoscopy

E. Exploratory laparotomy

ANSWER: B

COMMENTS: This patient has several sources of shock including hemorrhage from his thorax and likely intracranial and spinal injuries. He is too unstable to leave the resuscitation area to go for CT imaging, and an abdominal source of bleeding must be ruled out prior to the definitive management of his injuries. Diagnostic peritoneal tap with lavage is a very sensitive, but nonspecific, test that can be used for either blunt or penetrating trauma. In this situation, diagnostic peritoneal lavage (DPL) is used to determine an intraperitoneal injury. However, it will miss retroperitoneal bleeding. DPL is performed by introducing a catheter into the abdomen via the Seldinger technique and then infusing 1 L of 0.9% normal saline. The fluid is then returned by gravity and sent to the laboratory for analysis. A positive DPL is defined as one with greater than 100,000 red blood cells/mm^3, 500 white blood cells (WBCs)/mm^3, or the presence of bilious/particulate material. A limited version of this procedure is a diagnostic peritoneal tap in which a needle is passed into the peritoneal cavity. If blood or succus is aspirated by a 10-ml syringe, it is deemed positive. If this patient has a positive DPL, the next most appropriate step in management is exploratory laparotomy. Serial abdominal examinations in an unstable patient are not appropriate.

Ref.: 11, 12

7. A 20-year-old female presents after a motor vehicle crash. She complains of diffuse abdominal pain. Her HR is 140 beats/min, and blood pressure is 78/42 mmHg. FAST is positive. Which statement best describes the FAST examination?

A. A 3.5-MHz convex-array transducer should be used.

B. The hepatorenal space, known as the Morison pouch, is viewed between the 11th and 12th ribs in the right midaxillary line.

C. The splenorenal space is evaluated between the 9th and 11th ribs in the left posterior axillary line.

D. The bladder should preferentially be full before the examination to allow better visualization of fluid in the pelvis.

E. All of the above.

ANSWER: E

COMMENTS: Focused assessment for the sonographic examination of trauma patients is performed as part of the ATLS secondary survey. A 3.5-MHz convex-array transducer is used to evaluate for the presence of fluid in the abdomen. Four areas are to be examined. The first is the pericardial window, which is viewed with the transducer placed subxiphoid. The hepatorenal space is evaluated in the right midaxillary line, between the 11th and 12th ribs. The splenorenal space is evaluated in the right posterior axillary line, between the 9th and 11th ribs. The last area examined is the pouch of Douglas in the pelvis. This rectouterine/rectovesical space is evaluated with the transducer placed approximately 3 cm above the pubic symphysis. A full bladder aids in detecting the presence of blood in this space; therefore Foley catheters should be placed after FAST has been performed.

Ref.: 13

8. A 23-year-old male is brought by emergency medical services (EMS) with a stab wound to the chest 2 cm medial from the right nipple. He was intubated en route; carotid pulse was present but faint, and pupils were responsive to light. After transferring the patient onto the gurney, no palpable pulses are appreciated. What is the next step in management?

A. Right tube thoracostomy

B. Right anterolateral thoracotomy

C. Median sternotomy

D. Left anterolateral thoracotomy

E. Left posterolateral thoracotomy

ANSWER: D

COMMENTS: An ED thoracotomy is performed for a select group of patients, with the overall survival rate being dependent on the mechanism and ranging from 1.5% to 19%. It is least successful in patients with injuries caused by a blunt mechanism and is therefore usually reserved for those who initially have vital signs present but then lose these signs in the ED. In patients with a penetrating mechanism, a thoracotomy is indicated for those who have lost their pulse and blood pressure either in the ED after initial evaluation or during transport to the ED. Thoracotomy is best used when cardiac tamponade or severe thoracic hemorrhage is suspected. The thoracotomy is performed on the left side via an anterolateral approach, regardless of the supposed side of the injury, and allows the release of pericardial tamponade, open cardiopulmonary resuscitation, and aortic cross-clamping. Resuscitative endovascular balloon occlusion of the aorta (REBOA) is a newer, less invasive technique that is being utilized to control intraabdominal and pelvic hemorrhage. Outcomes are still inconclusive, and studies are ongoing to establish its routine use as an adjunct or alternative to current therapy.

Ref.: 14–16

9. A 29-year-old female is the driver of an automobile involved in a high-speed motor vehicle crash. She is 30 weeks pregnant. She complains of abdominal pain but does not have peritoneal signs. Her HR is 105 beats/min, and blood pressure is 108/66 mmHg. Which of the following statements is true regarding trauma in a pregnant patient?

A. Less than 5% of all pregnancies are affected by trauma.

B. The uterus is protected by the bony pelvis until the beginning of the second trimester.

C. A woman of 25 weeks' gestation will have a palpable fundal height at approximately the level of the umbilicus.

D. Blood volume during pregnancy increases by approximately 30%.

E. Hypotensive patients should be placed in the right lateral position.

ANSWER: B

COMMENTS: Trauma is the leading cause of death in women of childbearing age and thus understanding the physiologic changes throughout the progression of pregnancy is imperative. However, since approximately 10% of pregnant patients are unaware of their pregnancy, a pregnancy test is recommended for all women of childbearing age early in their resuscitation. The most common cause of fetal death is maternal death. Therefore the focus of all initial resuscitative effort is directed toward the mother. Although the primary and secondary surveys for a pregnant patient are virtually identical to those of a nonpregnant patient, it is important to perform a focused abdominal examination. Normal physiologic changes in pregnancy include an increase in HR by 10 to 15 beats/min, a 25% increase in cardiac output, mild hypotension with average systolic blood pressures of 100, increased minute ventilation with resulting respiratory alkalosis, relative anemia, and a hypercoagulable state. Blood volume may increase by as much as 50% during pregnancy, which means that a patient may not have the tachycardia and hypotension usually associated with acute blood loss until almost 30% of total blood volume is lost. The pelvis typically protects the uterus until about 12 weeks. At about 20 weeks' gestation, the fundal height of the uterus approximates the umbilicus, and for every week of gestation past this stage, the height increases roughly by 1 cm. During the advanced stages of pregnancy, the uterus causes compression on the inferior vena cava (IVC), thereby leading to a decreased central venous return. Hypotensive patients should be placed in the left lateral position, which even in patients with a suspected spinal injury can be accomplished by securing the patient firmly to the backboard, which can then be tilted to the left. Evaluation of the fetus is accomplished by fetal heart tone monitoring and pelvic ultrasound. Tachycardia, bradycardia, and decelerations with contractions are all signs of potential fetal distress.

Ref.: 17

10. A 32-year-old male presents after being assaulted by a bat to his head, face, and torso. He opens his eyes to sternal rub, localizes to pain, and is only making groaning sounds. What is this patient's GCS?

A. 7

B. 8

C. 9

D. 10

E. 11

11. The patient in the previous scenario now only has extensor posturing. What is the next best step in management?

A. CT scan of the head

B. Continue to perform primary and secondary surveys

C. Bolus of hypertonic saline

D. Elevation of the head of the bed 30 degrees

E. Endotracheal intubation

12. A CT of the head is obtained demonstrating a 3-cm right-sided subdural hematoma with a 1-cm midline shift. The patient is taken to the operating room, and the hematoma is evacuated. Postoperatively, he is admitted to the intensive care unit (ICU), intubated, and sedated with an ICP monitor in place. Which of the following treatment measures can be used to maintain adequate cerebral perfusion pressure (CPP)?

A. Hyperventilation to a $PaCO_2$ of 25 mmHg

B. Mannitol, 1 g/kg IV

C. Hydrocortisone, 100 mg IV every 8 h for 3 days

D. Strict blood pressure control to a systolic range of 90 to 100 mmHg

E. Reverse Trendelenburg positioning of the bed at all times

ANSWERS: C, E, B

COMMENTS: The GCS score allows multiple health professionals to follow a patient's neurologic status. It is based on the evaluation of three examinations—eyes, verbal, and motor—that are independently recorded and added together to obtain an overall score. Table 11.1 lists the GCS score that correlates to particular clinical exam findings. The best examination from each category is utilized. The motor component is the most important regarding prognosis. As with all trauma patients, repeated examinations with a focus on the fundamentals of airway, breathing, and circulation are key. This patient demonstrates a decline in GCS score, which should prompt an evaluation of his airway and intubation. A GCS score of 8 is often used as a marker for the need for intubation to secure an airway. Any patient with a GCS score ≤ 14 or loss of consciousness should get a CT of the brain without contrast to evaluate for an intracranial injury; however, this is secondary in this patient. The overall goal in treating patients with a traumatic head injury is maintaining adequate cerebral blood flow. An estimate of this flow is obtained by calculating CPP (CPP = mean blood pressure − ICP). The goal CPP in an adult is 60 to 70 mmHg. Therefore patients should be aggressively volume resuscitated or started on vasopressors to maintain adequate mean blood pressure. ICP monitors are indicated in patients with a GCS score of 3 to 8 and either (1) an abnormal finding on CT of the head or (2) any two of the following: (a) age older than 40 years, (b) posturing response to pain, or (c) systolic blood pressure less than 90 mmHg.

TABLE 11.1 Glasgow Coma Scale

Eye Response (4)	Verbal Response (5)	Motor Response (6)
		6 = obeys commands
	5 = oriented	5 = localizes pain
4 = open spontaneously	4 = confused	4 = withdraws from pain
3 = open to command	3 = inappropriate words	3 = flexion posturing
2 = open to pain	2 = incomprehensible sounds	2 = extension posturing
1 = no eye opening	1 = no verbal response	1 = no motor response

Overall, there is a 5% infection and 1% hematoma formation rate associated with ICP-monitoring catheters. Treatment measures used to decrease ICP include elevation of the head of the bed to 30 degrees or more, hyperventilation of patients to a $PaCO_2$ of 35 mmHg, barbiturates, and mannitol at a dose of 1 g/kg IV. $PaCO_2$ should not be kept below 30 mmHg to avoid worsening the cerebral ischemia. Steroids do not have a role in the treatment of acute traumatic head injury.

Ref.: 18–20

13. A 21-year-old male is brought in by EMTs on a backboard with a cervical collar in place after a bar fight that included falling over a stool. The patient is belligerent, and urine drug screen is positive for methamphetamines and alcohol. Primary survey is normal, and secondary survey reveals several facial fractures and multiple right hand fractures. What is the best way to evaluate this patient's c-spine and remove his collar?

A. Clinical examination

B. Radiographic series of the cervical spine—cross-table lateral, anteroposterior, and open-mouth view of the dens

C. Flexion–extension x-rays

D. Magnetic resonance imaging (MRI) cervical spine followed by clinical examination when appropriate

E. CT cervical spine followed by clinical examination when appropriate

ANSWER: E

COMMENTS: Clearance of cervical spine precautions relies on the patient's ability to participate in the examination. In an awake patient with minimal risk factors, clinical examination alone is appropriate. In an obtunded patient, many accepted algorithms are present to evaluate for injury. According to the Eastern Association for the Surgery of Trauma, obtunded patients should have a CT of the cervical spine. If no focal neurologic deficits are present and the patient is likely to be obtunded for greater than 72 h, the collar can be removed with a negative CT scan only. Alternatively, MRI evaluation can be added to the workup. If both studies are negative, the collar can be removed. If a person is likely to become appropriate within 24 h as determined by an alert mental state without distracting injuries, CT should be completed, and if negative, it should be followed by a clinical examination when the patient is appropriate. Prolonged use of a cervical collar has been linked to pressure ulcers, increased ICP, prolonged ICU stay, and pneumonia and should be avoided. CT allows for evaluation of the bony elements of the spine while MRI is best for soft tissue, the spinal cord, intervertebral disks, and ligaments. Patients with spinal cord injuries, especially in the cervical area, may require early intubation for airway protection and aggressive fluid resuscitation and vasopressors to counter the neurogenic shock due to the loss of autonomic innervation. These patients typically present with hypotension and relative bradycardia. Regardless of suspicion for the neurogenic cause of hypotension, full primary and secondary surveys should be completed to rule out the hemorrhagic shock.

Ref.: 21, 22

14. A 35-year-old male presents after being stabbed in the neck. A 3-cm wound is present at the base of the neck, just right of midline above the sternum. An expanding hematoma is noted. The patient is intubated for airway protection and taken to the operating room for exploration. What is the best initial incision to expose and control this injury?

A. Anterior border of the sternocleidomastoid muscle

B. Median sternotomy

C. Right anterolateral thoracotomy

D. Collar incision

E. Right infraclavicular incision

ANSWER: A

COMMENTS: The neck is divided into three zones, and management of penetrating injuries is based on the affected area. Zone 1 is most inferior from the base of the neck to the cricoid cartilage and is exposed with an incision along the anterior border of the sternocleidomastoid muscle with possible extension into a median sternotomy. Zone 2 extends from the cricoid cartilage to the angle of the mandible and is best approached with an incision along the anterior border of the sternocleidomastoid muscle. Zone 3 is most superior from the angle of the mandible to the skull base. It is very difficult to approach and may require nasotracheal intubation, division of the digastric muscle, and subluxation of the mandible. Endovascular techniques may be also utilized in this area. The aerodigestive tract, vascular system, and the spine all run through the neck and must be evaluated for injury. This can include a combination of a barium swallow followed by an esophagogastroduodenoscopy (EGD), bronchoscopy, a CT angiogram, or an MRI based on clinical symptoms.

Ref.: 23, 24

15. A 19-year-old male presents after a high-speed head-on motor vehicle crash into a tree. He was the unrestrained driver and hit the steering wheel with his chest. He has a sternal fracture, broken left clavicle, and a left pneumothorax. A left chest tube is placed with a resolution of the pneumothorax. What is the best initial evaluation for a blunt cardiac injury (BCI)?

A. Serial electrocardiogram (ECG) only

B. Serial troponins only

C. Echocardiogram only

D. Admission ECG and troponin

E. Admission echocardiogram and serial ECG

ANSWER: D

COMMENTS: The best way to evaluate for a significant BCI is an initial ECG and troponin. If these are both normal, BCI can be ruled out. Patients with significant blunt trauma to the anterior chest with associated injuries, including, but not limited to, rib and sternal fractures, pulmonary contusions, hemothorax, pneumothorax, and polytrauma, should be screened. Within this population, the incidence of BCI is 13%. Patients who have abnormal findings on EKG, an elevated troponin, or hemodynamic instability require telemetry monitoring for 24 h. These patients are at risk for a lethal arrhythmia, which may require immediate defibrillation. A transthoracic or transesophageal echocardiogram is also indicated. Most common findings include myocardial contusion and right ventricle and right atrial injuries. Left-sided, valvular, and coronary artery injuries are rare and may require cardiopulmonary bypass for repair. A subset of patients that will have abnormal ECG and elevated troponin are those who had an acute myocardial infarction immediately prior to or during their trauma. Cardiac CT or MRI can be used to distinguish these patients who may benefit from cardiac catheterization and anticoagulation.

Ref.: 25–27

16. A 26-year-old male presents with a stab wound to the right chest about 1 cm lateral to the sternum between the second and third ribs. The patient is awake but confused, his HR is 100 beats/min, and his blood pressure is 102/54 mmHg. He is taken to the operating room after initial resuscitation. What is the best approach to expose this injury?

A. Median sternotomy

B. Right anterolateral thoracotomy

C. Right posterolateral thoracotomy

D. Right supraclavicular incision

E. Incision over the stab wound

ANSWER: A

COMMENTS: Penetrating thoracic trauma is common, and the choice of incision can be critical in exposing and repairing the injury. For an unstable patient in the emergency room (ER), a left anterolateral thoracotomy that can be extended across the sternum onto the right chest can provide maximal exposure to the heart and pericardium, root of the ascending aorta, descending aorta to cross-clamp, and pulmonary hilum. A median sternotomy allows access to the ascending aorta, the innominate artery including the proximal right carotid and subclavian arteries, the left common carotid artery, and the heart. The distal right subclavian artery can be approached via a right supraclavicular incision with resection of the middle part of the clavicle. The proximal descending aorta and left subclavian artery are best exposed via a left posterolateral thoracotomy; however, this is not a favorable position in emergency surgery. Alternatively, a left third intercostal space anterolateral thoracotomy and a supraclavicular incision with resection of the middle part of the clavicle can be used. A median sternotomy can join these incisions, completing a trapdoor incision; however, this adds significant morbidity to the procedure. Placing a patient on cardiopulmonary bypass can assist with the repair of proximal thoracic vessels; however, this requires additional time and expertise.

Ref.: 14, 28

17. A 27-year-old female is brought in after a high-speed motor vehicle collision (MVC). The patient was intubated on scene for GCS 8. HR is 98 beats/min, blood pressure is 110/58 mmHg, and chest x-ray demonstrates a widened mediastinum. CT imaging demonstrates a 2-cm intracranial epidural hematoma with midline shift, a moderate amount of fluid in the abdomen, and a pseudoaneurysm of the descending thoracic aorta. What is correct regarding the management of a blunt aortic injury?

A. Repair of the aorta needs to be completed emergently to reduce the risk of rupture.

B. Mean arterial pressure should be maintained greater than 85 mmHg.

C. Open repair of the injury has less morbidity and mortality.

D. Most patients with a blunt aortic injury die on the scene.

E. The most common site for an aortic injury is at the root of the aorta.

ANSWER: D

COMMENTS: The reported incidence of a blunt thoracic aortic injury is approximately 0.5%; however, the real incidence is likely much higher due to the vast majority of patients dying prior to arrival to a hospital. The most common aortic injuries include pseudoaneurysms, dissections, intimal flaps, and transections. This occurs most often just distal to the takeoff of the left subclavian artery on the medial wall due to shear forces on a relatively fixed part of the aorta. Characteristic x-ray findings of a widened mediastinum, left apical capping, depression of left mainstem bronchus, and loss of aortic knob may initially be seen, raising suspicion for injury, and diagnosis can be confirmed with a CT angiogram of the chest. Treatment includes strict blood pressure control with restrictive fluid resuscitation and short-acting β-blockers such as esmolol titrated to maintain systolic blood pressures between 90 and 100 mmHg. This has reduced the incidence of rupture to less than 5% of patients who present to the hospital. Repair is now routinely delayed until other life-threatening injuries are definitively managed with minimum risk. Both open and endovascular techniques can be utilized, with recent literature demonstrating reduced morbidity and mortality with endovascular approaches. However, patients may suffer from complications such as endoleaks and access vessel injuries that may require additional procedures.

Ref.: 29, 30

18. A 41-year-old male falls from a 12-foot ladder and lands on his left side. He fractures left ribs 2 to 9 with a flail segment, resulting in pneumothorax. After the chest tube is placed, what is the next best step in management?

A. Pain control with an epidural

B. Incentive spirometer

C. Early ambulation

D. Conservative fluid management

E. All of the above

ANSWER: E

COMMENTS: Rib fractures are one of the most common injuries in trauma. Chest x-rays diagnose less than 50% of rib fractures, while CT scan detects nearly 100% of significant fractures. Fractures of ribs 1 to 3 can be associated with major thoracic vascular injuries, while fractures of ribs 9 to 12 can puncture intraabdominal organs such as the liver and spleen. The ideal treatment of rib fractures is centered on pain control and aggressive pulmonary toilet. Pain regimens include scheduled IV and per os (PO) medications, patient-controlled analgesia (PCA), intercostal blocks, and epidurals. Pulmonary toilet includes aggressive suctioning, deep breathing and coughing, incentive spirometer use, and early ambulation to decrease atelectasis. Conservative fluid management is encouraged to decrease pulmonary edema, which can worsen pulmonary contusions that are associated with rib fractures. Rib plating is making a resurgence with many proponents stating that early rib plating within 72 h can decrease many of the complications associated with severely displaced rib fractures, including prolonged need for ventilator support and pneumonia.

Ref.: 31, 32

19. A 37-year-old female comes in with a stab wound to the right chest just lateral to the sternal border. HR is 130 beats/min, blood pressure is 74/58 mmHg, and jugular venous distention is noted on examination with muffled heart sounds. Which option provides the appropriate diagnosis and treatment?

A. Tension pneumothorax: right thoracotomy

B. Tension pneumothorax: right tube thoracostomy

C. Tension pneumothorax: median sternotomy

D. Cardiac tamponade: pericardial window

E. Cardiac tamponade: left tube thoracostomy

ANSWER: D

COMMENTS: Many life-threatening injuries to the chest, such as a massive hemothorax, tension pneumothorax, open chest wound, and cardiac tamponade, must be identified on clinical examination and require prompt intervention. The clinical examination requires visual inspection of the chest rise for symmetry, open wound with air bubbles, paradoxical motion, and jugular venous distention. Palpation can detect crepitus and instability of ribs and sternum, while auscultation identifies absent or diminished breath sounds or dullness of heart tones. Extended FAST can also be used as part of the primary survey to detect a pneumothorax or pericardial effusion. Once the diagnosis is determined, immediate intervention must take place. A tension pneumothorax is classically described with absent breath sounds, hypotension, distended neck veins, and tracheal deviation and requires urgent chest tube placement. Many start with needle decompression; however, many times this intervention is done incorrectly, provides a false sense of security, and delays definitive treatment with tube thoracostomy. Cardiac tamponade presents with distended neck veins, muffled heart sounds, and hypotension due to fluid in the pericardial sac, decreased right atrial filling, and decreased venous return. This requires a pericardiocentesis or pericardial window.

Ref.: 1, 31

20. A 21-year-old man is taken to the ED with a gunshot wound to the right side of his chest. HR is 126 beats/min and blood pressure is 88/46 mmHg. A right-sided chest tube is placed, with the return of 1200 mL of blood. He is resuscitated with 2 L of lactated Ringer's solution, and his vital signs return to within normal limits. His chest tube output is rechecked 4 h later, and the total amount in the collection container is 2300 mL. What is the next most appropriate step in management?

A. Chest CT

B. Stat hemoglobin/hematocrit

C. Right thoracotomy

D. Left anterolateral thoracotomy

E. Admission to the ICU for continuous cardiac monitoring and pulse oximetry

ANSWER: C

COMMENTS: This patient has a massive hemothorax, which is defined as greater than 1500 mL of blood loss on initial placement of tube thoracostomy, continuing loss greater than 200 mL/h for 4 h, or a total of 2500 mL in 24 h after the initial placement. This is an indication that there is ongoing bleeding that requires surgical intervention. Additional indications for an urgent thoracotomy include tracheal, esophageal, great vessel, or lung injury. Penetrating injury to the lung parenchyma may present with a large and persistent air leak. This may be best managed with a tractotomy, which utilizes a stapler passed into the tract through the lung parenchyma to control the air leak and bleeding.

Ref.: 14, 31

21. A 38-year-old car mechanic is taken to the ED after having been pinned underneath a car. On chest radiography, multiple rib fractures are noted, as well as an air-fluid level consistent with the stomach being above the level of the left diaphragm. Which of the following statements regarding this injury is true?

A. Right-sided diaphragmatic rupture is more common than left-sided rupture.

B. There is a 30% incidence of coexisting pelvic fractures.

C. The best initial radiographic assessment for this type of injury is FAST.

D. In most acute diaphragmatic ruptures, repair can be completed with primary repair.

E. There is a 60% incidence of a coexisting thoracic aortic injury.

ANSWER: D

COMMENTS: Diaphragmatic injury/rupture occurs in 3%–5% of patients suffering major blunt abdominal trauma. Although this injury is uncommon, it is associated with a high incidence of coexistent injuries, including pelvic fractures (15%), hepatic and splenic injuries (40%), and rupture of the thoracic aorta (5%). The left side is affected three times more often than the right side. The use of CT imaging of these patients has significantly decreased the incidence of missed injury. Once a diagnosis of diaphragmatic rupture has been made, treatment is operative. In this situation, in which large diaphragmatic rupture is strongly suspected, laparoscopy is typically avoided because insufflation of the abdomen may cause a tension pneumothorax. However, laparoscopy may be useful to evaluate for a penetrating diaphragm injury. In the acute setting of a blunt diaphragmatic injury, laparotomy is the preferred operative approach. It allows reduction of any organs back into the abdominal cavity, as well as thorough inspection of all intraperitoneal contents. In the acute setting, even large defects can be closed primarily with a # 0- or # 1-monofilament or braided nonabsorbable suture. Diagnosing small diaphragmatic injuries can be difficult in as much as up to almost half of all patients have normal findings on physical examination at initial evaluation. Missed diaphragmatic injuries tend to enlarge over time, which may lead to herniation and strangulation of abdominal organs. Primary repair is not usually feasible because of the rapid atrophy of diaphragmatic muscle fibers. A thoracotomy is generally performed for a chronic diaphragmatic hernia since it provides better access to the adhesions usually found in the chest.

Ref.: 33, 34

22. A 46-year-old female presents after a high-speed head-on motor vehicle crash. The patient was wearing a seatbelt and is noted to have an abrasion across her neck and abdomen. CT of the abdomen demonstrates no solid organ injury and no pneumoperitoneum with trace free fluid in the pelvis. Abdominal examination is benign. What is the next appropriate management step?

A. Nil per os (NPO), admit for serial abdominal examinations

B. NPO, admit for serial CT scans

C. Diet and discharge home

D. Immediate repeat CT with PO contrast

E. Immediate exploratory laparotomy

ANSWER: A

COMMENTS: The incidence of a blunt small bowel injury is less than 1% of all traumatic injuries reported; however, it is associated with significant morbidity and mortality. A high index of suspicion must be used when evaluating for a blunt bowel injury. CT findings can be nonspecific with bowel wall thickening, fat stranding, mesenteric edema, and free fluid without solid organ injury. The presence of seatbelt sign or a lumbar vertebral body fracture significantly increases the risk of a small bowel injury. A patient without signs of peritonitis who is alert and appropriate can be monitored with clinical examinations. CT with oral contrast has not been shown to enhance the detection of these injuries and can lead to a delay of treatment and risk aspiration. If the patient has an unreliable examination, DPL may be attempted to look for amylase, bilirubin, particulates, or WBC > 500. Alternatively, a diagnostic laparoscopy or laparotomy may be completed.

Ref.: 1, 35

23. The patient from the previous scenario also has a CT angiogram of her neck performed. She is found to have a right carotid artery dissection. The patient has a normal neurologic examination with no deficits. No other injuries are present. What is the next step in management?

A. Operating room for neck exploration

B. Perform endovascular stenting

C. Anticoagulation with heparin and aspirin

D. No intervention, discharge home with follow-up CT angiogram in 1 week

E. Repeat imaging with formal angiogram to confirm known lesion

ANSWER: C

COMMENTS: Blunt cerebrovascular injury (BCVI) refers to injuries to the carotid and vertebral arteries. Patients at risk include those with a neck hematoma or arterial bleeding, bruit, neurologic deficit, CT brain with stroke, Lefort II or III fractures, basilar skull fracture involving the carotid canal, cervical spine fracture or ligamentous injury, diffuse axonal injury with GCS ≤ 6, and near-hanging with anoxia. These patients should be screened with a CT angiogram of the neck. Some may require a traditional angiogram if CT images are inadequate. Injuries are graded from I to V. Grade I injury is a dissection with <25% luminal narrowing, while grade II is ≥25% narrowing, a thrombus, or intimal flap. A pseudoaneurysm is a grade III lesion, and total occlusion is grade IV. These are all treated with systemic anticoagulation with heparin, with a partial thromboplastin time (PTT) goal of 40 to 50 and an antiplatelet agent, aspirin or clopidogrel. Anticoagulation has decreased the incidence of stroke in these patients, which most often occurs during the first week after injury. Grade V injuries are transections with free extravasation and require immediate operative or endovascular management. Repeat imaging is completed 7 to 10 days after the initial injury. If no lesion is seen, the injury has healed and antithrombotic therapy is stopped.

Ref.: 1, 36

24. An 8-year-old child hits a curb with his bicycle, which causes him to flip over the handlebars. He had no initial symptoms and was monitored at home by his parents. However, 2 days after the incident, he begins having nonbilious emesis. He is brought to the ED and undergoes CT of the abdomen and pelvis, which demonstrates a duodenal hematoma. What is the next step in management?

A. Initiation of NPO status and gastric decompression with a nasogastric tube

B. EGD to assess for luminal compromise

C. Drainage of the hematoma via laparoscopy

D. Drainage of the hematoma via laparotomy

E. Resection of the injured portion of the duodenum with primary anastomoses

ANSWER: A

COMMENTS: Blunt injuries to the duodenum can be difficult to diagnose. Duodenal hematomas typically occur up to 3 days after injury with a gastric outlet obstruction type of clinical picture. The duodenal lumen is narrowed because of the hematoma itself and the associated edema. CT with oral contrast enhancement and upper gastrointestinal studies are useful in diagnosing this condition. If no other indication exists for exploration, treatment is conservative and consists of placement of a nasogastric tube for decompression and parenteral nutrition. Typically, these hematomas and their symptoms resolve within 7 to 15 days after injury. Operative exploration is reserved for patients in whom the symptoms do not resolve within this period.

Ref.: 37

25. A patient with multiple gunshot wounds to the abdomen is taken to the operating room. On exploration she is found to have two small holes in the first part of the duodenum and a 2-cm lateral defect in the second part of the duodenum. The ampulla is intact and cannulated. Resulting pancreaticocholangiogram demonstrates normal anatomy. What is the best management for this patient?

A. Primary closure with internal drainage

B. Pancreaticoduodenectomy

C. Gastrojejunostomy

D. Omental patch only

E. Serosal patch only

ANSWER: A

COMMENTS: Management options for duodenal injuries include repair, reinforcement, intraluminal decompression, and enteric diversion. These can all be used in varying degrees depending on the nature of the injury and surgeon's preference. Two-layer primary repair may be completed for small injuries; however, with injuries involving the retroperitoneal duodenum or greater than 50% of the lumen, additional steps should be taken to prevent complications. Primary repairs can be reinforced with additional tissue such as a rotational flap of peritoneum from the abdominal wall, omentum, or a piece of small bowel (Thal patch). Internal drainage to reduce intraluminal pressure can be completed by passing a nasogastric tube postpyloric into the proximal duodenum or retrograde from the jejunum into the proximal duodenum. An enteric diversion while maintaining enteral nutrition can be completed with a Billroth II gastrojejunostomy or placement of a nasojejunal tube. A temporary alternative is a pyloric exclusion with a stapler or hand-sewn closure of the pylorus and a distal feeding jejunostomy; however, most open up within 4 weeks. Pancreaticoduodenectomy is only indicated in trauma if the damage to both the duodenum and pancreas is beyond repair and the patient is hemodynamically stable. Assessment of the pancreas and extrahepatic biliary tree is also mandated with duodenal injuries due to their close proximity to the duodenum.

Ref.: 32, 37

26. A 44-year-old male presents with a single gunshot wound to the abdomen. He is hemodynamically stable and taken to the operating room. On exploration, his injuries are found to be limited to four small bowel injuries 8 cm apart, each with destruction of 20% of the bowel wall, and a through-and-through injury to the ascending colon with destruction of 30% of the bowel wall. How should these injuries be managed?

A. Resection and anastomosis of the small bowel injuries and primary repair of the colon injury

B. Primary repair of both the small bowel and colon injuries

C. Primary repair of the small bowel injuries, primary repair of the colon injury, and creation of a diverting ileostomy

D. Resection of the small bowel injuries and exteriorization of the colon injury as a colostomy

E. Resection and anastomosis of all injuries

ANSWER: A

COMMENTS: Treatment of bowel injuries relies on the amount of damage to the viscera and stability of the patient. Patients who are hemodynamically stable and have injuries that involve less than 50% of the circumferential bowel with no vascular disruption can undergo primary repair without the need for diversion. Resection is indicated for injuries involving greater than 50% of the wall circumference, multiple injuries in a short segment, or both. Anastomosis can be hand-sewn or stapled. However, there may be a slight decrease in the number of complications with a hand-sewn technique. This can be completed with a running absorbable full-thickness suture for the inner layer and an interrupted silk suture for the outer seromuscular layer. Complications occur in approximately 10% of cases and include anastomotic leaks, deep space abscesses, and enterocutaneous fistulas. They are increased in damage control cases and those with other intraabdominal injuries, especially pancreaticoduodenal injuries. Broad-spectrum antibiotics should be given preoperatively and discontinued 24 h postoperatively.

Ref.: 11, 12, 35

27. A 42-year-old male unrestrained driver struck his steering wheel against his abdomen during a motor vehicle crash. He is hemodynamically stable but complains of abdominal pain. CT of the abdomen demonstrates a moderate amount of free fluid with no solid organ injuries. He undergoes an exploratory laparotomy, at which time complete transection of the pancreatic neck is found. What is the most appropriate management of this injury?

A. Roux-en-Y pancreaticojejunostomy to the distal end of the pancreas with oversewing of the proximal pancreatic stump
B. Distal pancreatectomy with oversewing of the proximal pancreatic stump
C. Primary repair and drainage of the pancreatic duct
D. Pancreaticoduodenectomy
E. Total pancreatectomy

ANSWER: B

COMMENTS: Operative management of pancreatic injuries centers on the location of the injury and whether the duct is involved. Approximately 50% of the pancreas is located on either side of the superior mesenteric artery. For pancreatic wounds with an intact duct, drainage of the area with soft closed suction drains suffices. If the main pancreatic duct is injured to the left of the mesenteric vessels, as in this patient, distal pancreatectomy with drainage of the proximal stump is indicated. The proximal pancreatic duct should be individually ligated with nonabsorbable suture, if possible, and the parenchymal tissue oversewn or stapled across with a stapler. The spleen should be preserved if the patient's hemodynamic status allows. Roux-en-Y pancreaticojejunostomy to the distal end of the pancreas with oversewing of the proximal pancreatic stump carries a high rate of leakage. A pancreaticoduodenectomy and total pancreatectomy would be reserved for injuries that involve extensive devitalization of the duodenum and pancreas. Primary repair is technically difficult and does not address the transected pancreatic tissue. Intraoperative cholangiography and pancreaticogram, or postoperative endoscopic retrograde cholangiopancreatography (ERCP) or magnetic resonance cholangiopancreatography (MRCP), can aid in defining critical anatomy.

Ref.: 37

28. During exploratory laparotomy in a patient with multiple gunshot wounds to the abdomen, a through-and-through gunshot wound is noted in the left lobe of the liver. Brisk bleeding is seen from the bullet track. Which is an appropriate operative maneuver for this injury?

A. Pringle maneuver
B. Tractotomy
C. Omental packing
D. Large mattress sutures traversing the bullet track
E. All of the above

ANSWER: E

COMMENTS: With regard to hepatic injuries, there are three overall goals of treatment: (1) control of hemorrhage, (2) debridement of nonviable tissue, and (3) adequate drainage. Multiple operative techniques can be used to establish control of bleeding, and often a combination of these techniques is used. The Pringle maneuver is direct compression of the portal triad, either manually or with a vascular clamp. This is helpful in identifying whether the bleeding source is from the hepatic artery or portal vein versus hepatic veins or retrohepatic vena cava. The clamping time should be minimized as much as possible with 5 min of flow for every 15 min clamped. These patients tend to be hypovolemic and, as a rule, do not tolerate hepatic ischemia well. Omental packing is performed by first creating a pedicle of omentum and then placing it across or in the defect. This creates a well-vascularized "packing" of the liver that also has its own natural hemostatic properties. Large mattress sutures using a 0-chromic on a blunt tipped needle work by compressing the bullet track with the surrounding liver parenchyma. A tractotomy is the act of opening the already present wound to fully examine the track and identify the bleeding vessels. This then allows directed individual vessel ligation. Historically, selective hepatic artery ligation has been used and involves ligation of the hepatic artery branch to the involved lobe. Although this is still a viable option, it is associated with a fairly high rate of abscess formation and hepatic necrosis.

Ref.: 38, 39

29. A 32-year-old female is a restrained passenger in a high-speed motor vehicle crash. Initial workup shows an HR of 95 beats/min, blood pressure of 110/82 mmHg, and hemoglobin of 12.2 g/dL. On FAST, a moderate amount of fluid is seen in the RUQ, between the liver, kidney, and diaphragm. A grade IV liver laceration is seen on CT with no active extravasation. Her vital signs 6 h after admission are an HR of 100 beats/min and blood pressure of 105/80 mmHg. What is the next most appropriate step?

A. Exploratory laparotomy
B. Angiography
C. Repeated FAST
D. Diagnostic laparoscopy
E. Repeated hemoglobin determination

ANSWER: E

COMMENTS: The overall success rate for nonoperative management of blunt hepatic injuries is about 90%. Patients with grade IV and V injuries are able to be treated without surgery between 75% and 80% of the time. Requirements for nonoperative therapy include hemodynamic stability, no signs or symptoms of peritonitis, and a transfusion requirement of no more than two to four units of packed red blood cells. This patient is hemodynamically stable, and therefore further imaging with CT is warranted. The initial CT can not only localize the injury but, in the case of solid organ injuries, also provide information regarding active hemorrhage. The patient should be closely monitored in an intensive care setting with serial abdominal examinations and hemoglobin determinations. Angiography is a helpful adjunct to nonoperative treatment, but it is usually reserved for situations in which active extravasation or a "blush" is seen on CT. Repeated CT is advised for patients who do experience a decrease in their hemoglobin to reevaluate the liver damage and to look for any active extravasation that would be amenable to angiographic embolization.

Ref.: 1, 38, 39

30. The patient in the previous scenario is discharged home on hospital day 4 without needing operative intervention. She returns to the clinic 2 months after discharge with persistent dull continuous RUQ pain. She denies any fevers or chills, and all laboratory studies, including a hepatic function panel, are within normal limits. CT of the abdomen and pelvis is performed and reveals a localized homogeneous fluid collection directly adjacent to the liver. What is the correct diagnosis and treatment?

A. Hemobilia: exploratory laparotomy and ligation of bleeding vessel
B. Hemobilia: ERCP with stent placement
C. Biloma: image-guided percutaneous drainage
D. Biloma: exploratory laparotomy with external drainage
E. Hepatic abscess: angiogram

ANSWER: C

COMMENTS: Because of the increasing number of patients with significant liver lacerations being treated nonoperatively, posttreatment complications are being encountered more often. Such complications include hemobilia, biloma, hepatic necrosis, and abscess. Hemobilia occurs when a connection exists between the biliary and arterial systems, and it is typically manifested as RUQ pain, melena, and jaundice. Hemobilia can be diagnosed by CT with IV contrast enhancement or upper endoscopy and is usually treated by angiography with embolization. Patients with hepatic necrosis or abscess (or both) typically have RUQ pain, fever, leukocytosis, and, at times, localized peritonitis. It can be appreciated on CT with IV contrast enhancement as nonperfused liver parenchyma sometimes associated with a heterogeneous fluid collection. This condition warrants laparotomy with debridement. Bilomas occur as a result of leakage of bile and typically close spontaneously over time. The fluid collections themselves are best treated with image-guided percutaneous drainage when localized, as in this patient. If the fluid collection is not amenable to percutaneous drainage, ERCP is recommended because biliary stents and sphincterotomy can reduce intrahepatic biliary pressure and increase healing.

Ref.: 1, 38, 39

31. A 22-year-old construction worker falls off of a ladder and lands on his left side. He fractures left ribs 6 to 12 and has a grade II splenic laceration. HR is 88 beats/min, and blood pressure is 110/76 mmHg. Hemoglobin is 12.3 g/dL. The patient is admitted to the ICU for serial hemoglobins and monitoring. Six hours later, the HR is 104 beats/min, blood pressure is 100/68 mmHg, and hemoglobin is 9.1 g/dL. What is the next step in management?

A. Exploratory laparoscopy
B. Exploratory laparotomy
C. Angiography
D. Continue serial examinations
E. Transfuse two units, and continue serial examinations

ANSWER: C

COMMENTS: The annual incidence of a blunt splenic injury is 40,000 patients, of which over 90% are managed without surgery. Nonoperative management, including observation, serial hemaglobins and abdominal examinations, limited blood transfusions, and angiography with possible embolization, is utilized for the remaining majority of patients. Although controversy exists regarding who should undergo angiography, the literature suggests that those with contrast blush or extravasation on initial CT or American Association for the Surgery of Trauma (AAST) grade III to V splenic injuries may benefit the most from intervention, reducing the need for delayed splenectomy. This strategy is limited to hemodynamically stable patients with reliable examinations. Complications associated with angiography and embolization include splenic abscesses, acute kidney injury, hematomas, and coil migration. Patients should be observed in the hospital or can be discharged home after 24 to 72 h of monitoring, with strict instructions to return to the hospital for any signs of bleeding. Most patients who fail nonoperative management require a splenectomy within 5 days of the injury. Transfusions of greater than two to four units of packed red blood cells, hypotension, tachycardia, or peritonitis are triggers to convert to operative management.

Ref.: 40, 41

32. The patient in the previous scenario is being monitored in the ICU. HR is now 122 beats/min, blood pressure is 88/56 mmHg, and hemoglobin is 8.2 g/dL. What is the next step in management?

A. Exploratory laparoscopy
B. Exploratory laparotomy
C. Angiography
D. Continue serial examinations
E. Transfuse two units, and continue serial examinations

ANSWER: B

COMMENTS: Patients with hypotension, tachycardia, or other injuries that limit reliable serial examinations should undergo urgent splenectomy. In this case scenario, the patient initially was appropriate for embolization but deteriorated despite intervention and became unstable, necessitating a trip to the operating room for a splenectomy. Although giving a transfusion is warranted, due to the significant drop in hemoglobin, tachycardia, and hypotension, surgical intervention is indicated.

Patients who respond to resuscitation and become relatively stable in the operating room with a limited splenic injury may benefit from splenorrhaphy or partial splenectomy. This can be completed by ligating the blood supply to the damaged part of the spleen, letting the tissue demarcate, and debriding nonviable tissue. The remaining spleen can be wrapped in an absorbable mesh or primarily repaired by approximating the splenic capsule with a pledgeted mattress suture. Patients who undergo splenectomy should be vaccinated against encapsulated organisms, specifically pneumococcus, meningococcus, and *Haemophilus influenzae*, prior to discharge. Immune function remains preserved after embolization.

Ref.: 42, 43

33. Which option provides the most appropriate management for the injury described?

A. Blunt mechanism: zone 3 nonexpanding retroperitoneal hematoma: exploration
B. Blunt mechanism: zone 2 expanding retroperitoneal hematoma: angiogram
C. Penetrating mechanism: zone 1 expanding hematoma: observation
D. Penetrating mechanism: zone 1 nonexpanding hematoma: exploration
E. Penetrating mechanism: zone 2 nonexpanding hematoma: angiogram

ANSWER: D

COMMENTS: The major abdominal vasculature is located in the retroperitoneum, which is divided into three zones. Management of injuries is based on the mechanism, blunt versus penetrating, if there is a concern for ongoing bleeding, and which zone is involved. Zone I is the central retroperitoneum and contains the aorta and its branches, the vena cava, and the proximal renal vessels. The lateral areas are zone II and contain the kidney, proximal collecting system, and distal renal vessels. Zone III is the pelvis and its contents including the iliac vessels. Most hematomas resulting from blunt trauma should not be explored other than zone 1 injuries or pulsatile expanding hematomas. All penetrating injuries must be explored due to the risk of injury to other retroperitoneal organs such as the duodenum, pancreas, colon, rectum, and bladder. The only exception is a stable retrohepatic hematoma. Obtaining proximal and distal control prior to exploration of a hematoma is ideal but not always possible. With blunt trauma, angiography with embolization may be used as an adjunct in nonexpanding hematomas.

Ref.: 1, 11

34. A patient presents with multiple gunshot wounds to the extremity and right lower quadrant. In the operating room, upon entry into the abdomen, a large amount of hemoperitoneum is encountered and all quadrants are packed immediately. Upon reinspection, the patient is noted to have an injury to the infrahepatic vena cava. How can you best expose this injury?

A. Transect the right renal artery
B. Right medial visceral rotation
C. Left medial visceral rotation
D. Transect the pancreas
E. All of the above

ANSWER: B

COMMENTS: Rapid exposure and control of abdominal vessels are critical in patients with life-threatening hemorrhage. The principles of proximal and distal control should always be attempted prior to entering a contained hematoma. However, once bleeding has started and the injury is identified, direct pressure with a finger may allow for temporary control. Left medial visceral rotation, which requires the division of the lateral attachments of the colon and spleen allowing for mobilization to the right toward midline, exposes the aorta and the left renal hilum. The distal aorta and iliac arteries can be exposed by lifting up the transverse colon and dissecting at the base of the mesocolon. The IVC and right renal hilum are best approached with right medial visceral rotation, which divides the colon and duodenum's lateral peritoneal attachments allowing for mobilization of the ascending and transverse colon, duodenum, and pancreas cephalad and to the left toward the midline. Suprahepatic IVC may require the division of the diaphragm or even a sternotomy for control within the pericardial sac. Supraceliac control of the aorta at the diaphragm can temporarily curb the bleeding when the patient is in extremis and can be used while attempting definitive vascular control. The vena cava can be controlled with sponge sticks placed proximal and distal to the injury. There are a few special maneuvers that can be utilized for repair of intraabdominal vascular injuries. Exposure of the back wall of the vena cava can be done through an anterior venotomy, allowing for repair. Superior mesenteric artery injuries may require transection of the pancreas for exposure, and the right iliac vein may require transection and subsequent repair of the right iliac artery for exposure.

Ref.: 28, 39

35. A 23-year-old male presents with multiple gunshot wounds to the abdomen and right leg. During exploration, the patient is found to have a grade IV liver laceration and multiple enterotomies. He also has a destructive injury to his proximal superficial femoral artery with no distal pulses. Anesthesia tells you that the patient's temperature is 36°C; he has received 10 units of product and is on vasopressors. Most recent arterial blood gas (ABG) shows a pH of 7.15 and a lactic acid that is twice the normal value. Which of these is a trigger to transition to damage control surgery in this patient?

A. Body temperature less than 37°C
B. Arterial pH less than 7.2
C. Base deficit greater than 6
D. Hemoglobin less than 7
E. Oxygen saturation less than 90%

ANSWER: B

COMMENTS: Damage control surgery is a staged resuscitation strategy with three phases that include the initial operation, resuscitation in the ICU, and return to the operating room for definitive treatment. Goals for the initial procedure include control of hemorrhage with sutures and packing, limiting fecal contamination and restoring critical blood flow. In the ICU, the patient is aggressively resuscitated with blood products, fluids, and vasopressors with the goal of obtaining a normal physiologic state. Once the patient is stable, a plan can be made to return to the operating room for definitive surgical management and evaluation for missed injuries. The trigger to employ a damage control strategy is metabolic failure defined by hypothermia, metabolic acidosis, and coagulopathy despite hemorrhage control. Published guidelines include an arterial pH of ≤ 7.2, lactic acid > 5 mmol/L, base deficit < -15 in a patient younger than 55 years or < -6 if older than 55 years, temperature < 35°C, and prothrombin time and/or PTT $> 50\%$ normal.

Ref.: 44, 45

36. In the previous scenario, what is the best treatment option for the superficial femoral artery injury?

A. Ligation of the artery
B. Placement of temporary intravascular shunt
C. Definitive repair with a reversed saphenous vein interposition graft from the contralateral leg
D. Definitive repair with an in situ saphenous vein interposition graft
E. Definitive repair with a polytetrafluoroethylene (PTFE) graft

ANSWER: B

COMMENTS: The patient in the above scenario is in extremis and requires a quick establishment of distal perfusion. Although ligation is an option, it puts the lower extremity at risk of ischemia and amputation. Placement of vascular shunts require proximal and distal control, debridement to clean edges, thrombectomy with a Fogarty catheter, regional heparinization, proper shunt selection, securing the distal end first with a 0 silk tie to allow for back bleeding, and then securing the proximal end to allow reestablishment of flow. Fasciotomy should be considered based on ischemia time.

This will allow perfusion and an increased chance for limb salvage while other life-threating injuries are being managed. Dwell times have ranged from 3 to 36 h and do not require systemic anticoagulation. They are routinely used for peripheral arterial injuries but have also been selectively used for extremity venous and truncal vascular injuries. Definitive repair can be completed during the next trip to the operating room with the best choice being a reversed saphenous vein interposition graft from the contralateral leg.

Ref.: 46

37. The patient is a 52-year-old male involved in a high-speed head-on motor vehicle crash. He arrives to the ED unstable with BP 80/60 mmHg and HR 125 beats/min. Initial x-ray workup reveals an open-book pelvis fracture. Despite 2 L of crystalloid, the patient remains tachycardic and hypotensive. What techniques can be used to control bleeding in this patient?

A. Interventional radiology (IR) angiogram
B. Preperitoneal packing
C. External fixator
D. Pelvic binder
E. All of the above

ANSWER: E

COMMENTS: Pelvic injuries are present in approximately 10% of blunt trauma patients. Pelvic fractures can be classified according to the force vector that caused the injury: anteroposterior compression, lateral compression, or vertical shear fractures. The overall mortality in these patients is 6%. However, it increases to greater than 30% when patients present with hemorrhagic shock. Bleeding is usually from branches of the internal iliac artery or the extensive venous plexus surrounding the sacrum. Early control of pelvic hemorrhage is critical. Placement of a pelvic binder or external fixator works by decreasing the volume of the pelvis and temporarily stabilizes the fractured bones, preventing additional injury. Preperitoneal packing completed through a low midline or suprapubic incision carried through the fascia allows for three rolled lap pads to be placed into the preperitoneal space on each side of the bladder, resulting in volume reduction and tamponade of bleeding. This can be done in the operating room in conjunction with a laparotomy being completed for other injuries through a separate incision. Bilateral internal iliac artery embolization with a temporary agent, such as gelatin material, is the preferred angiographic treatment in unstable patients. This provides quick control by limiting flow through the large number of collaterals feeding the pelvis and allowing time for a clot to form. REBOA is now being used in a limited number of centers as an adjunct for early control of pelvic bleeding and increasing mean arterial pressure in patients presenting in hemorrhagic shock with isolated pelvic trauma.

Ref.: 27, 47

38. For the patient in the previous scenario, a pelvic binder is placed and blood pressure and HR improves. A negative urethrogram is completed, and a Foley catheter is inserted. The urine output is bloody, and a cystogram demonstrates a bladder injury. Which combination of injury and management is correct?

A. Extraperitoneal bladder injury = operating room for primary repair
B. Extraperitoneal bladder injury = suprapubic catheter placement
C. Intraperitoneal bladder injury = operating room for primary repair
D. Intraperitoneal bladder injury = maintain Foley catheter
E. Intraperitoneal bladder injury = cystoscopy

ANSWER: C

COMMENTS: Approximately 5% of pelvic fractures will have an associated bladder injury. The majority of these will present with hematuria and can be diagnosed with a CT or traditional cystogram. Contrast extravasation into the retroperitoneum is seen as flame-shaped densities surrounding the bladder, which is characteristic of an extraperitoneal injury. With an intraperitoneal injury, contrast leaks into the abdomen, outlining loops of bowel. Approximately 80% of injuries are extraperitoneal and can be treated with a Foley catheter for 10 to 14 days. An intraperitoneal bladder injury requires operative exploration of the bladder, identification of ureteral orifices and bladder neck, and a two-layer repair with absorbable suture. A closed suction drain is left next to the repair, and the Foley catheter remains in place for 10 to 14 days. A repeat cystogram is completed at 10 days to evaluate the healing process. The Foley catheter can be removed at that time if no extravasation is noted.

Ref.: 27, 48

39. A 22-year-old man undergoes proctoscopy and exploratory laparotomy for a transpelvic gunshot wound. A 2-cm, partial-thickness laceration is found in the distal portion of the extraperitoneal rectum. What is the appropriate surgical management of this injury?

A. Resection of the injured area and anastomosis with a diverting colostomy
B. Primary repair with a diverting colostomy
C. Diverting colostomy only
D. Presacral drainage only
E. Primary repair only

ANSWER: C

COMMENTS: Repair of rectal injury largely depends on location, intraperitoneal versus extraperitoneal. The posterior rectum and distal third of the anterior rectum are not serosalized, and an injury in these regions is considered extraperitoneal. Extraperitoneal rectal injuries should be treated chiefly by fecal diversion. Nondestructive intraperitoneal lacerations that are less than 50% of the circumference of the rectal wall should be repaired primarily after debridement of any devitalized tissue in the absence of peritonitis. Presacral drainage, which historically had been used rather routinely, has been decreasing in use and has not been shown to decrease the complication rate.

Ref.: 1, 49

40. A 27-year-old female presents with multiple gunshot wounds to the abdomen. She is immediately taken to the operating room for an exploratory laparotomy. She is found to have a mid-ureter injury with a 2-cm segment loss. During the surgery, the patient becomes hypotensive, requiring vasopressors. What is the best damage control treatment option for an unstable patient with a ureteral injury?

A. Ligation of the injured ureter
B. Percutaneous nephrostomy
C. Ureteral drainage via a single-J stent, which is externalized to the skin
D. Placement of a bridging stent
E. All of the above

ANSWER: E

COMMENTS: When a trauma patient is unstable on the operating room table and damage control has been initiated, time should not be spent on primary repair of a ureteral injury. Surgical options for this type of situation consist of simple ligation of the ureter, placing a percutaneous nephrostomy through the renal parenchyma into the renal pelvis, inserting a catheter into the proximal end of the damaged ureter and bringing it out through the wound, or placing a catheter or stent in the proximal and distal ends of a small-segment ureteral injury. These methods will allow for urinary diversion until the patient is stable.

Ref.: 50, 51

41. A 30-year-old male is brought to the ED after being involved in a motorcycle crash. He is hemodynamically stable. Blood is noted at the urethral meatus. On portable pelvic radiographs, he is found to have bilateral pubic rami fractures. He has not yet voided since admission. Which of the following is the best next step?

A. Wait for the patient to void freely before attempting transurethral bladder catheterization.

B. Initially attempt gentle transurethral bladder catheterization but stop if resistance is encountered.

C. Obtain a urethrogram before attempting transurethral bladder catheterization.

D. Insert a suprapubic cystostomy tube.

E. Perform CT of the pelvis with three-dimensional reconstruction.

ANSWER: C

COMMENTS: Approximately 10% of all patients with a pelvic fracture have a concomitant urethral injury. Findings on physical examination, such as blood at the meatus, perineal ecchymosis or hematoma, or inability to void, should raise suspicion for a urethral injury. If any of these signs or symptoms is present, or there is a significant anterior pelvic fracture, a urethrogram should be obtained to exclude an injury before transurethral catheterization is attempted. Bladder decompression and drainage are the mainstays of treatment of urethral injuries, either via suprapubic cystostomy for complete disruption or with a bridging transurethral catheter for partial tears.

Ref.: 48

42. A 36-year-old male presents after a prolonged extrication from a motor vehicle crash. The patient has bilateral femur fractures and an open left tibia-fibula fracture with significant tissue loss and no distal pulses. Which statement is correct regarding the management of a mangled extremity?

A. This patient requires angiography prior to going to the operating room.

B. A mangled extremity severity score ≥ 5 is predictive of need for amputation.

C. In a hemodynamically unstable patient, the definitive vascular repair should be completed first.

D. Bony injury should be reduced prior to definitive vascular repair.

E. Optimal maximum time to surgery should be less than 24 h from injury.

ANSWER: D

COMMENTS: A significant injury to a limb requires assessment of multiple factors including bone, soft tissue, nerve function, vasculature, and overall hemodynamic status to assist with the decision for limb salvage versus amputation. Although multiple scoring systems, including the mangled extremity severity score (MESS) and the Ganga Hospital Score, have been created to help evaluate and manage mangled extremities, none have been predictive to determine which limb can be salvaged versus amputated. Despite these findings, experts recommend considering primary amputation with a MESS ≥ 7, delay of greater than 6 h to treatment, and in hemodynamically unstable patients. Imaging with CT angiogram or formal angiography may assist the surgeon. However, in the setting of "hard signs," including ongoing hemorrhage, expanding hematoma, a bruit or thrill, signs of ischemia, or absent pulses, patients should be taken directly to the operating room for exploration. Orthopedic injuries are reduced first and temporarily stabilized, which may unkink vessels and allow for reperfusion and better evaluation of a soft tissue injury.

Ref.: 52, 53

43. The patient in the previous scenario is taken to the ICU for postoperative monitoring. It is noted that his urine output has decreased in the past 2 h and is very dark. Urinalysis is positive for blood, but there are no red blood cells on microscopic analysis. What is true regarding his diagnosis?

A. Best treatment includes aggressive IV fluid resuscitation.

B. All patients with rhabdomyolysis require dialysis.

C. The renal failure from rhabdomyolysis typically resolves within 3 to 5 days.

D. Severe hyponatremia is a frequent complication.

E. Alkalinization to a pH between 8 and 9 is an important treatment goal.

ANSWER: A

COMMENTS: Rhabdomyolysis is the breakdown of muscles that causes a release of myoglobin. Myoglobin causes tubular obstruction and vasoconstriction, which leads to acute tubular necrosis and acute kidney injury. There are a variety of causes of rhabdomyolysis including crush injury, multiple trauma, seizures, illicit drugs, and several medications, including many antibiotics and antipsychotics. Creatine kinase is the most specific marker for diagnosis, and higher levels correlate with a greater injury. Additional tests show the described characteristic urinalysis, hyperkalemia, hypocalcemia, and elevated creatinine. Treatment includes preventing additional muscle breakdown, aggressive IV fluid resuscitation, and managing complications including electrolyte imbalances and renal failure, which may require renal replacement therapy. Indications for dialysis include hyperkalemia, metabolic acidosis, and hypervolemia. Treatment with bicarbonate infusion has been used to alkalinize urine to a pH of 6 to theoretically prevent myoglobin precipitation in the tubules; however, there are minimal data to support this practice. Overall prognosis with early and aggressive volume resuscitation is good, with most patients recovering to baseline renal function within 2 weeks to 3 months.

Ref.: 54, 55

44. A 34-year-old male presents with a gunshot wound to his left thigh with no pulses in his feet. The patient is taken immediately to the operating room, and a superficial femoral artery injury is repaired with a saphenous vein interposition graft. At the end of the surgery, the patient had equal pulses bilaterally and was neurologically intact. Five hours postoperatively, the left distal pulses are diminished and he begins to experience pain with passive dorsiflexion and extension. Which of the following statements is true regarding compartment syndrome in an extremity?

A. Fractures are the cause of approximately 30% of all compartment syndromes.

B. The lateral compartment of the lower part of the leg is the most commonly affected.

C. A compartment pressure of 25 mmHg negates a need for fasciotomy.

D. Loss of pulses is an early clinical development.

E. A four-compartment fasciotomy should be performed.

ANSWER: E

COMMENTS: Compartment syndrome of the extremity is an extremely important diagnosis to make as early as possible because of the significant risk for permanent limb dysfunction and potential loss. Causes of compartment syndrome include crush injury, reperfusion after a time of ischemia, and fractures, which account for 50% of cases. The anterior compartment of the lower part of the leg contains mostly type I (slow twitch) muscle fibers and is encased by dense fascia, thus making it most vulnerable to the development of ischemia. The diagnosis is largely clinical, with pain out of proportion to the findings on examination, pallor, paresthesias, paralysis, poikilothermia, pulselessness, and tense compartments being the hallmark symptoms. Because of the fact that even after an hour of ischemia, impulses can still be conducted through peripheral nerves, paresthesias are a late sign of compartment syndrome. In addition, even though compartment pressures of 30 mmHg or higher are classically quoted, lesser pressures do not prove that there is adequate tissue perfusion, and if other signs or symptoms of compartment syndrome are present, fasciotomies should still be performed.

Ref.: 28, 56, 57

45. A 24-year-old male presents after a motorcycle crash. He is found to have multiple left-sided rib fractures, a grade II splenic laceration, and a small 2-mm subdural hematoma. His GCS score is 15. The patient is admitted to the ICU for serial hemoglobin and neurologic checks. Clinical examination, hemoglobin, and repeat CT of the head at 48 h remain stable. What is the most appropriate deep vein thrombosis (DVT) prophylaxis to initiate at this time?

A. Early ambulation only

B. Sequential compression devices only

C. Retrievable IVC filter

D. Subcutaneous heparin 5000 units daily

E. Subcutaneous Lovenox 30 mg twice a day

ANSWER: E

COMMENTS: Trauma patients, especially those with multiple injuries, including intracranial hemorrhage, pelvic and extremity fractures, and spinal injuries, are at significant risk of having a DVT. This is also a population that has an increased risk of bleeding, and standard prophylaxis protocols have been modified to account for this. All patients should have sequential compression devices upon admission, and chemical prophylaxis with either heparin 5000 U three times per day or enoxaparin 30 U twice a day should be started as early as possible. LMWH has been shown to be superior in this patient population. Patients with truncal hemorrhage with stable hemoglobin values for 24 h are at minimal risk of bleeding with the initiation of chemical prophylaxis. Controversy has been placed around patients with traumatic brain injuries. Many recent studies have shown that it is safe to start chemical prophylaxis as early as 24 h after a stable brain CT without increased risk of progression of hematoma. Few patients will have contraindications to pharmacologic prophylaxis and should be considered for weekly extremity surveillance duplex ultrasound or placement of a retrievable IVC filter. Risks of placing an IVC filter include dislodgement, perforation, and thrombosis. These should be removed at the earliest occasion when pharmacologic prophylaxis becomes appropriate and the risk of bleeding is minimized.

Ref.: 58, 59

46. A 79-year-old female falls at home. In the ER, she is found to have a pelvic fracture with a large retroperitoneal hematoma. While waiting for angioembolization by Interventional Radiology (IR), the patient becomes hypotensive and is transfused with two units of packed red blood cells and two units of fresh-frozen plasma. After IR, the patient starts to complain of shortness of breath, has desaturations, and requires intubation. Which statement best describes a transfusion-related acute lung injury (TRALI)?

A. Onset occurs 24 h after a transfusion.

B. Onset occurs most often after transfusion with fresh-frozen plasma.

C. Clinical findings include dyspnea, hypertension, and bradycardia.

D. Treatment includes plasmapheresis.

E. Affected patients cannot receive blood transfusions in the future.

ANSWER: B

COMMENTS: The reported incidence of TRALI varies from 1% to 15% of patients receiving transfusions with a mortality rate of 5%–10%. It occurs 50 to 100 times more often in critically ill patients. It can occur after transfusion of any component of blood but is most associated with fresh-frozen plasma and red blood cells. Several hypotheses exist regarding its pathogenesis, including human leukocyte antigen–specific antibody in the donor directed against an antigen in the recipient, resulting in an inflammatory response causing damage to the endothelial lining of the lungs. Criteria for diagnosis include acute onset, usually within 6 h of transfusion, hypoxemia with a PaO_2/FiO_2 ratio less than 300, and bilateral infiltrates on chest x-ray in a patient with no alternative risk for lung injury. Symptoms include dyspnea, tachypnea, tachycardia, hypotension, and fever. Treatment is supportive, with approximately 70%–90% of patients requiring ventilator support. Being diagnosed with TRALI does not affect the ability to receive blood transfusions in the future. However, risk reduction maneuvers including restrictive transfusion policies and washing of stored blood products should be employed with future transfusions.

Ref.: 8, 60

47. A coal mine explodes in a rural part of the country. There is only one small local hospital, and critical patients will need to be airlifted to the closest Level 1 Trauma Center. Which patient should be triaged to the expectant category?

A. A 22-year-old male with a broken femur

B. An 18-year-old female with 90% total body surface area (TBSA) burns with agonal breathing

C. A 38-year-old male with multiple left rib fractures and decreased breath sounds

D. A 29-year-old female with a traumatic amputation of her right forearm

E. A 34-year-old male with a fractured thoracic spine and traumatic paralysis

ANSWER: B

COMMENTS: A mass casualty incident involves an influx of hundreds of casualties that overwhelms the capacity and resources of a hospital, resulting in suboptimal and delayed care. Field triage is defined as sorting casualties according to their needs, considering their chance of survival, and is key in providing the greatest benefit to the maximum number of patients in these emergencies. Sort, Assess, Lifesaving Interventions, Treatment/Transport (SALT) triage allows for quick determination of which patients will benefit the most from immediate hospital transfer. Approximately 15% of patients will be critically injured in any event, and limited resources such as ICU beds, ventilators, and operating rooms need to be directed toward these critical patients with a high likelihood of survival with intervention. Causalities defined as expectant will vary depending on casualty numbers, type and severity of injuries, and resource availability. To minimize a large resource expenditure on a patient with a low likelihood of survival, these patients are kept out of the hospital until the immediate surge subsides.

Ref.: 61, 62

REFERENCES

1. Martin RS, Meredith JW. Management of acute trauma. In: Townsend Jr CM, Beauchamp RD, Evers BM, Mattox KL, eds. *Sabiston Textbook of Surgery: The Biological Basis of Modern Surgical Practice*. 19th ed. Philadelphia: Elsevier; 2012.
2. Peck G, Buchman TG. Initial assessment and resuscitation of the trauma patient. In: Cameron JL, Cameron AM, eds. *Current Surgical Therapy*. 11th ed. Philadelphia: Elsevier; 2014.
3. Doben AR, Gross RI. Airway management: what every trauma surgeon should know, from intubation to cricothyroidotomy. In: Asensio JA, Trunkey DD, eds. *Current Therapy of Trauma and Surgical Critical Care*. 2nd ed. Philadelphia: Elsevier; 2016.
4. Galvagno Jr SM, Scalea TM. Airway management in the trauma patient. In: Cameron JL, Cameron AM, eds. *Current Surgical Therapy*. 11th ed. Philadelphia: Elsevier; 2014.
5. Lee PMJ, Lee C, Rattner P, et al. Intraosseous versus central venous catheter utilization and performance during inpatient medical emergencies. *Crit Care Med*. 2015;43:1233–1238.
6. Pasley J, Miller CHT, Dubose JJ, et al. Intraosseous infusion rates under high pressure: a cadaveric comparison of anatomic sites. *J Trauma Acute Care Surg*. 2015;78:295–299.
7. Holcomb JB, Tilley BC, Baraniuk S, et al. Transfusion of plasma, platelets, and red blood cells in a 1:1:1 vs a 1:1:2 ration and mortality in patients with severe trauma. The PROPPR randomized clinical trial. *JAMA*. 2015;313(5):471–482.
8. O'Keeffe T, Rhee P. Blood transfusion therapy in trauma. In: Cameron JL, Cameron AM, eds. *Current Surgical Therapy*. 11th ed. Philadelphia: Elsevier; 2014.
9. Frontera JA, Lewin JJ, Rabinstein AA, et al. Guideline for reversal of antithrombotics in intracranial hemorrhage. *Neurocrit Care*. 2016;24:6–46.
10. Pollack CV, Rielly PA, Eikelboom J, et al. Idarucizumab for dabigatran reversal. *N Engl J Med*. 2015;373:511–520.
11. Britt LD. Abdominal trauma. In: Cameron JL, Cameron AM, eds. *Current Surgical Therapy*. 11th ed. Philadelphia: Elsevier; 2014.
12. Pieracci FM, Jurkovich GJ. Penetrating abdominal trauma. In: Cameron JL, Cameron AM, eds. *Current Surgical Therapy*. 11th ed. Philadelphia: Elsevier; 2014.
13. Dente CJ, Rozycki GS. The surgeon's use of ultrasound in thoracoabdominal trauma. In: Cameron JL, Cameron AM, eds. *Current Surgical Therapy*. 11th ed. Philadelphia: Elsevier; 2014.
14. Mattox KL, Wall Jr MJ, Tsai P. Trauma thoracotomy: principles and techniques. In: Mattox KL, Moore EE, Feliciano DV, eds. *Trauma*. 7th ed. New York: McGraw-Hill; 2013.
15. Moore LJ, Megan B, Kozar RA, et al. Implementation of resuscitative endovascular balloon occlusion of the aorta as an alternative to resuscitative thoracotomy for noncompressible truncal hemorrhage. *J Trauma Acute Care Surg*. 2015;79:523–532.
16. Seamon MJ, Haut ER, Van Arendonk K, et al. An evidence-based approach to patient selection for emergency department thoracotomy: a practice management guideline from the Eastern Association for the Surgery of Trauma. *J Trauma Acute Care Surg*. 2015;79:159–173.
17. Knudson MM, Yeh DD. Trauma in pregnancy. In: Mattox KL, Moore EE, Feliciano DV, eds. *Trauma*. 7th ed. New York: McGraw-Hill; 2013.
18. Brain Trauma Foundation, American Association of Neurological Surgeons, Congress of Neurological Surgeons. Guidelines for the management of severe traumatic brain injury. *J Neurotrauma*. 2007;24(S1):1–106.
19. Cryer HG, Manley GT, et al. ACS TQUIP best practices in the management of traumatic brain injury. 2015.
20. Weingart JD. The management of traumatic brain injury. In: Cameron JL, Cameron AM, eds. *Current Surgical Therapy*. 11th ed. Philadelphia: Elsevier; 2014.
21. Bawa M, Fayssoux R. Vertebrae and spinal cord. In: Mattox KL, Moore EE, Feliciano DV, eds. *Trauma*. 7th ed. New York: McGraw-Hill; 2013.
22. Como JJ, Diaz JJ, Dunham CM, et al. Practice management guidelines for identification of cervical spine injuries following trauma: update from the Eastern Association for the Surgery of Trauma Practice Management Guidelines Committee. *J Trauma*. 2009;67:651–659.
23. Feliciano DV, Vercruysse GA. Neck. In: Mattox KL, Moore EE, Feliciano DV, eds. *Trauma*. 7th ed. New York: McGraw-Hill; 2013.
24. Maier RV, Marquardt DL. Penetrating neck trauma. In: Cameron JL, Cameron AM, eds. *Current Surgical Therapy*. 11th ed. Philadelphia: Elsevier; 2014.
25. Clancy K, Velopulos C, Bilaniuk JW, et al. Screening for blunt cardiac injury: an Eastern Association for the Surgery of Trauma practice management guideline. *J Trauma Acute Care Surg*. 2012;73:S301–S306.
26. Shah A, Balsara KR. Blunt cardiac injury. In: Cameron JL, Cameron AM, eds. *Current Surgical Therapy*. 11th ed. Philadelphia: Elsevier; 2014.
27. Velmahos GC, Karaiskakis M, Salim A, et al. Normal electrocardiography and serum troponin I levels preclude the presence of clinically significant blunt cardiac injury. *J Trauma*. 2003;54:45–51.
28. Pharaon KS, Trunkey DD. The management of vascular injuries. In: Cameron JL, Cameron AM, eds. *Current Surgical Therapy*. 11th ed. Philadelphia: Elsevier; 2014.
29. Demetriades D, Talving P, Inaba K. Blunt thoracic aortic injury. In: Rasmussen TE, Tai NRM, eds. *Rich's Vascular Trauma*. 3rd ed. Philadelphia: Elsevier; 2016.
30. Rabin J, DuBose J, Sliker CW, et al. Parameters for successful nonoperative management of traumatic aortic injury. *J Thorac Cardiovasc Surg*. 2014;147:143–150.
31. Coimbra R, Hoyt DB. Chest wall trauma, hemothorax, and pneumothorax. In: Cameron JL, Cameron AM, eds. *Current Surgical Therapy*. 11th ed. Philadelphia: Elsevier; 2014.
32. Pieracci FM, Lin Y, Rodil M, et al. A prospective, controlled clinical evaluation of surgical stabilization of severe rib fractures. *J Trauma Acute Care Surg*. 2016;80:187–194.
33. Ramsay PT, Feliciano DV. Diaphragmatic injuries. In: Cameron JL, Cameron AM, eds. *Current Surgical Therapy*. 11th ed. Philadelphia: Elsevier; 2014.
34. Schuster KM, Davis KA. Diaphragm. In: Mattox KL, Moore EE, Feliciano DV, eds. *Trauma*. 7th ed. New York: McGraw-Hill; 2013.

35. Zafar SN, Cornwell EE. Injuries to the small and large bowel. In: Cameron JL, Cameron AM, eds. *Current Surgical Therapy*. 11th ed. Philadelphia: Elsevier; 2014.
36. Biffl WL, Cothren CC, Moore EE, et al. Western Trauma Association critical decisions in trauma: screening for and treatment of blunt cerebrovascular injuries. *J Trauma*. 2009;67:1150–1153.
37. Duchesne JC, Simms ER. Norman McSwain Jr NE. Pancreatic and duodenal injuries and current surgical therapies. In: Cameron JL, Cameron AM, eds. *Current Surgical Therapy*. 11th ed. Philadelphia: Elsevier; 2014.
38. Fabian TC, Bee TK. Liver and biliary tract. In: Mattox KL, Moore EE, Feliciano DV, eds. *Trauma*. 7th ed. New York: McGraw-Hill; 2013.
39. Savage SA, Fabian TC. Inferior vena cava, portal, and mesenteric venous systems. In: Rasmussen TE, Tai NRM, eds. *Rich's Vascular Trauma*. 3rd ed. Philadelphia: Elsevier; 2016.
40. Ekeh AP, Khalaf S, Ilyas S, et al. Complications arising from splenic artery embolization: a review of an 11-year experience. *Am J Surg*. 2013;205:250–254.
41. Miller PR, Chang MC, Hoth JJ, et al. Prospective trial of angiography and embolization for all Grade III to V blunt splenic injuries: nonoperative management success rate is significantly improved. *J Am Coll Surg* 2014;218:644–651.
42. Wisner DH. Injury to the spleen. In: Mattox KL, Moore EE, Feliciano DV, eds. *Trauma*. 7th ed. New York: McGraw-Hill; 2013.
43. Zarzaur BL, Kozar R, Myers JG, et al. The splenic injury outcomes trial: an American Association for the Surgery of Trauma multi-institutional study. *J Trauma Acute Care Surg*. 2015;79:335–342.
44. Hicks CW, Haider A. Damage control operation. In: Cameron JL, Cameron AM, eds. *Current Surgical Therapy*. 11th ed. Philadelphia: Elsevier; 2014.
45. Wyrzykowski AD, Feliciano DV. Trauma damage control. In: Mattox KL, Moore EE, Feliciano DV, eds. *Trauma*. 7th ed. New York: McGraw-Hill; 2013.
46. Scott DJ, Rasmussen TE. Surgical damage control and temporary vascular shunts. In: Rasmussen TE, Tai NRM, eds. *Rich's Vascular Trauma*. 3rd ed. Philadelphia: Elsevier; 2016.
47. Costantini TW, Coimbra R, Holcomb JB, et al. Current management of hemorrhage from severe pelvic fractures: results of an American Association for the Surgery of Trauma multi-institutional trial. *J Trauma Acute Care Surg*. 2016 May;80(5):717–723; discussion 723–725.
48. Wessells H. Urologic complications of pelvic fracture. In: Cameron JL, Cameron AM, eds. *Current Surgical Therapy*. 11th ed. Philadelphia: Elsevier; 2014.
49. Ciesla DJ, Cha JY. The management of rectal injuries. In: Cameron JL, Cameron AM, eds. *Current Surgical Therapy*. 11th ed. Philadelphia: Elsevier; 2014.
50. Breyer BN, McAninch JW. Retroperitoneal injuries: kidney and ureter. In: Cameron JL, Cameron AM, eds. *Current Surgical Therapy*. 11th ed. Philadelphia: Elsevier; 2014.
51. Coburn M. Genitourinary trauma. In: Mattox KL, Moore EE, Feliciano DV, eds. *Trauma*. 7th ed. New York: McGraw-Hill; 2013.
52. Scalea TM, Dubose JJ, Moore EE, et al. Western Trauma Association critical decisions in trauma: management of the mangled extremity. *J Trauma*. 2012;72:86–93.
53. Stahel PF, Smith WR, Hak DJ. Lower extremity. In: Mattox KL, Moore EE, Feliciano DV, eds. *Trauma*. 7th ed. New York: McGraw-Hill; 2013.
54. Waxman K. Acute kidney injury. In: Cameron JL, Cameron AM, eds. *Current Surgical Therapy*. 11th ed. Philadelphia: Elsevier; 2014.
55. Zimmerman JL, Shen MC. Rhabdomyolysis. *Chest*. 2013;144(3): 1058–1065.
56. Ledgerwood AM, Lucas CE. The management of extremity compartment syndrome. In: Cameron JL, Cameron AM, eds. *Current Surgical Therapy*. 11th ed. Philadelphia: Elsevier; 2014.
57. Sise MJ, Shackford SR. Peripheral vascular injury. In: Mattox KL, Moore EE, Feliciano DV, eds. *Trauma*. 7th ed. New York: McGraw-Hill; 2013.
58. Farooqui A, Hiser B, Barnes SL, Litofsky NS. Safety and efficacy of early thromboembolism chemoprophylaxis after intracranial hemorrhage from traumatic brain injury. *J Neurosurg*. 2013;119:1576–1582.
59. Turney EJ, Lyden SP. The prevention of venous thromboembolism. In: Cameron JL, Cameron AM, eds. *Current Surgical Therapy*. 11th ed. Philadelphia: Elsevier; 2014.
60. Vlaar AP, Juffermans NP. Transfusion-related acute lung injury: a clinical review. *Lancet*. 2013;382:984–994.
61. Frykberg ER, Schecter WP. Disaster and mass casualty. In: Mattox KL, Moore EE, Feliciano DV, eds. *Trauma*. 7th ed. New York: McGraw-Hill; 2013.
62. Hirshberg A, Stein M. The surgeon's role in mass casualty incidents. In: Townsend Jr CM, Beauchamp RD, Evers BM, Mattox KL, eds. *Sabiston Textbook of Surgery: The Biological Basis of Modern Surgical Practice*. 19th ed. Philadelphia: Elsevier; 2012.

CHAPTER 12

BURNS

Charles Fredericks, M.D., James R. Yon, M.D., and Thomas A. Messer, M.D.

1. Select the true statement regarding the epidemiology of burn injury:
   A. Most burn injuries occur in occupational environments.
   B. Young adult men are the most likely to suffer burn injury.
   C. The most common cause of death after admission for a burn injury is airway occlusion.
   D. Scalding is the most common cause of burns in children younger than 5 years.
   E. Prevention has not had a significant impact on the incidence or mortality of burn injury.

ANSWER: D

COMMENTS: Approximately 1 million injuries are caused by thermal trauma yearly in the United States. The majority of burn injuries occur in the home (43%). In general, 65% of burns occur in non–work-related accidents, 17% in work-related accidents, and 5% each in recreational or in assault or abuse cases. House fires contribute to 75%–80% of deaths from burns. Burns occur in a bimodal distribution, with an increased risk occurring in children younger than 4 years and adults 65 years and older. African-Americans and Native Americans are disproportionately affected. Burns occur more frequently in vulnerable populations, including those with epilepsy, those with heavy alcohol use, the poor, and people living in substandard housing. Asphyxiation is a common cause of death at the scene of a fire, but the most common recorded cause of death in burn patients after admission is multi-organ failure. Other causes, in decreasing order of frequency, are shock, trauma, pulmonary failure or sepsis, cardiovascular failure, and burn wound sepsis. Hot-water scald injuries are the most common cause in children younger than 5 years, with flame burns becoming more frequent in those 5 years and older. Ordinances requiring water heaters to be set at no higher than 120°F have decreased the incidence of scald burns. Efforts at prevention have significantly decreased the number of burn injuries occurring in the United States, although disabled or impaired individuals are still at risk.

Ref.: 1–3

2. Which of the following regarding burn wound depth is true?
   A. First-degree burns heal rapidly but contribute significantly to the total body surface area (TBSA) burned in large, mixed-depth wounds.
   B. Second-degree burns characteristically cause erythema, pain, and blistering.
   C. Third-degree burns are generally painful and extremely sensitive to touch.
   D. Fourth-degree burns mandate amputation of the involved extremities.
   E. Superficial partial-thickness burn is the contemporary term for first-degree burns.

ANSWER: B

COMMENTS: The skin consists of two layers: epidermis and dermis. The epidermis is composed of five progressively differentiated layers of keratinocytes, the outermost of which, the stratum corneum, is relatively impermeable. The epidermis provides barrier functions and protects against infection, absorption of toxins, exposure to ultraviolet light, and fluid and heat loss. The dermis is a cellular and extracellular layer that provides the skin with durability and elasticity. Within the dermis, fibroblasts synthesize mesenchymal proteins, and inflammatory cells are present and contribute to the inflammatory responses to injury. Dermal papillae interdigitate with the epidermal rete ridges to form the dermal–epidermal junction, a site affected by some exfoliative diseases of the skin. Superficial, or first-degree, burns involve only the epidermis and are erythematous and painful. The damaged epidermis will slough off within 3 to 4 days and be replaced by regenerating keratinocytes. Most sunburns are first degree, and the treatment of superficial burns is similar to that of sunburns. Superficial burns do not contribute significantly to the systemic response to burn injury and are not counted in the percentage of TBSA (%TBSA) burned. Partial-thickness burns (second degree) involve both the epidermis and dermis and are subdivided into superficial partial thickness and deep partial thickness, depending on the depth of dermal involvement. Superficial partial-thickness burns involve the papillary dermis. Blistering occurs within 24 h of injury. The exposed underlying dermis is typically pink, blanching, moist, and tender to touch because the nerve endings are preserved. These burns heal within 2 to 3 weeks with little risk of scarring. Deep partial-thickness burns extend to the reticular dermis and may require more than 3 weeks to heal. These wounds blister and reveal mottled pink/white dermis. Sensation may be decreased, and the wounds may dry after initial observation. If deep partial-thickness wounds take longer than 3 weeks to heal, grafting may be required. Full-thickness (third-degree) burns extend through the entire dermis into subcutaneous tissue. Full-thickness burns may be dry, leathery, firm, and insensate. Even if mottled in appearance, they do not blanch and may be hemorrhagic. These wounds require excision of the burn eschar and skin grafting for closure. Indeterminate-depth wounds may be difficult to judge by initial appearance. Their potential to heal should be determined with serial observations because the initial evaluation may be inaccurate, even by experienced clinicians. Light reflectance techniques, fluorescein, thermography, and magnetic resonance imaging have not proved useful with respect to serial clinical evaluation. Noncontact laser Doppler imaging can be helpful but has not gained widespread clinical use. Fourth-degree burns extend to muscle, bone, or other deep structures. They are particularly common with electrical injuries or burns with prolonged contact occurring in impaired patients. These very deep burns pose serious reconstructive challenges, and amputation may be required when the extremities or digits are involved.

Ref.: 1–3

3. Which of the following statements regarding the order or description of the zones of injury is correct?

A. A zone of hyperemia inside a zone of stasis

B. A zone of hyperemia superficial to a zone of stasis, with a deeper zone of coagulation beneath

C. A zone of coagulation at the surface of a burn wound, a zone of stasis within the injured dermal layer, and a deep zone of hyperemia characterized by vasodilated subcutaneous vessels

D. A zone of coagulation, surrounded by a zone of stasis, which is surrounded by a zone of hyperemia

E. A zone of hemorrhagic burn that must be coagulated, a zone of stasis in which the depth of burn injury is already fixed, and a zone of hyperemia that may convert to coagulation

ANSWER: D

COMMENTS: Jackson's classification of zones of injury in 1953 referred to the varying depth of injury radiating outward from a burn wound and defined the pathophysiology of cutaneous thermal injury. The central zone of coagulation is necrotic and irreversibly damaged; it represents a full-thickness injury that will require excision and grafting. The zone of stasis refers to the immediately surrounding region and is characterized by constricted vessels and hypoxia. Initially viable, this tissue may convert to coagulation or a full-thickness injury as a result of edema, infection, or shock with decreased perfusion. The zone of stasis may remain viable if adequately perfused. In a patient with a large-TBSA burn, the viability of this zone may be critical in providing donor sites and reducing the total area that requires grafting. The **zone of hyperemia** surrounding this is characterized by vasodilation as a result of inflammatory mediators and is viable.

Ref.: 1

4. Select the most accurate statement regarding burn injury:

A. Contact burns occur commonly and rarely require grafting.

B. Intoxication is infrequently associated with deep burn injury.

C. Circumferential burns on both feet are seen in accidental bathing injuries in children.

D. Flash burns are generated by brief, intense heat, and articles of clothing are frequently protective.

E. Electrical burns are deeper than they appear because of the high flash temperatures generated by arcing.

ANSWER: D

COMMENTS: The mechanism of burn injury, if known, may aid in assessing the wound depth and predicting its capacity to heal. Flash burns are responsible for 50% of admissions to burn centers. Explosions caused by natural gas, propane, and gasoline vapors generate brief, intense heat. If not directly ignited, clothing is protective, with burns affecting only the exposed skin. The depth of injury can be variable; many flash burns heal without grafting. Flame burns generally result in a deep dermal or full-thickness injury because of the duration of exposure. Structure fires and ignition of bedding or clothing are common causes of flame burns, and burn depth is proportional to the time required to remove the burning or smoldering material from the victim. Intoxication or carbon monoxide (CO) poisoning occurring during a house fire increases the likelihood of deep flame burns. Scald burns are the second most common cause of burns in the United States. The depth of injury is related to the water temperature and the duration of contact. At 140°F (60°C), water causes a deep dermal injury in 3 s. Clothed areas may be scalded more deeply because of prolonged contact with the wet fabric before removal. Young children and elderly patients will scald faster and at lower temperatures. If not cautious, diabetic patients may accidentally scald themselves when soaking neuropathic or insensate feet in hot water. These burns are frequently deep partial to full thickness, and such patients are likely to have impaired healing as a result of their comorbid conditions. Hot oil and grease burns tend to be deep partial or full thickness because of the very high temperatures reached while cooking or heating oil. Contact burns result from direct contact with a heat source and often occur in work environments. The hot presses used in industrial applications can cause particularly devastating combined crush/burn injuries that may result in poor functional outcomes. Deep contact burns in domestic environments occur in children or impaired individuals (drugs, alcohol). Palmar or plantar surface burns generally deserve a period of observation because of the propensity of the thicker dermis of these surfaces to heal and less optimal results in terms of sensation and function obtained with split-thickness skin grafting in these areas. Electrical injuries may cause deep tissue destruction that belies the surface wound when current flows through the patient, but flash burns from electrical arcing without direct contact are similar to flash burns from other sources.

Ref.: 1

5. Which of the following patients do not meet the criteria for referral to a burn center?

A. A 50-year-old woman with a 1% TBSA partial-thickness burn on her left hand from a cooking accident

B. A 30-year-old construction worker with pain and blistering bilaterally on the knees after kneeling in wet cement all afternoon

C. A 25-year-old man with 7% TBSA partial-thickness burns on the chest

D. A 42-year-old woman with no cutaneous injury, found lying down at the scene of a house fire, and noted to have carbonaceous sputum after intubation in the field

E. An 18-year-old man in a motor vehicle collision with 30% TBSA burns on his chest and circumferential burns bilaterally on his arms

ANSWER: C

COMMENTS: The American Burn Association and the American College of Surgeons Committee on Trauma have published guidelines for patient referral to a burn center for care: (1) partial-thickness burns on greater than 10% of TBSA; (2) burns that involve the face, hands, feet, genitalia, perineum, or major joints;

(3) third-degree burns (any size) in any age group; (4) electrical burns, including lightning injury; (5) chemical burns; (6) inhalation injury; (7) burn injury in patients with preexisting medical disorders that could complicate management, prolong recovery, or affect mortality; (8) any patient with burns and concomitant trauma (such as fractures) in which the burn injury poses the greatest risk for morbidity or mortality (in such cases, if the trauma poses a greater immediate risk, the patient's condition may be stabilized initially in a trauma center before transfer to a burn center); (9) burned children in hospitals without qualified personnel or equipment for the care of children; and (10) burn injuries in patients who will require special social, emotional, or rehabilitative intervention. These criteria are not meant to be exclusive, and many centers will treat patients with wounds smaller than those mentioned in the guidelines. Many burn centers care for patients with exfoliative skin disorders, major wounds, necrotizing infections, and other diseases that require significant wound management and critical care.

Ref.: 4

6. A 25-year-old patient has been in the burn intensive care unit (ICU) intubated and sedated for 2 weeks after an 80% TBSA burn. He suddenly develops hypotension, tachycardia, and melena. What type of surgical problem is this patient most likely to have?

A. Curling's ulcer
B. Cushing's ulcer
C. Marjolin's ulcer
D. Dieulafoy's lesion
E. Boerhaave's syndrome

ANSWER: A

COMMENTS: Patients who are critically ill are at risk for a number of gastrointestinal emergencies as a result of their index injury. A Curling's ulcer is upper gastrointestinal bleeding in a burn patient, related to gastritis. Incidence is now decreased to 4% due to improved critical care, chemical ulcer prophylaxis, and early tube feeding. A Cushing's ulcer is similar, but presents in patients with severe neurologic injury and is likely related to increased intracranial pressure. Management of both types of ulcers is similar, with the patient receiving aggressive resuscitation, correction of coagulopathies, proton pump inhibitor administration, and endoscopic coagulation or clipping of any visible sources of bleeding. Selected arterial embolization can be used as an adjunct. Surgery is a last resort for patients who have persistent bleeding. A Marjolin's ulcer is the malignant transformation of a chronic wound (burn scars, hidradenitis suppurativa, venous stasis ulcers, fistula tracts, or any other chronic wound) into squamous cell carcinoma. This type of squamous cell carcinoma is very aggressive and will need wide local excision and metastatic workup. A Dieulafoy's lesion is a vascular malformation of large vessels (1 to 3 mm), in the stomach, usually along the lesser curve submucosa, and can result in massive blood loss. The mucosal defect overlying the vessel is often small, but the vessel itself is usually amenable to endoscopic clipping, which is successful >80% of the time. Boerhaave's syndrome is an esophageal perforation, usually distal, resulting from esophageal sphincter dysfunction caused by repeated vomiting.

Ref.: 2

7. A 45-year-old patient presents after being burned in a house fire. The patient has deep, dry, and painless circumferential burns around both legs, the anterior torso and abdomen, and the circumferential left arm. Additionally, the patient has painful erythema involving the circumferential right arm. What is this patient's %TBSA?

A. 63%
B. 72%
C. 45%
D. 81%
E. 36%

ANSWER: A

COMMENTS: The correct burn size estimation is crucial to burn care. The percentage of the TBSA burned guides all aspects including need for transfer, fluid administration, and prognosis. Overestimation can have negative effects, primarily overresuscitation and resultant problems of respiratory failure and compartment syndromes. Underresuscitation is also problematic as patients can progress into shock or renal failure. There are many different methods used to calculate TBSA, but the easiest and the most rapid assessment tool is called the "rule of nines," which divides the body into the following sections: head and neck, 9%; each upper extremity (front and back), 9%; anterior trunk, 18%; posterior trunk, 18%; anterior lower extremity (each), 9%; posterior lower extremity (each), 9%; and perineum/genitalia, 1%. Only partial-thickness (second degree) or full-thickness (third degree) burns should be included in the TBSA calculation; any areas of superficial, or first-degree, burns are not included. Another pitfall is using the adult "rule of nines" to calculate infant or pediatric TBSA. More detailed tools, such as the Lund-Browder chart, analyze the body surface area more accurately by smaller divisions and are adjusted for age (children have proportionally larger heads and smaller legs). Alternatively, small or scattered patches of burn can be estimated by using the surface of the patient's palm to represent 1% TBSA. Providers should also be cautioned that any scoring system is only an initial guideline for starting resuscitation and that fluid administration, hemodynamics, lab values, and urine output should be closely monitored to prevent over- or underresuscitation.

Ref.: 1, 2

8. A 22-year-old, 100-kg male presents with 70% TBSA burns. He initially presented directly from the scene to an outside hospital and has been getting a liter of normal saline an hour until he was able to be air-lifted to the burn center. In the 4 h since his burn, he has received 5 L of lactated Ringer's solution. He is currently hypotensive and oliguric. Which initial fluid administration plan is best for continued resuscitation of this patient?

A. Continue bolusing 1 L of normal saline each time the patient is hypotensive
B. Lactated Ringer's solution (LR) at 1125 mL/h for 8 h and then 875 mL/h for the following 16 h
C. Immediate transfusion of two units of packed red blood cells
D. LR at 2250 mL/h for 4 h and then 875 mL/h for the following 16 h
E. LR at 1750 mL/h for 8 h and then 875 mL/h for the following 16 h

ANSWER: D

COMMENTS: The **Parkland formula** (4 mL of lactated Ringer's solution × TBSA × weight in kg) is most commonly used to estimate the fluid resuscitation requirements for the first 24 h after a burn injury. This formula calls for 4 mL/kg per %TBSA burn to be given over a 24-h period. Half of the volume should be given over the first 8 h after injury and the remainder over the following 16 h. A common error is not taking into account fluid already administered prior to arrival, which can lead to overestimation of the amount of fluid needed. Another error is calculating the start time of fluid administration from presentation to the hospital, instead of the time of injury. For this patient, the initial calculation is 4 mL × 100 kg × 70 TBSA = 28,000 mL of lactated Ringer's solution to be given in the first 24 h after injury. Half (14,000 mL) should be given over the first 8 h, taking into account the 5000 mL administered prior to arrival for a remaining balance of 9000 mL to be given in the remaining 4 h (9000 mL/8 h = 2250 mL/h). The remainder should be given over the following 16 h (14,000 mL/16 h = 875 mL/h). Pediatric patients will need the normal weight-based rate of maintenance fluids with glucose due to their low glycogen stores and inability to concentrate urine. It is important to remember that any formula used to guide resuscitation is only the best estimate of the patient's needs. Many factors, including the patient's cardiovascular status, concomitant injuries from trauma, medical comorbidities, and age can all affect the response to volume administration. The patient's response to resuscitation should be monitored and IV fluids adjusted to the patient's urine output. The most useful marker of resuscitation is adequate hourly urine output, defined as 30 to 50 mL/h in adult patients and 1 mL/kg/h in children in the absence of myoglobinuria. Crystalloid boluses should be avoided unless required because of hypotensive episodes (mean arterial pressure persistently less than 60 mmHg) or to resuscitate blood loss from other traumatic injuries. Intravenous fluids are rapidly extravasated as a result of the capillary leakage that occurs in the first 48 h. Decreased urine output for 1 to 2 h would require increasing the hourly fluid rate. Adequate or excessive urine output may prompt the reduction of fluid administration rates. It is important to decrease fluid administration if not required because the morbidity (abdominal and extremity compartment syndromes, pulmonary edema) from massive volumes of resuscitation fluid is not insignificant.

Ref.: 1–3

9. Which of the following is correct regarding inhalation injury in burn patients?
   A. The admission chest radiograph is useful for ruling out inhalation injury on admission.
   B. Supraglottic inhalation injury may necessitate intubation even if gas exchange is initially unaffected.
   C. With proper pulmonary toilet, pneumonia is an unusual complication of smoke inhalation.
   D. Smoke inhalation is basically just a subset of acute respiratory distress syndrome (ARDS) seen in burn victims.
   E. Daily bronchoscopy is mandatory to monitor the evolution of inhalation injury.

ANSWER: B

COMMENTS: Inhalation injury occurs in up to a third of major burns and significantly increases mortality in patients when combined with cutaneous burns. Conceptually, inhalation injury can be divided into three types, all of which can coexist within any given patient: CO poisoning (and other toxic inhalation), upper airway thermal injury, and lower airway injury. Upper airway burns occur as a result of a thermal injury, as well as the toxic substances in smoke. The capacity for the oropharynx to absorb heat generally prevents the thermal injury from extending lower into the airway. Oropharyngeal thermal injury can be diagnosed by direct laryngoscopy and, if significant, is an indication for prophylactic endotracheal intubation to control the airway before life-threatening airway edema develops, particularly after large-volume resuscitation ensues. Endotracheal tubes may be difficult to secure if the patient has facial burns. They may be tied with cotton tape wrapped around the face. Airway edema occurs a maximum of 12 to 24 h after injury, and if airway protection is required, the patient may remain intubated for 72 h. Short courses of steroids may be considered in patients without significant burns, but they are contraindicated in those with large burns because of infectious and wound complications. Extubation may be performed when the patient has met weaning parameters and edema has subsided. Lower airway inhalation injury results from exposure of the respiratory epithelium to toxic irritants in smoke or steam. Chest x-ray findings on admission are typically normal because infiltrates and lung injury tend to develop in delayed fashion over the days following injury. Damage to the airway leads to inflammation, sloughing of mucosa, and impaired ciliary function, which results in edema, hemorrhage, bronchoconstriction, and bronchial obstruction. Pulmonary edema, ARDS, and pneumonia may complicate inhalation injury, with pneumonia occurring in up to 50% of patients. Lower airway inhalation injury is diagnosed most commonly by fiberoptic bronchoscopy, although nuclear medicine ventilation–perfusion scanning has been used. Treatment is primarily supportive and consists of aggressive pulmonary toilet, supplemental oxygen, and endotracheal intubation if required for either airway protection or oxygenation. Bronchoscopy may be used as an adjunct for pulmonary toilet if airway plugging leads to lobar collapse, but it is not always required for management. Aerosolized heparin is administered by some centers to aid mobilization of fibrin-rich casts, which contribute to airway obstruction. Laboratory and clinical research is ongoing for therapies dealing with smoke inhalation injury. Patients with severe inhalation injury may be extremely difficult to ventilate, and ventilatory strategies vary among burn centers. Low–tidal volume ventilation, high-frequency oscillatory ventilation, and even extracorporeal membrane oxygenation (ECMO) have been used by burn units.

Ref.: 1, 2

10. An 18-month-old boy presents to the burn unit after sustaining a scald burn to the buttocks. Which of the following burn patterns or components of the history is MOST suspicious for intentional burns in children?
    A. Irregular burn margin and depth
    B. Large TBSA of scald
    C. Scald injury sustained from spilling of nonwater hot liquid
    D. Symmetrical involvement of extremities
    E. Trunk, neck, or head involvement

ANSWER: D

COMMENTS: Intentional burns comprise assault burns and self-inflicted burns. It is important for the provider to be cognizant of the risk factors for intentional burns and to identify injury patterns characteristic of this type of injury. Vulnerable populations for intentional burns vary secondarily to geographic and cultural forces. In the United States, vulnerable populations include those with mental illness or history of drug abuse, victims of domestic violence, the elderly, and most often, children.

Maguire et al. published a systematic review of 26 studies to identify the injury patterns of intentional burns in children that were most suspicious for intentional motives. They found 15 unique characteristics of intentional burns grouped into mechanism (immersion), agent (hot tap water), pattern (clear upper margins, symmetrical scalding), distribution (isolated scald on the lower extremities, buttock, or perineum), and additional clinical features (history discordant with physical examination, associated injuries including fractures, introverted child on physical examination, and previous episodes of abuse). With any of these characteristics, the provider should rule out intentional injury.

Additional potential abuse-related burn patterns include skin fold sparing, stocking and glove distribution, and uniform scald depth. Characteristics not representative of intentional burns include spill/flowing water injury, scald from hot beverage, and irregular margin and depth. However, it is important for the provider to take the entire history and physical examination into account as low-risk characteristics do not entirely rule out intentional injury. No study has demonstrated large TBSA, child age, or gender as risk factors.

Ref.: 5

11. A 45-year-old man presents following a motor vehicle crash with 30% TBSA burns to the torso, face, and extremities. On presentation to the trauma bay, he is alert with a Glasgow coma score (GCS) of 15, but is hypotensive with diffuse abdominal pain. Which of the following is true regarding the management of combined trauma and burn victims?

A. Chest tubes should be placed through burned skin as the chest tube dressing serves as appropriate additional coverage for the burn.

B. In a patient with thoracic trauma and concern for pulmonary contusions and chest wall burns, patients should be deliberately underresuscitated to prevent an increase in pulmonary edema.

C. In patients with abdominal trauma and abdominal burns, a paramedian incision is recommended due to its lower rates of dehiscence.

D. The most common cause of combined trauma and burn injuries is from house fires and falling debris.

E. A neurologically impaired patient following automobile accident and fire must be quickly assessed for CO and cyanide poisoning as this can exacerbate traumatic brain injury.

ANSWER: E

COMMENTS: The simultaneous trauma and burn patient poses additional diagnostic and management challenges to the health care provider. Roughly 5%–7% of burn admissions will have additional traumatic injuries. In a large, 10-year retrospective study from Los Angeles County Burn Center, mortality for concomitant burn and trauma patients was 13% versus 6% of burns without additional trauma. Patients with inhalation injury were the highest-risk subgroup with a mortality of 41%. The origin of injury is most commonly from motor vehicle crashes, followed by falls from height in house fires.

The management of the combined burn and trauma patient begins similar to that of the monotrauma patient with assessment of the patient's airway, breathing, and circulation. In combined burn and trauma patients, each of the three components of the primary survey has nuanced features that focus on the diagnosis of burn-specific injuries, or those anatomic structures at increased risk of injury from burns and traumatic injury. For example, in the evaluation of the airway, the provider must assess for inhalation injury and progressive upper airway edema with careful attention to the cervical spine prior to manipulation of the neck during intubation or bronchoscopy.

During the assessment of the patient's ability to breathe, victims of automobile or structural fires are at risk for CO or cyanide poisoning, both of which can cause hypoxia and further exacerbate an existing traumatic brain injury. Treatment is 100% oxygen. Poor respiratory function may be secondary to a number of causes including inhalation injury, thoracic trauma, or ARDS. Judicious fluid administration, not deliberate underresuscitation, is indicated. A special subgroup of patients may require tube thoracostomy with overlying thoracic burns. These should be placed through healthy skin, if available, or otherwise through burn eschar.

Hypotension in the traumatically burned victim must be first ruled out as secondary to hemorrhage. Resuscitation begins with 2 L of crystalloid and assessment of the patient's hemodynamic response, followed by adequate resuscitation by calculation of the patient's 24-h volume requirements. For those who require laparotomy with abdominal burns, a paramedian incision has been associated with higher rates of dehiscence. Furthermore, special attention should be paid to the mode of abdominal wall closure in a burn patient who requires large-volume crystalloid resuscitation to prevent abdominal compartment syndrome.

Ref.: 6

12. An 88-year-old woman suffers 11% TBSA superficial partial-thickness burn as a result of scalding with hot soup. Which of the following is most correct regarding the topical antimicrobial agents that may be used?

A. Mafenide acetate is an undesirable choice because of metabolic alkalosis caused by carbonic anhydrase inhibition.

B. Silver nitrate solutions can lead to methemoglobinemia, which causes a shift of the oxygen–hemoglobin dissociation curve to the right.

C. Silver sulfadiazine should be discontinued if neutropenia occurs as a result of its use.

D. Silver sulfadiazine induces epithelial cell migration, but it is often painful on application.

E. Elemental silver-impregnated dressings must be moistened frequently with sterile water to retain the antimicrobial activity.

ANSWER: E

COMMENTS: Systemic antibiotics are not indicated for prophylaxis. Topical antimicrobial agents delay colonization and infection of wounds but have not changed mortality as much as early excision and grafting have. Silver sulfadiazine is the most commonly used agent for burns in the United States. Advantages include a broad spectrum of activity, soothing effect in most patients, and no significant metabolic activity. Silver sulfadiazine does not penetrate eschar, so it does not treat established wound infections. Many providers have implicated it as a cause of early postburn neutropenia, but this neutropenia is typically self-limited, and more current information suggests that it is more likely the result of margination of neutrophils rather than depletion by the topical agent. One other caution is the use of silver sulfadiazine in a sulfa-allergic patient. Mafenide acetate penetrates eschar and is therefore useful for the treatment of burn wound infections; it has a broad spectrum of activity against gram-negative organisms. It may be applied as a cream or a solution and is often used after grafting. Mafenide acetate is a carbonic anhydrase inhibitor that may cause metabolic acidosis when used on large areas. It is also painful on application, particularly to partial-thickness burns. Silver nitrate has a broad spectrum of activity and may be used for burn wound dressings. Dressings need to be repeatedly impregnated with an aqueous solution to prevent precipitation onto the wound. Concentrated silver nitrate may cause chemical burns and hyponatremia, along with the rare case of methemoglobinemia. Wounds, normal skin, linens, and the patient environment will be stained black by silver nitrate. Ointments of bacitracin, neomycin, and polymyxin B are commonly used for facial burns. Mupirocin has been used against methicillin-resistant *Staphylococcus aureus* (MRSA). Acticoat (Smith & Nephew, London, England) is a dressing impregnated with elemental silver that may be applied to burn wounds or grafts. Sheets of Acticoat are usually moistened in sterile water before application because sodium chloride will cause precipitation and inactivation of the silver ions. Silver disrupts bacterial cellular respiration, and silver dressings may be left in place for up to 7 days if necessary.

Ref.: 1–3

13. A 23-year-old man presents with diffuse skin sloughing after ingestion of trimethoprim-sulfamethoxazole. Which of the following is an independent risk factor for increased mortality in the SCORe of Toxic Epidermal Necrosis (SCORTEN) illness severity scale?

A. Age > 30

B. Serum bicarbonate > 20

C. Serum glucose > 150

D. Serum BUN > 28

E. Heart rate > 90 beats/min

ANSWER: D

COMMENTS: Stevens–Johnson syndrome (SJS) and toxic epidermal necrolysis (TEN) are systemic disease processes that cause varying degrees of epidermal sloughing, with mortality ranging from 5% to 30%. Commonly associated with drug ingestion with an immunologic basis, it is important for the provider to quickly identify and stop any potential culprit drug, as a delay in the cessation of drug administration decreases survival. Furthermore, early transfer of patients to a burn unit is the standard of care in initial management after the diagnosis of SJS/TEN is made.

The SCORTEN illness severity score was created and validated in the year 2000 as a predictor of mortality in patients with SJS/TEN. On multivariate analysis of 165 patients with SJS/TEN, prognostic risk factors, vitals, and laboratory values (corresponding odds ratios for mortality) are as follows: age > 40 years (2.7), associated malignancy (4.4), heart rate > 120 beats per min (2.7), serum BUN > 28 mg/dL (2.5), TBSA > 30% (3.3), serum bicarbonate < 20 mmol/L (4.3), and serum glucose > 252 mmol/L (5.3). Each independent predictor is attributed one point. Mortality ranges from 3.2% with one risk factor to over 90% with five or more risk factors. Treatment for SJS/TEN is supportive, with wound care and monitoring in the burn ICU to prevent additional superinfection.

Ref.: 7

14. A 35-year-old male comes in following an occupational injury in which he sustained 35% full-thickness burns to his torso and upper extremities. On hospital day #2, the decision is made to perform excision of his burns with split-thickness skin grafting. Which of the following is associated with early excision and grafting?

A. Decreased mortality

B. Decreased functional outcomes

C. Increased length of stay

D. Increased cost

E. Increased number of operations

ANSWER: A

COMMENTS: Early excision and grafting of deep burns has been one of the great advances in burn surgery. Although universally accepted now, early excision of a large burn during the initial-stage burn shock was initially considered to be prohibitively dangerous. In 1960, a paper concluded that early excision and grafting should only be used "in experienced hands, [sic] in so far as the risks require further investigation."

However, over the years research has clearly demonstrated the advantages of early excision of both small- and large-TBSA full-thickness burns. In 1982, researchers at the University of Washington demonstrated decreased rates of burn wound sepsis and hospitalization in patients treated by early excision (excision prior to 14 days) and grafting versus waiting for autoexcision of the eschar in TBSA burns of 20%–40%. This study was later corroborated by a 1989 prospective study by Herndon et al., which randomized patients with TBSA burns (>30%) into early excision or topical antibiotic treatment until autoexcision. Mortality in the early-excision group was 9% versus 45% in the delayed-excision cohort.

Additional studies have shown decreases in mortality, intensive care stays, and hospital expenditure. Theories on the survival advantage of the early removal of full-thickness burns include removal of a hyperinflammatory focus and prevention of secondary wound infection.

Ref.: 1–3, 8, 9

15. A 22-year-old man suffers partial- and full-thickness burns to 45% TBSA in a gas explosion while at work. Which of the following is most accurate regarding surgical management of his wounds?

A. Assessment of the depth of injury on admission is accurate enough for definitive surgery to be planned in more than 90% of cases.

B. Fascial excision allows grafts to be placed over a healthy muscle bed and is the preferred approach to burns on the hands and dorsal surface of the feet.

C. Sheet (unmeshed) grafting is preferred for areas subjected to repeated shear, thus making it the choice for extensive burns on dorsal surfaces.

D. Excision of burn wounds within 24 h of injury should not be performed due to the effects of hypothermia on coagulopathy and the time required to assess for adequacy of resuscitation.

E. Widely meshed grafts minimize the degree of wound contraction associated with the use of split-thickness grafts.

ANSWER: D

COMMENTS: Excision of deep partial- and full-thickness burn wounds should be done after resuscitation is complete and the patient is normothermic and hemodynamically stable. Although the advantages of early excision and grafting are well described, watchful waiting is appropriate to observe for healing in burns of indeterminate depth to avoid unnecessary grafting to those portions that will heal. Wounds expected to heal within 3 weeks are best treated with antimicrobial dressings, whereas full-thickness burns, as well as deep partial-thickness wounds with delayed healing, require grafting. Fascial excision refers to the removal of burned skin and subcutaneous tissue down to the level of the fascia, frequently with electrocautery. This approach provides a bed that readily takes graft and is usually easy to define. However, such deep debridement often results in fragile, esthetically displeasing grafts. Tangential excision involves sequentially cutting away eschar with a handheld knife with a depth guard until viable dermis or subcutaneous tissue is present as noted by diffuse punctate bleeding. Experience is important in judging the depth of excision required to support a graft. Hemostasis may be achieved with a combination of electrocautery, suture ligature, thrombin spray, direct pressure, and dilute epinephrine solution in gauze pads. Skin grafts may be full thickness for smaller grafts or split thickness for larger ones, depending on the amount of dermis present when harvested. Harvesting is most commonly done with a dermatome. Thinner grafts will heal with greater contraction, but thicker grafts come at the cost of loss of dermis at the donor site, which leads to prolonged times until healing and increased donor site scarring. Meshing of grafts (ranging from 1:1 to 4:1) may be used to allow egress of fluid from the wound bed through the graft and to increase the area covered when donor sites are limited. Widely meshed grafts are associated with prolonged healing, increased scarring, and more contraction than are less meshed or sheet grafts. A variety of dressings may be placed over grafted areas, the goal of which is to maintain contact of the graft with the wound bed to allow graft survival, prevent shearing, and facilitate subsequent vascular ingrowth into the graft.

Ref.: 1, 2

16. Which of the following is correct regarding the skin substitutes used in burn reconstruction?

A. Cultured epidermal autografts have dramatically increased survival in patients with nearly 100% TBSA burn injuries.

B. Allografting to burn wound sites is limited to temporary closure because of eventual rejection of the graft by the patient.

C. Porcine xenograft has the advantage of better early vascularization and engrafting after placement as a result of decreased antigenicity in comparison to most cadaveric human allografts.

D. Use of the Integra Dermal Regeneration Template is advantageous because of lower rates of wound infection than with early autografting in heavily colonized burn wounds.

E. Vascularization of porcine xenograft may be aided by the use of low-dose cyclosporine, provided that the patient is free of infectious complications at the time of placement.

ANSWER: B

COMMENTS: After debridement and excision of burn eschar, closure of the wound with immediate autografting, when possible, is preferred. Full-thickness skin grafts are the best possible cutaneous replacement, but they are not feasible for burns of significant size because the full-thickness donor site must be closed primarily. Meshed split-thickness grafts may be used to cover areas larger than the donor site harvested, but for large burns and patients with limited donor sites, even meshed autografts will not be able to cover all open wounds. Wounds not able to be autografted immediately may be covered with biologic dressings while awaiting donor site healing before reharvesting. Human allograft has been widely used as a temporary biologic dressing. It is usually meshed to allow drainage of fluid and applied in a similar fashion to other skin grafts. Allograft will vascularize and engraft, provide wound closure for 2 to 4 weeks, and subsequently be rejected and need to be replaced with new allograft or autograft if available. Sheets of allograft may be placed over widely meshed autograft at the time of surgery to protect grafts as the interstices epithelialize. Porcine xenograft is cheaper and more easily stored before use, but it does not vascularize and engraft. It may be used similar to allograft for temporary biologic coverage of burn wounds, as well as for exfoliative diseases of the skin (e.g., TEN). Cultured epidermal autografts grown from patient keratinocytes are promising as a skin substitute but are not yet in widespread availability and are associated with high cost and complexity. Dermal substitutes such as the Integra Dermal Regeneration Template (Integra Lifesciences, Plainsboro, NJ) have seen more clinical use. The Integra dermal template is a bilaminate composed of an outer silicone film that provides barrier function and an inner layer of type 1 collagen and chondroitin sulfate. This inner layer serves as a template for the ingrowth of autologous fibroblasts, endothelial cells, and other mesenchymal cells. After vascularization of the Integra, the silicone film is removed, and very thin autografts may be applied to the neodermis. Reported advantages include neodermis architecture similar to that of uninjured dermis, which results in improved cosmetic and functional results, as well as rapid healing of thin autograft donor sites. Disadvantages include wound infection and increased length of time and immobilization before final autograft closure.

Ref.: 1, 2

17. Which of the following statements is correct regarding surgical anatomy and technique in operations commonly performed by burn surgeons?

A. The main concept for incisions in torso escharotomies is separating the chest eschar down the midline, allowing free expansion of each side of the torso.

B. A dermatome must be held at a 0-degree angle to the skin when initiating skin grafting.

C. A hand escharotomy is performed on the palmar side of the hand between the metacarpals.

D. Effective mechanisms to control bleeding following tangential excision of burns include diluted dressings with epinephrine, or fibrinogen and thrombin spray.

E. Disadvantages of a fascial incision include increased blood loss compared with tangential incisions.

ANSWER: D

COMMENTS: Three common operations performed by burn surgeons are escharotomies, burn excision, and skin grafting. Escharotomies are performed for full-thickness burns causing life-threatening complications secondary to restricted peripheral blood flow or pulmonary compliance. Surgeons must be aware of the appropriate anatomy to perform a fully effective procedure. For burns of the chest wall, escharotomy incisions are made on bilateral posterior axillary lines with superior borders of clavicles to inferior borders of subcostal margins. For the hand, a hand escharotomy is performed on the dorsal side of the hand between the metacarpals.

Excision of full-thickness burns can be performed by fascial or tangential means by a variety of surgical instruments. A tangential excision will have greater blood loss than a fascial excision, which can be controlled using dressings diluted with epinephrine or fibrinogen and thrombin spray.

Skin grafting is performed in a split-thickness or full-thickness manner and must be performed appropriately for a successful graft take. Common donor sites include the thighs or back. After application of mineral oil, a dermatome is used to harvest a split-thickness skin graft.

Ref.: 1–3

18. A 22-year-old utility company employee is found down at a job site at the base of the ladder. He has a charred wound in the left temporal region with palpable shards of skull present. His left arm is waxy and fixed in flexion. There are full-thickness burns on his left flank, the lower part of his left leg is firm, and the toes of his left foot are burned and missing. Which of the following is the correct statement regarding electrical injury?

A. The cause of the dark, reddish urine noted in the urinary catheter will most likely be revealed by computed tomography of the abdomen.

B. Signs concerning for compartment syndrome should prompt urgent escharotomy of the affected limbs.

C. Neurologic deficits that develop in a delayed fashion, weeks to months after the injury, have a better prognosis.

D. Early fascial decompression of the extremities may be important in preserving limb function.

E. Myoglobinuria is addressed by maintaining an hourly urine output of 0.5 mL/kg in adults and 1 mL/kg in children less than 20 kg.

ANSWER: D

COMMENTS: Electrical injuries are classified in the medical literature into low-voltage, high-voltage (>1000 V), and lightning injuries (also termed ultra-high voltage). Patients injured by electricity may, in fact, have injuries by any of the three mechanisms: flash burns from the very high temperatures generated when high-voltage current arcs through the air, flame burns because of ignition of clothing, and true electrical injury as a result of conduction of electrical current through the patient's body. Low-voltage injuries may cause local tissue injury but rarely lead to systemic injury. High-voltage injuries may cause unpredictable patterns of local injury, including deep tissue destruction belied by the small size of the skin wounds, full-thickness cutaneous wounds at entry/exit sites and areas where arcing occurs across joints or flexor surfaces, and musculoskeletal injuries from severe tetanic contractions of the paravertebral and other muscle groups. Patients with an electrical injury are at particularly high risk for associated traumatic injuries because electrical exposures frequently occur in occupational settings and may involve falls from a height. In fact, the tetanic muscle contractions caused by alternating current tend to cause "hanging up" by workers who grasp an electrical source and pull themselves in; patients who hang up and survive may do so because they subsequently fall and break contact with the current, and can suffer other injuries as a result. Evaluation of patients suffering from a high-voltage electrical injury includes a full examination of the traumatic injury, radiographic studies, electrocardiogram, and bladder catheterization. Patients with no loss of consciousness at the scene, no history of arrhythmias during transport, and a normal admission electrocardiogram do not require cardiac monitoring unless the severity of the injury would otherwise require it. Deep tissue damage secondary to high-voltage current may result in unseen muscle swelling and necrosis. Neurovascular examination should document the extent of disability present at admission, and progressive deterioration in extremity function should prompt consideration of compartment release by fasciotomy. Compartment pressures may be measured if the patient is not likely to need compartment release, but fasciotomy should be prompted by clinical grounds if significant concern exists. Escharotomy refers to the division of band-like circumferential full-thickness burn eschars through to subcutaneous fat only. Fixed deficits or mummified extremities may not benefit from compartment release. Pigmented urine suggestive of myoglobinuria should be treated by fluid resuscitation sufficient to produce a urine output of 100 mL/h. Fasciotomies or even early debridement or amputation of necrotic muscle can be performed to avoid renal failure. Urine myoglobin assays are often not immediately available, but urine that is heme positive by dipstick with no red blood cells on microscopic examination may be presumed to be myoglobinuria resulting from rhabdomyolysis; hematuria found on urinalysis should additionally prompt reconsideration of occult genitourinary trauma. Toddlers may suffer electrical burns to the mouth from chewing on appliance cords. Full-thickness oral burns are typically treated conservatively with attention to preserving mouth opening, and families should be counseled about the possibility of delayed facial artery bleeding after the eschar softens and falls off. High-voltage injuries may result in progressive demyelinating injury and lead to sensory or motor loss weeks or months after the injury. Early cataract formation has been associated with high-voltage electrical exposure.

Ref.: 2

REFERENCES

1. Mulholland MW, Lillemoe KD, Doherty GM, et al., eds. *Greenfield's Surgery: Scientific Principles and Practice*. 4th ed. Philadelphia: Lippincott Williams & Wilkins; 2006.
2. Souba WW, Fink MP, Jurkovich GJ, et al., eds. *ACS Surgery: Principles and Practice*. 6th ed. New York: WebMD; 2007.
3. Herndon DN, ed. *Total Burn Care*. 4th ed. Philadelphia: WB Saunders; 2012.
4. Committee on Trauma. American College of Surgeons. Guidelines for the operation of burn centers: resources for optimal care of the injured patient. 2006:79–86. Available at http://www.ameriburn.org/Chapter14.pdf.
5. Maguire S, Moynihan S, Mann M, Potokar T, Kemp AM. A systematic review of the features that indicate intentional scalds in children. *Burns*. 2008;34(8):1072–1081.
6. Dougherty W, Waxman K. The complexities of managing severe burns with associated trauma. *Surg Clin North Am*. 1996;76(4):923–958.
7. Bastuji Garin S, Fouchard N, Bertocchi M, Roujeau JC, Revuz J, Wolkenstein P. SCORTEN: a severity-of-illness score for toxic epidermal necrolysis. *J Invest Dermatol*. 2000;115(2):149–153.
8. Gray DT, Pine RW, Harnar TJ, Marvin JA, Engrav LH, Heimbach DM. Early surgical excision versus conventional therapy in patients with 20 to 40 percent burns: a comparative study. *Am J Surg*. 1982;144(1):76–80.
9. Herndon DN, Barrow RE, Rutan RL, Rutan TC, Desai MH, Abston S. A comparison of conservative versus early excision therapies in severely burned patients. *Annals Surg*. 1989;209(5):547–552, discussion 552.

SECTION III

SOFT TISSUE, HERNIA, AND BREAST

CHAPTER 13

SKIN AND SOFT TISSUE

Rebecca A. Deal, M.D., and Andrea Madrigrano, M.D.

1. With regard to ultraviolet (UV) radiation, which of the following statements is correct?

A. Most of the UV radiation that reaches the earth is type B (UVB, wavelength of 290 to 320 nm).

B. Type A UV (UVA) radiation is responsible for most of the sun damage to human skin.

C. UVA is within the photoabsorption spectrum of DNA, whereas UVB is not.

D. The melanin content of the skin is the single best intrinsic factor for protecting the skin from the harmful effects of UV radiation.

E. UV radiation acts as a tumor promoter but not a tumor initiator.

ANSWER: D

COMMENTS: UV radiation comprises the middle of the electromagnetic spectrum and is divided into UVA (320 to 380 nm), UVB (290 to 320 nm), and type C UV (UVC) (240 to 290 nm), whereas visible light has a wavelength of 400 to 700 nm. UVC is virtually eliminated by stratospheric ozone and oxygen. Only 5% of solar UV emission is UVB, but it is the most carcinogenic part of the spectrum and is responsible for sunburn. Since UVB is partially eliminated by stratospheric ozone, a 1% decrease in stratospheric ozone increases UVB flux at the earth's surface by about 3%. More than 95% of the sun's UV radiation that reaches the earth's surface is UVA. Sunbeds for indoor recreational tanning emit predominantly UVA. UV light acts both by inducing direct DNA damage and by other mechanisms, such as alteration of cellular immunity and DNA repair mechanisms. Although UVB and UVC radiation is within the photoabsorption spectrum of DNA, UVA radiation contributes to the development of skin cancers mainly via non-DNA targets. It penetrates more deeply and affects dermal fibroblasts, which results in photoaging. Recent data suggest that UVA may also directly affect DNA; experimental studies have shown the UVA-induced development of the characteristic carcinogenic photoproduct (cyclobutane pyrimidine dimer) seen classically with DNA damage secondary to UVB. **Melanin** is the most important factor in protecting the skin from the harmful effects of UV light. Tightly woven clothing, sunscreen use, and avoidance of sun exposure also offer protection against the harmful effects of UV radiation. **UV radiation** can act as both a tumor initiator and a tumor promoter.

Ref.: 1–3

2. The most common histologic type of melanoma is:

A. Superficial spreading

B. Nodular

C. Lentigo maligna

D. Acral lentiginous

E. Desmoplastic

ANSWER: A

COMMENTS: Superficial spreading melanoma is the most common type; it accounts for 70% of melanomas and is characterized by some degree of radial growth (Fig. 13.1). **Nodular melanoma**, the next most common type, accounts for about 15% of melanomas and is characterized by vertical growth with a minimal to absent radial growth phase (Fig. 13.2). **Lentigo maligna melanoma**, about 10% of melanomas, is characterized by an extensive radial growth phase, most commonly occurring on sun-exposed body areas in older patients, and is generally diagnosed at a thinner stage (Fig. 13.3). **Acral lentiginous melanoma** is the most common type of melanoma in nonwhite individuals and is usually darkly pigmented (Fig. 13.4). The prognosis depends on the thickness of the lesion, not the histologic subtype per se.

Ref.: 2

3. Which statement correctly describes increased risk for the development of malignant melanoma?

A. Melanoma accounts for 50% of all skin cancer diagnoses but accounts for 10% of deaths due to skin cancer.

B. Populations that reside at further distances from the equator have a higher incidence of melanoma.

C. An adult patient with greater than 50 clinically normal-appearing nevi is at an increased risk for melanoma.

D. The *p16/CDKN2A* tumor suppressor gene, located on chromosome 9, is implicated in 40% of cases of familial melanoma.

E. A genetic component has been implicated in the pathogenesis of melanoma, with nearly 25% of all patients diagnosed with melanoma reporting a positive family history.

ANSWER: D

COMMENTS: Cutaneous melanoma accounts for only 4% of skin cancer diagnoses, yet accounts for nearly 75% of skin cancer–related

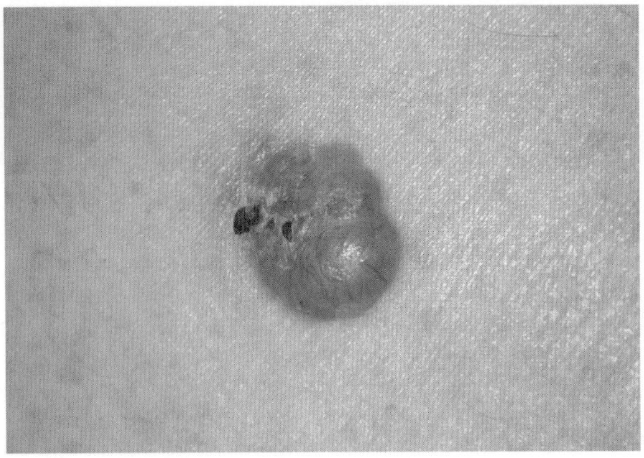

Fig. 13.1 Superficial spreading melanoma.

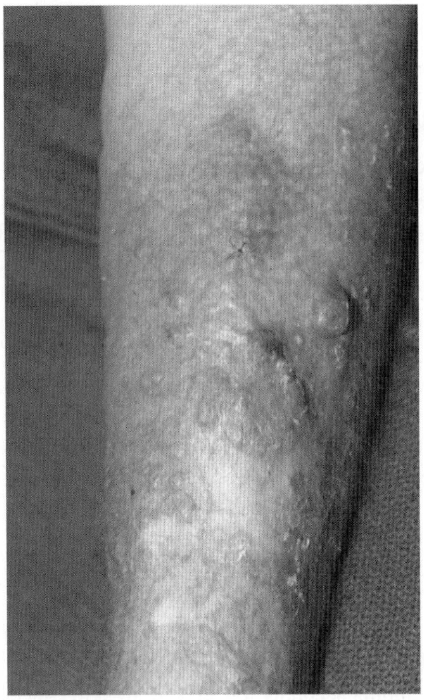

Fig. 13.2 Nodular melanoma.

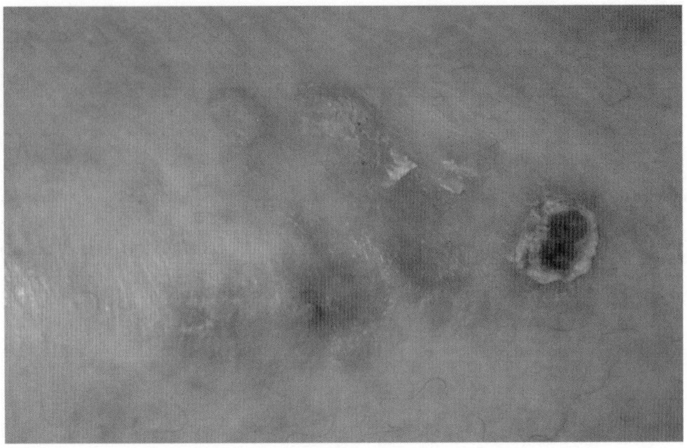

Fig. 13.3 Lentigo maligna melanoma.

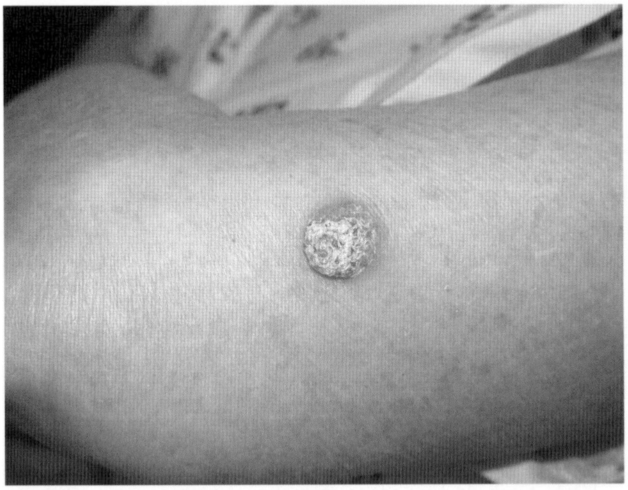

Fig. 13.4 Acral lentiginous melanoma.

deaths. Multiple environmental and genetic risk factors play a role in the development of cutaneous melanoma. Environmental factors associated with increased exposure to UVA and UVB radiations such as geographic location (closer to the equator), occupation, history of tanning bed use, and sensitivity to UV light are particularly important risk factors. Approximately 10%–15% of individuals with a prior history of melanoma develop a second primary melanoma, placing these patients at an increased lifelong risk of melanoma. A genetic link appears to exist, with 10%–15% of melanoma patients reporting a family history of the disease. Factors that increase the risk for melanoma include the presence of **dysplastic nevus syndrome** [familial atypical multiple mole melanoma syndrome or atypical mole syndrome], a clinical syndrome distinguished by the presence of numerous large dysplastic nevi usually over the trunk; xeroderma pigmentosum (characterized by mutations in genes responsible for the fidelity of DNA repair); familial retinoblastoma; and a family history of melanoma. Dysplastic nevus syndrome can be identified in adult patients with more than 100 clinically normal-appearing nevi or in children with more than 50 clinically normal-appearing nevi. Any patient with atypical or dysplastic nevi is at an increased risk for melanoma. Individuals at a high risk include those with two or more first-degree relatives with melanoma, two relatives of any degree if one exhibits signs of dysplastic nevus syndrome, and those with three relatives of any degree with melanoma. As with other familial cancers, **familial melanoma** is characterized by an earlier age at onset and multiple tumors. Germline mutations in the *CDKN2A* gene, which encodes the proteins p16/INK4A and p14ARF, are the most common cause of inherited risk for melanoma with high penetrance and may be identified in up to 40% of all melanoma families with three or more affected individuals. The penetrance of this gene is variable and varies significantly with geography, with melanoma penetrance of 0.13 (0.58) in Europe, 0.5 (0.76) in the United States, and 0.32 (0.91) in Australia by the age of 50 (80). Although commercial testing is available, testing may be premature at this time because of the risk for other cancers in *CDKN2A* families, and factors that modify penetrance are not yet well described. In addition, the lack of correlation between *CDKN2A* gene carriers and the phenotypic dysplastic nevus syndrome may falsely reassure family members. Mutations of the *CDK4* gene have been identified in a few melanoma kindreds. The most frequently identified gene that predisposes to melanoma is the *MC1R* gene associated with red hair and freckles. Variations in this gene are associated with an elevated risk for melanoma, even in patients without red hair, but such variations impart a weak susceptibility to melanoma (low penetrance) in white populations. The deleterious effect of *MC1R* variations is amplified by high sun exposure. Mutations in *PTC*, the human homolog of the *Drosophila* patched gene, have been identified in most patients with **basal cell nevus (Gorlin) syndrome**. Mutations have also been identified in a few sporadically occurring basal cell carcinomas.

Ref.: 2, 4–7

4. A 72-year-old female with a history of type 2 diabetes and obesity presents with 24 h of erythema and painful swelling of her right lower extremity. On examination, her temperature is 100.5°F, heart rate is 110 beats/minute (bpm), and blood pressure is 110/65 mmHg. Severe cellulitis is noted along the dorsal aspect of her right foot to her mid-calf. She has exquisite pain beyond the margins of the erythema that is out of proportion to her examination findings. No fluctuance, bullae, or crepitus is present. Lab values reveal white blood cell count of 22,000 cells/mm^3, hemoglobin 11 g/dL, C-reactive protein (CRP) 170 mg/dL, glucose 350 mg/dL, serum sodium 133 mmol/L, and serum creatinine 1.5 mg/dL. Which of the following is correct regarding her diagnosis?

A. They are most commonly classified as monomicrobial infections.

B. The Laboratory Risk Indicator for Necrotizing Fasciitis (LRINEC) score is used to diagnose necrotizing soft tissue infections (NSTIs).

C. Type I NSTIs are polymicrobial.

D. Confirmatory imaging studies [plain radiographs or computed tomography (CT)] should be obtained prior to surgical treatment.

E. Time between symptoms and antibiotic therapy is the most important factor contributing to morbidity and mortality.

ANSWER: C

COMMENTS: NSTIs are an uncommon diagnosis but a dangerous surgical emergency due to the significance of time and progression. The rapid progression of the disease and the systemic inflammatory response impart high morbidity and mortality if treatment is delayed. Approximately 80% of NSTIs are polymicrobial and classified as type I infections. Various species of gram-negative rods, gram-positive cocci, and anaerobes are typically isolated in type I NSTIs, with *Bacteroides fragilis* and *Escherichia coli* being the most common aerobic and anaerobic pathogens, respectively. The most common isolates from monomicrobial infections include *Streptococcus pyogenes* and *Clostridium perfringens.* Type II infections are caused by group A β-hemolytic *Streptococcus* sp. that may occur as a monomicrobial infection or in the presence of staphylococcal species. Type III NSTIs are rare, being caused by gram-negative marine organisms, most commonly *Vibrio vulnificus.* Definitive therapy for NSTI is aggressive surgical debridement of all devitalized tissue, keeping in mind that tissue necrosis extends beyond the borders of skin involvement. The most important factor contributing to morbidity and mortality is the delay in therapy related to the onset time of symptoms and the time period of operative therapy. Although antibiotics are an essential part of treating NSTIs, surgical therapy is necessary for patients' survival. The diagnosis of NSTI is primarily determined by a patient's history and physical examination. Signs and symptoms of early NSTI are similar to those of a cellulitis or abscess and may make the initial diagnosis difficult. Physical examination findings that should raise one's suspicion of NSTI include pain out of proportion to examination findings, bullae, crepitus, pain extending beyond lines of skin erythema, and manifestations of sepsis. Key components of a patient's history when considering NSTI include but are not limited to disruption of normal skin barriers (lacerations, ulcers, and surgical incisions), patient risk factors [diabetes mellitus (DM), chronic obstructive pulmonary disease (COPD), and congestive heart failure (CHF)], and environmental factors (exposure to salt/fresh water and animal/human bites). Although imaging studies such as CT and plain radiographs may show gas in soft tissues, the absence of gas does not rule out NSTI. Furthermore, obtaining radiographic studies may further delay treatment and thus should not be performed as a confirmatory test for NSTI. If NSTI is highly suspected based on clinical diagnosis, broad-spectrum antibiotics and surgical debridement are warranted. The LRINEC score may help increase a clinician's suspicion of NSTI but should not be used to diagnose or rule out NSTIs. The LRINEC score components include white blood cell count, hemoglobin, CRP, serum glucose, serum creatinine, and serum sodium.

Ref.: 8–13

5. Which of the following is true regarding benign cystic lesions of the skin?

A. An epidermal inclusion cyst lacks a fully mature epidermis with a granular cell layer.

B. The wall of a trichilemmal cyst, usually located on the scalp, is characterized by an epidermal lining that includes a granular cell layer.

C. The most common location of a ganglion cyst is on the dorsal aspect of the wrist.

D. Malignant degeneration may occur in a dermoid cyst.

E. A pilonidal cyst results from infection in a congenital coccygeal sinus.

ANSWER: C

COMMENTS: A number of **cystic lesions** occur in the skin. Complete excision of each of the lesions listed is curative, whereas incomplete excision may lead to recurrence. When an infection is present, primary incision plus drainage with secondary excision is preferred. The diagnosis can often be determined from the history and location of the cyst. **Epidermal inclusion cysts**, the most common type of cutaneous cyst, have a completely mature epidermis with a granular layer. The creamy material in the center of these cysts is keratin from desquamated cells. The wall of a **trichilemmal cyst**, the second most common type and often found on the scalp, does not have a granular layer. **Ganglions** are composed of connective tissue from the synovial membrane of a joint or tendon sheath and contain a thick jellylike mucinous material similar in composition to synovial fluid. Ganglions commonly occur over the tendons of the wrist, hands, and feet and may be congenital, related to trauma, or a result of arthritic conditions. They are more common in females. Sixty percent of ganglions occur on the dorsal aspect of the wrist and arise in the region of the scapholunate ligament. Asymptomatic ganglions may be treated expectantly. If treatment is needed, the initial approach can be aspiration with a large-bore needle, with or without steroid injection. Failure of this approach necessitates surgical excision, which should include removal of the pedicle of the ganglion from its origin at the involved joint or tendon sheath. **Dermoid cysts** are found along the body fusion planes and usually occur over the midline abdominal and sacral regions, over the occiput, and on the nose. Malignant degeneration has not been reported. Although in the past it was thought that **pilonidal cysts** result from the penetration of a congenital coccygeal sinus by an ingrown hair, which sets the stage for infection and cyst formation, most now believe that pilonidal cysts are acquired. The cysts result from embedded hairs in the intergluteal cleft but may occur at other locations in the body and are more common in hirsute persons. Males have a two to four times greater risk than females.

Ref.: 14–16

6. A 32-year-old man has multiple soft tissue masses over his trunk and extremities. He is noted to have axillary freckling and café au lait spots. Which of these statements most accurately describes his condition?

A. It is not associated with an increased risk for the development of central nervous system (CNS) tumors and lymphoma.

B. A malignant peripheral nerve sheath tumor (PNST) will develop in 50% of affected individuals.

C. Malignant PNSTs in these patients are more often multiple and occur at a younger age than do their sporadically occurring counterparts.

D. The gene responsible for this disorder is inherited in an autosomal recessive fashion.

E. It is not associated with an increased risk for the development of soft tissue sarcomas.

ANSWER: C

COMMENTS: Neurofibromatosis (NF) is a multisystem genetic disorder with characteristic cutaneous, neurologic, and bony manifestations. **Neurofibromatosis type 1** (NF1, von Recklinghausen disease) is an autosomal dominant disorder estimated to affect 1 in 3000 individuals. The *NF1* gene, located on chromosome 17q11.2, encodes a protein, neurofibromin, which is important for neuroectodermal differentiation and cardiac development. NF1 patients may have café au lait spots (six or more spots > 5 mm in children younger than 10 years or >15 mm in adults); neurofibromas (two or more); axillary or inguinal freckling; Lisch nodules (iris hamartomas, two or more); optic nerve gliomas; sphenoid dysplasia or long-bone abnormalities; cutaneous, subcutaneous, and visceral plexiform neurofibromas; and a first-degree relative with NF1. The presence of two or more of these eight characteristics confirms the clinical diagnosis of NF1. The most common tumor is a neurofibroma (a benign PNST), and benign schwannomas and neurilemomas may also be present. Although about half of malignant PNSTs develop in patients with NF1, affected individuals have a 3%–15% lifetime risk for the development of malignant tumors, including CNS tumors, Wilms tumor, soft tissue sarcomas, and lymphomas, as well as malignant PNSTs. These tumors often occur in association with major peripheral nerve trunks. Malignant tumors appear as enlarging soft tissue masses, variably associated with pain and other neurologic symptoms. NF1-associated malignant PNSTs may be multiple and tend to occur at a younger age than do their sporadic counterparts. Positron emission tomography (PET) may help differentiate benign neurofibromas and schwannomas from malignant tumors.

Ref.: 17–19

7. What condition is associated with the development of soft tissue sarcoma?

A. Familial retinoblastoma

B. Juvenile polyposis syndrome

C. von Hippel-Lindau syndrome

D. Asbestos exposure

E. Multiple endocrine neoplasia (MEN) type 1 syndrome

ANSWER: A

COMMENTS: Inherited syndromes, including retinoblastoma (also associated with osteosarcoma), Li-Fraumeni syndrome (also related to leukemia, brain, breast, and adrenocortical cancers), NF1, Gardner syndrome (familial adenomatous polyposis), Werner syndrome, and tuberous sclerosis, all confer an increased risk for **soft tissue sarcoma**. Ionizing radiation is a risk factor for soft tissue sarcomas, and such tumors tend to behave in an aggressive fashion. Exposure to vinyl chloride, arsenic, and thorium dioxide are associated with the development of hepatic angiosarcomas. Chronic lymphedema also predisposes to soft tissue sarcoma in the affected extremity, predominantly angiosarcoma. Stewart-Treves syndrome is an angiosarcoma that occurs due to chronic lymphedema after mastectomy with axillary lymph node dissection. Other acquired diseases that increase the risk for developing soft tissue sarcomas include the human immunodeficiency virus (HIV), which increases the risk of developing Kaposi's sarcoma. Juvenile polyposis syndrome is associated with polyps of the gastrointestinal (GI) tract as well as hereditary hemorrhagic telangiectasia. **Von Hippel-Lindau syndrome** is associated with renal cell carcinoma, as well as pheochromocytomas and hemangioblastomas (benign CNS tumors). Asbestos is associated with mesothelioma. MEN type 1 is associated with hyperparathyroidism, pancreatic and duodenal endocrine tumors, and pituitary adenomas, but it is not associated with an increased risk for sarcomas.

Ref.: 19–22

8. A 42-year-old woman has a mass in the posterior aspect of the upper part of her arm that was first noted 3 months earlier. It is not painful, and she has no associated symptoms. Magnetic resonance imaging (MRI) demonstrates a 5-cm neoplasm arising from the triceps. The best next step in the management of this patient is:

A. PET-CT
B. Fine-needle aspiration (FNA) biopsy
C. Percutaneous core needle biopsy
D. Incisional biopsy
E. Excisional biopsy

ANSWER: C

COMMENTS: See Question 8.

Ref.: 20, 21, 23, 24

9. After biopsy, a high-grade malignant fibrous histiocytoma is diagnosed in the patient in Question 8. Choose the best response regarding the outcome for this type of tumor.

A. Postoperative adjuvant radiotherapy improves outcome.
B. Preoperative chemotherapy improves outcome.
C. Lymph node dissection should be performed at the time of definitive surgical treatment.
D. Grade is a more important predictor of outcome than are tumor size and location.
E. Muscle compartment resection is necessary to maximize the chance for cure.

ANSWER: A

COMMENTS: Soft tissue sarcomas develop from mesenchymal tissues such as bone, muscle, fat, and other connective tissue. In addition, the disease accounts for less than 1% of adult and 15% of pediatric malignancies. The most common sites are the extremities, which account for more than 40% of the sites of occurrence. There are more than 50 histologic types of soft tissue sarcoma, with liposarcoma, malignant fibrous histiocytoma, and leiomyosarcoma being the most common. For lesions smaller than 4 cm, complete excision is an appropriate diagnostic procedure. Any subcutaneous solid soft tissue tumors greater than 4 cm should be evaluated by MRI before excision. In cases where imaging cannot be obtained, core needle biopsy is an appropriate alternative. If the imaging reveals a suspicious lesion, a core needle biopsy of the mass should be performed to determine pathology before a planned excision. When a soft tissue sarcoma of at least 4 cm is treated with an unplanned excision, the disease-free survival is lower than in those who were treated for an elective sarcoma excision. This is likely explained by a more aggressive approach for a known sarcoma with wide margins and function-sparing excisions. Although core needle biopsies should be the initial approach for obtaining the diagnosis of a soft tissue mass, an **incisional biopsy** may be considered if core needle biopsy yields nondiagnostic findings. When an incisional biopsy is necessary to achieve a diagnosis or when excising smaller tumors, it is important to plan the incision properly and avoid undue contamination of tissue planes so as not to interfere with definitive surgical treatment. An incision oriented on the long axis of the limb is preferred and should be performed so that the incision and remainder of the surgical field may be completely resected at the time of definitive surgical treatment. For the majority of soft tissue sarcomas in adults, complete surgical resection is the mainstay of treatment. Principles of surgical treatment include resection with approximately 2-cm margins of normal tissue (except vital structures) and avoidance of enucleation. Excision and amputation of muscle groups are no longer primary treatment modalities for most patients. The usual tumor node metastasis (TNM) staging system is modified for sarcomas because they rarely metastasize to lymph nodes and the tumor histologic grade has a significant prognostic value. Thus sarcomas are staged using the grade-tumor-node-metastasis (GTNM) system. Sentinel lymph node biopsy (SLNB) is not indicated for most sarcomas unless they are of a high-grade type. The histologic grade of soft tissue sarcomas is determined by cellular atypia, mitotic rate, and presence of tumor necrosis. Classification of soft tissue sarcomas is according to the tissues they mimic, not the type of tissue from which the tumor arises. When sarcomas are poorly differentiated such that no specific histogenesis can be determined, they are designated as spindle cell sarcomas or pleomorphic sarcomas. In addition to histopathology, it is important to evaluate the presence of any chromosomal translocations as these can be accurate diagnostic markers for soft tissue sarcomas. **Postoperative adjuvant radiotherapy** is beneficial in improving local control in patients with high-grade, large, and deep tumors, whereas it is probably unnecessary for patients with small (<5 cm), superficial, low-grade tumors treated by complete resection (microscopically negative margins). **Preoperative radiotherapy** permits a lower administered dose with a smaller treated field. However, it is associated with a higher incidence of postoperative wound complications, and treatment proceeds without knowledge of the final surgical histopathology. Preoperative radiotherapy is preferred for patients with marginally resectable, very large, high-grade tumors to maximize the chance of a microscopically margin-negative resection and functional preservation of the limb. With the exception of rhabdomyosarcoma and Ewing sarcoma, **neoadjuvant chemotherapy** is not generally beneficial. Limited data support neoadjuvant chemotherapy as justified in certain situations of carefully selected high-risk patients with large, high-grade tumors. In terms of distant recurrence and disease-specific survival, tumor size and tumor grade are equally important independent predictors of outcome.

Ref.: 20, 21, 23–25

10. A fair-skinned 68-year-old woman has a sharply demarcated 2-cm ulcerated skin lesion in an old burn scar on her forearm. What is the most appropriate treatment for this patient?

A. Topical chemotherapy
B. Topical biologic therapy
C. Surgical excision with frozen section
D. Mohs micrographic surgery
E. Radiotherapy

ANSWER: C

COMMENTS: Cutaneous squamous cell carcinoma (SCC) appears most frequently on sun-exposed areas, with two-thirds occurring on the head or neck; typical locations include exposed portion of the ears, the lower lip at the vermillion border, the paranasal areas, the maxillary skin, and the dorsum of the hands (Figs. 13.5 and 13.6). Risk factors for cutaneous SCC include fair skin; light-colored eyes; prior actinic keratosis; xeroderma pigmentosum; and exposure to nitrates, arsenicals, and hydrocarbons. Other risk factors associated with the disease are chronic excessive sun exposure, immunosuppression, previous trauma, and burns. The aggressiveness of these cancers is related to the underlying cause, location, and size of the lesion. It is increased in lesions arising in areas of previous burns (Marjolin ulcer) or trauma and in lesions of the lips and perineum. Excision of cutaneous SCC, generally with margins of 4 to 5 mm, should be accompanied by frozen section evaluation of the surgical margins. These tumors are radiosensitive. Surgery is preferred for tumors arising in scarred, traumatized, or previously irradiated skin. Large lesions may require adjuvant radiotherapy after surgical excision. Mohs surgery may be used for lesions with clinically indistinct margins. Regional lymph node dissection for SCC is performed for clinically evident (palpable) disease.

Ref.: 2, 26

11. Choose the correct statement regarding basal cell carcinoma.

A. It originates from the deep dermal appendages.

B. Intermittent intense exposure to UV light is a greater risk factor than exposure at a low dose per episode of a similar total dose.

C. Fifty percent of basal cell carcinoma occurs on the head and neck of an individual.

D. The risk for a second basal cell carcinoma is lower for men with index tumors on the trunk.

E. Most common type is superficial basal cell carcinoma.

ANSWER: B

COMMENTS: Basal cell carcinoma is the most common malignancy in the United States and accounts for about 80% of all skin cancers. It originates from the pluripotent basal keratinocytes of the epidermis and from hair follicles, not from the dermis. Exposure to UV radiation is a major risk factor for basal cell carcinoma, especially recreational exposure to the sun during childhood and adolescence. Although **cutaneous SCC** appears to be strongly related to cumulative sun exposure, the relationship between exposure to UV radiation and risk for basal cell carcinoma, like melanoma, is more complex. The timing, pattern, and amount of exposure are significant. Other risk factors are fair skin, light-colored hair and eyes, topical arsenic exposure, and immunosuppression. Eighty percent occur on the head or neck. The most common type of basal cell carcinoma is the nodular form, which accounts for 60% of cases, and it appears as a classic domed, pearly papule with surface telangiectasia (Fig. 13.7; E-Figures throughout this chapter are available online at www.expertconsult.inkling.com). Other types of basal cell carcinoma include superficial (15%), which usually appears as a minimally raised pink-red patch or papule, and morpheaform (sclerosing, infiltrative), which appears as a white scarlike plaque with indistinct margins. Some basal cell carcinomas are pigmented. Basal cell carcinomas rarely

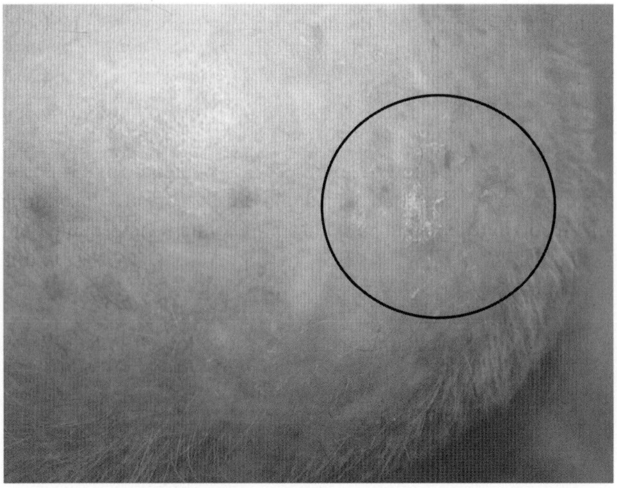

Fig. 13.5 Multiple squamous cell carcinomas.

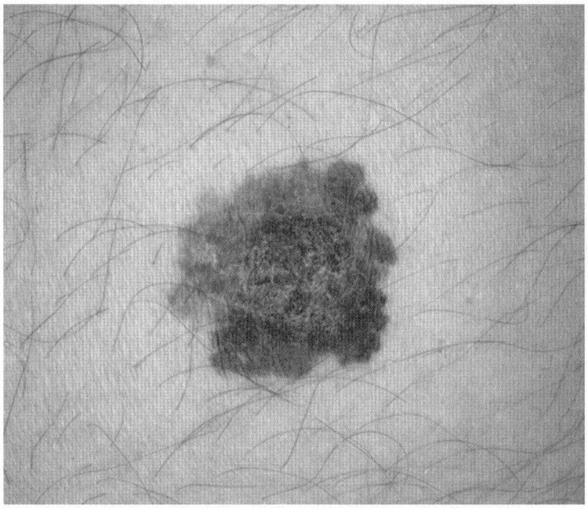

Fig. 13.6 Squamous cell carcinoma.

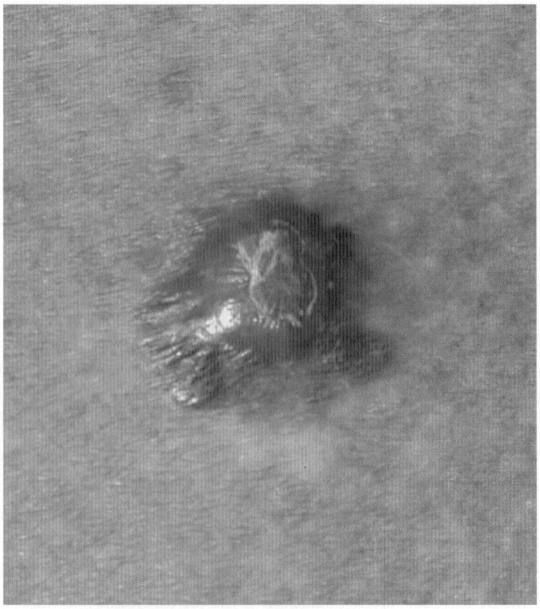

Fig. 13.7 Nodular basal cell carcinoma.

metastasize, but if they are neglected or recurrent, they can be locally destructive and require extensive local treatment and reconstruction. After an initial diagnosis of basal cell carcinoma, the risk for a second tumor is elevated tenfold. Male gender, truncal carcinomas, and older age increase a person's risk for the development of subsequent basal cell carcinomas.

Ref.: 26, 27

12. A 75-year-old man has a newly noted, raised 1.5-cm pearly nodule with surface telangiectasia on his cheek. What is the next most appropriate step in management?

A. Punch biopsy
B. Topical imiquimod
C. Curettage
D. Surgical excision
E. Radiation therapy

ANSWER: D

COMMENTS: Basal cell carcinoma may be treated surgically or nonsurgically. Surgical approaches include curettage, electrodesiccation, cryosurgery, excision, and Mohs micrographic surgery. The latter two have the benefit of histologic evaluation of the excised tumor. The cure rate after surgical excision is greater than 99% for primary lesions of any size on the neck, trunk, and extremities. Surgical excision is less efficacious for larger lesions of the head unless frozen section control of margins or **Mohs surgery** (fixation in vivo with repeated horizontal frozen section and excision to microscopic negative margins) is performed. Although recent randomized trial data show no significant difference in recurrence with primary or recurrent facial tumors, Mohs surgery is often used for these tumors and is probably beneficial for larger, poorly defined lesions in anatomically critical areas of the face. Treatment without histologic evaluation is acceptable for small, low-risk lesions. Nonsurgical approaches include radiotherapy, topical and injectable therapy, and photodynamic therapy. **Radiotherapy** is useful for tumors in difficult-to-treat locations and unresectable tumors, but it is potentially carcinogenic, has inferior cosmesis and efficacy, and is best avoided in patients younger than 60 years. Topical therapy includes 5-fluorouracil (5-FU) and imiquimod. Imiquimod, a nonspecific immune response modifier, was approved by the U.S. Food and Drug Administration (FDA) in 2004 for the treatment of superficial basal cell carcinomas smaller than 2.0 cm in nonimmunocompromised adults. Therapy for 5 days per week for 6 weeks results in histologic clearance rates greater than 80%.

Ref.: 26, 27

13. Which of the following is a potential premalignant precursor of melanoma?

A. Keratoacanthoma
B. Actinic keratosis
C. Seborrheic keratosis
D. Dysplastic nevus
E. Bowen disease

ANSWER: D

COMMENTS: Keratoacanthomas, characterized by rapid growth, rolled edges, and a crater filled with keratin, can mimic either squamous or basal cell carcinoma in appearance (Fig. 13.8). Although they often grow rapidly and then involute over a period of several months, a biopsy is usually performed. **Actinic (solar) keratosis** and **cutaneous horns** are premalignant lesions found on the sun-exposed areas of the skin in fair-skinned individuals, more commonly in those with prolonged exposure to the sun or to carcinogens (Fig. 13.9). These lesions may be treated with cryotherapy or topical agents. Raised lesions or lesions resistant to this treatment should be excised, although some may involute

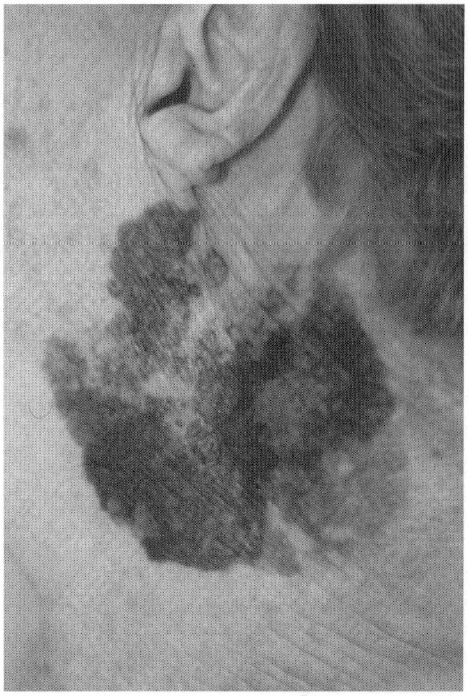

Fig. 13.8 Keratoacanthoma.

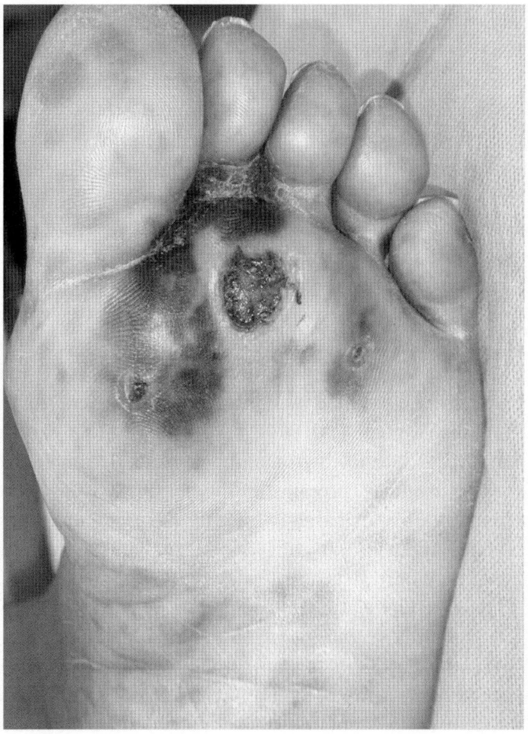

Fig. 13.9 Actinic keratosis.

spontaneously. The likelihood of progression to SCC is low (estimated to be 1 in 1000), with an associated lifetime risk of 5%–10%. **Bowen disease** is cutaneous SCC in situ. About 10% of these lesions progress to invasive SCC. They should be excised completely with negative margins. The presence of dysplastic nevi confers an increased risk for the development of melanoma. In addition, some dysplastic nevi represent true precursors of melanoma and may progress to invasive melanoma if untreated. They are usually reddish to brown, have scalloped edges and variegated pigmentation, are generally larger than 6 mm in diameter, and often appear on the trunk and other non–sun-exposed regions of the body.

Ref.: 2, 26

14. A 70-year-old retired male gardener presents with a rapidly growing, flesh-colored mass on his right forearm. On examination, a palpable lesion was noted, with a 2-cm, firm, nontender nodule having a smooth, shiny surface. A biopsy of the nodule demonstrates a cutaneous neuroendocrine tumor with keratin filaments. Which statement is true regarding his condition?

A. The SCC staging system should be used for this lesion.

B. A viral etiology may be responsible for this disease process.

C. Similar to melanoma, this type of cancer is not radiosensitive and thus radiation has no therapeutic role.

D. The presence of lymphovascular invasion is not a major prognostic factor for this lesion.

E. Unlike melanoma and nonmelanoma skin cancers, immunocompromised patients and those with long histories of sun exposure have no increased risk for developing this lesion.

ANSWER: B

COMMENTS: Merkel cell carcinoma (MCC) is a cutaneous neuroendocrine tumor derived from the neuroectoderm. The manifestation is known as a rapidly growing pink to red to blue to violaceous firm nodule and is often seen in elderly patients. MCC and melanoma share several clinical similarities—both occur on sun-damaged skin, lymphatic spread is common, and both can be staged with sentinel node biopsy. MCC has been noted to have an association with a polyomavirus that has been found integrated into the MCC genome, and infection may be the cause of this disease. After biopsy confirmation of the diagnosis, primary treatment consists of wide excision and histologic confirmation of negative margins. For tumors less than 2 cm in size, a 1 cm margin is acceptable, but for larger tumors (greater than 2 cm), a 2 cm margin should be obtained. MCC staging was previously combined with the staging system for SCC. However, the clinical and biologic profiles of the cancer are different; MCC has its own staging system. Lymphovascular invasion is a major prognostic factor for MCC. Although approximately 30% of patients initially have palpable regional lymph nodes, up to 70% of the remainder relapse in the regional lymph nodes within 2 years of diagnosis without nodal treatment. The Current National Comprehensive Cancer Network (NCCN) guidelines recommend SLNB with selective lymph node dissection for patients with clinically node-negative MCC; approximately 30% of patients will be found to have occult metastatic disease. Immunohistochemistry with pancytokeratin AE1/AE3, cytokeratin 20, and chromogranin A helps detect micrometastatic disease. This approach improves locoregional disease control, and sentinel node status is a significant indicator of prognosis. Unlike melanoma and SCC, MCC is fairly radio- and chemosensitive. Adjuvant radiotherapy is usually given to the primary site and may include the draining lymphatics and regional nodal basin for patients with node-positive disease. This improves the locoregional control over surgical treatment alone, and some studies have suggested a survival benefit as well. Overall survival is poor, with mortality rates of 50%–80% overall and of 30% at 5 years after diagnosis.

Ref.: 28–31

15. A 45-year-old female presents with a 0.5-mm lesion suspicious for melanoma. Which of the following principles should you follow when performing biopsies of lesions suspicious for melanoma?

A. Incisional biopsy can be performed on an area where skin is critical for cosmetics or function.

B. The specimen should be sent for frozen section.

C. Superficial shave technique should be performed.

D. Margins should be 0.5 to 1.0 mm.

E. Wide excision should be performed.

ANSWER: A

COMMENTS: Any lesion suspicious of melanoma should undergo a full-thickness excisional biopsy to the adipose tissue with 1- to 2-mm margins. Tumor depth is the most important determinant of prognosis and therapy for localized melanoma, and therefore accurate measurement of tumor thickness is vital. Partial-thickness and superficial shave biopsies would result in transection of the tumor and loss of tumor depth measurement. Wide local excision is not recommended as a biopsy technique as other lesions (benign and malignant) may mimic melanoma and wide excision would not allow for accurate SLNB. When a suspicious lesion is too large for complete excision or is located in an area critical to function or cosmetics, an incisional biopsy or punch biopsy can be performed to adipose tissue or deep dermis. Multiple incisional biopsies can be obtained throughout a large lesion with various morphologic features. Biopsies should be sent as formalin-fixed, paraffin-embedded permanent sections to determine tumor depth and histopathologic features. Frozen sections should not be used for cutaneous melanoma.

Ref.: 32–34

16. Which of the following is currently used in the TNM staging system used by the American Joint Committee on Cancer (AJCC) for melanoma?

A. Clark level of invasion

B. Location of primary tumor

C. Diameter of lesion

D. Serum lactate dehydrogenase (LDH)

E. Melanoma subtype (superficial spreading melanoma, nodular melanoma, acral lentiginous melanoma, or lentigo maligna melanoma)

ANSWER: D

COMMENTS: The five-stage system developed by the AJCC is based on prognosis and divides melanomas according to tumor characteristics (T), nodal stage (N), and presence of metastasis

(M). Stage 0 is melanoma in situ; stages I and II represent local disease; stage III encompasses regional nodal, in-transit, or satellite disease; and stage IV is distant metastases. Primary tumor characteristics for the T stage include tumor thickness (Breslow depth of invasion), presence of ulceration, and mitotic rate. Primary tumor diameter and Clark level of invasion are not used in the AJCC staging system. Although certain locations of primary melanoma are associated with poorer prognosis likely related to advanced disease due to late detection, this is not part of the TNM staging system. Four major subtypes of cutaneous melanoma exist based on clinical and histopathologic characteristics: superficial spreading melanoma, nodular melanoma, acral lentiginous melanoma, and lentigo maligna melanoma. Although each subtype has a varying prognosis for the risk of metastasis, the correlation of subtype to tumor depth is the basis for tumor behavior, not the tumor subtypes independently. Therefore tumor subtype is not used in the staging system. When staging patients with metastatic disease, elevated levels of LDH increase the M stage due to its association with worse prognosis.

Ref.: 35–37

17. A 75-year-old female presents to the clinic complaining of a chronic "rash" that has been enlarging over the past 3 months. On examination, she is noted to have a well-circumscribed, scaly, erythematous 5-mm plaque on her right lower back. She has no signs of a chronic wound or inflammation, draining sinus tract, or scar tissue. She has no history of radiation exposure. Biopsy reveals SCC in situ. What is the correct statement regarding her diagnosis?

A. Men are more affected by this disease than women.

B. Wide local excision is an appropriate therapeutic option.

C. The tissue adjacent to this lesion is not at an increased risk of neoplasia.

D. She will require radiation therapy.

E. Human papillomavirus (HPV) is not associated with this disease process.

ANSWER: B

COMMENTS: Several precursor lesions to **invasive SCC** exist; the most common of these are actinic keratoses and **Bowen disease**, the latter of which is represented in this clinical scenario. Bowen disease is SCC in situ of the skin and is clinically described as a slow-growing erythematous plaque with a scaling or crusted surface. The lesion is typically well-demarcated and in some cases can be pigmented or verrucous. Risk factors for this condition include sun exposure, chronic immunosuppression, and HPV. Men and women are equally affected by Bowen disease. Tissue adjacent to Bowen disease is at a higher risk for developing neoplasms. Although multiple therapeutic options exist for Bowen disease including cryotherapy, curettage, 5-FU, imiquimod, and photodynamic therapy, wide local resection is all that is required. If the disease is located in a critical area, radiation can be used to retard growth, but it is not the preferred treatment.

Ref.: 38–40

18. A 28-year-old female presents with a 4-cm mass in her right upper extremity and clinically suspicious lymph nodes in the right axilla. What is the most likely diagnosis?

A. Osteosarcoma

B. Synovial sarcoma

C. Malignant fibrous histiocytoma

D. Liposarcoma

E. Ewing sarcoma

ANSWER: B

COMMENTS: The majority of soft tissue sarcomas do not metastasize to lymph nodes, and thus exploration of lymph nodes is generally not warranted. However, when regional lymphadenopathy is discovered with concurrent sarcoma diagnosis, lymphadenectomy should be considered as tumor clearance may lead to better outcomes. The types of sarcoma that are more likely to have lymphatic spread include vascular sarcoma, clear cell sarcoma, rhabdomyosarcoma, epitheloid sarcoma, and synovial sarcoma. There is some evidence that SLNB may be considered in clinically node-negative disease for these subtypes of high-grade lymphomas given their propensity for lymphatic spread.

Ref.: 41–43

19. Adverse prognostic factors for clinically localized (stage I and II) melanoma include which of the following?

A. Male gender

B. Younger age

C. Decreased mitotic rate

D. Tumor location on extremity

E. Tumor regression

ANSWER: A

COMMENTS: Older age is a predictor of poorer **survival** as established in numerous studies and verified in retrospective reviews of recent clinical trials. Male patients fare worse than females. Tumor site (extremity better than the trunk or head or neck) is also prognostic. Tumor thickness is the most important predictor of outcome in patients with clinically localized melanoma, followed by ulceration (Fig. 13.10). A mitotic rate greater than or equal to 1 mm^2 carries a worse prognosis for the primary tumor. Although approximately half of **melanomas** show some degree of regression, the influence of regression on outcome is unclear; reports are variable regarding its significance, with some suggesting a favorable and others an adverse influence on outcome.

Ref.: 2, 44

20. A 33-year-old woman has a 2.1-mm-thick, nonulcerated nodular melanoma on her right thigh. The results of physical examination are otherwise normal. What is the most appropriate treatment?

A. Wide local excision with 1.0-cm margins

B. Wide local excision with 2.0-cm margins

C. Wide local excision with 2.0-cm margins and SLNB

D. Wide local excision with 2.0-cm margins, SLNB with frozen section, and possible inguinofemoral lymph node dissection

E. Wide local excision with 3.0-cm margins, SLNB with frozen section, and possible inguinofemoral lymph node dissection

ANSWER: C

COMMENTS: Treatment of **melanoma** involves complete excision of all skin and subcutaneous tissue down to the underlying fascia for a defined distance from the biopsy site, scar, or margins of the pigmented lesion, depending on tumor thickness.

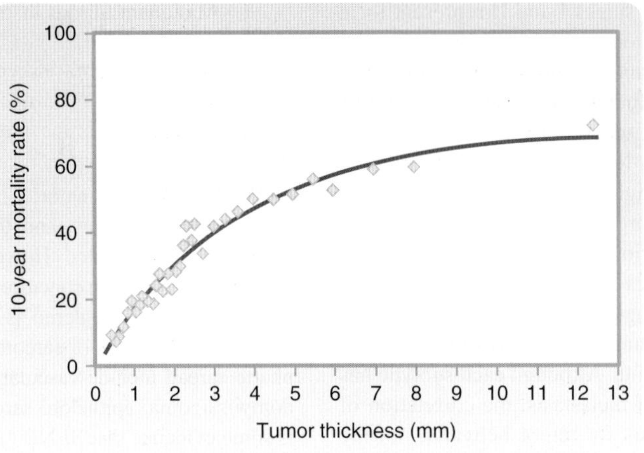

Fig. 13.10 Observed (*diamonds*) and predicted (*solid line*) 10-year mortality rate in patients with clinically localized melanoma. This is based on a mathematical model derived from the American Joint Committee on Cancer melanoma database of 15,230 patients. *(From Balch CM, Soong SJ, Gerschenwald JE, et al. Prognostic factors analysis of 17,600 melanoma patients: validation of the AJCC melanoma staging system.* J Clin Oncol. *2001;19:3622–3634.)*

Recommended margins, based on data from five randomized clinical trials, are 0.5 cm for melanoma in situ, 1.0 cm for thin melanomas, and 2.0 cm for melanomas thicker than 1.0 mm. Wider margins are considered for lesions thicker than 4 mm and those with satellite lesions. Margins may be adjusted for concerns regarding cosmesis and function (Table 13-1). Sentinel lymph node tumor burden is the most important prognostic factor for patients with early-stage melanoma. **Lymphatic mapping** (lymphoscintigraphy), **SLNB**, and selective lymph node dissection are recommended for all patients with melanomas greater than 1.0 mm in thickness with clinically negative lymph nodes. SLNB may be recommended for melanomas that are thinner (0.76 to 1.0 mm), ulcerated, diagnosed by incomplete biopsy, exhibiting regression, with a high mitotic rate, and occurring in younger patients. The likelihood of finding a positive sentinel lymph node is most strongly predicted by tumor thickness, with minimal risk for melanomas thinner than 0.76 mm, 5% for melanomas 0.76 to 1.0 mm, 8%–10% for melanomas 1.01 to 1.5 mm, 18%–30% for melanomas 1.51 to 4.0 mm, and 30%–40% for melanomas thicker than 4.0 mm. Although the use of the mitotic rate to classify thin melanomas as T1b was based on survival data, some data suggest that the likelihood of occult nodal disease increases with increasing mitotic rate. The use of immunohistochemistry (with at least one melanoma-specific marker such as HMB-45, Melan-A, or MART-1) will increase the sentinel lymph node positivity rate by approximately 10% over hematoxylin–eosin staining alone. Nomograms that incorporate patient age, site, thickness, level, and ulceration have been developed to help predict the likelihood of a positive sentinel lymph node. Results of the Multicenter Selective Lymphadenectomy Trial-1 (MSLT-1) confirmed SLNB to be a prognostic tool for melanoma. MSLT-1 randomized patients with intermediate-thickness melanoma (1.2 to 3.5 mm) to wide local excision alone or wide local excision plus SLNB with complete lymph node dissection (CLND) for positive sentinel lymph nodes. Patients assigned to observation underwent a therapeutic lymphadenectomy only if clinical evidence of nodal recurrence was present. In individuals assigned to the SLNB group, those who were discovered to have positive SLNBs had a significantly worse melanoma-specific 10-year survival compared with individuals who had a negative SLNB. Furthermore, MSLT-1 demonstrated a melanoma-specific survival advantage in patients who were diagnosed with lymph node involvement after SLNB and underwent early CLND compared with individuals who underwent wide local excision followed by observation and later underwent CLND after clinical recurrence. For lymph node–positive disease, the benefit of CLND on survival remains questionable. Currently, the MSLT-2 is underway to determine the survival benefit of CLND after positive SLNB compared with observation. The MSLT-2 is studying patients with positive sentinel lymph nodes but no clinical evidence of other lymph node involvement who are randomly assigned to immediate CLND or ultrasound examination of the remaining regional lymph nodes and CLND if signs of additional lymph node metastasis appear. For now, the standard of care is CLND for patients with positive SLNB. Frozen section examination of melanoma sentinel lymph nodes has been abandoned because of its low sensitivity (50%) and concern that tissue destruction may preclude an accurate diagnosis from permanent sections.

TABLE 13.1 Recommended Margins for Wide Local Excision of the Primary Site

Thickness	Margin	Note
Melanoma in situ	5 mm	Head and neck: consider preoperative margin assessment
Melanoma < 1 mm	1 cm	
Melanoma 1 to 4 mm	2 cm	1 cm acceptable in limited anatomic locations
Melanoma > 4 mm	2 cm	Consider 3 cm if easily obtained

Ref.: 2, 28, 45–49

21. The patient in Question 20 is found to have metastatic melanoma in an inguinal sentinel lymph node. Choose the correct response regarding her diagnosis.

A. On completion of lymphadenectomy, the likelihood of nonsentinel lymph node metastases is 1%–2%.

B. She should receive systemic interleukin-2 (IL-2) therapy.

C. Adequate inguinofemoral lymph node dissection implies removal of a minimum of 12 lymph nodes.

D. Adjuvant radiation therapy is beneficial for patients with more than three involved lymph nodes and when there is a breach of the nodal capsule with bulky nodal disease.

E. CLND is unnecessary for micrometastatic disease (<0.2-mm tumor within the sentinel lymph node).

ANSWER: D

COMMENTS: No prognostic factors or nomograms have been able to accurately and reproducibly identify a subset of sentinel lymph node–positive **melanoma** patients without risk of harboring additional metastatic lymph nodes. Approximately 20% of patients with positive sentinel lymph node disease are demonstrated to have further lymph node involvement (nonsentinel lymph node disease) after CLND. As mentioned previously, until the results of the MSLT-2 are released, **CLND** should be performed for all sentinel node–positive patients. The goals of surgery include control of regional disease and improved survival. The majority of patients who undergo CLND will not be found to have additional positive lymph nodes. However, examination of these nonsentinel lymph nodes is by necessity less rigorous than the stepwise examination of the sentinel lymph node, so small foci of disease may be missed. Unlike breast cancer, there is no lower limit of the size of metastatic **melanoma** within a lymph node that defines a positive lymph node. Retrospective studies suggest that patients with nodal disease less than 0.1 mm are at a substantially increased risk for relapse versus sentinel node–negative patients. Standard surgical oncology teaching defines CLNDs on the basis of anatomic boundaries. Recommendations based on expert opinion have suggested a minimum number of lymph nodes per region to define a CLND. A review by the Sidney Melanoma Unit based on more than 2000 regional lymph node dissections for melanoma suggested the following standard anatomic guidelines consisting of minimum (and target mean) **lymph node counts** of 10 (21) for the axilla, 7 (14) for inguinal and ilioinguinal dissections, and 20 (39) for cervical dissections involving four or more levels. The 2010 NCCN guidelines recommend CLND based on proper anatomic boundaries, which they recommend to be dictated into the operative note, but they do not set a target number of lymph nodes. A recent meta-analysis of **SLNB**–guided selective lymph node dissection versus observation with therapeutic lymph node dissection for nodal relapse demonstrated a significantly higher risk for death (hazard ratio of 1.6) among patients in the therapeutic lymph node dissection group. **Adjuvant radiotherapy** is considered for most patients with multiple cervical lymph node metastases and for those with bulky, large (metastatic nodes > 3 cm in size) or extracapsular disease at any site. Although no published randomized trials have compared surgery alone with surgery and postoperative radiotherapy, retrospective single-institution studies suggest improved regional control and disease-free survival.

Ref.: 2, 28, 45–50

22. A 38-year-old male presents with a 3-cm, blue-red, raised nodule over his right shoulder. He has noted the painless mass for several years but notes that it has slowly been enlarging. He has no other symptoms, and the rest of his physical exam is normal. Punch biopsy of the tumor reveals uniform spindle cells in the deep dermis arranged in a storiform pattern, and it is CD-34 positive. What is the next step in treatment for this patient?

A. Start systemic imatinib therapy

B. Wide local excision with SLNB

C. CT scan of chest, abdomen, and pelvis for staging

D. Radiation therapy

E. Wide local excision of mass with 3- to 5-cm margins

ANSWER: E

COMMENTS: Dermatofibrosarcoma protuberans (DFSP) is a rare, low-grade malignant neoplasm of the dermis. Its occurrence is rare; however, it is the most common dermal sarcoma. Clinically, these lesions appear as nodular or plaque-like and violaceous, red-blue, or brown in color. They are slow growing, confined to the dermis, and commonly found on the trunk and proximal extremities. DFSP most frequently affects middle-aged adults and exhibits high local recurrence rates after resection but minimal metastatic potential. Diagnosis is best achieved with a punch biopsy. If DFSP is suspected, excisional biopsy should be avoided as reexcision will require wide margins. Histologically, DFSP tumors are seen as spindle cells in the dermis with a storiform architecture, typically with a low mitotic rate, and tend to exhibit finger-like extensions of malignant cells at the borders of the tumor, making the status of the margins difficult to determine. On immunohistochemical staining, these tumors show CD 34 expression. Treatment of DFSP is surgical resection with 3- to 5-cm wide margins that are pathologically negative. Lymph node metastasis is rare, and other than a physical examination, no further assessment of lymphatic spread is necessary. As this is a relatively small tumor and its propensity to metastasize is small, a chest x-ray is the only imagining study required. In cases where tumors occur in locations where wide excision is not possible, Mohs micrographic surgery may be appropriate. Approximately 90% of DFSPs have a translocation between chromosome 17 and 22, leading to the upregulation of platelet-derived growth factor (PDGF). This has lead to the use of imatinib—a PDGF inhibitor—for metastatic and locally advanced disease in which the tumors exhibit this specific translocation. In this case, a wide local excision is all that is indicated and imatinib therapy should not be given. Radiation therapy may be used for unresectable disease or in cases where surgical margins are close or positive. Radiation therapy should not be used if complete resection with pathologically negative margins has been achieved.

Ref.: 51–55

23. Which of the following adjuvant therapies for node-positive melanoma patients has shown to improve disease-free survival?

A. Doxorubicin chemotherapy

B. Interferon-α2b (INF-α2b)

C. Cyclophosphamide chemotherapy

D. Injection with bacille Calmette–Guérin (BCG)

E. Tremelimumab

ANSWER: A

COMMENTS: Numerous randomized clinical trials of **chemotherapy**, nonspecific immune stimulants, and **vaccines** for high-risk stage II and stage III **melanoma** have been conducted but most have been underpowered and yielded negative results. The FDA-approved adjuvant therapy for node-positive melanoma patients is **INF-α2b**. Although randomized controlled clinical trials have demonstrated improved disease-free survival with adjuvant INF-α2b, there is a very modest effect on the overall survival, and associated side effects of the treatment are significant. Newer agents under study in the adjuvant setting include antiangiogenic therapy such as bevacizumab and the anti–CTLA-4 antibody ipilimumab. Because of the lack of effective adjuvant therapy with low toxicity, observation, either as a control arm of a clinical trial or in the absence of clinical trial enrollment, is acceptable. Melanoma has a limited response to chemotherapy. Dacarbazine, nitrosoureas, vinca alkaloids, and cisplatin are the most responsive chemotherapies for metastatic melanoma. Doxorubicin (Adriamycin) and cyclophosphamide are not effective for the treatment of melanoma. Although melanoma has been thought to be fairly radioresistant, in some cases radiation can be beneficial. Radiation can be employed for palliative care for bone metastases and metastatic disease to the brain. Adjuvant radiation therapy after CLND for node-positive disease is utilized in high-risk cases of nodal metastases: those with recurrent disease and four or more positive nodes and those with extracapsular extension. Prospective trials for adjuvant radiation therapy after CLND have shown an in-field recurrence of 7%; however, there was an increased morbidity without improvement in overall survival. Tremelimumab, formerly known as ticilimumab, has been shown to be an effective therapy for metastatic melanoma but has not been used in lymph node–positive disease.

Ref.: 2, 49, 50, 56–62

24. Which of the following is the most significant prognostic factor for patients with node-positive (stage III) melanoma?

A. Nodal size

B. Number of involved lymph nodes

C. Tumor thickness

D. Tumor ulceration

E. Patient gender

ANSWER: B

COMMENTS: The most significant prognostic factor for patients with **node-positive melanoma** is the number of involved lymph nodes. The next most significant prognostic factor is the nodal tumor burden (microscopic or clinically occult versus macroscopic or clinically apparent), followed by primary tumor ulceration and thickness. Nodal size is not a component of staging, nor has it been shown to have significant independent prognostic value. Gender does not have a significant effect on outcome in patients with node-positive melanoma.

Ref.: 35, 44

25. A 52-year-old man is evaluated for a palpable left inguinal lymph node 7 years after wide local excision of a thin melanoma on the ipsilateral right calf. No SLNB or other staging was done at the time of his initial diagnosis. What should be the next step in the care of this patient?

A. Excisional biopsy

B. Excisional biopsy with frozen section examination followed by immediate inguinofemoral lymph node dissection

C. Total-body PET-CT per melanoma protocol

D. FNA biopsy (cytology)

E. Measurement of serum S-100 protein and LDH

ANSWER: D

COMMENTS: Recurrence in the **regional lymph node** basin is the most common site of initial recurrence after treatment by wide local excision alone and can occur even in patients with thin primary **melanomas** and many years after the initial diagnosis. Evaluation of clinically palpable lymph nodes is most expeditiously performed by FNA, with or without ultrasound guidance. Core needle biopsy or excisional biopsy can be done if the FNA is negative or nondiagnostic. Frozen section evaluation of lymph node metastases of melanoma has low sensitivity, and freezing the tissue may destroy areas with metastatic disease; the diagnosis is generally deferred to evaluation of the permanent section. **Complete regional lymphadenectomy** will lead to durable long-term survival in approximately half of such patients. Once the diagnosis of nodal melanoma recurrence is established, given that the remainder of the patient's physical examination is unremarkable, a metastatic workup that includes liver function tests, PET-CT, and MRI of the head is appropriate before surgery to exclude the presence of clinically unsuspected metastatic disease. In this clinical scenario, evaluation with PET-CT is estimated to change treatment in 15%–30% of patients.

Ref.: 2, 63

26. Which of these treatments is indicated for the initial therapy of in-transit metastasis from cutaneous melanoma?

A. Mohs micrographic surgery

B. Isolated limb perfusion

C. Imatinib

D. Prednisone

E. Amputation

ANSWER: B

COMMENTS: In-transit metastases develop in about 2% of patients with cutaneous **melanoma** and appear as visible dermal or subcutaneous tumor nodules between the primary site and regional draining nodal basin. They arise from intralymphatic tumor spread. After evaluation for metastatic disease, treatment depends on the extent of the disease. Limited in-transit metastases amenable to excision may be treated by wide excision with 1-cm margins. Other local therapy options include laser ablation with healing by secondary intention and local immunotherapy with BCG or INF injection or topical application of imiquimod cream. Injection results in a response in approximately 80% of lesions, sometimes in neighboring lesions as well, and the toxicity is predominantly local (erythema, edema, ulceration). For extensive disease, **isolated limb perfusion** with a pump oxygenator circuit and regional chemotherapy (most commonly melphalan and sometimes the addition of tumor necrosis factor-α), with or without concomitant regional lymph node dissection, has limited indications but may be useful for locoregional control of disease. This involves surgical placement of arterial and venous cannulas in the affected extremity, which is excluded from the general circulation with a tourniquet. The reported complete response rate is 40%–80%, but the toxicity may be considerable and includes lymphedema, compartment syndrome, and neuropathy. Responses may not be durable, with 50% recurrence rates 18 months after infusion. Recently, isolated limb infusion with percutaneously placed cannulas has been proposed as an alternative, less-morbid therapy with complete response rates of approximately 30%. With these available therapies, major amputation is rarely required as a primary therapy for in-transit disease. As a secondary treatment, amputation may provide palliation, or regional control, for unmanageable progressive recurrences when other approaches fail. Indications are a usually intractable pain with loss of limb function (often associated with tumor fungation, bleeding, infection, gangrene, and severe lymphedema) in patients whose life expectancy is at least 3 months and who have reasonable performance status otherwise. In the absence of nodal metastases, patients with in-transit disease have 5- and 10-year overall survival rates of 69% and 52%, whereas those with concomitant regional nodal metastases have diminished 5- and 10-year overall survival rates of 46% and 33%, respectively. Imatinib can be used for the treatment of metastatic melanoma that is positive for *KIT* mutation and unresectable or metastatic DFSP. Prednisone would not be useful for treating in-transit melanoma.

Ref.: 64–69

27. A 37-year-old man is evaluated for a 4-month history of anemia and intermittent abdominal discomfort and distention 7 years after treatment of a stage I melanoma on his right forearm. The results of physical examination are normal, colonoscopy is negative, and CT demonstrates an area of invaginated jejunal mesentery with an adjacent dilated loop of small bowel. What is the next most appropriate step in the management of this patient?

A. Exploration and small bowel resection

B. Video capsule endoscopy

C. Systemic biochemotherapy

D. Whole-body PET-CT

E. Air-contrast small bowel barium study

ANSWER: A

COMMENTS: The small intestine is the most common site of **gastrointestinal tract metastases** from cutaneous **melanoma**, which are present in a high proportion of patients with melanoma at autopsy. Symptomatic patients most commonly have abdominal pain, chronic gastrointestinal bleeding, obstruction, and weight loss. Polypoid tumors arising from the submucosa may act as the lead point for an intussusception, as in this case. Surgical resection of solitary and even multiple small intestinal metastases is associated with improved survival over nonoperative therapy and is an effective treatment of associated obstruction. With complete resection of small intestinal disease, median survival times of 4 years are reported. Since this patient is symptomatic without evidence of other disease by physical examination or CT of the abdomen and pelvis, further preoperative radiologic workup is unlikely to alter the need for or benefit of surgery. Although the disease recurs in most patients at multiple sites and they are best treated with systemic therapy, those who are suitable candidates for resection of limited metastatic disease may experience long-term disease-free survival. In general, for stage IV melanoma, the site of the metastatic disease and the serum LDH level correlate with prognosis. One-year survival rates for those with cutaneous, subcutaneous, or distant nodal metastases (M1a) versus those with lung metastases (M1b) versus those with any other visceral metastases or any metastasis with an elevated serum LDH level (M1c) are estimated to be 62%, 53%, and 33%, respectively. Factors reported to be associated with improved outcome after resection of **melanoma metastases** include initial disease stage, disease-free interval after treatment of the primary melanoma, initial site of metastasis, solitary site of disease, and complete resection. Even when not performed with curative intent, palliative surgical treatment of metastatic melanoma may be beneficial for the treatment of symptomatic patients.

Ref.: 2, 35, 70

28. A 52-year-old female presents with metastatic melanoma to her lungs, liver, and spine. Match the appropriate treatment for metastatic melanoma with the correct target site.

A. INF-α and anticytotoxic T-lymphocyte–associated protein 4 (CTLA-4)

B. Vemurafenib and BRAF protein

C. Imatinib and MEK protein

D. Trametinib and immune response modulator

E. Ipilimumab and PD-1 protein

ANSWER: B

COMMENTS: Immunotherapy and targeted therapy both play roles in the management of metastatic melanoma. **IL-2** and **INF-α** act as general immune response modulators by acting as cytokines that activate T cells. More recent treatments are now targeting checkpoint inhibition proteins that act as immune modulators to increase the activity and number of T cells. **Pembrolizumab** and **nivolumab** are monoclonal PD-1 antibodies. PD-1 prevents T cells from being activated, and therefore blocking this protein will increase the immune response in a more specific manner compared with IL-2 and INF-α. **Ipilimumab** is a monoclonal antibody that targets CTLA-4, another protein that prevents T-cell activation. There are several therapies that target specific gene mutations that have been identified in melanoma. Approximately 40%–60% of advanced melanomas contain an activating mutation for **BRAF** within the mitogen-activated protein (MAP)-kinase pathway (MAPK). This mutation is most commonly caused by a single substitution of glutamic acid for valine at amino acid 600, known as the V600 mutation. **Vemurafenib** and **dabrafenib** both inhibit BRAF and are used as targeted therapies for advanced melanoma. MEK is another member of the MAPK pathway, and when inhibited, cell proliferation is blocked and apoptosis is induced. **Trametinib** acts as a MEK inhibitor and can be used with BRAF inhibitors in the presence of V600 BRAF mutation. C-kit mutations have been identified in 15%–20% of mucosal and acral melanomas. **Imatinib** inhibits tyrosine kinases that have been activated due to this c-kit mutation. Although early studies of imatinib treatment in unselected patients with advanced melanoma show minimal clinical efficacy, current studies are underway for selected patients with the c-kit mutation.

Ref.: 71–83

REFERENCES

1. Tran TT, Schulman J, Fisher DE. UV and pigmentation: molecular mechanisms and social controversies. *Pigment Cell Melanoma Res.* 2008;21:509–516.
2. Urist MM, Soong S-J. Melanoma and cutaneous malignancies. In: Townsend CM, Beauchamp RD, Evers BM, et al., eds. *Sabiston Textbook of Surgery: The Biological Basis of Modern Surgical Practice.* 18th ed. Philadelphia: WB Saunders; 2008.
3. Tyrrell RM. Ultraviolet protection. In: Lejeuene FJ, Chaudhuri PK, Das Gupta TK, eds. *Malignant Melanoma: Medical and Surgical Treatment.* New York: McGraw-Hill; 1994.
4. Siegel RL, Miller KD, Jemal A. Cancer statistics. *CA Cancer J Clin.* 2016;1:7–30.
5. Diepgen TL, Mahler V. The epidemiology of skin cancer. *Br J Dermatol.* 2002;146(61):1–6.
6. Bishop DT, Demenais F, Iles MM, et al. Genome-wide association study identifies three loci associated with melanoma risk. *Nat Genet.* 2009;41:920–925.
7. Bishop DT, Demenais F, Goldstein AM, et al. Geographical variation in the penetrance of CDKN2A mutations for melanoma. *J Natl Cancer Inst.* 2002;94:894–903.
8. Anaya DA, Dellinger EP. Necrotizing soft-tissue infection: diagnosis and management. *Clin Infect Dis.* 2007;5:705–710.
9. Brook I, Frazier EH. Clinical and microbiological features of necrotizing fasciitis. *J Clin Microbiol.* 1995;9:2382–2387.
10. Wong CH, Chang HC, Pasupathy S, et al. Necrotizing fasciitis: clinical presentation, microbiology, and determinants of mortality. *J Bone Joint Surg Am.* 2003;8:1454–1460.
11. Stevens DL, Bisno AL, Chambers HF, et al. Practice guidelines for the diagnosis and management of skin and soft tissue infections: 2014 update by the Infectious Diseases Society of America. *Clin Infect Dis.* 2014;2:147–159.

12. Wong CH, Khin LW, Heng KS, Tan KC, Low CO. The LRINEC (Laboratory Risk Indicator for Necrotizing Fasciitis) score: a tool for distinguishing necrotizing fasciitis from other soft tissue infections. *Crit Care Med*. 2004;7:1535–1541.
13. Hakkarainen TW, Kopari NM, Pham TN, Evans HL. Necrotizing soft tissue infections: review and current concepts in treatment, systems of care, and outcomes. *Curr Probl Surg*. 2014;8:344–362.
14. Netscher D, Fiore N. Hand surgery. In: Townsend CM, Beauchamp RD, Evers BM, et al., eds. *Sabiston Textbook of Surgery: The Biological Basis of Modern Surgical Practice*. 18th ed. Philadelphia: WB Saunders; 2008.
15. Cole P, Heller L, Bullocks J, et al. The skin and subcutaneous tissue. In: Brunicardi FC, Andersen DK, Billiar TR, et al., eds. *Schwartz's Principles of Surgery*. 9th ed. New York: McGraw-Hill; 2010.
16. Rakinic J. Modern management of pilonidal disease. In: Cameron JL, ed. *Current Surgical Therapy*. 9th ed. Philadelphia: CV Mosby; 2008.
17. Benz MR, Czernin J, Dry SM, et al. Quantitative F18-fluorodeoxyglucose positron emission tomography accurately characterizes peripheral nerve sheath tumors as malignant or benign. *Cancer*. 2010;116:451–458.
18. Pletcher BA. Neurofibromatosis type 1. In: eMedicine Clinical Knowledge Base, Neurology. Available at: www.emedicine.com. Accessed March 27, 2016.
19. Das Gupta TK, Chaudhuri PK. *Tumors of the Soft Tissues*. 2nd ed. Norwalk, CT: Appleton & Lange; 1998.
20. Singer S, Canter RJ. Soft tissue sarcoma. In: Cameron JL, ed. *Current Surgical Therapy*. 9th ed. Philadelphia: CV Mosby; 2008.
21. Singer S. Soft tissue sarcomas. In: Townsend CM, Beauchamp RD, Evers BM, et al., eds. *Sabiston Textbook of Surgery: The Biological Basis of Modern Surgical Practice*. 18th ed. Philadelphia: WB Saunders; 2008.
22. Hieken TJ. Genetic testing for cancer susceptibility. In: Saclarides TJ, Millikan KW, Godellas CV, eds. *Surgical Oncology: An Algorithmic Approach*. New York: Springer-Verlag; 2003.
23. Jemal A, Siegel R, Ward E, et al. Cancer statistics. *CA Cancer J Clin*. 2009;59:225–249.
24. Hueman MT, Thornton K, Herman JM, et al. Management of extremity soft tissue sarcomas. *Surg Clin North Am*. 2008;88:539–557.
25. Massengill AD, Seeger LL, Eckardt JJ. The role of plain radiography, computed tomography, and magnetic resonance imaging in sarcoma evaluation. *Hematol Oncol Clin North Am*. 1995;3:571–604.
26. Kazin R, Shermak MA. Skin and soft tissue. In: Cameron JL, ed. *Current Surgical Therapy*. 9th ed. Philadelphia: CV Mosby; 2008.
27. Rubin AI, Chen EH, Ratner D. Basal-cell carcinoma. *N Engl J Med*. 2005;353:2262–2269.
28. Edge SB, Byrd DR, Compton CC, et al., eds. Merkel cell carcinoma. In: *AJCC Cancer Staging Manual*. 7th ed. New York, NY: Springer; 2010:315–322.
29. Buethe D, Warner C, Miedler J, Cockerell CJ. Focus issue on squamous cell carcinoma: practical concerns regarding the 7th Edition AJCC Staging Guidelines. *J Skin Cancer*. 2010;2011:156391.
30. Wang TS, Byrne PJ, Jacobs LK, Taube JM. Merkel cell carcinoma: update and review. *Semin Cutan Med Surg*. 2011;1:48–56.
31. Fields RC, Busam KJ, Chou JF, et al. Five hundred patients with Merkel cell carcinoma evaluated at a single institution. *Ann Surg*. 2011;3:465–473. discussion 473–475.
32. Arca MJ, Biermann JS, Johnson TM, Chang AE. Biopsy techniques for skin, soft-tissue, and bone neoplasms. *Surg Oncol Clin North Am*. 1995;1:157–174.
33. Faries MB, Morton DL. Cutaneous melanoma. In: Cameron JL, ed. *Current Surgical Therapy*. 9th ed. Philadelphia: CV Mosby; 2008.
34. Criscione VD, Weinstock MA. Melanoma thickness trends in the United States, 1988-2006. *J Invest Dermatol*. 2010;130:793–797.
35. Balch CM, Gershenwald JE, Soong SJ, et al. Final version of 2009 AJCC melanoma staging and classification. *J Clin Oncol*. 2009;36:6199–6206.
36. Thompson JF, Soong SJ, Balch CM, et al. Prognostic significance of mitotic rate in localized primary cutaneous melanoma: an analysis of patients in the multi-institutional American Joint Committee on Cancer melanoma staging database. *J Clin Oncol*. 2011;16:2199–2205.
37. Gershenwald JE, Soong SJ, Balch CM. 2010 TNM staging system for cutaneous melanoma and beyond. *Ann Surg Oncol*. 2010;6:1475–1477.
38. Chute CG, Chuang TY, Bergstralh EJ, Su WP. The subsequent risk of internal cancer with Bowen's disease. A population-based study. *JAMA*. 1991;6:816–819.
39. Wang CY, Brodland DG, Su WP. Skin cancers associated with acquired immunodeficiency syndrome. *Mayo Clin Proc*. 1995;8:766–772.
40. Neubert T, Lehmann P. Bowen's disease: a review of newer treatment options. *Ther Clin Risk Manag*. 2008;5:1085–1095.
41. Blazer DG, Sabel MS, Sondak VK. Is there a role for sentinel lymph node biopsy in the management of sarcoma? *Surg Oncol*. 2003;3:201–206.
42. Al-Refaie WB, Andtbacka RH, Ensor J, et al. Lymphadenectomy for isolated lymph node metastasis from extremity soft-tissue sarcomas. *Cancer*. 2008;8:1821–1826.
43. Fong Y, Coit DG, Woodruff JM, Brennan MF. Lymph node metastasis from soft tissue sarcoma in adults. Analysis of data from a prospective database of 1772 sarcoma patients. *Ann Surg*. 1993;1:72–77.
44. Balch CM, Soong SJ, Gershenwald JE, et al. Prognostic factors analysis of 17,600 melanoma patients: validation of the American Joint Committee on Cancer melanoma staging system. *J Clin Oncol*. 2001;19:3622–3644.
45. Kachare SD, Brinkley J, Wong JH, Vohra NA, Zervos EE, Fitzgerald TL. The influence of sentinel lymph node biopsy on survival for intermediate-thickness melanoma. *Ann Surg Oncol*. 2014;11:3377–3385.
46. Morton DL, Thompson JF, Cochran AJ, et al. Final trial report of sentinel-node biopsy versus nodal observation in melanoma. *N Engl J Med*. 2014;7:599–609.
47. Morton DL, Hoon DS, Cochran AJ, et al. Lymphatic mapping and sentinel lymphadenectomy for early-stage melanoma: therapeutic utility and implications of nodal microanatomy and molecular staging for improving the accuracy of detection of nodal micrometastases. *Ann Surg*. 2003;4:538–549. discussion 549–550.
48. van der Ploeg AP, Haydu LE, Spillane AJ, et al. Outcome following sentinel node biopsy plus wide local excision versus wide local excision only for primary cutaneous melanoma: analysis of 5840 patients treated at a single institution. *Ann Surg*. 2014;1:149–157.
49. Paek SC, Griffith KA, Johnson TM, et al. The impact of factors beyond Breslow depth on predicting sentinel lymph node positivity in melanoma. *Cancer*. 2007;1:100–108.
50. Kirkwood JM, Strawderman MH, Ernstoff MS, Smith TJ, Borden EC, Blum RH. Interferon alfa-2b adjuvant therapy of high-risk resected cutaneous melanoma: the Eastern Cooperative Oncology Group Trial EST 1684. *J Clin Oncol*. 1996;14(1):7–17.
51. Liang CA, Jambusaria-Pahlajani A, Karia PS, Elenitsas R, Zhang PD, Schmults CD. A systematic review of outcome data for dermatofibrosarcoma protuberans with and without fibrosarcomatous change. *J Am Acad Dermatol*. 2014;4:781–786.
52. Foroozan M, Sei JF, Amini M, Beauchet A, Saiag P. Efficacy of Mohs micrographic surgery for the treatment of dermatofibrosarcoma protuberans: systematic review. *Arch Dermatol*. 2012;9:1055–1063.
53. McArthur G. Dermatofibrosarcoma protuberans: recent clinical progress. *Ann Surg Oncol*. 2007;10:2876–2886.
54. Noujaim J, Thway K, Fisher C, Jones RL. Dermatofibrosarcoma protuberans: from translocation to targeted therapy. *Cancer Biol Med*. 2015;4:375–384.
55. Rutkowski P, Dębiec-Rychter M, Nowecki Z, et al. Treatment of advanced dermatofibrosarcoma protuberans with imatinib mesylate with or without surgical resection. *J Eur Acad Dermatol Venereol*. 2011;3:264–270.
56. Sabel MS, Sondak VK. Pros and cons of adjuvant interferon in the treatment of melanoma. *Oncologist*. 2003;8(5):451–458.
57. Ballo MT, Bonnen MD, Garden AS, et al. Adjuvant irradiation for cervical lymph node metatases from melanoma. *Cancer*. 2003;97(7):1789–1796.
58. Ballo MT, Ang KK. Radiation therapy for malignant melanoma. *Surg Clin N Am*. 2003;83(2):323–342.
59. Burmeister BH, Mark Smithers B, Burmeister E, et al. A prospective phase II study of adjuvant postoperative radiation therapy following nodal surgery in malignant melanoma: Trans Tasman Radiation Oncology Group (TROG) study 96.06. *Radiother Oncol*. 2006;81(2):136–142.
60. Ribas A, Camacho LH, Lopez-Berestein G, et al. Antitumor activity in melanoma and anti-self responses in a phase I trial with the anti-CTLA-4 monoclonal antibody CP-675206. *J Clin Oncol*. 2005;23:8968–8977.
61. Attia P, Phan GQ, Maker AV, et al. Autoimmunity correlates with tumor regression in patients with metastatic melanoma treated with anti-CTLA4. *J Clin Oncol*. 2005;23:6043–6053.
62. Atkins MB, Hsu J, Lee S, et al. Phase III trial comparing concurrent biochemotherapy with cisplatin, vinblastine, dacarbazine, interleukin-2 and interferon alfa2b with cisplatin, vinblastine, and dacarbazine alone in patients with metastatic malignant melanoma (E3695): a trial coordinated by the Eastern Cooperative Oncology Group. *J Clin Oncol*. 2008;26(35):5748–5754.

63. Brady MS, Akhurst T, Spanknebel K, et al. Utility of preoperative (18)F fluorodeoxyglucose–positron emission tomography scanning in high-risk melanoma patients. *Ann Surg Oncol*. 2006;13:525–532.
64. Eggermont AMM, van Geel AN, de Wilt JH, ten Hagen TL. The role of isolated limb perfusion for melanoma confined to the extremities. *Surg Clin North Am*. 2003;83(2):371–384.
65. Lens MB, Dawes M. Isolated limb perfusion with melphalan in the treatment of malignant melanoma of the extremities: a systematic review of randomised controlled trials. *Lancet Oncol*. 2003;4(6):359–364.
66. Thompson JF, Kam PC, Waugh RC, Harman CR. Isolated limb infusion with cytotoxic agents: a simple alternative to isolated limb perfusion. *Semin Surg Oncol*. 1998;14:238–247.
67. Markowitz JS, Cosimi LA, Carey RW, et al. Prognosis after initial recurrence of cutaneous melanoma. *Arch Surg*. 1991;126:703–707.
68. Fraker DL. Management of in-transit melanoma of the extremity with isolated limb perfusion. *Curr Treat Options Oncol*. 2004;5(3):173–184.
69. Thompson JF, Kam PC. Isolated limb infusion for melanoma: a simple but effective alternative to isolated limb perfusion. *J Surg Oncol*. 2004;88(1):1–3.
70. Wargo JA, Tanabe K. Surgical management of melanoma. *Hematol Oncol Clin North Am*. 2009;23:565–581.
71. Moschos SJ, Edington HD, Land SR, et al. Neoadjuvant treatment of regional stage IIIB melanoma with high-dose interferon alfa-2b induces objective tumor regression in association with modulation of tumor infiltrating host cellular immune responses. *J Clin Oncol*. 2006;24(19):3164–3171.
72. Mocellin S, Pasquali S, Rossi CR, Nitti D. Interferon alpha adjuvant therapy in patients with high-risk melanoma: a systematic review and meta-analysis. *J Natl Cancer Inst*. 2010;102(7):493–501.
73. Long GV, Menzies AM, Nagrial AM, et al. Prognostic and clinicopathologic associations of oncogenic BRAF in metastatic melanoma. *J Clin Oncol*. 2011;29(10):1239–1246.
74. Eggermont AM, Chiarion-Sileni V, Grob JJ, et al. Adjuvant ipilimumab versus placebo after complete resection of high-risk stage III melanoma (EORTC 18071): a randomised, double-blind, phase 3 trial. *Lancet Oncol*. 2015;16(5):522–530.
75. Larkin J, Lao CD, Urba WJ, et al. Efficacy and safety of nivolumab in patients with BRAF V600 mutant and BRAF wild-type advanced melanoma: a pooled analysis of 4 clinical trials. *JAMA Oncol*. 2015;1(4):433–440.
76. Ribas A, Hamid O, Daud A, et al. Association of pembrolizumab with tumor response and survival among patients with advanced melanoma. *JAMA*. 2016;315(15):1600–1609.
77. Wellbrock C, Hurlstone A. BRAF as therapeutic target in melanoma. *Biochem Pharmacol*. 2010;80(5):561–567.
78. Smalley KS, Sondak VK. Melanoma—an unlikely poster child for personalized cancer therapy. *N Engl J Med*. 2010;363(9):876–878.
79. Larkin J, Ascierto PA, Dréno B, et al. Combined vemurafenib and cobimetinib in BRAF-mutated melanoma. *N Engl J Med*. 2014;371(20):1867–1876.
80. Hauschild A, Grob JJ, Demidov LV, et al. Dabrafenib in BRAF-mutated metastatic melanoma: a multicentre, open-label, phase 3 randomised controlled trial. *Lancet*. 2012;380(9839):358–365.
81. Flaherty KT, Robert C, Hersey P, et al. Improved survival with MEK inhibition in BRAF-mutated melanoma. *N Engl J Med*. 2012;367(2):107–114.
82. Ugurel S, Hildenbrand R, Zimpfer A, et al. Lack of clinical efficacy of imatinib in metastatic melanoma. *Br J Cancer*. 2005;92(8):1398–1405.
83. Wyman K, Atkins MB, Prieto V, et al. Multicenter phase II trial of high-dose imatinib mesylate in metastatic melanoma: significant toxicity with no clinical efficacy. *Cancer*. 2006;106(9):2005–2011.

CHAPTER 14

HERNIA

Kristine Makiewicz, M.D.

1. Match the hernia with the description:

A. Richter hernia	I: Hernia containing the appendix
B. Littre's hernia	II: Hernia containing the antimesenteric wall of the intestine
C. Lumbar hernia	III: Hernia in between the semilunar line and the rectus muscle
D. Spigelian hernia	IV: Hernia containing a Meckel's diverticulum
E. Amyand's hernia	V: Hernia through the superior or inferior lumbar triangle

ANSWER: A-II; B-IV; C-V; D-III; E-I

COMMENTS: A Richter hernia is an abdominal wall hernia that only contains the antimesenteric border of the small intestine. This type of hernia may be dangerous, because the incarcerated portion can strangulate without showing symptoms. A Littre's hernia is an abdominal wall hernia containing a Meckel's diverticulum. A lumbar hernia is a rare back hernia that can form through the superior or inferior lumbar triangles. The superior triangle has boundaries of the 12th rib, internal oblique muscle, and thoracic paraspinal muscle. The inferior triangle has boundaries of the iliac crest, external oblique muscle, and latissimus dorsi muscle. A spigelian hernia is a lateral abdominal wall hernia that forms between the semilunar line and the rectus muscle. These often form no noticeable bulge because the external oblique aponeurosis is intact. An Amyand's hernia is an abdominal wall hernia that contains the appendix.

Ref.: 1

2. Chronic groin pain following an inguinal hernia repair may be the result of:
   A. Division of the nerves during the surgical procedure
   B. Postoperative scar tissue
   C. Use of a mesh
   D. Injury from the use of tacks or staples
   E. All of the above

ANSWER: E

COMMENTS: Groin pain following an inguinal hernia repair is much more common than recurrence and has occurred at incidence as high as 29%–76% in several series. Transient pain with mild numbness inferior to the incision is common. Persistent, intense pain and loss of sensation suggest nerve injury or entrapment. In open repairs, the most common nerves involved are the ilioinguinal, iliohypogastric, or genital branch of the genitofemoral nerve. Injury to the lateral femoral cutaneous and genitofemoral nerves in laparoscopic repairs may occur from tack placement. Mesh inguinodynia, or post herniorraphy pain syndrome, has been reported to result from an inflammatory response to mesh or resultant scar tissue, or both. Although nerve blocks may be diagnostic or therapeutic, exploration may be necessary along with neurectomy, surgical removal of all or part of a nerve.

To prevent the problem from occurring, the best intervention is to be meticulous with identification and avoid entrapment of the aforementioned nerves in open repairs. In addition, tack placement should be avoided, particularly in the triangle of doom in laparoscopic procedures.

Ref.: 1

3. Which of the following statements is true regarding surgical technique?
   A. A Bassini repair can be used for femoral hernias.
   B. A Shouldice repair approximates the transversus abdominis aponeurosis to Cooper's ligament medially and the iliopubic tract laterally. It requires a relaxing incision.
   C. A total extraperitoneal repair (TEP) is a laparoscopic approach that stays in the preperitoneal space by using a balloon dissector.
   D. A Bassini repair uses a piece of mesh to reinforce the floor of the inguinal canal and recreate the internal ring in a tension-free manner.
   E. A McVay repair may never be used for femoral hernias.

ANSWER: C

COMMENTS: A McVay repair is described in answer E and can be used for femoral hernias. A transition stitch and a relaxing incision are needed for a McVay repair—medial to the edge of the femoral canal the transversus abdominis aponeurosis is stitched to Cooper's ligament, and lateral to the femoral canal the transversus abdominis is attached to the iliopubic tract. A Bassini repair is a tissue repair, and answer D describes a Lichtenstein repair. Since the Bassini repair is completely superior to the inguinal ligament, it cannot be used to repair a femoral hernia.

Ref.: 1

4. Which of the following statements are true regarding laparoscopic inguinal hernia anatomy?

A. The triangle of doom is bordered by the vas deferens, iliopubic tract, and gonadal vessels and contains the ilioinguinal and iliohypogastric nerves that must be avoided to prevent pain.

B. The lateral-most border of the dissection is the anterior superior iliac spine.

C. The femoral branch of the genitofemoral nerve and the lateral femoral cutaneous nerve are located medial and superior to the iliopubic tract.

D. The femoral canal cannot be accessed through a preperitoneal approach; therefore femoral hernias cannot be repaired laparoscopically.

E. A transabdominal preperitoneal repair (TAPP) approach uses a dissecting balloon to stay in the preperitoneal space throughout the procedure, and a TEP approach initially accesses the peritoneum before creating a peritoneal flap.

ANSWER: B

COMMENTS: Laparoscopic hernia repair is appropriate for femoral hernias and indicated for bilateral or recurrent inguinal hernias. There are two techniques to gain exposure to the inguinal region. A TEP uses an infraumbilical port and a balloon dissector in the preperitoneal space to expose the inguinal canal and hernia. A TAPP uses an infraumbilical port to gain access to the peritoneum. A peritoneal flap is created to expose the hernia. The lateral edge of the dissection is the anterior superior iliac spine in both approaches. The hernia is reduced, and a large mesh is placed over the defect. Important landmarks are the inferior epigastric vessels running along the edge of the rectus muscle dividing indirect and direct hernias. Tacks are placed medial to Cooper's ligament to secure the mesh in place. No tacks should be placed inferior to the iliopubic tract because the femoral branch of the genitofemoral nerve and the lateral femoral cutaneous nerve are located lateral and inferior. The triangle of pain contains the genitofemoral nerve and lateral cutaneous femoral nerve and is bound by the iliopubic tract superiorly and genital vessels inferiorly. The triangle of doom contains the external iliac vessels, and the femoral nerve is bound by the iliopubic tract superiorly, vas deferens medially, and spermatic vessels laterally.

Ref.: 1

5. Which of the following statements is false regarding the iliopubic tract?

A. It extends from the anterior superior iliac spine to the pubis.

B. It is a condensation of the transversalis fascia.

C. It is of anatomic interest but has little clinical significance.

D. It runs underneath the shelving portion of the Poupart's ligament.

E. Many branches of the lumbar plexus run inferior to the iliopubic tract.

ANSWER: C

COMMENTS: The transversalis fascia is the portion of the endoabdominal fascia that underlies the transversus abdominis muscle. It has several thickenings, the most important of which is the iliopubic tract, which arises from the iliopectineal arch, inserts on the anterior superior iliac spine, and extends over the femoral vessels to the pubis. Proper utilization of the transversalis fascia during the repair of an inguinal hernia is important to the success of operations not using the prosthetic material. The iliopubic tract has particular significance because of its importance as a landmark to laparoscopic surgeons. Many of the branches of the lumbar plexus run inferior to the tract, and damage to these nerves may be the result of aggressive dissection or the placement of tacks or staples to affix a mesh below this structure.

Ref.: 1–3

6. Which of the following statements is false regarding the incidence of abdominal wall hernias?

A. Two-thirds of all inguinal hernias are classified as indirect.

B. Femoral hernias are more common in females than in males.

C. Indirect hernias are common in females.

D. Hernias generally occur with equal frequency in males and females.

E. Premature babies have a 10% incidence of inguinal hernia.

ANSWER: D

COMMENTS: Approximately three-fourths of all abdominal wall hernias occur in the inguinal region, and roughly two-thirds of them are indirect inguinal hernias. Groin hernias are considered to be at least 25 times more common in males than in females. The incidence of inguinal hernias is increased by prematurity. The most common hernia in each gender is an indirect inguinal hernia. Femoral hernias are rare in men. On the other hand, direct hernias are uncommon in women. It has been estimated that inguinal hernias develop in 25% of males and 2% of females during their lifetime. Therefore hernias constitute a significant economic problem in terms of loss of time from work.

Ref.: 1–3

7. Which of the following statements is true regarding direct inguinal hernias?

A. Direct hernias are commonly congenital and found in younger patients.

B. The risk of incarceration of a direct hernia is high.

C. A direct hernia is solely a weakening of the inguinal floor and does not pass through the inguinal rings.

D. An indirect hernia may be present as well.

E. An indirect hernia will never be present with it.

ANSWER: D

COMMENTS: Through physical stress, the connective tissue breaks down. As a result, the strength of the transverse aponeurosis and fascia decreases from intraabdominal pressure, smoking, aging, connective tissue disease, and systemic illnesses. Therefore direct inguinal hernias are acquired from the "wear and tear" of daily life, including straining to urinate or defecate, chronic coughing, and heavy lifting. A decrease in the content of hydroxyproline in the aponeurosis of patients with hernias has been demonstrated, along with alterations in the ultrastructure of collagen. Large indirect hernias may weaken the floor of the Hesselbach's triangle and result in a functional direct component. Because the area of the Hesselbach's triangle is weaker without a narrow-necked sac, the risk for incarceration is low. Rarely, incarceration results when a direct hernia passes through the external ring posterior to the cord structures. The spermatic cord should be explored to rule out the presence of an indirect sac. A pantaloon hernia is composed of both direct and indirect inguinal hernias.

Ref.: 1–3

8. Which of the following statements about the management of inguinal hernias in infants and children is true?

A. Repair should be delayed until a child reaches school age since most inguinal hernia defects close spontaneously.

B. Repair usually requires a Bassini procedure.

C. The distal sac should be removed to prevent the formation of a secondary hydrocele.

D. Contralateral inguinal exploration is indicated routinely because of the high risk for bilaterality.

E. Intubation of the clinically apparent hernia sac with a laparoscope is one method of examining the contralateral side.

ANSWER: E

COMMENTS: Inguinal hernias in infants and children are nearly always indirect and result from the failure of obliteration of the processus vaginalis. Effective treatment requires only high ligation and transection of the sac with or without excision of the distal component. Repair need not be delayed unless the infant has associated medical problems. In fact, bowel obstruction and gonadal or intestinal infarction as a result of strangulation are most likely to occur during the first 6 months of life. Therefore the repair should be performed soon after the diagnosis is made. Exploration of the opposite side in children with a unilateral inguinal hernia is controversial. The incidence of a contralateral hernia following unilateral inguinal herniorrhaphy in children has been reported to be 10%–30%. Contralateral exploration should be performed routinely in the subset of patients most likely to have a clinically occult hernia: children younger than 2 years, girls younger than 3 years (higher bilateral rate), patients with ventriculoperitoneal shunts, and children younger than 2 years with a left-sided hernia. This last recommendation is based on the fact that most (60%) pediatric hernias are right sided. Intubation of the clinically apparent hernia sac with a laparoscope is one method of examining the contralateral side.

Ref.: 1–3

9. Which of the following hernias is most likely to recur after a primary repair?

A. Epigastric hernia

B. Spigelian hernia

C. Indirect hernia

D. Femoral hernia

E. Incisional hernia

ANSWER: E

COMMENTS: The primary repair of incisional hernias can be associated with a 30%–50% or higher recurrence rate, depending on the size of the hernia. Except for small incisional hernias, a prosthetic mesh is necessary to reduce recurrence rates to 10% or possibly less. Patients with incisional hernias usually have predisposing factors, such as obesity, chronic debilitating illness, diabetes, advanced age, and smoking. The predisposing factors also play a role in the failure of primary repair. Recurrence rates after the other listed hernia repairs should all be 5% or less.

Ref.: 1–3

10. Which of the following is a true statement regarding umbilical hernias?

A. They are the embryonic equivalent of a small omphalocele.

B. Repair in infants is usually deferred until approximately 1 year of age.

C. Repair in adults is generally indicated.

D. The "vest-over-pants" type of repair is stronger than simple approximation of fascial margins.

E. They are most common in white infants.

ANSWER: C

COMMENTS: Umbilical hernias are the result of a patent umbilical ring, whereas an omphalocele is the result of the failure of abdominal wall closure in the midline during early intrauterine life. Umbilical hernias are said to be present in 40%–90% of African-American infants. Incarceration is rare in infants. Unless the defect is large, most surgeons defer repair until the child is approximately 4 years of age because spontaneous closure does occur. In adults, however, repair should be carried out promptly because of the risk for incarceration. There is no convincing evidence that a "vest-over-pants" type of repair is structurally superior to a simple approximation of the fascial margins. Repair in adults may benefit from the use of prosthetic material, such as polypropylene, if the fascial defect is large or tension is present. There are several variations of mesh repairs with no evidence-based consensus of choice at this time.

Ref.: 1–3

11. A 75-year-old man is seen in the emergency department with a 2-h history of an incarcerated femoral hernia. He takes warfarin for a past history of atrial fibrillation and has an international normalized ratio (INR) of 3.1. Which of the following is the correct treatment?

A. Admit the patient for correction of the INR and repair the hernia in the morning.

B. Perform an emergency laparoscopic repair of the hernia.

C. Perform an emergency open repair of the hernia.

D. Attempt a reduction of the hernia in the emergency department after sedation.

E. Use a mesh in the repair of the hernia.

ANSWER: C

COMMENTS: The risk for strangulation in incarcerated femoral hernias is reported to be as high as 20%–40%. It is believed that the window for successful treatment to avoid bowel resection is 4 to 6 h. This clinical condition is considered a surgical emergency, and fresh-frozen plasma can be administered just before and during surgery. A laparoscopic repair can be challenging with an incarcerated hernia, and in addition there is a concern for increased bleeding in the patient. Laparoscopic repair also requires the use of a mesh, which may become infected. Although mesh decreases recurrence in femoral hernias, it is probably not advisable in this setting. An open approach is probably preferred and can be a tissue-to-tissue repair. Any attempt at reduction is probably contraindicated because of the high potential for strangulation. If the bowel drops into the abdomen during an open approach, insertion of a scope into the hernia sac may be useful in evaluating the integrity of the affected bowel.

Ref.: 1, 3

12. A 55-year-old man with liver failure and ascites has an enlarging umbilical hernia. He has never undergone diuretic therapy. The correct therapy is:

A. Open repair with a waterproof mesh

B. High-volume paracentesis immediately before repair

C. Deferring hernia repair until correction of the ascites by maximal medical therapy, transjugular intrahepatic portosystemic shunting, or liver transplantation

D. Laparoscopic repair with an inlay mesh

E. Repair of the hernia and use of an abdominal binder after the operation

ANSWER: C

COMMENTS: Repair of any hernia in a patient with ascites is a challenging problem. In general, any consideration of an elective repair should be deferred until the ascites is controlled with maximal medical therapy. If the ascites can be controlled, umbilical hernias should be repaired in patients with cirrhosis because of the high morbidity and mortality if the hernia ruptures. If there is skin breakdown and leakage of ascites, an urgent repair may be necessary to prevent peritonitis. Frequent paracentesis may be helpful in this difficult scenario with associated high morbidity.

Ref.: 3

13. Match the following Surgical Wound Classification with the hernia repair scenario:

A. Sterile	I: Explantation of infected mesh
B. Clean	II: Symptomatic reducible inguinal hernia
C. Clean contaminated	III: Strangulated inguinal hernia with ischemic bowel
D. Contaminated	IV: Not a surgical wound class
E. Dirty	V: Small bowel enterotomy during ventral hernia repair

ANSWER: A-IV; B-II; C-V; D-III; E-I

COMMENTS: A clean wound is only in contact with the normal skin flora and should have a surgical site infection rate of <2%. An elective inguinal hernia repair is a clean wound. A clean-contaminated wound enters a viscus in a controlled manner; the hernia has a surgical site infection risk of 2%–10%. Gynecologic cases, prepped colon or small bowel procedures, and head and neck cases are clean-contaminated cases. A contaminated wound has intestinal spillage without active signs of infection and has an infection rate of ~10% even with antibiotics. Examples of a contaminated wound are ischemic bowel and an unprepped colon. Dirty cases are surgeries with active infection such as an empyema and perforated appendicitis. During a hernia repair, the wound class is very important to help guide mesh placement. A synthetic mesh can be used with clean and clean-contaminated wounds. Biologic meshes are used for contaminated or dirty wounds if a mesh is needed. "Sterile" is not a part of the Surgical Wound Classification.

Ref.: 4

14. Which of the following statements is true regarding femoral hernias?

A. Femoral hernias should not be repaired through an infrainguinal approach.

B. If an incarcerated femoral hernia cannot be reduced intraoperatively, the insertion of the inguinal ligament can be cut from the pubic tubercle to allow more space.

C. Femoral hernias are more common than inguinal hernias in females.

D. A laparoscopic repair is an inappropriate choice for a femoral hernia repair.

E. Incarcerated femoral hernias can be observed and managed on an elective basis.

ANSWER: B

COMMENTS: Although femoral hernias are found more often in females than in males, inguinal hernias are still more common than femoral hernias. Femoral hernias with small orifices in women are repaired from below the inguinal ligament with a few sutures or plugged with a cone of polypropylene mesh because they are rarely associated with hernias above the inguinal ligament. Large femoral hernias can be repaired with the McVay Cooper's ligament procedure or even better with a preperitoneal permanent prosthesis placed either laparoscopically or using an open preperitoneal approach. Femoral hernias should be repaired promptly because the risk of incarceration is high. Viability of the intestine must be ensured since incarceration of the antimesenteric border of the intestine (Richter hernia) could result in infarction. The presence of bloody fluid in an otherwise empty sac mandates a careful examination of the intestine to rule out ischemia. The McVay repair may be preferred with incarcerated femoral hernias to avoid infection of the prosthetic mesh. If the hernia sac is too large to reduce through the hernia defect, the medial insertion of the inguinal ligament can be cut from the pubic tubercle to allow more space. After reduction, the inguinal ligament is reattached to the pubic tubercle or Cooper's ligament.

Ref.: 1–3, 5

15. Correct statements regarding the management of an incarcerated groin hernia include all of the following except:

A. A giant inguinal hernia is a chronically incarcerated hernia containing the majority of the bowel. After reduction, loss of abdominal domain and elevated intraabdominal pressures can be a concern.

B. Evaluation of the contents of the hernia sac is a step required in the repair of an incarcerated hernia.

C. Incarcerated femoral hernias can be repaired on an elective basis.

D. A hydrocele may mimic an incarcerated hernia.

E. Inadvertent reduction of incarcerated hernia contents during the induction of anesthesia does not ensure bowel viability.

ANSWER: C

COMMENTS: Incarceration with potential resultant strangulation of small bowel is a serious complication of groin hernias. If the patient has an incarcerated inguinal hernia and strangulation is not suspected, an attempt at reduction by using sedation, Trendelenburg positioning, and gentle sustained pressure over the groin mass is appropriate. Reduction en masse refers to the persistent nature of incarcerated tissue frequently through the external ring despite an apparently successful reduction. If there is any indication of strangulation, reduction should not be attempted preoperatively. Rather, the sac should first be opened before reduction to inspect the viability of the contents. The presence of bloody fluid in the peritoneal cavity should raise the question of intestinal viability. A delayed repair following a successful reduction may permit resolution of edema. A hydrocele can mimic an incarcerated hernia. Should physical examination fail to establish the diagnosis, a hydrocele will transilluminate clearly but a hernia will not. Ultrasound can confirm the presence of a hydrocele. In patients with a suspected strangulated hernia, spontaneous reduction of the hernia's contents could occur. However, the surgeon should not assume that the bowel is viable, and examination of the abdominal contents is mandatory. An incarcerated femoral hernia should always be repaired on an urgent basis, as the rate of strangulation is high. Giant inguinal hernias are often chronically incarcerated and can contain the majority of the intraabdominal contents. After reduction, the volume of the abdominal contents is increased enough that the abdominal wall closure can become problematic.

Ref.: 1–3, 6, 12

16. A 55-year-old obese woman returns to the office 2 weeks after an open incisional hernia repair with mesh complaining of increasing pain and redness. On examination, the wound is red and fluctuant consistent with a postoperative wound infection. Which of the following is true regarding wound infections?

A. Laparoscopic hernia repairs have lower rates of wound infections than open repairs.

B. Polytetrafluoroethylene (PTFE) mesh is an absorbable mesh that can be left in place even with a wound infection.

C. Suture ventral hernia repair has higher infection rates and recurrence rates than mesh ventral hernia repair.

D. Surgical site infections have no effect on the recurrence rate after a ventral hernia repair.

E. Closed and open repairs have high rates of systemic infections.

ANSWER: A

COMMENTS: The advantage of mesh in a hernia repair is that it decreases hernia recurrence from 8.2% to 2.7%, but has slightly high rates of infection. Mesh infection rates are 3%–10% after a hernia repair. Meta-analysis shows that a laparoscopic ventral hernia repair with a mesh has infection rates of 1%–2% compared with ~10% for an open ventral hernia repair with mesh, with no difference in the recurrence rate.

PTFE is a synthetic mesh that becomes encapsulated with no ingrowth of tissue; if infected, it must be explanted. Macroporous monofilament meshes are more resistant to infection because macrophages can enter the pores and combat infection. Surgical site infection is the most common reason that a mesh is explanted and leads to higher recurrence rates.

Ref.: 1, 7–9, 13

17. Which of the following developments has not led to a decrease in recurrence rates after a groin hernia repair?

A. Modifications of the Bassini repair

B. Routine use of prosthetic material

C. Widespread acceptance of the "tension-free" concept

D. Use of the preperitoneal space for hernia repair

E. Use of laparoscopy in hernia repair

ANSWER: A

COMMENTS: Recurrence rates for groin hernias vary from less than 1% to 30%. True recurrence rates are difficult to establish because of inadequate patient follow-up. The Bassini repair and its modifications (Shouldice and McVay) all create tension at the suture line and have been found to have recurrence rates between 10% and 30% when performed outside specialized centers. Several developments in the latter half of the 20th century have significantly influenced the currently accepted level of a recurrence rate of less than 5%. The routine uses of prosthetic material to perform a tension-free hernia repair became accepted by surgeons after being popularized by Lichtenstein in the 1980s. Others, such as Rutkow, Robbins, Kugel, Gilbert, Wantz, Stoppa, Millikan, and Nyhus, have used multiple prosthetic materials and approaches to continue to reduce the recurrence rate to below 1%. The most popular prosthetic materials are polypropylene, polyester fiber mesh, and PTFE. Use of the preperitoneal space also helped lower recurrence rates by allowing larger pieces of prosthetic material to be used and incorporating intraabdominal pressure to aid in keeping the mesh in place. Laparoscopy by itself has not helped lower recurrence rates below those achieved with open tension-free mesh repairs, but it has given the surgeon another option for accessing the preperitoneal space.

Ref.: 1, 9, 13

18. Which of the following is true regarding characteristics of mesh used in hernia repair?

A. Lightweight mesh, compared with heavyweight mesh, provokes an intense inflammatory reaction in the body causing scarring, pain, and shrinkage.

B. Synthetic meshes can never be placed into a contaminated field.

C. Polypropylene meshes have high adhesion risks, so they should not be placed directly next to bowel.

D. Biologic meshes are processed human, bovine, and porcine tissues composed of a collagen matrix and immune cells.

E. Use of a mesh reduces the rate of surgical site infections.

ANSWER: C

COMMENTS: Synthetic meshes are composed of PTFE, polypropylene, or polyester. Porosity is important in determining the flexibility and infection resistance of the mesh. Large pores decrease the inflammatory foreign body reaction and allow improved penetration by immune cells. Lightweight meshes have large pores with thinner filaments, and heavyweight meshes have small pores with thicker filaments leading to a denser material. Heavyweight meshes are less elastic, which can interfere with the abdominal wall compliance, and have more shrinkage than lightweight meshes. Polypropylene meshes have high rates of adhesion and cannot come into contact with bowel, and PTFE has less adhesion risk. Often composite materials are used with a polypropylene side to promote adherence to the abdominal wall and a PTFE side against the viscera. Biologic meshes are composed of acellular collagen matrices that have been derived from either porcine small intestine or human dermis.

Using mesh reduces the rate of recurrence but increases the rate of surgical site infections. Traditional teaching was that in a contaminated field (i.e., with a bowel resection or enterotomy), a synthetic mesh could never be used, but newer data show acceptable rates of surgical site infections in select circumstances.

Ref.: 1, 9

19. All of the following statements concerning the Lichtenstein repair are true except:

A. It is performed with local anesthesia in an outpatient setting.

B. Polypropylene is the most common prosthetic material used for the repair.

C. The medial edge of the mesh is sutured to the transversalis fascia, and the lateral edge is sutured to the inguinal ligament.

D. To reduce recurrence rates, the most cephalad tails of the mesh should extend 2 to 4 cm beyond the internal ring.

E. To reduce recurrence rates, the most caudal aspect of the mesh should extend at least 2 cm over the pubic tubercle.

ANSWER: C

COMMENTS: As commonly performed, the open herniorrhaphy technique is a tension-free repair popularized by Irving L. Lichtenstein and colleagues. The Lichtenstein repair is routinely performed in an outpatient setting with local anesthesia. A polypropylene mesh is most commonly sutured medially to the transversus abdominis arch, with the internal oblique being overlapped by approximately 2 cm. The latter edge of the mesh is sutured to the inguinal ligament. To reduce recurrence rates, Parviz Amid has described overlapping the mesh at least 2 cm over the pubic tubercle and 2 to 4 cm lateral to the internal ring. The Lichtenstein repair was one of the first prosthetic repairs to achieve approximately an overall 1% or lower recurrence rate in the United States.

Ref.: 1–3, 10

20. A morbidly obese man is in the ICU 12 h after a separation-of-components hernia repair for a large hernia with loss of abdominal domain. He is intubated and sedated. The nurse calls you to the bedside because of worsening abdominal distension. Which of the following is not a sign of developing an abdominal compartment syndrome?

A. Increasing peak airway pressures

B. Decreasing urine output

C. Increasing tidal volumes

D. Increasing bladder pressures

E. Decreased central venous pressure (CVP)

ANSWER: C

COMMENTS: Abdominal compartment syndrome is a serious complication that can develop after a separation-of-component hernia repair, especially if there was a large loss of abdominal domain preoperatively. Signs of increasing abdominal hypertension include elevated peak airway pressures, declining tidal volumes, increasing abdominal distension and firmness, decreasing urine output, and increasing bladder pressures. Intraabdominal hypertension is defined as sustained pressure > 12 mmHg, and abdominal compartment syndrome is sustained pressures > 20 mmHg with evidence of end-organ dysfunction. Since the measurement of intraabdominal pressure can be influenced by many factors, these numbers are taken within a clinical context. The concern is that with increasing abdominal pressure, intraabdominal organs will become ischemic, and it will be difficult to ventilate. The steps to reduce pressure and improve perfusion include deepening sedation, paralysis, and, as a last resort, reopening the abdomen.

Ref.: 11

21. Which of the following is not true regarding laparoscopic hernia repair?

A. Local anesthesia with sedation is the most common form of anesthesia used.

B. It could lead to injury to the genitofemoral nerve and the lateral femoral cutaneous nerve.

C. Transabdominal preperitoneal or total extraperitoneal approaches are commonly used.

D. Fixation devices for the mesh should not be placed below the iliopubic tract.

E. It is best suited for recurrent and bilateral hernias.

ANSWER: A

COMMENTS: Laparoscopic techniques for the repair of inguinal hernias were introduced in the 1990s and have gained mild-to-moderate acceptance, with less than 10% of all inguinal hernia repairs being performed via these approaches. The repairs are usually performed with the patient under general anesthesia, and the cost is considerably higher than that of an open approach with local anesthesia and sedation. Although there is controversy regarding its use for unilateral, newly diagnosed hernias, it seems ideally suited for recurrent and bilateral hernias, where the disability and technical difficulty associated with open (conventional) repairs cannot be overlooked. Laparoscopy can be performed totally extraperitoneally by dissecting within the preperitoneal space or transabdominally. In either case, a preperitoneal repair is performed. Mesh fixation devices placed below the iliopubic tract risk injury to the genitofemoral nerve and the lateral femoral cutaneous nerve. Placement of fixation devices is also avoided below the internal inguinal ring in an area known as the "triangle of doom." This triangle is bordered laterally by the spermatic vessels and medially by the vas deferens. Located within this triangle are the external iliac artery and vein and the femoral nerve.

Ref.: 1–3, 13

22. A 65-year-old man underwent sigmoid resection and end colostomy for perforated diverticulitis. One year after the surgery he presents to your office complaining of a bulge around his stoma and an inability to obtain a good seal on his appliance. Which of the follow is true regarding parastomal hernias?

A. Ileostomies develop parastomal hernias more often than colostomies.

B. Parastomal hernias are best prevented by making the fascial defect as small as possible during the initial operation and placing the intestine through the rectus sheath.

C. The only operative repair option is to relocate the stoma.

D. Parastomal hernias have large enough fascial defects that intestinal strangulation does not happen.

E. Every parastomal hernia should be repaired emergently to prevent high rates of strangulation.

ANSWER: B

COMMENTS: Parastomal hernias are a very common problem after stoma formation, affecting up to 30% of stomas. Colostomies are more likely to develop hernias than ileostomies. Hernias can be asymptomatic, painful, cause skin irritation from poorly fitting appliances, or lead to intestinal strangulation. Only symptomatic parastomal hernias should be repaired. Stomas should always be formed through the rectus sheath with the smallest defect necessary, and placement of a mesh at initial creation is not routine. There are three main methods to repair a parastomal hernia: relocation, keyhole mesh (either synthetic or biologic), or Sugarbaker repair—a single mesh is placed underneath the defect and the intestine is lateralized.

Ref.: 14

23. Which of the following urologic complications does not occur with hernia repair?

A. Ischemic orchitis

B. Transection of the vas deferens

C. Prostatitis

D. Testicular atrophy

E. Ovarian torsion within the hernia sac

ANSWER: C

COMMENTS: Transection of the vas deferens if identified intraoperatively should be repaired with interrupted fine monofilament suture. A crush injury and stretch can damage the vas as well without complete transection. There appears to be a small association between men who had a hernia repair as a child and adult infertility, but the exact mechanism is not defined. Testicular atrophy develops from ischemia caused by an incarcerated hernia or intraoperative injury. It occurs at a rate of 2.6%–5%, but testicles should only be removed for frank necrosis on intraoperative examination. Ischemic orchitis presents as postoperative testicular pain caused by venous thrombosis from the overaggressive handling of the pampiniform plexus. The occurrence is 1% and is managed conservatively with nonsteroidal antiinflammatory drugs (NSAIDs). Ovarian strangulation can be as high as 30% if found within an incarcerated hernia, primarily from ovarian torsion.

Ref.: 2, 15, 16

24. There are many different techniques to repair a ventral hernia. In the last few years, a new technique, the transversus abdominis muscle release (TAR), has been developed to repair large ventral hernias with the loss of domain. Which of the following is false regarding TAR?

A. TAR is a modification of the Rives-Stoppa retromuscular hernia repair.

B. TAR has higher wound complication rates than a traditional separation-of-components hernia repair.

C. To gain more abdominal wall length, the posterior rectus sheath is incised 0.5 to 1 cm medial to the linea semilunaris and the transversus abdominal muscle attachments are cut.

D. The transversus abdominis is mobilized from the costal margin to the space of Retzius.

E. A mesh can be placed in the retrorectus space to reinforce the hernia repair.

ANSWER: B

COMMENTS: A TAR is a newer modification of the Rives-Stoppa retromuscular hernia repair. Described by Rosen et al., the repair utilizes the retromuscular space. The posterior rectus sheath is entered and the posterior fascia dissected off the muscle laterally. At 0.5 to 1 cm medial to the linea semilunaris, the posterior rectus sheath is incised and the transversus abdominis muscle attachment is cut. The transversus abdominis is cut cranially to the costal margin and caudally into the space of Retzius. Releasing the transversus abdominis creates laxity of the abdominal wall allowing the posterior rectus fascia to be approximated along the midline. A large sublay mesh is placed into the retrorectus space and tacked in place with a few interrupted sutures. Drains are placed, the anterior rectus sheath is approximated, and the skin closed.

In comparison to the traditional separation-of-components technique, additional abdominal wall domain is gained without raising large subcutaneous flaps so the blood supply to the abdominal wall is preserved. This avoids the wound complications usually associated with a separation-of-components repair. In the initial study, the long-term recurrence rate was ~5%.

Ref.: 17

25. Which of the following statements is not true with regard to incisional ventral hernias?

A. Primary repairs are associated with a 30%–50% recurrence rate.

B. The incidence of incisional hernias is between 2% and 11% after laparotomy.

C. Prosthetic mesh repairs have reduced the recurrence rate to 20% or less.

D. Bilayer mesh can be placed safely in the intraabdominal cavity.

E. Comorbid conditions, such as diabetes, hypertension, and obesity, are uncommon in patients with incisional hernias.

ANSWER: E

COMMENTS: In the United States, approximately 2 million laparotomies are performed each year, with a reported incisional ventral hernia rate between 2% and 11%. The population of patients in whom wound dehiscence occurs tends to be obese, and they frequently might have one or more of the following: comorbidities of a smoking history, hypertension, and diabetes. Primary incisional ventral hernia repairs have been associated with recurrence rates of up to 50%. Prosthetic mesh repairs have lowered the recurrence rates to less than 10%. Recently, it has been found that a bilayer prosthesis composed of both polypropylene and PTFE can be placed safely in the abdominal cavity without the development of bowel obstruction or enterocutaneous fistulas. Intraabdominal placement of the mesh allows the greatest underlay of the fascial defect, thereby enabling the greatest amount of tissue ingrowth to occur. When polypropylene alone is placed in the intraabdominal cavity, bowel obstruction, enterocutaneous fistula, and difficult reentry to the abdomen occur with an unacceptable frequency.

There is increasing evidence of less recurrence with a laparoscopic incisional hernia repair using a mesh. This is typically an onlay with 3 to 5 cm overlap of the fascial defect. Local wound problems seem to be decreased. Lighter synthetic mesh is gaining in popularity. Again, expertise and experience in this advanced laparoscopic procedure are necessary to achieve low recurrence rates and avoid serious complications. A frequent but easily treated complication of a laparoscopic repair is seroma, which can occur in up to 30%–50% of patients. It is usually self-limited. The use of drains to avoid seroma formation is controversial, and it has not been associated with a decrease in its incidence. Aspiration of seromas is best accomplished under image guidance if they are symptomatic or concern about infection exists.

Ref.: 3, 18, 19

26. A 55-year-old man who runs marathons has a recurrent inguinal hernia. Which statement is correct?

A. The previous type of repair has no significance in the treatment plan.

B. A Shouldice repair is recommended.

C. He will have to stop running marathons after repair.

D. A repair can be performed with the patient under local anesthesia with a high likelihood of success.

E. Laparoscopic repair, if the previous repair was performed in an open manner with a mesh, is an evidence-based choice.

ANSWER: E

COMMENTS: The repair of a recurrent inguinal hernia can be challenging in terms of preventing recurrence and avoiding morbidity such as chronic pain. Tissue-to-tissue repairs may be repaired with an anterior mesh repair such as the Lichtenstein or plug-and-patch repair. Obtaining a prior operative report is strongly recommended to facilitate selection of the appropriate current repair. A laparoscopic repair for recurrence of a hernia after an open anterior mesh repair is supported by prospective trials. The caveat is that such results require expertise and experience in laparoscopic repair. A Shouldice repair is not generally recommended for recurrent hernias. A repair by an expert surgeon should allow resumption of all normal activity and is recommended for active individuals. A repair can be deferred if asymptomatic in selected patients.

Ref.: 19

27. A 30-year-old man presents to your office complaining of groin pain while playing sports. On examination, he has no palpable bulge but does experience tenderness with palpation over the pubic tubercle. Which of the following is true regarding a sports hernia or athletic pubalgia?

A. Athletic pubalgia is most common in long-distance runners.

B. Even though a hernia defect is not palpable on examination, it is clearly apparent on imaging.

C. There is no surgical role for the management of athletic pubalgia.

D. Operative management can be performed with open or laparoscopic hernia repair technique.

E. Athletic pubalgia is an acute traumatic tear of the inguinal ligament.

ANSWER: D

COMMENTS: The component of groin pain or a sports hernia treated by general surgeons is more precisely referred to as athletic pubalgia. This is a tear of the intersection of the rectus abdominis or adductor longus to the pubis from repetitive stress. The typical populations with athletic pubalgia are participants in sports with high-speed changes in direction and twisting such as hockey, soccer, wrestling, and football. They complain of pain with motion—especially hip adduction—but there is no visible bulge as there is no defect in the abdominal wall. On examination, there is point tenderness over the pubic tubercle. The inflammation and tear at the pubis can be identified on magnetic resonance imaging (MRI). Dynamic ultrasound shows laxity and bulge of the rectus muscle with no distinct hernia. Nonoperative management includes rest, physical therapy, and steroid injections. If nonoperative management fails, then an inguinal hernia repair (open or laparoscopic) can be used to resolve the pain. A hernia repair is thought to support the laxity of the pelvic floor and cause an inflammatory reaction reattaching the torn aponeurosis to the pubic tubercle. Some surgeons perform a nerve transection of the iliohypogastric and ilioinguinal nerves.

Ref.: 20, 21

28. The separation-of-components technique:

A. Is best for hernias with fascial defects of 3 cm or less

B. Has a recurrence rate of approximately 10%

C. May be used when there is contamination or bowel surgery is required

D. Is contraindicated for recurrent incisional hernias

E. Ideally avoids the use of a mesh

ANSWER: C

COMMENTS: Although a primary suture repair with mesh has acceptable recurrence rates for small incisional hernias, recurrence rates are disappointing when these techniques are used for very large hernias. In addition, more complications are associated with a mesh repair of very large hernias either by open or by laparoscopic technique.

The separation-of-components technique has demonstrated improved results in the repair of massive incisional hernias, with recurrence rates of approximately 20%. This technique can be used when there is contamination or bowel surgery is required, thereby avoiding the dreaded complication of mesh infection.

The separation-of-components technique can be used for failed mesh repairs. In selected cases, the addition of soft synthetic mesh has improved success with the technique.

Ref.: 22

REFERENCES

1. Malangoni M, Rosen MJ. Hernias. In: Townsend Jr C, Beauchamp R, Evers B, Mattox K, eds. *Sabiston Textbook of Surgery: The Biological Basis of Modern Surgical Practice*. 20th ed. Philadelphia: Elsevier Inc; 2017.
2. Fitzgibbons Jr R, Cemaj S, Quinn T. Abdominal wall hernias. In: Mulholland M, Lillemoe K, Doherty G, Maier R, Simeone D, Upchurch Jr G, eds. *Greenfield's Surgery: Scientific Principles and Practice*. 5th ed. Philadelphia: Wolters Kluwer; 2010:1159–1198.
3. Sherman V, Macho J, Brunicardi F. Inguinal hernias. In: Brunicardi F, Andersen D, Billiar T, eds. *Schwartz's Principles of Surgery*. 9th ed. New York: McGraw-Hill; 2010.
4. Mangram AJ, Horan TC, Pearson ML, Silver LC, Jarvis WR. Guideline for prevention of surgical site infection, 1999. Centers for Disease Control and Prevention (CDC) Hospital Infection Control Practices Advisory Committee. *Am J Infect Control*. 1999;27(2):97–132.
5. Robbins A, Rutkow I. Mesh plug repair and groin hernia surgery. *Surg Clin North Am*. 1998;78:1007–1023.

6. El Saadi AS, Al Wadan AH, Hamerna S. Approach to a giant inguinoscrotal hernia. *Hernia*. 2005;9(3):277–279.
7. Arita NA, Nguyen MT, Nguyen DH, et al. Laparoscopic repair reduces incidence of surgical site infections for all ventral hernias. *Surg Endosc Other Interv Tech*. 2015;29(7):1769–1780.
8. Hawn MT, Gray SH, Snyder CW, Graham LA, Finan KR, Vick CC. Predictors of mesh explantation after incisional hernia repair. *Am J Surg*. 2011;202(1):28–33.
9. Brown CN, Finch JG. Which mesh for hernia repair? *Ann R Coll Surg Engl*. 2010;92(4):272–278.
10. Amid P. How to avoid recurrence in Lichtenstein tension-free hernioplasty. *Am J Surg*. 2002;184:259–260.
11. Veronikis D. Surgery of hernia. In: Fischer J, Jones D, Pomposelli F, et al., eds. *Fischer's Mastery of Surgery*. 6th ed. Philadelphia: Lippencott Williams & Wilkins; 2012.
12. Millikan K, Doolas A. A long-term evaluation of the modified meshplug hernioplasty in over 2000 patients. *Hernia*. 2008;12:257–260.
13. Millikan K, Deziel D. The management of hernia: considerations in cost effectiveness. *Surg Clin North Am*. 1996;76:105–116.
14. Sands L, Marchetti F. Intestinal stomas. In: Beck D, Roberts P, Saclarides T, Senagore A, Stamos M, Wexner S, eds. *The ASCRS Textbook of Colon and Rectal Surgery*. 2nd ed. New York: Springer; 2011.
15. Glick P, Boulanger S. Inguinal hernias and hydroceles. In: Coran A, Adzick N, Krummel T, Laberge J, Schamberger R, Caldamone A, eds. *Pediatric Surgery*. 7th ed. Philadelphia: Elsevier; 2012.
16. Nelson E. Prolene hernia system—hernia repair. In: Evans S, ed. *Surgical Pitfalls: Prevention and Management*. 1st ed. Philadelphia: Elsevier; 2009.
17. Novitsky YW, Elliott HL, Orenstein SB, Rosen MJ. Transversus abdominis muscle release: a novel approach to posterior component separation during complex abdominal wall reconstruction. *Am J Surg*. 2012;204(5):709–716.
18. Millikan K, Baptista M, Amin B. Intraperitoneal underlay ventral hernia repair utilizing bilayer expanded polytetrafluoroethylene and polypropylene mesh. *Am Surg*. 2003;69:287–292.
19. Itani KMF, Hur K, Kim LT, et al. Comparison of laparoscopic and open repair with mesh for the treatment of ventral incisional hernia: a randomized trial. *Arch Surg*. 2010;145(4):322–328.
20. Nam A, Brody F. Management and therapy for sports hernia. *J Am Coll Surg*. 2008;206(1):154–164.
21. Ellsworth AA, Zoland MP, Tyler TF. Athletic pubalgia and associated rehabilitation. *Int J Sports Phys Ther*. 2014;9(6):774–784.
22. Ko J, Wang E, Salvay D. Abdominal wall reconstruction: lessons learned from 200 "components separation" procedures. *Arch Surg*. 2009;144:1047–1055.

CHAPTER 15

BREAST

Tara Spivey, M.D., Katherine Kopkash, M.D., Ruta Rao, M.D., Thomas Witt, M.D., and Andrea Madrigrano, M.D.

1. A 35-year-old woman visits her physician after her initial mammogram, which was normal, and asks what her lifetime chance for the development of breast cancer is. She has no personal or family history of breast disease. Her menarche occurred at age 13, and her first child was born when she was 22. She has never taken oral contraceptives. Which of the following is not a factor in estimating the Gail risk?

A. Age
B. History of a previous breast biopsy
C. Prior history of radiation exposure
D. Age at menarche
E. Age at first live birth

ANSWER: C

COMMENTS: The American Cancer Society (ACS) estimated in 2008 that there would be 179,920 new cases of breast cancer in the United States and 40,730 deaths. The lifetime probability for the development of breast cancer is now estimated to be 1 in 8 (12.5%). After continuously increasing for more than two decades, breast cancer incidence rates in women have decreased by 3.5% per year from 2001 to 2004. This is due in part to a slight decline in mammography utilization and a reduction in the use of hormone replacement therapy.

The **Gail model** is a validated breast cancer risk assessment tool that is primarily based on nonmodifiable breast cancer risk factors. It is a multivariate statistical model that uses age, age at menarche, age at first live birth, family history of breast cancer, and number of breast biopsies to estimate the breast cancer risk in individuals without a previous history of breast cancer. When used in large groups, it has been shown to accurately estimate the proportion of women in whom breast cancer will develop. However, it performs poorly in discriminating between individual women in whom breast cancer will and will not develop. Although previous thoracic radiation therapy does increase the breast cancer risk, it is not a part of the Gail model. Other significant risk factors for breast cancer in women include previous biopsy specimens revealing atypical hyperplasia or lobular carcinoma in situ (LCIS), personal history of breast cancer, family history of breast cancer, and being a known carrier of a mutation in the *BRCA1* or *BRCA2* genes or a first-degree relative of an individual with a mutation.

Ref.: 1–5

2. A 55-year-old woman is found on examination to have a 3-cm breast mass with palpable axillary lymph nodes. A modified radical mastectomy is performed, and the pathologic evaluation reveals a 3.2-cm infiltrating ductal carcinoma, with 5 of 15 axillary nodes positive for metastasis. Her review of systems is otherwise negative, and findings on laboratory studies and basic imaging are normal. What is her tumor-nodes-metastasis (TNM) stage?

A. T2N1M0
B. T1N2M1
C. T2N2M0
D. T4N1M0
E. T3N2M0

ANSWER: C

COMMENTS: Breast cancer stage is determined by the results of pathologic evaluation of surgical resection specimens and imaging studies. It is classified with the **TNM classification system**, which is based on a description of the primary tumor (T), the status of regional lymph nodes (N), and the presence of distant metastasis (M). The most widely used system is that of the American Joint Commission for Cancer. T1 designates tumors up to 2 cm in size, T2 is used for those between 2 and 5 cm, T3 indicates tumors larger than 5 cm, and T4 is used for tumors of any size with extension to the chest wall or skin. N1 indicates metastasis to 1 to 3 axillary nodes or clinically occult internal mammary nodes (or both); N2 includes metastasis to 4 to 9 axillary nodes or clinically positive internal mammary nodes (without axillary metastasis); and N3 is used for metastasis to 10 or more axillary nodes, a combination of axillary and internal mammary nodes, or paraclavicular nodes. M1 designates evidence of distant metastasis.

Ref.: 5

3. Which of the following 5-year survival rates by stage for treated breast cancer is incorrect?

A. Stage I: 95%–100%
B. Stage II: 80%–90%
C. Stage III: 50%–70%
D. Stage IV: 1%–5%
E. Stage Tis: 98%–100%

ANSWER: D

COMMENTS: The wide range of survival rates in patients with the same stages of breast cancer reflects the variability in biologic behavior among the differing subtypes of breast cancer within a given stage. Because of increasingly effective systemic therapies, patients with stage IV disease now have up to a 20% 5-year relative survival rate.

Ref.: 5

4. Which of the following is not true regarding magnetic resonance imaging (MRI) for evaluation of breast abnormalities?

A. It is useful for finding the primary breast lesion in patients with positive axillary nodes but no mammographic evidence of a breast tumor.

B. It is more accurate than mammography in establishing the extent of disease in invasive lobular cancer.

C. It is more accurate than mammography in assessing the tumor extent in older women.

D. Its sensitivity in detecting invasive cancer is greater than 90%.

E. Its use as a screening tool is still under investigation.

ANSWER: C

COMMENTS: MRI is increasingly being used for the evaluation of breast abnormalities. It is useful in finding the primary breast lesion in patients with malignant axillary nodes but no palpable or mammographic evidence of a primary breast tumor. MRI may be more accurate than mammography in assessing the extent of the primary tumor, particularly in young women with dense breast tissue, and in diagnosing invasive lobular cancer; it may help determine the eligibility for breast conservation. Use of MRI as a screening tool is still under investigation, but it appears promising for early detection of malignancy in patients with *BRCA* gene mutations. The sensitivity of MRI for invasive cancer is greater than 90%, but it is only 60% or less for ductal carcinoma in situ (DCIS).

Ref.: 5

5. With regard to breast carcinoma in men, which statement is true?

A. It is detected most commonly in men aged 60 to 70 years.

B. Gynecomastia is a risk factor.

C. It is commonly associated with a mutation in the *BRCA1* gene.

D. The prognosis is worse stage for stage than for women.

E. Sentinel lymph node biopsy (SLNB) is contraindicated.

ANSWER: A

COMMENTS: Breast cancer infrequently occurs in **men**; it accounts for just 0.8% of all breast cancers and less than 1% of all newly diagnosed cancers in men. The median age at diagnosis is 68 years, 5 years older than that in women. Risk factors include increasing age, radiation exposure, factors related to abnormalities in estrogen and androgen balance (testicular disease, infertility, obesity, and cirrhosis), and genetic predisposition, including **Klinefelter syndrome**, family history, and ***BRCA2*** **gene mutations**. Ninety percent of male breast cancers are **invasive ductal carcinomas**. The majority of men with breast cancer have a breast mass, and when matched for age and stage, survival is similar to that in women. Treatment of carcinoma in the male breast is similar to that in the female breast, and prognostic factors include nodal involvement, tumor size, histologic grade, and hormone receptor status.

Ref.: 5

6. Modern therapy for breast cancer focuses on molecular markers to help guide treatment strategies. Which of the following statements is correct?

A. Carriers of the *BRCA2* mutation are more likely to have triple-negative cancers.

B. Human epidermal growth factor receptor (HER)-2–positive cancers are unlikely to respond to treatment with trastuzumab.

C. Estrogen receptor (ER)-positive/HER-2–negative patients should be treated with endocrine therapy.

D. All breast cancers are sensitive to endocrine therapy.

E. Basal-like cancers are triple-positive cancers.

ANSWER: C

COMMENTS: Before the discovery of the ER, all breast cancers were thought to be sensitive to endocrine therapy. Clinical trials and laboratory research established that only cancers containing ER (ER-positive cancers) respond to endocrine treatments. Furthermore, because binding of **estrogen** to its receptor induces **progesterone receptor (PR)** expression, the presence of PR correlates with response to endocrine therapy. The presence of both receptors in a tumor is associated with an almost 80% chance of favorably responding to hormone blockade. Recently, the uniqueness of tumors that are ER negative, PR negative, and HER-2 negative has been investigated, and these **triple-negative cancers** express proteins in common with myoepithelial cells at the base of mammary ducts and therefore are also called **basal-like cancers**. Women who carry a disease-associated mutation in ***BRCA1*** (but not *BRCA2*) are much more likely to contract a *basal-like cancer* than other subtypes. **HER-2** (or the **erb-B-2/neu protein**) is a product of the *erb-B2* gene and is amplified in about 20% of human breast cancers. Trastuzumab is a humanized antibody directed against the extracellular domain of the surface receptor and is an effective treatment for HER-2–positive tumors.

Ref.: 5

7. A 40-year-old woman has a mammogram showing extensive microcalcifications involving the entire upper aspect of her right breast. Stereotactic biopsy is performed, and pathologic analysis reveals grade 3 DCIS with comedo features. What is the appropriate management?

A. Total mastectomy with SLNB

B. Wide local excision alone

C. Modified radical mastectomy

D. Wide local excision with radiotherapy

E. Radiotherapy alone

ANSWER: A

COMMENTS: See Question 8.

Ref.: 5,6

8. In the patient in Question 7, the operating surgeon performed a total mastectomy. Final pathologic review of the breast showed extensive DCIS and multiple foci of infiltrating ductal carcinoma, with the largest focus being 1.5 cm. What is the next best step in the management of this patient?

A. SLNB

B. Chemotherapy

C. Tamoxifen alone

D. Axillary dissection

E. Radiotherapy

ANSWER: D

COMMENTS: DCIS is a heterogeneous lesion morphologically, and pathologists have recognized four broad categories: **papillary**, **cribriform**, **solid**, and **comedo**. DCIS is recognized as discrete spaces surrounded by a basement membrane; these spaces are filled with malignant cells and usually with an identifiable, basally located cell layer made up of presumably normal myoepithelial cells. The solid and comedo types of DCIS are generally higher-grade lesions and probably invade over a shortened natural history. DCIS frequently coexists with invasive cancers. In current practice, reasons to select total mastectomy for the treatment of DCIS include the following: diffuse suspicious mammographic calcifications suggestive of extensive disease, inability to obtain clear margins on wide excision, likelihood of a poor cosmetic result after wide excision of involved tissue, patient not motivated to preserve her breast, and contraindications to radiation therapy. Sentinel node biopsy is currently recommended when mastectomy is performed for DCIS because up to 10% of patients with DCIS on diagnostic biopsy will be found to have invasive cancer in their mastectomy specimen. The addition of SLNB to mastectomy adds minimal morbidity, and because sentinel node mapping is no longer possible after mastectomy, it may avoid the need for axillary dissection if invasive cancer is identified later. If the axillary lymph nodes are found to be positive for cancer, this patient should undergo chemotherapy. Because her tumor is ER positive, she is also a candidate for adjuvant endocrine therapy, such as tamoxifen.

Ref.: 5

9. Which patient would not benefit from postmastectomy radiotherapy?

A. A 49-year-old patient with inflammatory breast cancer

B. A 25-year-old patient with DCIS

C. A 57-year-old patient with a T1N2 infiltrating ductal carcinoma

D. A 48-year-old patient with a 2.5-cm breast mass involving the underlying pectoral muscle

E. A 42-year-old patient with a 3.0-cm primary tumor and one lymph node positive that has extracapsular extension

ANSWER: B

COMMENTS: Three large prospective randomized trials addressing the role of **postmastectomy irradiation** have found that in addition to the expected benefit of reducing locoregional recurrences, it also resulted in a significant improvement in the overall survival in all three studies. Postmastectomy irradiation has been found to reduce the risk for local or regional recurrence by approximately two-thirds and to reduce breast cancer in all three studies. Nodal irradiation is recommended after mastectomy for patients with four or more positive nodes, with large cancers (>5 cm) or very aggressive histology (diffuse vascular invasion), and with the extranodal extension of breast cancer. Other indications include positive surgical margins; inflammatory breast cancer; or involvement of the skin, pectoral fascia, or skeletal muscle. Radiation therapy is not indicated after mastectomy for DCIS, regardless of its size.

Ref.: 5

10. A 45-year-old woman had a recent stereotactic biopsy revealing atypical ductal hyperplasia. What is the next most appropriate step in her management?

A. Bilateral prophylactic mastectomies

B. Tamoxifen

C. Wire-localized excisional biopsy of the area

D. *BRCA* mutation testing

E. Mammography in 6 months

ANSWER: C

COMMENTS: Certain forms of benign breast disease can be important risk factors for the eventual development of breast cancer. The classification scheme for **benign breast disease** usually includes **nonproliferative lesions**, proliferation of breast epithelium without atypia (**hyperplasia**), and **proliferation with atypia**. The relative risk for cancer in women with either atypical ductal hyperplasia or atypical lobular hyperplasia is between four and five times the risk for development of breast cancer in a control population of women. If there is a positive family history with the existence of atypical hyperplasia, the risk is increased to nearly nine times that of the general population. **Tamoxifen** (20 mg/day for 5 years) is considered as a preventive option in women found to have atypical hyperplasia. This patient should undergo a wire-localized excisional biopsy of the area because there is up to a 15% chance of having a higher-stage lesion in the area (such as DCIS or invasive cancer) when the surrounding tissue is examined.

Ref.: 5

11. Which of the following factors does not influence the choice of systemic adjuvant therapy for invasive breast cancer?

A. Tumor size

B. DNA ploidy

C. HER-2/neu

D. Axillary node status

E. ER status

ANSWER: B

COMMENTS: Metastatic disease is the primary cause of death from breast cancer. Patients who benefit from chemotherapy or hormonal therapy for early-stage disease do so because metastasis is prevented, cured, or delayed. Currently, the recommendation for adjuvant systemic therapy is based on consideration of tumor size, HER-2/neu status, nodal status, ER status, and age or menopausal status. In patients with **node-negative cancer**, certain groups may suffer higher relapse rates, and the absolute benefits of chemotherapy are greater. **Poor prognostic signs** include tumor size greater than 2 cm, poor histologic and nuclear grade, absence of hormone receptors, high proliferative fraction, and overexpression of certain oncogenes such as HER-2/neu. When **trastuzumab (Herceptin)** is used in patients with HER-2–positive breast cancers, there is a 50% reduction in recurrence. In general, all **node-positive** tumors require chemotherapy. In women with ER-positive breast cancers, 5 years of tamoxifen or an **aromatase inhibitor** after surgical treatment nearly halves their recurrence rate and reduces breast cancer mortality by a third. Oncotype DX is a diagnostic test that assesses the tumor tissue and predicts chemotherapy benefit and the likelihood of distant breast cancer recurrence. Aneuploid versus diploid characteristics of the tumor are not currently considered in the choice of systemic therapy.

Ref.: 5

12. A 44-year-old woman has a tender, movable mass in the 12-o'clock position of her left breast. A mammogram shows a 2.5-cm, well-circumscribed density in the palpable area of concern. Ultrasound shows an anechoic, well-circumscribed mass with increased through-transmission. What would you recommend to the patient?

A. Excisional biopsy

B. Ultrasound-guided core needle biopsy

C. Tamoxifen

D. Fine-needle aspiration

E. Magnification and compression mammographic views of the lesion

ANSWER: D

COMMENTS: Cysts within the breast are fluid-filled, epithelium-lined cavities that may vary in size from microscopic to large, palpable masses. A palpable cyst develops in at least 1 in every 14 women. Cysts are influenced by ovarian hormones, a fact that explains their variation with the menstrual cycle. Most cysts occur in women older than 35 years. A palpable mass can be confirmed to be a cyst by aspiration or ultrasound. Cyst fluid can be straw colored, opaque, or dark green and may contain flecks of debris. On **ultrasound**, cysts are round with smooth borders, have a paucity of internal sound echoes, and exhibit increased through-transmission of sound with enhanced posterior echoes. If the palpable mass disappears completely after aspiration and the cyst contents are not grossly bloody, the fluid need not be sent for cytologic analysis. If the cyst recurs, sending fluid for cytologic evaluation is justified. Surgical removal of a cyst is usually indicated if the cytologic findings are atypical or suspicious for malignancy or if the cyst continues to recur.

Ref.: 5

13. Which of the following is associated with the appearance of invasive lobular carcinoma on mammography?

A. Discrete bilateral masses

B. Partially cystic appearance

C. Asymmetric density on mammogram

D. Masses with microcalcifications

E. Branching pleomorphic microcalcifications

ANSWER: C

COMMENTS: When compared with invasive ductal carcinoma, **invasive lobular carcinoma** tends to be more indistinct and difficult to visualize on mammograms. The extent of the tumor is often underestimated on the mammogram and may be more accurately appreciated by ultrasound imaging or **MRI**. Nonetheless, recurrence and survival rates for invasive lobular carcinoma are equivalent to those for ductal carcinoma, stage for stage.

Ref.: 5

14. With regard to breast development, which of the following statements is true?

A. Breast enlargement in male neonates is indicative of an underlying estrogen-secreting adrenal tumor.

B. Accessory nipples can be found anywhere from the axilla to the groin.

C. Extramammary breast tissue is not under the influence of the hormonal status of the patient.

D. Inverted nipples in children suggest underlying breast cancer.

E. Gynecomastia in a prepubertal boy requires excision.

ANSWER: B

COMMENTS: If the embryologic mammary ridge extending from the axilla to the groin fails to involute fully, accessory nipples (**polythelia**) can appear along this route. Accessory breast tissue (**polymastia**) is also seen frequently in the axilla and may enlarge during pregnancy and lactation, as well as during the response to normal fluctuations in the patient's hormonal status during her menstrual cycle. **Accessory breast tissue** can be detected on mammography and may present differential diagnostic difficulties for both the mammographer and the clinician. Shortly after birth, both males and females may exhibit unilateral or bilateral breast enlargement, which is attributed to high levels of circulating maternal estrogen. These changes regress spontaneously during the neonatal period. In female infants, failure of one or both nipples to evert following birth and into adulthood leads to functional problems related to future breastfeeding but is unrelated to future breast cancer. **Gynecomastia** in prepubescent boys is usually a transient condition.

Ref.: 5, 6

15. Which of the following clinical characteristics of breast masses on physical examination is more suggestive of a malignant than a benign disease?

A. Indistinct borders blending into surrounding breast tissue

B. Excessive mobility within breast tissue

C. Tenderness over a soft mass

D. Tethering to underlying muscular structures

E. Variability through the menstrual cycle

ANSWER: D

COMMENTS: Although there are many exceptions to the classic physical findings of breast cancer, the typical breast carcinoma is hard and has fairly distinct borders. Fixation to deeper structures is highly suggestive of malignancy. A smooth, rubbery, mobile mass is more suggestive of **fibroadenoma**. **Fibrocystic disease** may be manifested as a disk-like or polynodular thickening, with one or more of the borders blending indistinctly into the surrounding breast tissue. Tenderness over a soft breast mass is often found with breast cysts. Variability over the **menstrual cycle** is a benign feature.

Ref.: 5, 6

16. A 57-year-old woman with a 1.5-cm infiltrating ductal carcinoma and a clinically negative axilla is found to be ER negative, PR negative, and HER-2/neu positive. She comes to your office to discuss treatment options. What would you recommend?

A. Modified radical mastectomy alone

B. Wide local excision, radiation therapy, and tamoxifen

C. Simple mastectomy, SLNB, trastuzumab (Herceptin), and tamoxifen

D. Modified radical mastectomy and adjuvant chemotherapy

E. Wide local excision, SLNB, radiation therapy, and adjuvant chemotherapy with trastuzumab

ANSWER: E

COMMENTS: In current practice, **lumpectomy** (wide local excision) is considered in cases in which the tumor can be excised to clear margins and leave an acceptable cosmetic result. Randomized trials have studied breast conservation for tumors up to 5 cm in size. Patients who undergo lumpectomy followed by radiation therapy have the same survival rate as do those who undergo modified radical mastectomy. **SLNB** is an acceptable method of staging the axilla in breast cancer patients without clinically suspicious lymph nodes. Because the patient is ER and PR negative, she would not derive any benefit from treatment with tamoxifen. However, she is HER-2/neu positive and would therefore benefit from treatment with **trastuzumab**. Recent studies have shown that the addition of trastuzumab to conventional adjuvant chemotherapy significantly reduces the rate of recurrence (almost a 50% reduction).

Ref.: 5

17. A 58-year-old woman has a chronic erythematous, oozing, eczematoid rash involving her left nipple and areola. There are no palpable breast masses, and the findings on a recently obtained mammogram are normal. Which of the following recommendations is appropriate?

A. Referral to a dermatologist

B. Oral vitamin E and topical aloe and lanolin

C. Punch biopsy

D. Trial of cortisone

E. Routine clinical and mammographic follow-up in 1 year because findings on the current mammogram are normal

ANSWER: C

COMMENTS: Paget's disease accounts for 1% or less of breast malignancies and is characterized clinically by nipple erythema and irritation with associated itching and may progress to nipple crusting and ulceration. A manifestation of this sort is very concerning, and therefore a biopsy of the nipple is necessary. Delay in the diagnosis of Paget's disease of the breast is common because of the mistaken presumption that the findings represent a benign dermatologic condition. Pathologically, Paget cells are large, pale-staining cells with round or oval nuclei and large nucleoli and are located between the normal keratinocytes of the nipple epidermis. More than 97% of patients with Paget's disease have an underlying DCIS or invasive breast carcinoma, but there is an accompanying mass in only 54% of patients. The treatment of Paget's disease includes mastectomy with axillary staging or wide excision of the nipple and areola and underlying retroareolar tissue to achieve clear margins, possibly axillary staging, and radiation therapy.

Ref.: 5, 6

18. Which of the following is not a characteristic of medullary breast cancer?

A. Lymphocytic infiltrate

B. Benign appearance on ultrasound

C. High rate of lymph node metastasis

D. Statistically better than average prognosis

E. Usually manifested as a palpable mass

ANSWER: C

COMMENTS: Medullary breast cancer accounts for approximately 5% of breast cancers. It is usually manifested as a palpable mass with smooth borders on imaging that can mimic benign conditions. On ultrasound, medullary carcinoma often has smooth contours, homogeneous interior echogenicity, and posterior enhancement, which are the same findings that one would expect with a fibroadenoma. These tumors are characterized by an infiltrate of small mononuclear lymphocytes, are less likely to be associated with axillary node metastasis, and have a better than average prognosis.

Ref.: 5, 6

19. With regard to phyllodes tumor of the breast, which statement is incorrect?

A. It is histologically characterized by epithelial cyst-like spaces.

B. Examination reveals it as a firm, mobile, well-circumscribed mass.

C. Ten percent to 15% of these tumors are malignant.

D. The benign version can grow aggressively and recur locally.

E. It commonly metastasizes to lymph nodes.

ANSWER: E

COMMENTS: Although only approximately 10% of all **phyllodes tumors** are malignant, they are still the most common primary sarcoma of the breast. They are classified as benign, borderline, or malignant. The benign and malignant varieties may be differentiated by counting the number of **mitoses** seen per high-power field, in addition to observing other features. If the tumor is histologically benign, wide local excision is considered an adequate treatment. Even when benign, phyllodes tumors have a high frequency of local recurrence, and therefore a careful, long-term follow-up is essential. In the malignant variety, lymph node involvement is uncommon because these tumors usually metastasize via hematogenous spread, most often to the lung. Therefore **total mastectomy** without axillary dissection may be indicated, although for small malignant lesions, wide excision with 1-cm margins may be appropriate. Malignant cystosarcoma has no significant incidence of multicentricity within the breast (unlike ductal or lobular carcinoma).

Ref.: 5–7

20. Which of the following is not an indication for postmastectomy radiotherapy?

A. T3 tumors

B. Multicentric DCIS larger than 6 cm

C. Four or more positive axillary lymph nodes

D. Inflammatory breast cancer

E. Gross extranodal extension

ANSWER: B

COMMENTS: For most patients with breast cancer, mastectomy provides an effective local control and radiation therapy is not required. However, certain subsets remain at an increased risk for local and regional recurrences and benefit from the ability of radiation to control any microscopic residual tumor. **Adjuvant radiation therapy** after mastectomy does decrease locoregional recurrences by up to two-thirds, and some studies have shown an improvement in overall survival. Radiation therapy has many potential side effects as a result of irradiation of the chest wall, including skin ulceration, arm edema, rib fracture, radiation-induced pneumonitis, chest wall sarcoma, and cardiac toxicity. Therefore most centers now recommend chest wall and nodal irradiation after mastectomy only for patients at an increased risk for recurrence. This category includes those with four or more positive lymph nodes and patients with large cancers (>5 cm), aggressive histology (diffuse vascular invasion), and extranodal extension of breast cancer. Other indicators include positive surgical margins; **inflammatory breast cancer**; or involvement of the skin, fascia, or skeletal muscle. Extensive DCIS is not an indication for radiation therapy, provided that the margins of the mastectomy specimen are not involved.

Ref.: 5, 7

21. Which of the following is most likely to be associated with breast pain?

A. Breast cancer

B. LCIS

C. DCIS

D. Sclerosing adenosis

E. Breast cysts

ANSWER: E

COMMENTS: Although **breast pain** common, it is rarely associated with carcinoma. Normal ovarian hormonal influences on breast glandular elements frequently produce **cyclic mastalgia**. Occasionally, a simple cyst may cause a noncyclic breast pain, and aspiration of the cyst ends the evaluation. Frequently, lifestyle and dietary changes result in improvement of **mastalgia**. Decreasing caffeine intake and the use of bras with better support are the first steps in the management of breast pain. Medications such as **danazol**, **primrose oil**, and nonsteroidal antiinflammatory drugs have been shown to be occasionally effective in refractory cases. In many cases, patients report a lessening of the pain after being reassured that the pain is not associated with cancer.

Ref.: 5, 7

22. A 32-year-old woman who is 10 weeks pregnant has a palpable 2.5-cm mass in the upper outer quadrant of her right breast. The mass is not visualized on ultrasound. Which of the following management options is appropriate?

A. Reassurance of the patient that this is probably benign in nature

B. Reexamination 1 month after delivery

C. Cyst aspiration and, if no fluid is obtained, reassurance of the patient

D. Palpation-guided core needle biopsy

E. Simple mastectomy

ANSWER: D

COMMENTS: See Question 23.

Ref.: 5, 7

23. Core needle biopsy in the pregnant patient in Question 22 demonstrates an infiltrating ductal carcinoma, which is grade 3, ER negative, and HER-2/neu negative. Further evaluation reveals a suspicious, palpable 1.5-cm right axillary mass that is positive on fine-needle biopsy. What is the most appropriate next step in her treatment?

A. Immediate neoadjuvant chemotherapy followed by mastectomy with SLNB

B. Modified radical mastectomy followed by chemotherapy

C. Lumpectomy, axillary dissection, and radiation therapy delayed until after delivery

D. Simple mastectomy with SLNB and chemotherapy

E. Lumpectomy, axillary dissection, and immediate radiation therapy

ANSWER: B

COMMENTS: Stage for stage, the **prognosis of breast cancer** is the same in pregnant as in nonpregnant women. However, the overall prognosis for **pregnant women** is worse because they tend to initially be seen with a more advanced stage. Reluctance to evaluate breast masses in pregnant women on the part of both the patient and her physician is a contributing factor. The evaluation and treatment of breast masses must not be delayed because of pregnancy. Diagnostic mammograms can be performed safely in pregnant women with proper shielding of the uterus. However, radiation therapy, even with proper shielding, is associated with a significant incidence of fetal injury and is contraindicated. Mastectomy is usually appropriate during early and middle pregnancy. During the third trimester, breast preservation may be considered if early delivery after confirmation of fetal maturity would facilitate prompt commencement of whole-breast irradiation. This patient has a suspicious axillary node and is therefore not a candidate for SLNB. It is worth noting that there have been no reported consequences to either the mother or the fetus from injections of technetium sulfur colloid or isosulfan blue, which are the two agents that may be injected during SLNB. This does not imply that there is no risk, simply that none has been reported to date. Chemotherapy has been administered safely to patients in the second trimester. For patients in the second and third trimester in whom breast cancer is diagnosed, breast conservation therapy can be an option, with radiation therapy delayed until after delivery.

Ref.: 5, 7

24. A 39-year-old woman with no family history of breast cancer underwent excisional biopsy of a 2-cm breast mass that was deemed discordant on core needle biopsy. Histologic sections showed the presence of fibrosis, ductal ectasia, atypical lobular hyperplasia, and multiple foci of LCIS at the medial, superior, and inferior margins. Which of the following statements is false?

A. At a minimum, she needs to undergo reexcision to achieve negative margins.

B. Tamoxifen can decrease the risk for the future development of invasive cancer by 50%.

C. If breast cancer develops, it would most likely be a ductal carcinoma.

D. LCIS is typically not visible on mammography but is discovered incidentally on a biopsy.

E. LCIS is often multicentric and bilateral.

ANSWER: A

COMMENTS: LCIS is a histologic finding that is usually seen in tissue from a biopsy specimen of some other lesion. It represents a risk marker that predicts up to a ninefold increase in the chance for the development of breast cancer. **Atypical lobular hyperplasia** alone increases the risk fourfold. Acquisition of free margins is not necessary since LCIS is now not considered to be a malignant lesion but more of a risk factor for the development of breast cancer. Either infiltrating lobular or infiltrating ductal carcinoma may develop in this patient, with the latter being the more likely type. Less aggressive management is typically performed for this kind of lesion and consists of close follow-up with periodic physical examination and bilateral mammograms or the use of tamoxifen as chemoprevention, which has resulted in a nearly 50% reduction in the risk for the development of breast cancer. LCIS is usually multicentric and often found in both breasts.

Ref.: 5, 7

25. With regard to asymptomatic, nonpalpable, mammographically detected breast masses, which of the following statements is true?

A. The mass should be excised if it is found in a woman older than 40 years.

B. Unless the mass is painful, it can be followed with a mammogram in 6 months.

C. Ultrasound is helpful in further defining breast lesions.

D. Imaging-guided biopsy is contraindicated.

E. Masses with a small, well-defined border on both mammogram and US can be observed

ANSWER: C

COMMENTS: Mammographic abnormalities that cannot be detected by physical examination include clustered microcalcifications and areas of abnormal density (masses, architectural distortions, and asymmetries). The **Breast Imaging Reporting and Data System (BI-RADS)** is used to categorize the degree of suspicion of malignancy for a mammographic abnormality. To avoid unnecessary biopsies for low-suspicion mammographic findings, probably benign lesions are designated BI-RADS 3 and are monitored with a schedule of short-interval mammograms over a 2-year period. An **image-guided biopsy** is performed only for lesions that progress during follow-up; this can be done by image-guided core needle biopsy or image-guided wire localization followed by surgical excision. **Ultrasound** is useful in establishing whether a lesion detected by other modalities is solid or cystic and in determining the contour and internal properties of a lesion. Smooth, rounded masses cannot be assumed to be benign even if previous mammograms demonstrate a stable appearance over a long period. Some malignant tumors, including mucinous and medullary carcinoma or cystosarcoma phyllodes, can have a benign appearance on both ultrasound imaging and mammography.

Ref.: 5, 7

26. Which of the following is not true regarding skin-sparing mastectomy?

A. Involves the removal of 30%–50% of breast skin

B. May be appropriate for a central tumor that would require removal of the nipple/areola complex

C. May be used for multifocal, minimal breast cancers

D. Includes skin excision with 1-cm margins around the previous biopsy site or scar overlying the index neoplasm

E. Requires skin excision (marginal only) of the nipple/areola complex

ANSWER: A

COMMENTS: In traditional mastectomies without reconstruction, 30-50% of the breast skin is removed. **"Skin-sparing" mastectomy**, or limited skin excision, can be defined as excision of the nipple/areola complex, the skin around the biopsy site, and the skin within 1 to 2 cm of the tumor margin. This technique usually sacrifices only 5%–10% of the breast skin, and the excision is usually closed primarily or in association with breast reconstruction. The extent of breast skin excision required with mastectomy has decreased as locoregional control measures have improved over the last 60 years. Patients who are not candidates for lumpectomy and postoperative radiation therapy but are candidates for skin-sparing mastectomy include those with multicentric disease, invasive carcinoma associated with an extensive intraductal component, T2 tumors with difficult-to-interpret mammograms, and central tumors that would require removal of the nipple/areola complex. The skin-sparing mastectomy may include SLNB as indicated and, if histologically positive, axillary lymph node dissection to be completed synchronously.

Ref.: 7

27. What factor(s) increase(s) the risk for the development of lymphedema?

A. High body mass index (BMI)

B. Postoperative infection

C. Radiation

D. All of the above

E. A and B

ANSWER: D

COMMENTS: The incidence of **lymphedema after axillary node dissection** ranges from 15% to 30%, depending on the definition used. Greatest incidence is in the first 2 years. The probability of lymphedema increases with greater dissection and level of nodes removed, the tumor burden in the axilla, the presence of lymphedema before surgery, and whether radiation is applied to the field after surgery. Postoperative infection also increases the risk. With the advent of SLNB, the rate of lymphedema has been shown to be much lower, in the range of 2%–4%.

Ref.: 7

28. Radiation delivered to the breast after a right lumpectomy and SLNB for a 1.2-cm node-negative infiltrating ductal carcinoma is likely to be associated with which of the following?

A. Decreased risk for systemic recurrence

B. Can be used in lieu of chemotherapy in early-stage breast cancers

C. Increased risk for lymphoma

D. Decreased risk for local recurrence

E. Cardiac toxicity

ANSWER: D

COMMENTS: The addition of **breast irradiation** after **breast conservation** has been shown in multiple randomized trials to decrease the incidence of local tumor recurrence but is considered controversial in terms of survival benefit. Radiation is used for local control, and chemotherapy is a modality for systemic control; the decision for chemotherapy is made independently and is based on the presence of tumor factors and risk for distant disease. Lymphoma is not associated with breast irradiation. The risk for cardiac toxicity in right-sided lesions with modern techniques of radiation therapy planning and dosimetry is very low.

Ref.: 7

29. In which population is the incidence of *BRCA* mutations highest?

A. Ashkenazi Jews

B. Patients with a history of radiation therapy for Hodgkin disease

C. Patients with a first-degree relative with breast cancer

D. A woman with a Gail score of 2.3%

E. A woman with a prior diagnosis of uterine cancer

ANSWER: A

COMMENTS: The ***BRCA*** mutation rate is highest in **Ashkenazi Jews** and ranges from 1% to 3%. The incidence of breast cancer in those who have undergone mantel irradiation for Hodgkin disease is five times that of the general population. A person with a first-degree relative with postmenopausal breast cancer has a relative risk 1.8 times that of the general population. **Ovarian cancer** increases the risk for breast cancer in a woman, but uterine cancer has not been linked to breast cancer.

Ref.: 7

30. A 47-year-old woman with a history of breast pain has a recent onset of nonspontaneous, bilateral, green nipple discharge from multiple ducts. She has generalized bilateral tenderness and no palpable mass on breast examination. The discharge is Hemoccult negative. Findings on mammography and ultrasound are unremarkable. Which of the following is the most appropriate first step in management?

A. Schedule an MRI

B. Perform an ultrasound-guided core biopsy

C. Reassure the patient

D. Obtain a galactogram

E. Excise the major retroareolar ducts

ANSWER: C

COMMENTS: Nipple discharge and breast tenderness are common complaints associated with **mammary duct ectasia** and **fibrocystic change**. Bilateral versus unilateral, multiple ducts versus single duct, expressible (nonspontaneous) versus spontaneous, and colored (nonbloody) versus clear or bloody fluid are all strongly suggestive of a benign cause of the discharge. Accordingly, surgery would be inappropriate in this case. Reassurance is the appropriate management decision in this context, particularly in light of the clinical characteristics of the nipple discharge and the negative mammographic and physical examination findings. If the drainage is bloody, serous, or watery, further diagnostic workup is indicated to determine the cause of the discharge. Although such discharges demand evaluation, the cause is often benign (commonly an intraductal papilloma or papillomatosis). Although some surgeons prefer a preoperative contrast-enhanced radiograph of the involved duct (a **galactogram**) as a guide, the blood-distended duct is usually identifiable and can be removed through a circumareolar incision or lacrimal probe-guided terminal duct excision. If either preoperative or intraoperative ultrasound imaging is available, this modality can be used in real time to facilitate identification of the distended duct and to precisely map the area of operative excision.

Ref.: 7

31. With regard to pure tubular carcinoma, which of the following is true?

A. Lymph node involvement is seen in 25% of cases.

B. It is a highly aggressive, frequently fatal carcinoma.

C. It tends to be ER negative.

D. Neoadjuvant chemotherapy should be strongly considered.

E. Stage for stage, it has a more favorable prognosis than other forms of ductal carcinoma.

ANSWER: E

COMMENTS: When **tubular carcinoma** is present in its pure form, the distant metastatic potential is very low. The diagnosis is made when characteristic angulated tubules, composed of cells with low-grade nuclei, constitute at least 90% of the carcinoma. Tubular carcinoma has a better prognosis than other varieties of infiltrating ductal cancer, and one classic study showed that all the studied patients whose carcinoma was composed purely of the characteristic low-grade, angulated tubules survived at least 15 years, regardless of the tumor size. Tubular carcinoma represents only about 3%–5% of all invasive carcinomas, has the biologic correlates of a low-grade cancer (ER positive, diploid, low S phase, and no expression of c-erbB-2), and is more likely to occur in older patients. The survival of patients with tubular carcinoma is generally similar to that of the general population, and systemic adjuvant therapy may be avoided in these patients. For selected cases of pure tubular carcinoma removed with an adequate negative margin, mastectomy, radiation therapy, or even axillary lymph node staging may be unnecessary.

Ref.: 7

32. A 13-year-old girl is referred to a breast surgeon for breast asymmetry secondary to a rapidly growing right breast mass. Physical examination reveals an 8-cm central right breast mass. She underwent menarche 1 year ago. Breast cancer was diagnosed in her mother at age 38. What is the appropriate next step?

A. Mastectomy
B. Incisional biopsy
C. Mammogram
D. Ultrasound
E. Reassurance to the patient and her mother that this is a normal breast development

ANSWER: D

COMMENTS: See Question 33.

Ref.: 7

33. Regarding the patient in the Question 32, ultrasound reveals an 8-cm hypoechoic solid mass with rounded edges. What is the next appropriate step in the management of this patient?

A. Excisional biopsy
B. Mastectomy
C. Cyst aspiration
D. Bilateral mastectomies
E. Reassurance to the patient and the mother

ANSWER: A

COMMENTS: This patient most likely has a **juvenile fibroadenoma**. Fibroadenoma may be regarded as a generic term and refers to any benign, confined tumor of the breast that has a mixture of glandular and mesenchymal elements; juvenile fibroadenoma is considered a variant. These lesions tend to occur in women in the younger age range and are characterized by increased cellularity of stroma or epithelium. Juvenile fibroadenomas are notable for their rapid growth and large size and tend to occur around the time of menarche. They often have a common ductal pattern of epithelial hyperplasia and defining stromal hypercellularity. The initial imaging modality for a young woman is ultrasound because it is accurate in evaluating the dense breast tissue common in younger women, involves no radiation exposure, and is essentially painless. A rounded hypoechoic solid mass on ultrasound is indicative of fibroadenoma, and excisional biopsy would be considered an appropriate treatment at this time.

Ref.: 7

34. Which is not true regarding chronic granulomatous mastitis?

A. Tuberculosis should be a strong consideration in the differential diagnosis.
B. Chronic granulomatous mastitis includes variants of ductal ectasia.
C. Treatment can include immunosuppression.
D. It may be a sign of a systemic disorder.
E. Treatment is primarily surgical.

ANSWER: A

COMMENTS: Chronic granulomatous mastitis is a broad descriptive designation that includes variants of ductal ectasia, granulomatous infectious diseases, and idiopathic granulomatous conditions. It may be difficult to distinguish chronic granulomatous mastitis from ductal ectasia or from infectious granulomatous mastitis. Specific granulomatous infections such as tuberculosis may occur in the breast, although this is very uncommon; tuberculosis is responsible for approximately 0.025%–0.1% of all surgically treated diseases of the breast. Recognition of granulomatous inflammation at the time of frozen section should prompt a search for the etiologic agent through culture. Granulomatous mastitis may be the initial sign of a systemic disorder such as **Wegener's granulomatosis**. **Sarcoidosis** is another diagnostic consideration when granulomas are found in the breast. These conditions are often treated with corticosteroid therapy, with promising results.

Ref.: 7

35. Which of the following is not a germline mutation associated with a higher incidence of breast cancer?

A. Hereditary papillary renal carcinoma (HPRC)
B. *BRCA1*
C. *PALB2*
D. *p53*
E. *PTEN*

ANSWER: A

COMMENTS: All of the choices are **germline mutations**. A germline mutation is a mutation that exists in every cell of the body and is therefore capable of being passed to the offspring via the sperm or egg. The predominant genes responsible for hereditary breast cancer are *BRCA1* and *BRCA2*. Women who carry a germline mutation in either of these genes have about an 85% likelihood of breast cancer developing by the age of 70, although most cancers occur before 50 years of age. Women with these mutations also have an increased risk (20%–40%) for the development of ovarian cancer. Inherited mutations of the *p53* gene result in **Li-Fraumeni syndrome**, which is associated with the development of a number of malignancies, including breast cancer, sarcomas, brain tumors, adrenocortical carcinomas, and leukemia. Germline mutations in the *PTEN* gene are associated with **Cowden disease**, which is a hereditary disorder (also known as **multiple hamartoma syndrome**) inherited as an autosomal dominant trait and is characterized by distinctive mucocutaneous lesions and cancer of the breast, thyroid, and female genitourinary tract. *PALB2* gene mutations are associated with an increased risk for breast cancer. The lifetime risk for breast cancer in women carrying a *PALB2* gene mutation is partially dependent on her family history of breast cancer. The breast cancer risks found in a study published in the *New England Journal of Medicine* in August 2014 were 14% risk by the age of 50 and 35% risk by the age of 70 for a woman who has no family history of breast cancer. Women who have one or more first-degree relatives with a history of breast cancer may have up to a 58% lifetime risk for breast cancer compared with the general population risk of approximately 12% for a woman to develop breast cancer in her lifetime. *PALB2* has also been shown to have a link to an increased risk for male breast cancer and pancreatic cancer; however, these risks are not well defined. HPRC is an autosomal dominant disorder related to the MET protooncogene. These papillary renal carcinomas tend to be multifocal and bilateral.

Ref.: 7

36. A germline mutation in *BRCA1* or *BRCA2* is associated with all of the following characteristics except:

A. Autosomal dominant transmission
B. High incidence of breast and ovarian cancer in women
C. Higher than average incidence of breast cancer in men
D. Incomplete penetrance
E. Late-onset breast cancer

ANSWER: E

COMMENTS: Mutations in ***BRCA1*** or ***BRCA2*** result in a higher incidence of breast and **ovarian cancers**. The risk for breast cancer is about 85% in individuals who carry the mutation and have a family history of breast cancer. The risk for ovarian cancer is about 40% with *BRCA1* mutations and 20% with *BRCA2* mutations. Breast cancer will develop in about 10% of males with *BRCA2* mutations. These genes are incompletely penetrant; that is, some mutation carriers can live to old age without the development of cancer. The mutation is autosomal dominant; therefore a mutation in only one of the pair of chromosomes usually produces the disease. Although postmenopausal breast cancer can develop in women who carry germline mutations of these genes, cancer will develop in most of these carriers at a younger age.

Ref.: 7

37. A 75-year-old woman has a 1.2-cm mass in her right breast on physical examination that is found to be an infiltrating ductal carcinoma, and ER/PR positive, on core biopsy. Her axilla is clinically negative, as is her review of systems. She has multiple medical problems and wants to have as little done as possible. Which factor is not significantly associated with lymph node metastasis in elderly patients?

A. Age
B. Tumor location
C. Tumor size
D. Lymphovascular invasion
E. HER-2/neu status

ANSWER: B

COMMENTS: Nodal evaluation in elderly women with breast cancer remains controversial. The risk associated with lymph node evaluation must be balanced with the benefit of staging and local control. A recent large, prospective, multicenter trial found that on multivariate analysis, patient age, tumor size, and lymphovascular invasion were significant factors predicting **lymph node metastasis**. Patient race, palpable tumor, tumor grade, histologic subtype, and tumor location were not found to be significant. These findings suggest that some **elderly breast cancer** patients with a low likelihood of lymph node metastasis may be spared lymph node evaluation. The HER-2/neu status is not an indicator of the lymph node status.

Ref.: 10

38. A 24-year-old woman who is 9 months postpartum and still lactating has a tender, fluctuant area in her right breast near the areolar border. She denies fever or chills and has no other medical problems. Ultrasound demonstrates a hypoechoic collection with no associated vascularity and with acoustic enhancement. What is the most appropriate treatment?

A. Surgical incision and drainage
B. Needle aspiration
C. Multidrug antibiotics
D. Core needle biopsy to exclude malignancy
E. Needle aspiration and antibiotics

ANSWER: E

COMMENTS: Infections of the breast fall into two general categories: **lactational infections** (such as in this patient) and **chronic subareolar infections** associated with **ductal ectasia**. Lactation-related infections are thought to arise from the entry of bacteria through the nipple and into the duct system and are characterized by erythema, tenderness, and, less often, fever and leukocytosis. They are most frequently due to ***Staphylococcus aureus***. In the past, these abscesses were often drained surgically, but the more recent literature supports antibiotics and needle aspiration of the abscess.

Ref.: 5, 10, 11

39. With regard to the current therapy for stage I and stage II breast cancer, which statement is true?

A. The Halsted radical mastectomy has resulted in a cure rate superior to that of other surgical treatment options.
B. Lumpectomy and radiation therapy are associated with a local recurrence rate of 25%.
C. Tumor genomic testing assists in making decisions regarding the benefit of chemotherapy in early-stage (stages I–III) ER-positive breast cancers.
D. Node-negative patients who undergo modified radical mastectomy have a survival advantage over those who choose lumpectomy, SLNB, and radiation therapy.
E. There is no role for nipple-sparing mastectomy in the treatment of invasive cancers.

ANSWER: C

COMMENTS: The two most commonly used modalities of definitive therapy for stage I and II breast cancers are (1) **modified radical mastectomy**, which preserves the pectoralis major muscle while excising all breast tissue, including the nipple and axillary nodal basin, and (2) wide local excision of the breast tumor (**lumpectomy/partial mastectomy**) and axillary evaluation (**SLNB** or **axillary dissection**, or both) in conjunction with postoperative whole-breast irradiation. A number of large randomized trials have shown no significant disease-free survival advantage for the more radical (pectoralis-removing) Halsted mastectomy. Lumpectomy plus radiation therapy is associated with a local recurrence rate of 14%. **Genomic testing currently consists of assays that predict the risk for tumor recurrence based on tumor biology. Genomic testing** is increasingly being used to determine the aggressiveness of certain cancers and can therefore help guide decisions regarding adjuvant therapy. The **National Surgical Adjuvant Breast and Bowel Project B-06 (NSABP B-06) trial** showed that regardless of the nodal status, there was no difference in the overall survival between patients undergoing modified radical mastectomy and those undergoing lumpectomy with surgical axillary staging and radiation therapy. A nipple-sparing mastectomy can be performed for invasive cancer if immediate reconstruction is planned, and the tumor is remote from the nipple–areolar complex (>2 cm) and does not have a detrimental effect on long-term survival or local recurrence rates.

Ref.: 6–8, 12

40. Which of the following is true regarding breast reconstruction following mastectomy for breast cancer?

A. Coverage by insurance carriers is variable.
B. Immediate reconstruction has a detrimental effect on local recurrence rates.

C. Reconstruction must be delayed in patients who might require postmastectomy radiation therapy.
D. BMI plays no role in complication rates.
E. Autogenous tissue usually provides better symmetry than an implant.

ANSWER: E

COMMENTS: Breast reconstruction may be performed as immediate reconstruction (same day as mastectomy) or as delayed reconstruction (months or years later). Immediate reconstruction is facilitated by preserving the maximum amount of breast skin, and it offers the advantages of combining the recovery period for both procedures and avoiding a period without reconstruction. In a recent study, 75% of reconstructions were performed immediately. Clinical trials have shown that there is no increased risk for cancer recurrence and no increased difficulty with surveillance for recurrence of breast cancer after immediate reconstruction. Reconstruction may be delayed in patients who might require postmastectomy radiation therapy and is usually delayed in patients with locally advanced cancer. Reconstructive options can be divided into two main types: those using an autogenous tissue and those requiring alloplastic material. In general, autogenous tissue will usually provide better symmetry than an implant. One study showed that only 35% of **transverse rectus abdominus myocutaneous (TRAM) flap** reconstructions required a symmetry procedure versus 55% of **implant** reconstructions.

Ref.: 12

41. A 53-year-old woman with no family history of breast cancer detects a well-defined, 2-cm mass in the upper outer quadrant of her right breast. Mammography reveals only dense breast tissue, and findings on ultrasound are unremarkable. What is the next step in the management of this patient?

A. Mammography and ultrasonography are extremely sensitive; therefore you can reassure her that the lesion is benign.
B. Advise her to return for reevaluation in 3 months.
C. Perform a core needle biopsy in the office.
D. Order a breast MRI.
E. Schedule her for an excisional biopsy.

ANSWER: C

COMMENTS: Most patients with breast cancer do not have a family history; therefore any **palpable mass** requires investigation. Either needle aspiration or core needle biopsy of a solid mass would be acceptable as an initial diagnostic step. A major goal of modern breast medicine is to minimize the number of patients with benign lesions who undergo open surgical breast biopsy for diagnosis. There are relatively few patients for whom excisional biopsy should be the initial procedure for diagnosis. For patients with a diagnosis of breast cancer, the goal is to make the diagnosis with a needle and to go to the operating room one time for definitive treatment. A definitive diagnosis of breast cancer made from a minimally invasive **needle biopsy** specimen permits optimal preoperative workup, patient counseling, and surgical planning. Percutaneous histologic tissue acquisition techniques include large-core biopsy (typically 12 to 14 gauge) and vacuum-assisted biopsy (typically 7 to 11 gauge). Dense breast tissue decreases the diagnostic sensitivity of mammography and can easily obscure a carcinoma. The absence of mammographic visualization in the presence of a palpable mass does not diminish the need for tissue diagnosis. In fact, up to 10% of breast cancers are found in women with a "negative" mammogram. Delaying the evaluation of a well-defined mass for 3 months is ill advised. **MRI** is a very sensitive diagnostic tool, but at this point in evaluation of this lesion, a negative MRI result would not obviate the need for a biopsy.

Ref.: 7, 13

42. A 45-year-old woman has an abnormal diagnostic mammogram revealing a cluster of indeterminate microcalcifications in the upper outer quadrant of her left breast. Physical examination reveals normal findings. The patient denies any risk factors for breast cancer. Which of the following is the most appropriate initial management?

A. Stereotactic-guided core needle biopsy
B. Ultrasound-guided core needle biopsy
C. Reassurance and continuation of yearly mammography
D. Excisional biopsy
E. Repeat mammography of the left breast in 6 months

ANSWER: A

COMMENTS: One of the goals of modern breast medicine is to reduce the number of unnecessary open surgical breast biopsies for benign lesions. Image-guided **percutaneous needle biopsy** is the diagnostic procedure of choice for image-detected breast abnormalities. It should be readily available to all patients with image-detected lesions. The presence of **indeterminate microcalcifications** is a suspicious finding on mammography that warrants a tissue diagnosis; therefore reassurance or close follow-up is not an appropriate management option. Ultrasound is the preferred biopsy guidance method for sonographically visible lesions, but this lesion was found on mammography, and therefore stereotactic guidance would most likely be the initial choice for a biopsy.

Ref.: 13

43. A 33-year-old asymptomatic woman is referred to the clinician with abnormal findings on a mammogram. No masses are palpable in either breast. The mammogram shows a tight cluster of microcalcifications at the 2-o'clock position in her left breast. Magnification compression views show at least 20 tiny, irregular calcifications in a 2-cm area that vary in shape and density with no associated mass lesion. There are no other calcifications present in either breast. What is the next appropriate step?

A. Wire-localized excision
B. Follow-up imaging in 6 months
C. Reassurance of benign pathology
D. Stereotactic biopsy
E. Ultrasound-guided biopsy

ANSWER: D

COMMENTS: See Question 44.

Ref.: 7, 14

44. Which of the following is the most likely diagnosis?

A. LCIS
B. Fibroadenoma
C. Infiltrating ductal carcinoma
D. DCIS (intraductal)
E. Fibrocystic changes

ANSWER: D

COMMENTS: Mammographic calcifications without an associated mass lesion are the hallmark of early breast cancer, particularly DCIS; however, the common causes of calcifications identified on mammography are varied. Specific patterns have been identified that are often associated with and predictive of these pathologic processes. Parenchymal calcifications (i.e., those indicative of a pathologic breast process) occur in the lobar ductal system and in the terminal ductal lobular unit. Certain patterns of ductal calcification are almost pathognomonic of **DCIS**, as is a specific bilateral pattern seen with **plasma cell mastitis**. One mammographic feature common to both high-grade DCIS and plasma cell mastitis is the appearance of calcium in a linear, branching pattern. Evenly scattered calcifications, more often than not bilateral, are indicative of a lobular process. This pattern is the one most commonly encountered and is indicative of either active or involutional fibrocystic change. **Clustered calcifications**, whether single or multiple, present a diagnostic dilemma because of the varied pathologic processes that give rise to this pattern. A close scrutiny of these areas on magnification views is required to delineate the finer characteristics of the calcifications. Coarse, granular-appearing calcifications are seen with partially calcified fibroadenomas and papillomas, fibrocystic change, and low- to intermediate-grade DCIS. Powdery calcifications are seen with sclerosing adenosis, with or without atypia, and low-grade DCIS. Large, coarse calcifications (popcorn-like) are classically associated with a degenerating fibroadenoma and are readily discernible on mammography. **LCIS** and **invasive lobular carcinoma** are typically not associated with microcalcifications. The clustered geographic distribution and characteristics of the calcifications described in this scenario make a diagnosis of DCIS more likely than that of an invasive carcinoma, which often has an associated mass lesion seen on mammography.

Ref.: 7, 14

45. Which of the following statements is true regarding breast conservation surgery?

A. Sixty percent of locally recurrent breast cancers develop at or near the site of the original breast cancer.

B. Intraoperative radiotherapy (IORT) targeted to the tumor bed permits breast-conserving surgery and radiotherapy to be completed in one sitting.

C. IORT is significantly more expensive than MammoSite balloon catheter brachytherapy.

D. One known disadvantage of delivering radiotherapy at the time of breast cancer resection is increased toxicity to adjacent tissues.

E. IORT can be repeated as needed.

ANSWER: B

COMMENTS: The targeted intraoperative radiation therapy **(TARGIT) trial** is a phase III, prospective, randomized trial comparing single-fraction targeted **IORT** with conventional whole-breast external beam radiotherapy for the management of early-stage invasive breast cancer. Inclusion criteria for the trial include age 35 years and older and operable invasive breast cancer (T13, N01, M0) suitable for breast-conserving surgery. The principal objective of the trial is to determine whether single-fraction IORT targeted to the tumor bed provides equivalent local control as conventional therapy. In June 2010, the first-phase initial results showed that IORT was equally effective at controlling recurrence. Toxicity was lower in the target group. However, the trial was limited to patients older than 45, and the tumor size was 3 cm or less. Randomized trials have shown that approximately 90% of locally recurrent breast cancers develop at or near the site of the original breast cancer. IORT is a form of accelerated partial breast irradiation in which the entire radiotherapy dose is given intraoperatively, typically at the time of tumor removal. Spherical applicators are used that conform the breast tissue around the radiation source to permit the delivery of a uniform field of radiation to a prescribed tissue depth. Chest wall and skin can be protected by tungsten-impregnated silicone barriers, which provide 93% shielding and minimize pulmonary, cardiac, and skin toxicity. Other advantages of IORT include convenience in that breast-conserving surgery and radiotherapy are completed in one sitting while the patient is still under anesthesia, accurate dose delivery because the radiation dose is directed to the surgical margins, and lower cost (IORT has one-third the cost of MammoSite balloon catheter brachytherapy). Important limitations of IORT are the possible need for additional radiotherapy (repeated IORT is not permitted; therefore if inadequate surgical margins are found after IORT, external beam therapy may be required), lack of pretreatment pathologic review, and concern that this modality may be subtherapeutic and leave patients at an elevated risk for local recurrence.

Ref.: 15

46. Which of the following statements regarding the HER-2 gene is false?

A. It controls normal cell growth.

B. It is amplified in 25% of all breast cancers.

C. Trastuzumab is an antibody against the HER-2/neu receptor.

D. Prior to the use of HER-2–directed therapies, HER-2 positivity was an independent predictor of poor outcome in breast cancer.

E. HER-2 status is hereditary.

ANSWER: E

COMMENTS: HER-2/neu (**c-erbB-2**) is a protooncogene that is found on the surface of some normal cells in the body; however, it is overexpressed or amplified in 25% of all breast cancers. It is a member of the **epidermal growth factor** family and is a transmembrane receptor with **tyrosine kinase** activity. Studies have shown that HER-2/neu overexpression is found in more aggressive cancers and is a negative prognostic factor. Women with node-negative, but HER-2/neu–positive, lesions have up to a 15% chance of having a higher-stage lesion compared with those with node-negative, HER-2/neu–negative lesions. Trastuzumab is a humanized murine monoclonal antibody raised against the erbB-2 or HER-2 surface receptor. The use of trastuzumab with chemotherapy has been shown to improve the overall survival of patients with metastatic HER-2–positive breast cancers and reduce the risk of distant recurrence in patients with early-stage HER-2–positive breast cancers. Pertuzumab is a newer recombinant monoclonal antibody against the Her-2 receptor that prevents dimerization. When combined with trastuzumab, there is a greater signal blocking of the Her-2 receptor, resulting in higher complete pathologic response rates. The HER-2 status is not considered as a hereditary trait.

Ref.: 7, 16

47. Which of the following patients is considered an appropriate candidate for breast-preserving therapy?

A. A 40-year-old woman with a history of active scleroderma and a T1N0 infiltrating ductal carcinoma of her right breast

B. A 45-year-old woman with a T1N1 infiltrating ductal carcinoma of her left breast after lumpectomy, negative surgical margins, and axillary lymph node dissection with 5 of 12 lymph nodes positive

C. A 37-year-old woman with a T2N0 infiltrating ductal carcinoma of her right breast who has a history of Hodgkin disease treated with 36 Gy to a mantle field 15 years earlier

D. All of the above

E. None of the above

ANSWER: B

COMMENTS: The **NSABP B-06 trial** demonstrated that lumpectomy followed by radiation therapy to the breast is an appropriate treatment for patients with primary tumors 4 cm or less in diameter and either positive or negative axillary lymph nodes. Several other trials have confirmed these results for patients with stage I and II breast cancers. The 20-year results from the NSABP B-06 trial showed an equal overall survival and disease-free survival for all patients whether they were treated by breast preservation or mastectomy. However, the cohort of patients treated by lumpectomy alone without irradiation suffered a 35% recurrence rate in the ipsilateral breast. This recurrence rate is considered unacceptably high when compared with the 10% risk for **ipsilateral breast recurrences** in patients who underwent radiation therapy of the breast following lumpectomy. Several series have shown that patients with certain collagen vascular diseases may incur increased toxicity from radiation therapy. Although excessive complications have not been consistently shown with all types of collagen vascular disorders, severe fibrosis and soft tissue necrosis have been associated with scleroderma, thus suggesting that patients with scleroderma may be better served with a mastectomy. Patients with active **systemic lupus erythematosus** and **rheumatoid arthritis** may also be at an increased risk for toxicity from radiation therapy. Mastectomy is recommended for patients who have had previous radiation therapy to the chest or to a mantle field (which includes the neck, axilla, mediastinum, and pulmonary hila) because the radiation tolerance of regional normal tissues may be exceeded and result in excessive toxicity.

Ref.: 17, 18

48. A 15-year-old girl is brought to the office by her mother because of asymmetrical breast development. Physical examination reveals normal breast development on the left and a hypoplastic breast on the right, with hypoplasia of the pectoralis major muscle also seen on the right. Which of the following conditions is this an example of?

A. This is a normal situation in this age group since breast tissue often develops at different rates and is slightly asymmetrical during adolescence.

B. This is an example of Poland syndrome.

C. This is an example of Li-Fraumeni syndrome.

D. This is an example of amazia.

E. This is an example of fragile X syndrome.

ANSWER: B

COMMENTS: This patient is demonstrating **Poland syndrome**, which is characterized by unilateral hypoplasia of the breast, pectoral muscles, and chest wall caused by diminished blood flow to the subclavian artery during fetal development. **Li-Fraumeni syndrome** is one of the inherited breast cancer syndromes in which there is an increased incidence of breast cancer, soft tissue sarcoma and osteosarcoma, brain tumors, adrenocortical cancer, and leukemia in the same family. Nearly 30% of the tumors in these families occur before the age of 15. **Amazia** refers to a condition in which the nipple is present, but the breast mound is absent.

Ref.: 19

49. A 57-year-old woman undergoes image-guided biopsy of a 1.5-cm spiculated, centrally dense mass. The pathologic review shows benign breast parenchyma. Which of the following is the most appropriate recommendation at this point?

A. Routine screening mammography in 1 year

B. Additional imaging with contrast-enhanced MRI

C. Short-term follow-up in 4 to 6 months

D. Wire-localized excisional biopsy

E. Tamoxifen

ANSWER: D

COMMENTS: When mammographic changes are highly suspicious for malignancy but a **negative core biopsy** is obtained, these results must be viewed with caution because the possibility of sampling error is considered discordant. Definitive wide excision with wire localization in such circumstances would then be warranted. The reasons for the initial core biopsy in such suspicious cases are multiple and include the value of having a tissue diagnosis (rather than just a "suspicion") when discussing diagnosis and management options with the patient. Negative MRI findings would not preclude additional biopsy of this mammographically suspicious lesion.

Ref.: 19

50. A 47-year-old woman undergoes a modified radical mastectomy for a T2N2 infiltrating ductal carcinoma. She arrives at her first postoperative visit complaining of hypoesthesia of the upper posteromedial aspect of the ipsilateral arm. What might explain this finding?

A. Lymphatic fibrosis

B. Medial pectoral pedicle injury

C. Second intercostal brachial cutaneous nerve injury

D. Axillary vein thrombosis

E. Thoracodorsal pedicle injury

ANSWER: C

COMMENTS: A number of neurovascular structures that are at risk of injury are identified and dissected during axillary dissection. The axilla is rich in lymphatic vessels draining the ipsilateral arm. Some of these lymphatics are disrupted during axillary dissection, but continued fibrosis of the remaining lymphatics, especially in cases in which the dissected axilla has been irradiated, may lead to progressive **lymphedema** of the arm, which can begin years after therapy. The possibility of an unsightly and disabling **lymphedema**

occasionally developing has led to a generally more conservative surgical approach toward axillary dissection for breast cancer in recent years. The medial pectoral pedicle contains the principal motor nerve and partial blood supply to the **pectoralis major** muscle. Injury leads to atrophy but not ischemia because the blood supply to this muscle is derived from many different sources. The second intercostal **brachial cutaneous nerve** provides sensation to the upper lateral chest wall and medial and posterior aspects of the upper part of the arm. It passes transversely across the axilla about 1 to 2 cm caudal to the axillary vein. In the past, it was routinely sectioned to allow a cleaner en bloc removal of the axillary contents, but many surgeons now choose to preserve it in cases in which it is not in close proximity to clinically suspicious lymph nodes. The **axillary vein** can be narrowed or ligated as a result of a surgical error during the procedure or can undergo acute spontaneous thrombosis during the immediate postoperative period. Because collateral channels have not had a chance to develop, the resulting swelling of the ipsilateral arm is usually acute and painful. The **thoracodorsal** pedicle contains the motor nerve and the principal artery and vein serving the **latissimus dorsi** muscle. Injury to the nerve leads to atrophy, but this is rarely clinically significant, except in athletes. Loss of the vascular pedicle distal to its branch to the serratus muscle, however, would lead to ischemic loss of the latissimus dorsi myocutaneous rotation flap, one of the principal sources of autologous tissue for breast reconstruction and for the closure of soft tissue deficits of the chest wall. The **long thoracic nerve** is also at risk for injury during axillary surgery; such injury can cause loss of function of the serratus anterior muscle and in turn lead to winging of the scapula.

Ref.: 19

51. An ultrasound image of a 45-year-old patient's breast reveals a 2-cm simple cyst. Aspiration yields clear straw-colored fluid, and there is complete resolution on postprocedure ultrasound imaging. What should the clinician's next step be?

A. Order repeat ultrasound imaging in 3 months.
B. Have the fluid sent to the laboratory for Hemoccult testing, cytologic studies, and assessment of tumor markers.
C. Perform wire-localized excision of the cavity.
D. Prescribe antibiotics for the patient.
E. Advise the patient to continue with routine clinical breast examinations and mammograms.

ANSWER: E

COMMENTS: A simple **cyst** that completely resolves after aspiration of straw-colored fluid needs no further diagnostic or surgical evaluation and confers no increased risk for future cancer. Routine follow-up with clinical examination and scheduled mammograms is indicated. If the cyst recurs, especially in the postmenopausal setting, surgical excision should be considered.

Ref.: 19

52. What is the approximate false-negative rate (FNR) for SLNB?

A. 1%
B. 8%
C. 15%
D. 20%
E. 25%

ANSWER: B

COMMENTS: The SLNB technique has a learning curve of approximately 30 cases before proficiency is attained. In experienced hands, the FNR ranges from 4% to 12%. The use of tracer **blue dye** versus **technetium-labeled sulfur colloid**, or both, has not been shown to affect the detection rate or FNR if the surgeon is proficient. However, **isosulfan blue** dye is associated with a small incidence of anaphylactic reactions.

Ref.: 7, 19

53. For which of the following patients is an aromatase inhibitor, such as anastrozole (Arimidex) or letrozole (Femara), considered to be useful?

A. A 57-year-old woman with T1N0 ER-positive breast cancer
B. A 35-year-old woman with LCIS
C. A 65-year-old woman with T2N1, ER-negative breast cancer
D. A 42-year-old woman with DCIS
E. A 45-year-old woman who is a known carrier of the *BRCA* mutation

ANSWER: A

COMMENTS: Aromatase inhibitors are useful only in the **postmenopausal** setting for women with invasive cancers. In postmenopausal women, the ovaries stop producing estrogen, but low levels of estrogen remain because aromatase converts other steroid hormones into estrogen in the peripheral fat. The **ATAC trial** (Arimidex, tamoxifen, alone or in combination) showed that in postmenopausal women with invasive breast cancer, taking **anastrozole** led to a lower recurrence rate, a lower chance for the development of a new primary, and less toxicity than in women taking tamoxifen. A subset analysis of this trial showed that the advantage of anastrozole was seen only in women with steroid receptor–positive breast cancer. **Tamoxifen** may be indicated for chemoprevention in high-risk patients, such as those with LCIS or DCIS or those carrying a *BRCA* mutation.

Ref.: 7, 19

54. What additional treatment should a 42-year-old patient with a 2-cm focus of ER-positive DCIS < 0.1 mm from the inferior margin by lumpectomy receive?

A. Radiation therapy alone
B. Tamoxifen alone
C. Surgical reexcision alone
D. Radiation and tamoxifen alone
E. Surgical reexcision, radiation therapy, and tamoxifen

ANSWER: D

COMMENTS: If ductal carcinoma has been transected at the margin of resection, its rate of recurrence is unacceptably high in both the noninvasive and invasive forms. **Reexcision** to clear margins is the standard of care. Subsequent radiation therapy significantly reduces local recurrence and is recommended for all but the smallest of tumors. The addition of tamoxifen has been shown to further decrease the incidence of recurrent DCIS and new invasive breast cancer. Recent studies have shown that this benefit is best seen in women with ER-positive DCIS.

Ref.: 7, 19

55. Which statement is false regarding radial scars?

A. Usually detected as a stellate lesion on mammography

B. Extensive elastosis is common

C. May be associated with or contain atypical ductal hyperplasia or DCIS

D. Increase the risk for the future development of breast cancer by 20%

E. Benign proliferative disease of the breast

ANSWER: D

COMMENTS: Radial scars are benign breast lesions of uncertain etiology and behavior. They have a characteristic low-power stellate architecture with cystically dilated glands encircling the periphery. The mostly acellular core is composed of connective tissue and elastin surrounded by radiating bands of compressed ducts and lobules that demonstrate dual myoepithelial and epithelial layers. Proliferative epithelial lesions, including sclerosing adenosis, hyperplasia, and papillomas, are often seen within radial scars. One large review study found that radial scars do not confer an increased risk for subsequent breast cancer over that of other proliferative lesions, although there is a slightly increased association between radial scars and atypical hyperplasia. The growth pattern in radial scars can resemble a malignancy and is difficult to distinguish from invasive carcinoma on mammography, which prompts a biopsy of these lesions. When diagnosed by core biopsy, excision of the lesion is usually recommended.

Ref.: 20

56. A 34-year-old woman underwent wide local excision, axillary dissection, and radiation therapy (5000 cGy over a 5-week period) in her left breast for a node-positive, ER-negative, 2-cm infiltrating ductal carcinoma 3 years earlier. She received eight cycles of adjuvant chemotherapy with cyclophosphamide (Cytoxan), doxorubicin (Adriamycin), and Taxol at that time. The surgeon now performs a biopsy of a new 2-cm mass in the same breast, and it shows infiltrating ductal carcinoma. She has no other evidence of local, regional, or distant disease on imaging studies and clinical examination. Which of the following treatment plans is most appropriate?

A. Left total mastectomy

B. Reexcision to free margins

C. A sentinel lymph node biopsy and a third-generation chemotherapy

D. Left total mastectomy followed by chemotherapy

E. Reexcision and 5000-cGy boost to the breast followed by chemotherapy

ANSWER: D

COMMENTS: The **NSABP B-06 trial** found that approximately 8.8% of patients treated using lumpectomy, axillary dissection, radiation therapy, and chemotherapy had a local recurrence within 10 years of initial treatment. A **mastectomy** is usually required in these situations and results in a long-term survival similar to that of patients who had a mastectomy performed as the primary operation. In the absence of palpable nodes, a second surgical axillary evaluation is unnecessary and hazardous. The effects of ionizing irradiation are cumulative and do not diminish with time; therefore additional radiation would lead to excessive toxicity in normal tissue in the irradiated area. Because local control is needed for this tumor, chemotherapy alone would be an inappropriate treatment option.The population of patients with isolated locoregional recurrences was studied in a multiinstitutional randomized controlled trial published in 2014, the chemotherapy for isolated locoregional recurrence of breast cancer (CALOR) trial, aiming to determine whether adjuvant chemotherapy improves survival in this patient population. Patients were randomized to chemotherapy versus no chemotherapy. There was a statistically significant disease-free survival benefit in the chemotherapy arm. Adjuvant chemotherapy for recurrence was of even greater benefit in the patients with ER-negative breast cancer.

Ref.: 5, 7, 8, 21

57. In which patient should MRI be used as an adjunct to mammography for breast cancer screening purposes?

A. A 27-year-old woman whose mother was diagnosed with breast cancer at age 52

B. A 52-year-old woman with moderately dense breasts

C. A 72-year-old woman with a history of DCIS

D. A 31-year-old woman whose sister carries the *BRCA* mutation but has declined genetic testing for herself

E. A 55-year-old woman who received radiation treatments at age 50 for uterine cancer

ANSWER: D

COMMENTS: MRI uses magnetic fields to produce detailed cross-sectional images of tissue structures and provides very good soft tissue contrast. The ACS has recommendations for breast MRI screening as an adjunct to mammography based on certain levels of evidence. The ACS recommends annual MRI screening (based on evidence from nonrandomized screening trials and observational studies) for patients with the *BRCA* mutation, those with first-degree relatives who are *BRCA* carriers but are themselves untested, and those with a lifetime risk of 20%–25% or greater for the development of breast cancer, as defined by BRCAPRO or other models that are largely dependent on family history. The ACS recommends annual MRI screening (based on expert consensus opinion and evidence of lifetime risk for breast cancer) for patients with irradiation of the chest between 10 and 30 years of age, patients and their first-degree relatives with **Li-Fraumeni syndrome**, and patients and their first-degree relatives with **Cowden disease** and **Bannayan-Riley-Ruvalcaba syndrome**. There is insufficient evidence to recommend for or against MRI screening in the following subgroups: patients with a lifetime risk of 15%–20%, as defined by BRCAPRO or other models that are largely dependent on family history; those with LCIS or atypical lobular hyperplasia; those with atypical ductal hyperplasia; women with heterogeneously or extremely dense breasts on mammography; and women with a personal history of breast cancer, including DCIS. The ACS recommends against MRI screening for women with less than a 15% lifetime risk for breast cancer.

Ref.: 21

58. A 42-year-old woman underwent lumpectomy and SLNB for a 2-cm, moderately differentiated, ER-negative infiltrating ductal carcinoma. Pathologic examination revealed adequate margins, and one of the three lymph nodes was found to be positive for carcinoma. Which of the following treatment plans is most appropriate?

A. Axillary dissection followed by radiation
B. Axillary dissection, chemotherapy, and whole-breast radiation
C. Chemotherapy and radiation therapy
D. Chemotherapy, radiation therapy, and tamoxifen
E. Chemotherapy alone

ANSWER: C

COMMENTS: Multiple randomized prospective studies have shown both disease-free and overall survival benefit for **adjuvant chemotherapy** in node-positive premenopausal women, with the greatest advantage occurring in those with one to three positive nodes. Postmenopausal node-positive women have generally shown a more modest benefit. Multiple-drug therapy has consistently been more effective than single-drug therapy. Adding **tamoxifen** to the chemotherapy for node-positive premenopausal patients confers an additional benefit when the cancer is ER positive, but it is not beneficial in ER-negative cancers. The use of radiation therapy in conjunction with surgery has allowed dramatic reductions in the extent of surgery required for local control of breast cancer. At 20 years of follow-up, local recurrence rates are approximately 8.8% for lumpectomy plus radiation compared with 44% for lumpectomy alone. The landmark ACOSOG Z0011 trial has also provided evidence that in early-stage breast cancer (stages I and II) in patients who undergo breast conservation therapy, axillary lymph node dissection does not improve locoregional control or survival. This trial has demonstrated the safety of limiting axillary surgery to the SLNB without performing formal axillary dissection for sentinel node positivity. The ability to forgo axillary lymph node dissection in this subset of early breast cancer patients allows avoidance of the significant associated morbidity of the axillary dissection. In this scenario, the patient should receive adjuvant chemotherapy and radiation therapy. This early-stage breast cancer patient would not gain additional locoregional control by an additional axillary dissection, based on the results of the Z0011 trial.

Ref.: 5–7, 22

59. Which of the following patients are eligible for a nipple-sparing mastectomy based on the Memorial Sloan-Kettering criteria?

A. A 53-year-old female with a left breast nonpalpable 1.5-cm invasive ductal carcinoma whose breast cancer was discovered after she presented to her primary care provider with unilateral bloody nipple discharge
B. A 62-year-old female with a 5.2-cm right breast invasive ductal carcinoma located in the upper outer quadrant 6.1 cm from the nipple
C. A 57-year-old female initially diagnosed with left mammary Paget's disease whose workup also revealed an underlying invasive ductal carcinoma located in the left upper outer quadrant
D. A 66-year-old female with a small 0.7-cm invasive ductal carcinoma found on screening mammogram in the lower inner quadrant of her right breast located 0.9 cm from the nipple
E. A 55-year-old female with a 1.8-cm invasive ductal carcinoma located in her left inner upper quadrant 3.2 cm from the nipple

ANSWER: E

COMMENTS: Because of the successes in outcomes in breast cancer patients receiving skin-sparing mastectomies, the natural progression was for investigators to consider nipple-sparing mastectomies. Nipple-sparing mastectomies have been found to be technically feasible and, with careful patient selection, have also shown promising oncologic results. Surgeons at Memorial Sloan-Kettering have published their results of nipple-sparing mastectomies and, together with a review of the literature, have devised a set of guidelines that are used at many institutions to select patients eligible for nipple-sparing mastectomy. In order to be a candidate for a nipple-sparing mastectomy: (1) there must be no clinical involvement of the nipple–areolar complex including no nipple discharge, (2) the tumor must be less than 5 cm in size (or no greater than T2), and (3) the tumor-to-nipple distance must be greater than or equal to 2 cm.

Ref.: 23

60. A 75-year-old woman underwent a lumpectomy with SLNB with pathology showing infiltrating ductal carcinoma, grade 2, 2 cm, node negative, ER and PR positive, and Her-2 negative with a low Ki 67. Adjuvant treatment recommendations include:

A. No adjuvant treatment indicated
B. Chemotherapy, radiation, and antihormonal therapy
C. Radiation or antihormonal therapy
D. Chemotherapy and radiation
E. No additional treatment

ANSWER: C

COMMENTS: The CALBG 9343 trial demonstrated that radiation therapy could be safely omitted in patients older than 70 with ER-positive tumors treated with breast-conserving surgery who are managed with endocrine therapy. Criteria include size less than 3 cm and being node negative. Although survival was not impacted with the omission of radiation, there is a lower absolute risk of locoregional recurrence compared with no RT.

Ref.: 24

61. A 57-year-old woman elects breast conservation treatment for a T1N0 infiltrating ductal carcinoma. The surgical pathology reveals negative margins with a close lateral margin of 1 mm. What is the next step in management?

A. Reexcision of lateral margin to achieve greater negative margins prior to radiation treatment
B. Completion of mastectomy followed by radiation
C. Completion of mastectomy without radiation
D. Radiation treatment
E. Reexcision of all margins

ANSWER: D

COMMENTS: Negative margins, or "no ink on tumor," is the acceptable standard in breast oncology. Negative breast cancer margins have traditionally been defined as any degree of a negative margin; this controversial topic was scrutinized in 2014 when a panel of experts with representatives from the Society of Surgical Oncology (SSO), the American Society for Radiation Oncology (ASTRO), the American Society of Clinical Oncology (ASCO), the American Society of Breast Surgery (ASBS), and the College of

American Pathologists (CAP) reported a new consensus guideline on margins necessary for breast conservation surgery in stages I and II breast cancer. The guideline included evidence from 33 studies to support the conclusion that no ink on tumor or any degree of negative margins is sufficient and that wider margin widths do not significantly lower the risk of tumor recurrence. The routine practice to obtain wider negative margin widths, which incur compromised cosmetic outcomes, higher health care costs, and no clinical benefit, is not recommended.

In this scenario, the patient's pathology has negative margins; therefore no further surgery is indicated. Her next step in management is radiation therapy to complete her breast conservation treatment.

Ref.: 25

62. Which of the following risks is not elevated with the use of tamoxifen?

A. Stroke

B. Deep vein thrombosis (DVT)

C. Cataracts

D. Ischemic heart disease

E. Endometrial cancer

ANSWER: D

COMMENTS: Although tamoxifen is highly effective in preventing the recurrence of ER-positive breast cancer in premenopausal women, it does have side effects. Common side effects include mood swings, nausea, low libido, hot flashes, and vaginal dryness. More concerning risks of tamoxifen include stroke, DVT/pulmonary embolism (PE), and endometrial cancer (1% risk for blood clots and 0.1% risk for endometrial cancer). There is also an association with increased risk for cataracts. In a major study evaluating the use of tamoxifen to prevent breast cancer in high-risk women, 13,388 women were randomly assigned to receive placebo or tamoxifen for 5 years. The rate of invasive breast cancer was reduced from 42.5 per 1000 women in the placebo group to 24.8 per 1000 women in the tamoxifen group. Relative risks of stroke, DVT, PE, endometrial cancer, and cataracts were increased with tamoxifen. Relative risks for ischemic heart disease and death were not increased with the use of tamoxifen. Of note, the use of tamoxifen is also associated with a decrease in osteoporotic fractures by 32%.

Ref.: 26

63. A large-breasted, 44-year-old female noticed a 2 × 3 cm firm, round mass in her left lower, outer breast a few months ago, which has doubled in size over the past month. Her mammogram is only remarkable for this mass and no other findings. The mass was biopsied, with pathology consistent with a cellular fibroepithelial lesion. What should you offer the patient?

A. Close surveillance

B. Excisional biopsy

C. Wide local excision

D. Mastectomy

E. Bilateral mastectomy

ANSWER: C

COMMENTS: See Question 64.

Ref.: 27

64. The patient in Question 63 comes back to your office 9 months later with a firm round growth beneath her incision. Mammogram and ultrasound reveal the single mass in question without other findings. Core needle biopsy results are consistent with either a fibroadenoma or a phyllodes tumor. What is the next step in management?

A. Excisional biopsy

B. Chest imaging and if no evidence of metastatic disease, wide excision for >2-cm margins

C. Close surveillance with follow-up physical examination in 3 months

D. Chest imaging and if no evidence of metastatic disease, wide excision for >1-cm margins

E. Chest imaging and if no evidence of metastatic disease, wide excision for >2-cm margins with SLNB

ANSWER: D

COMMENTS: It is often difficult to distinguish between fibroadenoma and phyllodes tumor based on core biopsy or fine-needle aspiration. Therefore when the suspicion is high for a phyllodes tumor, for example, in the case of a rapidly growing large tumor, wide local excision is the most appropriate surgery. The difference between an excisional biopsy and a wide local excision is that in excisional biopsy, the goal is excision of the lesion without the intent of obtaining surgical margins, whereas in wide excision, the intent is to obtain surgical margins, which are >1 cm in the case of a suspected phyllodes tumor.

In the case of locally recurrent phyllodes, as is suspected in this case, chest imaging should be pursued to rule out evidence of metastatic disease. The majority of phyllodes tumors are benign, and surgery is curative. In the case of malignant phyllodes, these tumors behave like soft tissue sarcomas and spread hematogenously, discounting the need for nodal staging. Common sites of metastasis include lung, bone, abdominal viscera, and mediastinum. Metastatic phyllodes tumors should be treated like a sarcoma.

In this case of a recurrent phyllodes tumor, chest imaging should be pursued, and after evidence of metastasis has been ruled out, wide excision should be the next step in management to achieve surgical margins >1 cm.

Ref.: 5, 27

65. Which of the following is FALSE regarding nipple discharge?

A. If it is bilateral and milky, it may be associated with hormone-related causes including recent lactation or increased prolactin levels.

B. The most common cause of unilateral bloody nipple discharge is intraductal papilloma.

C. Intraductal papillomas are most commonly located close to the nipple and are polyps of-lined breast ducts.

D. Ductography is not universally employed in the workup of nipple discharge.

E. Approximately half of the patients who present with nipple discharge have serious underlying pathology.

ANSWER: E

COMMENTS: Of patients referred to physicians for breast concerns, 6.8% are for nipple discharge, and of those patients, a mere 5% have a serious underlying disease. Although largely benign in nature, nipple discharge must be carefully evaluated to rule out concerning diagnoses such as breast cancer or pituitary tumors.

It is important to determine whether nipple discharge is unilateral or bilateral and to determine the character of the fluid—bloody, serous, milky, purulent, or green. First, rule out if galactorrhea is associated with recent lactation. If no recent lactation, it may be associated with increased prolactin production. Thyroid-stimulating hormone and a prolactin should be ordered as initial workup. Nipple discharge not considered to be galactorrhea is caused by a ductal condition, such as ductal ectasia, fibrocystic breast changes, intraductal papilloma, intraductal carcinoma, and invasive ductal carcinoma. Ductal ectasia is characterized by dilatation of the major ducts along with inflammation and fibrosis around the ducts. Discharge is usually dark green or black, and for this type of multiduct nipple discharge, surgery is not necessary and surveillance is sufficient. If only one duct is involved, a diagnostic excisional biopsy is recommended. Fibrocystic disease typically results in serous or light-green multiduct discharge. Patients with fibrocystic disease complain of cyclic breast pain and premenstrual breast lumpiness, and examination reveals a diffuse fine nodularity. Mammography and ultrasound are confirmatory and show dense breast tissue with nodularity and presence of cysts.

The most common cause of bloody single duct discharge is intraductal papilloma. Discharge is usually spontaneous, and palpation can usually localize to a single duct. Mammography is typically negative, and ultrasound may show a dilated duct with an intraluminal lesion. Most intraductal papillomas occur near the areolar edge. Treatment of intraductal papilloma is duct excision.

Intraductal and invasive ductal carcinoma are only rarely associated with nipple discharge in the absence of an abnormal mammogram or palpable mass. DCIS and papillary carcinoma cause most cancer-associated nipple discharges. Occasionally, bloody discharge occurs with Paget's disease.

Ref.: 28

66. A 36-year-old patient is diagnosed with T2N1M0 invasive breast cancer and undergoes breast conservation. The pathology result shows a grade III invasive ductal carcinoma that is ER positive, PR positive, and Her-2 negative with the presence of LCIS at the anterior margin and 1- to 2-mm margins for invasive cancer on all sides. Regarding the margin status:

A. No reexcision indicated

B. Reexcision indicated based on the LCIS-positive margin

C. Reexcision indicated based on narrow negative margins for invasive cancer in a very young patient

D. Reexcision indicated based on young age, narrow negative margins for invasive cancer, and positive margins for LCIS

E. Prophylactic bilateral mastectomy is the only option given the presence of LCIS

ANSWER: A

COMMENTS: Negative margins, or "no ink on tumor," is the acceptable standard in breast oncology. The presence of LCIS at the margin is not an indication for reexcision. There is increased risk for local recurrence in young patients (<40 years old) after breast conservation therapy; however, there are no data to support that wider negative margins decrease this risk. If there were an invasive carcinoma or DCIS at the inked tumor margin, this would be an indication for reexcision of positive margins as it is associated with at least a twofold increase in local recurrence. The increased risk of local recurrence for invasive cancer positive margins is not nullified by the use of adjunctive treatment, such as hormonal therapy, chemotherapy, boost radiation therapy, or favorable tumor biology, and therefore requires reexcision to achieve negative margins. Prophylactic bilateral mastectomy is not the only option for LCIS; in fact, given the large impact of this surgery, it is a highly individualized decision. Other more common treatment alternatives for LCIS are risk reduction strategies that include hormonal therapy, such as tamoxifen, and increased surveillance.

Ref.: 25

67. A 55-year-old female presents for surgical consultation after receiving neoadjuvant chemotherapy for a 4-cm, node-positive, infiltrating carcinoma that is ER negative, PR negative, and Her-2 positive. Posttreatment MRI demonstrates no visible disease. What is your surgical plan?

A. Modified radical mastectomy

B. Partial mastectomy and SLNB and axillary dissection if cancer is found in the lymph node

C. No surgery is indicated; proceed with radiation

D. Partial mastectomy and SLNB with axillary dissection only if carcinoma is found in 3/3 lymph nodes

ANSWER: B

COMMENTS: The associated risk and morbidity involved with axillary node dissection has led the pursuit for trials to determine when formal axillary dissections are necessary. Axillary lymph node staging is highly important information to guide treatment decisions. Sentinel lymph node biopsies have proven to be a reliable method to evaluate patients presenting with clinically node-negative disease. In 2013, a multicenter, randomized controlled trial was published to determine the reliability of sentinel lymph node biopsies in patients who initially present with biopsy-proven clinical N1 breast cancer following chemotherapy. In this trial, 756 women with node-positive breast cancer were enrolled, and after neoadjuvant chemotherapy was completed, at the time of surgery, these patients underwent SLNB followed by axillary node dissection to determine the FNR of SLNB in this population. The study sought to evaluate if the FNR of SLNB was less than 10% or equivalent to the FNR in the cN0 patient population. When two or more sentinel lymph nodes were evaluated in cN1 patients after neoadjuvant chemotherapy, the FNR was higher than the 10% threshold, with an FNR of 12.6%. However, this trial demonstrated that this FNR could be lowered by using dual sentinel lymph node mapping modalities and recovering greater than three sentinel lymph nodes. On the basis of this evidence, patients who present with cN1 breast cancer after neoadjuvant chemotherapy should receive a SLNB with the usage of dual mapping modalities and attempts to retrieve three or more sentinel lymph nodes before simply moving toward a formal axillary dissection.

It is important to use biopsy clips at the time of initial diagnosis to allow the possibility of breast conservation after neoadjuvant chemotherapy because it is not uncommon to find no evidence of disease after chemotherapy.

Ref.: 29

68. Given the current ASTRO guidelines, who would be a suitable candidate for partial breast irradiation with accelerated partial breast irradiation?

A. A 25-year-old patient with multicentric grade III, ER-negative DCIS

B. A 65-year-old patient with a 1-cm, grade II, infiltrating ductal carcinoma, ER positive, PR positive, Her-2 negative, and node negative

C. A 65-year-old patient with a 1-cm, grade I, infiltrating lobular carcinoma, ER positive, PR positive, Her-2 negative, and node negative

D. A 55-year-old patient with a 3.2-cm, grade II, infiltrating carcinoma, ER positive, PR positive, Her-2 negative, and node negative

E. B and C

ANSWER: B

COMMENTS: The current ASTRO guidelines have set forth criteria for suitable candidates for accelerated partial breast irradiation:

Patient factors:

- Age greater than or equal to 60
- Not a *BRCA* mutation carrier

Pathologic factors:

- Tumor size less than or equal to 2 cm
- T1 tumor stage
- Negative tumor margins by at least 2 mm
- Any grade
- No lymph-vascular space invasion
- ER positive
- Unicentric only
- Clinically unifocal with total size <2.0 cm
- Histology: invasive ductal or other favorable subtypes
- Cannot be pure DCIS
- Cannot have extensive intraductal component
- Associated LCIS

Nodal factors:

- N0
- Must have SLNB or axillary dissection

Treatment factors:

- Neoadjuvant therapy not allowed

Ref.: 30

69. A 45-year-old female presents with the complaint of a single duct, spontaneous bloody nipple discharge and normal mammogram and ultrasound findings. What would you do next?

A. Review her medications and draw a prolactin level

B. Reassurance and continue with yearly mammography

C. Counsel the patient that this places her at an elevated risk for the future development of breast cancer

D. Recommend duct excision

E. Send discharge for cytology and excise only if atypical cells are identified

ANSWER: D

COMMENTS: Of patients referred to physicians for breast concerns, 6.8% are for nipple discharge, and of those patients, a mere 5% have a serious underlying disease. Although largely benign in nature, nipple discharge must be carefully evaluated to rule out concerning diagnoses such as breast cancer or pituitary tumors. It is important to determine whether nipple discharge is unilateral or bilateral and whether the fluid is bloody, contains blood, is green or serous, or is milky (galactorrhea). First, rule out if galactorrhea is associated with recent lactation. If no recent lactation, it may be associated with increased prolactin production. Thyroid-stimulating hormone and a prolactin should be ordered as initial workup. Nipple discharge not considered to be galactorrhea is caused by a ductal condition, such as ductal ectasia, fibrocystic breast changes, intraductal papilloma, intraductal carcinoma, and invasive ductal carcinoma. Ductal ectasia is characterized by dilatation of the major ducts along with inflammation and fibrosis around the ducts. Discharge is usually dark green or black, and for this type of multiduct nipple discharge, surgery is not necessary and surveillance is sufficient. If only one duct is involved, a diagnostic excisional biopsy is recommended. Fibrocystic disease typically results in serous or light-green multiduct discharge. Patients with fibrocystic disease complain of cyclic breast pain and premenstrual breast lumpiness, and examination reveals a diffuse fine nodularity. Mammography and ultrasound are confirmatory and show dense breast tissue with nodularity and presence of cysts.

The most common cause of bloody uniductal discharge is intraductal papilloma. Discharge is usually spontaneous, and palpation can usually localize to a single duct. Mammography is typically negative, and ultrasound may show a dilated duct with an intraluminal lesion. Most intraductal papillomas occur near the areolar edge. Treatment of intraductal papilloma is duct excision.

Intraductal and invasive ductal carcinoma are only rarely associated with nipple discharge in the absence of an abnormal mammogram or palpable mass. DCIS and papillary carcinoma cause most cancer-associated nipple discharges. Occasionally, bloody discharge occurs with Paget's disease.

Ref.: 31

REFERENCES

1. American Cancer Society. 2008. Available at: www.cancer.org.
2. DevCan: Probability of developing or dying of cancer software, version 6.2.1, Statistical Research and Applications Branch, NCI, 2007. Available at: http://surveillance.cancer.gov/devcan/.
3. National Cancer Institute. Surveillance, epidemiology, and end results program, delay-adjusted incidence database: SEER incidence delay-adjusted rates, 9 Registries, 1975–2004, 2007.
4. Gail MH, Brinton LA, Byar DP, et al. Projecting individualized probabilities of developing breast cancer for white females who are being examined annually. *J Natl Cancer Inst*. 1989;81(24):1879–1886.
5. Iglehart JD, Smith BL. Diseases of the breast. In: Townsend CM, Beauchamp RD, Evers BM, et al., eds. *Sabiston Textbook of Surgery: The Biological Basis of Modern Surgical Practice*. 18th ed. Philadelphia: WB Saunders; 2008.
6. Hunt KK, Newman LA, Copeland EM, et al. The breast. In: Brunicardi FC, Anderson DK, Billiar TR, et al., eds. *Schwartz Principles of Surgery. Newman LA, Copeland EM.* 9th ed. New York: McGraw-Hill; 2010.
7. Bland KI, Copeland EM, eds. *The Breast: Comprehensive Management of Benign and Malignant Disorders*. 3rd ed. St. Louis: WB Saunders; 2004.
8. Fisher B, Jeong JH, Anderson S, Bryant J, Fisher ER, Wolmark N. Twenty-five-year follow-up of a randomized trial comparing radical mastectomy, total mastectomy, and total mastectomy followed by irradiation. *N Engl J Med*. 2002;347:567–575.

9. Chagpar AB, McMasters KM, Edwards MJ. Can sentinel node biopsy be avoided in some elderly breast cancer patients? *Ann Surg*. 2009;249(3):455–460.
10. Tan SM, Low SC. Non-operative treatment of breast abscesses. *Aust N Z J Surg*. 1998;68(6):423–424.
11. Wilhelmi BJ, Phillips LG. Breast reconstruction. In: Townsend CM, Beauchamp RD, Evers BM, et al., eds. *Sabiston Textbook of Surgery: The Biological Basis of Modern Surgical Practice*. 18th ed. Philadelphia: WB Saunders; 2008.
12. The American Society of Breast Surgeons. 2008. Available at: www.breastsurgeons.org.
13. Tabar L, Dean PB. *Teaching Atlas of Mammography*. New York: Thieme; 2001.
14. Holmes DR, Baum M, Joseph D. The TARGIT trial: targeted intraoperative radiation therapy versus conventional postoperative whole-breast radiotherapy after breast-conserving surgery for the management of early-stage invasive breast cancer (a trial update). *Am J Surg*. 2007;194(4):507–510.
15. Slamon DJ, Godolphin W, Jones LA, et al. Studies of the HER-2/neu proto-oncogene in human breast and ovarian cancer. *Science*. 1989;244(4905):707–712.
16. Fisher B, Anderson S, Redmond CK, Wolmark N, Wickerham DL, Cronin WM. Reanalysis and results after 12 years of follow-up in a randomized clinical trial comparing total mastectomy with lumpectomy with or without irradiation in the treatment of breast cancer. *N Engl J Med*. 1995;333(22):1456–1461.
17. Perez CA, Taylor ME. Breast: stage Tis, T1 and T2 tumors. In: Perez CA, Brady LW, eds. *Principles and Practice of Radiation Oncology*. 3rd ed. Philadelphia: Lippincott-Raven; 1998.
18. Harris J, Lippman M, Morrow M, et al. *Diseases of the Breast*. Philadelphia: Lippincott Williams & Wilkins; 2004.
19. Berg JC, Visscher DW, Vierkant RA, et al. Breast cancer risk in women with radial scars in benign breast biopsies. *Breast Cancer Res Treat*. 2008;108(2):167–174.
20. Saslow D, Boetes C, Burke W, et al. American Cancer Society guidelines for breast screening with MRI as an adjunct to mammography. *CA Cancer J Clin*. 2007;57(2):75–89.
21. Aebi S, Gelber S, Anderson SJ, et al. Chemotherapy for isolated locoregional recurrence of breast cancer (CALOR): a randomized trial. *Lancet Oncol*. 2014;15(2):156–163.
22. Guiliano AE, McCal L, Beitsch P, et al. Locoregional recurrence after sentinel lymph node dissection with or without axillary dissection in patients with sentinel lymph node metastases. The American College of Surgeons Oncology Group Z0011 Randomized Trial. *Ann Surg*. 2010;252(3):426–432.
23. Garcia-Etienne CA, Cody HS, Disa JJ, et al. Nipple-sparing mastectomy: initial experience at the Memorial Sloan-Kettering Cancer Center and a comprehensive review of literature. *Breast J*. 2009;15(4): 440–449.
24. Hughes KS, Schnaper LA, Bellon JR, et al. Lumpectomy plus tamoxifen or anastrozole with or without irradiation in women age 70 years or older with early breast cancer: long term follow up of CALBG 9343. *J Clin Oncol*. 2013;31(19):2382–2387.
25. Moran MS, Schnitt SJ, Guiliano AE, et al. Society of Surgical Oncology–American Society for Radiation Oncology Consensus Guideline on Margins for Breast-Conserving Surgery with Whole-Breast Irradiation in Stages I and II Invasive Breast Cancer. *Am Surg Oncol*. 2014;21:704–716.
26. Fisher B, Costantino JP, Wickerham DL, et al. Tamoxifen for the prevention of breast cancer: current status of the National Surgical Adjuvant Breast and Bowel Project P-1 study. *J Natl Cancer Inst*. 2005;97(22):1652–1662.
27. National Comprehensive Cancer Network. NCCN Clinical Practice Guidelines in Oncology (NCCN Guidelines) Version 2. 2016. Available at: https://www.nccn.org/professionals/physician_gls/pdf/breast.pdf.
28. Santen RJ, Mansel R. Benign breast disorders. *N Eng J Med*. 2005;353:275–285.
29. Boughey JC, Suman VJ, Mittendorf EA. Sentinel lymph node surgery after neoadjuvant chemotherapy in patients with node-positive breast cancer. *JAMA*. 2013;310(14):1455–1461.
30. Smith BD, Arthur DW, Buchholz TA, et al. Accelerated partial breast irradiation consensus statement from the American Society for Radiation Oncology (ASTRO). *Int J Radiat Oncol Biol Phys*. 2009;74(4): 987–1001.
31. Santen RJ, Mansel R. Benign breast disorders. *N Eng J Med*. 2005;353:275–284.

SECTION IV

ENDOCRINE SURGERY

CHAPTER 16

THYROID

Samer R. Rajjoub, M.D., and Shabirhusain S. Abadin, M.D.

1. When performing a thyroidectomy, which of the following anatomic considerations is incorrect:
   A. The middle thyroid veins drain into the internal jugular vein.
   B. The inferior thyroid artery arises directly from the external carotid artery.
   C. The thyroidea ima artery arises directly from the aorta in 1%–4% of patients.
   D. The ligament of Berry is located near the entry point of the recurrent laryngeal nerve (RLN).
   E. Venous drainage of the thyroid gland is via the superior, middle, and inferior branches.

ANSWER: B

COMMENTS: The **arterial blood supply** of the thyroid gland is provided by two main arterial branches. The superior thyroid artery arises from the external carotid artery and gives off multiple branches that are collectively referred to as the superior pole vessels. The inferior thyroid artery is given off as a branch of the thyrocervical trunk, which originates from the subclavian artery. The ligament of Berry is a condensation of the thyroid capsule located on the posterior surface of the gland. It is a tough band of tissue that passes either anterior or posterior to the course of the RLN as it travels into the cricothyroid membrane. The superior, middle, and inferior thyroid veins drain the thyroid gland. The superior and middle thyroid veins eventually drain into the internal jugular vein, while the inferior thyroid veins drain into the innominate and brachiocephalic veins. The distal end of the thyroglossal duct persists in approximately 50% of people. This remnant is anatomically referred to as the pyramidal lobe.

Ref.: 1, 2

2. A 45-year-old woman has chronic neck pain and a newly diagnosed posterior pharyngeal neck mass found on magnetic resonance imaging (MRI) (see image of transoral examination—Fig. 16.1). The next best step in the appropriate management of this patient is:
   A. Computed tomography (CT)
   B. Cervical ultrasound
   C. Physical examination with observed swallowing
   D. Radioiodine uptake scan
   E. Observation

ANSWER: C

COMMENTS: The most likely diagnosis in this patient is a **lingual thyroid**. This abnormality arises when the thyroid fails to descend normally into the standard cervical position. In some patients, this may be the only thyroid tissue present. It originates from the base of the tongue in the region of the foramen cecum. The diagnosis is best made by a physical examination that demonstrates a midline anterior cervical mass that moves with protrusion of the tongue as opposed to deglutition. Cervical ultrasound demonstrating an absence of thyroid tissue is also highly suggestive of a lingual thyroid. A radioactive uptake scan demonstrates the uptake of iodine within the mass. If the gland is enlarged, patients may have obstructive symptoms such as dysphagia, choking, or airway obstruction. Management of these patients is typically excision.

Ref.: 1, 2

3. A 46-year-old male is undergoing an anterior cervical disk fusion. Which of the following is correct with regard to the RLN?
   A. The left RLN loops around the subclavian artery and ascends medially into the neck.
   B. The right RLN loops around the inferior thyroid artery, ascends laterally to medially, and enters the cricothyroid membrane.
   C. The right inferior laryngeal nerve is nonrecurrent in 0.5%–1% of patients.
   D. The RLNs innervate the true vocal cords and the cricothyroid muscles.
   E. The medial branch of the RLN is primarily sensory.

ANSWER: C

COMMENTS: The **RLN** arises from the vagus nerve after passing into the mediastinum. The left RLN encircles the aortic arch at the ductus arteriosus and then ascends medially in the neck within the tracheoesophageal groove. The right RLN encircles the right subclavian artery and ascends laterally to medially toward the tracheoesophageal groove. Once in the central aspect of the neck, the RLN nerve can branch into medial and lateral components. The medial branch typically carries the motor fibers and is at risk for injury along its course toward the cricothyroid membrane if not identified as a separate structure relative to the lateral sensory branch. The laryngeal nerves can be

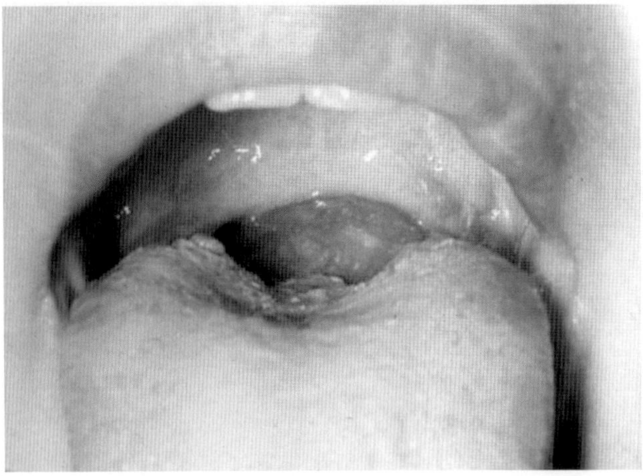

Fig. 16.1 Lingual thyroid. Originates from the base of the tongue and is often associated with dysphagia, airway obstruction or pain.

nonrecurring in approximately 0.5%–1% of patients. In this case, the nerve originates from the cervical position of the vagus nerve. The risk for injury during cervical procedures is higher when the nerve is nonrecurrent because it travels perpendicular rather than parallel to the tracheoesophageal groove. It is more common on the right and is most often associated with the presence of aberrant cervical vascular anatomy such as a retroesophageal subclavian artery. On the left, it is rarer as it is associated with situs inversus and a right-sided aortic arch. The RLN innervates all of the intrinsic muscles of the larynx except the cricothyroid muscle, which is innervated by the external branch of the superior laryngeal nerve.

Ref.: 1, 2

4. With regard to thyroid hormone synthesis and uptake, which of the following is correct?

A. Iodine trapping involves endocytosis of circulating iodine particles.

B. In the euthyroid state, Triiodothyronine (T_3) is the main hormone produced by the thyroid.

C. Thyroid peroxidase is responsible for the peripheral conversion of T_4 to thyroxine (T_3).

D. Thyroglobulin is a glycoprotein synthesized in the rough endoplasmic reticulum of the thyrocyte.

E. The primary site of peripheral deiodination of T_4 to the active form T_3 occurs in the adrenal gland.

ANSWER: D

COMMENTS: The synthesis and uptake of thyroid hormones consists of several steps. It begins with iodine trapping via adenosine triphosphate–dependent transport across the basement membrane of the thyrocyte. **Thyroglobulin**, a glycoprotein synthesized in the rough endoplasmic reticulum, then becomes iodinated by an intracellularly located catalytic enzyme called thyroid peroxidase. Two diiodotyrosines are coupled to form T_4. Peripherally, T_4 is converted to the active thyroid hormone T_3. In the euthyroid state, T_4 is the predominant hormone produced by the thyroid gland. Peripheral deiodination of T_4 to the active form T_3 occurs in the liver, muscle, kidney, and anterior pituitary. T_3 is transported in the serum bound to circulating carrier proteins such as thyroxine-binding globulin (TBG) and albumin.

Ref.: 1, 2

5. Hypothyroidism can be associated with all of the following pharmacologic therapies except:

A. Lithium

B. Amiodarone

C. Interleukin-2

D. Propylthiouracil (PTU)

E. Cimetidine

ANSWER: E

COMMENTS: Hypothyroidism has been associated with a number of pharmacologic therapies, the most frequent being lithium. The mechanism involves blockage of the cyclic adenosine monophosphate–dependent pathway of hormone synthesis. It is also seen with other agents, including amiodarone, cytokines, and antithyroid medications. No relationship has been demonstrated between hypothyroidism and cimetidine.

Ref.: 1, 2

6. With regard to the pharmacologic treatment of hyperthyroidism, which of the following is incorrect?

A. PTU works by inhibiting organic binding of iodine and coupling of iodotyrosines.

B. PTU is associated with agranulocytosis.

C. PTU is the preferred treatment in pregnant patients.

D. Methimazole can worsen exophthalmos in patients with Graves' disease.

E. Methimazole has a longer half-life and only requires once-daily dosing.

ANSWER: D

COMMENTS: The two most commonly prescribed antithyroid medications in the treatment of Graves' disease are **methimazole** and **PTU**. Both agents work by blocking organic binding of iodine and coupling of iodotyrosines. PTU also inhibits peripheral conversion of T_4 to T_3. Both have a side-effect profile that includes hepatotoxicity and reversible granulocytopenia. Methimazole is favored since it requires once-daily dosing as a result of its longer half-life. Both cross the placenta during pregnancy, but PTU appears to exhibit less transplacental transfer and has a lower toxicity profile. Radioactive iodine therapy, an alternative to surgery or medical therapy, can worsen **exophthalmos** following treatment, but neither antithyroid medication alters the degree of the eye findings associated with Graves' disease.

Ref.: 1, 2

7. All of the following are extrathyroidal manifestations of Graves' disease except:

A. Vitiligo

B. Pretibial myxedema

C. Exophthalmos

D. Myxedema coma

E. Acropachy

ANSWER: D

COMMENTS: Graves' disease is an example of an organ-specific autoimmune disease. It has been associated with other autoimmune diseases such as pernicious anemia, vitiligo, alopecia, angioedema, and myasthenia gravis. The extrathyroidal manifestations of Graves' disease include exophthalmos, pretibial myxedema, acropachy, and vitiligo. Patients with severe hypothyroidism may present with myxedema coma and can require initial emergency treatment with high doses of IV T_4.

Ref.: 1, 2

8. Which of the following antibodies is diagnostic of patients with Graves' disease?

A. Thyroglobulin antibodies (anti-Tg)

B. Thyroid peroxidase antibodies (anti-TPO)

C. Anticardiolipin antibodies

D. Thyroid-stimulating antibodies (anti-TSH)

E. Antimicrosomal antibodies

ANSWER: D

COMMENTS: A common feature of autoimmune thyroid disease is the presence of immunoreactivity toward specific thyroid antigens. More than 90% of patients with Graves' disease will express elevated **thyroid-stimulating antibodies** (anti-TSH), which is considered diagnostic. Thyroid antibodies also include thyroid peroxidase antibodies (anti-TPO) and **thyroglobulin** antibodies (anti-Tg), which typically indicate an autoimmune thyroiditis, but not thyroid function. Rarely in Graves' disease do patients have antinuclear antibodies such as anti-Ro, anti-dsDNA, or anticardiolipin antibodies.

Ref.: 1, 2

9. A 42-year-old woman complains to her physician of symptoms associated with hyperthyroidism. On examination she has a palpable nodule, but no evidence of exophthalmos. She does have pretibial myxedema. Her laboratory workup reveals a suppressed thyroid stimulating hormone (TSH) level with elevated free T_3. What is the next best step in the management of this patient?

A. Radioactive ^{123}I uptake scan

B. Thyroid peroxidase antibodies (anti-TPO)

C. PTU

D. Fine-needle aspiration (FNA)

E. Cervical ultrasound

ANSWER: A

COMMENTS: See Question 10.

Ref.: 1, 2

10. Which of the following is not an acceptable indication for surgical treatment of hyperthyroidism of the patient in Question 9?

A. A nodule confirmed or suspicious for malignancy

B. Pretibial myxedema

C. Noncompliance with medical management

D. Age younger than 15 years

E. Severe Graves' ophthalmopathy

ANSWER: B

COMMENTS: A diagnosis of **thyrotoxicosis** is suspected in this patient. Of the tests listed, the one most likely to yield a diagnosis is a radioactive uptake scan. The initial workup of a thyroid nodule should not include a **thyroid uptake scan** unless the patient exhibits signs or symptoms of **hyperthyroidism**. Elevated uptake with a diffusely enlarged gland confirms the diagnosis of **Graves' disease** and assists in differentiating it from other forms of hyperthyroidism. In this patient, the palpable mass on examination could instead be a toxic nodule, and the radioactive uptake scan would illustrate a "hot" nodule in the setting of a suppressed gland. A **thyroid uptake scan** is useful in determining whether the patient has a toxic nodular goiter as a potential explanation of her hyperthyroid state. Cervical ultrasound depicts thyroid anatomy, but does not indicate thyroid function. The most useful test in the initial screening of patients for hyperthyroidism is TSH since the suppression of TSH below normal is a sensitive indicator of excess circulating thyroid hormone. It would not be appropriate to initiate therapy for hyperthyroidism, however, until the cause of the hyperthyroidism is established. **Thyroid peroxidase antibodies (anti-TPO)** are commonly found in Graves' disease, but are not diagnostic. A biopsy by FNA would be appropriate if the nodules were found to have no uptake on a radioiodine uptake scan. Treatment of hyperthyroidism includes medical therapy, radioactive iodine, and surgical resection. Presently, the majority of patients with thyrotoxicosis are treated with pharmacologic agents or, alternatively, ablation with radioactive iodine. Surgical treatment is recommended for patients who have (1) a large goiter with a low radioiodine uptake, (2) noncompliance with medical management, (3) suspicion of malignancy, (4) severe exophthalmos, (5) pregnancy, and (6) age younger than 15 years (because of the risks associated with exposure to radiation).

Ref.: 1, 2

11. With regard to Hashimoto's thyroiditis, which of the following is correct?

A. The majority of patients are transiently hypothyroid but with time return to a euthyroid state.

B. It is primarily treated surgically.

C. Radioactive iodine is useful in the treatment of Hashimoto's thyroiditis.

D. Thyroid microsomal antibodies are detected in the serum of patients.

E. Hashimoto's thyroiditis is more common in men than in women.

ANSWER: D

COMMENTS: Hashimoto's disease is a type of autoimmune thyroiditis. Histologically, the gland exhibits a dense lymphocytic infiltrate associated with a dense fibrosis. When the disease is active, patients can experience symptoms associated with either hypothyroidism or hyperthyroidism. The natural progression of the disease is the eventual development of a multinodular goiter associated with hypothyroidism. Surgery is rarely indicated except in the setting of (1) debilitating symptoms of thyroid dysfunction, (2) compressive symptoms from multinodular goiter, and (3) suspicion of malignancy. The presence of a nodular disease mandates FNA to rule out lymphoma or papillary thyroid carcinoma. Hashimoto's thyroiditis is more common in women than in men (4 to 10:1 female preponderance).

Ref.: 1, 2

12. All of the following statements regarding Hürthle cell carcinoma are correct except:

A. It represents a subtype of papillary thyroid carcinoma.

B. It is associated with a higher mortality rate.

C. It is more likely to be multifocal compared with follicular carcinoma

D. It demonstrates poor radioactive iodine uptake.

E. It is more likely than follicular carcinoma to have lymph node metastases.

ANSWER: A

COMMENTS: Hürthle cell carcinoma is considered a subtype of follicular carcinoma and, similarly, is characterized by vascular or capsular invasion. Hürthle cell carcinomas account for approximately 3% of all thyroid malignancies. Different from follicular carcinoma, Hürthle cell carcinomas are more often multifocal and bilateral, have a higher rate of local nodal metastases (25%), and demonstrate a poor radioactive iodine uptake. Hürthle cell carcinomas have also been associated with higher mortality than follicular carcinomas (approximately 20% at 10 years). Previous radiation exposure has been correlated with an increase in bilateralism and multicentricity of Hürthle cell neoplasms, as well as an increased incidence of contralateral non–Hürthle cell malignant thyroid lesions.

Ref.: 1, 2

13. A patient is undergoing a planned total thyroidectomy for bilateral thyroid nodules, of which the right nodule was consistent with a follicular neoplasm with Hürthle cell features on FNA. During initial mobilization of the gland on the right side, the right RLN was unintentionally transected. What is the best next step in the management of this patient?

A. Repair RLN primarily.

B. Perform a frozen section of the contralateral nodule and proceed with total thyroidectomy only if the biopsy specimen suggests malignancy.

C. Perform right lobectomy and isthmusectomy.

D. Perform left subtotal lobectomy.

E. Perform right lobectomy with nodulectomy of the lesion located on the left.

ANSWER: C

COMMENTS: Injury to the **RLN** occurs in less than 1% of patients. The risk is higher with low-volume surgeons, **reoperative surgery**, irradiated necks, and invasive cancers. Transient **neurapraxia** can occur as a result of excessive stretch on the nerve, but typically recovers following the procedure. In such cases, there can be a loss of signal with intraoperative nerve monitoring, just as would be seen if the nerves were completely transected. One should repair the nerve primarily or using a nerve graft if necessary, typically from ansa cervicalis, in order to decrease tension on the repair at the same operation. The goal of repairing the nerve is to maintain tone to the false vocal cords, thereby preventing it from atrophying over time. This, however, should be completed after the ipsilateral lobe of the thyroid is removed to prevent the repair from being disturbed. If this problem is encountered in a patient such as this one in whom the intended operation is not yet complete, the best decision is to complete the procedure on the side where the nerve has been injured and not to proceed to the unaffected side since a diagnosis of malignancy has not yet been established. After the recovery period, the patient should undergo a formal vocal cord evaluation and have a lengthy discussion regarding the risks and benefits of proceeding with the subsequent portion of the operation if necessary. Intraoperative laryngoscopy is of no use because the patient is unresponsive, and a functional vocal cord evaluation is very limited while the patient is still intubated.

Ref.: 1, 2

14. With regard to the pathologic features of thyroid carcinoma, which of the following is correct?

A. Psammoma bodies are a feature of medullary thyroid carcinoma (MTC).

B. Hürthle cell carcinoma represents a subtype of anaplastic thyroid carcinoma.

C. Amyloid deposits are a characteristic of papillary thyroid carcinoma.

D. MTC typically spreads hematogenously.

E. Nuclear grooves and inclusions are a characteristic feature of papillary thyroid carcinoma.

ANSWER: E

COMMENTS: The pathologic characteristics of **papillary thyroid carcinoma** include nuclear grooves and inclusions. **Psammoma bodies** are also pathognomonic of papillary thyroid carcinoma. Papillary thyroid carcinoma spreads via the lymphatics, while follicular thyroid carcinoma spreads hematogenously. MTC spreads via the lymphatics initially. Amyloid deposits represent collections of calcitonin within the thyroid specimen. **Hürthle cell carcinoma** is a subtype of follicular thyroid carcinoma that has a more aggressive phenotype.

Ref.: 1, 2

15. A 72-year-old woman with Hashimoto's thyroiditis is evaluated for a rapidly enlarging neck mass. The patient takes levothyroxine replacement. Despite no change in her medication dosage, she has been experiencing fevers, night sweats, and weight loss. Ultrasound reveals a 4-cm left thyroid mass with a pseudocystic pattern. FNA is nondiagnostic. What is the next step in the management of this patient?

A. Nonsteroidal antiinflammatory drugs

B. Repeated FNA

C. Radioactive iodine

D. Open or core biopsy

E. Increased dose of levothyroxine with follow-up ultrasound in 6 months

ANSWER: D

COMMENTS: Primary **thyroid lymphoma** is rare (<1% of all thyroid malignancies). There is an increased association between lymphoma and Hashimoto's thyroiditis. The initial workup of a newly diagnosed thyroid mass should be completed. FNA can be diagnostic, but flow cytometry is needed to establish the diagnosis. On ultrasound, the thyroid will classically have a pseudocystic pattern. In the current patient, the presence of Hashimoto's thyroiditis, a rapidly enlarging mass, and the constitutional symptoms are highly suggestive of primary thyroid lymphoma. If FNA fails to yield a diagnosis on the first attempt, it has been shown that repeated FNA is unlikely to be diagnostic in subsequent attempts. Observation is not an appropriate step in the management of any patient with a rapidly enlarging neck mass. Performing open or core biopsy is a feasible option in these circumstances and would more likely provide an adequate cell yield to complete flow cytometry and establish monoclonality. Treatment varies between chemotherapy and surgical ablation. Resection is typically reserved for patients who fail to respond to chemotherapy or have completed their course of adjuvant therapy and demonstrated incomplete regression of disease. If surgery is planned, total thyroidectomy should be performed, followed by chemotherapy.

Ref.: 1, 2

16. Which of the following genes has been associated with a less favorable prognosis in patients with papillary thyroid carcinoma?

A. *RET* protooncogene

B. *Ras*

C. *BRAF*

D. *Menin*

E. *p53*

ANSWER: C

COMMENTS: Papillary thyroid carcinoma is the most common type of thyroid malignancy. Patients have an overall predicted 5-year survival rate greater than 95%. Several clinical factors are currently used as prognosticators of a patient's clinical outcome. **B-type RAF** (*BRAF*) is part of the Raf kinase family and plays a fundamental role in the classic intracellular signaling mitogen-activated protein kinase (MAPK) pathway. *BRAF* mutations occur in papillary and anaplastic tumors, but not in follicular thyroid carcinomas. *BRAF* mutations are associated with an increased risk for LN metastasis, extrathyroidal invasion, and advanced tumor stages. ***RET*** is the gene found to be mutated in patients with MTC. *RET* can also fuse with other genes, and such fusion products have been implicated in the pathogenesis of papillary thyroid carcinoma. *Menin* is mutated in patients with multiple endocrine neoplasia type I. Both ***p53*** and ***RAS*** have not been identified as genetic prognosticators in patients with papillary thyroid carcinoma.

Ref.: 1, 2

17. An 82-year-old female with a long-standing history of a neck mass presents because of sudden rapid painful neck enlargement associated with a change in her voice and dysphagia. FNA biopsy reveals giant and multinucleated cells. All of the following are appropriate steps in the management of this patient except:

A. Immediate tracheostomy

B. Total thyroidectomy with LN dissection for intrathyroidal tumors

C. Cytotoxic chemotherapy

D. Adjuvant radiation if performance status permits

E. En bloc resection for tumors with extrathyroidal extension

ANSWER: A

COMMENTS: Approximately 1% of thyroid malignancies in the United States are discovered to be **anaplastic thyroid carcinoma**. Elderly women are more commonly affected. The tumors are often large and may be fixed to surrounding structures with areas of necrosis that can be visualized on MRI. Diagnosis is confirmed with the above FNA biopsy result. All patients should undergo a preoperative laryngoscopy to assess the status of the vocal cords. A total thyroidectomy with LN dissection is recommended for intrathyroidal masses. En bloc resection should be considered if an R1 resection can be achieved for tumors with extrathyroidal extension. Cytotoxic chemotherapy is typically given along with adjuvant radiation for patients with a good performance status and no evidence of metastatic disease. Tracheostomy should be avoided for as long as possible unless there is impending airway loss.

Ref.: 1, 2

18. With regard to thyroid metastases, which of the following malignancies most commonly spreads to the thyroid?

A. Renal cell carcinoma

B. Breast cancer

C. Colon cancer

D. Lung cancer

E. Melanoma

ANSWER: A

COMMENTS: Metastases to the thyroid are rare. The most common metastases to the thyroid are from renal cell carcinoma, and they can develop several years after the initial diagnosis. Other types of cancer that metastasize to the thyroid include lung and breast cancers. Management depends on the state of the primary disease in other locations and the predicted overall survival.

Ref.: 1, 2

19. All of the following are considered an increased risk factor for cancer in a patient with a thyroid mass except:

A. Age younger than 45 years

B. Rapid growth

C. Family history

D. Hot nodules on thyroid uptake scan

E. Male gender

ANSWER: D

COMMENTS: There is an associated increased risk for thyroid malignancy in patients with thyroid nodules and any of the following features: radiation exposure, rapid growth during observation, family history of thyroid cancer, cold nodule on radioactive uptake scan, male gender, and age older than 45 years. **Hot nodules** on a thyroid uptake scan generally indicate hyperfunctioning growth associated with such conditions as toxic multinodular goiter or Graves' disease.

Ref.: 3

20. A 57-year-old female presents with a new diagnosis of a thyroid nodule. Routine workup includes all of the following except:

A. Physical examination

B. TSH

C. Cervical ultrasound

D. Thyroglobulin

E. Total thyroxine (T_4)

ANSWER: D

COMMENTS: The initial workup of a new thyroid nodule involves obtaining a thorough history and physical examination, with particular attention to the sequelae of hyper- and hypothyroidism, symptoms of compression, and signs of malignancy. The physical examination focuses on palpation of the thyroid and cervical lymphadenopathy. Ultrasonography should be performed to document whether a nodule is suspicious and warrants further workup before surgery. If a diagnosis of malignancy is made, the extent of surgery (subtotal versus complete versus LN dissection) can be determined preoperatively. **Thyroid dysfunction** involves measurement of TSH. The thyroid production of T_4 is assessed by measuring both free and total T_4. Total T_4 is the amount of both free and protein-bound hormone. Thyroglobulin is not routinely measured as part of the initial assessment of thyroid function. Obtaining a family history of thyroid dysfunction or malignancy and a history of radiation are other key aspects of the history taking and physical examination.

Ref.: 1–3

21. Calcitonin is produced by the parafollicular cells of the thyroid gland. Measurement of calcitonin is most useful in what disease process?

A. Pheochromocytoma

B. Follicular thyroid carcinoma

C. Hashimoto's disease

D. MTC

E. Papillary thyroid carcinoma

ANSWER: D

COMMENTS: Calcitonin is produced by the parafollicular cells of the thyroid gland. This 32–amino acid polypeptide is the principal hormone responsible for lowering serum calcium levels during states of hypercalcemia. The action of calcitonin takes place on the surface receptors of osteoclasts, which work to inhibit bone resorption and thus reduce serum calcium levels. **MTCs** are tumors of the parafollicular cells that produce calcitonin. The resulting hypercalcitoninemia seen in these patients can be a measure of tumor burden. Carcinoembryonic antigen (CEA) may also be elevated in some patients with MTC. Calcitonin doubling times of greater than 2 years are associated with a better long-term prognosis than the doubling times of less than 6 months. The American Thyroid Association (ATA) provides a web-based calculator to monitor the levels of calcitonin and CEA to aid in the follow-up and management of patients with MTC.

Ref.: 1, 2, 4

22. In the management of thyrotoxicosis, which of the following is correct?

A. Iodine given in large doses stimulates the release of thyroid hormone.

B. A euthyroid state should be achieved through the use of antithyroid drugs before surgery.

C. Corticosteroids stimulate the peripheral conversion of T_4 to T_3.

D. β-Blockers potentiate the effects of thyroid hormone through adrenergic stimulation of thyroid receptors.

E. Supersaturated potassium iodide (SSKI) should not be administered preoperatively.

ANSWER: B

COMMENTS: Preoperatively, patients with Graves' disease should have their **thyrotoxic state** controlled through the use of **antithyroid medications**. Without this, induction of anesthesia can induce a thyroid storm. Many endocrine surgeons advocate giving patients a 7- to 10-day preoperative course of either **Lugol's solution** or SSKI to help diminish the hypervascularity of the gland and minimize operative blood loss, although some studies have shown that preoperative administration of concentrated iodide preparations can also induce hypertrophy of the gland and should possibly be avoided in patients with diffusely enlarged toxic goiters. When given in concentrated doses, iodine can inhibit the release of thyroid hormone. This process of "thyroid stunning" is referred to as the **Wolff–Chaikoff effect**. It is sometimes seen in patients who have a diagnostic radioactive iodine scan and then demonstrate minimal uptake of radioactive iodine when the therapeutic dose is given. In preparing hyperthyroid patients for surgery, administration of potassium iodide solutions has been shown to treat hyperactivity and decrease intraoperative blood loss during thyroidectomy. This stunning effect is transient and is thus not used for the long-term management of hyperthyroid patients. Concentrated potassium iodide (**Lugol's solution**) should be used with caution in this setting since it will aggravate the hyperthyroidism after its initial effect wears off. **β-Blockers** are used to mitigate the symptoms of adrenergic stimulation but are not given to all patients with Graves' disease preoperatively unless they exhibit signs of thyrotoxic-induced tachycardia. **β-Blockers** do not directly inhibit synthesis of thyroid hormone, but they do counteract some of the peripheral effects of its action on the cardiovascular system. Corticosteroids not only inhibit peripheral conversion of T_4 to T_3 but also suppress the production of TSH. In **acute severe hyperthyroid states**, corticosteroids can help in the initial treatment.

Ref.: 1, 2, 5

23. A 25-year-old woman at 10 weeks' gestation has increasing shortness of breath and anxiety. The clinician wishes to screen her for hyperthyroidism. Which of the following statements is relevant to the interpretation of thyroid function in pregnant patients?

A. TBG is decreased and thus levels of total T_4 and T_3 are increased.

B. Decreased renal iodine clearance causes a reciprocal decrease in total T_3.

C. Increased plasma volume decreases the total T_4 and T_3 levels measured in serum.

D. A first-trimester increase in human chorionic gonadotropin (hCG) causes a reciprocal decrease in TSH levels.

E. Thyrotoxicosis is relatively common in the first and second trimesters of pregnancy.

ANSWER: D

COMMENTS: **Thyrotoxicosis** occurs in approximately 0.1%–0.4% of pregnancies in the United States. If not recognized and treated promptly, severe complications can arise in both the mother and the fetus. The hormonal changes and fluctuating metabolic demands during pregnancy have an important impact on thyroid physiology. These changes can make interpretation of laboratory tests of thyroid function in pregnant patients extremely challenging. During pregnancy, there is a rise in **TBG**, which in turn causes an increase in the total serum T_4 and T_3. The degree of change in TBG levels is dependent on the particular trimester. By 16 to 20 weeks, serum TBG levels have in most cases risen to double the nonpregnant values. Additionally, hCG shares structural similarity with TSH and has been shown to have weak thyroid-stimulating activity. This fact may explain why thyroid nodules often increase in size during pregnancy. The mimicked activity of TSH allows hCG to provide negative feedback in such a way that TSH levels during pregnancy are always lower than is reflective of the true thyroid functional state. Thus if normal ranges of TSH that are specific to pregnancy are not used, hyperthyroidism can be inappropriately diagnosed. Additionally, in pregnancy, renal clearance of iodine is increased, and thus patients will have increased baseline 24-h radioactive iodine uptake when compared with nonpregnant patients. The increased renal clearance has no direct effect on the circulating levels of total T_3. In fact, pregnant patients have increased T_4 and T_3 levels because of their increased total plasma volumes.

Ref.: 1, 2, 6

24. A 37-year-old woman has an incidentally discovered thyroid mass on CT performed during a recent visit to the emergency department for workup of a fall at work. The patient undergoes neck ultrasonography. Which of the following features is less likely to be a malignant lesion?

A. Incomplete halo

B. Peripheral calcifications

C. Hypoechoic lesion

D. Irregular margins

E. Size smaller than 2 cm

ANSWER: B

COMMENTS: In a clinically euthyroid patient, the initial test of choice should be cervical ultrasound followed by **FNA** of any suspicious nodules discovered on clinical or radiographic examination. FNA has a false-negative rate of approximately 3% and a false-positive rate of 4%. A TSH level should be ordered to document thyroid function. Not all calcifications on thyroid ultrasound are associated with a malignant lesion. Typical benign cystic lesions will exhibit a complete halo (intact capsule) and peripheral calcifications. Size is not generally thought to be a consistent predictor of malignancy. However, lesions greater than 1 cm are believed to be amenable to fine-needle biopsy. Table 16.1 lists some of the **ultrasonographic** features associated with benign and malignant disease.

Ref.: 1, 2, 7, 8

25. The patient in Question 16 is found to have a 2-cm dominant nodule located in the right thyroid lobe. Cytologic evaluation of an FNA biopsy specimen reveals "atypia of undetermined significance." All of the following are acceptable next steps in her management except:

A. Right thyroid lobectomy

B. Observation with repeat ultrasound and FNA in 6 months

C. Right thyroid lobectomy with an intraoperative frozen section

D. Radioactive iodine ablation

E. Gene expression analysis of thyroid nodule FNA aspirate

ANSWER: D

COMMENTS: A finding of follicular neoplasm on **FNA** carries approximately 15%–30% risk of harboring a malignancy. At a minimum, the patient should undergo a right lobectomy with or without a frozen resection. Surgical excision is necessary because **follicular neoplasms** cannot be diagnosed as malignant or benign without microscopic examination of the nodule's capsule. In patients who have additional risk factors for thyroid cancer (e.g., family history and exposure to radiation), total thyroidectomy should strongly be considered to avoid the need for reoperative surgery given the higher likelihood of finding a malignant nodule. Only patients with atypia of undetermined significance should be offered the option of observation and repeated imaging in 6 months. Expression arrays, which are being used to investigate microRNAs that have been implicated for their role in carcinogenesis, are sometimes used to aid in the determination of the risk of malignancy for inconclusive FNA biopsies although their utility has yet to be definitely established.

Ref.: 1, 2, 9

26. Overall, papillary thyroid carcinoma carries a favorable prognosis. Which of the following is not a prognostic risk factor in the tumor/node/metastasis (TNM) staging system?

A. LN metastases

B. Synchronous bone metastases

C. Serum thyroglobulin level

D. Extranodal extension

E. Vascular invasion

ANSWER: C

COMMENTS: Papillary thyroid carcinoma carries a very favorable prognosis with a 10-year survival of greater than 95%. **Risk stratification** is a fundamental aspect of how treatment and surveillance algorithms are developed. For well-differentiated thyroid carcinomas, the TNM staging is divided into those younger than 45 years old and those 45 years or older. For those younger than 45 years, stage I includes any T or N and M0 and stage II includes any T or N and M1. For those 45 years or older, stage I includes T1, N0, and M0; stage II includes T2 or T3, N0, and M0; stage III includes T4, N0, M0, and any T, N1, M0; and stage IV includes any T or N, and M1. All undifferentiated or anaplastic carcinomas are stage IV. In addition to the **TNM** staging system, other frequently used systems include **AGES** (age, grade, extrathyroidal extension, and size) and **AMES** (age, metastases, extension, and size). Although each of these staging systems does a reasonable job of predicting cancer-specific survival, none have any prognostic value in assessing the risk of recurrence. Thyroglobulin levels are not a part of any of the current staging systems and are most useful in the surveillance for recurrence of thyroid cancer after thyroidectomy and/or radioactive iodine therapy.

Ref.: 1, 2, 10

TABLE 16.1 Ultrasonographic Features of Thyroid Nodules

Variable	Benign	Malignant
Calcifications	Peripheral and coarse	Microcalcifications
Vascularity	Hypovascular	Hypervascular
Margins	Smooth, well defined	Irregular, infiltrative
Peripheral halo	Complete halo	Incomplete halo
Echogenicity	Anechoic or hyperechoic	Hypoechoic
Size	<1 cm	>1 cm
Shape	Symmetrical	More tall than wide

27. A 35-year-old man is newly diagnosed with MTC and is found to have an elevated calcitonin. In regard to the management of this patient, all are correct except:

A. Preoperative ultrasound for LN mapping of the lateral and central compartments should be performed routinely.

B. Biochemical screening for associated endocrinopathies (e.g., hyperparathyroidism or pheochromocytoma) is part of the preoperative workup.

C. Treatment consists of total thyroidectomy with bilateral central node dissection.

D. Measurement of CEA is not a useful marker of disease burden.

E. Genetic counseling and screening should be offered to the patient and his immediate family members.

ANSWER: D

COMMENTS: **MTC** arises from the parafollicular cells of the thyroid. Its serum tumor marker is **calcitonin**. Patients with diffuse and advanced disease can have symptoms of calcitonin excess (diarrhea, flushing, and abdominal cramping). More than 80% of cases of MTC are sporadic and thus have no hereditary association. That being said, every patient in whom MTC is newly diagnosed should be referred for genetic counseling and evaluation for a *RET* protooncogene mutation because there are identifiable genetic mutations that predict the prognosis and aggressiveness of the disease. The overall survival of patients with MTC is determined largely by the completeness of resection and the presence of persistent disease. Thus surgical treatment of MTC tends to favor aggressive therapy. All patients with biopsy-confirmed MTC and no evidence of nodal or distant metastases should undergo a minimum **total thyroidectomy with bilateral central node dissection**. Whether lateral compartment dissection is performed is dependent on whether there is radiographic or operative evidence of gross disease. Current 2015 ATA guidelines for MTC recommend that all patients with findings on FNA or a calcitonin level suggestive of MTC should undergo preoperative neck ultrasonography for the evaluation of LN metastases. Biochemical screening for associated manifestations (e.g., hyperparathyroidism and pheochromocytoma) should also be performed by obtaining a serum calcium level and measurement of either plasma metanephrines or 24-h urine catecholamines. CEA and calcitonin are useful tumor markers in predicting disease burden and recurrence in patients with MTC.

Ref.: 1, 2, 10

28. Recent studies have shown that the incidence of thyroid cancer has nearly doubled in the last two decades. Plausible explanations given by epidemiologists include all of the following except:

A. Childhood radiation exposure

B. Iodine deficiency

C. Estrogen hormone

D. Increased use of diagnostic imaging modalities

E. Increased use of thyroid function tests

ANSWER: E

COMMENTS: According to the *2016 Cancer Facts and Figures* published by the American Cancer Society, the incidence of thyroid cancer has not only been rising worldwide over the past few decades but is now the most rapidly increasing cancer in the United States. In the United States, rates have increased by over 5% per year from 2003 to 2012. Current evidence supports the fact that the increase is most likely multifactorial, including radiation exposure, environmental, hormonal, and genetic factors. The rise is also partly attributed to increased detection as a result of both an increased use of imaging and more sensitive diagnostic modalities. The iodine status does appear to influence the subtype of thyroid cancer that populations are at risk for. There is a reported increased risk for thyroid cancer in iodine-replete areas, mainly papillary thyroid carcinoma, whereas iodine-deficient areas show a slightly increased incidence of follicular thyroid carcinoma. The utilization of thyroid function tests is not directly associated with the rise in the incidence of thyroid cancer.

Ref.: 1, 2, 11

REFERENCES

1. Hanks JB, Salomone LJ. Thyroid. In: Townsend CM, Beauchamp RD, Evers BM, et al., eds. *Sabiston Textbook of Surgery: The Biological Basis of Modern Surgical Practice*. 19th ed. Philadelphia: WB Saunders; 2012.
2. Lal G, Clark OH. Thyroid, parathyroid and adrenal. In: Brunicardi FC, Andersen DK, Billiar TR, et al., eds. *Schwartz's Principles of Surgery*. 10th ed. New York: McGraw-Hill; 2015.
3. Hall SF, Walker H, Siemens R, Schneeberg A. Increasing detection and increasing incidence in thyroid cancer. *World J Surg*. 2009;33:2567–2571.
4. American Thyroid Association. Calcitonin and carcinoembryonic antigen (CEA) doubling time calculator. Available at: http://www.thyroid.org/professionals/calculators/thyroid-cancer-carcinoma/. Accessed on May 24, 2016.
5. Erbil Y, Ozluk Y, Giris M, et al. Effect of Lugol solution on thyroid gland blood flow and microvessel density in the patients with Graves' disease. *J Clin Endocrinol Metab*. 2007;92:2182–2189.
6. Stagnaro-Green A, Abalovich M, Alexander E, et al. Guidelines of the American Thyroid Association for the diagnosis and management of thyroid disease during pregnancy and postpartum. *Thyroid*. 2011;21:1081–1125.
7. Frates MC, Benson CB, Charboneau JW, et al. Management of thyroid nodules detected at US: Society of Radiologists in Ultrasound consensus conference statement. *Radiology*. 2005;237:794–800.
8. Castro MR, Gharib H. Continuing controversies in the management of thyroid nodules. *Ann Intern Med*. 2005;142:926–931.
9. Cibas ES, Ali SZ. NCI Thyroid FNA State of the Science Conference. The Bethesda system for reporting thyroid cytopathology. *Am J Clin Pathol*. 2009;132(5):658–665.
10. Haugen BR, Alexander EK, Bible KC, et al. 2015 American Thyroid Association Management Guidelines for Adult Patients with Thyroid Nodules and Differentiated Thyroid Cancer: The American Thyroid Association Guidelines Task Force on Thyroid Nodules and Differentiated Thyroid Cancer. *Thyroid*. 2016;26(1):1–133.
11. American Cancer Society. Cancer facts, figures 2016. Available at: http://www.cancer.org/acs/groups/content/@research/documents/document/acspc-047079.pdf. Accessed May 27, 2016.

CHAPTER 17

PARATHYROID

Samer R. Rajjoub, M.D., and Shabirhusain S. Abadin, M.D.

1. With regard to parathyroid anatomy, which of the following is incorrect?
   A. The superior parathyroid glands are lateral and posterior to the recurrent laryngeal nerve (RLN).
   B. Parathyroid glands derive the majority of their blood supply from branches of the superior thyroid artery.
   C. The inferior parathyroid glands are medial and anterior to the RLN.
   D. Parathyroid glands are drained by the superior, middle, and inferior thyroid veins.
   E. Branches from the thyroidea ima may provide arterial blood supply to the parathyroid glands.

ANSWER: B

COMMENTS: There are typically four parathyroid glands. Supernumerary glands have been found in up to 13% of people on autopsy. They are typically light brown in appearance, measure 7 mm in size, and each weighs 50 mg. The superior glands are dorsal and lateral to the RLN, while the inferior glands are ventral and medial to the RLN. Parathyroid glands primarily derive their blood supply from the inferior thyroid artery. Branches of the superior thyroid artery can provide up to 20% of the blood supply of the superior glands. Branches from the thyroidea ima, in addition to vessels to the trachea, esophagus, larynx, and mediastinum, may also be found.

Ref.: 1, 2

2. With regard to calcium homeostasis, which of the following statements is incorrect?
   A. Calcium is the most abundant cation in human beings.
   B. Approximately 50% of calcium is free or ionized and is metabolically active.
   C. Hypoalbuminemia can make the measured total calcium concentration appear artificially low.
   D. Hypoventilation can decrease ionized calcium levels and in turn exacerbate symptoms of hypocalcemia.
   E. Calcium is bound to citrate and is biologically inactive.

ANSWER: D

COMMENTS: Calcium is the most abundant cation in the human body. As much as 99% of calcium is stored in the musculoskeletal system. The remainder is present in serum and exists in three forms: (1) 45% is bound to albumin and is biologically inert, (2) 50% is ionized and metabolically active, and (3) a small percentage is complexed with citrate and is also biologically inactive. Hypoalbuminemia means that more of the total serum calcium will be free and metabolically active. Although total serum calcium may be low, the patient may not be metabolically hypocalcemic. Ionized calcium levels are inversely affected by the pH of blood. A one-unit rise in pH will decrease the ionized calcium level by 0.36 mmol/L. Hypoventilation would cause a drop in pH and thus a subsequent rise in the ionized calcium level.

Ref.: 1, 2

3. Vitamin D synthesis begins in the skin keratinocytes. What is the next step of activation in vitamin D synthesis?
   A. Hydroxylation in the kidney to yield 1,25-dihydroxyvitamin D
   B. Hydroxylation in the liver to yield 25-hydroxyvitamin D
   C. Decarboxylation in the liver to yield 25-hydroxyvitamin D
   D. Decarboxylation in the kidney to yield 25-hydroxyvitamin D
   E. Decarboxylation in the periphery to yield 25-hydroxyvitamin D

ANSWER: B

COMMENTS: Vitamin D synthesis begins in the keratinocytes of the skin. Subsequently, hydroxylation occurs in the liver to yield 25-hydroxyvitamin D. The final step in the conversion of vitamin D to its active form occurs in the kidney, where a second hydroxylation reaction takes place to yield 1,25-dihydroxyvitamin D. Sunlight plays a key role in the initial synthesis step in the skin. Persons who are not exposed to sunlight require supplemental vitamin D through dietary intake.

Ref.: 1, 2

4. Calcitonin helps mediate calcium homeostasis by which of the following actions?
   A. Stimulates osteoblast-mediated bone formation and inhibits renal resorption of calcium and phosphate
   B. Directly inhibits secretion of parathyroid hormone (PTH)
   C. Inhibits intestinal absorption of calcium
   D. Stimulates hydroxylation of vitamin D
   E. Stimulates osteoclast-mediated bone resorption

ANSWER: A

COMMENTS: Calcitonin is produced by the parafollicular cells (C cells) of the thyroid gland and works to oppose the actions of PTH. It helps lower ionized calcium levels in primarily two ways. First, it inhibits osteoclast-mediated bone resorption. Second, it inhibits resorption of calcium and phosphate by the kidney. Calcitonin has no direct effects on intestinal absorption or osteoblast-mediated bone formation. It is also used in the treatment of hypercalcemic crisis (4 IU/kg subcutaneously/intramuscularly). It acts quickly (24 to 48 h) and is more effective when used in combination with glucocorticoids. Finally, calcitonin is a useful marker with regard to surveillance in medullary thyroid carcinoma.

Ref.: 1, 2

5. With regard to PTH, which of the following statements is incorrect?

A. PTH blocks calcium excretion at the ascending limb of the loop of Henle.

B. PTH stimulates osteoclast resorption of calcium and phosphate.

C. PTH cells express G protein–coupled calcium-sensing receptors.

D. PTH inhibits calcium excretion at the distal convoluted tubule of the kidney.

E. PTH enhances renally mediated hydroxylation of 25-hydroxyvitamin D.

ANSWER: A

COMMENTS: PTH has a variety of actions and targets to help increase serum calcium levels. The parathyroid cells express a G protein–coupled membrane receptor that senses serum calcium levels. When calcium levels fall below appropriate levels, the receptor stimulates the release of PTH into the circulation. PTH has a half-life of about 2 to 4 min in the circulation. Before its rapid clearance, it first targets osteoclasts and stimulates them to resorb calcium and phosphate from bone. In the kidney, PTH blocks calcium excretion at the distal convoluted tubule. It indirectly promotes intestinal absorption of calcium by enhancing the renally mediated activation of vitamin D.

Ref.: 1, 2

6. What is the cause of hypercalcemia?

A. Sarcoidosis

B. Tuberculosis

C. Histoplasmosis

D. Malignancy in hospitalized patients

E. All of the above

ANSWER: E

COMMENTS: A number of conditions can cause hypercalcemia, including granulomatous disorders such as sarcoidosis, tuberculosis, and histoplasmosis. Medications can falsely elevate the serum calcium level. Examples include thiazide diuretics, lithium, and vitamin A or D. Other conditions include Paget's disease, immobilization, and malignancy. In hospitalized patients, malignancy is the most common cause of hypercalcemia.

Ref.: 1, 2

7. Routine workup of a patient with suspected primary hyperparathyroidism (PHPT) includes ruling out familial hypocalciuric hypercalcemia (FHH). Which of the following excludes FHH?

A. Nephrolithiasis

B. 24-h urine calcium

C. T-score of −3.0 at distal radius

D. Intact PTH

E. Negative sestamibi

ANSWER: B

COMMENTS: In a patient with suspected PHPT, it is important to document normal renal function before the interpretation of parathyroid function tests. The minimum testing that should be performed includes intact PTH, serum calcium, blood urea nitrogen (BUN), creatinine, and vitamin D levels. In addition, a 24-h urine calcium excretion should be measured to exclude FHH. Measuring PTH-related protein (PTHrp) is unnecessary unless metastatic cancer is suspected. FHH should be strongly considered in patients who have a family history of hypercalcemia and no previous history of normal calcium levels.

Ref.: 1, 2

8. All of the following are consistent with the diagnosis of secondary hyperparathyroidism except:

A. History of chronic kidney disease (CKD)/chronic renal insufficiency (CRI)

B. Elevated serum calcium level

C. Vitamin D deficiency

D. Elevated PTH level

E. History of gastric bypass

ANSWER: B

COMMENTS: The pathophysiology of secondary hyperparathyroidism is multifactorial and can result from phosphorous retention, altered vitamin D metabolism and resistance, altered metabolism of PTH, impaired calcemic response to PTH, and possible genetic mutations. The condition most commonly occurs in patients with a history of chronic renal failure. Gastric bypass has also been an increasingly recognized cause of altered vitamin D metabolism. Patients will commonly have an elevated PTH level and normal serum calcium. In such a setting, vitamin D levels should be measured and, if low, treated for a minimum of 6 weeks with supplemental vitamin D.

Ref.: 1, 2

9. All of the following are indications for surgical treatment of secondary hyperparathyroidism except:

A. Calcium phosphate product of ≤70

B. Uremic pruritus

C. Osteitis fibrosa cystica

D. Calciphylaxis

E. Tumoral calcinosis

ANSWER: A

COMMENTS: Secondary hyperparathyroidism is most commonly managed medically with the use of calcimimetic agents (e.g., cinacalcet), phosphate binders, adequate calcium intake, and vitamin D replacement. Cinacalcet works by binding the calcium-sensing receptors on the chief cells of the parathyroid gland and increasing its sensitivity to extracellular calcium. Surgical treatment is indicated in patients with (1) renal osteodystrophy, (2) calciphylaxis, (3) calcium phosphate product of ≥70, (4) soft tissue calcium deposition and tumoral calcinosis, and (5) calcium level greater than 11 mg/dL with an inappropriately high level of PTH. Renal osteodystrophy is a major issue in hemodialysis patients. The aluminum present in the dialysate bath accumulates in the bone and contributes to the development of osteomalacia. Osteitis fibrosa cystica, a type of renal osteodystrophy, is characterized by marrow fibrosis and increased bone turnover. Bone cysts, osteopenia, and decreased bone strength develop. To halt the progression of this disease process, these patients with secondary hyperparathyroidism are treated surgically. Calciphylaxis is a rare vascular disorder in which calcium is deposited in the media of small- to medium-sized arteries. As a result, ischemic damage to the dermal and epidermal structures develops. The ulcerated lesions are extremely painful and can become infected with subsequent sepsis, and eventually death. Patients with early signs of calciphylaxis should undergo an urgent parathyroidectomy, although there is some evidence that aggressive management of serum calcium and parathyroid levels with cinacalcet may be beneficial. Care should be taken in wound care management because aggressive debridement can lead to chronic nonhealing wounds since wound healing is very poor in these patients. Uremic pruritus is characterized by severe itching that is thought to result from increased deposition of calcium salt in the dermis without the visible lesions of calciphylaxis. Parathyroidectomy seems to alleviate these symptoms and halts progression to the more serious skin and vascular complications seen with calciphylaxis.

Ref.: 1, 2

10. With regard to PHPT, which of the following statements is true?

A. PHPT is more common in men than in women.

B. A common feature of PHPT is polyuria.

C. A history of nephrolithiasis is present in 80% of patients with PHPT.

D. Five percent of patients with PHPT can have multiple glands affected.

E. Familial hypercalcemic hypocalciuria is associated with PHPT.

ANSWER: B

COMMENTS: PHPT is a relatively common disorder that affects 0.3% of the human population, most commonly women. The exact cause of PHPT is unknown. In 80% of patients only a single adenoma is present, but multiple adenomas or hyperplasia can be present in up to 15%–20%. Patients with PHPT can have symptomatic or "asymptomatic" disease. Some degree of renal dysfunction is present in up to 80% of patients. Nephrolithiasis, however, is far less common, with an incidence of approximately 20%–25%. The clinical manifestations of PHPT vary widely across patients, but if a detailed history is taken, many will complain of polydipsia and polyuria from the calciuresis associated with the disease. Although PHPT occurs sporadically in the majority of patients, in a small percentage it is part of a familial syndrome. Multiple endocrine neoplasia type I (MEN-I) results from a germline mutation in the *menin* gene located on chromosome 11q12-13. Patients with MEN-I are susceptible to the development of pancreatic neuroendocrine tumors, pituitary adenomas, and PHPT. MEN-IIA is an autosomal dominantly inherited condition caused by a germline mutation on chromosome 11 that is associated with PHPT, pheochromocytoma, and medullary thyroid cancer. Patients with familial jaw tumor syndrome have a higher risk for the development of parathyroid carcinoma. Familial hypercalcemic hypocalciuria is associated with elevated calcium levels and low urinary excretion of calcium. The primary defect is the abnormal sensing of calcium in blood by the parathyroid gland and the renal tubules, which causes inappropriate secretion of PTH and excessive renal reabsorption of calcium.

Ref.: 1, 2

11. In 2014, the fourth international workshop released guidelines for the surgical management of asymptomatic PHPT, outlining indications for the surgical treatment of this disease. All of the following are part of the criteria except:

A. PHPT in a patient younger than 50 years

B. Calcium elevated to greater than 1 mg/dL above normal

C. Creatinine clearance < 60 mL/min

D. Nephrolithiasis

E. 24-h urine for calcium > 200 mg/day

ANSWER: E

COMMENTS: Guidelines for surgery in asymptomatic PHPT include age less than 50 years old; a serum calcium measurement 1.0 mg/dL (0.25 mmol/L) above the upper limit of normal; bone mineral density by dual-energy x-ray absorptiometry (DXA) with a T-score < −2.5 at lumbar, spine, total hip, femoral neck, or distal 1/3 radius, vertebral fracture on x-ray, computed tomography (CT), magnetic resonance imaging (MRI), 24-h urine for calcium > 400 mg/day (>10 mmol/day) and increased risk of stone on biochemical stone risk analysis, or the presence of nephrolithiasis or nephrocalcinosis on x-ray, ultrasound, or CT. For patients with PHPT who do not undergo surgery, monitoring guidelines include at minimum obtaining an annual serum calcium, DXA every 1 to 2 years, and annual estimated glomerular filtration rate (eGFR)/serum creatinine.

Ref.: 3, 4

12. A 54-year-old woman has proximal muscle weakness, polyuria, and a depressed mood. Laboratory workup reveals a serum calcium level of 11.2 mg/dL and a PTH level of 110 ng/L. Which of the following is the least sensitive preoperative localization study to identify an abnormal parathyroid gland?

A. MRI

B. Single-photon emission computed tomography (SPECT)

C. Technetium-99m–labeled sestamibi scan

D. Neck ultrasound

E. Four-dimensional CT (4D-CT)

ANSWER: A

COMMENTS: Although all of these imaging studies have been used to identify the location of a parathyroid adenoma, MRI is the least sensitive of those listed. Routine preoperative localization in patients with PHPT includes neck ultrasound and technetium-99m–labeled sestamibi scan. Sestamibi scan has a reported sensitivity as high as 90%. Ultrasound is slightly less sensitive (75%), but the ease of in-office use makes it a useful tool for the general surgeon. SPECT, when used with planar sestamibi, is very good at locating potential ectopic glands such as those in the mediastinum. 4D-CT incorporates contrast perfusion in hyperfunctioning parathyroid tissue over time. This additional layer provides functional information in addition to the anatomic information provided by a standard

CT scan. In a recent study, 4D-CT has shown improved sensitivity over all other modalities, especially when used in combination with ultrasound.

Ref.: 1, 2

13. Of the following, which patient is the least likely to have multigland disease?

A. A 65-year-old lady with a PTH level of 110 ng/L and calcium level of 10.5 mg/dL

B. A 22-year-old woman with a PTH level of 140 ng/L, a calcium level of 10.1 mg/dL, and MEN-I

C. A 75-year-old man with a 10-year history of renal failure

D. A 44-year-old woman with a diagnosis of secondary hyperparathyroidism

E. A 39-year-old woman 6 years after a gastric bypass for morbid obesity

ANSWER: A

COMMENTS: No study has yet identified a reliable predictor for determining which patients with sporadic hyperparathyroidism will have multigland disease. The exception is in familial, secondary, and tertiary hyperparathyroidism. Because of the nearly uniform incidence of four-gland hyperplasia, all these patients are managed with bilateral neck exploration and either total parathyroidectomy with autotransplantation or three-and-a-half gland parathyroidectomy. Although some surgeons believe that patients with higher preoperative PTH or calcium levels (or both) are more likely to have multigland disease, this has not been proved to be true in clinical studies.

Ref.: 1, 2

14. A 55-year-old woman with a diagnosis of hyperparathyroidism wishes to undergo focused parathyroidectomy. Which of the following would preclude a patient from being a candidate for this approach?

A. PHPT

B. Lack of availability of intraoperative PTH (IOPTH)

C. Preoperative imaging of a solitary lesion on only one of two localization studies

D. Previous neck surgery

E. Secondary hyperparathyroidism

ANSWER: B

COMMENTS: Focused parathyroidectomy is the preferred approach in patients who have a solitary lesion that is imaged conclusively by ultrasound, sestamibi, or other appropriate imaging modalities. If the surgeon is not attempting to visualize all four glands, the use of IOPTH to determine whether all hyperfunctioning tissue has been removed and to document an appropriate drop in PTH levels after the removal of the suspected gland is the standard of care. The most common criterion used is a 50% or greater reduction in the PTH level from the baseline 10 min after parathyroidectomy. The best clinical marker of single-gland disease is concordant preoperative imaging in combination with an appropriate correction of IOPTH levels. Previous neck surgery or lack of concordant imaging on two types of studies is not a contraindication to attempting focused parathyroidectomy. Patients suspected of having multigland disease are managed by four-gland exploration via a smaller incision.

Ref.: 1, 2

15. A pregnant mother in her first trimester comes to her clinician's office with a diagnosis of PHPT. What is the correct management?

A. Parathyroidectomy during the second trimester

B. Parathyroidectomy during the third trimester

C. Prescribing a calcimimetic agent to help reduce hypercalcemia until after delivery, when definitive surgery can be offered safely

D. Close observation and parathyroidectomy following delivery

E. Weekly injections of calcitonin until delivery, when definitive surgery can be offered safely

ANSWER: A

COMMENTS: Hyperparathyroidism during pregnancy is often unrecognized and is associated with a 3.5-fold increase in miscarriage. Loss of the pregnancy most often occurs during the late second trimester. The incidence of hyperparathyroidism in pregnancy is 0.7%. Maternal complications include hyperemesis, nephrolithiasis, and pancreatitis. Fetal complications include spontaneous abortion and growth retardation. In those who reach delivery, neonatal complications include hypocalcemic crisis within the first few days of life. Calcimimetic medications have not been used in the setting of hyperparathyroidism in pregnancy. Calcitonin has no role in the management of hyperparathyroidism.

Ref.: 1, 2

16. A patient is undergoing focused exploration for PHPT. A single large parathyroid gland is found adjacent to the left superior thyroid pole. The baseline PTH level was 300 ng/L, and the pre–pedicle clamp level was 400 ng/L. Five and 10 min after the removal of the gland, the PTH level is measured to be 200 and 175 ng/L, respectively. All are appropriate next steps in the management of this patient except:

A. Repeated PTH measurement

B. Frozen-section confirmation of the removed parathyroid gland

C. Four-gland exploration

D. Drawing blood from the contralateral jugular vein to determine the PTH level

E. Conclusion of the operation given the 50% drop from the highest preremoval level

ANSWER: E

COMMENTS: Although this patient did experience a 50% drop from the highest preremoval level, 200 ng/L is still quite elevated. When the surgeon is going to accept a 50% drop, the final level should either approach normal or be following a kinetic trend toward normal. A preexcision level that is within a few-fold elevation of the upper limit of normal should demonstrate normal kinetics and rapidly approach normal levels within two to three half-lives of the hormone after the adenoma is removed. The first steps in this situation should be to repeat the PTH level 15 to 20 min following gland removal and send off a frozen section for confirmation of the candidate gland removed. It would then be appropriate to either await the results of these two tests or proceed with the four-gland exploration. The use of intraoperative PTH monitoring has revolutionized how parathyroid surgery is performed. It has allowed surgeons to perform directed operations and, before leaving the operating room, document whether a biochemical cure has been achieved with relative certainty. Many surgeons include determination of a preincision PTH level, a stimulated (pre–pedicle ligation) level, and subsequent postremoval levels at 5-min intervals until a normal level is achieved. In patients with secondary or tertiary hyperparathyroidism and stimulation levels as high as 2000 ng/L, a 90% decrease has been suggested as being indicative of cure.

Ref.: 1, 2

17. The patient in Question 16 has a repeated PTH value of 200 ng/mL (ng/L). Frozen section of the removed left superior candidate gland shows "hyperplastic parathyroid tissue." On further exploration, no gland can be identified in the left inferior location. The right side is explored, both glands are biopsied, and "hyperplastic parathyroid tissue" is confirmed on frozen section. Blood is drawn from the left internal jugular vein to determine the PTH level, which is found to be 600 ng/L. All of the following include appropriate steps in the management of this patient except:

A. Cervical thymectomy

B. Exploration of the left carotid sheath

C. Left thyroid lobectomy

D. Left lateral neck dissection

E. Exploration of the retroesophageal space

ANSWER: D

COMMENTS: The left inferior parathyroid gland has not been identified in this patient. "Hyperplastic parathyroid tissue" has been confirmed on frozen section in the three identified glands. Failure to find a normal parathyroid gland among those identified should alert the surgeon that the patient probably has four-gland hyperplasia. Failure to find the remaining gland places the patient at a high risk for persistent hyperparathyroidism. Most lower parathyroid glands are found in proximity to the lower thyroid pole. If not found at this location, the thyrothymic ligament and thymus should be explored. If the IOPTH level does not normalize after this maneuver, intraoperative ultrasound of the left thyroid lobe versus left lobectomy should be performed. Finally, *central* neck dissection and exploration of the left carotid sheath are performed. The procedure is terminated after these steps, and further imaging and localization studies should be undertaken if the patient has persistent hyperparathyroidism.

Ref.: 1, 2

18. The most common site of an ectopic parathyroid gland in a patient with persistent or recurrent hyperparathyroidism is:

A. Paraesophageal

B. Mediastinal

C. Intrathymic

D. Intrathyroidal

E. In the carotid sheath

ANSWER: D

COMMENTS: The most common causes for persistent and recurrent hyperparathyroidism include ectopic parathyroids, unrecognized hyperplasia, or supernumerary glands. The most common ectopic location is paraesophageal (28%), followed by mediastinal (26%), intrathymic (25%), intrathyroidal (11%), carotid sheath (9%), and high cervical or undescended (2%). Less common causes include missed adenoma in a normal position, incomplete resection of an abnormal gland, parathyroid carcinoma, and parathyromatosis.

Ref.: 2

19. All of the following have been associated with an increased risk for hungry bone syndrome after parathyroidectomy except:

A. Graves' disease

B. Tertiary hyperparathyroidism

C. Preoperative PTH level

D. Age

E. Large single adenomas

ANSWER: C

COMMENTS: "Hungry bone syndrome" is characterized by post-parathyroidectomy hypocalcemia and hypophosphatemia. Patients most at risk are those with four-gland hyperplasia from secondary or tertiary hyperparathyroidism. The postoperative calcium level in these patients can drop critically low and necessitate intravenous calcium supplementation. During this period both serum calcium and phosphate levels must be monitored closely. In some patients it can take more than 4 to 5 days for serum calcium and phosphate levels to stabilize. Other patients shown to have increased risk for this condition are those who are older or have concomitant thyrotoxicosis or a large single adenoma. The preoperative PTH level has not been found to be an independent predictor of whether "hungry bone syndrome" will develop postoperatively.

Ref.: 1, 2

20. A patient comes to the emergency department with increasing confusion, muscle weakness, nausea, vomiting, and fatigue. The serum calcium level is 16.4 mg/dL. A previously measured calcium level was 11 with a PTH of 247. The first step in the management of this patient should be:

A. Emergency parathyroidectomy

B. Aggressive intravenous hydration

C. Initiation of furosemide infusion

D. Continuous calcitonin infusion

E. Initiation of bisphosphonates

ANSWER: B

COMMENTS: The first step in the management of this patient with hypercalcemia should be aggressive immediate IV hydration with 0.9% saline solution and a goal urine output above 100 mL/h. After an adequate urine output is established, a loop diuretic should be given to facilitate the renal clearance of calcium. Other adjuncts include the use of bisphosphonates, calcitonin, mithramycin, gallium nitrate, and glucocorticoids. Table 17.1 lists therapies used to treat hypercalcemic crisis, along with the onset of action, advantages, and disadvantages of each treatment.

Ref.: 1, 2

21. Which of the following is the first sign or symptom of hypocalcemia?

A. Shortened QT interval

B. Trousseau sign

C. Circumoral numbness

D. Anxiety

E. Laryngospasm

TABLE 17.1 Management Options for Hypercalcemic Crisis

Treatment	Onset	Advantages	Disadvantages
Saline hydration	Hours	These patients are usually dehydrated	Volume overload in cardiac-sensitive patients
Diuretics	Hours	Rapid action	Should not be started if the patient is severely volume depleted
Bisphosphonates	1 to 2 days	High potency	Medications may be tolerated poorly in some patients
Calcitonin	Hours	Rapid onset	Rapid tachyphylaxis
Intravenous phosphate	Hours	Rapid action, useful in patients with cardiac and/or renal decompensation	Can cause renal damage or fatal hypocalcemia
Glucocorticoids	Days	Oral therapy, good for chronic management	Side effects of glucocorticoids
Dialysis	Hours	Especially useful in patients with renal failure, immediate reversal of life-threatening hypercalcemia	Invasive

ANSWER: C

COMMENTS: Postoperative hypocalcemia following parathyroidectomy is not unusual. The majority of patients are asymptomatic and identified only when routine postoperative laboratory tests are obtained. In asymptomatic patients, oral calcium and vitamin D should be initiated promptly. Symptomatic patients will most commonly complain of circumoral numbness first followed by tingling in their extremities. These two features are early signs of hypocalcemia. PTH and calcium levels should be drawn. If the patient is hypocalcemic, high doses of calcium should be started. If PTH is undetectable, 1, 25-dihydroxy vitamin D (calcitriol) should be started 0.25 to 0.5 μg twice a day. On examination, these patients may have carpopedal spasm elicited by occlusion of blood flow to the forearm (Trousseau sign) or contraction of the facial muscles elicited by tapping on the facial nerve (Chvostek sign). However, nearly 20% of the general population has a positive Chvostek sign. If the condition is allowed to worsen, tetany, laryngeal stridor, or tonic–clonic seizures can develop, all of which can be fatal. These patients should be treated immediately with intravenous calcium.

Ref.: 1, 2

22. A 34-year-old woman has undergone three operations for hyperparathyroidism. She states that in each previous operation the surgeon has removed pathologically confirmed hyperplastic parathyroid tissue in the central portion of her neck and nodules within various muscles of her neck. Nonetheless, she continues to have elevated parathyroid levels associated with progressive bone loss. What is the most likely diagnosis in this patient?

A. Missed parathyroid adenoma
B. Multigland disease
C. Parathyromatosis
D. Familial hyperparathyroidism
E. Vitamin D deficiency

ANSWER: C

COMMENTS: This scenario is a classic description of a patient with parathyromatosis. This rare condition is manifested clinically as recurrent or persistent hyperparathyroidism following multiple attempts at resection. On exploration, patients will have several small nodules of hyperfunctioning parathyroid tissue throughout the neck and possibly the mediastinum. It can be difficult to distinguish this condition from parathyroid carcinoma or an "atypical adenoma." Parathyromatosis is believed to result from either a low-grade parathyroid malignancy, fracture of the parathyroid adenoma capsule at the original procedure, or overgrowth of embryologic rests of parathyroid tissue. Management of these patients involves either serial debulking of the disease when it can be radiographically identified or pharmacologic treatment. Patients are rarely cured with surgery.

Ref.: 1, 2

23. A 54-year-old woman arrives for surgical evaluation with a PTH level of 280 ng/L and serum calcium level of 14.5 mg/dL. She has a past medical history of mild renal failure (creatinine, 1.9 mg/dL) and jaw tumor syndrome. The most likely diagnosis in this patient is:

A. Parathyromatosis
B. Missed adenoma
C. Parathyroid carcinoma
D. Secondary hyperparathyroidism
E. Tertiary hyperparathyroidism

ANSWER: C

COMMENTS: A preoperative serum calcium level greater than 14 mg/dL, a palpable nodule, and adherence to surrounding tissues have all been found to be useful predictors of parathyroid carcinoma. Additionally, patients with familial hyperparathyroidism with jaw tumor syndrome, which is associated with tumor suppressor locus HRPT2 (parafibromin or CDC73) on chromosome 1, have an increased risk for parathyroid cancer. Parathyroid carcinoma is rare and represents just 1% of all cases of PHPT. The prognosis is extremely poor, and most patients have advanced disease when initially seen. Parathyroid carcinoma should be suspected in a patient with a preoperative calcium level greater than 14 mg/dL or a serum PTH level two to three times the upper limit of normal. Intraoperatively, parathyroid cancers are typically large and less brown than a benign parathyroid adenoma. Invasion or adherence to the surrounding tissues should also raise suspicion for parathyroid carcinoma. Appropriate surgical management of this condition entails en bloc resection of the tumor with ipsilateral thyroid lobectomy. It is *not* necessary to perform a total thyroidectomy. A compartment-oriented lymph node dissection is necessary only if there is gross evidence of lymph node involvement.

Ref.: 1, 2

24. Which of the following is not part of the standard workup of a patient with persistent or recurrent hyperparathyroidism?

A. Selective venous sampling
B. SPECT
C. Technetium-Tc-99m-sestamibi scanning
D. Ultrasound
E. Positron emission tomography (PET)

ANSWER: E

COMMENTS: Persistent hypercalcemia is characterized by hypercalcemia that fails to correct after parathyroidectomy. Recurrent hyperparathyroidism occurs less frequently and is defined by the development of postoperative hypercalcemia at least 6 months after having achieved normocalcemia. Preoperative localization is the mainstay of treatment algorithms for patients with persistent or recurrent hyperparathyroidism. The tests available can be divided into those that are noninvasive versus invasive. The noninvasive tests include ultrasound, sestamibi scanning, SPECT, MRI, standard CT, and 4D-CT. Invasive testing includes selective venous sampling and intraoperative radioprobe guidance. Patients receive intravenous technetium-99m in the morning of the surgery, and then the radioprobe is used intraoperatively to identify the parathyroid gland. One limitation of this technology is a high background level, which can prevent the identification of an intrathyroidal parathyroid gland. PET has yet to have any defined role in parathyroid localization.

Ref.: 1, 2

REFERENCES

1. Hanks JB, Salomone LJ. The parathyroid glands. In: Townsend CM, Beauchamp RD, Evers BM, et al., eds. *Sabiston Textbook of Surgery: The Biological Basis of Modern Surgical Practice*. 19th ed. Philadelphia: WB Saunders; 2012.
2. Lal G, Clark OH. Thyroid, parathyroid and adrenal. In: Brunicardi FC, Andersen DK, Billiar TR, et al., eds. *Schwartz's Principles of Surgery*. 10th ed. New York: McGraw-Hill; 2015.
3. Udelsman R, Åkerström G, Biagini C, et al. The surgical management of asymptomatic primary hyperparathyroidism: proceedings of the Fourth International Workshop. *J Clin Endocrinol Metab*. 2014;99:3595–3606.
4. Bilezikian JP, Brandi ML, Eastell R, et al. Guidelines for the management of asymptomatic primary hyperparathyroidism: summary statement from the Fourth International Workshop. *J Clin Endocrinol Metab*. 2014;99:3561–3569.

CHAPTER 18

ADRENAL

Samer R. Rajjoub, M.D., and Shabirhusain S. Abadin, M.D.

1. Which of the following statements regarding the anatomy of the adrenal glands is incorrect?
   A. They are retroperitoneal organs.
   B. The right adrenal gland is semilunar in shape.
   C. They are yellow or sulfur in appearance.
   D. The left adrenal is closely associated with the spleen and tail of the pancreas.
   E. The adrenal medulla is derived from the neural crest tissue.

ANSWER: B

COMMENTS: The adrenal glands are retroperitoneal organs located superior and medial to the kidneys. The right gland is pyramidal in shape (resembling a Witch's hat), and the left gland is semilunar in shape. The adrenal gland is divided into two parts, a cortex and a medulla, which account for approximately 80%–90% and 10%–20% of the gland's volume, respectively. Histologically, the cortex is divided into the outer zona glomerulosa, the middle zona fasciculata, and the inner zona reticularis. The adrenal medulla is composed of chromaffin cells derived from the neural crest tissue.

Ref.: 1, 2

2. In regard to the vascular anatomy of the adrenal gland, which of the following statements is incorrect?
   A. The superior arterial supply arises from branches of the inferior phrenic artery.
   B. The left adrenal vein, joined by the inferior phrenic vein, drains into the left renal vein.
   C. The right adrenal vein enters directly into the inferior vena cava (IVC).
   D. The inferior arterial supply arises from branches originating from the aorta.
   E. The adrenal vein is longer on the left side.

ANSWER: D

COMMENTS: The arterial supply of the adrenal gland arises from three sources. Superiorly, branches arise from the inferior phrenic artery, whereas the middle branches originate from the aorta. Along the medial and inferior aspect of the gland are contributory branches given off by the ipsilateral renal artery. The anatomy of the venous drainage of the left and right adrenal gland differ. The inferior phrenic vein joins the left adrenal vein before it drains into the left renal vein and can measure 2 cm in length. Variably, the left inferior phrenic vein will drain separately into the left renal vein. On the right, the adrenal vein enters directly into the IVC posteriorly and is shorter and broader than the left one. This shorter configuration can make ligation technically more challenging.

Ref.: 1, 2

3. What is the rate-limiting enzyme of catecholamine synthesis?
   A. Tyrosine hydroxylase
   B. Monoamine oxidase
   C. Dopamine β-hydroxylase
   D. Dopa decarboxylase
   E. Phenylethanolamine-*N*-methyltransferase (PNMT)

ANSWER: A

COMMENTS: Tyrosine hydroxylase is the rate-limiting enzyme in catecholamine synthesis. The first step in catecholamine synthesis involves the conversion of L-tyrosine into dihydroxyphenylalanine (L-dopa) by the enzyme tyrosine hydroxylase. Dopa decarboxylase then converts L-dopa into dopamine. Dopamine is subsequently converted to norepinephrine by the enzyme dopamine α-hydroxylase. PNMT is the enzyme located exclusively in the adrenal gland and is responsible for the conversion of norepinephrine into epinephrine.

Ref.: 1, 2

4. What enzyme is responsible for the conversion of norepinephrine to epinephrine?
   A. Tyrosine hydroxylase
   B. Monoamine oxidase
   C. Catechol *O*-methyltransferase
   D. PNMT
   E. Dopamine β-hydroxylase

ANSWER: D

COMMENTS: Histologically, the adrenal gland is divided into two components: the centrally located medulla and the peripherally located cortex. The adrenal cortex arises from the mesoderm and accounts for approximately 90% of the total adrenal mass. Histologically, the cortex is made up of three zones: the glomerulosa, fasciculata, and reticularis. Each zone corresponds to the synthesis of mineralocorticosteroids, corticosteroids, and sex steroids, respectively. The medulla is composed of chromaffin cells derived from ectodermal neural crest cells. The chromaffin cells are innervated by sympathetic fibers traveling from the sympathetic chain.

They secrete the vasoactive catecholamines, epinephrine and norepinephrine. Norepinephrine is converted to epinephrine by the enzyme PNMT. This enzyme is exclusively located within the adrenal medulla and is not found in ectopic adrenal medullary tissue. Thus ectopic pheochromocytomas are incapable of producing epinephrine since they lack this enzyme.

Ref.: 1, 2

5. Aldosterone secretion is under the control of all of the following except:

A. Potassium

B. Adrenocorticotropic hormone (ACTH)

C. Angiotensin II

D. Heparin

E. Epinephrine

ANSWER: E

COMMENTS: Aldosterone synthesis is under the control of angiotensin II, potassium, and, to a lesser extent, ACTH. Its synthesis is inhibited by somatostatin, dopamine, atrial natriuretic factor, and heparin. Aldosterone synthase (CYP11B2) is restricted to the zona glomerulosa, where aldosterone is primarily synthesized. Angiotensin II and potassium stimulate aldosterone secretion by increasing the transcription of CYP11B2. ACTH increases aldosterone secretion by no more than 10%–20% over baseline values and does so by stimulating the earlier pathways of adrenal steroidogenesis. Epinephrine plays no direct regulatory role in aldosterone synthesis.

Ref.: 1, 2

6. Congenital adrenal hyperplasia (CAH) is most commonly caused by a deficiency of which of the following enzymes?

A. 21-Hydroxylase

B. 17α-Hydroxylase

C. 11β-Hydroxylase

D. 5α-Reductase

E. 21β-Hydroxylase

ANSWER: A

COMMENTS: The most common cause of CAH is mutations or deletions of *CYP21A2*, the gene that encodes for 21-hydroxylase. This enzyme defect accounts for more than 90% of the cases of CAH. In most patients, it is manifested as a salt-wasting form in which lack of the 21-hydroxylase enzyme impedes the downstream synthesis of aldosterone. Clinically, this becomes apparent within the first few months of life with the development of hypovolemia and hyperkalemia. There is excess production of ACTH because of the lack of negative feedback on steroid synthesis. Upstream precursors accumulate as a result of lack of the 21-hydroxylase enzyme and are then shunted into the sex steroidogenesis pathway. This leads to the presence of ambiguous genitalia in females. The diagnosis is made by finding elevated levels of 17-hydroxyprogesterone, the 21-hydroxylase substrate, and by genetic testing.

Ref.: 1, 2

7. A 75-year-old male patient is currently being treated in the surgical intensive care unit for urosepsis following partial colectomy. His laboratory values are as follows: hemoglobin, 8 g/dL; white blood cell count, 8 × 103 cells/μL; and blood glucose, 34 mg/dL. In postoperative week 2, increasing pressor requirements develop suddenly in this patient, whose sepsis had been resolving despite broadening his antibiotic coverage and blood cultures being negative. You suspect adrenal insufficiency. What is the most definitive diagnostic test?

A. Serum chemistry panel

B. Morning serum cortisol

C. Cosyntropin stimulation test

D. Morning salivary cortisol

E. Mixed venous oxygen saturation

ANSWER: C

COMMENTS: Acute adrenal insufficiency is a life-threatening emergency. In the critically ill patient population it can develop in either the acute or chronic phase of the illness. In the intensive care setting, if acute hypotension that is not cardiogenic in origin and is refractory to pressor support develops suddenly, acute adrenal insufficiency should be excluded. The cosyntropin stimulation test is the definitive means of diagnosing adrenal insufficiency. This test, however, can take up to 24 h to return. In the acute setting, evidence of hyperkalemia, hyperglycemia, and refractory hypotension is sufficient to begin empirically treating these patients with steroids until the diagnosis can be confirmed. Morning salivary cortisol concentration higher than 5.8 ng/mL or morning serum cortisol concentration higher than 15 ug/dL rule out adrenal insufficiency as the cause.

Ref.: 1, 2

8. The patient described in Question 7 has worsening hypotension despite an escalation in intravenous (IV) norepinephrine. What is the best next step in the management of this patient?

A. Addition of vasopressin

B. IV fluids

C. Cosyntropin stimulation test

D. Hydrocortisone injection

E. Blood transfusion

ANSWER: B

COMMENTS: The first step in the management of a hypotensive patient suspected of having adrenal insufficiency is volume resuscitation followed by empirical steroid replacement. Corticosteroid replacement in patients with acute adrenal insufficiency should include the IV administration of either hydrocortisone 100 mg every 6 to 8 h or dexamethasone 4 mg every 24 h. Dexamethasone is long acting and does not interfere with the administration of a cosyntropin stimulation test. Blood transfusion will not reverse this patient's condition and is not generally recommended for patients with a hemoglobin level greater than 7 g/dL.

Ref.: 1, 2

9. A 30-year-old female with type I diabetes presents with nausea, vague abdominal pain, and skin hyperpigmentation. Important principles in the management of this disease include all of the following except:

A. Mimic endogenous rhythm

B. Simple monitoring and dose titration

C. Use standard treatment dose

D. Minimize the risk of overtreatment

E. Treat with glucocorticoids/mineralocorticoids

ANSWER: C

COMMENTS: In 1855, Thomas Addison described a clinical condition that involved salt wasting, skin hyperpigmentation, and histopathologic destruction of the adrenal gland. Additional clinical symptoms of the disorder can include nausea and vague abdominal pain, musculoskeletal complaints, and postural dizziness. The most characteristic feature of Addison disease is hyperpigmentation of the skin and mucous membranes. When Addison disease was first described, tuberculous adrenalitis was the most common cause of primary adrenal insufficiency. As a result of the decreased incidence of advanced tuberculosis, the current most common cause is an autoimmune reaction known as Addison disease. Autoimmune Addison disease is typically associated with other autoimmune disorders such as type 1 diabetes mellitus.

In patients with chronic adrenal insufficiency, maintenance therapy can be achieved with short-acting glucocorticoids (e.g., hydrocortisone—multiple recommended regimens), which are preferred as they better mimic the normal diurnal rhythm, longer-acting glucocorticoids (e.g., prednisone), which may be useful in noncompliant patients, and the mineralocorticoid fludrocortisone, usual dose 0.1 mg/day. Treatment regimens should be tailored to each individual patient and monitored on a regular basis. Supplemental corticosteroids are required during physiologic stress such as illness, trauma, anesthesia, and surgical procedures. One standard dose should not be applied to all patients with adrenal insufficiency, but should rather be individualized to account for the amount of glucocorticoids the patient is taking and the procedure or stress they are undergoing.

Ref.: 1, 2

10. The most common endogenous cause of Cushing syndrome is:

A. Adrenocortical carcinoma (ACC)

B. ACTH-hypersecreting pituitary adenoma

C. Cortisol-hypersecreting adrenal adenoma

D. Ectopic ACTH-producing tumor

E. Adrenal hyperplasia

ANSWER: B

COMMENTS: Overall, the most common cause of Cushing syndrome is the exogenous use of corticosteroids. Among the endogenous types of Cushing syndrome, an ACTH-hypersecreting pituitary adenoma is the most common (70%). Adrenal adenomas and ectopic ACTH-producing tumors each account for 10% of the endogenous causes of Cushing syndrome.

Ref.: 1, 2

11. A 58-year-old man is involved in a motor vehicle accident and presents to the trauma bay with a Glasgow Coma Scale score of 7 for which he is intubated. Use of which pharmacologic agent can lead to adrenal insufficiency?

A. Succinylcholine

B. Propofol

C. Ketamine

D. Midazolam

E. Etomidate

ANSWER: E

COMMENTS: Etomidate, a commonly used induction agent for general anesthesia, is a potent inhibitor of the 11-hydroxylase enzyme. It is the only inhibitor of steroid synthesis that can be given parenterally and can lead to the development of adrenal insufficiency. It is the treatment of choice in critically ill patients with hypercortisolism who are unable to take oral medications. Its onset of action is very rapid (<1 min), and its half-life is only 3 to 5 h. The medication is administered as a continuous infusion, with nonhypnotic doses ranging between 0.2 and 0.6 mg/kg per h. The infusion is titrated according to the decline in serum cortisol levels. Once the cortisol levels are brought within a physiologic range, some patients may require hydrocortisone supplementation to avoid the development of adrenal insufficiency.

Ref.: 1, 2

12. On workup, a patient is found to have elevated free cortisol and plasma ACTH levels. Further testing reveals that both low- and high-dose dexamethasone administration fail to suppress cortisol production. What is the most likely diagnosis?

A. Bilateral adrenal hyperplasia

B. Pituitary tumor

C. Adrenal adenoma

D. Ectopic ACTH-producing tumor

E. Exogenous corticosteroids

ANSWER: D

COMMENTS: Failure to suppress the cortisol production after the administration of high-dose dexamethasone concomitant with elevated plasma ACTH levels suggests that the hypothalamic-pituitary-adrenal axis is not intact. This scenario suggests the presence of an ectopic source of ACTH. Ectopic ACTH-producing tumors account for 10%–15% of cases of Cushing syndrome. Thoracic tumors are more common than abdominal tumors as a cause of ectopic ACTH syndrome. Of those arising in the mediastinum, primary lung carcinoids are the most common. Following in frequency are small cell lung cancer and thymic tumors. In approximately 20% of patients, the site of ACTH production is never found.

Ref.: 1, 2

13. A 26-year-old female with a history of deep vein thromboses presents to the office with hypertension, facial plethora, and truncal obesity. Which of the following additional features is not associated with this syndrome?

A. Hyperglycemia

B. Decreased libido

C. Hyperkalemia

D. Nephrolithiasis

E. Proximal muscle weakness

ANSWER: C

COMMENTS: Patients with Cushing syndrome can have a wide variety of symptoms. Classically, patients will have newly diagnosed or poorly controlled hypertension, glucose intolerance, and truncal obesity. Additional signs and symptoms include easy bruising, proximal muscle weakness, decreased libido, nephrolithiasis, and a flushed facial appearance (facial plethora). Nephrolithiasis occurs in up to 50% of patients with Cushing syndrome. The underlying pathogenesis is not yet clearly defined. There is evidence that patients with Cushing syndrome have elevated urinary uric acid secretion, which could contribute to increased stone formation. Additionally, there is a documented increased risk of 1.9% for deep venous thrombosis in patients with Cushing syndrome in the nonoperative setting. In postoperative Cushing patients, the risk for venous thromboembolism ranges between 0% and 5.6%. Chronic glucocorticoid excess produces a metabolic syndrome that is associated with increased morbidity and mortality. The elevated risk for venous thromboembolic disease is thought, in part, to be due to the increased prevalence of cardiovascular disease, glucose intolerance, and obesity. Some researchers have postulated that hypercortisolism is associated with a hypercoagulable state independent of these associated risk factors. Hyperkalemia is not a feature of Cushing syndrome; in fact, hypokalemia is more likely to occur given the weak mineralocorticoid effect of cortisol.

Ref.: 1, 2

14. A 37-year-old-female presents to the emergency department with complaints of abdominal pain and weight loss. On physical examination, she is found to have facial plethora, purple striae, and truncal obesity. Computed tomography (CT) scan reveals a 5.7-cm right adrenal mass with invasion into the IVC. There are no demonstrable sites of metastases. Which of the following is the best treatment option?

A. Neoadjuvant therapy with mitotane

B. Laparoscopic right adrenalectomy

C. Right adrenal biopsy

D. Observation

E. Open right adrenalectomy with tumor thrombus extirpation and IVC reconstruction

ANSWER: E

COMMENTS: Adrenal cortical carcinomas are rare with a worldwide incidence of 2 per 1 million. Size is the most important criteria to help diagnose malignancy. The majority are sporadic, but they are also associated with Li-Fraumeni syndrome and multiple endocrine neoplasia type 1. Approximately half are nonfunctioning, while the other half secretes cortisol (30%), androgens (20%), estrogens (10%), aldosterone (2%), and multiple hormones (35%). Adequacy of resection is the most important predictor of survival. Those who undergo complete en bloc resection with involved lymph nodes and other surrounding organs (e.g., diaphragm, kidney, pancreas, liver, or IVC) have 5-year survival rates ranging from 32% to 48%. Mitotane has adrenolytic activity and can be used for the treatment of metastatic or unresectable disease. Systemic chemotherapeutic agents can also be used but provide inconsistent responses. There is a role for neoadjuvant therapy in those with borderline resectable cases.

Ref.: 1, 2

15. Which of the following is least likely to metastasize to the adrenal glands?

A. Pancreatic tumors

B. Thyroid carcinoma

C. Lung carcinoma

D. Breast carcinoma

E. Melanoma

ANSWER: B

COMMENTS: The rich vascular supply of the adrenal glands predisposes them to metastases. Approximately 25% of patients with carcinomas will eventually develop adrenal involvement. The primary cancers are those of the gastrointestinal tract, lung, breast, pancreas, kidney, and skin (melanoma). It remains essential to complete a functional workup for adrenal incidentalomas even in a patient with a prior history of malignancies. If, however, the functional workup is negative and clinical suspicion is high for a metastatic adrenal lesion, in contrast to primary adrenal lesions, biopsy of the adrenal gland may be warranted to aid in establishing a diagnosis.

Ref.: 1, 2

16. A 13-year-old female presents to the office complaining of frequent headaches, anxiety, and facial flushing. Her family history is significant for acquired blindness. Which of the following conditions is not associated with her disease process?

A. Angiomatosis

B. Hypoglycemia

C. Renal cell carcinoma

D. Hemangioblastomas

E. Pheochromocytoma

ANSWER: B

COMMENTS: This patient has Von Hippel-Lindau disease with an associated pheochromocytoma. Pallor, headache, and a sense of impending doom are all relatively common symptoms of patients with pheochromocytoma. Hyperglycemia is also a relatively common feature in such patients. The insulin-producing islet cells of the pancreas are under inhibitory control by α_2-receptors. Thus with catecholamine excess, a relative hypoinsulinemia can develop and lead to hyperglycemia. Flushing, nausea, and fever can occur rarely.

Elevated plasma-free metanephrine and normetanephrine levels are the most sensitive biochemical tests to diagnose a pheochromocytoma. However, its specificity (risk for false-positive results) is lower than that of urinary epinephrine, urinary norepinephrine, urinary vanillylmandelic acid, and urinary total metanephrines. The specificity of plasma-free metanephrines can be improved by using a cutoff value of at least four times the upper limit of normal. Table 18.1 illustrates the specificity of other biochemical tests performed for the evaluation of pheochromocytoma.

Ref.: 1, 2

TABLE 18.1 Biochemical Tests for Pheochromocytoma

Test	Sensitivity (%)	Specificity (%)
Plasma-free metanephrines and normetanephrines	99	85 to 89
Urinary total metanephrines	71 to 77	93 to 99
Urinary epinephrine	29	99
Urinary norepinephrine	50	99
Urinary dopamine	8	100
Urinary vanillylmandelic acid	64	95

17. The initial biochemical screening tests for incidentally discovered adrenal nodules include all of the following except:

A. High-dose dexamethasone test
B. Plasma aldosterone concentration (PAC)
C. Low-dose dexamethasone test
D. Plasma renin activity (PRA)
E. Plasma-free catecholamines

ANSWER: A

COMMENTS: The workup of an incidental adrenal mass includes screening and secondary confirmatory testing. Screening tests include (1) a low-dose dexamethasone test or a 24-h urine cortisol (or both), (2) a morning PAC and PRA, (3) plasma-free metanephrine and normetanephrine or 24-h total and fractionated urinary metanephrines (or both), and (4) a late-night salivary cortisol test. Confirmatory tests are done when the results of initial testing are equivocal and include, but are not limited to, a high-dose dexamethasone test and a salt-loading aldosterone suppression test. Measurement of the serum ACTH level is performed once a diagnosis of hypercortisolism is established. Cortisol levels follow a circadian rhythm, which explains why random cortisol levels are not useful in the screening of these patients. When there is normal diurnal variation, cortisol should be at its lowest at late night. In patients suspected of having Cushing syndrome, an elevated serum cortisol level at 11 pm can be an early, albeit not definitive, factor in the diagnosis of the condition. For its simplicity, measurement of late-night salivary cortisol levels has increased in popularity and has a sensitivity and specificity approaching 90%–95%. A low or suppressed level of ACTH or dehydroepiandrosterone sulfate (DHEAS) concentration further supports the diagnosis of subclinical Cushing syndrome. In recent years, DHEAS has been obtained when there is a suspicion for ACC as well, as this can be elevated.

Ref.: 1–3

18. A 43-year-old woman has a 5-year history of poorly controlled hypertension, fatigue, and myalgias. She is taking three different medications, including a diuretic and β-blocker. What is the next best step in establishing the diagnosis of surgically correctable hypertension?

A. CT of the abdomen and pelvis
B. 24-h total and fractionated urinary metanephrines
C. PAC and PRA
D. Renal ultrasound
E. Saline suppression testing

ANSWER: C

COMMENTS: The most likely diagnosis in this patient is primary hyperaldosteronism. There is a general consensus that all patients with young age, poorly controlled hypertension, and a history of hypokalemia should undergo evaluation for an aldosterone-secreting adenoma. Hypokalemia can be associated with myalgias, constipation, and fatigue. The initial step is measuring the aldosterone-to-renin ratio. This test should be performed after discontinuing such interfering medications as spironolactone. An aldosterone-to-renin ratio of greater than 20 (e.g., a serum aldosterone level of ≥10 ng/dL with a renin level of <0.5 ng/mL) is suggestive of the diagnosis. The diagnosis is then confirmed by doing a 24-h urine aldosterone, sodium, and potassium test with the patient ingesting a high-salt diet. A 24-h urinary aldosterone level greater than 12 μg in 24 h is considered positive. After establishing the biochemical diagnosis, the next step is to determine whether there is laterality of the disease. Only at this time should diagnostic imaging be ordered.

Ref.: 1–3

19. Biochemical testing confirms the diagnosis of primary hyperaldosteronism in the patient in Question 18. The next step in the management should be:

A. Imaging repeated in 6 months
B. Long-term management with spironolactone
C. Bilateral cortical-sparing adrenalectomies
D. Selective venous sampling
E. Laparoscopic ultrasound

ANSWER: D

COMMENTS: After establishing the biochemical diagnosis, the next step is to determine whether there is laterality of the disease. Selective venous sampling is indicated when patients are >40 years old, have bilateral adrenal lesions, or no visible adrenal lesion on imaging. Adrenal vein sampling (AVS) is done by performing simultaneous measurements of serum cortisol and aldosterone in the cannulated adrenal veins and the peripheral circulation. Confirmation of successful cannulation is established by documenting a greater than five-fold elevation in cortisol concentration relative to the peripheral circulation. Lateralization is confirmed by an unbalanced ratio of aldosterone to cortisol when comparing one side with the other. Corrected aldosterone/cortisol ratios (i.e., aldosterone/cortisol ratio of one side to aldosterone/cortisol ratio of the other side) of greater than 4:1 are indicative of a unilateral source of aldosterone excess.

Ref.: 1–3

20. The patient in Question 18 undergoes diagnostic imaging. What is the most likely finding on imaging?

A. Bilateral idiopathic adrenal hyperplasia
B. Unilateral adenoma
C. Normal-appearing adrenal glands
D. Bilateral adrenal adenomas
E. Unilateral adrenal hyperplasia

ANSWER: A

COMMENTS: The most common cause of primary hyperaldosteronism is bilateral idiopathic hyperplasia (60%–70%). The second most common cause is an aldosterone-producing adenoma (35%), also known as Conn's syndrome. The remaining subtypes include unilateral adrenal hyperplasia (2%), carcinoma (<1%), and familial hyperaldosteronism types I and II (<1%). It is important to distinguish which subtype of hyperaldosteronism a patient has because some types, including bilateral idiopathic hyperplasia, are managed nonoperatively.

Secondary hyperaldosteronism is the result of increased renin production by the kidney. This condition can be the consequence of reduced intravascular volume as is seen in congestive heart failure, cirrhosis, nephrosis, renovascular hypertension, Bartter syndrome, and pregnancy. Adrenal function is normal, and treatment is directed at the underlying condition.

Ref.: 1, 2

21. A 55-year-old male smoker with no previous medical history comes to the surgical clinic after having recently undergone CT for nonspecific abdominal pain. A 2.5-cm left adrenal mass was identified on CT. What is the next step in the management of the incidental adrenal mass in this patient?

A. Magnetic resonance imaging (MRI)

B. CT-guided fine-needle aspiration (FNA) biopsy

C. Biochemical workup

D. Observation and follow-up CT in 6 months

E. CT of the lung

ANSWER: C

COMMENTS: Despite no previous history suggesting an underlying biochemical syndrome, the first step in the management of an incidental adrenal lesion is to complete a functional evaluation. If the lesion is nonfunctional, the next step in the management is to distinguish benign from malignant disease. MRI can be useful in this regard, but most times an index of suspicion for a malignant process can be garnered from CT alone. An image-guided biopsy is *not* believed to be useful in helping differentiate benign from malignant adrenal lesions. According to the National Institutes of Health State-of-the-Science Conference on the workup of adrenal incidentalomas, FNA is recommended in patients with a history of malignancy and no other signs of metastases. Before percutaneous biopsy, it is imperative that the presence of a pheochromocytoma be excluded since a life-threatening pheochromocytoma crisis can occur with this intervention. Metastatic lung cancer should be considered in the differential diagnosis, but CT of the lung should not be the initial step in this patient.

Ref.: 1–3

22. A 66-year-old woman has a 3.8-cm left adrenal mass noted on CT. On review of the CT scan, which of the following suggests a benign lesion?

A. Mass larger than 4 cm

B. Contrast washout of less than 50% at 10 min

C. Unilateral lesion

D. Heterogeneous enhancement

E. Less than 10 Hounsfield units (HU)

ANSWER: E

COMMENTS: In the evaluation of nonfunctional tumors, there are a number of radiographic findings that can assist the clinician in determining whether a lesion is likely to be benign or malignant (Table 18.2). Measurement of HU on CT is a commonly used parameter and is associated with acceptable rates of specificity and sensitivity when other features such as size, shape, or growth are considered. Less than 10 HU on noncontrast CT is indicative of a benign lesion. When IV contrast material is administered and delayed imaging is performed, the rapidity of washout of the contrast agent can be measured. Benign lesions typically demonstrate rapid washout, with a greater than 50% loss of initial attenuation on delayed imaging at 10 to 15 min. Less than 50% washout suggests malignancy or pheochromocytoma. Lipid-poor adenomas may have values of 20 to 40 HU on noncontrast CT but will demonstrate >50% washout at 10 to 15 min.

Ref.: 1–3

23. The patient in Question 22 undergoes repeat CT in 1 year, followed by MRI. CT shows the lesion has grown from 3.8 to 4.1 cm during that period. Characteristics on CT reveal a low-attenuation lesion of less than 10 HU. MRI shows a hyperintense lesion on T1-weighted in-phase MRI. What is the probable diagnosis in this patient?

A. Adrenocortical adenoma

B. Pheochromocytoma

C. ACC

D. Myelolipoma

E. Aldosteronoma

ANSWER: D

COMMENTS: The imaging characteristics described are typical of myelolipoma. These lesions are composed of erythroid, myeloid, and an abundant amount of adipose tissue. On noncontrast CT, they are of low attenuation and consist of nearly pure fat. On MRI, they are hyperintense on T1-weighted images. On T2-weighted images, malignant lesions are typically hyperintense, as are pheochromocytomas, while benign lesions are isointense relative to the liver. In comparison, aldosteronomas rarely get this large and are slower growing. Myelolipomas are not indicated for surgical removal unless they are causing symptoms of compression or pain.

Ref.: 1–3

24. According to the most current recommendations, at what size should operative intervention of adrenal incidentalomas be considered?

A. 2 cm

B. 3 cm

C. 4 cm

D. 5 cm

E. 6 cm

TABLE 18.2 Imaging Characteristics of Adrenal Incidentalomas

Variable	Adrenal Adenoma	Adrenal Cortical Carcinoma	Metastatic Lesion
Size	Small, <4 cm	Large, ≥4 cm	Variable
Shape	Round, smooth	Irregular	Variable
Enhancement	Homogeneous	Heterogeneous	Heterogeneous
Hounsfield units (HU) on noncontrast CT scan	<10 HU or 20 to 40 HU for lipid-poor adenomas	>20 HU	>20 HU
Rapidity of contrast washout on IV contrast CT scan	>50% at 10 to 15 min	<50% at 10 to 15 min	<50% at 10 to 15 min
Magnetic resonance imaging	Isointense relative to the liver on T2-weighted images	Hyperintense relative to the liver on T2-weighted images	Hyperintense relative to the liver on T2-weighted images
Growth	Stable, <1 cm/year	Rapid, >1 cm/year	Variable

ANSWER: C

COMMENTS: The American Association of Clinical Endocrinologists (AACE)/American Association of Endocrine Surgeons (AAES) medical guidelines for the management of adrenal incidentalomas recommend that surgical resection be considered for any nonfunctional adrenal incidentaloma 4 cm or larger. Observation is appropriate for lesions smaller than 4 cm. In distinguishing between a malignant tumor and a benign lesion, size alone was associated with a 93% sensitivity and 24% specificity using the cutoff of 4 cm. With improved imaging and the use of laparoscopy in adrenal surgery, more benign tumors are being removed.

Ref.: 3

25. A 22-year-old man with a history of multiple endocrine neoplasia type IIA (MEN-IIA) is found on biochemical surveillance to have elevated serum catecholamines. CT reveals a 1-cm left adrenal mass and right adrenal fullness, but no discrete mass. What is not an appropriate management of this patient?

A. Bilateral adrenalectomy

B. Left adrenalectomy with a cortical-sparing right adrenalectomy

C. Left adrenalectomy

D. Bilateral cortical-sparing adrenalectomy

E. Cortical-sparing left adrenalectomy

ANSWER: A

COMMENTS: Considerable controversy exists around the appropriate surgical management of pheochromocytomas in patients with MEN. If at initial evaluation only one side shows evidence of a mass and a unilateral adrenalectomy is performed, the chance of a contralateral pheochromocytoma developing over an interval of 12 years is 52%. Patients with MEN type II should not undergo prophylactic removal of the contralateral side if no mass or presence of pheochromocytoma is confirmed. When the laterality of the pheochromocytoma is at question and the patient's disease is relatively asymptomatic, some surgeons favor observation in young patients as nearly a fourth of patients will experience at least one episode of acute adrenal insufficiency requiring hospitalization. This is a special concern in young patients, in whom the reliability of taking medications regularly or adjusting for physiologic stressors is highly variable. Alternatively, surgeons have begun performing laparoscopic cortical-sparing procedures in these patients, in whom the success rate of avoiding exogenous steroid dependence is reported to be between 65% and 100%. Thus in the patient described here, it would be appropriate to perform a left cortical-sparing adrenalectomy, a left adrenalectomy, a left adrenalectomy with the cortical-sparing removal of the right, or a bilateral cortical-sparing adrenalectomy. AVS in these patients preoperatively can be a useful adjunct to assess the prevalence of bilateral pheochromocytomas when imaging is not able to lateralize the side of an active disease.

Ref.: 2, 4

26. A 44-year-old man is due to undergo a laparoscopic adrenalectomy for a pheochromocytoma. Which of the following is not an appropriate optimization strategy prior to surgery?

A. α-Blockade

B. Dysrhythmia control with medications

C. Calcium channel blockers with plan for IV magnesium infusion intraoperatively

D. Cardioversion of arrhythmia

E. β-Blockade as needed

ANSWER: D

COMMENTS: Preoperative catecholamine receptor blockade is done to reduce the incidence and magnitude of intraoperative fluctuations in blood pressure and the development of arrhythmias. A α-blocker such as atenolol should never be administered before the use of an α-blocker because α-blockade can cause severe vasoconstriction and hypertension from inhibition of the vasodilator action of epinephrine. Prazosin and phenoxybenzamine are both α-blockers and have been used routinely for preoperative α-blockade in patients with pheochromocytoma. The use of calcium channel blockers has become more popular as they are better tolerated by patients, readily available, and less costly, and can be used as a substitute or as an adjunct to an α-blocker. Intraoperative magnesium sulfate infusion is used for its cardiovascular-stabilizing properties. The benefit of these agents is that coronary vasospasm is reduced and, when given in conjunction with an α-blocker, they can reduce the dosage of the α-blocker needed.

Ref.: 1, 2, 5

27. The patient in Question 26 demonstrates signs of confusion and complains of sweating and headache several hours following his operation. His blood pressure is 130/65 mmHg, heart rate is 85 beats/min, and respiratory rate is 12 breaths/min. What is the most likely cause of his symptoms?

A. Dehydration

B. Postoperative bleeding

C. Hypoglycemia

D. Narcotic overdose

E. Incomplete removal of the pheochromocytoma

ANSWER: C

COMMENTS: In the postoperative setting, patients with pheochromocytoma should be monitored closely for signs or symptoms associated with hypoglycemia. Profound hypoglycemia can develop in these patients as a result of the rebound hyperinsulinemia that occurs with the removal of the inhibitory catecholamine effect. Liver glycogen stores may be severely depleted in these patients because catecholamines promote glycogen breakdown. Thus the patient's ability to respond acutely to the hypoglycemia is impaired. It is unpredictable in which patient the hypoglycemia will develop, so those with pheochromocytoma are usually administered a prophylactic dextrose infusion postoperatively.

Ref.: 1, 2

REFERENCES

1. Lal G, Clark OH. Thyroid, parathyroid and adrenal. In: Brunicardi FC, Andersen DK, Billiar TR, et al., eds. *Schwartz's Principles of Surgery*. 10th ed. New York: McGraw-Hill; 2015.
2. Hanks JB, Salomone LJ. The adrenal gland. In: Townsend CM, Beauchamp RD, Evers BM, et al., eds. *Sabiston Textbook of Surgery: The Biological Basis of Modern Surgical Practice*. 19th ed. Philadelphia: WB Saunders; 2012.

3. Zeiger MA, Thompson GB, Duh Q-Y, et al. American Association of Clinical Endocrinologists and American Association of Endocrine Surgeons medical guidelines for the management of adrenal incidentalomas: executive summary of recommendations. *Endocrine Pract.* 2009;15(5):450–453.
4. Wells Jr SA, Asa SL, Dralle H, et al. Revised American Thyroid Association guidelines for the management of medullary thyroid carcinoma. *Thyroid.* 2015;25:567–610.
5. Siddiqi H, Yang H, Laird A, et al. Utility of oral nicardipine and magnesium sulfate infusion during preparation and resection of pheochromocytomas. *Surgery.* 2012;152:1027–1036.

CHAPTER 19

METABOLIC AND BARIATRIC SURGERY

John F. Tierney, M.D., and Minh B. Luu, M.D.

1. Which of the following definitions regarding body mass index (BMI) and obesity is not correct?

A. BMI is calculated as weight in kilograms divided by the square of height in meters.

B. Obese individuals have a BMI of 30 or higher.

C. Normal weight is a BMI of 25 to 30.

D. Morbid obesity is a BMI of 40 or greater.

E. Morbid obesity is defined as being either 100 lb above the ideal body weight or twice the ideal body weight.

ANSWER: C

COMMENTS: BMI is calculated by the equation BMI = weight (kg)/height (m)^2. Normal BMI ranges from 18.5 to 24.9; individuals with a BMI less than 18.5 are classified as underweight. Overweight individuals have a BMI of 25 to 29.9 kg/m^2. Obesity is defined as a BMI of 30 or higher. Obesity is divided into four classes by BMI. Class I obesity is defined by a BMI of 30 to 34.9; class II obesity, 35 to 39.9; class III obesity (severely or morbidly obese), 40 to 49.9; and class IV obesity (super obese), >50.

Ref.: 1, 4

2. Which of the following statements about the epidemiology of obesity is true?

A. 15% of the US population is classified as morbidly obese.

B. The prevalence of morbid obesity in the United States equals that in Europe.

C. 50% of adolescents in the United States are obese.

D. The life expectancy of a 25-year-old morbidly obese man is 12 years shorter than that of a normal-weight man of the same age.

E. More people die of breast and colon cancer combined than of complications of obesity.

ANSWER: D

COMMENTS: In 2006, 5.9% of the US population was classified as morbidly obese, which is defined as 100 lb above the ideal body weight, twice the ideal body weight, or, most commonly, a BMI > 40 kg/m^2. The prevalence of morbid obesity is higher in the United States than in Europe; 35% of US adolescents and 20% of European adolescents are obese, defined as weighing 40% more than the ideal body weight. Each year, 300,000 people die of complications of obesity in the United States compared with a combined 90,000 deaths from breast and colon cancer. Only tobacco causes more preventable deaths in the United States than obesity.

Ref.: 4

3. Which of the following statements concerning the hormone ghrelin is true?

A. It is produced mainly by the arcuate nucleus of the hypothalamus.

B. Plasma levels increase after meals.

C. Plasma levels are increased after gastric bypass.

D. Plasma levels are increased in individuals following a low-calorie diet.

E. Plasma levels are unchanged after sleeve gastrectomy.

ANSWER: D

COMMENTS: Ghrelin is a 28–amino acid peptide predominantly secreted by the oxyntic glands of the proximal part of the stomach with lesser amounts produced by the bowel, pancreas, and hypothalamus. Ghrelin is a potent orexigenic circulating hormone that causes the release of growth hormone and influences the insulin signaling mechanism. Ghrelin secretion is increased by weight loss and by caloric restriction. Ghrelin levels are decreased after gastric bypass and sleeve gastrectomy. The rise in ghrelin levels with caloric restriction contributes to the failure of dieting to promote weight loss in obese individuals.

Ref.: 1, 4

4. Which of the following is not associated with morbid obesity?

A. Metabolic syndrome

B. Asthma

C. Uterine cancer

D. Lung cancer

E. Hypercholesterolemia

ANSWER: D

COMMENTS: Medical problems associated with obesity affect nearly every organ system. Most commonly, **arthritis** and degenerative **joint disease** affect more than 50% of patients seeking treatment. The **metabolic syndrome** is a constellation of medical conditions consisting of type 2 diabetes, impaired glucose tolerance, dyslipidemia, and hypertension. Other common comorbid conditions include obstructive sleep apnea, asthma, hypertension, diabetes, and gastroesophageal reflux disease (GERD). Additionally, accumulating evidence suggests an association between obesity and **multiple cancers**, including an increased risk for breast, colon, endometrial, renal, and esophageal cancers. The International Agency for Research on Cancer Working Group noted a similar association with gallbladder, liver, and pancreatic cancers. Furthermore, a linear relationship seems to exist between increasing BMI and higher mortality in patients with colon, renal, and esophageal cancers. No relationship has been identified between morbid obesity and lung cancer.

Ref.: 1, 4, 5

5. All of the following statements about medical therapy for obesity are true except:

A. Low-calorie diets (800 to 1500 calories/day) are as effective as very-low-calorie diets in promoting weight loss.

B. A daily energy deficit of 500 kcal leads to a loss of 1 lb of fat per week.

C. Only 3% of morbidly obese patients are able to reduce their BMI below 35 with diet and exercise alone.

D. Orlistat decreases lipid absorption in the intestine.

E. Behavior modification programs that reward patients for meeting dietary and exercise requirements promote lasting weight loss after the reward ceases.

ANSWER: E

COMMENTS: Behavior modification programs in which patients receive a nonfood desirable reward for meeting dietary and exercise requirements have been shown to lead to weight loss in the short term. Although 60% of patients are able to sustain a 10% weight loss for 40 weeks, only 8.6% can sustain this weight loss for 1 year. Low-calorie diets and very-low-calorie diets are equally effective in promoting weight loss, but very-low-calorie diets are associated with increased vitamin and nutrient deficiencies. Orlistat inhibits gastric and pancreatic lipase; it leads to a 6%–10% weight loss in the first year of taking the medication, but patients regain their weight after they stop taking the drug. Sibutramine blocks the presynaptic uptake of both norepinephrine and serotonin, thereby potentiating their anorexic effect in the central nervous system, but is also ineffective in promoting lasting weight loss in morbidly obese patients. Medical therapy alone has been shown to be ineffective in promoting weight loss in patients with a BMI > 30. It is unsuccessful in treating morbid obesity, as only 3% of morbidly obese patients lose enough weight to achieve a BMI < 35 kg/m^2.

Ref.: 3, 4

6. Which of the following patients meets criteria for bariatric surgery?

A. A 37-year-old woman with poorly controlled type 2 diabetes (HbA1c = 11.7) and a BMI of 34

B. A 42-year-old man with well-controlled depression and type 2 diabetes (HbA1c = 6.7) and a BMI of 38

C. A 68-year-old man with New York Heart Association class III heart failure and a BMI of 37

D. A 19-year-old man with Prader-Willi syndrome and a BMI of 48

E. A 28-year-old female with asthma, hyperlipidemia, alcohol abuse, and a BMI of 42

ANSWER: B

COMMENTS: Patients with a BMI > 40 or a BMI > 35 with comorbidities of obesity are eligible for bariatric surgery, according to the National Institutes of Health consensus guidelines. Patients must also have failed dietary attempts at weight loss, be psychiatrically stable without substance abuse problems, have knowledge about the operation and its sequelae, and be medically able to safely undergo a surgical procedure. The patient in option B has a BMI greater than 35 with a comorbidity of obesity, so he would benefit from bariatric surgery. His depression is well controlled and should not disqualify him from bariatric surgery, as psychiatric instability would. He would be expected to lose at least 50% of his excess body weight and achieve resolution of his diabetes; his depression might also be improved with weight loss. The patient in option A has a comorbidity of obesity, but her BMI is not greater than 35. The patient in option C has severe heart failure that would classify him as an American Society of Anesthesiologists (ASA) class IV patient, which is a contraindication to bariatric surgery; he is also less likely to benefit from a weight-loss surgery because of his advanced heart failure, which is already a late-stage complication of obesity. The patient in option D has Prader-Willi syndrome, which is a genetic disorder that leads to chronic hunger and overeating; it is an absolute contraindication to bariatric surgery because surgery will not adequately restrict this patient's appetite. Active alcohol abuse is also a contraindication to bariatric surgery (patient in option E).

Ref.: 1, 3, 4

7. Which of the following statements regarding bariatric operations is not correct?

A. Laparoscopic adjustable gastric banding (LAGB) is a restrictive procedure.

B. Biliopancreatic diversion (BPD) is mainly a malabsorptive procedure.

C. The Roux-en-Y gastric bypass is mainly a restrictive procedure with a malabsorptive component.

D. Vertical sleeve gastrectomy is a malabsorptive procedure.

E. Vertical banded gastroplasty is a restrictive procedure.

ANSWER: D

COMMENTS: Bariatric operations are categorized according to their mechanism of action: restriction of oral intake and malabsorption of ingested food. Examples of restrictive procedures include the **adjustable gastric band**, **vertical sleeve gastrectomy**, and **vertical banded gastroplasty**. Malabsorptive procedures function by creating a long intestinal channel that extends from the stomach or gastric pouch to a distal anastomosis between the small intestine and the biliopancreatic limb. This results in the malabsorption of ingested food proximal to the common channel where bile and pancreatic enzymes digest the nutrients for absorption. An example of a malabsorptive procedure with a mild restrictive component is **BPD**. The **Roux-en-Y gastric bypass** is a combined procedure that functions by creating a small restrictive pouch in addition to a malabsorptive Roux limb. The length of the Roux limb used varies from 75 to 150 cm depending on the severity of obesity. All of the aforementioned procedures can be performed through a laparoscopic or open approach. Advantages of the laparoscopic approach include a reduced rate of incisional hernias and shorter hospitalization.

Ref.: 1, 3, 4

8. A 34-year-old woman with a history of a laparoscopic adjustable gastric band placement 8 years ago presents to the emergency department with sudden-onset food intolerance 2 months after her last band adjustment. An abdominal x-ray shows a horizontally oriented gastric band. Which of the following is associated with the lowest risk of this complication?

A. Using an open surgical approach
B. Fixing the band to the stomach with anterior imbricating sutures
C. Using the perigastric technique
D. Securing the port to the abdominal wall fascia
E. Using the pars flaccida technique

ANSWER: E

COMMENTS: This patient has suffered from a slipped gastric band. Such patients most commonly present with sudden-onset food intolerance. A band in proper position should be oriented diagonally along the 1:00–7:00 axis on x-ray; a slipped band is oriented horizontally. The surgical technique for the correct laparoscopic placement of an adjustable band requires careful retraction of the left lateral lobe of the liver followed by division of the peritoneum overlying the angle of His and the pars flaccida of the gastrohepatic omentum. The right crus of the diaphragm is identified, and a tunnel is made from the lesser curvature of the stomach to the angle of His; the band is pulled through this tunnel and buckled into place, around both the pars flaccida and the stomach. The pars flaccida technique is associated with a 4% risk of band slippage compared with a 15% risk for the perigastric technique in which the band is fixed directly around the stomach itself.

Ref.: 3, 4

9. Which of the following is false about the laparoscopic gastric band?

A. A gastric band is first placed without any saline in the band.
B. Saline is initially added to the band to maintain a weight loss of approximately 1 to 2 kg/week.
C. Band adjustments may be performed under fluoroscopy.
D. Patients often require iron supplementation following gastric band surgery.
E. The gastric band was shown to resolve type 2 diabetes in nearly half of the patients.

ANSWER: D

COMMENTS: Nutrient deficiencies following a gastric band procedure are rare, as surgery does not lead to malabsorption. The LAGB was shown to resolve diabetes in 47.9% of patients and to improve diabetes in 80.8%. The band is placed without any saline; the port can be accessed for adjustments several weeks postoperatively using a noncoring needle. Saline is added to the band to increase restriction of the stomach to maintain a weight loss of approximately 1 to 2 kg/week.

Ref.: 3, 4

10. A 37-year-old woman is seen in your office 2 years after the placement of an LAGB. She has lost 80 lb, and her BMI is down to 28 kg/m^2. She states that her port site is tender and red. Her last adjustment took place 3 months earlier. What is the next step in the management?

A. Upper endoscopy
B. Computed tomography (CT) of abdomen with IV and PO contrast
C. Reassurance
D. Prescribe a 1-week course of clindamycin
E. Ultrasound of the port site

ANSWER: A

COMMENTS: The mortality associated with **LAGB** ranges from 0.02% to 0.1%, which is significantly lower than that associated with bypass (0.3%–0.5%) or the malabsorptive operations (0.9%–1.1%). The rate of perioperative complications with LAGB is 1.5%, with late complications occurring in up to 15% of patients: band slippage or prolapse (13.9%), erosion (3%), and port access problems (5.4%). Band slippage occurs when the fundus of the stomach herniates up through the band and causes obstruction; preferential use of the **pars flaccida technique** over the perigastric technique has resulted in a decrease in band slippage rates from 15% in early studies to 4% in recent studies (see Question 9). **Port access site problems** are the most common complications after LAGB and include leakage of the access tubing, kinking of the tubing as it passes through the fascia, or port flip. Most port site problems can be repaired with the patient under local anesthesia. **Port site infection** is rare (<1%) but should be evaluated with upper endoscopy because it may be indicative of band erosion. This phenomenon involves erosion of the band into the lumen of the stomach and may increase with the passage of time. The incidence remains low at 1%, and it may be manifested as abdominal pain or port access site infection. It may be caused by placement of a band that is too tight or by imbrication sutures placed too close to the buckle of the band. Treatment involves removal of the band and repair of the stomach.

Ref.: 4

11–14. A 42-year-old woman with a 20-year history of morbid obesity wants to have a "gastric bypass" because her neighbor has undergone the procedure. She stands 5 ft 5 in. tall and weighs 280 lb with a BMI of 46.6 kg/m^2. She has a history of medication-controlled hypertension and hyperlipidemia. The patient has undergone several commercial and physician-directed diet and exercise programs with weight fluctuations from 260 to 295 lb.

11. Which of the following is true regarding gastric bypass?

A. The incidence of postoperative gallstone or sludge formation is about 5%.
B. The greater curvature of the stomach is removed.
C. The gastric pouch is completely divided from the distal part of the stomach.
D. Three anastomoses are required in the Roux-en-Y reconstruction.
E. A common channel of 100 cm is created by measuring proximal to the ileocecal valve.

ANSWER: C

COMMENTS: The essential components of **gastric bypass** include creating a 10- to 15-mL proximal gastric pouch based on the upper lesser curvature of the stomach to prevent dilation and minimize acid production, complete division of the gastric pouch from the distal end of the stomach by creating a Roux limb at least 75 cm in length and constructing an enteroenterostomy that avoids stenosis or obstruction, and closure of all potential spaces for internal hernias. A gastrojejunostomy is created in an antecolic or retrocolic fashion depending on surgeon preference. Incomplete division of the gastric pouch from the distal part of the stomach remnant has been associated with gastrogastric fistula formation and weight-loss failure. A **gastrojejunostomy** and a **jejunojejunostomy** are the two anastomoses in the **Roux-en-Y** reconstruction after gastric bypass (Fig. 19.1). The incidence of gallstone or sludge formation after gastric bypass is approximately 30%. Answer B refers to sleeve gastrectomy. Answer E describes BPD/duodenal switch (DS) and accounts for the malabsorptive component of the procedure.

Ref.: 4, 6

12. The patient undergoes a laparoscopic Roux-en-Y gastric bypass. On postoperative day 5, she is tachycardic with a pulse of 130 beats/min, tachypneic, and oliguric. What clinical scenario are you most concerned about?

A. Hypovolemia
B. Postoperative bleeding
C. Pulmonary embolism (PE)
D. Anastomotic leak
E. Inadequate pain control

ANSWER: D

COMMENTS: Complications after gastric bypass can be classified as early (<30 days) or late (>30 days) and vary depending on reporting. The most-feared early complication specific to gastric bypass is a **leak at the gastrojejunostomy**. It is generally manifested as tachycardia, along with tachypnea and oliguria. Fever or signs of peritonitis may be absent. Leak rates were previously reported at 2%–3%, but a more recent study shows them to be as low as 0.3%. Imaging will show free fluid, air, or extravasation of contrast material. **PE** is another leading cause of death in the early postoperative period. It may be manifested as tachycardia, tachypnea, and hypoxia. There are no data to support a superior prophylaxis regimen, but many centers use a combination of early ambulation, sequential compression devices, and subcutaneous administration of fractionated or unfractionated heparin.

Ref.: 1, 3, 4

13. At her 3-month postoperative clinic visit, she reports that after her initial weight loss of 50 lb, she has not lost any weight in a week. She is tolerating a general diet but has vomited three times after eating steak since the operation. She is fatigued and has two to three loose bowel movements per day. Which of the following is the likely cause of her most concerning symptom?

A. Iron deficiency anemia from malabsorption of iron
B. A short Roux limb preventing adequate weight loss
C. A partial gastric outlet obstruction from a marginal ulcer
D. Thiamine deficiency
E. B_{12} deficiency

ANSWER: A

COMMENTS: Fatigue is a symptom of iron deficiency anemia, which is present in 20% of patients who undergo gastric bypass; iron deficiency without anemia is present in up to 40% of patients.

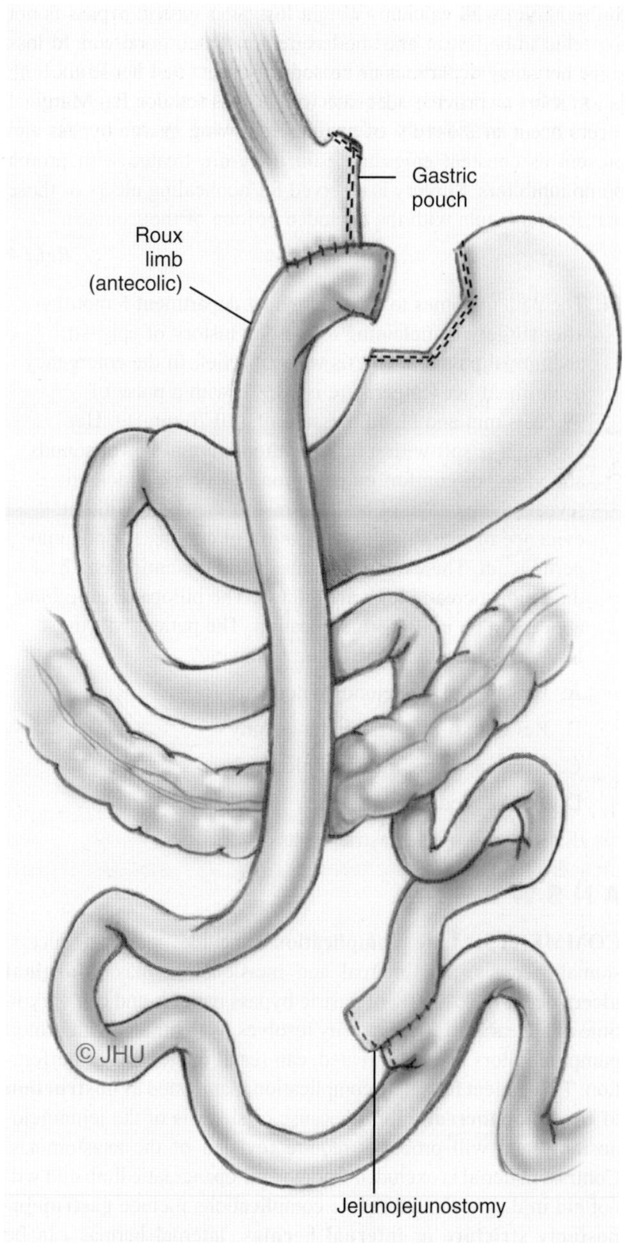

Fig. 19.1 Roux-en-Y Gastric Bypass

Iron is preferentially absorbed in the duodenum and jejunum, which are bypassed in a Roux-en-Y gastric bypass, leading to iron deficiency. It is usually effectively treated with oral ferrous gluconate. B_{12} deficiency can also occur after gastric bypass, but it is less common than iron deficiency. B_{12} is absorbed in the terminal ileum, but it must first be conjugated with intrinsic factor (IF), which is produced in the fundus and body of the stomach. Gastric bypass delays the mixing of IF and B_{12}, which decreases absorption. A several years' supply of B_{12} is stored in the liver, so B_{12} malabsorption would not manifest as anemia at a 3-month postoperative visit. Thiamine deficiency (choice D) results from persistent vomiting, which this patient does not have. Thiamine deficiency must be treated with parenteral thiamine to prevent the development of Wernicke's encephalopathy. Other potential nutrient deficiencies after gastric bypass include calcium, vitamin D, and protein; patients should be counseled on a high-protein diet preoperatively and should be prescribed a multivitamin with calcium. Weight loss after gastric bypass is not expected to be linear, and she has demonstrated good weight loss since her surgery; there is no reason to suspect that her Roux limb is too short to provide adequate weight loss (choice B). Marginal ulcers occur in 2%–10% of patients following gastric bypass and present as constant epigastric pain; they are treated with proton pump inhibitors. Surgery is reserved for nonhealing ulcers or those that form a fistula with the excluded portion of the stomach.

Ref.: 4

14. The patient comes to the emergency department 6 months after surgery complaining of a 2-day history of epigastric abdominal pain and emesis without relief. In the emergency department her temperature is 98.9°F with a pulse of 99 beats/min and blood pressure of 140/70 mmHg. Her abdomen is soft with mild distention, normal bowel sounds, and vague discomfort on palpation. CT of the abdomen reveals the passage of oral contrast to the colon without evidence of free fluid, extravasation of contrast, or pneumoperitoneum. The excluded stomach and the entire length of the biliopancreatic limb are dilated. The biliopancreatic limb appears to be in its normal location. The patient will most likely require which one of the following?

A. Revision of the jejunojejunostomy

B. Revision of the gastrojejunostomy

C. Excision of the marginal ulcer

D. Hernia repair with a mesh

E. Reversal of the gastric bypass

ANSWER: A

COMMENTS: Late complications include marginal ulcers, stomal stenosis, and internal and incisional hernias. **Marginal ulcers** occur in 2%–10% of gastric bypass patients and can vary in time of appearance. The majority resolves by treatment with proton pump inhibitors but, if untreated, can result in stenosis or perforation. This patient has a late complication manifested as **obstruction of the biliopancreatic limb** because of stenosis of the jejunojejunostomy and will probably require revision of the anastomosis. Contrast material is excluded from the biliopancreatic limb and will not aid in diagnosis. Other late complications include **gastrojejunostomy stricture** or **internal hernias**. Internal hernias can be difficult to diagnose but are repaired by reduction and primary closure. Many surgeons advocate closure of all mesenteric defects at the time of the original operation to reduce the risk for internal hernia formation.

Ref.: 1, 4

15. Advantages of a laparoscopic Roux-en-Y gastric bypass over the open approach include all of the following except:

A. Decreased postoperative pneumonia rate

B. Decreased deep venous thrombosis (DVT) and PE rate

C. Decreased wound infection rate

D. Decreased incisional hernia rate

E. Decreased internal hernia rate

ANSWER: E

COMMENTS: Laparoscopic Roux-en-Y gastric bypass is associated with decreased respiratory complications, including pneumonia, atelectasis, and PE. It is also associated with decreased wound complications, including wound infection and incisional hernias, and shorter length of stay. Laparoscopic Roux-en-Y gastric bypass is associated with a higher rate of internal hernias, likely because of decreased intraabdominal adhesion formation. Patients with a history of a Roux-en-Y gastric bypass who develop a bowel obstruction need an urgent operation because the high rate of internal hernias increases the likelihood of a strangulating bowel obstruction.

Ref.: 3, 4

16. A 35-year-old man with long-standing morbid obesity is evaluated for bariatric surgery. He is 5 ft 8 in. tall, weighs 475 lb with a BMI of 72.2 kg/m^2, and has limited mobility requiring the assistance of a walker. His medical history is significant for hypertension, type 2 diabetes, sleep apnea, and GERD. Which of the following is true when discussing BPD as an option for this patient?

A. Malabsorption of fat-soluble vitamins is rare.

B. Protein malnutrition is the most significant long-term complication seen after BPD.

C. Postoperative diarrhea is uncommon.

D. Long-term weight-loss results are not as good as with gastric bypass.

E. A portion of the stomach is divided but not removed from the patient.

ANSWER: B

COMMENTS: BPD involves performing a hemigastrectomy that is drained by a Roux limb anastomosed to the biliopancreatic limb 50 to 150 cm proximal to the ileocecal valve (Fig. 19.2). Malabsorption is the essential weight-loss mechanism with this approach. **DS** is an American adaptation of the BPD that involves tubularizing the stomach with a vertical sleeve gastrectomy and preserving the pylorus (rather than performing a hemigastrectomy) in an effort to decrease the incidence of marginal ulcers after BPD. This provides a restrictive component to the operation. The pylorus is then connected to the Roux limb with a downstream construction similar to the original BPD (Fig. 19.3). In addition to decreased marginal ulcers, preservation of the pylorus results in reduced dumping syndrome and improved iron homeostasis. In patients with BMIs greater than 60 kg/m^2, some surgeons recommend a two stage procedure in which sleeve gastrectomy only is performed during the first operation to decrease operative risk. The remainder of the operation is performed in a delayed time frame after initial weight loss from the sleeve gastrectomy. The most significant long-term complication following BPD/DS is **protein malnutrition**, which occurs in up to 12% of the patients. **Malabsorption of fat-soluble vitamins** is another major problem following surgery, with depressed levels of vitamins A, D, and K occurring in 63%–69% of patients. Mortality rates have been reported at 1.1%, along with a 5.9% wound complication rate, 1.8% leak rate, and 4.2% reoperation rate. Following BPD/DS, three to four loose bowel movements a day, excessive flatulence, and foul-smelling stool may be normal and are results of the malabsorptive nature of the procedure. Difficulty in managing the protein and vitamin deficiencies coupled with the technical difficulty in performing BPD/DS has prevented its wide acceptance in the United States. Nonetheless, the procedure does result in significant weight loss, with studies demonstrating 70%–78% loss of excess body weight up to 12 years after surgery.

Ref.: 1, 4

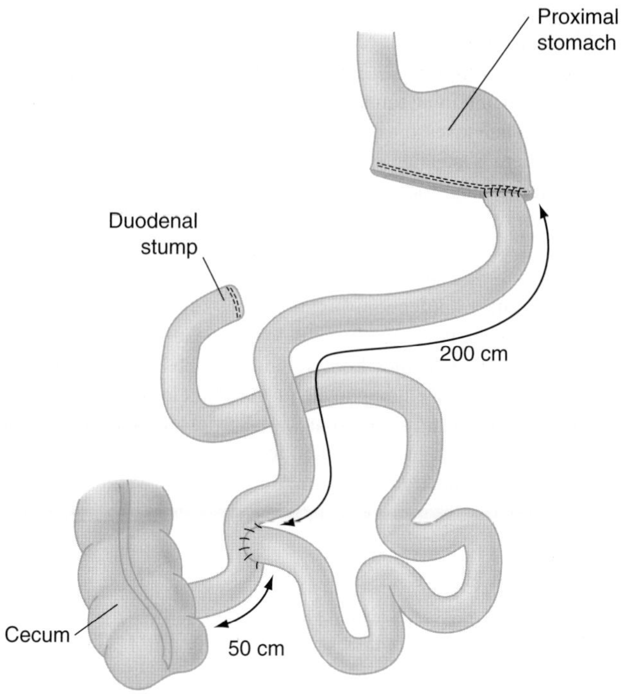

Alimentary channel = 250 (± 50) cm
Common channel = 50 cm

Fig. 19.2 Biliopancreatic Diversion

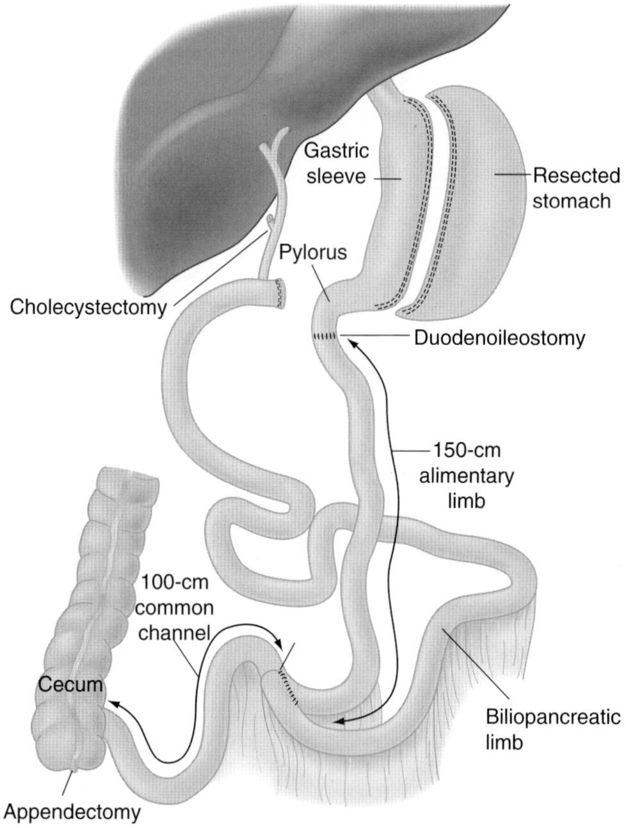

Fig. 19.3 Biliopancreatic Diversion with Duodenal Switch

17. Which of the following is true about sleeve gastrectomy?

A. It is both a restrictive and malabsorptive procedure.

B. It can be converted into a Roux-en-Y gastric bypass if greater weight loss is desired.

C. It reduces circulating ghrelin hormone levels because the antrum is removed.

D. It originated as the first part of a two-stage gastric bypass operation.

E. Weight loss with a gastric sleeve is equal to weight loss with a gastric band.

ANSWER: B

COMMENTS: Sleeve gastrectomy leads to weight loss in two ways: it restricts the size of the stomach and decreases circulating levels of ghrelin, a hormone produced in the fundus that leads to a sensation of hunger. Sleeve gastrectomy does not promote malabsorption. It originated as the first part of a two-stage BPD operation in patients with a BMI > 60 kg/m^2 to decrease morbidity. Some patients lost enough weight after the sleeve gastrectomy that the BPD stage was deemed unnecessary. A gastric sleeve can be converted to a gastric bypass if more weight loss is desired. Randomized control trials have shown superior weight loss and better satiety following sleeve gastrectomy compared with a gastric band.

Ref.: 4

18. Which of the following complications is increased in sleeve gastrectomy compared with Roux-en-Y gastric bypass?

A. Late anastomotic leak

B. Fat-soluble vitamin deficiency

C. Iron deficiency

D. Wernicke's encephalopathy

E. Internal hernias

ANSWER: A

COMMENTS: The late anastomotic leak rate is increased following sleeve gastrectomy compared with gastric bypass. A sleeve gastrectomy creates a gastric conduit with high intraluminal pressure, which increases the risk of staple line leaks. A sleeve that is too narrow at the incisura will increase the pressure proximally and the risk of leak from the proximal staple line. Proximal staple line leaks may occur early or late (greater than 6 weeks postoperatively). Early leaks are seen after all bariatric surgeries, but late leaks are seen primarily following sleeve gastrectomy. Treatment of proximal staple line leaks must include decreasing the intraluminal pressure by either endoscopic dilation or stenting of the distal obstruction. Leaks at the distal staple line occur early and are caused by a mechanical failure of the staples; they are adequately treated by oversewing the staple line. Vitamin and nutrient deficiencies are less common after sleeve gastrectomy because the surgery does not lead to malabsorption.

Ref.: 3

19. Which of the following comorbidities of obesity is not improved by sleeve gastrectomy?

A. Type 2 diabetes

B. Hypertension

C. GERD

D. Obstructive sleep apnea

E. Hyperlipidemia

ANSWER: C

COMMENTS: Patients may experience worsening of their GERD symptoms after sleeve gastrectomy. The operation of choice for morbidly obese patients with severe GERD is a Roux-en-Y gastric bypass, which resolves GERD immediately in 90% of cases. Other comorbidities of obesity, including diabetes, are adequately treated with sleeve gastrectomy. Nutritional deficiencies following sleeve gastrectomy are less common than after Roux-en-Y gastric bypass because the sleeve operation does not include a malabsorptive component. Most surgeons continue to recommend B_{12}, iron, and multivitamin supplementation.

Ref.: 3

20. All of the following conditions associated with obesity improve after bariatric surgery except:

A. Cholelithiasis

B. Venous stasis ulcers

C. Pseudotumor cerebri

D. Nonalcoholic fatty liver disease

E. Polycystic ovarian syndrome

ANSWER: A

COMMENTS: Following bariatric surgery, gallstone formation occurs in 30% of the patients and the rate is higher after a malabsorptive operation. Many surgeons will perform a preoperative ultrasound to assess for cholelithiasis and will perform a cholecystectomy at the time of a Roux-en-Y gastric bypass if gallstones are present. A 6-month course of ursodiol reduces the rate of gallstone formation after gastric bypass to 4%, but compliance to this therapy is difficult because of associated nausea, diarrhea, and pruritus. One reason to consider cholecystectomy at the time of a gastric bypass in patients with cholelithiasis is that postoperatively, the biliary system is not accessible by endoscopic retrograde cholangiopancreatography (ERCP). Choices B to E are improved by weight loss with bariatric surgery.

Ref.: 3

21. The most common indication for revision surgery after gastric bypass is:

A. Perforation

B. Protein deficiency

C. Failure to lose weight

D. Dumping syndrome

E. Anastomotic bleeding

ANSWER: C

COMMENTS: Approximately 10% of gastric bypass patients fail to lose or maintain adequate weight loss and often seek **revision surgery**. When assessing these patients, it is important to determine whether there is an anatomic defect (dilated gastric pouch, enlarged gastrojejunostomy, and gastrogastric fistula) that might be the cause of the failure. Reoperation on a patient who fails to lose weight with an anatomically intact and well-constructed gastric bypass is likely to be unsuccessful. Revision surgery is associated with an increased rate of infection, organ injury, and leakage. Revision bariatric surgery is relatively rare; 4.4% of the operations logged in the Bariatric Outcomes Longitudinal Database were performed for complications (including inadequate weight loss) and only 1.9% were conversions to a different bariatric procedure. A revision operation for an indication other than weight loss should both correct the complication and allow for continued weight loss.

Ref.: 4, 7

REFERENCES

1. Lamond KG, Lidor AO. Morbid obesity. In: Cameron JL, ed. *Current Surgical Therapy*. 11th ed. Philadelphia: Elsevier; 2014.
2. Schauer PR, Schirmer B. The surgical management of obesity. In: Brunicardi F, Andersen DK, Billiar TR, et al., eds. *Schwartz's Principles of Surgery*. 10th ed. New York, NY: McGraw-Hill; 2014.
3. Townsend CM, Beauchamp RD, Evers M, Mattox KL. Morbid obesity. In: Townsend CM, ed. *Sabiston Textbook of Surgery*. 19th ed. Philadelphia: Elsevier; 2012.
4. International Agency for Research on Cancer Working Group on Evaluation of Cancer-Preventive Strategies. *Weight Control and Physical Activity*. Lyon, France: IARC Press; 2002.
5. Zuberi KA, Magnuson T, Schweitzer MA. Laparoscopic surgery for morbid obesity. In: Cameron JL, ed. *Current Surgical Therapy*. 11th ed. Philadelphia: Elsevier; 2014.
6. Townsend CM, Beauchamp RD, Evers M, Mattox KL. Morbid obesity. In: Townsend CM, ed. *Sabiston Textbook of Surgery*. 20th ed. Philadelphia: Elsevier; 2017.

SECTION V

ALIMENTARY TRACT

CHAPTER 20

ESOPHAGUS

Ryan C. Knoper, M.D., Benjamin R. Veenstra, M.D., and Minh B. Luu, M.D.

1. Which of the following is true regarding the anatomy of the esophagus?

A. The narrowest point of the esophagus is at the level of the bronchoaortic constriction.

B. The Meissner's plexus is located in the submucosa.

C. The Auerbach's plexus is located between the longitudinal muscle and the adventitia.

D. The serosa is the strongest layer of the esophagus.

E. The outer longitudinal layer is an extension of the cricopharyngeus muscle.

ANSWER: B

COMMENTS: The esophagus is a two-layered muscular tube, and it is approximately 25 to 30 cm in length. The esophagus is unique from the other parts of the alimentary tract in its lack of a serosal layer. The inner circular muscle is an extension of the cricopharyngeus muscle. Two nerve plexuses, the Meissner's and Auerbach's plexuses, are found in the submucosa and between the muscle layers of the esophagus, respectively. They comprise the intrinsic autonomic nerve system of the esophagus and are responsible for peristalsis. Three distinct anatomic constrictions of the esophagus occur at the level of the cricopharyngeus muscle (approximately 14 mm), left mainstem bronchus (15 to 17 mm), and the diaphragmatic hiatus (16 to 19 mm), in order of increasing diameter.

Ref.: 1

2. Which of the following is true of the esophageal sphincters?

A. The upper esophageal sphincter (UES) is mainly composed of the inferior constrictor muscle.

B. The mean resting pressure of the UES is approximately 20 to 30 mmHg.

C. The lower esophageal sphincter (LES) is approximately 2 to 5 cm in length.

D. The LES can be identified by an area of hypertrophic muscle.

E. The LES resting pressure is between 6 and 26 mmHg and can be overcome by normal peristalsis.

ANSWER: C

COMMENTS: The upper and **LESs** are high-pressure zones rather than actual anatomic landmarks. The cricopharyngeus muscle is thought to be the main contributor to the upper high-pressure zone. When swallowing, UES pressure can reach 90 mmHg and return to an average resting pressure of 60 mmHg. The **LES** is characterized by a resting pressure zone of approximately 6 to 26 mmHg and measures 2 to 5 cm in length. Vagus-mediated relaxation of the LES occurs during normal food transit. Gastrin and motilin increase LES pressure, whereas cholecystokinin and secretin decrease LES pressure.

Ref.: 1, 2

3. The blood supply to the cervical esophagus arises from the:

A. Bronchial arteries

B. Direct branches from the aorta

C. Inferior thyroid arteries

D. Left gastric artery

E. Short gastric arteries

ANSWER: C

COMMENTS: The blood supply to the cervical esophagus arises from the inferior thyroid arteries, a branch from the thyrocervical trunk of the right subclavian artery. The proximal thoracic esophagus receives its blood supply from the bronchial arteries. The distal thoracic esophagus receives its blood supply from direct branches arising from the aorta. The intraabdominal esophagus receives its blood supply from the inferior phrenic arteries. The short gastric arteries cross the gastrosplenic ligament arising from the end of the splenic artery and anastomosing with the branches of the left gastric and left gastroepiploic arteries.

Ref.: 3

4. Esophageal contractions are coordinated in the:

A. Midbrain

B. Pons

C. Hypothalamus

D. Medulla

E. Cerebellum

ANSWER: D

COMMENTS: Esophageal contractions are controlled by the swallowing center located in the **medulla**. Swallowing is a complex series of coordinated events, which can be broken down into the oral, pharyngeal, and esophageal phases. The oral phase is voluntary and controlled by the medial temporal lobes and limbic system of the cerebral cortex. When a food bolus is passed to the pharyngeal phase, it becomes involuntary. This phase involves the closure of the larynx, protecting the airway, via elevation of the hyoid among other coordinated events. The food bolus eventually passes through the UES to begin the esophageal phase. Esophageal peristalsis is separated into primary, secondary, and tertiary peristalsis as delineated on manometry. **Primary** peristalsis is triggered voluntarily after swallowing but becomes involuntary after initiation. Waves travel the entire length of the esophagus and work to propel the food bolus toward the stomach. **Secondary** peristalsis is involuntary and triggered by esophageal distension or irritation. They are thought to have defensive purposes working to propel reflux contents back toward the stomach. **Tertiary** peristalsis involves uncoordinated waves that are nonprogressive and nonperistaltic, representing smooth muscle contractions and related to motility disorders and spasm.

Ref.: 4

5. Lifestyle modifications are thought to help with mild symptoms of gastroesophageal reflux disease (GERD). Cigarette smoking is thought to contribute to GERD by:

A. Decreasing LES pressure and impairing contractility
B. Increasing acid production
C. Decreasing the esophageal clearance of acid
D. Increasing secondary peristalsis
E. Increasing saliva production

ANSWER: A

COMMENTS: A number of lifestyle factors have been found to be associated with GERD, including acidic liquids and foods, smoking, drinking, obesity, supine sleeping, and certain medications. Although modification of these associated risk factors is plausible and has proven benefits in symptoms of GERD patients, they are limited and often provide inconsistent relief. **Smoking** has been proven to cause decreased pressure of the LES on high resolution manometry immediately after smoking; the pressure returns to baseline several minutes after completion. Cigarettes also lead to decreased saliva production and decreased contractility, leading to prolonged acid secretion, and impair the pharyngeal/UES reflex during deglutition.

Ref.: 5

6. Which of the following is the least important when performing a Nissen fundoplication for reflux disease?

A. Use of pledgets to prevent suture tears
B. Lengthening the intraabdominal esophagus
C. Division of the short gastric vessels
D. Hiatal dissection and closure
E. Short and floppy fundoplication around the esophagus with a bougie

ANSWER: A

COMMENTS: The principles of **antireflux surgery** (ARS) that have been studied and accepted are hiatal dissection and closure, lengthening of the intraabdominal esophagus, division of the short gastric vessels, creation of a short (2 cm) and floppy fundoplication, and the use of a bougie. Common techniques often used by many surgeons but not well established are fixation of wrap, use of pledgets, bougie size, and number of sutures used.

Ref.: 6

7. Which of the following findings is a contraindication to ARS?

A. Presence of severe esophagitis on endoscopy
B. A DeMeester score of 55
C. Type III hiatal hernia seen on an esophagogram
D. Barrett's esophagus with high-grade dysplasia
E. A shortened esophagus

ANSWER: D

COMMENTS: The indications for **ARS** are severe esophageal injury, incomplete resolution of symptoms with medical therapy, patient preference against long-term pharmacologic therapy, or complications from a hiatal hernia. The success of ARS depends on the accuracy of diagnosing GERD, which can be enhanced by monitoring pH. The DeMeester score is used to assess the degree of abnormality (>14) of the pH study. The presence of a short esophagus requires a lengthening procedure such as a Collis gastroplasty in addition to fundoplication, but it is not a contraindication to ARS. The presence of high-grade dysplasia within a Barrett's esophagus requires resection and is a contraindication to ARS.

Ref.: 2, 6

8. Seven years after her initial ARS, a patient undergoes a reoperation for recurrence of symptoms. During the reoperation, what is the most likely finding?

A. Disrupted wrap
B. Loose wrap
C. Herniated wrap
D. Slipped wrap
E. Stricture

ANSWER: C

COMMENTS: The long-term success rate of ARS approaches 90% with approximately a 1%-per-year failure rate. The most common operative finding on repeated **fundoplication** is a herniated fundoplication (33%) above the diaphragm, followed by a disrupted wrap (18%), a tight wrap (13%), and a slipped wrap (10%) onto the body of the stomach.

Ref.: 6, 7

9. Several endoscopic options exist as alternatives to surgical ARS. Transoral incisionless fundoplication (TIF) is an endoscopic wrap. Which of the following is true regarding TIF?

A. Approved for use with hiatal hernias larger than 2 cm
B. Performs a complete 360-degree wrap
C. Provides good symptom relief in the majority of patients for up to 1 year
D. Requires radiofrequency ablation to bulk LES with fibrosis
E. Can perform a cruroplasty at the same time

ANSWER: C

COMMENTS: **TIF** is a totally endoscopic procedure for performing a partial fundoplication using T-bar fasteners. This wrap is usually performed as a 270-degree to 290-degree wrap. It is not approved as a modality to treat hiatal hernias > 2 cm but is approved to reduce hernias < 2 cm. This is performed using a suction traction device to pull the stomach downward. Several studies with 12-month follow-up data have reported more than 90% of patients remaining off proton pump inhibitors

(PPIs). No trial has compared TIF to surgical ARS, and longer-term follow-up studies are required. ARS remains an option after TIF if the wrap has failed. Radiofrequency ablation is a therapeutic modality utilized in the treatment of Barrett's esophagus with high-grade dysplasia and is an endoscopic treatment option (Stretta). This technique is thought to bulk the LES with fibrotic reaction changes thus decreasing reflux. TIF does not provide a cruroplasty as part of the repair of small hiatal hernias.

Ref.: 8, 10-13

10. Which of the following is true regarding hiatal hernia repair?

A. A 5- to 6-cm wrap is recommended.

B. Mobilization of intrathoracic esophagus is required to the level of the aortic arch.

C. Permanent synthetic mesh is preferred for large crural defects.

D. Iatrogenic pneumothorax during laparoscopic repair often requires tube thoracostomy.

E. Shortened esophagus can be lengthened with a Collis gastroplasty.

ANSWER: E

COMMENTS: A 2-cm floppy wrap is recommended, providing adequate control of reflux. Longer wraps may control reflux better but have been associated with increased symptoms of dysphagia. The intrathoracic esophagus is mobilized to lengthen the intraabdominal portion in an attempt to relocate the LES at its physiologic level. This typically requires at least 2 to 3 cm of mobilization. Pneumoperitoneum during laparoscopic dissection can artificially make this length appear longer intraoperatively. Use of **mesh** to buttress hiatal hernia repairs is typically used in large defects, defined as >5 cm, or when crural dissection has left much of the peritoneum stripped. There is no consensus on the use of mesh; however, the use of permanent mesh has been largely abandoned due to problems with erosion. Often, dissection of large hernias results in the entering of one or both of the pleural spaces. Carbon dioxide is rapidly resorbed and does not require repair or tube thoracostomy. **Shortened esophagus** is relatively uncommon in smaller hiatal hernias with a higher incidence in large hiatal hernias, peptic strictures, and reoperative ARS. Insufficient mobilization of intraabdominal esophagus can result in high rates of recurrence, up to 40% in large and giant hernias. Creation of a tension-free wrap then requires lengthening of the esophagus via Collis gastroplasty. This involves excising a portion of the cardia, creating a "neo-esophagus," and thus moving the gastroesophageal junction (GEJ) and angle of His into the abdominal cavity.

Ref.: 9

11. A 53-year-old male has typical symptoms of GERD refractory to medical management and is referred to your clinic to discuss surgical options. He has previously had a distal pancreatectomy/splenectomy from a gunshot wound and three subsequent laparotomies for adhesive bowel obstruction. What surgical option allows for satisfactory control of reflux while avoiding the abdomen?

A. Toupet

B. Hill

C. Dor

D. Belsey Mark-IV

E. Gastropexy

ANSWER: D

COMMENTS: The **Belsey Mark-IV** operation recreates the LES while reducing an intrathoracic stomach and closing a hiatal defect. This operation is approached via a left thoracotomy, allowing the surgeon to avoid a hostile abdomen and is typically reserved for redo situations in the current era of laparoscopic **Nissen** fundoplication. This approach can also be useful in the dissection of large and giant chronic paraesophageal hernias. The Belsey Mark-IV provides a 240-degree partial wrap, imbricating cardia against the distal esophagus. Each of the other operations requires an abdominal approach. The **Toupet** is a 270-degree, posterior partial wrap, while the **Dor** is a 180-degree anterior partial wrap. The **Hill** operation focuses on the creation of a gastroesophageal flap valve in an attempt to recreate normal anatomy. **Gastropexy** is reserved for the highest-risk patients with hernias at risk for volvulus and can include a percutaneous endoscopic gastrostomy tube. This, however, should not be considered in patients with significant abdominal surgical histories.

Ref.: 14

12. A 55-year-old man is evaluated for dysphagia and chest pain. A barium esophagogram shows a 3-cm smooth filling defect in the distal end of the esophagus. Which of the following is true of his condition?

A. Cystic transformation or central necrosis is often associated with these lesions.

B. Patients often have hematemesis or chronic anemia because of ulceration.

C. Endoscopic ultrasound (EUS) will show a hypoechoic mass in the submucosa.

D. Endoscopic biopsy should be performed to rule out malignancy.

E. Esophagectomy is recommended for lesions larger than 2 cm.

ANSWER: C

COMMENTS: Benign tumors of the esophagus are rare and represent less than 1% of esophageal neoplasms. **Leiomyomas** account for 60% of these lesions and are often found in the distal two-thirds of the esophagus. Most of these tumors are asymptomatic. Pain and dysphagia are the most common complaints. They have a characteristic smooth filling defect on contrast-enhanced study and are described as a hypoechoic mass within the submucosa or muscularis propria on EUS. Recently, they have been classified as a gastrointestinal stromal tumor. Most of these tumors occur from mutations of the c-*KIT* oncogene. Leiomyomas are removed by enucleation, and biopsy should be avoided because of the increased risk for perforation.

Ref.: 1

13. Which of the following most likely contributes to GERD?

A. Intraabdominal LES length of 3 cm

B. LES resting pressure of 12 mmHg

C. Thirty percent tertiary waveforms

D. Total LES length of 5 cm

E. Attachment of the phrenoesophageal ligament 4 cm above the GEJ

TABLE 20.1 Manometric Features of Primary and Nonspecific Esophageal Motility Disorders

	Normal	Achalasia	Vigorous Achalasia	Hypertensive LES	Diffuse Esophageal Spasm	Nutcracker Esophagus	Ineffective Esophageal Motility	Nonspecific Esophageal Motility Disorder
Symptoms	None	Dysphagia Chest pressure Regurgitation	Dysphagia Chest pain	Dysphagia	Chest pain Dysphagia	Dysphagia Chest pain	Dysphagia Heartburn Chest pain	Dysphagia Chest pain
Esophagography	Normal	Bird's beak Dilated esophagus	Abnormal	Distal obstruction	Corkscrew esophagus	Normal progressive contractions	Slow transit Incomplete emptying	Slow transit Incomplete emptying
Endoscopy	Normal	Patulous esophagus	Normal	Normal	Hyperperistalsis	Hyperperistalsis	Nonspecific	Nonspecific
LES pressure	15 to 25 mmHg	Hypertensive (>26 mmHg)	Normal or hypertensive	Hypertensive (>26 mmHg)	Normal or slightly elevated	Normal	Normal or low	Normal
LES relaxation	Follows swallowing	Incomplete Residual pressure (<5 mmHg)	Partial or absent	Normal	Normal	Normal	Normal	Incomplete (>90%) Residual pressure (>5 mmHg)
Amplitude pressure	50 to 120 mmHg	Decreased (<40 mmHg)	Normal	Normal	Normal	Hypertensive (>180 mmHg) (>400 mmHg)	Decreased (<30 mmHg)	Decreased (<35 mmHg)
Contraction waves	Progressive	Simultaneous Mirrored Pressurized	Simultaneous Repetitive	Normal	Simultaneous Repetitive	Long duration (>6 s)	Nontransmitted (>30%)	Nontransmitted (>20%) Triple-peaked, retrograde Prolonged (>6 s)
Peristalsis	Normal	None	None	Normal	None	Hypertensive peristalsis	Abnormal	Abnormal

LES, Lower esophageal sphincter.

ANSWER: C

COMMENTS: Factors that contribute to the failure of the intrinsic antireflux mechanism are intraabdominal **LES** length less than 1 cm, LES resting pressure less than 6 mmHg, the presence of esophageal dysmotility, LES total length less than 2 cm, and a low attachment of the phrenoesophageal ligament.

Ref.: 1, 2, 5, 9

14. A 28-year-old male presents with symptoms of dysphagia to solids and liquids with regurgitation. Esophogography shows distal narrowing to a point. What is the most likely finding on high-resolution manometry?

A. Aperistalsis without relaxation of the LES with deglutition

B. Uncoordinated peristalsis

C. Esophageal pressure of 250 mmHg

D. Contraction wave of 9 s

E. LES pressure 20 mmHg

ANSWER: A

COMMENTS: This patient has **achalasia**, an esophageal motility disorder affecting 1 in 10,000. Its exact etiology is unknown, and it results from an uncontrolled balance of excitatory and inhibitory signals. Symptoms may be vague but typically involve dysphagia, regurgitation, and weight loss. Its diagnosis can be made by a characteristic distal narrowing on esophagogram, creating the classic "bird's beak" appearance. Manometry is required to confirm the diagnosis and typically displays aperistalsis with a hypertensive resting LES that fails to relax with deglutition (Table 20.1 and Fig. 20.1). High-amplitude waves, pressure, and prolonged contraction waves are characteristic of **Nutcracker** esophagus. These waves result in typically complete propagation and in LES relaxation. Uncoordinated peristalsis is present in **diffuse esophageal spasm (DES)**. The normal resting pressure of the LES is between 15 and 25 mmHg.

Ref.: 15

15. The above patient decides to undergo surgical therapy for his diagnosis. Which of the following is true regarding the surgical management of achalasia?

A. Nonsurgical therapy results in durable relief of dysphagia.

B. Myotomy should extend at least 5 cm cephalad and 2 cm caudad onto the stomach.

C. Addition of antireflux component to operation is not required.

D. Accidental esophagostomy can be repaired primarily with continued use of the same myotomy site.

E. Only the longitudinal muscle fibers are incised.

ANSWER: B

COMMENTS: Heller myotomy remains the most common surgical treatment for achalasia. This can be performed open or laparoscopically and begins with hilar dissection and mobilization of intrathoracic esophagus for visualization. A myotomy is performed to release the LES to provide symptomatic relief and typically begins just proximal to the GEJ anteriorly and extends a minimum of 5 cm cephalad and 2 to 3 cm caudad. It is important that both longitudinal (outer) and circular (inner) muscle layers be released. An antireflux component is routinely added as postoperative reflux can be disabling after myotomy. Typically, a partial wrap, either the Dor or Toupet, is used because of fear of recurrent dysphagia with complete Nissen wrap, although this has been successfully utilized. No wrap has been proven to be superior. Entrance into the

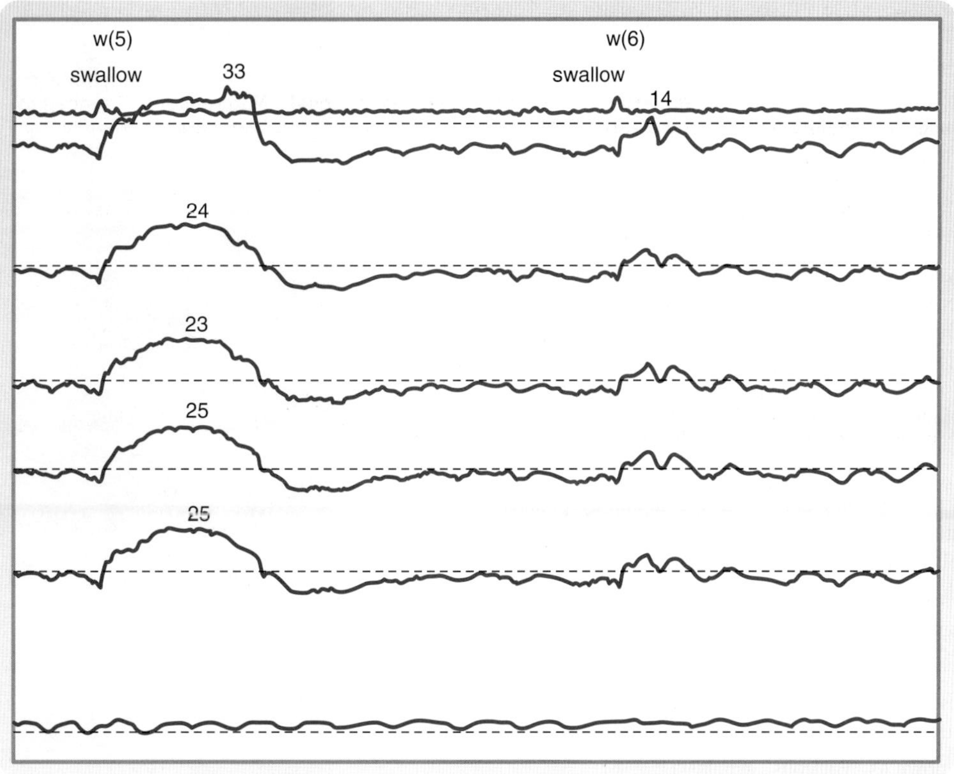

Fig. 20.1 Esophageal motility in a patient with achalasia. *(From Bremner CG, DeMeester TR, Bremner RM, et al. Esophageal Motility Testing Made Easy. St. Louis: Quality Medical Publishing; 2001:75.)*

esophageal lumen requires repair with the creation of a new myotomy site. Nonsurgical options include **Botox** injections and **pneumatic dilation**. Botox injections provide good relief but lack durability with recurrent symptoms typically occurring 1 to 4 months after injection. Additionally, Botox can significantly increase the difficulty of surgical myotomy and should only be reserved for nonsurgical candidates. Pneumatic dilation provides good relief of dysphagia but lacks durability, often requiring repeat dilations with up to half of the patients at 5 years having recurrent symptoms. The most devastating complication of dilation is esophageal perforation, and it occurs in up to 4% of patients. Peroral endoscopic myotomy, POEM, is an interesting endoscopic approach to performing a surgical myotomy and has been shown to have good results.

Ref.: 15

16. A patient arrives at the emergency department 8 h after balloon dilation of her esophagus with complaints of dysphagia and chest pain. She was found to be febrile, tachycardic, and normotensive. Esophagography showed "bird's beak" narrowing and a leak at the distal end of the esophagus with contrast material in the left side of the chest. After fluid resuscitation and antibiotics, which of the following is the most appropriate management?

A. Nasogastric tube decompression and observation

B. Endoscopic evaluation of the injury and stenting

C. Left thoracotomy, primary repair, myotomy, and drain placement

D. Laparotomy, primary repair, and gastrostomy tube placement

E. Laparotomy, esophagectomy, and cervical esophagogastrostomy

ANSWER: C

COMMENTS: The rate of esophageal perforation after **endoscopic pneumatic dilation** is low (4%). Early diagnosis plus treatment of esophageal perforation is associated with improved survival. In stable patients with a contained perforation, there is a role for nonoperable management consisting of nothing by mouth and intravenous antibiotics. If the perforation is because of an underlying pathology that causes distal obstruction (e.g., achalasia, esophageal cancer, or stricture), the operative treatment must address the underlying disease. A **myotomy** should be performed in patients with achalasia and esophagectomy considered only in those with a sigmoid esophagus or megaesophagus.

Ref.: 1, 16

17. A 42-year-old female presents with symptoms of dysphagia. Thus far, a workup has included a normal esophagogastroduodenoscopy (EGD), esophagogram, and manometry. She is frustrated with the lack of answers and is referred to your clinic by her gastroenterologist. You order a computed tomography (CT) of chest, which helps diagnose her with *dysphagia lusoria.* What findings would be present on the CT scan?

A. Left pulmonary artery arising from the right pulmonary artery

B. Right subclavian artery arising from the descending thoracic aorta

C. Double aortic arch

D. Left common carotid arising from the brachiocephalic artery

E. Late, posterior takeoff of the brachiocephalic artery

ANSWER: B

COMMENTS: Vascular rings are a known cause of tracheoesophageal compressive symptoms. They typically present the children as diet is transitioned from milk to solids but can vary widely in presentation. A left pulmonary artery arising from the right pulmonary artery and a double aortic arch may form a sling around the esophagus and cause symptoms of dysphagia but typically present at a younger age. The left common carotid arising from the brachiocephalic artery is a normal variant of arch anatomy; it is asymptomatic and referred to as a bovine arch. An aberrant right subclavian artery that arises from the descending aorta and travels posterior to the esophagus can present as dysphagia in the adult. Surgical correction is required in the symptomatic patient and involves ligation at its origin and reimplantation on the right common carotid artery.

Ref.: 17

18. A 40-year-old woman complains of chest pain and dysphagia. Manometric studies show simultaneous multipeaked contractions of 140 mmHg, lasting 4 to 5 s, and normal LES relaxation. Which of the following is true of her disease?

A. Esophagography will show a "corkscrew esophagus."

B. It can be caused by infection with *Trypanosoma cruzi.*

C. It is the result of fibrous replacement of the esophageal smooth muscle.

D. It is also known as "vigorous" achalasia.

E. Bougie dilation is the first-line treatment.

ANSWER: A

COMMENTS: DES is a poorly understood motility disorder of the esophagus. Chest pain and dysphagia are often present. The diagnosis is made by esophagography demonstrating a classic picture of a corkscrew esophagus (Fig. 20.2). **Manometry** will show simultaneous multipeaked contractions similar to those seen in achalasia; however, the LES will have normal receptive relaxation. A variant of achalasia in which amplitude pressure is normal or elevated is also known as vigorous achalasia. Pharmacotherapy (nitrates, calcium channel blockers, and phosphodiesterase inhibitors) aimed at smooth muscle relaxation is the first-line treatment of DES. Bougie or pneumatic dilations are used with variable results for severe dysphagia with documented LES hypertension. Surgery, which involves a long **esophagomyotomy** from the level of the aortic arch to the LES, is reserved for patients who fail pharmacologic and endoscopic therapies.

Ref.: 1, 2

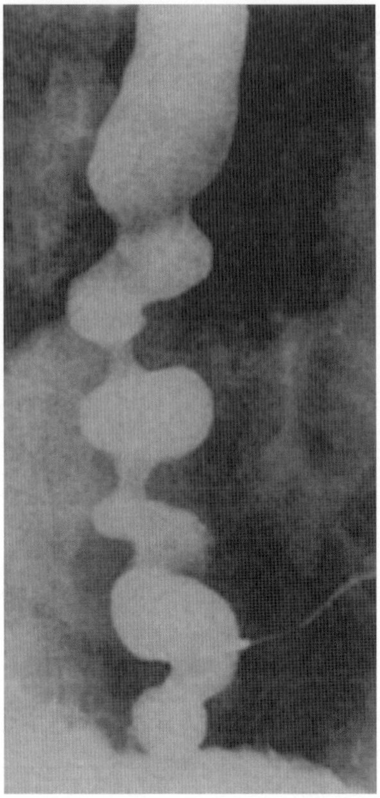

Fig. 20.2 Barium esophagogram of diffuse esophageal spasm. *(Modified from Peters JH, DeMeester TR. Esophagus and diaphragmatic hernia. In: Schwartz SI, Shires TG, Spencer FC, eds. Principles of Surgery. 7th ed. New York: McGraw-Hill; 1999:1129.)*

19. A 68-year-old male presents with symptoms of dysphagia and halitosis. An esophagogram displays outpouching at the cricothyroid on lateral view. Which of the following is true regarding his condition?

A. It is a true diverticulum.

B. Endoscopic esophagodiverticulostomy is best for small, <2 cm, diverticula.

C. Diverticulectomy alone is sufficient.

D. It is caused by a traction mechanism.

E. Diverticulopexy and myotomy are preferred approaches.

ANSWER: E

COMMENTS: Esophageal diverticula may be classified by type (true or false), location, and pathophysiology (traction or pulsion). **Parabronchial** diverticula are the only true diverticula and result from traction associated with inflamed mediastinal lymph nodes. **Epiphrenic** diverticula are false resulting from pulsion and occur in the distal esophagus. **Zenkers**, or pharyngoesophageal, diverticula occur in Killian's triangle at the level of the cricopharyngeus and are thought to be the result of increased pressure and pulsion during swallowing. Symptoms involve dysphagia, halitosis, and regurgitation. Symptomatic Zenkers requires surgical therapy. **Diverticulopexy** and **myotomy** remain the preferred approaches, minimizing potential salivary fistulas that **diverticulectomy** predisposes. For small diverticula, myotomy alone has proven sufficient. Videoendoscopic stapling via **esophagodiverticulostomy** combines the myotomy and enlarges the pouch but is contraindicated in diverticula < 3 cm. This is because there is insufficient room for placement of the stapler jaws.

Ref.: 18

20. A 65-year-old man with a 10-year history of heartburn undergoes an endoscopy with a distal esophageal biopsy, which shows intestinal columnar metaplasia. Which of the following is true of his condition?

A. The metaplastic cells are more prone to reflux injury than the squamous epithelium.

B. The condition is found in 50% of patients with GERD.

C. *Helicobacter pylori* is associated with the condition.

D. More than 70% of cases are found in men in their fifth and sixth decades.

E. The condition is associated with a fivefold increase in the risk for adenocarcinoma.

ANSWER: D

COMMENTS: Esophageal mucosal injuries result from reflux of gastric juice that may contain bile salts from the duodenum. Within a pH range of 2 to 6.5, bile salts are soluble and nonionized; they are therefore better absorbed by esophageal mucosa cells and cause the greatest cell damage. **Barrett's esophagus** is a condition in which intestinal columnar epithelium replaces the esophageal squamous epithelium as a result of inflammation secondary to chronic reflux. The metaplastic cells are more resistant to injury from reflux but are more prone to malignant transformation. Barrett's esophagus is found in 10% of patients with GERD, and more than 70% of cases are found in men aged 55 to 63 years. Patients with Barrett's esophagus have a 40-fold increased risk for esophageal carcinoma.

Ref.: 1

21. The patient in the above question is found to have high-grade dysplasia on follow-up surveillance. Which of the following is true regarding Barrett's esophagus with high-grade dysplasia?

A. Surveillance endoscopy every 6 months is acceptable.

B. Photodynamic therapy (PDT) is superior to radiofrequency ablation.

C. Surveillance protocol dictates four-quadrant biopsies at the z-line.

D. ARS is indicated.

E. His risk of progression to adenocarcinoma is 6% per year.

ANSWER: E

COMMENTS: The treatment of Barrett's esophagus varies depending on the presence or absence of dysplasia and whether it is low or high grade. The differentiation between low-grade dysplasia (LGD) and high-grade dysplasia (HGD) is purely histologic and subjective with reported interobserver variability (LGD < 50% agreement vs. HGD 85% agreement). Barrett's without dysplasia may be observed every 3 to 5 years via endoscopy with biopsies. Treatment consists of managing the acidic reflux and includes medical therapy with PPI and ARS. **LGD** requires initial 6-month **surveillance** endoscopies with biopsies performed in four quadrants every 1 cm with subsequent endoscopies yearly. **HGD** should be treated; if it is not treated, it should be surveilled every 3 months. Endoscopic therapies for dysplasia include **radiofrequency ablation** and **PDT**; however, no head-to-head trial has been performed to show superiority. Endoscopic mucosal resection, **EMR**, is a less invasive option for evaluation of the depth of lesions as well as resection of HGD and early adenocarcinoma, T1a lesions < 2 cm. The risk of progression of HGD to adenocarcinoma is 6% per year; for nondysplastic Barrett's esophagus, it is approximately 0.5% per year, which is similar to colon polyps.

Ref.: 19

22. An otherwise healthy 40-year-old man seeks treatment in the emergency department because of hematemesis after a night of binge drinking and retching. Which of the following is true of his condition?

A. It is caused by a pulsion diverticulum.

B. Endoscopy should not be performed because of the increased risk for perforation.

C. The bleeding is from an arterial source.

D. Surgical resection is often required.

E. *H. pylori* infection is a known risk factor.

ANSWER: C

COMMENTS: Mallory-Weiss tears are linear tears in the esophagogastric mucosa that cause bleeding in patients with repeated emesis. The diagnosis is made by endoscopy, and most bleeding stops spontaneously. Because the source of the bleeding is arterial, pressure tamponade is not helpful and may lead to perforation of the esophagus. For refractory bleeding, endoscopic injection or cautery can be used, but definitive treatment requires a gastrotomy and suture ligation.

Ref.: 20

23. A 60-year-old man has GERD and episodic dysphagia. An upper gastrointestinal contrast-enhanced study shows a type I hiatal hernia and thin band-like narrowing of the distal end of the esophagus. Which of the following is true of his condition?

A. Oral dilation is the treatment of choice.

B. It is the result of hypertrophy of the circular muscle layer.

C. Endoscopic mucosal resection is recommended.

D. There is squamous mucosa above and below the narrowing.

E. Surgical resection is indicated.

ANSWER: A

COMMENTS: Schatzki rings are concentric constrictions of the distal end of the esophagus (Fig. 20.3) occurring at the squamocolumnar junction; as a result, there is esophageal mucosa above and gastric mucosa below. The rings consist of muscularis mucosa, connective tissue, and submucosal fibrosis. Treatment involves oral dilation, which can provide relief for up to 18 months. Excision of the rings should be avoided because the esophageal strictures that result from resection are much more difficult to manage.

Ref.: 1

24. With regard to squamous cell carcinoma of the esophagus, which of the following is true?

A. Worldwide, it is the most common type of esophageal cancer.

B. It affects mainly Caucasian males.

C. It has a strong association with columnar epithelial metaplasia.

D. There is no proven association with alcohol or tobacco.

E. The male-to-female ratio is 15:1.

ANSWER: C

COMMENTS: Esophageal cancer is the sixth most common malignancy and has an incidence of 20 per 100,000 in the United States. Worldwide, squamous cell carcinoma is the most common type; however, in the United States, adenocarcinoma accounts for up to 70% of patients with esophageal cancer. The male-to-female ratio is 3:1 for squamous cell carcinoma and 15:1 for adenocarcinoma. In addition, squamous cell carcinoma mainly affects African-American men, whereas adenocarcinoma mainly affects white men. Alcohol and tobacco smoking increase the risk for esophageal cancer fivefold

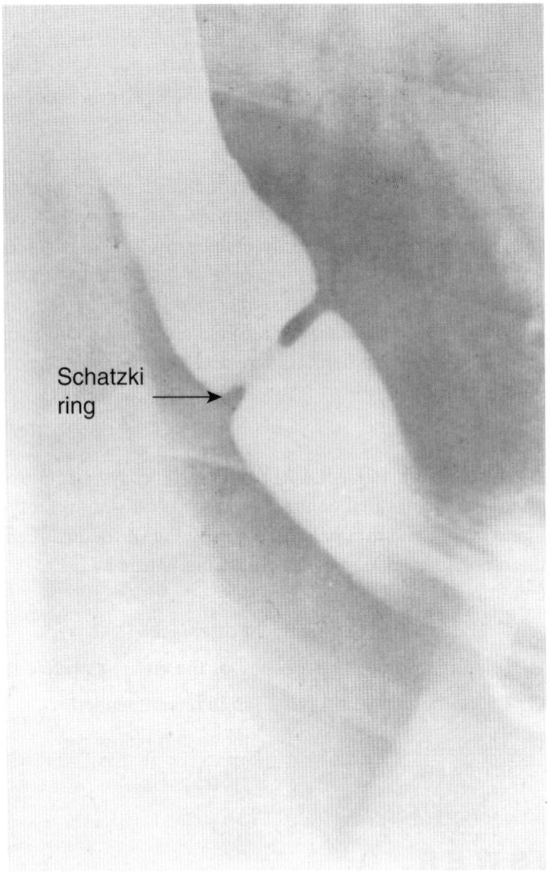

Fig. 20.3 Barium esophagogram of a Schatzki ring. *(Modified from Wilkins Jr EW. Rings and webs. In: Pearson FG, Cooper JD, Deslauriers J, et al., eds. Esophageal Surgery. 2nd ed. New York: Churchill-Livingstone; 2002:298.)*

each and 25-fold to 100-fold in combination. Additives such as nitrosamines in pickled and smoked foods have been implicated in the risk for cancer.

Ref.: 21, 22

25. A 75-year-old white man with a history of alcohol abuse, 40-pack-per year tobacco use, and long-standing GERD controlled by antacids is evaluated for dysphagia and weight loss. Esophagography shows an apple core lesion at the distal end of the esophagus. Which of the following is true regarding further workup?

A. Endoscopic biopsy should be avoided because of the risk for perforation.

B. CT is excellent for tumor staging.

C. Positron emission tomography (PET) is an excellent tool for staging and can be used as a single diagnostic modality.

D. Magnetic resonance imaging (MRI) is a poor imaging modality for liver metastasis.

E. EUS is more sensitive than CT for evaluating the celiac lymph nodes.

ANSWER: E

COMMENTS: Many imaging modalities are available for the characterization of esophageal cancers. Barium esophagography is a good first test for patients with dysphagia and a history suspicious for cancer. Although CT is accurate for M staging, it is only 57% accurate for T staging. PET is an excellent tool that can be used to evaluate N and M staging but should not be used as a single diagnostic modality. MRI is excellent for detecting metastatic and T4 lesions. **EUS** is the most important diagnostic tool in esophageal cancer staging. Tissue samples can be obtained from lymph nodes, as well as from the primary lesion. EUS is more sensitive and specific than CT in evaluating the celiac lymph nodes.

Ref.: 1, 21

26. The patient in Question 25 underwent EUS that showed a T2 lesion. The biopsy specimen is positive for adenocarcinoma of the esophagus. His chance of having a positive lymph node is:

A. 20%

B. 40%

C. 60%

D. 80%

E. 100%

ANSWER: C

COMMENTS: The risk of lymph node involvement is directly proportional to tumor depth or **T stage**. The incidence of positive lymph nodes is 18% for T1a intramucosal, 55% for T1b submucosal, 60% for T2 not beyond the muscularis propria, 80% for T3 with the involvement of paraesophageal tissue but not adjacent structures, and 100% for T4 with the involvement of adjacent structures. This is related to the anatomy of lymphatic drainage in the esophagus. The lymph channels travel within the submucosa in an axial fashion, allowing cancer to travel significant distances in cranial and caudal directions before causing an obstruction or draining beyond the muscularis.

Ref.: 1

27. The patient in Question 25 undergoes neoadjuvant chemoradiation therapy. Which of the following is true regarding multimodality therapy?

A. A complete histologic response occurs in approximately 25% of patients.

B. Squamous cell carcinoma and adenocarcinoma cell types have similar response rates to radiation therapy.

C. Survival beyond 5 years has not been reported in patients with stage IV disease.

D. Cisplatin-based combination therapy is no longer used because of the high rate of neuropathy.

E. Radiation therapy alone is an option for stage I disease.

ANSWER: A

COMMENTS: Treatment of esophageal cancer is complex, and multiple modalities are often necessary. The decision regarding treatment options depends on whether the intent is curative or palliative. **Squamous cell carcinoma** is much more radio responsive than adenocarcinoma, although with the latter, a complete histologic response is seen in approximately 25% of patients undergoing neoadjuvant chemoradiation therapy. Neoadjuvant radiation therapy is limited to 4500 cGy to avoid the surgical morbidity associated with high-dose radiation. Cisplatin, in combination with 5-fluorouracil and epirubicin, is an established chemotherapy regimen, but the use of mitomycin C, etoposide, and paclitaxel as third agents is gaining favor. Stage I disease is best treated with curative surgical resection.

Ref.: 1, 23

28. The patient in Question 25 undergoes transhiatal esophagectomy. Which of the following is true of the procedure?

A. Three incisions are required: cervical, thoracic, and abdominal.

B. A gastric conduit is preferred, and the blood supply is based on the right gastroepiploic artery.

C. More lymph nodes can be harvested than with en- bloc esophagectomy.

D. A substernal route of the replacement conduit is preferred because of the shorter route and improved function.

E. Cervical anastomotic leak rates are lower than thoracic leak rates but carry the same morbidity.

ANSWER: B

COMMENTS: Transhiatal esophagectomy was first described by Wolfgang Denk in 1913 and popularized by Orringer in the 1980s. Incisions on the left side of the neck and abdomen are used, and a thoracotomy is avoided. The esophagus is bluntly dissected, and the tabularized stomach is pulled through the posterior mediastinum to create a cervical esophagogastric anastomosis. The blood supply to the gastric conduit is based on the right gastroepiploic artery. A gastric pull-up procedure, based on the right gastroepiploic artery, in the posterior mediastinal position has the best functional result. Alternative routes (subcutaneous, substernal, or right pleural space) or conduits (colon or jejunum) can be used but result in an inferior function. Thoracic anastomosis, as the result of an **Ivor-Lewis** esophagectomy, results in a lower leak rate but carries a much higher morbidity and mortality as a result of associated mediastinitis. Thoracic esophagectomy is also associated with a greater lymphadenectomy due to direct access of the mediastinum for dissection. This has not been equivocally proven to yield improved disease-free or overall survival. When all three incisions are combined (cervical, thoracotomy, and laparotomy), this is referred to as a three hole, or a **McKeown**.

Ref.: 1, 21, 24, 25

29. An 88-year-old female with known advanced adenocarcinoma of the midesophagus presents with progressive dysphagia and is found on esophagogram to have a severe narrowing of her distal esophageal lumen. Which of the following is true regarding palliation of dysphagia in esophageal carcinoma?

A. Covered stents have less migration than uncovered stents.

B. PDT provides good relief in bulky, deeply penetrating tumors.

C. Neodymium:yttrium-aluminum-garnet (Nd:YAG) laser ablation is effective in proximal lesions.

D. Chemoradiation provides immediate relief.

E. Cervical esophagostomy (spit fistula) is a first-line therapy.

ANSWER: C

COMMENTS: The goal of **palliative care** is to relieve suffering and improve the overall quality of life by reducing tumor burden and restoring nutritional access. Chemotherapy, radiation therapy, PDT, laser treatment, stenting, and feeding tubes are options for palliation. Dysphagia is the most common initial symptom of patients with esophageal cancer, especially in those with advanced disease. **Endoscopic laser** fulguration with the Nd:YAG laser is 75%–80% successful in treating dysphagia, but multiple treatments may be required, and the risk of perforation is highest at 10%. **PDT**, an alternative form of laser therapy, is also an excellent tool for palliation in patients suffering from dysphagia. A photosensitizing drug [porfimer (Photofrin)] is injected intravenously before treatment and is selectively taken up by neoplastic cells. Activation of Photofrin with a red light at 630 nm releases singlet oxygen, which kills the host cell. The depth of penetration is limited to 5 mm and thus not great for deep lesions or extrinsic compression. Self-expanding metal **stents** (SEMS) provide good immediate relief from dysphagia. Covered stents prevent ingrowth of cancer into the stent, which can lead to subsequent recurrent stenosis. Covered stents also have a high incidence of migration compared with uncovered stents. In general, stents cannot be used for cervical lesions due to difficulty in swallowing after placement and for GEJ lesions due to severe reflux after placement. PDT may work best for GEJ lesions, and Nd:YAG ablation works well in cervical lesions that cannot be stented. **Chemotherapy** is used to treat systemic disease and reduce overall tumor burden but needs to be administered with radiation therapy to control local disease and can take weeks to be effective. As such it should be reserved for patients with a longer life expectancy.

Ref.: 25

30. The patient in the above question undergoes serial dilation and Nd:YAG ablation. She is observed overnight for symptoms. The next morning, she complains of chest pain, is febrile to 102.4°F, and has a heart rate of 128 beats/min. Esophagogram confirms extravasation of contrast. What is the most common cause of esophageal perforation?

A. Iatrogenic

B. Trauma

C. Cancer

D. Boerhaave's syndrome

E. Caustic injury

ANSWER: A

COMMENTS: Iatrogenic causes account for the largest cause of esophageal perforation, typically as the result of instrumentation including esophagoscopy, transesophageal echocardiography, and dilation (pneumatic and bougie). Boerhaave's syndrome is the most common cause of spontaneous esophageal perforation, accounting for 15% of cases. Cancer only accounts for 1% of esophageal perforations.

Ref.: 16

31. Which of the following is true regarding the management of esophageal perforation?

A. The distal esophagus is best approached through the right chest.

B. Cervical perforations occur most commonly at the thoracic inlet.

C. Primary repair alone is sufficient in early perforation.

D. Diversion and wide drainage are best in high-risk patients.

E. Resection is required in perforation with achalasia.

ANSWER: D

COMMENTS: Esophageal perforation carries a high morbidity and between a 10% and 40% mortality. Traditional teaching is that repair of esophageal perforation should only occur if identified early; however, modern studies have reported great success with repair of delayed injuries as well. Esophageal **repair** should involve a two-layer repair with an onlay buttress, typically of pericardium, pleural fat, or a pedicle intercostal muscle flap. The cervical esophagus is best approached via a left neck incision anterior to the sternocleidomastoid. Perforations here are most commonly found at the cricopharyngeus/UES as this is the highest pressure zone. The upper two-thirds of the thoracic esophagus is best approached via a right thoracotomy and the distal one-third via a left thoracotomy. The intraabdominal esophagus is best approached via an upper midline laparotomy. In achalasia, most perforations are the result of pneumatic dilation and can be managed with repair and myotomy at a different location; however, resection is not required. For patients with perforation associated with a malignancy, resection should be considered if feasible. Recently covered stent placement with wide mediastinal drainage allows temporization and an oncologic operation to occur under more elective circumstances. Cervical esophagostomy as a **diversion** with wide mediastinal drainage and feeding tube placement should be reserved for those with prohibitive risk to resection, short life expectancy, or significant gross contamination and sepsis.

Ref.: 16

32. A 45-year-old man arrives at the emergency department after ingesting lye in a suicide attempt. Which of the following is true?

A. Injury to the esophagus is the result of coagulative necrosis.

B. Endoscopy should not be performed within the first 72 h because of the risk for perforation.

C. The lye should be neutralized with milk or egg whites if the patient is seen within the first hour of ingestion.

D. Before reepithelialization, dilations should be performed to decrease the long-term stricture rate.

E. For a long-segment interposition graft, the colon is the preferred conduit.

ANSWER: E

COMMENTS: Caustic injury to the esophagus can be attributed to the ingestion of acidic or alkaline liquids. Alkaline substances (lye) produce liquefactive necrosis of tissue and can cause deep tissue penetration. If diagnosed within the first hour of ingestion, half-strength vinegar or citrus juice can be used to neutralize the ingested alkali. After careful examination of the oropharynx, airway, chest, and abdomen, endoscopy should be performed to grade the burn. Serial esophagograms should be performed to evaluate for stricture formation rather than waiting for symptoms of obstruction to develop. Early stent placement or bougie dilation is effective in preventing long-term strictures; however, dilation should be performed only after reepithelialization has been confirmed with endoscopy. For long-segment strictures requiring resection, colonic interposition is the preferred graft.

Ref.: 1, 26, 27

REFERENCES

1. Maish MS. Esophagus. In: Townsend TM, Beauchamp RD, Evers BM, Mattox KL, eds. *Sabiston Textbook of Surgery: The Biological Basis of Modern Surgical Practice*. 19th ed. Philadelphia: Saunders; 2012.
2. Carrott PW, Mann JA, Kozower BD. Esophageal function tests. In: Cameron JL, Cameron AM, eds. *Current Surgical Therapy*. 11th ed. Philadelphia: Elsevier Saunders; 2014.
3. Liebermann-Meffert D. Clinically oriented anatomy, embryology and histology. In: Patterson GA, Cooper JD, Deslauriers J, et al., eds. *Pearson's Thoracic and Esophageal Surgery*. 3rd ed. Philadelphia: Churchill-Livingstone; 2008.
4. Duranceau A. Physiology of the esophagus and classification of esophageal motor abnormalities. In: Patterson GA, Cooper JD, Deslauriers J, et al., eds. *Pearson's Thoracic and Esophageal Surgery*. 3rd ed. Philadelphia: Churchill-Livingstone; 2008.
5. Richter JE. Medical treatment of gastroesophageal reflux disease. In: Patterson GA, Cooper JD, Deslauriers J, et al., eds. *Pearson's Thoracic and Esophageal Surgery*. 3rd ed. Philadelphia: Churchill-Livingstone; 2008.
6. Petersen RP, Pellegrini CA, Oelschlager BK. Hiatal hernia and gastroesophageal reflux disease. In: Townsend TM, Beauchamp RD, Evers BM, Mattox KL, eds. *Sabiston Textbook of Surgery: The Biological Basis of Modern Surgical Practice*. 19th ed. Philadelphia: Saunders; 2012.
7. Carlson MA, Frantzides CT. Complications and results of laparoscopic antireflux procedures: a review of 10,489 cases. *J Am Coll Surg*. 2001;193:428–439.
8. Edmundowicz S. Endoscopic management of reflux. In: Patterson GA, Cooper JD, Deslauriers J, et al., eds. *Pearson's Thoracic and Esophageal Surgery*. 3rd ed. Philadelphia: Churchill-Livingstone; 2008.
9. Irshod K, Pennathur A, Luketich JD. Evaluation and surgical treatment of hiatal hernias and gastroesophageal reflux. In: Patterson GA, Cooper JD, Deslauriers J, et al., eds. *Pearson's Thoracic and Esophageal Surgery*. 3rd ed. Philadelphia: Churchill-Livingstone; 2008.
10. Poulose BK, Richards WO. Endoluminal approaches to gastroesophageal reflux disease. In: Cameron JL, ed. *Current Surgical Therapy*. 9th ed. Philadelphia: CV Mosby; 2008.
11. Fry LC, Monkenmuller K, Malfertheiner P. Systematic review: endoluminal therapy for gastro-esophageal reflux disease: evidence from clinical trials. *Eur J Gastroenterol Hepatol*. 2007;19:1125–1139.
12. Torquati A, Richards WO. Endoluminal GERD treatments: critical appraisal of current literature with evidence-based medicine instruments. *Surg Endosc*. 2007;21:697–706.
13. Cadiere GB, Rajan A, Germay O, et al. Endoluminal fundoplication by a transoral device for the treatment of GERD: a feasibility study. *Surg Endosc*. 2008;22:333–342.
14. Lerut TEMR, Hiebert CA. Belsey Mark IV repair. In: Patterson GA, Cooper JD, Deslauriers J, et al., eds. *Pearson's Thoracic and Esophageal Surgery*. 3rd ed. Philadelphia: Churchill-Livingstone; 2008.
15. Markar SD, Low DE. The management of achalasia of the esophagus. In: Cameron JL, Cameron AM, eds. *Current Surgical Therapy*. 11th ed. Philadelphia: Elsevier; 2014.
16. Fergusun CM. Esophageal perforation. In: Cameron JL, Cameron AM, eds. *Current Surgical Therapy*. 11th ed. Philadelphia: Elsevier Saunders; 2014.
17. Duncan BW, Krakovitz P, Arruda MJ. Vascular tracheoesophageal compression: vascular rings, pulmonary artery sling, and innominate artery compression of the trachea. In: Patterson GA, Cooper JD, Deslauriers J, et al., eds. *Pearson's Thoracic and Esophageal Surgery*. 3rd ed. Philadelphia: Churchill Livingstone; 2008.
18. Lerut TE, Luketich JD, Bizekis C. Esophageal diverticula. In: Patterson GA, Cooper JD, Deslauriers J, et al., eds. *Pearson's Thoracic and Esophageal Surgery*. 3rd ed. Philadelphia: Churchill-Livingstone; 2008.
19. Teran MD, Brock MV. The management of Barrett's esophagus. In: Cameron JL, Cameron AM, eds. *Current Surgical Therapy*. 11th ed. Philadelphia: Elsevier Saunders; 2014.
20. Harbison SP, Dempsey DT. Mallory-Weiss syndrome. In: Cameron JL, ed. *Current Surgical Therapy*. 9th ed. Philadelphia: CV Mosby; 2008.
21. Lada MJ, Peters JH. The management of esophageal carcinoma. In: Cameron JL, Cameron AM, eds. *Current Surgical Therapy*. 11th ed. Philadelphia: Elsevier Saunders; 2014.
22. Maish MS. Esophagus. In: Townsend TM, Beauchamp RD, Evers BM, Mattox KL, eds. *Sabiston Textbook of Surgery: The Biological Basis of Modern Surgical Practice*. 19th ed. Philadelphia: Saunders; 2012.

23. Rizk NP. Neoadjuvant and adjuvant therapy of esophageal cancer. In: Cameron JL, Cameron AM, eds. *Current Surgical Therapy*. 11th ed. Philadelphia: Elsevier Saunders; 2014.
24. Orringer MB. Transhiatal esophagectomy without thoracotomy for carcinoma of the thoracic esophagus. *Ann Surg*. 1984;200:282–288.
25. Litle VR, Christie NA. Palliation of esophageal cancer. In: Patterson GA, Cooper JD, Deslauriers J, et al., eds. *Pearson's Thoracic and Esophageal Surgery*. 3rd ed. Philadelphia: Churchill-Livingstone; 2008.
26. Jobe BA, Hunter JG, Peters JH. Esophagus and diaphragmatic hernia. In: Brunicardi FC, Andersen DK, Billiar TR, et al., eds. *Schwartz's Principles of Surgery*. 9th ed. New York: McGraw-Hill; 2010.
27. Fischer AC. Chemical esophageal injuries. In: Cameron JL, ed. *Current Surgical Therapy*. 9th ed. Philadelphia: CV Mosby; 2008.

CHAPTER 21

STOMACH AND DUODENUM

Lia Jordano, M.D., and Minh B. Luu, M.D.

1. One month after an antrectomy with Billroth II reconstruction, a patient presents with colicky abdominal pain, distention, bilious emesis, and failure to pass gas. This most likely represents:

A. Blind loop syndrome

B. Afferent loop syndrome

C. Reflux gastritis

D. Efferent loop syndrome

E. Vitamin deficiency

ANSWER: D

COMMENTS: See Question 3.

Ref.: 1

2. As opposed to the above condition, the patient presents with chronic vague abdominal discomfort and cramping with postprandial explosive bilious emesis, which relieves the pain. He continues to be able to pass gas. What is the best management for this patient?

A. Dietary modification to reduce the meal size

B. Emergent surgery to reduce the internal hernia

C. Iron and calcium supplementation

D. Conversion to a Roux-en-Y with a longer afferent limb

E. Conversion to a Roux-en-Y with a shorter afferent limb

ANSWER: E

COMMENTS: See Question 3.

Ref.: 1

3. Following a Billroth II reconstruction, a patient presents with epigastric abdominal pain, bilious emesis that does not relieve the pain, and weight loss. Which of the following tests would reveal the diagnosis?

A. Hydroxy iminodiacetic acid (HIDA) scan

B. Computed tomography (CT) scan

C. Barium swallow

D. Kidney, ureter, and bladder (KUB) test

E. Gastric emptying study

ANSWER: A

COMMENTS: Postgastrectomy complications range from nutritional deficiencies to mechanical malfunctions requiring surgical intervention. The most common metabolic disturbance is **anemia**, either iron deficiency or megaloblastic secondary to B_{12} deficiency. Loss of a significant portion of the stomach reduces the amount of intrinsic factor that is required to absorb vitamin B_{12}. **Calcium deficiencies** are also observed, leading to osteoporosis and osteomalacia, as calcium is primarily absorbed in the duodenum. All of these conditions are treated with supplementation. **Afferent loop syndrome** occurs as a result of a partial or complete obstruction in the afferent limb. It can be acute or chronic and progress to **blind loop syndrome** in which bacterial overgrowth occurs. In the case of blind loop syndrome, megaloblastic anemia can develop due to bacterial consumption of vitamin B_{12}. The presentation of afferent loop syndrome includes postprandial pain and fullness with eventual purely bilious emesis, which relieves the pain. Diagnosis is made with a CT scan. Treatment consists of antibiotics for bacterial overgrowth and conversion to a Roux-en-Y with a short afferent limb. **Efferent loop obstruction** presents the same as a small bowel obstruction. Diagnosis can be established by demonstrating a lack of filling of the efferent limb on barium swallow or by CT scan. Operative management consists of correction of the cause for the obstruction be it adhesions, internal herniation, etc. Finally, **alkaline reflux gastritis** most commonly plagues patients who have undergone a Billroth II reconstruction and consists of bile refluxing into the stomach remnant. Patients present with bilious emesis that does not tend to relieve their pain. Diagnosis can be made with a HIDA scan, demonstrating biliary secretion into the stomach. The surgical management of this condition involves conversion to a Roux en-Y with a Roux limb that is greater than 40 cm in length.

Ref.: 1

4. Which of the following pairs of diagnostic measures and their role in the management of a patient with gastric cancer is correct?

A. Physical examination/identify occult metastatic disease

B. Esophagogastroduodenoscopy (EGD) with endoscopic ultrasound (EUS)/examine for locoregional staging

C. CT scan/monitor for response to neoadjuvant therapy

D. Positron emission tomography (PET) scan/detect intraabdominal metastatic disease

E. Diagnostic laparoscopy/resect intraabdominal metastases

ANSWER: B

COMMENTS: The workup of a patient with gastric cancer begins with a thorough **physical examination** in which care is taken to identify signs of advanced disease. Prominent supraclavicular or periumbilical nodes, hepatomegaly, ascites, palpable ovaries on pelvic examination, or a firm Blumer's shelf on rectal examination all represent possible metastasis. After an initial examination, patients should undergo an **EGD with EUS** for locoregional staging purposes and a **CT scan** for the detection of intraabdominal metastatic spread. **PET scans** do not have a reliable role in the staging workup of a patient; however, they have been used to track response to neoadjuvant therapy. Because CT scan has an overall detection rate of 85% for intraabdominal spread and only 50% for peritoneal metastasis, **diagnostic laparoscopy** can be utilized to identify the occult metastatic disease. In a 2007 study that included 106 patients with gastric cancer, 33% of patients previously thought to be resection candidates based on preoperative imaging were found to have CT occult disease on laparoscopy. There is no role for the laparoscopic resection of intraabdominal metastases.

Ref.: 1

5. Which of the following is true regarding dumping syndrome?

A. Late dumping syndrome is the result of a massive influx of high osmolarity contents into the intestines.

B. It is more common after Billroth I reconstructions versus Billroth II.

C. It can include cardiovascular effects such as palpitations, diaphoresis, fainting, and flushing.

D. Early dumping syndrome is made worse by high-carbohydrate foods.

E. Most patients require long-acting octreotide agonists to control their symptoms.

ANSWER: C

COMMENTS: Dumping syndrome can be divided into early and late phases, with the early occurring 20 to 30 min after eating and the late 2 to 3 h after eating. Early dumping occurs when high osmolarity contents enter the intestines at a rapid rate, inducing a large shift of extracellular fluid into the lumen. Symptoms include cramping, nausea and vomiting, epigastric fullness, and diarrhea. Late dumping occurs when contents high in carbohydrates enter the intestines, stimulating an overcompensatory insulin release that, in turn, results in profound hypoglycemia. Cardiovascular effects occur with both types; however, they are more common with late dumping. Most patients find effective relief with dietary modification alone including smaller portions, slower eating, avoiding foods high in sugars, and separating liquids from solids. Octreotide agonists are reserved for the few who do not respond to these measures. Overall, dumping is more common after Billroth II reconstructions.

Ref.: 1

6. Which of the following is true concerning the pharmacologic regulation of acid secretion?

A. Proton pump inhibitors (PPIs) exert their effect at a final common pathway of acid secretion.

B. H_2 blockers inhibit the release of histamine from the enterochromaffin-like (ECL) cells.

C. PPIs function as reversible receptor antagonists.

D. H_2 blockers have a more prolonged inhibition of gastric acid secretion than do PPIs.

E. Antisecretory agents do not affect serum gastrin levels.

ANSWER: A

COMMENTS: Both H_2 blockers and PPIs work to decrease acid secretion by parietal cells. H_2 blockers function as histamine receptor antagonists at the level of the parietal cell but do not influence the release of histamine from the ECL cells. PPIs more completely inhibit acid secretion by irreversibly inhibiting the final common pathway, the proton pump. For the recovery of acid secretion to occur, new proton pumps need to be synthesized, giving them a longer duration of action than H_2 blockers. All antisecretory agents result in the elevation of serum gastrin levels and hyperplasia of the G cells and ECL cells.

Ref.: 1

7. A patient presents after several episodes of violent emesis, which eventually turned bloody. Which of the following is the best diagnostic tactic?

A. Upright chest x-ray

B. Placement of a nasogastric (NG) tube

C. Barium swallow

D. CT of the chest and abdomen

E. Endoscopy

ANSWER: E

COMMENTS: Mallory-Weiss tears are the result of violent retching, vomiting, or coughing. They generally occur high on the **lesser curvature** and involve only the **mucosa**, not a full perforation. They comprise around 15% of upper gastrointestinal (GI) hemorrhages. The majority of patients can be effectively diagnosed and managed with **endoscopy** alone. In the rare case that endoscopic control is unsuccessful, operative intervention can be carried out via an **anterior gastrotomy** and oversewing of the injury with **mucosal reapproximation**. None of the other answers would accurately diagnose this condition.

Ref.: 1

8. Concerning duodenal diverticula, which of the following statements is false?

A. They are twice as common in women as in men.

B. Duodenal diverticula are the second most common congenital diverticula of the intestine after Meckel's diverticulum.

C. The majority of duodenal diverticula are found in the periampullary region.

D. Most of them are asymptomatic and found incidentally.

E. They can result in cholangitis and pancreatitis from the obstruction of the biliary or pancreatic ducts, respectively.

ANSWER: B

COMMENTS: Duodenal diverticula are false diverticula containing only mucosa and submucosa, as opposed to a true diverticulum, which contains all layers of the intestinal wall (e.g., Meckel's diverticulum). Duodenal diverticula are the second most common cause of acquired diverticula after those in the colon. They are more commonly seen in women than in men (2:1) and usually occur later in life, similar to colonic diverticula. The majority of these diverticula (~75%) are found within a 2-cm radius from the ampulla of Vater and generally protrude through the medial wall of the duodenum. These duodenal diverticula are rarely symptomatic and do not require intervention. Surgery is reserved for those that are symptomatic and in which complications develop. Symptoms are usually the result of hemorrhage, perforation, blind loop syndrome, cholangitis, or pancreatitis from the obstruction of the biliary or pancreatic ducts. Juxtapyloric diverticula have been noted to be associated with choledocholithiasis. Their presence increases the difficulty of successful completion of endoscopic retrograde cholangiopancreatography (ERCP). When treatment is required, surgical excision (**diverticulectomy**) is recommended.

Ref.: 1

9. A 23-year-old thin (92 lb) woman with a history of surgical correction of her scoliosis is evaluated for symptoms of postprandial epigastric pain, fullness, nausea, and vomiting. Her physical examination is unremarkable except for her thin physique/stature. Barium upper GI series showed a dilated duodenum and stomach with minimal flow of barium into the jejunum. Which of the following is the operative management of choice for this patient's condition?

A. Segmental duodenectomy
B. Pancreaticoduodenectomy
C. Gastrojejunostomy
D. Duodenojejunostomy
E. Roux-en-Y hepaticojejunostomy

ANSWER: D

COMMENTS: The patient in this scenario has compression of the third portion of the duodenum by the superior mesenteric artery (SMA) as it passes over it. This rare condition is known as **SMA syndrome** or **Wilkie syndrome**. This syndrome is usually seen in young asthenic females with predisposing conditions of weight loss, scoliosis or corrective surgery for it, supine mobilization, and placement of a body cast. The diagnosis is usually made with either a barium upper GI series or a CT, with oral and intravenous (IV) contrast enhancement demonstrating a dilated duodenum and stomach with an abrupt or nearly complete cutoff of contrast agent at the third portion of the duodenum and minimal flow into the jejunum. Conservative management consisting of nutritional supplementation can be tried initially. In patients who fail medical management, the operative treatment of choice is **duodenojejunostomy**.

Ref.: 1

10. Which hormone is matched with the correct diagnostic/therapeutic function?

A. Cholecystokinin (CCK)/treatment of esophageal variceal bleeding
B. Somatostatin/relief of spasm of the sphincter of Oddi
C. Gastrin/measurement of maximal gastric acid secretion
D. Glucagon/provocative test for gastrinoma
E. Secretin/stimulation of gallbladder contraction

ANSWER: C

COMMENTS: GI hormones or their analogues have been used clinically as diagnostic or therapeutic agents. **CCK** is used to **stimulate gallbladder contraction**. This is useful in identifying patients with **biliary dyskinesia** or acalculous cholecystitis with the help of CCK cholescintigraphy. **Pentagastrin**, a **gastrin analogue**, is used to measure gastric acid secretion. **Somatostatin** or its analogues are used in various conditions as a result of their universal inhibitory function. Because they inhibit the release of GI hormones, somatostatin analogues are used for various endocrine neoplasms such as **Zollinger-Ellison syndrome**, **VIPoma**, **insulinoma**, and **carcinoid tumors**. They are also useful in patients with **pancreatic fistulas**, **pancreatic ascites**, and **enterocutaneous fistulas** by decreasing GI secretions. Additionally, they have been used as a treatment to decrease bleeding from the GI tract. **Glucagon** is used by endoscopists to **relax the sphincter of Oddi** to facilitate ERCP. **Secretin**, which inhibits acid secretion, causes a paradoxical increase in serum gastrin levels in patients with gastrinoma. **Pancreatic polypeptide** (PP) is predominantly secreted in the pancreatic head. PP serum levels drop following the Whipple procedure and may be related to the delayed gastric emptying observed after pyloric-preserving pancreatoduodenectomy. In addition, PP secretion necessitates intact vagal nerve function; thus a blunt response to stimulation by sham feedings has been used to evaluate intact vagal nerve function, particularly in patients suspected of having iatrogenic vagus nerve injury.

Ref.: 1, 2

11. A patient with gastric outlet obstruction and prolonged vomiting has which of the following metabolic abnormalities?

A. Hypochloremic, hyperkalemic metabolic alkalosis
B. Hyperchloremic, hypokalemic metabolic acidosis
C. Hyponatremic, hypokalemic metabolic acidosis
D. Hypochloremic, hypokalemic metabolic alkalosis
E. Hyperchloremic, hyperkalemic metabolic acidosis

ANSWER: D

COMMENTS: The most common cause of gastric outlet obstruction is malignancy. The classic metabolic abnormality resulting from gastric outlet obstruction and prolonged **vomiting** is **hypochloremic, hypokalemic metabolic alkalosis**. Initial loss of hydrochloric acid causes hypochloremia and mild alkalosis compensated for by renal excretion of bicarbonate. Therefore in the early stages, the urine is alkaline. Continued vomiting produces a severe extracellular fluid deficit and sodium deficit from both renal and gastric losses. The kidneys begin to conserve sodium and, in exchange, excrete hydrogen and potassium cations to accompany bicarbonate. The kidneys are the predominant site of potassium loss, and the urine is paradoxically acidic. Urine chloride content is reduced throughout and is eventually absent. Serum ionized calcium levels are decreased because calcium is mildly alkaline and shifts to its nonionized form to reduce alkalosis. Treatment of this metabolic situation is accomplished primarily by the administration of isotonic saline solution, which replenishes the deficits in volume, sodium, and chloride. Potassium is replaced once the renal function is optimized.

Ref.: 1, 2

12. Which of the following statements is true with regard to the arterial blood supply of the stomach?

A. The left gastroepiploic artery is the main blood supply to the gastric conduit used in esophagectomies.
B. Ligation of the left gastric artery can result in acute left-sided hepatic ischemia.
C. The stomach is susceptible to ischemia because of poor collateral circulation.
D. The inferior phrenic and short gastric arteries provide significant blood supply to the body of the stomach.
E. A replaced right hepatic artery may originate from the left gastric artery.

ANSWER: B

COMMENTS: The arterial blood supply of the stomach is derived primarily from the **celiac artery**. The **left gastric artery** comes off of the celiac artery and supplies the stomach along the lesser curvature. An aberrant/replaced **left hepatic artery** originates from the left gastric artery (15%–24%) and can represent the only arterial blood supply to the left hepatic lobe. This aberrant/replaced left hepatic artery runs in the gastrohepatic ligament. The **right gastric artery** typically arises from the common hepatic artery distal to the gastroduodenal artery. The **right and left gastroepiploic arteries** usually originate from the gastroduodenal artery and splenic artery, respectively. It is the **right estroepiploic** artery that functions as the main blood supply to the gastric conduit used in esophagectomies. The short gastric arteries arising from the splenic artery and inferior phrenic arteries also contribute significant blood volume to the proximal part of the stomach. The stomach is well protected from ischemia and can easily survive with ligation of three of four arteries because of its rich collateral circulation.

Ref.: 1, 2

13. Choose the correct type of vagotomy with the appropriate level of vagal transection from the pairs listed below:

A. Truncal vagotomy/criminal nerve of Grassi

B. Highly selective vagotomy/anterior and posterior vagal trunks below the celiac and hepatic branches

C. Selective vagotomy/anterior and posterior vagal trunks above the celiac and hepatic branches

D. Parietal cell vagotomy/terminal branches of the nerve of Latarjet

E. Highly selective vagotomy/hepatic branches

ANSWER: D

COMMENTS: In the chest, the vagal trunks are situated to the right and left of the esophagus. At the level of the cardia, the left vagal trunk is found anterior and the right vagal trunk is found posterior secondary to the embryonic gastric rotation. The anterior vagal trunk divides into hepatic and anterior gastric (anterior nerve of Latarjet) branches. The posterior vagus divides into the posterior nerve of Latarjet and celiac branches. One of the proximal posterior branches of the posterior vagal trunk is known as the **criminal nerve of Grassi** and is identified as a possible cause of recurrent ulcers if left undivided during selective vagotomy. **Truncal vagotomy** is conventionally performed at or just above or below the diaphragmatic esophageal hiatus before it gives off **celiac and hepatic branches**. In contrast, a **selective vagotomy** is performed distal to this location and spares the celiac and hepatic branches. **Highly selective vagotomy** (also known as **proximal gastric or parietal cell vagotomy**) divides individual **terminal branches of the nerve of Latarjet** in the fundus and corpus of the stomach but spares the vagal branches to the antrum and pylorus, which control gastric motility and emptying—thus obviating the need for a drainage procedure.

Ref.: 1, 2

14. Concerning the treatment of patients with Zollinger-Ellison syndrome, which of the following statements is true?

A. Operative treatment of associated hyperparathyroidism takes precedence over abdominal surgery.

B. Pancreatic tumors should not be removed by enucleation.

C. Duodenal tumors usually require pancreaticoduodenectomy.

D. Antrectomy is indicated if the tumor cannot be localized.

E. Resection of liver metastases is not indicated.

ANSWER: A

COMMENTS: Treatment of **Zollinger-Ellison syndrome** is two pronged and aimed at both resecting the tumor when possible and protecting the gastric end organ. Therapy must be individualized. Patients with known endocrine tumors should undergo careful evaluation for other potential endocrine tumors. In patients with **gastrinoma** and **hyperparathyroidism**, **parathyroidectomy** should be performed first to eliminate hypercalcemia. Abdominal surgery is not urgent with the current antisecretory medications. Although gastrinomas are often multiple and are usually metastatic, long-term survival is possible. Aggressive attempts to localize and resect tumors can provide a cure in 5%–20% of patients and can diminish gastrin secretion in others. Digital palpation through a duodenotomy and intraoperative ultrasound are useful operative adjuncts. Both pancreatic and duodenal gastrinomas can be resected by **enucleation** when appropriately located. Blind pancreatic resections are not generally indicated. When complete tumor removal is not possible, a gastric operation may be appropriate. Proximal gastric vagotomy may be useful, but **total gastrectomy** still provides the best long-term quality of life for some patients. Life-long pharmacologic treatment with antisecretory agents may control the ulcer diathesis in some patients, but problems with high doses, compliance, and side effects may occur. Resection or ablation of metastatic disease, although not curative, can provide important palliation and decrease the need for drug therapy.

Ref.: 1–3

15. Which of the following clinical conditions is not associated with delayed gastric emptying?

A. Hypocalcemia

B. Scleroderma

C. Hyperglycemia

D. Myxedema

E. Zollinger-Ellison syndrome

ANSWER: E

COMMENTS: Disorders of gastric emptying can be divided into rapid or delayed emptying, both of which can be significantly disabling conditions. **Delayed gastric emptying** is the more frequently encountered problem of gastric motility. Excluding mechanical obstruction, important causes of delayed gastric emptying include **metabolic derangements** (e.g., **myxedema** and **hyperglycemia**), **electrolyte abnormalities** (e.g., **hypokalemia** and **hypocalcemia**), **drugs** (e.g., **narcotics** and **anticholinergics**), and **systemic diseases** (e.g., **diabetes mellitus** and **scleroderma**). Up to 40% of **postvagotomy** patients experience delayed gastric emptying. **Rapid gastric emptying** is less commonly observed. Causes of rapid gastric emptying include previous **gastric resection**, conditions with **impaired fat absorption** resulting in the loss of the inhibition of gastric emptying (e.g., **pancreatic insufficiency** and **short bowel syndrome**), and conditions with **hypergastrinemia** such as **Zollinger-Ellison syndrome**.

Ref.: 1–3

16. Which of the following conditions is not associated with *Helicobacter pylori* infection?

A. Duodenal ulcer

B. Gastric cancer

C. Mucosa-associated lymphoid tissue (MALT) lymphoma

D. Gastroesophageal reflux disease

E. Chronic gastritis

ANSWER: D

COMMENTS: ***H. pylori*** is a curved or S-shaped, gram-negative microaerophilic motile bacterium whose natural habitat is the human stomach. *H. pylori* infection has been demonstrated to be associated with 90% of **duodenal ulcers** and 75% of **gastric ulcers**. After eradication of the organism as a part of ulcer treatment, recurrence of ulcer is extremely rare. In addition, *H. pylori* has been associated with **chronic atrophic gastritis**, which in turn leads to **gastric atrophy** and **intestinal metaplasia**, a suspected precursor of **gastric cancer**. *H. pylori* infection also increases the risk for low-grade **MALT lymphoma**; eradication of *H. pylori* results in the resolution of MALT lymphomas in most cases. There appears to be a negative association between *H. pylori* infection and **GI reflux disease**.

Ref.: 1, 2, 4

17. With regard to *H. pylori*–negative duodenal ulcer disease, which of the following statements is true?

A. Nonsteroidal antiinflammatory drugs (NSAIDs) are not a cause of duodenal ulcers in patients who are *H. pylori* negative.

B. Because of the high prevalence of *H. pylori*–positive duodenal ulcers, patients should be treated for *H. pylori* without confirmatory testing.

C. In contrast to *H. pylori*–positive duodenal ulcers, NSAID-induced ulcers are frequently associated with chronic active gastritis.

D. *H. pylori*–negative duodenal ulcers are usually large ulcers that are not often associated with bleeding.

E. Older age, multiple comorbid conditions, and sepsis are independently associated with *H. pylori*–negative duodenal ulcers.

ANSWER: E

COMMENTS: Initial studies have demonstrated that ***H. pylori*** infection is present in more than 90% of patients with duodenal ulcers. However, more recently, it has been shown that the prevalence of *H. pylori*–associated duodenal ulcers is only 75% and is found to be decreasing. Thus it is important to first make the diagnosis of an active *H. pylori* infection rather than initiating **empirical therapy**. ***H. pylori*–negative duodenal ulcers** are independently associated with **NSAID use**, **older age**, **multiple medical problems**, and **sepsis**. Use of NSAIDs is the major cause of duodenal ulcers in patients who are *H. pylori* negative. **Bleeding** is the initial manifestation in these patients, and they have large and multiple ulcers.

Ref.: 1, 6

18. If the patient in Question 21 was found to have a perforated gastric ulcer instead of a duodenal ulcer, which additional procedure would need to be conducted during the operative intervention besides closure of the perforation?

A. Feeding jejunostomy

B. Gastrojejunostomy

C. Gastrostomy tube placement

D. Excision or biopsy of the ulcer

E. Pyloroplasty

ANSWER: D

COMMENTS: The preferred treatment of a **perforated duodenal ulcer** is resuscitation and prompt surgery. Nonoperative management is reserved for old contained perforations or for terminally ill patients who otherwise cannot undergo surgery. The diagnosis is a presumptive one based on clinical grounds and should not be excluded if pneumoperitoneum cannot be demonstrated, because about 20% of patients with perforations do not have this typical radiographic feature. Operative management requires the closure of the perforation, which is generally best accomplished with an **omental (Graham) patch**. Closure of the perforation is usually sufficient in patients with duodenal ulcers; however, excision of the ulcer is necessary to rule out malignancy in patients with gastric ulcers before closure. Following simple repair alone, the traditional natural history has been that about one-third of patients have no further ulcer problems, one-third have ulcer recurrence amenable to medical management, and one-third require a subsequent operation for ulcer disease. It is not clear how precisely this applies to patients with *H. pylori* infection or those with NSAID-induced ulcers. Definitive operations should be performed only in stable patients and in those with documented failure after appropriate *H. pylori* eradication. **Truncal vagotomy** can be performed expeditiously but has a greater incidence of side effects. Highly selective vagotomy is an excellent choice but is time consuming and requires a surgeon with the expertise to perform it. Resective procedures are generally avoided in the setting of perforation because of higher morbidity. Following surgery, ulcerogenic drugs should be withheld, and any concomitant *H. pylori* infection should be treated.

Ref.: 1, 6

19. A 45-year-old man requires surgery for an intractable duodenal ulcer. Which operation best prevents ulcer recurrence?

A. Subtotal gastrectomy

B. Truncal vagotomy and pyloroplasty

C. Truncal vagotomy and antrectomy

D. Selective vagotomy

E. Highly selective vagotomy

ANSWER: C

COMMENTS: See Question 20.

Ref.: 1, 2, 6

20. Which operation for duodenal ulcer is least likely to produce undesirable postoperative symptoms?

A. Subtotal gastrectomy

B. Truncal vagotomy and pyloroplasty

C. Truncal vagotomy and antrectomy

D. Selective vagotomy

E. Highly selective vagotomy

ANSWER: E

COMMENTS: The goal of surgical therapy for **duodenal ulcers** is to reduce acid production in a manner that is safe and has the fewest possible side effects. Acid can be reduced by eliminating vagal stimulation, removing the antral source of gastrin, and removing the parietal cell mass. Traditionally, subtotal two-thirds gastrectomy has carried the highest mortality rate. **Truncal vagotomy with antrectomy** has the lowest recurrence rate. Procedures involving antrectomy, pyloroplasty, or truncal vagotomy may be complicated by diarrhea, postprandial dumping, or bile reflux. **Selective vagotomy**, which preserves the hepatic and celiac vagal branches, has been associated with a lower rate of diarrhea than truncal vagotomy. **Highly selective vagotomy**, also known as parietal cell vagotomy, aims to denervate the parietal cell–bearing portion of the stomach but preserves innervations to the pyloroantral region and thus maintains more normal gastric emptying. This operation carries the lowest mortality rate and the lowest incidence of side effects, but the highest recurrence rate, which ranges from 5% to 15%.

Ref.: 1, 2, 6

21. A 75-year-old man taking NSAIDs for arthritis has an acute abdomen and pneumoperitoneum. His symptoms are 6 h old, and his vital signs are stable after the infusion of 1 L of normal saline solution. What should be the next step in the management of this patient?

A. CT of the abdomen

B. EGD

C. Antisecretory drugs, broad-spectrum antibiotics, and surgery if he fails to improve in 6 h

D. Antisecretory drugs, antibiotics for *H. pylori*, and surgery if he fails to improve in 6 h

E. Surgery

ANSWER: E

COMMENTS: See Question 18.

Ref.: 1, 2, 6

22. During an operation for a bleeding duodenal ulcer, three-point "U" stitches are placed to ligate which of the following arteries after longitudinal pyloroduodenotomy?

A. Common hepatic, right gastric, and gastroduodenal arteries

B. Proximal and distal gastroduodenal and transverse pancreatic arteries

C. Right gastric, gastroduodenal, and right gastroepiploic arteries

D. Right gastric and anterior and posterior inferior pancreaticoduodenal arteries

E. Common hepatic, gastroduodenal, and superior mesenteric arteries

ANSWER: B

COMMENTS: Massive bleeding is usually the result of posterior erosion of a duodenal ulcer into the gastroduodenal artery. Emergency surgical intervention is indicated when bleeding is refractory to endoscopic therapy or in the presence of hemorrhagic shock. After expeditious preoperative resuscitation, the abdomen is entered and a **longitudinal pyloroduodenotomy** is performed. Digital pressure is applied over the ulcer base to temporize the bleeding and allow resuscitation before suture control is obtained. Proper control of bleeding requires three-point suture ligation of the duodenal ulcer. These "U" stitches are placed superior and inferior to the site of penetration to ligate the proximal and distal **gastroduodenal artery**. A third suture is placed on the medial aspect of the ulcer to control the **transverse pancreatic branch** coming off the gastroduodenal artery. After the bleeding is controlled, biopsy of gastric mucosa should be performed for histologic analysis of *H. pylori.* The longitudinal pyloroduodenotomy is then closed transversely (**Heineke-Mikulicz** or **Weinberg pyloroplasty**).

Ref.: 1, 2, 4, 6

23. Which gastric ulcer corresponds with the correct recommended surgical management?

A. Type I/Billroth I or II reconstruction

B. Type II/truncal vagotomy and pyloroplasty

C. Type III/Csendes gastrectomy with Roux-en-Y gastrojejunostomy or Pauchet gastrectomy and Billroth I reconstruction

D. Type IV/Billroth I or II reconstruction with truncal vagotomy

E. Type IV/total gastrectomy

ANSWER: A

COMMENTS: Benign **gastric ulcers** have been classified in terms of their anatomic location. **Type I** ulcers are the most common (50%) and occur in the body of the stomach along the lesser curvature. These ulcers are associated with low to normal acid secretion. **Type II** gastric ulcers (25%) also occur in the body of the stomach but have associated duodenal ulcers. **Type III** gastric ulcers (20%) are located in the prepyloric region. Both type II and type III ulcers are associated with excessive acid secretion. **Type IV** ulcers are the least common (<10%) and occur near the GE junction along the lesser curve. Like type I ulcers, they are associated with low or normal acid secretion. Surgical intervention is indicated for patients who have failed maximal medical therapy (12 weeks), for those in whom complications develop, or for those in whom malignancy cannot be ruled out. Surgical therapy for benign gastric ulcers depends on the type of ulcer and its associated acid secretion. Type I ulcers are usually well treated with antrectomy or hemigastrectomy (including removal of the ulcer) without vagotomy. Type IV ulcers do not require vagotomy either. Type IV ulcers near the GE junction can be treated by modifications of distal gastrectomy that include ulcer excision. Distal gastrectomy with extension along the lesser curvature to include the ulcer (**Pauchet procedure**) and Billroth I reconstruction can be performed for ulcers that are 2 to 5 cm from the GE junction. For type IV ulcers at the GE junction, subtotal gastrectomy with Roux-en-Y jejunal reconstruction (**Csendes procedure**), a rotational **Tanner** gastrectomy, or a **Kahler-Muhlenberg** procedure should be performed. Because type II and type III ulcers are associated with acid hypersecretion, they are treated as duodenal ulcers. Truncal vagotomy with Billroth I or II reconstruction is the preferred surgical therapy because it accomplishes both goals of a decrease in acid secretion and excision of the ulcer.

Ref.: 1, 4, 6

24. Which of the following tests is best to document eradication of *H. pylori* infection in patients with peptic ulcer disease (PUD)?

A. Urea breath test

B. Histologic examination of mucosa

C. Rapid urease test

D. Culture and sensitivity testing

E. *H. pylori* serology

ANSWER: A

COMMENTS: It is important to document the presence or absence of ***H. pylori*** to adequately treat patients with PUD. Both invasive and noninvasive tests are available for the diagnosis of *H. pylori* infection. **Invasive tests** require endoscopic mucosal biopsy and include **histologic examination**, **rapid urease test**, and **culture**. **Noninvasive tests** include the **urea breath test** and **serology**. Histologic examination can accurately diagnose *H. pylori* with two biopsy specimens with high sensitivity and specificity (90%). The rapid urease test on a mucosal biopsy specimen uses a change in pH resulting from the breakdown of urea by a urease enzyme produced by *H. pylori*. This test is considered the initial test of choice because of its simplicity, accuracy, and rapid results. Culture of *H. pylori* has the most specificity (100%) but is difficult to perform and is currently not widely available. Cultures should usually be reserved for research purposes or for patients with suspected antibiotic resistance. The urea breath test is a noninvasive test that analyzes breath for labeled carbon dioxide produced by bacterial urease from the conversion of ingested labeled urea. Because of its noninvasiveness plus high sensitivity and specificity (95%), the urea breath test is considered the test of choice for documentation of *H. pylori* eradication. Serologic tests are quick and inexpensive but cannot differentiate between active infection and previous exposure. Serology is useful for the initial diagnosis of *H. pylori* infection in patients in whom endoscopy is not indicated.

Ref.: 1, 5, 6

25. Which of the following conditions is not associated with gastric cancer?

A. Chronic atrophic gastritis

B. *H. pylori* infection

C. Hereditary nonpolyposis colorectal cancer

D. Adenomatous gastric polyps

E. Fundic gland polyps

ANSWER: E

COMMENTS: Certain gastric lesions have a significant association with gastric adenocarcinoma and can be considered precursors to malignancy. **Chronic atrophic gastritis**, of which several forms are recognized, underlies most gastric cancers. The epithelial changes of intestinal metaplasia and dysplasia are premalignant. Autoimmune chronic gastritis involves the body and fundus of the stomach. It is associated with pernicious anemia, achlorhydria, very high gastrin levels, and a high risk for cancer. Hypersecretory chronic gastritis involves the gastric antrum and is associated with PUD but not malignancy. ***H. pylori*** infection may be the most important risk factor for gastric adenocarcinoma worldwide. The immunoglobulin (Ig)G antibody positivity in various populations correlates with the local incidence of gastric cancer. **Hereditary nonpolyposis colorectal cancer** is an inheritable risk factor for gastric cancer. **Adenomatous gastric polyps** have malignant potential similar to colonic adenomatous polyps. The risk increases with increasing size of the polyp. **Fundic gland polyps** are benign and have no malignant potential.

Ref.: 1, 6, 7

26. With regard to the surgical treatment of gastric adenocarcinoma, which of the following statements is true?

A. Total gastrectomy for antral lesions results in longer survival than does partial gastrectomy.

B. Routine splenectomy does not improve survival rates.

C. Extended lymph node dissection improves survival rates in patients with stages I and II lesions.

D. Total gastrectomy for palliation is contraindicated.

E. Linitis plastica should be resected to histologically negative margins.

ANSWER: B

COMMENTS: Gastric adenocarcinoma is preferably treated by resection, although resection usually proves to be **palliative**. The general strategy for curative resection is to remove as much of the stomach as necessary to obtain free margins and to perform limited node dissection. Although data from Japan support the benefit of extended nodal dissection (celiac, mesenteric, hepatic, and paraaortic), studies in the United States have not generally confirmed this benefit. Furthermore, these extended dissections can be associated with substantial morbidity. Most resections entail distal subtotal gastrectomy. Total gastrectomy is appropriate for locally extensive tumors, proximal tumors (to avoid esophageal anastomosis to the distal stomach remnant), and even palliation if necessary. Extending clear margins on a distal tumor by total rather than subtotal gastrectomy is of no benefit. Resections for **linitis plastica** are palliative, usually necessitate total gastrectomy, and are carried out to grossly negative margins only. **Splenectomy** is performed according to the location of gastric resection, but its routine performance does not improve the survival rate. The number of lymph nodes resected, the number of positive nodes, and the ratio of positive to the total number of lymph nodes have important staging implications. Furthermore, a minimum number of 15 lymph nodes should routinely be examined.

Ref.: 1, 6, 7

27. With regard to gastrointestinal stromal tumors (GISTs), which of the following statements is incorrect?

A. A combination of cellular morphology on hematoxylin–eosin staining and KIT immunohistochemistry are required for the diagnosis of GIST.

B. After the small intestine, the stomach is the second most common location for GISTs, followed by the colon and rectum.

C. The majority of GISTs have an activating mutation in the *KIT* oncogene.

D. GISTs are usually resistant to conventional chemotherapy and radiation therapy.

E. Complete surgical resection is the standard of treatment.

ANSWER: B

COMMENTS: GI stromal tumors are the most common mesenchymal neoplasms of the GI tract. The majority of these GISTs occur in the stomach (60%), followed by the small bowel (30%), esophagus (1%–5%), and colon and rectum (5%). The diagnosis of GIST is based on the presence of characteristic pathologic findings on hematoxylin–eosin staining and expression of the **KIT receptor** on immunohistochemistry. Rarely, KIT might not be overexpressed, and in such cases molecular evaluation may be necessary. These tumors do not usually metastasize to lymph nodes. Complete surgical resection is the standard of treatment of primary, localized GISTs. The majority of GISTs have an activating mutation in the *KIT* protooncogene that can be effectively inhibited by tyrosine kinase inhibitors such as **imatinib mesylate** (**Gleevec**). GISTs are resistant to conventional chemoradiation therapy. Laparoscopic resection is increasingly being used, provided that a negative margin can be obtained. Both the size and number of mitoses per 50 high-power field have been used to categorize tumor aggressiveness. Tumor location may have prognostic implications in that extragastric tumors may carry a worse prognosis. Large or unresectable tumors that show KIT overexpression may initially be treated with Gleevec.

Ref.: 1, 8

28. Which of the following statements regarding Crohn's disease of the duodenum is false?

A. Duodenal Crohn's disease accounts only for 2%–4% of all patients with Crohn's disease.

B. Because of its location, operative intervention is frequently needed for duodenal Crohn's disease.

C. When an operation is required, a bypass such as gastrojejunostomy is performed rather than duodenal resection.

D. In well-selected patients, strictureplasty can be carried out with good results.

E. Adenocarcinoma is the leading cause of disease-specific death in patients with Crohn's disease.

ANSWER: B

COMMENTS: Crohn's disease of the duodenum is not common and is seen in only 2%–4% of patients with Crohn's disease. Medical therapy remains the mainstay of treatment of duodenal Crohn's disease, with surgical intervention being reserved for patients who do not respond to medical therapy or in whom a complication such as obstruction or perforation develops. In patients who do need a surgical procedure, bypass is preferred over duodenal resection. In a few select patients, their anatomy might be amenable to **strictureplasty**.

Irrespective of the location of Crohn's disease, GI cancer remains the leading cause of death in patients with Crohn's disease.

Ref.: 1, 9, 10

29. With regard to gastric volvulus, which of the following statements is true?

A. The Borchardt's triad includes acute epigastric pain, retching without vomiting, and inability to pass an NG tube.

B. Its symptoms consist of severe nausea with bilious emesis.

C. It more frequently involves rotation around the axis that bisects the greater and lesser curvatures.

D. Its surgical management is via a transthoracic approach.

E. Surgical management of volvulus without a diaphragmatic defect involves only detorsion of the stomach.

ANSWER: A

COMMENTS: Gastric volvulus is a serious complication of **paraesophageal hernia**. Two types of gastric volvulus may occur, depending on the axis of rotation. **Organoaxial** volvulus, the more common type, involves rotation around the axis of a line connecting the cardia and pylorus. **Mesenteroaxial** volvulus is not associated with a diaphragmatic defect and involves rotation around the line that bisects the greater and lesser curvatures. Combined types have also been described. Patients classically present with **Borchardt's triad**, which includes acute epigastric pain, violent retching without vomiting, and the inability to pass an NG tube. Acute gastric volvulus is a surgical emergency and requires prompt reduction via a transabdominal approach. Repair of the diaphragmatic defect should follow with possible fundoplication. In the setting of volvulus without an associated diaphragmatic defect, detorsion of the stomach and either gastropexy or tube gastrostomy is performed to reduce the risk for recurrence.

Ref.: 1, 11

30. In a patient who presents with intractable ulcer disease, which of the following statements is true?

A. A fasting serum gastrin level of >200 pg/mL is diagnostic of a gastrinoma.

B. A CT scan may demonstrate a mass within the tail of the pancreas.

C. In the setting of Zollinger-Ellison syndrome, endoscopy would demonstrate atrophic gastric mucosa.

D. The most sensitive and specific diagnostic test for Zollinger-Ellison syndrome is the secretin stimulation test.

E. Testing for associated multiple endocrine neoplasia II (MEN II) endocrine tumors should be considered.

ANSWER: D

COMMENTS: Intractable ulcer disease is defined as that occurring after an adequate duration of antacid therapy, documentation of eradication of *H. pylori* infection, and elimination of NSAID use. In these patients, malignancy must be ruled out and a serum gastrin level should be drawn to evaluate for a gastrinoma. **Zollinger-Ellison syndrome** is the triad of gastric acid hypersecretion, severe PUD, and non–beta islet cell tumors of the pancreas. Gastrinomas occur most commonly within the **gastrinoma triangle** as defined by the confluence of the cystic and common bile duct, the junction of the second and third portions of the duodenum, and the junction of the neck and body of the pancreas. They are found almost equally within the wall of the duodenum as the head of the pancreas but not in the tail of the pancreas. Endoscopy often reveals **prominent rugal folds**, which result from the trophic effect of the hypergastrinemia. Fasting serum gastrin levels are usually elevated above 200 pg/mL, but a value greater than 1000 pg/mL is diagnostic. In the setting of equivocal gastrin levels, the most sensitive test is the secretin stimulation test. A rise in gastrin levels of greater than 200 pg/mL above baseline is specific for gastrinoma. Gastrinomas are associated with MEN I syndrome, not MEN II syndrome. Testing for associated endocrine tumors should be performed.

Ref.: 1, 11

31. Which of the following is true with regard to gastric carcinoid neoplasms?

A. The incidence is decreasing.

B. They commonly present with abdominal pain, bleeding, and carcinoid syndrome.

C. The subtypes associated with low acid states have a better prognosis.

D. Long-term use of PPIs has not been shown to increase the risk for developing a gastric carcinoid neoplasm.

E. The treatment is based largely on nonsurgical management with somatostatin analogues.

ANSWER: C

COMMENTS: Long thought to be a rare location for carcinoid malignancies, **gastric carcinoid neoplasms** (or neuroendocrine tumors, NET) are increasing in incidence. Many patients are asymptomatic and **diagnosed incidentally** during endoscopy, though rarely they can present with abdominal pain, bleeding, and symptoms of carcinoid syndrome. The rise in the use of endoscopy has been postulated to account for some of the increase in incidence; however, the increase in the **long-term use of PPIs** may also play a part as it has been shown to be an independent risk factor for the development of gastric carcinoid tumors. There are three types of gastric carcinoids. The majority of these are type 1 and are associated with a **low acid state** (normally from atrophic gastritis), resulting in **hypergastrinemia**, which in turn is thought to cause **ECL cell hyperplasia** and eventual dysplasia. This type carries a better prognosis than sporadic types, type 3, not associated with low acid states. The final type is type 2, which is associated with Zollinger-Ellison syndrome and high gastrin levels. Treatment is based on **complete resection** whether accomplished via endoscopic removal, wedge resection, or total gastrectomy, depending on the extent of the disease. **Somatostatin analogues** can serve to decrease tumor burden and address symptoms of carcinoid syndrome in patients with recurrent or metastatic disease.

Ref.: 1, 11

32. On the cellular level, which of the following is true regarding acid secretion?

A. Acid secretion is stimulated only by gastrin.

B. Acid secretion is stimulated by gastrin and secretin.

C. The final common pathway of acid secretion is the hydrogen-potassium adenosine triphosphatase (H^+, K^+-ATPase).

D. Histamine activates acid secretion via increases in intracellular calcium.

E. Acid secretion is stimulated by CCK.

ANSWER: C

COMMENTS: It is important to have the knowledge of the cellular basis for parietal cell acid secretion to understand the pharmacologic control of acid. The **parietal cell** has three specific plasma membrane receptors that stimulate acid secretion: **acetylcholine**, **histamine**, and **gastrin** receptors. All three receptors eventually activate the **H^+, K^+-ATPase** pump via different mechanisms, which results in the secretion of a hydrogen ion for potassium. Acetylcholine- and gastrin-stimulated secretion depends on increases in **intracellular calcium levels**, with subsequent **phosphorylase kinase**–induced phosphorylation and H^+, K^+-ATPase activity. Histamine activates the **adenylate cyclase** pathway. **Somatostatin**, **CCK**, and **secretin** inhibit acid secretion.

Ref.: 1, 11

33. Which of the following statements is true regarding the gross or microscopic anatomy of the stomach?

A. The angularis incisura marks the transition from the body of the stomach to the antrum along the greater curvature.

B. The angle of His is formed by the junction of the fundus with the left diaphragmatic crus.

C. The cardia is dominated by mucus-secreting cells.

D. The majority of the parietal cells exist in the fundus and the proximal body.

E. The GE junction is normally found at the diaphragmatic hiatus.

ANSWER: C

COMMENTS: The most proximal region of the stomach is the **cardia**. This is dominated by **mucus-secreting cells**, which provide a mechanical barrier to injury. Gastric ulcers in this area are deemed type IV ulcers and are associated with a breakdown of this mucus barrier. The uppermost part of the stomach is the **fundus**. The junction of the fundus and the left margin of the esophagus forms the **angle of His**. The **GE junction** is normally found about 2 to 3 cm below the diaphragmatic esophageal hiatus. The extension of the esophagus into the abdominal cavity creates an anatomically important pressure differential between the distal esophagus within the positive pressure abdomen and the midesophagus within the negative pressure thoracic cavity that helps to prevent reflux. This relationship is disturbed in patients with type I hiatal hernias. The **body** is bound by the lesser curvature on the right and greater curvature on the left. **Parietal cells** exist primarily within the body, with few in the fundus and antrum and none in the cardia or prepyloric antrum. As the lesser curvature meets the pylorus, it angles abruptly to the right, identifying the **angularis incisura**.

Ref.: 1, 11

34. Which of the following statements is true regarding the management of upper GI bleeding?

A. The return of clear fluid from an NG lavage rules out upper GI bleeding.

B. Primary hemostasis is only achieved in 60% of patients by endoscopy alone.

C. The majority of upper GI bleeding will require intervention.

D. Patients with an upper GI bleed should undergo endoscopy within 24 h of presentation.

E. All patients should be placed on PPI and octreotide infusions.

ANSWER: D

COMMENTS: The majority of upper GI bleeding requires no intervention and ceases spontaneously. However, if it persists, it is associated with a mortality rate of 6%–8%. Initial management should include IV access, fluid resuscitation, and blood products as indicated. Placement of an NG tube can confirm upper GI bleeding with return of bloody or coffee ground lavage; however, only return of bilious lavage can effectively rule out an upper GI source of a bleed. Regardless of the degree of severity, patients who present with upper GI bleeding should undergo endoscopy within 24 h of presentation for both diagnostic and therapeutic purposes. Endoscopic control results in primary hemostasis in approximately 90% of patients. Patients should be closely monitored in an intensive care unit (ICU) setting in case of persistent bleeding, and all high-risk patients should be placed on PPI infusion. Octreotide infusions are reserved for upper GI bleeding as a result of esophageal varices.

Ref.: 1, 11

35. Which cell type is matched with the appropriate secretory product?

A. Chief cell/gastrin

B. Delta cell/somatostatin

C. Parietal cell/pepsin

D. G cell/histamine

E. ECL cell/intrinsic factor

ANSWER: B

COMMENTS: See Question 36.

Ref.: 1, 2, 11

36. Which cell type is matched with the correct primary anatomic location?

A. Chief cell/gastric antrum

B. G cell/gastric cardia

C. D cell/gastric fundus

D. Parietal cell/gastric fundus

E. Endocrine cell/gastric body

ANSWER: E

COMMENTS: The gastric mucosa consists of surface columnar epithelial cells and glands containing various cell types. The mucosal cells vary in their anatomic location and secretory function. Within the cardia, the glands contain primarily mucus-secreting cells and the pits are short. In the body of the stomach, the glands retain their mucus-secreting cells at their luminal end but the pits extend deeper and begin to include other secretory cells. Parietal and chief cells are located predominately in the body. **Parietal cells** produce **hydrochloric acid** and **intrinsic factor**, whereas **chief cells** secrete **pepsinogen**. The **G cells** of the antrum are the primary source of **gastrin**. **Somatostatin** is synthesized and stored in **delta cells** located in the gastric corpus and antrum. **Ghrelin**, produced by **endocrine cells** of the gastric body, probably plays a role in the neuroendocrine response to changes in nutritional status and has been shown to enhance appetite and increase food intake. Removal of a significant portion of the gastric body resulting in decreased ghrelin levels is thought to be the mechanism of appetite control after a sleeve gastrectomy.

Ref.: 1, 2, 11

37. Which of the following statements is true regarding gastric MALT lymphoma?

A. Negative histologic *H. pylori* testing confirms an *H. pylori*–negative MALT lymphoma.

B. Less than 10% of gastric lymphomas have associated *H. pylori* infection.

C. Upper GI endoscopy with gastric biopsy for the determination of the presence of *H. pylori* and the histologic type of lymphoma is the diagnostic test of choice.

D. Surveillance includes repeat endoscopy in 6 months to document clearance of the infection.

E. CT of the abdomen, chest radiography, bone marrow biopsy, and diagnostic laparoscopy are required for complete staging.

ANSWER: C

COMMENTS: Gastric MALT lymphoma is associated with chronic ***H. pylori*** infection in more than 90% of cases. Chronic infection with *H. pylori* results in monoclonal B-cell proliferation and development of lymphoid tissue resembling Peyer's patches in the stomach. Treatment directed toward *H. pylori* eradication results in the resolution of MALT lymphomas in 75% of cases. **Upper endoscopy with biopsy** is the diagnostic test of choice. Gastric biopsies are used to evaluate the presence of *H. pylori* and the histologic type of lymphoma. The depth of gastric wall invasion and the presence of nodal involvement can be determined with the help of **endoscopic ultrasonography**. Histologically, *H. pylori*–negative MALT lymphomas should be confirmed as such with serologic testing. Staging is completed with a chest radiograph, bone marrow biopsy, and CT of the abdomen. Surveillance is achieved with repeat endoscopy in 2 months with biopsy to document clearance of infection and subsequent endoscopy every 6 months for 3 years. Certain genetic translocations, large cell phenotype, nodal involvement, or transmural tumor extension all predict failure of *H. pylori* eradication alone.

Ref.: 1, 6, 11

38. Which of the following statements about high-grade gastric lymphoma is true?

A. Diffuse large B-cell lymphoma is the second most common gastric lymphoma after MALT lymphoma.

B. The addition of surgery to chemotherapy alone has been shown to improve outcomes.

C. Hemorrhage is a frequent complication of chemotherapy.

D. Surgical treatment is usually reserved for patients with limited gastric disease, localized persistent lymphoma, or complications associated with nonsurgical treatment.

E. Perforation is a frequent complication after chemotherapy.

ANSWER: D

COMMENTS: Diffuse large B-cell lymphoma is the most common type of gastric lymphoma, with MALT lymphoma being the second most common. High-grade gastric lymphoma is generally treated with chemotherapy or chemoradiation. Compared with surgical treatment, patient survival has been shown to be equivalent or better with nonsurgical treatment in several prospective clinical trials (randomized and nonrandomized). It was previously believed that surgery was superior to chemotherapy due to the risk for complications such as **perforation** and **hemorrhage** with chemotherapy. However, these risks have been found to be only approximately 5%. It is postulated that these risks may be increased with full-thickness involvement of the gastric wall. EUS can be used to determine the depth of invasion, and this information can be offered to the patient when discussing risks and benefits of treatment options. Operative intervention is therefore largely reserved for limited gastric disease in which R0 resection is a reasonable goal, patients undergoing chemoradiation with treatment failure, or for the management of rare complications of nonsurgical treatment including perforation, hemorrhage, and obstruction.

Ref.: 1, 6, 11

39. Regarding gastric varices, which of the following is false?

A. Gastric varices develop via increased flow and pressure transmitted through the short and posterior gastric veins.

B. Isolated gastric varices are the result of splenic vein thrombosis.

C. Gastric varices are more often associated with generalized portal hypertension than with splenic vein thrombosis.

D. Isolated gastric varices should be managed with endoscopic banding and sclerotherapy.

E. Gastric varices associated with portal hypertension should be managed with endoscopic banding and sclerotherapy.

ANSWER: D

COMMENTS: There are two types of **gastric varices**: those that occur in the setting of portal hypertension and those that are secondary to **splenic vein thrombosis (isolated gastric varices)**. To establish the diagnosis of isolated gastric varices, there must be no evidence of portal hypertension, cirrhosis, or esophageal varices on endoscopy. In either type, an increased flow and pressure is transmitted via the **short and posterior gastric veins**. For isolated gastric varices, **splenectomy** is curative. Splenectomy is neither curative nor indicated when the varices are associated with portal hypertension. Rather, this type is best managed similarly to esophageal varices with endoscopy, banding, and sclerotherapy.

Ref.: 1, 12

40. Regarding the gross anatomy of the duodenum, which of the following is true?

A. The length of the duodenum is approximately 20 cm.

B. The second, third, and fourth portions of the duodenum are retroperitoneal.

C. The SMA marks the transition point between the second and third portions.

D. Lack of collateral blood supply puts the duodenum at a high risk for ischemia.

E. The minor papilla is located in the first portion of the duodenum and the major in the second.

ANSWER: A

COMMENTS: The duodenum is the first portion of the small intestine and the most distal foregut-derived structure. It is approximately 20 cm in length and is divided into four portions, of which the second and third are found retroperitoneally. Although the minor papilla is found superiorly to the major, they are both located within the second portion. The acute angle between the aorta and the SMA marks the transition point between the third and fourth portions. The blood supply to the duodenum is via the superior and inferior pancreaticoduodenal arteries, both of which have posterior and anterior divisions and constitute a rich bed of vascular collaterals. The anastomosis of these two vessels also represents the only connection between celiac and SMA blood supply.

Ref.: 1, 13

41. With regard to adenocarcinoma of the small bowel, which of the following statements is false?

A. Small bowel adenocarcinoma is found in decreasing order of frequency in the ileum, jejunum, and duodenum.

B. Villous adenomas of the small bowel are commonly found in the duodenum around the ampulla of Vater.

C. Adenocarcinoma of the duodenum usually occurs earlier than small bowel adenocarcinoma elsewhere in the jejunum and ileum.

D. Villous adenomas of the duodenum are frequently associated with familial adenomatous polyposis (FAP).

E. Operative resection is the treatment modality of choice and has curative potential.

ANSWER: A

COMMENTS: Small bowel adenocarcinoma accounts for the majority (35%–50%) of small bowel malignant neoplasms, followed by carcinoid tumors, lymphomas, and sarcomas. Adenocarcinoma of the small bowel is more common in the duodenum, whereas **carcinoid tumors** and **lymphoma** are more frequently seen in the ileum. Small bowel adenocarcinoma is found in decreasing order of frequency in the duodenum, jejunum, and ileum. Most patients have nonspecific symptoms initially; however, adenocarcinoma of the duodenum is manifested earlier with signs and symptoms of obstructive jaundice, gastric outlet obstruction, and abdominal pain. Operative resection (pancreaticoduodenectomy and local excision) is the treatment of choice, depending on the size and location of the adenocarcinoma, the patient's health, and the surgeon's expertise. Although rare in the small bowel, **villous adenomas** are frequently found in the duodenum and are associated with **FAP syndrome** (31%–92%). These villous adenomas have high malignant potential, especially if they are larger than 5 cm or are accompanied by bleeding or obstruction. The Spigelman criteria are used to grade duodenal polyposis seen in FAP. They consist of five incremental stages of severity (0 to IV). Points are earned for the number of polyps, size of polyps, histology, and grade of dysplasia. This classification also correlates with the risk for malignancy as follows: stage II, 2.3% risk; stage III, 2.4% risk; and stage IV, 36% risk. Pancreaticoduodenectomy is recommended for stage IV.

Ref.: 1, 2, 6, 14

REFERENCES

1. Mercer DW, Robinson EK. Stomach. In: Townsend CM, Beauchamp RD, Evers BM, et al., eds. *Sabiston Textbook of Surgery: The Biological Basis of Modern Surgical Practice*. 18th ed. Philadelphia: WB Saunders; 2008.
2. Dempsey DT. Stomach. In: Brunicardi FC, Andersen DK, Billiar TR, et al., eds. *Schwartz's Principles of Surgery*. 9th ed. New York: McGraw-Hill; 2010.
3. Rice-Townsend SE, Norton JA. Zollinger-Ellison syndrome. In: Cameron JL, ed. *Current Surgical Therapy*. 9th ed. Philadelphia: CV Mosby; 2008.
4. Winkleman BJ, Usatii A, Ellison EC. Duodenal ulcer. In: Cameron JL, ed. *Current Surgical Therapy*. 9th ed. Philadelphia: CV Mosby; 2008.
5. Fisher WE, Brunicardi FC. Benign gastric ulcer. In: Cameron JL, ed. *Current Surgical Therapy*. 9th ed. Philadelphia: CV Mosby; 2008.
6. Bland KI, Büchler MW, Csendes A, Garden OJ, Wong J. *General Surgery: Principles and International Practice*. 2nd ed. New York: Springer-Verlag; 2008.
7. Cho CS, Brennan MF. Gastric adenocarcinoma. In: Cameron JL, ed. *Current Surgical Therapy*. 9th ed. Philadelphia: CV Mosby; 2008.
8. Efron DT. Gastrointestinal stromal tumors. In: Cameron JL, ed. *Current Surgical Therapy*. 9th ed. Philadelphia: CV Mosby; 2008.
9. Mintz Y, Talamini MA. Crohn's disease of the small bowel. In: Cameron JL, ed. *Current Surgical Therapy*. 9th ed. Philadelphia: CV Mosby; 2008.
10. Tavakkolizadeh A, Whang EE, Ashley SW, Zinner MJ. Small intestine. In: Brunicardi FC, Andersen DK, Billiar TR, et al., eds. *Schwartz's Principles of Surgery*. 9th ed. New York: McGraw-Hill; 2010.
11. Mulholland M. Stomach and duodenum. In: Mulholland M, Lillemoe K, Doherty GM, et al., eds. *Greenfield's Surgery: Scientific Principles and Practice*. 5th ed. Ann Arbor: Lippincott Williams & Wilkins; 2010.
12. Fraker D. The spleen. In: Mulholland M, Lillemoe K, Doherty GM, et al., eds. *Greenfield's Surgery: Scientific Principles and Practice*. 5th ed. Ann Arbor: Lippincott Williams & Wilkins; 2010.
13. Drake R, Vogl A, Mitchell A. *Gray's Anatomy*. 2nd ed. Philadelphia: Churchill Livingstone Elsevier; 2010.
14. Groves CJ, Saunders BP, Spigelman AD, Phillips RKS. Duodenal cancer in patient with familial adenomatous polyposis (FAP): results of a 10-year prospective study. *Gut*. 2002;50:636–641.

CHAPTER 22

SMALL BOWEL AND APPENDIX

A. Small Bowel

Donnamarie Packer, M.D.

1. The small intestine typically reabsorbs what percentage of the fluid that passes through its lumen?

A. 10

B. 20

C. 40

D. 50

E. 80

ANSWER: E

COMMENTS: The intestine has a remarkable ability to absorb and secrete large quantities of fluid. Absorption of water is a net result of fluxes into and out of the intestinal lumen. An average person consumes approximately 1 to 1.5 liters (L) of water per day. The gastrointestinal tract (GI) secretes an additional 5 to 10 L, including 1 to 2 L of saliva, 2 to 3 L of gastric secretions, 0.5 L of biliary secretions, 1 to 2 L of pancreatic juice, and 1 L of intestinal secretions. The small intestine reabsorbs nearly 80% of the fluid that passes through it. A rapid bidirectional movement of fluid in the intestinal lumen accomplishes this dynamic process. A total of 6 to 11 L of water enters the duodenum every day, but only 1 to 1.5 L arrives in the colon. Alterations in this fine balance caused by either impaired absorption or augmented secretion can result in overall net secretion of water and result in diarrhea.

Ref.: 1

2. With regard to ileostomy physiology, which of the following statements is true?

A. Daily output from an established ileostomy is approximately 1500 mL.

B. Ileostomy output can increase by 50% at times of dietary indiscretion.

C. With dehydration, the concentration of sodium output from the ileostomy rises.

D. Compared with normal ileal fluid, ileostomy effluent contains a 100-fold increase in aerobes and a 2500-fold increase in coliform bacteria.

E. The microbiologic flora of ileostomy output is similar to that of normal ileal fluid.

ANSWER: D

COMMENTS: The daily output from an established ileostomy is typically 500 to 1000 mL. Although there is a great deal of variation in daily output among individuals, the output in a given patient varies only about 20% with changes in diet or with episodes of gastroenteritis. The usual ileostomy sodium concentration is 115 mEq/L, although the concentration rises and falls with changes in total body sodium. With dehydration, the sodium concentration falls and the potassium level rises as a result of the ability of the terminal ileum to conserve sodium in times of salt depletion. Normally, the sodium-to-potassium ratio is about 12:1. The microbiologic flora of ileostomy output is markedly different from that of normal ileal fluid. The total number of bacteria is 80 times greater, and there is a 100-fold increase in the number of aerobes, a 2500-fold increase in the number of coliform bacteria, and an increase in the total number of anaerobes.

Ref.: 1

3. A patient undergoes a contrast radiograph of the small bowel for evaluation of intestinal pseudo-obstruction. The average transit time from the duodenum to the cecum is:

A. 30 min

B. 1 h

C. 3 h

D. 5 h

E. 7 h

ANSWER: B

COMMENTS: In healthy humans, the transit time of barium contrast from the duodenum to the terminal ileum varies greatly, from 30 min to 5 h. The average (>80%) transit time is approximately 1 h. However, the composition of the meal affects the rate of occurrence and propagation of contractions during the postprandial period. The frequency of contraction is greatest with meals containing glucose and least after meals high in fat. Therefore transit is regulated to optimize absorption of nutrients.

Ref.: 2

4. Which of the following statements about small bowel motility is true?

A. Oral feeding stimulates the production of migrating motor complexes (MMCs).

B. If motility is impaired, absorption of nutrients is similarly affected.

C. MMCs are peristaltic contractions occurring at 10- to 20-min intervals.

D. Vagotomy-induced diarrhea is the result of increased secretion secondary to denervation.

E. Segmental bowel resection causes a temporary interruption of MMCs, but the clinical results are usually insignificant.

ANSWER: E

COMMENTS: MMCs are sets of propagated aboral peristaltic contractions occurring at 90-min intervals during fasting. They are one of the most recognizable and reproducible GI motility activities. The activity fronts of MMCs usually originate high in the stomach, propagate distally, and end in the ileum, usually at the mid-ileal level. Oral feeding inhibits MMCs and results in irregular, nonpropagating contractions throughout most of the small intestine. This postprandial inhibition generally persists for 3 to 4 h after a meal and is most pronounced with lipids. Although this motility pattern appears to be disorganized, there is a distal progression of chyme. Absorption is not affected by intestinal motility. Enteral feedings can therefore be used safely and efficiently in postoperative patients in whom motility may be altered.

Both gastric and small bowel motility can be affected by exogenous conditions. The small bowel is less sensitive than the stomach to general anesthesia and laparotomy, each of which decreases the frequency of MMCs. The frequency of MMCs returns to normal within 6 to 24 h in the absence of peritonitis or abscess formation. The tone of the stomach is affected more than that of the small bowel by general anesthesia and laparotomy and may take longer than 24 h to normalize. This may explain the occurrence of postoperative nausea and emesis. Vagotomy-induced diarrhea is a result of persistence of the sustained, organized wave of MMCs during the postprandial state due to loss of vagal parasympathetic inhibition of MMCs.

Segmental small bowel resection or denervation temporarily reduces the frequency of MMCs with a resultant temporary impairment of motility. Resection or denervation does not produce long-term sequelae provided that intestinal length is sufficient.

Ref.: 3

5. A 27-year-old man with a long-standing history of Crohn's disease is noted to have several extraintestinal manifestations of Crohn's disease including erythema nodosum, arthritis, ankylosing spondylitis, anemia, and episodes of pancreatitis. During evaluation of his right lower quadrant pain, he is found to have a segment of thickened ileum causing obstruction. Which extraintestinal manifestations of his Crohn's disease would you not expect to subside after resection of the involved segment of bowel?

A. Erythema nodosum

B. Arthritis

C. Ankylosing spondylitis

D. Anemia

E. Pancreatitis

ANSWER: C

COMMENTS: The extraintestinal manifestations of Crohn's disease are listed in Table 22A.1. They are not a primary indication for surgery in most patients with this disease. Indications for surgery include obstruction, perforation, abscesses, internal or cutaneous fistulas, and perianal disease. However, if the involved bowel were resected, most extraintestinal manifestations would improve except for ankylosing spondylitis and hepatic changes.

Surgery is not held to be curative in Crohn's disease since it is a systemic disorder. Surgery is indicated when medical therapy fails or when the side effects of medications (such as steroids) are significant. Bowel-conserving approaches are important since the majority of patients will require multiple surgeries in their lifetime. Resection is limited to the offending segment(s). If adjacent areas of bowel are affected but are not the cause of perforation, obstruction, or fistula formation, they should be spared and managed medically. Obstruction due to fibrotic stricturing is the most common indication for abdominal surgery in patients with Crohn's disease. Options for obstructed segments of the bowel include segmental resection and primary anastomosis or ostomy, stricturoplasty, and, rarely, bypass procedures. Repeated wide resections of small bowel may lead to a short gut syndrome. Stricturoplasty is beneficial in patients with multiple short areas of narrowing separated by normal intestine. Perforation occurs in 15%–20% of patients and usually results in the formation of a contained abscess, phlegmon, or an internal fistula to the bowel, bladder, or vagina. Enterocutaneous fistulas rarely occur in patients without previous operation, but they are common after surgery. Free perforations into the peritoneal cavity with peritonitis are rare. Anemia is common, but frank hemorrhage is rare. It may occur if an ulcer erodes into a large blood vessel.

Anorectal disease occurs in 50% of patients with Crohn's disease and may be the presenting problem in 5% of patients. Perirectal abscesses and/or fistulas develop in up to 30% of patients with Crohn's disease of the small bowel and are separate from the diseased segment of small bowel.

Patients with Crohn's disease have an increased risk for the development of cancer in comparison with the general population, but the risk for colon cancer does not approach the level seen in patients with chronic ulcerative colitis. This difference may be related to the segmental nature of Crohn's disease involving a smaller proportion of the colon and the shorter average period between diagnosis and colectomy in Crohn's disease. The risk, however, is not considered high enough to warrant prophylactic resection. However, colonoscopic surveillance is indicated. Most cases of small bowel cancer associated with Crohn's disease occur

TABLE 22A.1 Extraintestinal Manifestations of Crohn's Disease

Skin	Eyes	Joints	Blood	Liver	Kidneys	Pancreas	General
Erythema multiforme	Iritis	Peripheral arthritis	Anemia	Nonspecific triad inflammation	Nephrotic syndrome	Pancreatitis	Amyloidosis
Erythema nodosum	Uveitis	Ankylosing spondylitis	Thrombocytosis	Sclerosing cholangitis	Amyloidosis		
Pyoderma gangrenosum	Conjunctivitis		Phlebothrombosis				
			Arterial thrombosis				

in patients with long-standing disease and are most commonly found in a previously bypassed segment of bowel or at the site of a chronic small bowel stricture.

Ref.: 2

6. A patient with Crohn's disease and obstructing chronic fibrotic small bowel strictures not responding to medical therapy is taken to the operating room. Appropriate surgical management includes:

A. Resecting the diseased segments with frozen section evaluation of the margins

B. Avoiding bowel resection for long strictures

C. Resecting bowel to palpably normal tissue

D. Resecting only the obviously obstructing segment and preserving as much bowel as possible

E. Performing no more than two stricturoplasties during a single operation

ANSWER: C

COMMENTS: Proximal and distal margins of resection are determined by gross visual examination and palpation to soft pliable tissue. Frozen sections should not be routinely performed. Resecting to areas without microscopic evidence of inflammation does not reduce recurrence rates or decrease complications such as leaks and may lead to unnecessary loss of small bowel length. All areas of significant stricturing must be addressed during the operation since leaving any will often result in rapid recurrence of symptoms and the need for additional surgery. Bowel resection for strictures is the most common abdominal procedure performed in Crohn's disease; however, stricturoplasty is preferred for short obstructing segments since no normal bowel is sacrificed at the margins. The length of a stricture acceptable for stricturoplasty is debatable. Different surgeons have advocated for various types of stricturoplasty to manage longer segments. However, the commonly accepted approach is to perform the now standard Heineke–Mikulicz type of stricturoplasty for strictures up to 3 to 4 cm long. There is no defined limit for the number of strictures that can be treated during one operation; some studies have shown up to 19 stricturoplasties done at once without increased morbidity. Remarkably, there is a low leak rate, and the disease at these sites usually resolves.

Ref.: 2, 4

7. Which of the following statements is true of the microscopic appearance of Crohn's disease?

A. The disease is confined to the mucosa and submucosa.

B. Identification of noncaseating granulomas is required for diagnosis.

C. Granulomas demonstrating caseation without acid-fast bacilli confirm the diagnosis.

D. Submucosal fibrosis occurs secondary to bacterial invasion.

E. Marked lymphangiectasia is a prominent microscopic feature.

ANSWER: E

COMMENTS: Several microscopic features characterize but are not specific for Crohn's disease. These features progress from an early to a late phase of involvement and can be described as a granulomatous fibrotic inflammation progressing through all layers of the bowel wall.

In the early phase, edema of the entire bowel wall is seen, accompanied by lymphangiectasia and hyperemia and an increased proportion of goblet cells in an otherwise normal mucosa.

In the intermediate phase, thickening is caused by fibrosis of the submucosal and subserosal areas of the bowel. Focal mucosal ulcers become numerous, and in 60% of patients, sarcoid-like granulomas appear, particularly in the submucosa, subserosa, and regional lymph nodes. These granulomas contain epithelioid giant cells, do not caseate, and do not contain acid-fast bacilli. The absence of granulomas does not exclude the diagnosis of Crohn's disease. Lymphangiectasia remains visible throughout the intermediate and late phases.

In the late phase, the dense fibrosis exceeds that expected from the simple healing of an inflammatory insult and produces a fixed stenosis and partial obstruction of the lumen. The mucosa is denuded over wide areas, with occasional islands of intact mucosal cells (pseudopolyps). Glands deep in the mucosa resemble those of the pyloric region and are termed aberrant pyloric glands or Brunner gland metaplasia. The ulcers can be deep, and progression through the bowel wall may result in abscess and/or fistula formation.

Ref.: 2, 4

8. Diarrhea is one of the common clinical manifestations of Crohn's disease. Which of the following statements is true regarding this manifestation?

A. Most patients experience intermittent bloody diarrhea.

B. Diarrhea is the result of segmental inflammation, leading to decreased small bowel absorption.

C. Decreased bile salt absorption in the diseased terminal ileum produces choleretic diarrhea.

D. Diarrhea is frequently described as mucus or pus like.

E. Bloody diarrhea almost always produces anemia.

ANSWER: C

COMMENTS: Only 10% of patients with Crohn's disease are initially seen in an acute stage, usually with symptoms similar to those of appendicitis. In most patients, the onset is insidious, with intermittent pain or discomfort being the most frequent and sometimes the only symptom. The pain is often precipitated by a dietary indiscretion. With advanced disease, the pain may become associated with signs and symptoms of partial obstruction. Symptoms worsen with eating, and many patients resort to a liquid diet. Constant, localized pain, especially if associated with a palpable mass, suggests the presence of a phlegmon, abscess, or enteric fistula.

Diarrhea is the next most frequent symptom, and, unlike diarrhea in patients with chronic ulcerative colitis, it rarely contains mucus, pus, or blood. Diarrhea is the result of several factors. The inflamed segment of small bowel has a decreased capacity to absorb intestinal contents. In addition, the obstruction produced by this involved segment alters the absorptive capacity of the proximal part of the bowel. Decreased absorption of bile salts in the diseased terminal ileum leads to bile salt–induced damage to the absorptive cells of the colonic mucosa and produces choleretic diarrhea.

One-third of patients initially have a fever, and about 50% experience weight loss, weakness, and fatigue. Although the diarrhea is usually not bloody, persistent occult loss of blood frequently produces iron deficiency anemia, which may be aggravated by the deficiency of vitamin B_{12}, which is absorbed in the terminal ileum. Hypoproteinemia occurs because of increased loss of protein from the inflamed bowel mucosa. Vitamin and mineral deficiencies are the results of decreased ingestion, altered metabolism, and decreased absorption.

Ref.: 2, 4

9. A 26-year-old woman with a history of Crohn's disease is experiencing a flare of her disease. She is 6 weeks pregnant. Which of the following is true regarding the use of corticosteroids in patients with inflammatory bowel disease?

A. Corticosteroids are unsafe to use in pregnant patients with an acute flare of Crohn's disease.

B. Corticosteroids effectively maintain remission of Crohn's colitis and ulcerative colitis during pregnancy.

C. Corticosteroids used in enema (topical) form are not absorbed into the systemic circulation and therefore have no systemic side effects.

D. Therapy every other day is effective in pregnant patients during acute flares.

E. Intravenous corticosteroids and adrenocorticotropic hormone (ACTH) are equally effective in patients with acute severe ulcerative colitis that is refractory to oral treatment during pregnancy.

ANSWER: E

COMMENTS: The use of steroids in patients with an acute flare of Crohn's colitis or ulcerative colitis during pregnancy has been shown to be not only effective but also safe for the mother and fetus. This is also true of sulfasalazine.

Corticosteroids have never been shown to maintain remission of Crohn's colitis or ulcerative colitis, and prolonged use often results in major side effects. Sulfasalazine and other 5-acetylsalicylic acid (5-ASA) products including mesalamine and coated 5-ASA compounds are effective in maintaining remission only in patients with ulcerative colitis.

Topical steroids in foam or enema preparations may be absorbed in small amounts (10%–20%). Alternate-day dosing has not been effective in patients with inflammatory bowel disease.

Intravenous ACTH is preferred instead of intravenous hydrocortisone by some, but controversy still exists regarding whether ACTH is more effective, even for previously untreated ulcerative colitis. An ACTH dose of 40 to 60 units over an 8-h period appears to be as effective as 300 to 400 mg/day of hydrocortisone. ACTH use has waned in the face of newer medical therapies.

The duration of steroid therapy varies depending on the severity of the disease, but it should always be tapered on an individual basis with the goal of discontinuation. Although some patients (10%–15%) are kept on a low maintenance dose when complete elimination leads to flare-up, steroid therapy should not be continued as maintenance in patients who have achieved complete remission. Failure to achieve remission after 2 months of administering more than 15 mg of prednisone may be an indication for surgical management.

Ref.: 5

10. During resection of the terminal ileum and ascending colon for Crohn's disease, a 38-year-old man had 3 feet of small bowel removed. Six months later, he presents complaining of persistent diarrhea. Contrast studies and endoscopy are normal. The most likely etiology is:

A. Malabsorption of bile salts

B. Reactivation of Crohn's disease

C. Gastric acid hypersecretion

D. Bacterial overgrowth

E. Partial bowel obstruction

ANSWER: A

COMMENTS: The most likely etiology of diarrhea in this patient is malabsorption of bile salts. Bile salts and vitamin B_{12} are absorbed in the terminal ileum. After resection of the terminal ileum, bile salt reabsorption may be compromised and it enters the colon in much higher concentrations than normal. Bile salts irritate the colonic mucosa and interfere with absorption of fluid and electrolytes, leading to increased frequency and watery stools. Treatment for bile salt–induced diarrhea is oral cholestyramine, a bile salt–binding resin.

Reactivation of Crohn's disease is common following surgery. Rates vary from 28% to 73% at 1 year and from 77% to 85% at 3 years after ileal resection. The lowest rates of recurrence are in patients with disease limited to the colon after total colectomy (20%). Endoscopic recurrence rates are higher than symptomatic recurrence rates. Most colonic and terminal ileal recurrences may be seen with colonoscopy.

Bacterial overgrowth is more frequently associated with a nonfunctioning portion of bowel that leads to stasis. Examples include dilated proximal bowel above a stenotic obstruction, intestinal diverticula, and diversion or bypass surgery. Bacteria consume vitamins and nutrients. Symptoms include nausea, vomiting, bloating, and diarrhea. The diagnosis is made with an abnormal D-xylose breath test. Symptoms generally improve with antibiotics, although repeated courses or maintenance may be needed if the situation is not surgically corrected.

Gastric acid hypersecretion is associated with short gut syndrome. Short gut syndrome will most likely occur in patients with less than 100 cm bowel and no ileocecal valve or in those with less than 50 cm bowel and an ileocecal valve. This patient has had approximately 90 cm of bowel removed, leaving behind enough bowel that short gut syndrome is unlikely.

Ref.: 5

11. Nutritional support may be beneficial in patients with inflammatory bowel disease refractory to medical treatment. Which of the following statements is true?

A. Bowel rest and parenteral nutrition are the primary therapy for Crohn's colitis.

B. In those with Crohn's disease and a high-output fistula, total parenteral nutrition (TPN) promotes closure of the fistula.

C. TPN helps prevent the need for total colectomy in patients with ulcerative colitis.

D. In patients with Crohn's ileitis, TPN is superior to enteral nutrition for providing an adequate caloric replacement.

E. An elemental diet is the primary therapy for exacerbation of Crohn's disease.

ANSWER: B

COMMENTS: TPN has no role as a primary therapy for ulcerative colitis, but it may help maintain a satisfactory nutritional state during bowel rest. TPN does not prevent the need for colectomy in refractory cases. The role of TPN in patients with Crohn's colitis is not well established, but in those with Crohn's colitis and small bowel involvement, TPN may improve remission rates and promote fistula closure. Elemental diets have been sporadically shown by some to be effective in inducing remission of active Crohn's disease. The patient's tolerance may be poor, however, and the results are not superior to those obtained with corticosteroids and sulfasalazine. Peripheral parenteral alimentation (PPN) rarely provides adequate caloric replacement and may induce venous sclerosis and phlebitis. Enteral nutrition is preferable to TPN, when possible, since complications are much lower and nutritional balance is better. Nutrition delivered through the GI tract appears to preserve normal GI function, benefit normal immune function, and decrease systemic inflammation.

Ref.: 6

12. A 30-year-old woman has a bowel obstruction secondary to Crohn's disease. She has undergone multiple previous small bowel resections. At laparotomy, multiple strictures are noted throughout her bowel. Which of the following statements is true?

A. Stricturoplasty should be considered only for patients with an isolated stricture.

B. Segmental bowel resections are preferable to stricturoplasty for the current laparotomy.

C. Restricture at the stricturoplasty site has been seen in less than 5% of patients.

D. Anastomotic leakage and fistula formation following stricturoplasty have been seen in 50% of cases.

E. Because residual disease is left behind, reoperation for Crohn's disease is more likely with stricturoplasty than with bowel resection.

ANSWER: C

COMMENTS: Stricturoplasty for Crohn's disease was first performed in 1981 by Emanuel Lee based on his experience with patients with intestinal tuberculosis in India. The procedure was popularized by Victor Fazio and his colleagues at the Cleveland Clinic. Experience since then has shown it to be a safe alternative to resection in properly selected patients. Stricturoplasty should be considered in any patient who has had extensive previous resections of diseased bowel and in whom further resection might create short bowel syndrome (SBS) and in those with multiple separated fibrotic small bowel strictures. Many strictures can be treated safely by a single laparotomy. The entire small bowel must be inspected to avoid overlooking strictures that are not obvious. This can be accomplished by passing a long intestinal tube through one of the stricturoplasty sites. The catheter is passed both proximally and distally through the entire length of small bowel. The balloon on the catheter is inflated to 2 cm, and then the catheter is gradually withdrawn, identifying all significant strictures that are marked with a suture. A longitudinal incision is made over the stricture and extended for 2 cm proximally and distally beyond the stricture. A biopsy is performed to rule out neoplasia. The enterotomy is then closed transversely with a single layer of interrupted absorbable sutures. The site is marked with a metal clip. If a single stricture or several strictures close together are encountered at a patient's first surgery, resection rather than stricturoplasty is preferable because it eliminates the diseased bowel and establishes the diagnosis. Patients treated by stricturoplasty have been compared with patients treated by resection. The need for reoperation at the original site is similar. Postoperative complications are infrequent. At the Cleveland Clinic, anastomotic leakage, abscesses, or fistulas have occurred in 9% of patients treated by stricturoplasty. Restricture at the stricturoplasty site occurred in only 2%.

Ref.: 1

13. A 54-year-old man is being assessed for colicky abdominal pain and occasional nonbilious emesis. He denies fevers and does not have leukocytosis. He has a history of melanoma that was resected from his arm 5 years earlier. His upper GI (UGI) radiograph is shown in Fig. 22A.1. What is the next best step in this patient's management?

A. Barium enema with pneumatic decompression

B. Exploratory laparotomy and manual reduction

C. Exploratory laparotomy, manual reduction, and resection of the involved segment

D. Nasogastric tube placement, intravenous fluid, and a trial of nonoperative management

E. Exploratory laparotomy and intestinal bypass

ANSWER: C

COMMENTS: Intussusception is the telescoping of one portion of an intestinal segment onto the lumen of an adjacent segment (Fig. 22A.2). It is commonly seen in children. The lead point is commonly a Meckel's diverticulum or ileal lymphoid hyperplasia. It is the most frequent cause of pediatric bowel obstruction.

It is rare in adults, in whom it accounts for less than 5% of cases of bowel obstruction. Most cases of intussusception in adults

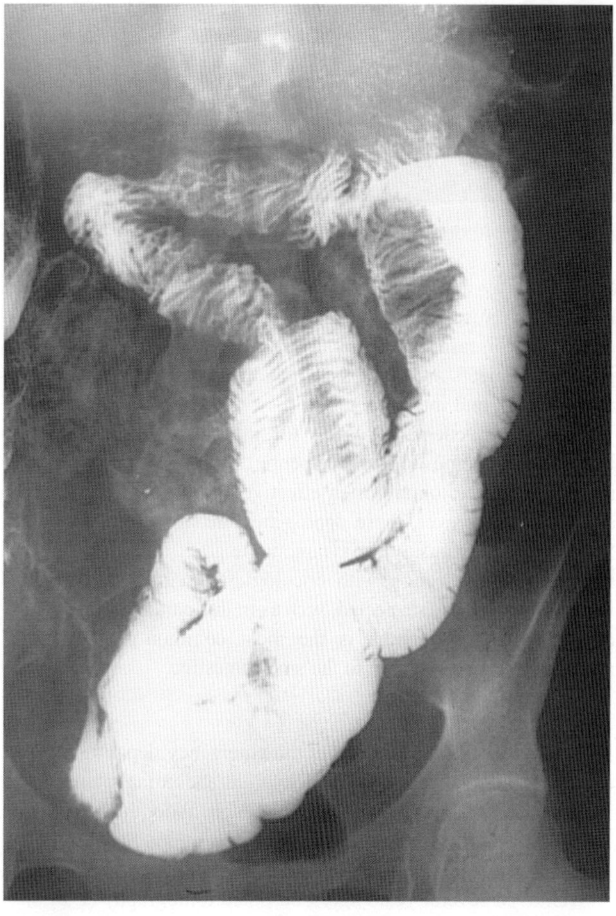

Fig. 22A.1 Upper gastrointestinal radiograph. *(Courtesy of Melvyn H. Schreiber, M.D., The University of Texas Medical Branch.)*

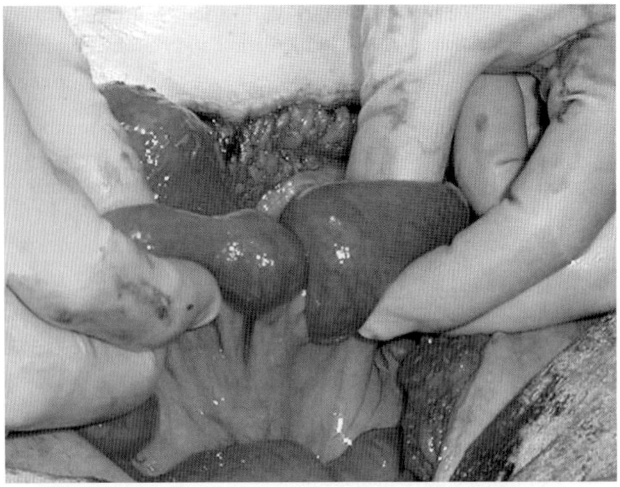

Fig. 22A.2 Intussusception. *(Courtesy of Steven Williams, M.D., Nampa, Idaho.)*

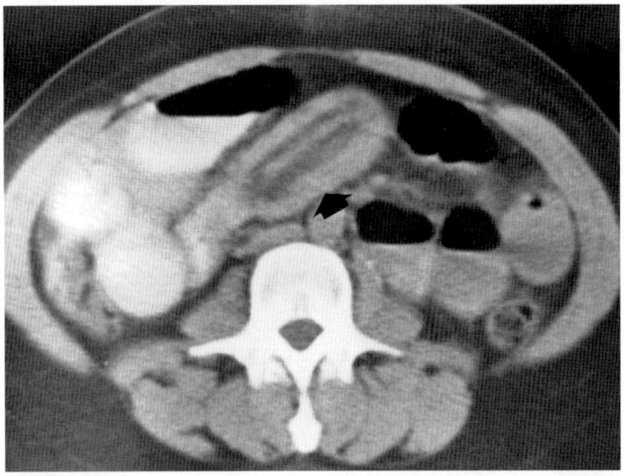

Fig. 22A.3 Abdominal computed tomographic scan.

are caused by a specific lead point, whereas only 8%–20% are idiopathic. Causes of intussusception in adults include inflammatory bowel disease, adhesions, Meckel's diverticulum, neoplasms including cancers and polyps such as those in Peutz-Jeghers syndrome (PJS), and intestinal tubes.

A barium enema is useful for intussusception in children because it is diagnostic and therapeutic. Barium enemas and pneumatic decompression are often effective at reduction of the intussusception. However, these approaches are not useful in adults. Surgery is the mainstay for symptomatic adult intussusception. A formal bowel resection with oncologic principles is warranted when malignancy is suspected, such as in this patient with a history of melanoma. Melanoma is the most common nonabdominal malignancy to metastasize to the small intestine.

Ref.: 3, 7

14. A 26-year-old man arrives at the emergency department with a complaint of recurrent, colicky, mid-abdominal pain. Physical examination reveals a palpable abdominal mass and several areas of increased pigmentation on his lips, palms, and soles. He states that his father had a colon polyp removed several years ago. Computed tomography (CT) of the abdomen was performed (Fig. 22A.3). PJS is suspected. Which of the following is true of PJS?

A. It is a sex-linked recessive familial disease characterized by intestinal polyposis and mucocutaneous hyperpigmentation.

B. Polyps are most frequently located in the jejunum and ileum but can also be found in the stomach, duodenum, colon, and rectum.

C. Surgical treatment includes resecting all bowel containing polyps.

D. Peutz-Jeghers polyps have a high malignant potential.

E. Peutz-Jeghers polyps are typically adenomatous.

ANSWER: B

COMMENTS: PJS is an autosomal dominant familial disease characterized by intestinal polyposis and mucocutaneous hyperpigmentation. The polyps are hamartomas that are most frequently located in the jejunum and ileum, but they can also be found in the stomach, duodenum, colon, and rectum. It is generally believed that their malignant potential is fairly low. PJS can cause intussusception or hemorrhage. Up to one-third of patients initially have abdominal pain and a palpable mass. Symptoms may be self-limited as the intussusception comes and goes. The diagnosis of intestinal polyps may be made with UGI and small bowel follow-through contrast studies, pill endoscopy, or at the time of surgery. Magnetic resonance (MR) enterography may prove to be useful as this modality becomes more refined. Surgery is indicated for persistent obstruction, frequent recurrences, or bleeding. Surgical treatment is limited to conservative resection of the polyps through enterotomies or limited resection. Only larger or intussuscepting polyps need to be removed. Intraoperative total endoscopy is the most accurate method of polyp identification.

Ref.: 8

15. Which of the following statements is true concerning the causes of intestinal obstruction?

A. Among adults, 20% of intussusception cases are associated with a pathologic process, most commonly a tumor.

B. A leading cause of bowel obstruction is early postoperative adhesions.

C. In the United States, adhesions account for more than 50% of cases of small bowel obstruction.

D. Richter's hernia cannot lead to complete obstruction.

E. Hernias are the leading cause of obstruction in the United States.

ANSWER: C

COMMENTS: Peritoneal adhesions account for more than 50% of cases of small bowel obstruction in the United States. Obstruction immediately after abdominal operations, however, is uncommon, occurring among only 1% of patients in the 4 weeks after laparotomy. Hernias of all types are second only to adhesions as the most frequent cause of obstruction. External hernias such as inguinal or femoral hernias can present with symptoms of obstruction. Femoral hernias are particularly prone to incarceration and bowel necrosis because of the small size of the hernia inlet. An important consideration is Richter hernia. In this variant, only a portion of the bowel wall is incarcerated. Richter hernia most frequently occurs in association with femoral or inguinal hernia. Yet complete obstruction can occur if more than one-half to two-thirds of the bowel circumference is incarcerated. Approximately 5% of cases of intussusception occur among adults. Intussusception occurs when one segment of bowel telescopes into an adjacent segment. The result is obstruction and ischemic injury to the intussuscepting segment. Of adult cases of intussusception, 90% are associated with pathologic processes. Tumors, benign and malignant, can act as a lead point causing the intussusception in more than 65% of cases among adults.

Ref.: 2, 7

16. Which of the following is true concerning postoperative ileus (POI)?

A. The presence of peritonitis at the time of surgery delays return of normal function.

B. The use of metoclopramide hastens the return of motility.

C. Contrast radiographic studies have no role in differentiating early postoperative bowel obstruction from POI.

D. The judicious use of intravenous patient-controlled analgesia has no effect on the return of small bowel motor activity.

E. Alvimopan has not been shown to affect the return of small bowel motor activity.

ANSWER: A

COMMENTS: The term "ileus" reflects underlying alterations in motility of the gastrointestinal tract that lead to functional (not mechanical) obstruction. Differentiating normal POI and the prolonged course of paralytic ileus is based primarily on the time since operation and the clinical circumstances. Besides the location of the previous operation (upper abdominal, lower abdominal, pelvic), the nature of the previous operation and the findings may contribute. Peritonitis or spillage of noxious material delays the return of normal bowel function. Differentiating paralytic ileus from mechanical obstruction often is difficult. Abdominal radiographs will reveal gas in segments of both the small and large bowels in POI. Occasionally, UGI contrast radiography or CT can be helpful in discriminating the cause. Early postoperative obstruction is uncommon and is particularly rare for upper abdominal surgery. Most cases occur after operations on the colon, particularly abdominoperineal resection. There has been little success in the use of active prokinetic agents, such as metoclopramide, to shorten recovery times after lower abdominal procedures; however, alvimopan has been shown to significantly decrease the incidence of POI. Alvimopan competitively binds to mu-opioid receptors on the bowel. If given prior to the use of narcotics, it reduces the motility-slowing effects of these commonly used medications. Thus recovery after POI can take longer with the use of intravenous narcotics than with epidural pain control. Enhanced recovery after surgery protocols commonly include the use of alvimopan starting before surgery, epidurals, nonnarcotic pain medications, and regional blocks for pain control and may demonstrate improvement in time-to-recovery of bowel function.

Ref.: 2

17. Which of the following is true regarding the initial treatment of patients with acute, complete small bowel obstruction?

A. Immediate surgery is warranted as soon as the diagnosis is made.

B. Nasogastric decompression should be used for as long as possible in patients with complete small bowel obstruction to allow resolution.

C. The presence of fever, tachycardia, localized pain, or leukocytosis suggests strangulation and warrants prompt surgery.

D. All patients with complete small bowel obstruction require blood and plasma for resuscitation.

E. If a small bowel resection must be performed, a stoma and mucous fistula are necessary because of the high risk of anastomotic failure.

ANSWER: C

COMMENTS: Timing an operation for a small bowel obstruction requires considerable clinical judgment. The duration of initial resuscitation must be balanced against the need to prevent gangrene by prompt intervention. Severe intravascular volume depletion can occur as a result of fluid sequestration (as much as 6 L) in the lumen of the bowel and peritoneal cavity. Sodium, chloride, and potassium depletion frequently accompanies bowel obstruction. Blood loss is unusual unless strangulation is present. Before induction of general anesthesia, fluid and electrolyte replacement should be instituted with isotonic saline solution to normalize the heart rate, blood pressure, and urine output. Potassium repletion should begin once adequate urine output is established. Surgery is delayed until the patient is stabilized. Nasogastric decompression is an important component of supportive therapy; nausea and vomiting are controlled by this measure, and the risk for aspiration is reduced. Swallowed air is evacuated, thus further limiting intestinal distention.

In patients with adhesive partial bowel obstruction and no signs of strangulation (i.e., fever, tachycardia, localized abdominal pain, or leukocytosis), a 24- to 48-h period of bowel rest and nasogastric decompression is warranted. Most patients with a partial obstruction will resolve spontaneously with the above measures. Delay in surgical intervention for a complete small bowel obstruction is not recommended (beyond 1 to 2 days) because the likelihood of strangulation and ischemia increases and is higher than with partial bowel obstruction.

There is no increase in the anastomotic leakage rate of small bowel anastomoses in urgent versus elective small bowel resections, provided that the segment of bowel used for the anastomosis is healthy and not overly distended. Therefore a proximal stoma and mucous fistula are seldom necessary following uncomplicated small bowel resection for obstruction.

Ref.: 2, 4

18. An 85-year-old woman has severe abdominal pain and distention. She is tachycardic, oliguric, and acidotic. Abdominal radiographs show pneumobilia and a mass (Fig. 22A.4). What is the best surgical management for this patient during an exploratory laparotomy?

A. Resection of the mass

B. "Milking" the mass distally past the obstruction

C. Cholecystectomy, enterotomy, and removal of the mass

D. Enterotomy and removal of the mass

E. Hepaticojejunostomy

ANSWER: D

COMMENTS: This patient has gallstone ileus. Gallstone ileus accounts for only 1% of all intestinal obstructions but is widely discussed. It is caused by the passage of a large stone through a biliary–enteric fistula (commonly the duodenum) thus producing a bowel obstruction. Thus the name "gallstone ileus" is a misnomer since it is

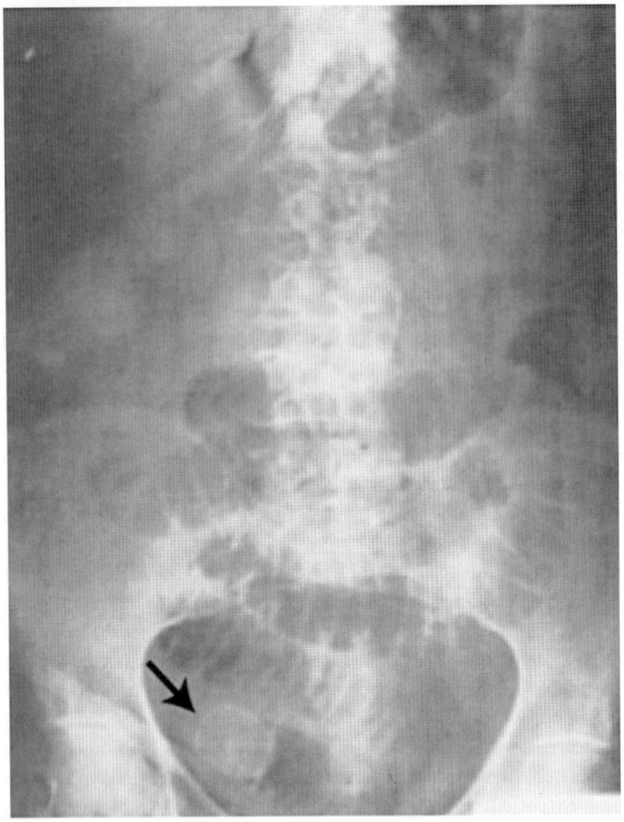

Fig. 22A.4 Abdominal radiograph showing pneumobilia and a mass (*arrow*).

a true obstruction and not an ileus. The most common site of obstruction in patients with gallstone ileus is the terminal ileum because of the narrow lumen at the ileocecal junction. The most common manifestations of gallstone ileus are nausea, vomiting, and abdominal pain. About 50% of patients will have gallbladder-related symptoms. Plain abdominal radiographs can reveal pneumobilia, dilated loops of small bowel, and a calcified stone outside the gallbladder.

Gallstone ileus is treated surgically. Obstruction is relieved by milking the stone in a retrograde fashion and removing it through a proximal enterotomy. The segment of bowel at the site of impaction should be inspected for evidence of ischemia and necrosis. If an ischemic compromise has occurred, the ischemic bowel should be resected. Takedown of the biliary–enteric fistula and cholecystectomy may be done during the initial laparotomy. However, in patients who are not able to tolerate a prolonged operation, this may be deferred. Although many surgeons recommend cholecystectomy and fistula repair at some point, it is not clear that this is absolutely necessary, particularly in elderly or infirm patients.

Ref.: 2

19. A 4-year-old male presents with blood per rectum. Technetium-99 pertechnetate scintigraphy suggests a bleeding Meckel's diverticulum. Which of the following is the appropriate treatment?

A. Ileal segmental resection with primary reanastomosis

B. Diverticulectomy

C. Medical management with proton pump inhibitor and octreotide

D. Angiography for embolization

E. Push enteroscopy for endoscopic treatment

ANSWER: A

COMMENTS: See Question 20.

20. A woman is undergoing an open incisional hernia repair through a previous cesarean section incision. During the operation, this structure (Fig. 22A.5) is noted about 60 cm from the ileocecal valve. What is true regarding this incidental finding?

A. It is a true diverticulum.

B. This lesion may be found in various anatomic forms in 50% of the population.

C. Pancreatic tissue is the most common ectopic tissue found in this diverticula.

D. Most complications occur in the elderly.

E. Diverticulitis is the most common complication.

ANSWER: A

COMMENTS: A Meckel's diverticulum, the most frequently encountered diverticulum involving the small intestine, occurs in 2%–4% of the general population. It is a true diverticulum containing all layers of the bowel wall and arises from the antimesenteric border of the ileum, 50 to 75 cm from the ileocecal valve. The diverticulum is a result of abnormal regression of the embryonic vitelline duct. Frequently, there is a persistent band of tissue extending from the tip of the diverticulum to the umbilicus.

The rule of 2's states that it usually presents by the age of 2, is 2 feet from the ileocecal valve, occurs in 2% of the population, and may contain one of the 2 types of heterotopic mucosa. The diverticulum may contain ectopic gastric mucosa capable of producing peptic ulceration and bleeding in the adjacent ileal mucosa. This ectopic gastric mucosa can be visualized with ^{99m}Tc-labeled scans. Gastric tissue is the most common ectopic tissue and is found in 50% of these lesions. Pancreatic tissue is the next most common, although colonic mucosa has been found rarely.

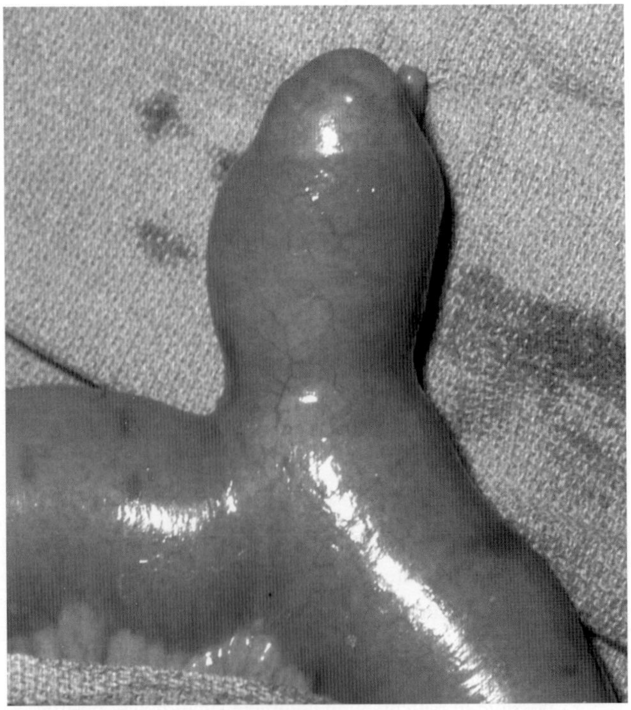

Fig. 22A.5 Meckel's diverticulum.

Clinical problems are most often seen in the young pediatric population. The most frequent complications are bleeding, intussusception, and obstruction. The latter is generally caused by volvulus or twisting around the persistent band. The least common complication is diverticulitis, which is clinically manifested as lower abdominal pain and is usually thought to be appendicitis on presentation. Therapy consists of diverticulectomy for uncomplicated diverticulitis and segmental ileal resection for complicated diverticulitis or bleeding since the ulcer is usually outside of the diverticulum.

Prophylactic diverticulectomy for an incidentally found Meckel's diverticulum is still somewhat controversial. Some clinicians recommend not removing the diverticulum when found incidentally unless there is evidence of ectopic gastric mucosa or the neck of the diverticulum is narrow. The rate of complication from a Meckel's diverticulum is about 6.4% over a lifetime and becomes smaller as a person ages. Other clinicians argue that postoperative complications after prophylactic removal are rare, and they should be removed when found. In an otherwise uncomplicated procedure, particularly in a younger person, prophylactic diverticulectomy is reasonable.

Ref.: 2, 4

21. Which of the following statements is true regarding duodenal, jejunal, and ileal diverticula?

A. Duodenal diverticula are true diverticula.

B. Duodenal diverticula are often multiple, whereas jejunal diverticula are often solitary.

C. Asymptomatic duodenal diverticula should be resected to avoid potentially serious complications.

D. Duodenal diverticula usually cause symptoms and are found during specific workup.

E. Asymptomatic jejunal diverticula do not require therapy.

ANSWER: E

COMMENTS: Small bowel diverticula are not terribly uncommon and may be found in the duodenum in 3%–5% of individuals and in the jejunum and ileum in 1%–2% on radiographs, endoscopy, and autopsies. Most duodenal, jejunal, and ileal diverticula are asymptomatic and are found incidentally. Diverticula of the duodenum, jejunum, and ileum are most commonly false (pulsion) diverticula and lack muscularis propria.

Duodenal diverticula are usually solitary and project medially toward the head of the pancreas. Although most are asymptomatic, 10% of patients may have nonspecific epigastric symptoms, such as pain and bloating. They also may bleed and perforate. In instances of contained perforation, the abscess should be drained. Gastrojejunostomy is the operation most often applicable, although biliary decompression is occasionally necessary when the duct is compressed. When there is bleeding without inflammation, diverticulectomy is indicated, either from a dorsal approach using the Kocher maneuver or via a duodenotomy.

Jejunal and ileal diverticula are often multiple and project from the mesenteric border of the bowel into the leaves of the mesentery. This type of diverticulum is more common in the jejunum than in the ileum. Bacterial overgrowth may be treated with antibiotics. Bleeding and perforation are treated with segmental resection.

Asymptomatic diverticula of the duodenum, jejunum, or ileum do not require therapy.

Ref.: 4

22. What is the most common finding with small bowel tumors?

A. Hematemesis

B. Abdominal pain

C. Perforation

D. Intussusception

E. Anemia

ANSWER: B

COMMENTS: See Question 23.

23. What is the most common symptomatic small bowel tumor?

A. Lipoma

B. Gastrointestinal stromal tumor (GIST)

C. Hamartoma

D. Hemangioma

E. Adenoma

ANSWER: B

COMMENTS: The most frequent symptom of small bowel tumors is abdominal pain. Common benign lesions of the small intestine include gastrointestinal stromal tumors, adenoma, hemangioma, and lipoma. The most common benign small bowel tumor is an adenoma. The most common symptomatic small bowel tumors are GISTs. Symptoms associated with small bowel tumors are often vague and nonspecific such as anorexia, dyspepsia, and abdominal pain. Patients may also have signs of obstruction that are usually related to intussusception but may also be due to malignant narrowing. Occult bleeding is also a common initial symptom. When small bowel neoplasms are suspected, a barium small bowel follow-through study is indicated and is generally diagnostic. CT or MR enterography may also be useful.

GISTs arise from the interstitial cells of Cajal. They express CD117 and CD34. These tumors grow intramurally and can cause obstruction. At times, these tumors can reach considerable size and outgrow their blood supply, which results in GI bleeding. Mitotic rates higher than 5 per 50 high-power fields increase the risk for recurrence. Lipomas are now included in the GIST category.

There are three types of small bowel adenomas: tubular adenomas, villous adenomas, and Brunner gland adenomas (usually in the duodenum). Most of these lesions are asymptomatic and found incidentally at the time of autopsy. Adenomas present with bleeding or obstruction. Polypectomy may be performed in the duodenum if the tumor is histologically benign. Jejunal and ileal lesions are treated with segmental resection.

Hamartomas of the small bowel are usually associated with PJS. Patients also have 1- to 2-mm pigmented lesions located in the circumoral region of the face, buccal mucosa, palms, soles, and perianal region. The most common initial symptom is a colicky abdominal pain, usually as a result of intermittent intussusception.

Hemangiomas are malformations consisting of a submucosal proliferation of blood vessels. They can occur anywhere along the GI tract, with the jejunum being the most common small bowel segment involved. Bleeding is the most frequent symptom. Angiography and ^{99m}Tc-labeled red blood cell scanning are useful diagnostic studies.

When identified, small bowel tumors should be excised because of the risk for complications, to establish the diagnosis, and to exclude cancer. Small lesions can be excised with an enterotomy and primary closure. Larger or suspicious lesions should be treated with segmental resection with primary anastomosis.

Ref.: 2, 9

24. What is the most common primary malignant small bowel tumor?

A. Leiomyosarcoma

B. Carcinoid

C. Lymphoma

D. GIST

E. Adenocarcinoma

ANSWER: E

COMMENTS: See Question 25.

25. What is the most common finding in patients with malignant small bowel tumors?

A. Hematemesis

B. Perforation

C. Abdominal pain

D. Intussusception

E. Anemia

ANSWER: C

COMMENTS: Malignant tumors of the small bowel account for 2% of all GI malignancies. The most frequent primary type is adenocarcinoma, followed in decreasing frequency by carcinoid, GIST, and lymphoma. Although adenocarcinoma occurs with equal frequency in the duodenum, jejunum, and ileum, the other types tend to occur most often in the ileum. In contrast to benign lesions, malignant lesions of the small intestine are usually accompanied by pain and weight loss. Other clinical manifestations may include diarrhea, obstruction, or chronic blood loss with anemia. Obstruction from malignant lesions is usually because of tumor infiltration, stricturing, and adhesion. The preferred therapy is wide resection with regional lymphadenectomy. For each entity, survival is dependent on a number of factors and is variable, but in general, GISTs have a 5-year survival rate that ranges from 7% to 56%, lymphomas have a 5-year survival rate of about 40%, and adenocarcinoma has the lowest survival, at about 20%. Postoperative chemotherapy and radiation therapy can be useful in treating a patient with lymphoma but are not useful adjuncts for adenocarcinoma or sarcoma. Histiocytic lymphoma may develop in patients with long-standing celiac sprue and has a worse prognosis than do conventional small bowel lymphomas. The Mediterranean-type lymphoma, a variant associated with monoclonal alpha heavy chains and a dense plasma cell tumor infiltration, also carries a poor prognosis.

Ref.: 2, 4, 9

26. A 35-year-old man presents with obstructive symptoms and, on exploration, is found to have a mid-jejunal mass. Frozen section reveals a GIST. Which of the following is true regarding GISTs?

A. GISTs originate from the interstitial cells of Cajal.

B. The most frequent site of GISTs is the small bowel.

C. Nodal status is the most reliable predictor of aggressive behavior.

D. Postoperative imatinib mesylate is used in all patients to reduce recurrence.

E. On endoscopy, a GIST typically appears as an ulcerating mucosal lesion.

ANSWER: A

COMMENTS: GISTs are the most common nonepithelial neoplasms of the small bowel. They originate from the interstitial cells of Cajal. GISTs are most common in the stomach (60%), followed by the small bowel (30%). On endoscopy, GISTs classically appear as submucosal lesions. The majority express the CD117 antigen of the KIT transmembrane receptor tyrosine kinase, which is the product of the KIT protooncogene. Mutation in *KIT* leads to abnormally activated KIT protein and enables oncogenic signaling in the cell. This discovery led to the development of systemic therapy with imatinib mesylate (Gleevec), which blocks KIT signaling and inhibits tumor proliferation. Postoperative imatinib has been shown to prolong recurrence-free survival and is considered standard following resection of GIST tumors larger than 3 cm. The clinical behavior of GISTs is highly variable, but GISTs > 1 cm have increased malignant potential. Tumor size and mitotic rate are the two major criteria used to define aggressive behavior.

Ref.: 9, 10

27. A 54-year-old man reports with a 2-month history of abdominal pain and significant weight loss. Upper endoscopy, colonoscopy, and CT were all normal. A barium upper GI study with small bowel follow-through identified a mass in his mid-ileum. At surgical exploration, a carcinoid tumor, confirmed by frozen section, was found in the mid-ileum. Which statement is true regarding his condition?

A. Prognosis is primarily related to lymph node status.

B. The cell of origin is the Kulchitsky cell.

C. The ileum is the most common site of origin.

D. A 1-cm distal ileum carcinoid tumor should be treated with a formal right hemicolectomy.

E. Resection is not indicated in patients with metastatic disease.

ANSWER: B

COMMENTS: The origin of carcinoid tumors is the Kulchitsky cell, which is thought to arise from the neural crest. Carcinoids can occur anywhere in the GI tract. The most frequent site is the appendix, followed by the ileum and rectum. Extraintestinal sites include the bronchus and ovaries. Small bowel carcinoid tumors tend to be multiple in 30% of cases, and a second GI tumor of another histologic type can be found in 30% of patients. The prognosis is a function of the size of the tumor and its site of origin. Ileal carcinoids tend to metastasize more commonly than those that originate in the appendix.

The usual submucosal location of carcinoid tumors often makes them difficult to find on radiographic examination or with cursory palpation during an exploratory laparotomy. The tumors may incite an intense fibrotic reaction in the surrounding soft tissue and mesentery, which can cause luminal narrowing. Mesenteric lymph node and liver metastases can be large in comparison with the primary tumor. Tumors less than 1 cm in diameter and without demonstrable metastases can be treated by excision or segmental resection. Those larger than 1 cm or with regional metastases should be excised widely along with lymph node clearance; right hemicolectomy is indicated for >1-cm lesions of the distal ileum and appendix. For patients with metastases (local or distant) and in whom carcinoid syndrome is present, removal of the primary tumor and debulking of metastatic disease can provide considerable palliation.

Ref.: 2, 4, 11

28. Which of the following is true of carcinoid syndrome?

A. Cardiac manifestations commonly affect the mitral and aortic valves.

B. 5-Hydroxyindoleacetic acid (5-HIAA) is the active metabolite leading to carcinoid syndrome symptoms.

C. Diarrhea affects less than 30% of patients.

D. The most useful diagnostic test for suspected carcinoid syndrome is the determination of serum serotonin levels.

E. Functional carcinoid tumors divert dietary tryptophan into the production of serotonin.

ANSWER: E

COMMENTS: Episodic manifestations of carcinoid syndrome include flushing, diarrhea, and asthma. The cutaneous manifestations are the most common and consist of episodes of flushing of the face, neck, arms, and upper part of the trunk, occasionally accompanied by vasomotor collapse. Diarrhea is significant in more than 80% of patients and is usually sudden in onset, watery, and accompanied by cramping pain and borborygmi. Asthmatic attacks occur in 25% of patients. Manifestations of long-standing involvement include the development of facial hyperemia with telangiectasias on the cheeks, nose, and forehead; development of the cutaneous lesions of pellagra; and valvular heart disease. The valves most commonly involved are the tricuspid and pulmonic, although the mitral and aortic valves are sometimes affected. Peripheral edema is present in about 70% of patients and can occur in the absence of valvular disease.

Functioning carcinoid tumors divert up to 60% of dietary tryptophan into the production of serotonin, thereby contributing to the development of pellagra and protein deficiency. Serotonin is metabolized in the liver to 5-HIAA, which is excreted in urine. For this reason, the most useful diagnostic test in patients suspected of having a carcinoid tumor is the determination of 5-HIAA levels in a 24-h collection of urine. 5-HIAA is inactive and does not cause carcinoid syndrome. Carcinoid syndrome is produced by release of serotonin into the systemic circulation either by liver metastases or by tumors located outside the portal distribution.

Although it is generally believed that patients with carcinoid syndrome have tumors that produce serotonin, the role of serotonin in the mediation of the syndrome is not clear. Not all patients with elevated production of serotonin have the syndrome. Some patients with the syndrome have normal levels of 5-HIAA in urine, and injection of pure serotonin does not create all of the manifestations of the disease. It is likely that carcinoid tumors have the capacity to produce a number of biologically active peptides, which accounts for the variability of the syndrome and discrepancies between a patient's serotonin levels and the clinical findings. Other substances produced by carcinoid tumors include histamine, dopamine, kallikrein, substance P, prostaglandins, and neuropeptide K. Treatment of carcinoid crisis includes intravenous octreotide, intravenous antihistamine, and hydrocortisone.

Ref.: 2, 4, 11

29. During a routine appendectomy, a 1-cm mass is found at the tip of the appendix. Frozen section is concerning for carcinoid tumor. What is the best treatment option for this patient?

A. Right hemicolectomy

B. Medical therapy with octreotide

C. Neoadjuvant therapy with streptozotocin and 5-fluorouracil

D. Appendectomy

E. Ileocecectomy

ANSWER: D

COMMENTS: See Question 30.

30. On abdominal exploration for a suspected carcinoid tumor, a 2-cm mass is found in the terminal ileum. No liver lesions were detected on preoperative imaging or with intraoperative palpation. What is the best treatment option for this patient?

A. Appendectomy

B. Right hemicolectomy

C. Medical therapy with octreotide

D. Neoadjuvant therapy with streptozotocin and 5-fluorouracil

E. Ileocecectomy

ANSWER: B

COMMENTS: Treatment of small bowel carcinoid is based on tumor size and the presence or absence of metastatic disease. Segmental resection is adequate for tumors smaller than 1 cm without regional lymph node metastasis. Wide excision is indicated for lesions larger than 1 cm, multiple tumors, or regional lymph node metastasis. Right hemicolectomy is indicated for lesions of the terminal ileum or base of the appendix. Debulking is indicated for metastatic carcinoid tumors. This may involve liver resection. Hepatic artery ligation or percutaneous embolization has also produced good results in controlling the carcinoid symptoms produced by liver metastasis.

Medical therapy for patients with malignant carcinoid is directed at relieving symptoms. Octreotide, a somatostatin analogue, helps relieve symptoms in most patients. Regression of tumor with the use of octreotide has been reported. Interferon-alfa has also been shown to relieve symptoms. Chemotherapeutic agents such as streptozotocin and 5-fluorouracil have had limited success in treating malignant carcinoid. They are used mostly in patients with metastatic disease who are symptomatic and unresponsive to other therapies.

Ref.: 2

31. Somatostatin has emerged as a safe and effective agent with a broad range of applications. Which of the following is true about the use of somatostatin in patients with carcinoid tumors?

A. Somatostatin may be used as a provocative agent before measuring 5-HIAA levels.

B. Somatostatin receptor scintigraphy is more effective than CT or magnetic resonance imaging (MRI) in localizing primary and metastatic carcinoid tumors.

C. Somatostatin is ineffective for the management of carcinoid crisis.

D. Somatostatin therapy improves survival in patients with carcinoid syndrome.

E. Administration of somatostatin can be used as a provocative diagnostic test.

ANSWER: B

COMMENTS: Somatostatin was first identified in 1973. Since then, a great deal of interest has been directed at characterizing and identifying its physiologic effects and the clinical utility of somatostatin and its analogues. Somatostatin is a 14–amino acid protein with several analogues of shorter lengths that maintain clinical effectiveness. The general effects of somatostatin are those of an inhibitory hormone. Several provocative agents may be used before conducting tests for neuroendocrine tumors, including pentagastrin, secretin, and calcium infusion. Somatostatin is not effective as a provocative agent.

Somatostatin receptor scintigraphy uses indium-111 and a gamma camera. This study has several advantages over conventional imaging (CT or MRI). Its sensitivity is higher (90% vs. 70%) for metastatic disease, it is more effective in identifying the primary tumor site, and it visualizes the entire body to detect occult metastases. Carcinoid tumors visible by somatostatin receptor scintigraphy suggest that these particular tumors have somatostatin receptors and are therefore subject to the inhibitory effects of somatostatin.

Carcinoid crisis is a life-threatening event that may develop during episodes of flushing, anesthesia, or surgery. Severe hypotension and bronchospasm may occur during carcinoid crises, and they may be refractory to the usual supportive care. The reported incidence of such crises is variable and ranges from 2% to 50%. Somatostatin may be administered preoperatively as a prophylactic agent or during a carcinoid crisis as a therapeutic agent. It is usually successful in reversing the condition.

Somatostatin has also been found to be highly effective in relieving the symptoms of carcinoid syndrome. It has been suggested that chronic octreotide therapy results in longer survival in patients with carcinoid syndrome than in those treated with chemotherapy, but this hypothesis remains to be proven by randomized, controlled trials.

Ref.: 2, 11

32. A 62-year-old woman complains of abdominal pain and weight loss. She undergoes a small bowel follow-through study (Fig. 22A.6). Her past medical and surgical history includes a stable small right lung nodule, removal of a skin lesion on her right leg, and an endoscopic polypectomy of a gastric polyp. She has a strong family history of breast cancer. If the lesion noted in the stomach is metastatic, what is the most likely primary cancer?

A. Squamous cell skin cancer

B. Lymphoma

C. Lung cancer

D. Breast cancer

E. Melanoma

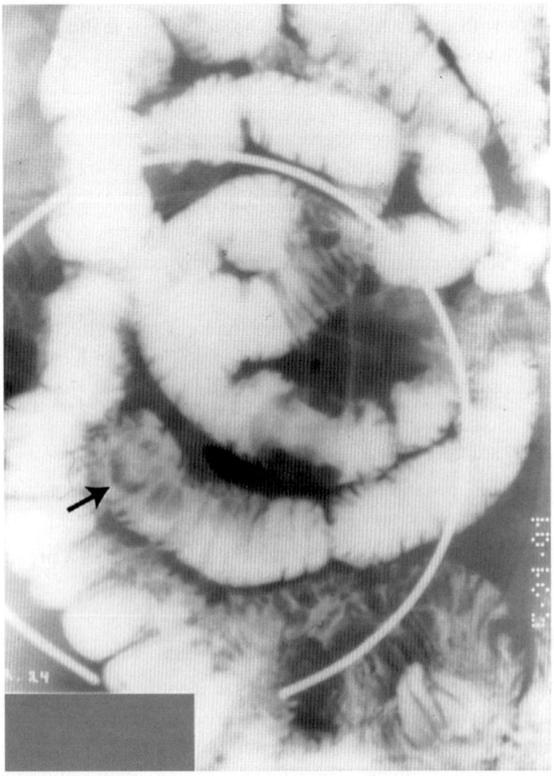

Fig. 22A.6 Small bowel study showing a lesion (*arrow*). *(Courtesy of Melvyn H. Schreiber, M.D., The University of Texas Medical Branch.)*

ANSWER: E

COMMENTS: Metastatic tumors of the small bowel are more common than primary tumors. The most common metastases to the small bowel are primary tumors arising from other intra abdominal organs. In these cases, small bowel involvement occurs by either direct extension or implantation of tumor cells. Extra abdominal metastasis to the small bowel is rare. Cutaneous melanoma is the most common extra abdominal source of metastasis to the small bowel. Other extra abdominal sources include breast and lung cancers. Treatment is palliative resection or bypass if the metastatic tumor is not amenable to resection.

Ref.: 2

33. A 56-year-old woman had a right hemicolectomy for villous adenoma of the cecum. Five days after surgery her surgical wound becomes red and tender. She underwent pelvic radiation therapy 5 years ago for cervical cancer. The surgeon opens her wound with immediate drainage of purulent fluid. The drainage persists as a continuous brown liquid discharge over the next day. Which of the following is the most likely diagnosis?

A. Simple wound infection

B. Clostridial infection

C. Anastomotic leakage with an enterocutaneous fistula

D. Dehiscence

E. Cellulitis

ANSWER: C

COMMENTS: Most fistulas are iatrogenic and result from anastomotic leakage, inadvertent injury to the bowel during the operation, laceration of the bowel during an abdominal closure, or retained foreign bodies. Less than 2% of fistulas are the result of diseased bowel. When they are, the most common contributing factors are preoperative radiation therapy, intestinal obstruction, and inflammatory bowel disease. Although small bowel fistulas occasionally lead to generalized peritonitis, they most commonly produce a walled-off abscess manifested as an infection of the operative incision. The initial drainage may be purulent, but if the infection is caused by anastomotic leakage of the small bowel, the drainage becomes enteric within 1 to 2 days.

Ref.: 2

34. For the patient described in Question 33, which of the following is the most appropriate initial management?

A. Packing of the subcutaneous tissue with wet-to-dry dressings

B. Packing of subcutaneous tissue with dry, absorbent dressings

C. Immediate return to the operating room for exploration

D. Skin protection and appliance placement to collect the drainage

E. Sutured closure of the fascial defect

ANSWER: D

COMMENTS: The initial management of a small bowel fistula includes the administration of appropriate intravenous fluids, proximal decompression with nasogastric suction, control and quantification of the output of the fistula, and protection of the surrounding skin.

Fistulas are classified according to their locations and the volumes of their output. Proximal fistulas tend to have higher output and lead to more severe electrolyte and fluid imbalances. Nasogastric suction can be helpful in diminishing the output of proximal intestinal fistulas, but the output of those more distal in the gut may not be influenced by this maneuver. Sump catheters can provide a means of controlling and quantifying high-output fistulas, especially early in their formation. Maintaining proper position of the catheter in the wound can be problematic. Once the fistula tract is established, suction catheters should be promptly replaced with a stoma appliance fixed to the edges of the fistula. Enteric contents are highly corrosive, and the skin surrounding the fistula opening should be protected carefully. Gauze dressings are generally ineffective at absorbing all the drainage and protecting the skin. Therefore their use is generally avoided. Most well-established fistulas do not produce sepsis, but in patients with persistent fever, systemic administration of antibiotics and a careful search for an undrained abdominal abscess are indicated.

Early in the workup of this patient and before the GI tract has been filled with contrast material (from conventional GI radiographs), CT should be performed to look for areas of abscess formation or fluid accumulation. It may also identify the site of the fistula. If CT does not show the site, fistulography is helpful. If one is concerned about distal obstruction, a small bowel follow-through study may provide information, if this issue was not satisfactorily answered by CT or fistulography.

Ref.: 4

35. Diagnostic workup of the woman described in Question 34 reveals that she has a distal ileal fistula that is communicating with a small cavity. Daily output of the fistula is 100 mL. Which of the following is appropriate therapy?

A. Prompt exploration and division of the fistula tract

B. Prompt exploration and bypass of the fistula

C. Prompt exploration and resection of the involved ileum with primary anastomosis

D. Six weeks of intravenous hyperalimentation

E. Two weeks of low-residue or elemental enteral alimentation

ANSWER: E

COMMENTS: Knowing the location of the fistula is of important prognostic and therapeutic value. The overall mortality rate for small bowel fistulas is 20%; the rate is higher for jejunal fistulas and lower for those of the ileum. With proper supportive care, such as intravenous or enteral alimentation, and in the absence of distal obstruction, up to 40% of small bowel fistulas close spontaneously. Enteral alimentation has the advantage of avoiding the possible hepatic and septic complications associated with prolonged TPN. Even if there is a slight increase in fistula output after the start of enteral nutrition, the fistula may still close. Fistulas of the proximal jejunum may require transnasal insertion of a long tube through the stomach and duodenum and just beyond the fistula before starting enteral alimentation. Surgery should be avoided for 4 to 6 weeks to permit spontaneous closure and allow the local inflammation to subside, thereby facilitating subsequent surgery. The preferred operation for correcting a persistent fistula is resection of the fistula in continuity with the segment of involved bowel, followed by primary anastomosis. Alternative therapies include complete or partial exclusion with primary anastomosis.

Ref.: 4

36. One year after undergoing antrectomy and Billroth II reconstruction for peptic ulcer disease, a patient is being evaluated for anemia. The patient is also noted to have vague epigastric pain that is relieved by projectile bilious emesis without food particles. Which statement is true regarding this patient's condition?

A. Medical management with tetracycline and vitamin B_{12} can definitively correct the condition.

B. Bacteria successfully compete for vitamin B_6, which may lead to megaloblastic anemia.

C. Bacterial deconjugation of bile salts can lead to steatorrhea.

D. The addition of intrinsic factor in the Schilling test causes urinary vitamin B_{12} excretion to return to normal.

E. The addition of tetracycline in the Schilling test causes urinary vitamin B_6 excretion to return to normal.

ANSWER: C

COMMENTS: The blind loop syndrome is caused by stasis of the intestinal contents with subsequent bacterial overgrowth. This stasis can be caused by a number of abnormalities, including stricture, stenosis, fistula, diverticulum, or the formation of a blind pouch (as noted in a Billroth II operation). Steatorrhea, diarrhea, anemia, weight loss, abdominal pain, multiple vitamin deficiencies, joint pains, and occasionally neurologic disorders characterize the syndrome. The steatorrhea is the result of bile salt deconjugation in the stagnant fluid in the blind loop of bowel. Megaloblastic anemia is probably a result of successful competition by bacteria for vitamin B_{12}. The Schilling test reveals a type of urinary excretion of vitamin B_{12} similar to that seen with pernicious anemia except that it is corrected, not by the addition of intrinsic factor, but by the use of oral tetracycline. Although the administration of tetracycline and parenteral vitamin B_{12} can correct megaloblastic anemia, only surgical correction of the cause of the bowel stasis is curative. Surgical correction includes converting the Billroth II to a Billroth I operation or the creation of Roux-en-Y limb gastrojejunostomy with a vagotomy to prevent marginal ulceration.

Ref.: 2

37. Which of the following statements regarding SBS is true?

A. Resection of up to 70% of the bowel can be tolerated if the terminal ileum and ileocecal valve are preserved.

B. Diarrhea is best controlled by the administration of medium-chain triglycerides.

C. The administration of oral bile salts is of central importance in controlling steatorrhea.

D. Vagotomy and pyloroplasty and reversal of a segment of bowel are the two most important operations for the early management of SBS.

E. Relative gastric hyposecretion, with increased intestinal pH in conjunction with interruption of the enterohepatic bile salt circulation, is the cause of steatorrhea.

ANSWER: A

COMMENTS: SBS may be diagnosed when there is significant malabsorption of vitamins and minerals or an inability to maintain caloric enteral nutrition in the setting of extensive small bowel resection. The usual quoted rule that less than 100 cm of intact small bowel results in SBS is not terribly useful since SBS may develop in a variety of situations and amounts of residual bowel. The normal length of small bowel from the ligament of Treitz to the ileocecal valve is about 500 cm, but a wide range was found, from 250 to 850 cm, in a recent study. The entire jejunum can be resected without adverse nutritional sequelae. The entire ileum can be resected without harm as long as vitamin B_{12} is administered regularly afterward. Up to 70% of the small bowel can be resected safely if the terminal ileum and ileocecal valve are left intact. If they are resected, however, loss of 50%–60% of the small bowel can lead to severely compromised nutrition.

The deficiencies created by extensive resection of the small bowel are vitamin B_{12} malabsorption (terminal ileum), altered fat absorption, and fluid and electrolyte problems. Vitamin B_{12} malabsorption leads to vitamin B_{12} deficiency and megaloblastic anemia. Altered fat absorption produces steatorrhea as a result of several factors. First, massive small bowel resection leads to gastric hypersecretion because decreased bowel pH stimulates the intestine, thereby shortening transit time and interfering with the absorption of ingested fat. Second, interruption of bile salt resorption interferes with micelle formation. Third, the unabsorbed fats are irritating to the colonic mucosa, thereby increasing diarrhea and steatorrhea associated with the syndrome. Fluid and electrolyte problems are a function of the shortened transit time and diarrhea that results from loss of small bowel absorptive area.

Treatment of SBS centers on control of diarrhea and parenteral maintenance of nutrition. With time (2 to 3 years), the mucosa of as little as 30 to 45 cm of small bowel may undergo enough hypertrophy to allow withdrawal of intravenous alimentation and the start of carefully modified oral feedings. Treatment with growth hormone, glutamine, and fiber has shown some promise in stimulating gut regeneration. Diarrhea can be controlled with agents such as Lomotil or codeine that slow intestinal motility. Oral calcium carbonate is also useful and acts by neutralizing hydrochloric acid and free fatty acids. When oral intake is resumed, dietary fat is restricted to 30 to 50 g daily. Some patients benefit from the use of medium-chain triglycerides. Oral bile salts are tolerated and aid in the formation of micelles in some patients, whereas in others, they cause increased diarrhea. Cholestyramine, an agent that sequesters bile acids, is useful in patients who have had less than 100 cm of small bowel resected.

There is no standard approach to the resumption of oral intake, and treatment must be highly individualized. Although some patients ultimately do well with a modified oral diet, others remain dependent on permanent parenteral nutrition. There are no operative procedures that reliably correct SBS. Therefore operative treatment should be considered only in patients who cannot maintain their body weight within 30% of normal without intravenous supplementation. Operations that may be useful are reversal of a segment of intestine, creation of a recirculating loop of small bowel, creation of an artificial sphincter, vagotomy and pyloroplasty, correction of bowel obstruction, and placing all bowel in continuity (i.e., reversal of preexisting stomas). Vagotomy and pyloroplasty have rarely been performed for SBS since the introduction of H_2 blockers and proton pump inhibitors. Allotransplantation of small bowel in humans has been performed successfully, but has a high failure rate and is only available in a few specialized centers.

Ref.: 2, 4, 12

38. During a small bowel resection, you have finished your anastomosis and have just closed the mesenteric defect. As you are closing the midline wound, you see a large hematoma in the area of the mesenteric defect. Choose the best treatment option.

A. Observation alone

B. If hematoma is expanding, open, explore, and obtain hemostasis

C. Resect the involved segment and redo the anastomosis

D. Proceed with closure if the hematoma is expanding but the anastomosis appears perfused

E. Evacuate the hematoma under all circumstances

ANSWER: B

COMMENTS: The hematoma should be observed for several minutes to evaluate if it is expanding. If there is no evidence of expansion or ongoing bleeding, one can proceed with closing. Not every hematoma requires intervention. If the hematoma is large or expanding, the mesentery should be opened and explored. Hematomas can expand and tamponade the veins, leading to arterial inflow obstruction and poor blood flow to the anastomosis. Only if you cannot adequately control the hematoma should the involved segment be resected and the anastomosis redone.

Ref.: 13

39. Peyer's patches are primarily responsible for the local synthesis of:

A. IgD

B. IgE

C. IgG

D. IgM

E. IgA

ANSWER: E

COMMENTS: Nodules of lymphoid tissues found throughout the small intestine and colon are known as Peyer's patches. IgA is elaborated by plasma cells and is unique in that this immunoglobulin is transcytosed directly across enterocytes or hepatocytes for secretion directly into the intestinal contents or bile. Peyer's patches are part of the mucosal-associated lymphoid tissue (MALT).

Ref.: 14

40. Which of the following statements regarding tuberculous enteritis is incorrect?

A. Primary infection usually results from the ingestion of nonpasteurized milk contaminated with *Mycobacterium bovis.*

B. Secondary infection results from the ingestion of bacilli contained in contaminated sputum.

C. The duodenum is the site of involvement in 85% of patients.

D. Infection may be indistinguishable from Crohn's disease or cancer.

E. Approximately one-half of patients with colonic or ileocolonic disease may be treated medically without surgery.

ANSWER: C

COMMENTS: Primary enteral tuberculosis is rare in the United States, but is still common in underdeveloped countries where ingestion of unpasteurized milk occurs more commonly. Usually, it causes minimal symptoms, but occasionally, it results in stricturing and stenosis in the ileocecal area. The radiographic findings may be indistinguishable from those of carcinoma of the colon. Although it may be necessary to resect bowel because of high-grade obstruction, it is not appropriate to do so simply to establish the diagnosis. This can be accomplished with biopsy alone. Treatment with isoniazid, *p*-aminosalicylic acid, and streptomycin usually suffices.

Ulcerative tuberculosis is a form that develops secondary to pulmonary disease and is more common than the primary form of this disease in the United States. Symptoms are nonspecific and variable, but most often consist of pain and diarrhea. Suspicion should be raised in Asian patients, particularly those coming from the Indian subcontinent. The most common laboratory findings are anemia and an elevated C-reactive protein. The diagnosis can be strongly suggested by barium examination, CT with intravenous (IV) and per os (po) contrast, or MR enterography. Confirmation is obtained by a positive tuberculin skin test, although a negative test does not rule out the diagnosis. Not infrequently, the diagnosis is made by open or laparoscopic exploration and biopsies. An appropriate response to antitubercular therapy also confirms the diagnosis. Surgery is best reserved for complications such as perforation, obstruction, or hemorrhage.

Ref.: 15

41. Which of the following statements regarding typhoid enteritis is true?

A. Culturing *Salmonella typhi* from blood or stool can make the diagnosis.

B. Chloramphenicol is the preferred treatment.

C. Bleeding requiring operative intervention occurs in 10%–20% of patients.

D. Steroids have no use in treating typhoid enteritis.

E. Hyperplasia and ulceration of Peyer's patches and mesenteric lymphadenopathy are rare findings.

ANSWER: A

COMMENTS: Typhoid enteritis, a systemic infection caused by *S. typhi*, is accompanied by fever, headache, coughing, maculopapular rash, abdominal pain, and leukopenia. Hyperplasia and ulceration of Peyer's patches, mesenteric lymphadenopathy, and splenomegaly also occur. Chloramphenicol is not the drug of choice because of the emergence of resistant strains of bacteria and the risk for marrow toxicity. Currently, trimethoprim-sulfamethoxazole (Bactrim) is preferred. Patients who remain in a toxic state after 1 week of therapy often benefit from a short course of prednisone. Bleeding occurs in 10%–20% of patients and is usually treated by transfusion. Perforation through ulcerated Peyer's patches occurs in 2% of patients and is most often free, solitary, and located in the terminal ileum. Operative closure and appropriate peritoneal toilet are required. Occasionally, the perforations are multiple, which necessitates intestinal resection with primary anastomosis.

Ref.: 4

REFERENCES

1. Gordon PH, Nivatvongs SH. *Principles and Practice of Surgery for the Colon, Rectum, and Anus*. St. Louis: Quality Medical; 1999.
2. Evers BM. Small intestine. In: Townsend CM, Beauchamp RD, Evers BM, et al., eds. *Sabiston Textbook of Surgery: The Biological Basis of Modern Surgical Practice*. 18th ed. Philadelphia: WB Saunders; 2008.
3. Matthews JB, Hodin RA. *Acute Abdomen and Appendix. Greenfield's Surgery: Scientific Principles and Practice*. 4th ed. Philadelphia; Lippincott Williams & Wilkins; 2006.
4. Tavakkolizadeh A, Whang EE, Ashley SW, et al. Small intestine. In: Brunicardi FC, Andersen DK, Billiar TR, et al., eds. *Schwartz's Principles of Surgery*. 9th ed. New York: McGraw-Hill; 2010.
5. Sleisenger MH, Fordtran JS. *Gastrointestinal and Liver Disease: Pathophysiology, Diagnosis, Management*. 4th ed. Philadelphia: WB Saunders; 1989.
6. Wilson JD, Braunwald E, Isselbacher KJ, et al. *Harrison's Principles of Internal Medicine*. 12th ed. New York: McGraw-Hill; 1991.
7. Marinis A, Yiallourou A, Samanides L, et al. Intussusception of the bowel in adults: a review. *World J Gastroenterol*. 2009;15:407–411.
8. Fry RD, Mahmoud N, Maron DJ. Colon and rectum. In: Townsend CM, Beauchamp RD, Evers BM, et al., eds. *Sabiston Textbook of Surgery: The Biological Basis of Modern Surgical Practice*. 18th ed. Philadelphia: WB Saunders; 2008.
9. Greenson JK. Gastrointestinal stromal tumors and other mesenchymal lesions of the gut. *Mod Pathol*. 2003;16:366–375.
10. Mahvi D, Krantz S. Stomach. In: Townsend CM, Beauchamp RD, Evers BM, et al., eds. *Sabiston Textbook of Surgery: The Biological Basis of Modern Surgical Practice*. 18th ed. Philadelphia: WB Saunders; 2008.
11. Memon MA, Nelson H. Gastrointestinal carcinoid tumors: current management strategies. *Dis Colon Rectum*. 1997;40:1101–1118.
12. Teitelbaum ER, Vaziri K, Zettervall S, Amdur RL, Orkin BA. Intraoperative small bowel length measurements and analysis of demographic predictors of increased length. *Clin Anat*. 2013;26(7):827–832.
13. Britt LD, Pickleman JR. *Small and Large Bowel Obstruction. Fischer's Mastery of Surgery*. 6th ed. Philadelphia: JB Lippincott; 2012.
14. Liu C, Crawford JM. The gastrointestinal tract. In: Kumar V, Abbas AK, Aster JC, et al., eds. *Robbins and Cotran Pathologic Basis of Disease*. Philadelphia: Elsevier Saunders; 2005. Chapter 17.
15. Corman ML. *Colon and Rectal Surgery*. 5th ed. Philadelphia: JB Lippincott; 2005.

B. Appendix

Robin Alley, M.D.

1. Which of the following is true regarding the location of the appendix?

A. The base of the appendix can always be found at the confluence of the cecal taenia.

B. The tip of the appendix is found in the pelvis in the majority of cases.

C. The appendix is often retrocecal and extraperitoneal.

D. After the fifth gestational month of pregnancy, the appendix is shifted posteriorly and laterally by the gravid uterus.

E. The position of the tip of the appendix does not determine the symptoms of the patient with appendicitis.

ANSWER: A

COMMENTS: The **appendix**, along with the ileum and ascending colon, is a derivative of the **midgut**. Following developmental rotation, the cecum becomes fixed in the right lower quadrant, and this determines the final location of the appendix. The appendiceal orifice and therefore the base of the appendix are always found at the antimesenteric confluence of the cecal **taeniae**. The anterior taenia, in particular, may be used as a landmark to find the appendix at surgery. Although the base of the appendix is found in a constant location, the position of the tip varies. The tip of the appendix is found retrocecally in the majority of patients (65%), in the pelvis in approximately 30%, and in a retroperitoneal position in approximately 7%. In **pregnancy**, the gravid uterus tends to push the appendix superiorly and the tip medially. The various locations of the tip of the inflamed appendix determine the location of physical findings produced by irritation of the parietal peritoneum, but the prodromal symptoms remain the same.

Ref.: 1, 2

2. Which of the following statements regarding the appendix is false?

A. The average length of an adult appendix is 9 cm.

B. The blood supply to the appendix is from the appendicular artery, a branch of the ileocolic artery.

C. Innervation of the appendix is derived from the somatic nervous system.

D. The appendix contains large amounts of lymphoid aggregates, but it has no significant exocrine function.

E. The lymphatic drainage of the appendix goes through the ileocolic nodes.

ANSWER: C

COMMENTS: The length of the appendix varies from 2 to 20 cm, with an average length of 9 cm in adults. The blood supply to the appendix is from the appendicular artery, which is a branch of the ileocolic artery. The innervation of the appendix, like other visceral organs, is derived from the autonomic nervous system. As appendicitis progresses, irritation of the surrounding parietal peritoneum activates the somatic pain fibers, which localizes pain to the right lower quadrant. The appendix contains large amounts of lymphoid tissue in aggregates but has no known significant exocrine function. The lymphatic drainage of the appendix is the same as the cecum and follows that of the ileocolic nodes. These nodes are often enlarged and hyperplastic in acute appendicitis.

Ref.: 1, 3

3. Which of the following statements regarding the pathogenesis of appendicitis is false?

A. The antimesenteric border has the poorest blood supply and is usually the site of the perforation.

B. Fecaliths are commonly responsible for appendicitis in children.

C. Viral or bacterial infections can precede an episode of appendicitis.

D. Obstruction of venous outflow and then arterial inflow results in gangrene.

E. Obstruction of the lumen may occur as a result of inspissated stool or a foreign body.

ANSWER: B

COMMENTS: In most instances of appendicitis, luminal obstruction leads to bacterial overgrowth, active secretion of mucus, and increased luminal pressure. Increased pressure leads to decreased venous return and, later, decreased arterial inflow, which results in gangrene, bacterial translocation, and perforation. The midportion of the antimesenteric border of the appendix has the poorest blood supply and most frequently shows evidence of perforation. The cause of the obstruction is usually lymphoid hyperplasia in younger patients and fecaliths in adults. Fecaliths are responsible for approximately 30% of cases in adults and have been identified in 90% of patients with gangrenous appendicitis with rupture. However, luminal obstruction does not occur in all cases. In some patients, the lumen of the appendix is found to be patent during radiologic, gross, and histologic examinations. The pathogenesis in these cases remains unclear. It is thought that either viral or bacterial infection, such as *Salmonella*, *Shigella*, or infectious mononucleosis, can precede appendicitis. These infections probably cause lymphoid hyperplasia in the appendix and subsequent obstruction.

Ref.: 1, 2

4. A 27-year-old man has a 1-day history of right lower quadrant pain and leukocytosis. Probable nonperforated acute appendicitis is diagnosed. What is the best antibiotic and surgical management for this patient?

A. Operate and then await the results of peritoneal fluid cultures to tailor the selection of antibiotics.

B. Administer cefazolin perioperatively to reduce the risk of wound infection and then operate.

C. Begin ceftriaxone and metronidazole (Flagyl), monitor the patient with serial abdominal examinations, and operate if he fails to improve.

D. Administer ceftriaxone and metronidazole (Flagyl) and proceed with surgery.

E. Begin clindamycin perioperatively, because *Bacteroides fragilis* is the most common organism involved in acute appendicitis, and proceed with surgery.

ANSWER: D

COMMENTS: Antibiotics play an important role in the treatment of appendicitis. The flora of the normal appendix is similar to that of the colon. There is a mixture of aerobic (*Escherichia coli*, most common) and anaerobic bacteria (*Bacteroides*, most common). If early nonperforated appendicitis is suspected, an appendectomy is warranted. Perioperative antibiotics help prevent wound infection and should cover both anaerobes and aerobes. Ceftriaxone plus metronidazole is the antibiotic regimen presented that is most appropriate. Peritoneal cultures in patients with acute nonperforated appendicitis are frequently negative. Peritoneal cultures in patients with perforated appendicitis usually reveal multiple colonic bacteria with predictable sensitivities. Therefore antibiotic choice is not based on peritoneal cultures. Currently, nonoperative management of appendicitis is controversial in the United States. Most surgeons agree that appendectomy is preferred for nonperforated cases.

Ref.: 2

5. A 62-year-old female presents with a 5-day history of right lower quadrant abdominal pain and nausea. A computed tomography (CT) of the abdomen and pelvis shows perforated appendicitis with a 5-cm abscess. She was started on broad-spectrum antibiotics and underwent percutaneous drainage of the abscess. In 72 h she was afebrile, and her leukocytosis and symptoms had resolved. What should the next treatment step be?

A. Appendectomy prior to discharge

B. Continue broad-spectrum antibiotics until drain removal

C. Schedule a colonoscopy and consider an interval appendectomy in 8 weeks

D. Interval appendectomy in 4 weeks

E. Ileocecectomy in 6 weeks

ANSWER: C

COMMENTS: Patients who present with perforated appendicitis with an abscess or phlegmon are best treated nonoperatively with broad-spectrum intravenous antibiotics and drainage of any intraabdominal abscess larger than 4 to 5 cm. This decreases the morbidity and risk of injury to adjacent structures due to inflammation during appendectomy. Most patients respond within 24 to 48 h. The duration of antibiotic treatment varies, but the maximum duration of course is 7 to 10 days. Some physicians believe that once the patient is afebrile, tolerating a diet, and has resolution of leukocytosis, antibiotics are no longer needed. If the patient has persistent fever, leukocytosis, or ileus, antibiotics should be adjusted to cover *Pseudomonas* and the CT should be repeated. Surgery may be warranted. Interval appendectomy is somewhat controversial. Recurrent appendicitis without appendectomy occurs in about 10% of patients, usually by 6 months. Factors such as age, comorbidities, and prior abdominal operations should be considered in the decision to proceed with an interval appendectomy. Surgery is usually performed 6 to 10 weeks after initial presentation. Adults who have not had a recent colonoscopy should undergo one because up to 5% of patients have a cecal neoplasm.

Ref.: 1–4

6. A 27-year-old man is suspected of having acute appendicitis. On physical examination his abdomen is soft and nondistended. He does not have pain with coughing or reproduction of tenderness in the right lower quadrant when palpated in the left lower quadrant. He experiences abdominal pain during extension of the right thigh while lying on his left side. He does not have pain with passive rotation of his right hip in a flexed position. Where do you suspect the location of the tip of his appendix to be?

A. Displaced to the right upper quadrant

B. Extraperitoneal and lying anterior to the cecum

C. In the pelvis

D. In the left lower quadrant

E. Retrocecal over the psoas muscle

ANSWER: E

COMMENTS: Variations in the location of the appendix can account for variations in the classic location of somatic pain. McBurney's point in the right lower quadrant, one-third of the distance between the anterior superior iliac spine and the umbilicus, is the typical site of maximal tenderness. Pain exaggerated by coughing is called the Dunphy's sign and is associated with peritoneal irritation. The Rovsing's sign is elicited by palpating the left lower quadrant that causes pain to be felt in the right lower quadrant, a finding suggestive of peritoneal irritation. The psoas sign is elicited by extension of the right thigh with the patient lying in the left lateral decubitus position. The stretched psoas muscle may irritate an inflamed overlying appendix and suggest retrocecal appendicitis. The obturator sign is elicited with passive external rotation of the flexed right hip. If positive, the obturator sign suggests that the inflamed tip is lying in the pelvis.

Ref.: 1–3

7. With regard to appendicitis in the elderly, which statement is false?

A. Elderly patients tend to present later in the course of acute appendicitis.

B. Elderly patients have a higher rate of perforation because of omental atrophy.

C. Perforation has an associated mortality rate of 50%.

D. Appendicitis may mimic bowel obstruction.

E. Symptoms of appendicitis along with anemia should raise suspicion for a concomitant cecal neoplasm.

ANSWER: C

COMMENTS: Acute appendicitis in the elderly may not be accompanied by the typical signs and symptoms of appendicitis. Fever, leukocytosis, and right lower quadrant pain may be minimal or absent. The absence of typical symptoms often results in a delay in diagnosis and an increase in the perforation rate (up to 60%–90%). A mortality rate of approximately 15% has been reported for perforated appendicitis in elderly patients.

The atrophic omentum is less capable of walling off a perforated appendix; therefore diffuse peritonitis or a distant intraabdominal abscess is more common in elderly than in younger patients. Physical examination is characterized by a paucity of findings. Abdominal distention is prominent, and symptoms and signs mimicking bowel obstruction such as nausea and vomiting are not uncommon. Occasionally, a patient has a painless palpable mass in the right lower quadrant because of a gangrenous appendix and a surrounding phlegmon. Anemia, particularly in elderly patients, should raise suspicion for carcinoma of the cecum. If found or strongly suspected, a right hemicolectomy may be appropriate.

Ref.: 1, 2

8. A 30-year-old, 28-week pregnant female presents to the emergency department with a 24-h history of right upper quadrant abdominal pain. The white blood cell (WBC) count is 18,000. An ultrasound was done showing a normal gallbladder and viable fetus. The appendix was not visualized. What is the next best step?

A. Obtain a CT abdomen/pelvis.

B. Treat with antibiotics in an attempt to avoid an operation.

C. Proceed with laparoscopy after delivery.

D. Obtain a magnetic resonance imaging (MRI) and proceed with an appendectomy if positive.

E. Admit the patient for serial abdominal examinations and repeat lab tests in the morning.

ANSWER: D

COMMENTS: Appendicitis occurs with equal frequency in both pregnant and nonpregnant women. Peritonitis may result in fetal loss. Diagnosing appendicitis during pregnancy can be difficult because abdominal pain, nausea, vomiting, and elevated WBC count are common during pregnancy. Additionally, as the uterus enlarges, the location of the appendix is shifted superiorly and medially. Delayed diagnosis and therefore delay in the treatment leading to perforated appendicitis increases the risk of fetal loss to about 30%. Ultrasound is helpful in establishing the diagnosis. In cases where ultrasound is equivocal, an MRI can be performed for further evaluation without the risk of radiation exposure to the developing fetus. A fairly aggressive approach with early laparoscopic exploration is a reasonable option in pregnant women with suspected appendicitis. The risk of maternal and/or fetal morbidity is quite low with a negative laparoscopy and appendectomy.

Ref.: 1, 2, 5

9. You are performing a laparoscopic appendectomy on a 35-year-old male who presented with classic acute appendicitis. During the operation, you note that the appendix is necrotic and perforated at the base. What is the best way to proceed with the appendectomy?

A. Perform a limited cecal resection using a stapling device.

B. Staple across the necrotic base of the appendix making sure the perforation is closed.

C. Place an endoloop around the base of the appendix.

D. Irrigate and place a drain with plans to perform an interval appendectomy in 6 weeks.

E. Perform an ileocecectomy.

ANSWER: A

COMMENTS: Using the standard appendectomy technique of stapling across or placing an endoloop at the base of an appendix that is acutely inflamed and necrotic or perforated increases the risk for failure and subsequent leak or abscess markedly. A limited cecal resection using a stapler or inverting the closed appendiceal stump and oversewing the cecal wall will decrease the risk of leak. Inverting and oversewing the appendiceal stump laparoscopically requires advanced laparoscopic skills, and therefore a limited, stapled cecectomy through healthy appearing tissue is best during laparoscopy. A formal ileocolic resection is rarely necessary.

Ref.: 5

10. A 20-year-old woman is operated on through a right lower quadrant incision for presumed appendicitis, but the appendix is normal. At this point, which of the following would be an appropriate treatment?

A. Exploration and appendectomy if no other pathology is found

B. Exploration, treatment of any associated pathologic condition, as indicated, and avoiding removal of a healthy appearing appendix

C. Exploration and diverticulectomy if a Meckel's diverticulum is present and is normal by inspection and palpation

D. Midline laparotomy for complete exploration if no pathology can be seen through the right lower quadrant incision

E. Exploration and ileal resection if the terminal ileum appears acutely inflamed

ANSWER: A

COMMENTS: If appendicitis is not found at the time of surgery, careful exploration for other pathologic conditions must be carried out. The accuracy of a preoperative diagnosis of appendicitis should be at least 85% (90% in men and 70% in women). In general, appendectomy is performed whether or not the appendix is inflamed, except when ileal or cecal Crohn's disease is found. In this case, the bowel is not violated, and the patient is started on a medical therapy soon after surgery. The pelvic organs, gallbladder, colon, and gastroduodenal areas should be inspected. A laparoscopic approach may allow better evaluation of other areas than can be accomplished through a limited right lower quadrant incision.

The differential diagnosis of appendicitis is basically that of an acute abdomen. The surgeon must be prepared to treat other pathologic entities should they be found. Such differential diagnoses include acute mesenteric adenitis, gastroenteritis, diverticulitis, epiploic appendagitis, gynecologic problems, and cancer.

Acute mesenteric adenitis is most often confused with appendicitis in children. Frequently, an upper respiratory tract infection precedes or is present at the onset of diffuse abdominal pain. Generalized lymphadenopathy or relative lymphocytosis, when present, can be of help. At surgery, the mesenteric lymph nodes are assessed. If they are enlarged, a biopsy is performed. The lymph nodes are examined histologically for granulomas (including Crohn's disease), and tissue is cultured for mycobacteria and *Yersinia*. Infection with *Yersinia* may cause mesenteric adenitis, ileitis, colitis, and acute appendicitis.

Acute gastroenteritis is characterized by cramping pain followed by watery stools, nausea, and vomiting. Laboratory results are usually normal. Diagnosis of a specific bacterial infection (e.g., *Salmonella* or typhoid fever) is made by stool culture.

The small intestine is inspected in a retrograde manner for evidence of inflammatory bowel disease or an inflamed Meckel's diverticulum. The incidence of perforation or peritonitis with Meckel's diverticulitis is about 50%. Resection of a Meckel's diverticulum is indicated if diverticulitis is present. An asymptomatic Meckel's diverticulum found incidentally during a laparotomy in adults may be removed with low risk in the absence of other pathology. Diverticulitis of the cecum may be impossible to distinguish from acute appendicitis or cancer clinically. Both may be manifested as a right lower quadrant mass with evidence of infection and peritonitis. Sigmoid diverticulitis may also mimic appendicitis if a mobile, inflamed sigmoid colon is located in the right lower quadrant.

Epiploic appendagitis usually results from infarction of the appendage secondary to torsion. The pain is short-lived and well-localized, recovery is fairly rapid, and patients do not appear ill.

If no pathology is found and a right lower quadrant incision is made, an appendectomy should be performed to eliminate potential confusion in the management of right lower quadrant abdominal pain in the future.

Ref.: 1, 2

11. With regard to appendicitis in immunocompromised patients, which of the following statements is false?

A. Immunocompromised patients with appendicitis often have a fever, a normal WBC count, and nonspecific abdominal pain.

B. Typhlitis often mimics acute appendicitis.

C. CT is particularly useful in immunocompromised patients.

D. Unusual infections such as those caused by mycobacteria, protozoa, and fungi do not usually mimic appendicitis.

E. Cytomegalovirus (CMV) infections and Kaposi sarcoma can occlude the appendiceal orifice and cause acute appendicitis.

ANSWER: D

COMMENTS: Appendicitis in immunocompromised patients can be difficult to diagnose. These patients cannot mount the normal immune response to infection and so the signs and symptoms may be diffuse, vague, and blunted. However, these patients may also progress to sepsis and critical illness. Therefore a heightened level of awareness must be maintained. The patient often has nonspecific findings on abdominal examination, fever, and a normal WBC count. The differential diagnosis in an immunocompromised patient with abdominal pain includes CMV enteritis, typhlitis, and unusual infections, including those caused by mycobacteria, protozoal species, and fungi. Typhlitis, or neutropenic colitis, often mimics appendicitis in these patients since the cecum is the most common location. Treatment with antibiotics and recovery of immune function usually obviate surgery. CT can be particularly useful in helping establish the diagnosis. Acute appendicitis secondary to luminal obstruction in a patient with acquired immunodeficiency syndrome (AIDS) may be the result of a fecalith, CMV bodies, or Kaposi sarcoma. Approximately 30% of cases of acute appendicitis in patients with AIDS are caused by conditions particular to AIDS.

Ref.: 1, 2

12. A patient suspected of having acute appendicitis underwent exploration. An inflamed terminal ileum consistent with Crohn's disease was found. Which of the following is true?

A. The normal appendix should always be removed.

B. All grossly involved bowel, including the appendix, should be resected.

C. An inflamed appendix, cecum, and terminal ileum should be resected.

D. Perforated bowel and advanced Crohn's disease with obstruction should be resected.

E. Only the tip of the appendix should be resected if the base is found to be involved with Crohn's disease.

ANSWER: D

COMMENTS: If a normal appendix is found at the time of laparotomy, other causes should be sought. If Crohn's disease is encountered and the cecum and base of the appendix are normal, an appendectomy should be performed. If the base is involved with Crohn's disease, appendectomy should be avoided as the rate of fistula formation is high after an appendectomy in patients with Crohn's disease. If the areas involved with Crohn's disease are not complicated by perforation or obstruction, bowel resection is not indicated, and medical therapy should be instituted. However, in the setting of perforation or high-grade obstruction from a fibrotic segment, the involved bowel should be resected. Ileostomy and deferred anastomosis may be appropriate in some cases.

Ref.: 1, 2, 5

13. Which of the following is true regarding appendiceal carcinoid tumors?

A. Carcinoid tumor is the second most common tumor of the appendix.

B. For tumors greater than 2 cm, a formal right hemicolectomy is indicated.

C. All tumors less than 2 cm that do not involve the appendiceal base can be treated with an appendectomy alone.

D. Nearly 75% of appendiceal carcinoid tumors are located in the proximal one-third of the appendix.

E. Carcinoid tumors arise from the smooth muscle within the appendiceal wall.

ANSWER: B

COMMENTS: Carcinoid tumors arise from neural crest cells and are derived from enteroendocrine cells. Fifty percent of carcinoid tumors within the gastrointestinal cells arise within the appendix. Nearly 75% of appendiceal carcinoid tumors are located in the distal one-third of the appendix. Tumors less than 1 cm are usually treated with an appendectomy alone. Treatment of tumors between 1 and 1.9 cm is based on the risk of recurrence. Tumors with poor prognostic indicators should be treated with a formal right hemicolectomy. Thirty to sixty percent of appendiceal carcinoid tumors greater than 2 cm are associated with nodal disease or distant metastases. Therefore all tumors greater than 2 cm should be treated with a formal right hemicolectomy.

Ref.: 1, 6

14. A 35-year-old male underwent a laparoscopic appendectomy. On final pathology, he was found to have a 1.4-cm carcinoid tumor in the mid-appendix with direct extension to the mesoappendix, negative margins, and no lymphovascular invasion. What is the best treatment plan?

A. No further treatment needed

B. Ileocecectomy

C. Right hemicolectomy

D. Medical treatment with octreotide

E. Chemotherapy

ANSWER: C

COMMENTS: Carcinoid tumors between 1 and 1.9 cm must be treated based on the risk of recurrence. Poor prognostic indicators include high-grade lesions with a high mitotic rate, direct extension into the mesoappendix, lymph node involvement, lymphovascular invasion, positive margins, or mucin-producing tumors. If any of these are present, a formal right hemicolectomy is warranted. Octreotide is used for metastatic disease, and chemotherapy has very limited benefit for either local or metastatic carcinoid tumors.

Ref.: 3, 6

15. A 57-year-old male with a complaint of watery diarrhea underwent a colonoscopy and was found to have a mass within the appendiceal orifice. This was biopsied and the pathology was consistent with a carcinoid tumor. A CT of the chest, abdomen, and pelvis showed a 3-cm appendiceal base mass and two liver lesions. Which of the following is true?

A. Appendiceal carcinoid tumors with metastases to the liver are fast growing and have a 5-year survival rate of only 10%.

B. Octreotide decreases metastatic tumor progression and improves survival rates.

C. Carcinoid syndrome occurs when the primary tumor becomes larger than 2 cm and secretes hormones.

D. Hepatic resection of liver metastases is not recommended as a method for tumor debulking and symptom control.

E. Synchronous treatment with a right hemicolectomy and radiofrequency ablation of the liver metastases is appropriate.

ANSWER: E

COMMENTS: Rarely, appendiceal carcinoids are associated with liver metastases. Appendiceal carcinoid tumors with metastases are slow growing and have 5- and 10-year survival rates approaching 60%. Carcinoid syndrome occurs when the tumor produces hormones, most commonly serotonin, which reaches the systemic circulation. Typically, carcinoid syndrome only occurs with gastrointestinal tumors when they metastasize to either the liver or the retroperitoneum. The liver contains monoamine oxidase, which deactivates serotonin. Therefore to develop carcinoid syndrome, the patient must have a tumor that does not drain primarily through the portal venous system. The clinical manifestations of the carcinoid syndrome include episodic flushing, wheezing, nonbloody watery diarrhea, abdominal pain, and right-sided heart failure. Flushing is the most common symptom, occurring in 80% of patients with carcinoid syndrome, followed by watery diarrhea in 75% and cardiac manifestations in 60% to 70%. Management of carcinoid syndrome is multimodal, using surgical, medical, and radiologic treatment. Surgical debulking may improve symptoms and prolong life. This includes excision of the primary tumor and debulking of hepatic metastases. Hepatic artery embolization and radiofrequency ablation of hepatic metastases are also options for disease control and symptom relief. Somatostatin analogues (octreotide) are effective at controlling symptoms and decreasing tumor progression, but no overall survival benefit has been demonstrated.

Ref.: 1, 6

16. When a mucocele of the appendix is found at the time of surgery, which of the following is an appropriate initial therapy?

A. Incisional biopsy with subsequent appendectomy if malignancy is confirmed by frozen section

B. Routine right hemicolectomy with lymph node dissection

C. Needle aspiration of cystic fluid for cytologic examination

D. Appendectomy

E. Closure and observation

ANSWER: D

COMMENTS: Appendectomy is an adequate treatment of a mucocele, but care must be taken to avoid rupture, because pseudomyxoma peritonei has been reported following rupture and peritoneal dissemination of the appendiceal contents, even if the appendix was free of cancer. Histologically, mucoceles can be categorized as a benign type, which is the result of occlusion of the proximal lumen of the appendix, or a malignant type, which is a variant of a mucous papillary adenocarcinoma. Treatment of an appendiceal *adenocarcinoma* is right hemicolectomy.

Ref.: 1, 2

17. Which of the following is true regarding adenocarcinoma of the appendix?

A. Appendectomy is an adequate treatment for tumors less than 1 cm without lymph node involvement and clear margins.

B. Fifty percent of patients have metastatic disease at the time of diagnosis.

C. Right hemicolectomy is required for all appendiceal adenocarcinomas.

D. A second primary adenocarcinoma is rarely found elsewhere in the gastrointestinal tract at the time of diagnosis.

E. Adenocarcinoma is the most common tumor of the appendix.

ANSWER: B

COMMENTS: Primary adenocarcinoma of the appendix is very rare. Approximately 50% of patients present with metastatic disease at the time of diagnosis. Early lesions confined to the mucosa or submucosa (T0–T1) may be treated with a simple appendectomy as long as there are clear margins. Any more invasive lesions require a formal right hemicolectomy. Staging and treatment for appendiceal adenocarcinoma are similar to colon adenocarcinoma. A second primary adenocarcinoma is found in 35% of patients with an appendiceal adenocarcinoma, most often involving other areas of the gastrointestinal tract. Therefore thorough evaluation of the abdominal cavity and bowel should be performed at the time of operation.

Ref.: 1

18. During an exploratory laparotomy on a 46-year-old male with a small bowel obstruction, mucinous ascites is found throughout the abdomen along with a large cystic-appearing appendiceal mass. What is the most likely diagnosis?

A. Malignant peritoneal mesothelioma

B. Appendiceal carcinoid tumor

C. Perforated acute appendicitis

D. Metastatic melanoma

E. Pseudomyxoma peritonei

ANSWER: E

COMMENTS: Pseudomyxoma peritonei is malignant mucinous ascites that usually arises from a ruptured ovarian or mucinous appendiceal adenocarcinoma. The peritoneal surfaces are coated with a diffuse, mucus-secreting tumor that often fills the peritoneal cavity. It may cover any of the abdominal cavity surfaces including the abdominal wall, liver, spleen, bowel, uterus, ovaries and tubes, bladder, and diaphragm. It occurs in equal frequency in men and women and is most common between the ages of 40 and 50 years. Patients are often asymptomatic until they have advanced disease. Symptoms are nonspecific and may include abdominal pain, bloating, distention, loss of appetite and weight, and wasting. CT scanning often does not identify the problem. Vague thickening or nodularity of surfaces and ascites may be seen. The diagnosis is usually made at laparotomy. Treatment involves debulking resection of as much of the tumor as possible (cytoreduction) and heated intraperitoneal chemotherapy. Cytoreduction includes omentectomy, stripping of the involved peritoneum, resection of involved organs, and right hemicolectomy. Successful cytoreduction leaves no residual tumor nodules larger than 2 mm to allow for better penetration of the intraperitoneal chemotherapy. These operations may be very long and tedious. For best results, these patients should be treated at a center and by surgeons that specialize in peritoneal malignancies. Complication rates are high (25%–35%), but significant prolongation of life is possible in many patients. The best approach for the operating surgeon who is not prepared to do a formal cytoreduction operation is to establish the diagnosis by the least invasive procedure (appendectomy or biopsies), relieve any intestinal obstruction, close, and refer the patient to a specialized center.

Ref.: 7

REFERENCES

1. Matthews JB, Hodin RA. Acute abdomen and appendix. In: Mulholland MW, Lillemoe KD, Doherty GM, et al., eds. *Greenfield's Surgery: Scientific Principles and Practice*. 5th ed. Philadelphia: Lippincott Williams & Wilkins; 2011.
2. Maa J, Kirkwood KS. The appendix. In: Townsend CM, Beauchamp RD, Evers BM, et al., eds. *Sabiston Textbook of Surgery: The Biological Basis of Modern Surgical Practice*. 19th ed. Philadelphia: Elsevier Saunders; 2012.
3. Lowry SF, Davidov T, Shiroff AM. Appendicitis and appendiceal abscess. In: Fischer JE, Jones DB, Pomposelli FB, et al., eds. *Fischer's Mastery of Surgery*. 6th ed. Philadelphia: Lippincott Williams & Wilkins; 2012.
4. Stewart D. The management of acute appendicitis. In: Cameron JL, Cameron AM, eds. *Current Surgical Therapy*. 11th ed. Philadelphia: Elsevier Saunders; 2014.
5. Eubanks S, Phillip S. Laparoscopic appendectomy. In: Fischer JE, Jones DB, Pomposelli FB, et al., eds. *Fischer's Mastery of Surgery*. 6th ed. Philadelphia: Lippincott Williams & Wilkins; 2012.
6. Bonshey RP, Moloo H. Miscellaneous neoplasms. In: Beck DE, Roberts PL, Saclarides TJ, et al., eds. *The ASCRS Textbook of Colon and Rectal Surgery*. 2nd ed. New York: Springer; 2011.
7. Turnage RH, Badgwell B. Abdominal wall and umbilicus. In: Townsend CM, Beauchamp RD, Evers BM, et al., eds. *Sabiston Textbook of Surgery: The Biological Basis of Modern Surgical Practice*. 19th ed. Philadelphia: Elsevier Saunders; 2012.

CHAPTER 23

COLON, RECTUM, AND ANUS

A. Colon and Rectum

Tara Spivey, M.D., Vidya Fleetwood, M.D., and Jose Cintron, M.D.

1. A 77-year-old man is admitted with bright red blood per rectum. He takes warfarin for atrial fibrillation and has hypertension, aortic stenosis, and chronic obstructive pulmonary disease. The patient's initial hemoglobin upon presentation is 6.7 g/dL, and his international normalized ratio (INR) is 2.2. Initially, his blood pressure is 86/56, which improves to 112/74 with infusion of two units of packed red blood cells (RBCs), four units of fresh frozen plasma, and crystalloids. A nasogastric tube is placed, and lavage reveals bilious contents and no blood. Rectal examination reveals gross blood in the rectal vault but no hemorrhoids or fissures. Colonoscopy reveals blood throughout the colon but no identifiable source. What should be the next step in management?

A. Tagged RBC scan
B. H2 blocker
C. Mesenteric angiography
D. Exploratory laparoscopy
E. Total abdominal colectomy

ANSWER: C

COMMENTS: The workup of this patient has revealed probable lower gastrointestinal (GI) bleeding given the negative nasogastric lavage and the presence of blood throughout the colon on colonoscopy. The source of this bleed, however, has not yet been localized. Fifteen percent of cases of upper GI bleeding may present as lower GI bleeding because of rapid transit through the GI tract. As is often the case with GI bleeding, this patient has a very high perioperative risk for an acute coronary event and even death. A tagged RBC scan is often helpful in localizing the region of slower or recurrent bleeding, but it is not therapeutic for an unstable patient who continues to bleed. Suppression of gastric acid secretion with an H2 blocker or a proton pump inhibitor (PPI) is not indicated in this setting. Mesenteric angiography would be the next step in managing this patient since it can be both diagnostic and therapeutic. Mesenteric angiography can pinpoint the site of active bleeding that may be treated with superselective embolization. Although a concern in the past, the risk of intestinal ischemia is low with this approach. Whenever possible, the site or at least the region of intestinal bleeding should be identified prior to surgery. Laparoscopy is not useful in identifying the source of bleeding. Emergency total abdominal colectomy is rarely necessary and should be a last resort since it is associated with significant morbidity and mortality in elderly and vasculopathic patients.

Ref.: 1

2. With regard to the anatomy of the colon and rectum, which of the following statements is true?

A. The colon has a complete outer longitudinal and an incomplete inner circular muscle layer.
B. The haustra are separated by plicae circulares.
C. The ascending colon and descending colon are usually fixed to the retroperitoneum.
D. The rectum is totally invested by three complete muscle layers.
E. The distal part of the rectum begins at the point where the taeniae coli merge.

ANSWER: C

COMMENTS: A thorough understanding of anatomy is integral to the surgical management of problems of the colon and rectum. The colon has two muscle layers: an outer longitudinal layer and an inner circular layer. The inner layer completely encircles the colon. The outer layer, unlike in the small intestine, is in the form of three grossly recognizable longitudinal strips, or taeniae coli, that do not cover the full circumference of the colon. At the rectosigmoid junction, the three taeniae coli spread out and fuse together to cover the rectum circumferentially with a longitudinal coat. This explains why acquired diverticula do not form in the rectum.

The plicae semilunares are spaced, transverse, crescentic folds that separate the tissue between the taeniae coli and form haustra. They produce a characteristic, intermittently bulging pattern that radiologically permits differentiation of the colon from the small intestine, which has circular mucosal folds known as plicae circulares or valvulae conniventes. In contrast to the plicae semilunares, the plicae circulares go all the way around the small bowel lumen, thereby facilitating radiographic distinction.

Usually, the ascending and descending portions of the colon are fused to the retroperitoneum, whereas the transverse and sigmoid portions are free. However, developmental anomalies of fixation, as seen with malrotation and in some cases of volvulus, are not uncommon. Cecal volvulus, for example, could not occur unless incomplete fixation to the retroperitoneum makes it possible for a mobile cecum to rotate around a narrow mesenteric pedicle.

Surgeons have traditionally placed the upper border of the rectum at the peritoneal reflection, but this is an external and unreliable landmark. Indeed, the peritoneum may only cover the upper anterior portion of the rectum or may go all the way down to the pelvic floor, creating a deep cu-de-sac. A better definition is the point at which the taeniae have completely merged. The rectum therefore lacks taeniae and appendices epiploicae. This is generally easy to recognize intraoperatively. Posteriorly, the upper rectal mesentery may be narrow since it is a continuation of the sigmoid mesentery and derived from the inferior mesenteric vessels. The rectal mesentery spreads out laterally as it descends and then narrows and thins out as it reaches the anorectal ring. All of this must be removed when operating for middle and lower rectal cancers, the so-called total mesorectal excision (TME).

Ref.: 1

3. A 22-year-old man in whom Crohn's disease has recently been diagnosed has just recovered from his first Crohn's flare-up. Currently, he has no perianal involvement. What medical therapy is not used as a first-line agent to *maintain remission*?

A. 6-Mercaptopurine

B. Metronidazole

C. Mesalamine

D. Infliximab

E. Prednisone

ANSWER: E

COMMENTS: Currently, there is no cure for Crohn's disease. It is felt to be a systemic autoimmune disease. There is early evidence of genetic predisposition and a weak inheritance pattern, but this seems to require an additional push for the patient to develop the clinical picture of Crohn's disease (the two-hit theory). This push might be an infection or exposure to an allergen to which the immune system responds. Normally, the immune response will decrease after the inciting event passes and will return to homeostasis. In Crohn's disease, this ability to downregulate seems to be abnormal and inadequate, leading to persistent inflammation. Medical therapy for Crohn's disease is aimed at general or targeted control of the immune system and inflammation. Most medications such as steroids and many of the older immunosuppressants like azathioprine, 6-mercaptopurine, and methotrexate have broad effects on the immune system and many have deleterious side effects, such as increased risk of infections. Steroids such as prednisone are well known for their very high complication rates when used for the long term, even in the young. These include osteoporosis; aseptic joint necrosis; adrenal insufficiency; GI, hepatic, and ophthalmologic effects (glaucoma); hyperlipidemia; growth suppression; central obesity and peripheral wasting; striae; poor healing; Cushingoid facies; buffalo hump; amenorrhea; irritability and wide mood swings; acne; and possible congenital malformations.

Sulfasalazine is commonly used for Crohn's disease. Its active component is 5-aminosalicylic acid (5-ASA). It has been shown to be beneficial in patients with colitis and ileocolitis, but its effectiveness for Crohn's disease limited to the small bowel is controversial. Sulfasalazine alone has not been proved to maintain remission. Many patients are allergic to the sulfa component of this medication, and so it is not used as much today because of newer options. Mesalamine is a newer drug that also releases 5-ASA. It is available in several oral forms as well as a suppository. Mesalamine is considered a first-line therapy for Crohn's disease and is also often used in combination with a corticosteroid. Corticosteroids, such as prednisone and budesonide, are very useful in the induction of remission of active Crohn's disease. Corticosteroids alone are ineffective in maintaining remission and should not be used for longer than 6 months, if at all possible. Tapering of steroids and transition to other maintenance medications is part of the standard approach to therapy.

Antibiotics have been used as adjuncts to other medications. Metronidazole is the most commonly used antibiotic for Crohn's disease in the setting of perianal disease, enterocutaneous fistulas, or active colonic disease. It seems to have both antimicrobial and immunologic effects, although the mechanism is unclear.

Several newer medications have been developed over the last decade, which have had major effects on treatment paradigms. Most of these medications target specific points in the immune inflammatory cascade. These are anti–tumor necrosis factor-α (anti-TNF-α) antibodies that block the TNF-α receptor, which in turn decreases inflammation. It is used to reduce the signs and symptoms of inflammatory bowel disease (IBD) and maintain remission. Infliximab (Remicade) was the first in this class. It has proved to be very useful in treating patients with Crohn's disease and has some effect on related fistulas. Other options now include adalimumab (Humira), certolizumab pegol (Cimzia), and vedolizumab (Entyvio). Although initially not used as a first-line therapy for Crohn's disease, these targeting medications are now being added earlier and earlier because of superior response and possible maintenance of remission. Yet, even these medications have potentially serious consequences including the development of lymphoma and infections. Although much discussed, the risk of lymphoma is actually quite low. Attempts to estimate the actual incidence is confounded by the concomitant use of other immune modulators and reliance on retrospective and limited data.

Surgical therapy is reserved for consequences of the disease that cannot be well managed medically or to reduce the need for high-risk medications, particularly steroids. Typical surgical indications include fibrotic obstruction, abscesses, perforation, fistulas, anorectal disease, cancer, and the rare instance of life-threatening bleeding. Even with high-quality medical management, 50% of patients with Crohn's disease will require an operation at some time in their life, and many will need more than one. Most medications have not yet proven to be particularly effective for maintaining remission after surgery.

Ref.: 1

4. Which of the following statements is true regarding colon physiology?

A. Transit time through the colon is independent of the fermentability of nonstarch polysaccharides such as lignin, cellulose, and pectins.

B. The left colon is the segment of colon where bacteria are the most metabolically active in the fermentation process. The right colon is the site of storage and dehydration of stool.

C. Fifty percent of the daily energy expenditure is obtained from the absorption of short-chain fatty acids by the colon; this energy is used to stimulate blood flow, regulate the pH of the colonic environment, and renew colonic mucosal cells.

D. Butyrate is a short-chain fatty acid and a bacterial fermentation product that is the main fuel for colonic epithelial cells.

E. Colonic epithelium can use various fuels, but it prefers glutamine over n-butyrate, glucose, or ketone bodies.

ANSWER: D

COMMENTS: The colon plays an important role in the digestive process for fluids and electrolytes. In healthy subjects, the colon normally absorbs 1 to 2 L of water and up to 200 mEq of sodium and chloride per day. This absorptive capacity can increase up to 5 to 6 L/day, thereby protecting against severe diarrhea and dehydration. The cecum and right colon absorb sodium and water the most rapidly, whereas the rectum is impermeable to sodium and water. Sodium is actively absorbed against chemical and electrical gradients in the colon. Butyrate plays a role in stimulating sodium absorption in the colon. Potassium and chloride are secreted by the colon through sodium-potassium adenosine triphosphatase (Na^+, K^+-ATPase) and sodium/potassium/chloride ($Na^+/K^+/Cl^-$) cotransporters. Chloride ions are actively absorbed at the expense of bicarbonate, which is secreted in exchange. The absence of luminal chloride inhibits secretion of bicarbonate. The main anions in stool include the short-chain fatty acids butyrate, acetate, and propionate. The host and the colonic bacterial flora have a symbiotic relationship: the host promotes bacterial proliferation with energy substrates from the diet and cellular debris, whereas bacteria provide the host with butyrate, a bacterial fermentation product and short-chain fatty acid that fuels colonic epithelial cells. Nonstarch polysaccharides, or dietary fiber such as lignin, cellulose, and fruit pectins, are the main substrates for bacterial fermentation. Fermentation takes place mostly in the right colon, with the cecum being the colonic segment where bacteria are the most metabolically active. Colonic transit time and bulking of stool are dependent on the fermentability of nonstarch polysaccharides. The transit time of stool through the colon is also dependent on stool pH, the autonomic nervous system, and the gastrocolic reflex (postprandial increase in electrical activity and colonic tone).

Ref.: 1, 2, 4

5. A 20-year-old healthy, active man with no previous medical problems is being evaluated for chronic constipation. His electrolyte levels are normal. He denies recent travel and is not currently taking any medications. Plain radiographs show a dilated colon. Transit studies are abnormal with slow transit times. What is the next best step in the management of this patient?
   A. Flexible sigmoidoscopy
   B. Modification of diet and antibiotics
   C. Placement of a rectal tube proximal to the normal-caliber aganglionic bowel to decompress the dilated nondiseased bowel
   D. Anal manometry, rectal biopsy, and barium enema
   E. Exploratory laparotomy

ANSWER: D

COMMENTS: This patient should be evaluated for Hirschsprung's disease. Megacolon may be congenital or acquired. Both forms are characterized by dilation, elongation, and hypertrophy of the colon proximal to a segment of nonperistaltic collapsed bowel causing obstruction. Both are associated with an increased risk for volvulus. Infection with *Trypanosoma cruzi* (Chagas disease), Hirschsprung's disease, and neuronal intestinal dysplasia should all be considered in a patient with slow transit constipation and megacolon.

Hirschsprung's disease is caused by congenital absence of ganglion cells in the myenteric plexus of the bowel, which results in the loss of peristaltic activity in that segment of the intestine. The rectosigmoid region is most frequently involved, with the variable extension of the disease proximally. There is a transition zone from normal bowel, which is dilated, to abnormal bowel, which is aganglionic, aperistaltic, and of normal or decreased caliber. Although Hirschsprung's disease is primarily a disease of infants and children, occasionally patients with Hirschsprung's disease will present later in life if an ultrashort distal rectal segment is involved. In these cases, patients usually relate a history of constipation dating back to infancy. In most cases, the diagnosis is apparent during the first 24 h of life when the infant fails to pass meconium. A rectal biopsy is diagnostic. In adolescents and young adults, Hirschsprung's disease can be diagnosed by anal manometry. If the disease is present, the rectoanal inhibitory reflex (relaxation of the internal sphincter in response to rectal distention) is lost because of the absence of normal ganglion cells, necessary for this myenteric reflex. Treatment of Hirschsprung's disease is surgical. The effected segment plus any markedly dilated bowel above it is resected, and a coloanal anastomosis is constructed.

Acquired megacolon may be seen in patients with protozoal colon infections with *T. cruzi*, which is endemic in South and Central America. This condition has not been reported in North America. *T. cruzi* causes widespread destruction of the intramural nervous system. Acquired megacolon may also occur in patients with colonic dilation due to chronic constipation because of the loss of voluntary defecatory muscles (e.g., in paraplegia), extreme inactivity (e.g., in poliomyelitis), or voluntary inhibition of defecation (e.g., in psychotic disorders). Resection of the excessive redundant colon is occasionally justified in the latter group of patients.

Ref.: 1, 3

6. A screening colonoscopy identifies a broad sessile villous-appearing lesion of the rectum beginning 4 cm above the anal verge and extending 5 cm proximally. Biopsies show a villous adenoma with dysplasia. Endorectal ultrasound (EUS) shows that the muscularis propria is not involved. No suspicious lymph nodes are seen. Which of the following approaches is the most appropriate for the management of this patient?
   A. Repeated biopsies
   B. Fulguration
   C. Transanal excision
   D. Abdominoperineal resection (APR)
   E. Intracavitary radiotherapy

ANSWER: C

COMMENTS: A villous adenoma with the dimensions given has a 30%–50% chance of harboring cancer. An endoscopic biopsy represents a very limited sample size and is not an adequate proof of the lesion's precise histologic characteristics. In this instance, the finding of dysplasia suggests a high probability of cancer elsewhere in the adenoma. A complete, full-thickness transanal excision of the lesion should be performed so that if a carcinoma is present, its depth of penetration can be assessed accurately. If there is no invasive cancer, the patient is monitored by interval endoscopic examinations because the risk for recurrence is approximately 10%, even though the initial lesion was benign. If invasive cancer is found, the need for further treatment is determined on the basis of the depth of penetration. A T1 cancer is adequately treated by transanal excision, provided that the tumor is not poorly differentiated and lacks vascular or lymphatic invasion and the margins of excision are clear. T2 or T3 cancers should be treated by radical resection because of the much higher rate of lymphatic spread. Radiation therapy is not used for benign lesions and is not necessary for T1 lesions. Some patients may refuse radical resection for a T2 or T3 lesion; radiation with or without chemotherapy may be offered, but this is not the standard of care. Fulguration of these lesions can be performed in very poor-risk patients in whom precise histologic staging is not essential. However, this is not the standard of care for good-risk patients. If there is a local recurrence after the transanal excision of a benign lesion, reexcision, endoscopic fulguration, or argon plasma coagulation may be considered. APR is rarely indicated for benign polyps because many less radical treatment options are now available. Intracavitary radiotherapy was performed for superficially invading malignant lesions earlier, but the unit has not been made for many decades now and so is rarely available. Lesions extending above 6 to 8 cm from the anal verge are best excised with either transanal endoscopic microsurgery (TEM) or transanal minimally invasive surgery (TAMIS). TEM excision has been shown to be much more precise and reliable than transanal excision with standard operating anoscopes. Long-term data on TAMIS is not yet available.

Ref.: 1, 3, 7, 8

7. In which of the following settings should a low anterior resection (LAR) be performed?

A. A 56-year-old male with a circumferential villous adenoma beginning at the dentate line and extending 8 cm proximally

B. Palliation of obstructing rectal cancer just above the dentate line with minimal liver metastases in a 60-year-old female

C. An 80-year-old male with a large rectal cancer that produces anal pain and tenesmus and involves the anal sphincter

D. A 45-year-old female with an anastomotic recurrence after LAR of a distal rectal cancer

E. A 75-year-old male with urinary incontinence and a rectal cancer 5 cm above the dentate line

ANSWER: E

COMMENTS: APR of the sigmoid, rectum, and anus with a permanent colostomy was originally described by William Ernest Miles in his landmark paper from 1908. It is frequently performed for cancers of the distal part of the rectum and for recurrent or persistent anal cancer. Miles showed that there are three routes of lymphatic spread from rectal cancer: superiorly along the inferior mesenteric artery (IMA) chain, laterally along the middle rectal vessels to the pelvic and iliac chains, and inferiorly along the pudendal and inguinal pathways. At that time, most cancers presented in advanced stages. Subsequently, it has been found that virtually all spread of rectal adenocarcinoma is through the superior route. Spread in the other two directions only occurs when the superior route is obstructed by advanced disease.

The APR is a large operation and is associated with many complications such as sexual and urinary dysfunction and poor healing of the perineal wound, especially after radiation. Most benign lesions of the rectum including large and even circumferential rectal adenomas may be removed with a variety of transanal techniques that preserve the sphincter muscles and fecal continence. Curative resection of cancers in the mid and even distal portions of the rectum in some patients can be performed by LAR and either colorectal or coloanal anastomosis without the need for a permanent colostomy. Many studies from the 1940s to the 1960s showed that cure rates were equivalent when comparing APR with LAR as long as margins were not compromised and a complete mesenteric resection was performed. Limiting factors include the need for a distal mural margin of 2 cm, adequate mesorectal excision, and good sphincter function. The end-to-end surgical stapling devices introduced through the rectum have greatly facilitated anastomoses deep in the pelvis. Concerns that local recurrence rates would be higher as a result have not been borne out. Recurrence rates after stapled and hand-sewn anastomoses are the same.

APR is usually performed with curative intent, although it may be justified for symptomatic patients (palliative) with a minimal metastatic disease who are expected to survive 6 months or longer. A cancer that produces anal pain and tenesmus usually involves the sphincter muscle or is obstructing. Recurrent cancer following low resection of a distal cancer usually mandates APR. Fecal incontinence if already present will probably worsen following LAR and a deep pelvic anastomosis because of the loss of normal rectal compliance and capacity.

Ref.: 1, 3

8. With regard to ulcerative colitis, which of the following statements is true?

A. The entire colon is involved with skip areas in at least one-half of patients.

B. Crypt abscesses on pathology are diagnostic of ulcerative colitis and are not seen with other inflammatory conditions of the bowel.

C. The course of the disease is most commonly a chronic relapsing one, with acute fulminant colitis in only 10%–15% of patients.

D. Cancers arising in association with ulcerative colitis tend to be located in the rectum and sigmoid colon, similar to sporadic colorectal cancers (CRCs).

E. Histologic demonstration of granulomas reliably confirms the diagnosis.

ANSWER: C

COMMENTS: Ulcerative colitis is usually limited to the mucosal and submucosal layers of the colon and rectum. The rectum is almost always involved with continuous spread proximally to varying lengths of the colon. The entire colon is involved in at least one-half of patients. The characteristic pathologic finding is crypt abscesses and not noncaseating granulations that are seen in about one-third of patients with Crohn's disease. Crypt abscesses are disruptions of the epithelium and lamina propria at the base of the colonic crypts of Lieberkühn. They are characterized by sloughing epithelial cells and infiltration of neutrophils and eosinophils in the epithelium and lamina propria. Crypt abscesses are always present with ulcerative colitis but may also be seen with other inflammatory conditions of the colon such as radiation colitis and certain infections. Therefore they are not pathognomonic for ulcerative colitis. An additional common pathologic finding is goblet cell depletion, as opposed to Crohn's disease, in which the goblet cells are preserved.

Ulcerative colitis is most commonly chronic and relapsing in character, although in 10%–15% of patients the disease runs an acute and fulminant course that may present as toxic colitis.

Cancers associated with ulcerative colitis are often advanced when diagnosed because the signs and symptoms may be confused with an inflammatory relapse. For this reason, these cancers are associated with a poorer prognosis. Studies have shown that contrary to what was previously believed, cancers in colitis patients do not behave more aggressively than sporadic cancers when similar stages are compared. Cancers associated with ulcerative colitis are more evenly distributed throughout the colon than sporadic cancers that are more common in the rectum and sigmoid, have a higher incidence of proximal involvement, and are frequently multiple.

Ref.: 1, 3

9. A 39-year-old man with a history of mild, long-standing ulcerative colitis controlled with sulfasalazine recently underwent routine colonoscopy that showed a lesion in the sigmoid colon. Pathologic evaluation reveals high-grade dysplasia. Which of the following is the best management option?

A. Sigmoid colectomy, provided that the rectum is minimally involved

B. Proctocolectomy with ileal pouch–anal anastomosis (IPAA)

C. Total abdominal colectomy with ileorectal anastomosis (IRA)

D. Total proctocolectomy with Brooke ileostomy

E. Polypectomy and frequent surveillance colonoscopy to remove further polyps

ANSWER: B

COMMENTS: Cancer develops in approximately 5%–6% of patients with ulcerative colitis. Patients with pancolitis or disease of long-standing duration (> 8 to 10 years) are at the highest risk.

Sigmoid colectomy is not a reasonable option since the finding of high-grade dysplasia is indicative of a high risk for cancer anywhere in the colon, not just where the biopsy was taken. Abdominal colectomy with IRA does not eradicate the disease or remove all of the mucosa at risk for malignant transformation. IRA is now rarely performed for ulcerative colitis because of the presence of persistent disease in the rectum, the risk of neoplasia in the rectum, and poor function because of poor rectal compliance and tenesmus. Historically, the risk for subsequent rectal cancer after an IRA is approximately 20% after 25 years, even with close surveillance. Therefore over 50% of patients will require completion proctectomy because of cancer, dysplastic changes, refractory proctitis, or poor function.

Total proctocolectomy with permanent end ileostomy (TPC) is an acceptable operation, particularly when a one-step approach is preferred or when the patient is a poor candidate for a sphincter-preserving procedure because of age, c-morbidities, or poor sphincter function. Healthy, motivated patients who require surgery for ulcerative colitis generally prefer a proctocolectomy with sphincter preservation and IPAA.

The continent ileostomy procedure (Kock pouch) with the creation of an internal distal ileal reservoir and an invaginated nipple valve was described in the late 1960s for urinary diversion and then adapted as an alternative for the standard end ileostomy. The pouch must be intubated with a rigid plastic tube multiple times each day to stent the valve open and allow the pouch to empty. Even in the best of hands, these require revision surgery in 25%–30% of patients because of slippage of the nipple valve and incontinence or obstruction. This procedure has been largely replaced by the IPAA operation.

The combination of proctocolectomy, an ileal reservoir (J pouch), and IPAA offers advantages over proctocolectomy and permanent ileostomy because not only is the diseased mucosa eliminated but so is the need for a permanent abdominal stoma. The straight ileoanal operation was originally described by Mark Ravich, M.D., and David Sabiston, M.D., in 1947 but was not pursued because of copious diarrhea and frequency. The technique has undergone many modifications, most notably the addition of an ileal pouch proximal to the IPAA. The pouch may be S or J shaped, which increases stool storage capacity and decreases frequency. A temporary diverting ileostomy is usually required for 2 to 3 months while the pouch heals. The procedure is currently recommended for the majority of patients with ulcerative colitis and for patients with familial polyposis. It is not indicated for Crohn's disease because of the high risk for recurrence within the pouch that may lead to complex fistulas and septic complications. Although advanced age is not an absolute contraindication, elderly patients with multiple comorbid conditions may be better served by a TPC with a permanent ileostomy. For appropriately selected patients, the functional results are good, with preservation of the autonomic innervation to the bladder and genitalia. Fecal sensation and continence are retained in most patients. Daytime incontinence occurs in about 5% and nocturnal incontinence or soiling occurs in 20% of patients. Over 95% of patients retain the pouch over the long term.

Ref.: 1, 3

10. Enteric fistulas may be a complication of diverticulitis. Which of the following statements is true?

A. Colocutaneous fistulas frequently occur spontaneously.

B. Suspected colovesical fistulas are best confirmed with barium enema.

C. Coloenteric fistulas may be totally asymptomatic.

D. Surgical correction of enteric fistulas is best accomplished in stages.

E. Colonic fistulas occur in about 30% of complicated cases of diverticulitis.

ANSWER: C

COMMENTS: Enteric fistulas occur in about 5% of acute cases of colonic diverticulitis. Fistulas usually develop as a consequence of localized abscess formation with perforation into an adjacent hollow organ, typically the bladder, uterus, vagina (after hysterectomy), or small bowel. Most spontaneous diverticular complications occur with the first episode of diverticulitis. Colocutaneous fistulas rarely form spontaneously. They are most commonly seen as a postoperative complication in which they drain through operative incisions or drain tracts.

Colovesical fistulas are most frequently the result of diverticular disease, followed in frequency by cancer, Crohn's disease, radiation-induced colitis, and foreign bodies. The primary symptoms of fecaluria and pneumaturia are associated with the urinary tract. The patient may relate a history of abdominal pain and fever before the development of the fistula. Although a barium enema may give information regarding the site and extent of involvement of the colon with diverticulosis, the fistula is demonstrated in only one-half of the cases. Cystoscopy is often very useful and may demonstrate the fistula opening into the bladder with stool, gas, or mucous passage or erythema and edema of the wall of the bladder, a finding consistent with a fistula. Computed tomography (CT) may reveal a constellation of findings, including air in the bladder, a thickened loop of bowel lying against the bladder, and enteric contrast in the bladder (before intravenous contrast material has been administered). CT has become the diagnostic test of choice. Coloenteric fistulas may cause no symptoms or may produce diarrhea, depending on which segments of bowel are involved with the fistula.

Most stable fistulas can be corrected with a one-stage operation, which is the preferred treatment. If bowel preparation is inadequate or there is extensive local inflammation or abscess formation beyond the immediate vicinity of the colon or its mesentery, a staged approach may be required. The first stage includes a Hartmann's resection of the involved bowel with a colostomy and distal closure along with repair of the bladder. The second stage involves colostomy take down and colorectal anastomosis.

Ref.: 1, 3

11. A 54-year-old man underwent right hemicolectomy for colon cancer. Pathologic analysis showed invasion of the tumor into the muscularis propria, with 2 of 18 lymph nodes positive for tumor. What is his pathologic staging?

    A. Dukes A
    B. Astler-Coller A
    C. T2N1 (stage IIIA)
    D. T2N1 (stage IIB)
    E. T3N2 (stage IIIA)

ANSWER: C

COMMENTS: The Dukes classification (1932) was the original standardized method for staging CRC. In subsequent years, however, confusion arose because of numerous modifications.

The American Joint Committee on Cancer (AJCC) standardized the tumor-nodes-metastasis (TNM) classification that is now used globally (Table 23A.1). The TNM classification stages a tumor according to the depth of tumor invasion into the bowel wall (T), the presence or absence of lymph node involvement (N), and distant metastases (M). A T1 tumor penetrates only into the submucosa, whereas a T2 tumor partially invades the muscularis propria. Transmural penetration imparts a T3 designation, a T4a lesion comes through to the serosal surface of the bowel, and a T4b tumor invades into an adjacent structure. An N0 lesion has not metastasized to regional nodes, an N1 lesion involves three or fewer lymph nodes, and an N2 lesion has metastasized to four or more lymph nodes. The designations M0 and M1 indicate whether there are distant metastases. It is recommended that a minimum of 12 lymph nodes should be examined for reliable nodal staging. Stage I is T1 or T2 only, stage II is T3 or T4 only, stage III is any lymph node involvement (or tumor deposits separate from the primary), and stage IV is any distant metastases (Table 23A.1).

Prognosis is clearly differentiated by these stages, and survival has gradually improved over time with better surgery and better adjuvant therapy. Stage I colon cancer patients have a 5-year disease-free survival (DFS) rate of about 90%. Stage II patients who have had appropriate surgical resection have a 5-year DFS of about 75%. Stage III cancer patients treated by surgery alone have a 5-year survival of about 30%, but with adjuvant therapy the 5-year survival will rise to 60%–70%. Stage IV colon cancer carries a poor prognosis, with a 5-year survival rate of 5%. Some patients with disease limited to the liver or the lungs may be treated for cure.

Ref.: 1, 3

TABLE 23A.1 TNM Classification of Colon Cancer

Primary tumor (T)	
TX	Primary tumor cannot be assessed
T0	No evidence of primary tumor
Tis	Carcinoma in situ: intraepithelial or invasion of lamina propria
T1	Tumor invades submucosa
T2	Tumor invades muscularis propria
T3	Tumor invades through the muscularis propria into the pericolorectal tissues
T4a	Tumor penetrates to the surface of the visceral peritoneum
T4b	Tumor directly invades or is adherent to other organs or structures
Regional lymph nodes (N)	
NX	Regional lymph nodes cannot be assessed
N0	No regional lymph node metastasis
N1	Metastasis in one to three regional lymph nodes
N1a	Metastasis in one regional lymph node
N1b	Metastasis in two to three regional lymph nodes
N1c	Tumor deposit(s) in the subserosa, mesentery, or nonperitonealized pericolic or perirectal tissues without regional nodal metastasis
N2	Metastasis in four or more lymph nodes
N2a	Metastasis in four to six regional lymph nodes
N2b	Metastasis in seven or more regional lymph nodes
Distant metastasis (M)	
M0	No distant metastasis
M1	Distant metastasis
M1a	Metastasis confined to one organ or site (e.g., liver, lung, ovary, nonregional node)
M1b	Metastases in more than one organ/site or the peritoneum

Stage	T	N	M
0	Tis	N0	M0
I	T1	N0	M0
	T2	N0	M0
IIA	T3	N0	M0
IIB	T4a	N0	M0
IIC	T4b	N0	M0
IIIA	T1–T2	N1/N1c	M0
	T1	N2a	M0
IIIB	T3–T4a	N1/N1c	M0
	T2–T3	N2a	M0
	T1–T2	N2b	M0
IIIC	T4a	N2a	M0
	T3–T4a	N2b	M0
	T4b	N1–N2	M0
IVA	Any T	Any N	M1a
IVB	Any T	Any N	M1b

12. Cecal diverticula are different from sigmoid diverticula in that:

    A. Sigmoid diverticula are true diverticula while cecal diverticula are false diverticula.
    B. Cecal diverticulitis is usually distinguishable from cancer.
    C. Cecal diverticula are considered congenital in origin.
    D. Asymptomatic cecal diverticula found on barium enema or colonoscopy should be treated operatively because of the high incidence of complications.
    E. Feculent peritonitis from perforation of a cecal diverticulum may be treated with resection and primary anastomosis in most cases.

ANSWER: C

COMMENTS: True diverticula contain all layers of the bowel wall and are generally congenital. False diverticula lack the muscularis propria and are acquired. Sigmoid diverticula are acquired false diverticula. Isolated cecal diverticula are usually true or congenital. However, acquired diverticulosis may affect all parts of the colon (pan-diverticulosis). Cecal diverticulitis is relatively uncommon, and 80% of cases are initially diagnosed as acute appendicitis or, occasionally, perforated cancer. It is more common in patients of Asian descent. In patients with repeated attacks, the cecal inflammation and subsequent fibrotic scarring may be indistinguishable from cancer. Such an inflammatory mass of the sigmoid colon may resemble a cancer at laparotomy.

Treatment depends on symptoms, complications, and the number and severity of recurrent episodes. Incidentally found asymptomatic diverticula do not require surgery. Surgical options depend on the extent of inflammation. If the inflammation is minimal and limited, segmental resection and anastomosis may be performed. If there has been perforation with frank feculent peritonitis, a Hartmann's resection with a proximal ostomy and distal closure is performed. A middle of the road option is resection with anastomosis and proximal diverting loop ileostomy. Closure of the loop ileostomy is a much smaller operation than closure after a Hartmann's procedure.

Ref.: 3

13. A 21-year-old woman is noted to have persistent bloody diarrhea, abdominal cramps, and fever. Stool studies are negative for infectious diarrhea. Colonoscopy reveals friable mucosa in a continuous manner from the rectum to the sigmoid colon. No granulomas are found on biopsy. Which of the following statements is true regarding the most likely diagnosis in this patient?

A. Pseudopolyps and cobblestoning are common colonoscopic findings.

B. Surgery is curative for this diagnosis.

C. Rectal sparing is commonly seen on colonoscopy.

D. Perianal fistulas are commonly found on rectal examination.

E. Small bowel involvement is common.

ANSWER: B

COMMENTS: This patient's presentation is most consistent with ulcerative colitis. In ulcerative colitis, the anus is spared, whereas in Crohn's disease, the anal or perianal disease is the first manifestation in up to 25% of patients. The anal disease ultimately develops in 50%–70% of patients with Crohn's colitis. Rectal involvement can be seen with both of these inflammatory diseases of the colon but is more common in ulcerative colitis (95% vs. 50%). The small bowel is extensively involved in approximately 50% of patients with Crohn's disease, whereas "backwash ileitis," a nonspecific dilation of the terminal ileum, occurs in about 10% of patients with ulcerative colitis and has no prognostic or physiologic implications.

The clinical features of these two entities are similar: chronic diarrhea, cramping, abdominal pain, and fever. Bloody stools are quite common with ulcerative colitis and are much less frequent with Crohn's disease. Removing the entire colon and rectum is curative in ulcerative colitis, whereas there is no curative operation for Crohn's disease since it may involve any part of the intestinal tract. Total proctocolectomy for isolated colonic involvement of Crohn's disease has the lowest recurrence rate of any operation for that disease, yet recurrence in the small bowel is still seen in more than 25% of patients. Moreover, one-third of patients require additional surgery for such recurrence.

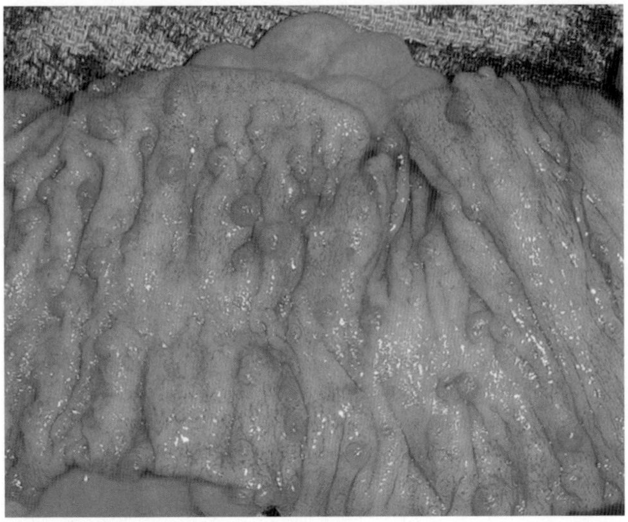

Fig. 23A.1 Postcholecystectomy colonoscopic findings. *(Source: BAOrkin.)*

Toxic megacolon can be an emergency, life-threatening complication of either ulcerative colitis or Crohn's disease, although it is more common in ulcerative colitis. Surgery for ulcerative colitis has two goals: eliminate the disease and provide reasonable GI function. Common surgical options today are total proctocolectomy with end ileostomy or proctocolectomy with sphincter preservation and IPAA. Yet, even when clinical and pathological findings confirm ulcerative colitis, recurrence or development of Crohn's disease in the small bowel and especially in the pouch or anus occurs in about 5% of patients after proctocolectomy.

Ref.: 3

14. A 27-year-old man after cholecystectomy has recently undergone colonoscopy for recurrent blood per rectum. His colonoscopic findings are seen in Fig. 23A.1. Which of the following is the most likely explanation for the endoscopic findings?

A. Diet high in fiber

B. Diet low in animal fat and protein

C. Ulcerative colitis

D. Familial polyposis

E. Previous cholecystectomy

ANSWER: D

COMMENTS: In the United States, CRC is second only to lung cancer as the leading cause of death from cancer when both genders are considered. Environmental factors, particularly dietary habits, may explain the wide variation in the geographic distribution of colon cancer. This patient has familial polyposis. Genetic factors play a definite role in carcinogenesis, and mutational abnormalities have been identified in patients with familial polyposis and hereditary nonpolyposis colorectal cancer (HNPCC) syndromes. Cancer develops in almost 100% of patients with familial polyposis, usually by the age of 40 years, if the colon is left untreated. In HNPCC syndrome, the lifetime risk for the development of colorectal cancer approaches 80%. Diets low in fiber and high in animal fats and protein are associated with an increased risk for colon cancer. The mechanisms may include alterations in intestinal transit time and an increase in the formation of carcinogenic compounds as a result of bacterial metabolism of dietary components. Gallstone disease appears to be more common in areas where colon cancer is prevalent. Some studies have suggested that cholecystectomy is associated with a higher incidence of subsequent colon cancer, particularly that involving the right colon. A proposed mechanism for this relationship is related to the carcinogenic potential of secondary bile acids, to which the intestinal mucosa is increasingly exposed after cholecystectomy as a result of increased enterohepatic cycling. However, evidence supporting this association is conflicting, and any association that may exist is minimal.

Risk factors for the development of cancer in patients with ulcerative colitis include disease of long duration (the incidence increases by 1%–2% per year after 10 years) and total colonic involvement. An increased risk for cancer has also been seen in patients with Crohn's disease of both the small and large intestines, particularly in bypassed segments. The aforementioned notwithstanding, familial polyposis, HNPCC syndrome, and ulcerative colitis account for only a small percentage of the total cases of CRC; most colon cancers occur sporadically without a genetic or inflammatory predisposition.

Ref.: 1, 5

15. Which disease is correctly matched to the appropriate treatment?

A. Actinomycosis: penicillin and drainage

B. Lymphogranuloma venereum: penicillin and steroids

C. Tuberculous enteritis: isoniazid and colectomy

D. *Yersinia* infections: metronidazole and appendectomy

E. *Entamoeba histolytica*: metronidazole and right hemicolectomy

ANSWER: A

COMMENTS: Actinomycosis is a suppurative, granulomatous disease caused by *Actinomyces israelii*, an anaerobic, gram-positive bacterium that produces chronic inflammatory induration and sinus formation. Although the causative organism is often part of the normal oral flora, infections may occur in the cervicofacial area, thorax, or abdomen. The cecal region is the most frequent site of abdominal infection. A pericecal mass, abscesses, and sinus tracts may be seen. Rectal strictures have been reported as well. Treatment consists of surgical drainage and penicillin or tetracycline.

Lymphogranuloma venereum is a sexually transmissible disease caused by *Chlamydia trachomatis*. It occurs most frequently in men who have sex with men. It starts as proctitis with symptoms of tenesmus, discharge, and bleeding. Perianal and rectovaginal fistulas and rectal strictures may develop. The diagnosis is made with the Frei intracutaneous test when it is available. Otherwise, the diagnosis may be confirmed by a complement fixation test. Tetracycline is curative, and steroids are occasionally recommended.

Tuberculous enteritis is seen most commonly in the ileocecal region and occasionally leads to stenosis of the distal ileum, cecum, and ascending colon; the endoscopic and radiographic features produced may be indistinguishable from those of Crohn's disease. Surgery is reserved for patients with obstruction. A triple-drug therapy consisting of isoniazid, *p*-aminosalicylic acid, and streptomycin usually heals the intestinal lesions.

Yersinia infections are caused by a gram-negative rod that is transmitted through food contaminated by feces or urine. It is often associated with eating undercooked pork. It produces a clinical picture frequently indistinguishable from that of acute appendicitis with fever and right lower quadrant abdominal pain. *Yersinia* may also cause acute diarrheal gastroenteritis. It primarily affects the ileocecal region. Diagnosis is made by stool cultures or a polymerase chain reaction (PCR) probe. Scanning often shows inflammation and thickening of the terminal ileum. *Yersinia enterocolitis* may be self-limited. When suspected or diagnosed, it generally responds promptly to treatment with tetracycline, streptomycin, ampicillin, or kanamycin.

Amebic colitis is caused by the protozoan *E. histolytica*. It primarily affects the colon and rectum and may secondarily infect other organs such as the liver. Up to 10% of the American population are asymptomatic carriers. Transmission of the disease is through food or water contaminated with feces containing *Entamoeba* cysts. The disease can assume an acute or a chronic form. Treatment is metronidazole, 750 mg three times a day for 10 days.

Ref.: 1, 3, 5

16. At the time of surgery for left colon obstruction, you find a thickened segment of colon with a narrow lumen and proximal bowel impacted with stool. There are no liver masses palpated. Which of the following is not an appropriate operative strategy for this patient?

A. Stricturoplasty

B. Left hemicolectomy and primary anastomosis following intraoperative colonic irrigation

C. Initial decompressive colostomy, bowel washout, and resection within 7 to 10 days

D. Primary left colectomy, colostomy, and either a Hartmann's pouch or mucous fistula

E. Primary subtotal colectomy and ileocolic anastomosis

ANSWER: A

COMMENTS: CRC is the leading cause of colon obstruction in industrialized countries, and left-sided tumors in particular are susceptible to obstruction because of the more formed consistency of the stool. This scenario may also be seen with other types of primary or metastatic cancer, diverticular disease, and radiation- or ischemia-induced stricturing. For left-sided tumors producing obstruction, the traditional surgical approach was an initial decompressive transverse colostomy, followed by resection within 7 to 10 days, and often a third-stage operation for the closure of colostomy. Initial treatment by decompressive colostomy alone is still appropriate for poor-risk or debilitated patients and for those with a marked colon dilation. The most common approach today is the Hartmann's procedure—primary resection of the obstructing pathologic entity, colostomy, and distal closure. The distal side may also be brought out as another ostomy (mucous fistula) for decompression, to provide a route for distal washout, and when the viability of the end may be in question. The colostomy (and mucous fistula, when present) is taken down, and an anastomosis is constructed at a second stage.

Some surgeons advocate primary subtotal or total colectomy with an ileocolic or IRA as a one-stage procedure for left-sided obstruction. However, this may result in diarrhea and incontinence, especially in older patients. Most right and transverse colon cancers with obstruction can be treated safely by primary resection and reanastomosis as a one-stage procedure as long as the ileum is minimally distended and healthy.

In the absence of peritonitis or perforation, an alternative approach consists of resection followed by intraoperative colonic irrigation and then primary anastomosis if the proximal bowel is not compromised. Colonic irrigation to wash out the lumen is performed by placing either a cecostomy or an appendicostomy tube, mobilizing the proximal colon margin site enough to hang it over the lateral abdominal wall, and creating a controlled conduit for the effluent to exit through a large-caliber anesthesia tubing or a long plastic sleeve fixed in the lumen. Several liters of saline solution are washed through the colon while manually breaking up stool and milking it down the lumen. This process is rather arduous and time consuming. Anastomoses created with this technique have a clinical leak rate of 5%–7% or more. It is not appropriate when the patient is not stable or when the bowel is at all compromised. This technique is not used very often.

Endoscopically placed colon stents are now commonly used to decompress patients with both malignant and benign strictures. Stents may be used for palliation of a patient with an extensive metastatic disease or as a bridge to surgery. They cannot be used in low rectal cancers since they protrude for several centimeters below the tumor and may cause considerable pain if ending in the very low in the rectum or anal canal.

Stricturoplasty has no role in managing colon obstruction. It is used primarily for patients with benign fibrotic small bowel strictures due to Crohn's disease.

Ref.: 1, 3, 5

17. Which statement is correct concerning intestinal polyposis syndromes?

A. Hamartomas are found in patients with both juvenile polyps and Peutz-Jeghers syndrome (PJS).

B. Familial polyposis syndrome often includes extraintestinal manifestations.

C. Turcot syndrome often includes small bowel polyps.

D. PJS, Gardner syndrome, and Turcot syndrome are inherited in an autosomal recessive pattern.

E. Familial polyposis and Turcot syndrome are benign conditions without malignant potential.

ANSWER: A

COMMENTS: PJS is a disorder characterized by intestinal hamartomatous polyps along with skin and mucosa pigmentation or "cafe-au-lait" spots. It is due to a mutation in the *STK11* gene on chromosome 19 and is inherited as an autosomal dominant trait. Hamartomas are lesions in which normal tissue is found in an abnormal structural configuration. Hamartomatous polyps are found primarily in the jejunum and ileum, with involvement of the colon and rectum in one-third and the stomach in one-fourth of patients. The polyps may cause obstruction, intussusception, or bleeding. The pigmented spots are found on the oral mucosa, lips, palms of the hands, and soles of the feet. There is an increased incidence of many cancers in PJS, including those in the pancreas, liver, lungs, breast, ovaries, uterus, and testicles. However, the polyps themselves do not become cancerous very often. Gastric and colon polyps are usually treated by polypectomy. Small bowel polyps may be seen on capsule endoscopy. Symptomatic small bowel polyps may be localized with intraoperative total endoscopy, marking of each site, and serial enterotomy with surgical polypectomy when symptomatic.

Sporadic **juvenile polyps** in children are solitary 70% of the time, and in 60% of cases they are located within 10 cm of the anal verge. They are thought to be a developmental abnormality and may bleed or prolapse. The syndrome of **juvenile polyposis** is characterized by the presence of multiple hamartomatous polyps in the stomach, small bowel, or colon, with large "mucous lakes" on pathology. Mutations in the *BMPR1A* and *SMAD4* are usually found. It has an autosomal dominant inheritance pattern. Signs and symptoms of anemia, anergy, hypoproteinemia, and failure to thrive may be seen. Solitary juvenile polyps seem to have little propensity for malignancy; however, up to 40% of patients with juvenile polyposis will develop a CRC.

Cronkhite-Canada syndrome (CCS) is a sporadically occurring polyposis syndrome not thought to be inherited. It is diagnosed mostly in patients of Japanese descent, but it can occur in any ethnic group. The polyps are hamartomas, often have an inflammatory component, and may be anywhere along the GI tract. In addition, there are pigmented skin areas, alopecia, and atrophy of the fingernails and toenails. The syndrome may be due to an autoimmune disorder since there are elevated levels of immunoglobulin (Ig)G4, and it often responds to treatment with steroids and immunosuppressives. There seems to be an increased risk of colorectal neoplasia, but because of its rarity, the level of risk is not clear. Nevertheless, regular screening is recommended.

Familial adenomatous polyposis (FAP) is the best characterized inherited CRC syndrome and is due to an autosomal dominant mutation in the adenomatous polyposis coli (*APC*) gene. Patients develop hundreds to thousands of polyps by their early teens. Although most are in the colon, many patients also develop duodenal and jejunal polyps, which can be very difficult to manage. Periampullary cancer is a significant risk. Most patients with FAP do not have extraintestinal manifestations; however, Turcot and Gardner syndromes are variants that do. Patients with Turcot syndrome develop central nervous system tumors, and patients with Gardner syndrome develop osteomas, exostoses, and desmoid tumors, which may be quite debilitating.

Ref.: 1, 3, 5

18. With regard to ischemic colitis, which of the following statements is true?

A. The most common symptoms are lower abdominal pain and bright red rectal bleeding.

B. Occlusion of the major mesenteric vessels is the cause of ischemia in most cases.

C. The splenic flexure and hepatic flexure are the most vulnerable areas of the colon.

D. Nonoperative management is not justified because of the significant rates of perforation and peritonitis.

E. Griffith's point at the rectosigmoid junction is the most vulnerable area.

ANSWER: A

COMMENTS: Ischemic colitis should be considered in the differential diagnosis of any elderly patient with lower abdominal pain. It can also be found in individuals of any age in association with hypercoagulable states, periarteritis nodosa, systemic lupus erythematosus, rheumatoid arthritis, polycythemia vera, and scleroderma. Ischemic colitis may be manifested as three distinct clinical syndromes, depending on (1) the extent and duration of vascular occlusion, (2) the adequacy of the collateral circulation, and (3) the extent of septic complications.

Approximately 80% of the blood flow to the wall of the colon reaches the mucosa and submucosa, and the remaining 20% supplies the muscularis. Despite the extensive collateral vessels to the colon, it receives only about 50% of the blood flow that the small intestine does. The colon is therefore more sensitive to ischemic injury during acute reductions in blood flow. In contrast to other areas of the body, an increase in functional motor activity of the colon does not result in a parallel increase in absolute colonic blood flow.

Ischemic colitis appears to be a disease of the small arterioles. Although this disease can occur in any segment of the large bowel, it is seen most commonly in the splenic flexure or distal sigmoid colon. A plausible explanation is that these areas may receive suboptimal blood flow since they are positioned between two vascular systems ("watershed areas") that rely on an intact but meandering artery for their blood supply. Sudeck's point is the area between the blood supply from the last sigmoid artery and the superior rectal artery. However, the clinical significance of Sudeck's point is questionable because of retrograde flow from the middle and inferior rectal arteries. Griffith's point is the vulnerable area at the splenic flexure that is positioned between areas of the colon perfused by the left branch of the middle colic artery and the ascending branch of the left colic artery. The diagnosis is often made by an endoscopic examination that reveals cyanotic, edematous mucosa that may be covered with exudative membranes. Barium enema may show the typical "thumbprinting" of the edematous bowel wall. Injection angiography or CT angiography may be helpful in the questionable patient. However, if gangrenous colitis is suspected on the basis of ominous physical findings, such as involuntary guarding and rebound tenderness and shock, these studies are contraindicated and prompt laparotomy is mandatory.

Transient ischemic colitis without full-thickness necrosis usually responds to nonoperative management. Parts of the mucosa may slough, but the muscularis remains intact. Late consequences include ischemic strictures that may be resected electively with primary anastomosis after the initial ischemic episode has subsided. If surgery is needed for peritonitis and gangrenous colitis, resection with end colostomy is the preferred operation (Hartmann's procedure or double-barreled colostomy).

Ref.: 1, 3, 5

19. Which of the following colonoscopic screening recommendations is correct?

A. A patient whose father had CRC at age 64—start screening at age 40, repeat every 10 years

B. A patient whose father had colorectal polyps at age 58—start screening at age 50, repeat every 10 years

C. A patient whose mother had colorectal polyps at age 58—start screening at age 40, repeat every 5 years

D. A patient with HNPCC—start screening at age 30, repeat every 5 years

E. A patient with ulcerative colitis—annual screening after initial diagnosis

ANSWER: A

COMMENTS: Although screening recommendations initially involve utilizing stool guaiac and flexible sigmoidoscopy, most patients are still screened by colonoscopy. Determining the initiation and timing of screening colonoscopies requires physicians to take a thorough personal and family history of colorectal and other diseases. Briefly, the timing of screening initiation varies by the patient's history of IBD or genetic predisposition to the disease and by the family history of disease. The interval is determined by the age of onset of disease in the patient's family history as a surrogate for the aggressiveness of disease. All recommendations are a guideline and may be adjusted to more frequent intervals if a colonoscopy reveals positive findings.

It is important to note that these recommendations exist only for screening colonoscopy; should a patient present with changes in bowel habits, rectal bleeding, or other concerning symptoms, the colonoscopy is considered diagnostic and is obtained immediately without regard to the screening age.

The screening recommendations for colonoscopy are as follows:

- Patients with no family history of CRC or polyps—begin at age 50 and repeat at 10-year intervals
- Patients with a first-degree relative with CRC or polyps at age 60 or older (or two first- or second-degree relatives of any age)—begin at age 40, or 10 years before the earliest diagnosed age, and repeat at 10-year intervals
- Patients with a first-degree relative with CRC or polyps at age 60 or *younger* (or two first-degree relatives of any age)—begin at age 40, or 10 years before the earliest diagnosed age, and repeat at 5-year intervals
- Patients with known HNPCC—begin at age 20 to 25 years and repeat at 1- to 2-year intervals
- Patients with a known family history of FAP—begin flexible sigmoidoscopy at puberty and perform annually until 25 or until the colon and rectum are removed. If negative at 25, perform colonoscopy every 10 years
- Patients with known ulcerative colitis—begin at 8 to 10 years after the onset of the disease and repeat annually
- Patients with known Crohn's colitis—similar to ulcerative colitis

Ref.: 9

20. A 54-year-old man is referred by his physician for the evaluation of rectal bleeding. He admits to a recent history of constipation and rectal fullness. Colonoscopy showed a 3-cm mass starting 2 cm above the dentate line. Biopsies are consistent with a neuroendocrine cancer that contains a large amount of amine precursor (5-hydroxytryptophan). Which statement is correct regarding this tumor?

A. This tumor occurs at equal frequency in the colon and rectum.

B. The incidence of invasive malignancy and metastases correlates with the location of the tumor.

C. This tumor in the rectum frequently causes flushing, diarrhea, and heat intolerance.

D. These lesions are treated by enucleation.

E. Rectal lesions larger than 2 cm are best treated by radical resection.

ANSWER: E

COMMENTS: This patient has a carcinoid tumor of the rectum. This is a neuroendocrine tumor. This group of tumors includes a wide and diverse set of neoplasms that range from small, completely benign lesions to large, poorly differentiated cancers with an extremely dismal prognosis. These neoplasms have the potential of storing large amounts of an amine precursor (5-hydroxytryptophan), and through the amine precursor uptake and decarboxylation (APUD) system, these lesions may produce several biologically active amines including serotonin.

Carcinoids may be found anywhere along the GI tract and in the pulmonary tree and may occasionally be found elsewhere. They are generally divided into foregut, midgut, and hindgut. The most common locations are the appendix and ileum (midgut), rectum and colon (hindgut), and stomach (foregut). Rectal carcinoids are fairly common and account for 12%–15% of lesions, while colon carcinoids are relatively rare and account for only 2.5% of all GI lesions. The incidence of invasive malignancy and metastases to regional lymph nodes correlates well with the size of the carcinoid for both colonic and rectal lesions. Carcinoids larger than 2 cm are malignant 90%–95% of the time, while lesions smaller than 2 cm are malignant only 5% of the time.

GI carcinoids typically arise in the submucosa. Rectal lesions smaller than 2 cm rarely invade the muscularis or spread to the lymph nodes and very rarely secrete metabolically active substances. Therefore they are not associated with carcinoid syndrome and symptoms of flushing, diarrhea, and heat intolerance. They may be locally excised transanally. Enucleation is not appropriate. Recurrence is rare if margins are clear. Rectal lesions larger than 2 cm or those that have penetrated into the rectal muscularis are usually aggressive neuroendocrine cancers. Metastatic evaluation is necessary. If widespread metastases are not present, these malignancies are best treated by APR and colostomy or LAR with anastomosis if higher in the rectum. These tumors are not particularly radiosensitive, and no specific chemotherapy regimens have been shown to be particularly effective. However, large series are lacking because of the relative rarity of these lesions, and radiation and chemotherapy are used selectively for palliation.

Malignant colon carcinoids are treated by formal oncologic resection with wide lymphatic clearance. Up to two-thirds of patients with neuroendocrine cancers of the colon are found to have either local spread or systemic metastases at the time of diagnosis. If disseminated disease is present, resection of the primary lesion is still recommended to alleviate symptoms and avoid bleeding and obstruction. Carcinoids of the colon infrequently produce carcinoid syndrome, although occasional lesions that have metastasized to the liver will do so.

Ref.: 9

21. Which of the following findings warrants APR?

A. A fixed circumferential adenocarcinoma just above the dentate line

B. An ulcerating adenocarcinoma whose lower edge is 7 cm from the dentate line, with infiltration and expansion of the second hypoechoic layer seen on ultrasound imaging

C. A 2-cm mobile adenocarcinoma arising in a villous adenoma 3 cm from the dentate line, with an intact second hypoechoic band seen on ultrasound imaging

D. A circumferential adenocarcinoma 12 cm from the anal verge

E. A 1.5-cm submucosal carcinoid tumor 5 cm from the dentate line

ANSWER: A

COMMENTS: The most important determinant of the type of operation to perform for a rectal cancer is the location of the lesion within the rectum. Tumors located 0 to 5 cm from the anal verge, especially those that involve the sphincter muscle and are producing pain, are best treated by APR. Approximately 10%–15% of tumors within this region can be considered for local excision if they are minimally invasive (Tis or T1—no deeper than the submucosa), are not poorly differentiated, and do not have a lymphovascular or perineural invasion. A coloanal anastomosis can be performed when the distal margin is 2 cm after mobilization, although functional results are often poor. Lesions in the upper part of the rectum (10 to 15 cm) are amenable to anterior resection, with the restoration of intestinal continuity by colorectal anastomosis.

Lesions located in the mid-rectum (5 to 10 cm) are treated by a variety of operations, depending on the skill of the surgeon and the patient's body habitus. Most cancers in this region can be treated by LAR with colorectal anastomosis or coloanal anastomosis. A temporary loop ileostomy is often used to protect the low colorectal anastomosis, especially in radiated patients because of the higher risk of anastomotic leak. Impaired fecal continence has been noted in 10%–35% of patients after coloanal anastomosis. Part of the degradation in the function is due to the loss of the rectum's capacity and storage function. Techniques such as the construction of a colonic J pouch or performance of a coloplasty to widen and increase the compliance of the distal colon may improve function but have not been adopted widely. The decision to perform a sphincter-saving operation must be individualized, and safety is a primary concern. If the patient is obese or debilitated; if the pelvis is long, narrow, and angulated; if a satisfactory anastomosis cannot be performed; or if sphincter function is poor, an APR may be the best choice.

Low rectal carcinoids larger than 2 cm should be treated with radical resection (APR or LAR) and lymphadenectomy. Smaller lesions may be treated with local excision.

Ref.: 9

22. Which of the following is the appropriate operation for a sigmoid cancer that has not metastasized?

A. Segmental resection of the sigmoid with 5-cm margins and high ligation of the sigmoid branch of the IMA

B. Resection of the entire sigmoid from the distal descending colon to the rectosigmoid junction, sparing the main left colic artery

C. Resection of the sigmoid and the descending colon, with high ligation of the IMA at its origin

D. Resection of the entire colon proximal to the lesion with IRA

E. Resection of the entire sigmoid with wide iliac lymph node dissection and prophylactic oophorectomy

ANSWER: B

COMMENTS: The amount of colon resected when operating with the intent to cure colon cancer is based more on the need for removal of the draining mesenteric lymph nodes that parallel the vascular supply to that area of the colon. The IMA arises from the aorta 3 to 4 cm above the aortic bifurcation. The left colic artery splits off about 3 cm below the origin of the IMA and ascends in the mesentery to meet the marginal artery of Drummond that communicates with the left branch of the middle colic artery and the superior mesenteric artery distribution. Below the left colic artery, the IMA gives off several sigmoidal branches and finally terminates as the left and right superior rectal arteries. Sigmoid cancers should be resected with at least a 5-cm margin and usually much more since this is not the determining factor. The need for wide mesenteric clearance is important since up to one-third of patients with involved lymph nodes are cured by proper resection alone. Adequate lymph node clearance also provides a large number of nodes for sampling to determine the stage. At least 12 lymph nodes must be evaluated, but a comprehensive pathologic examination will often identify 30 nodes or more. The more nodes evaluated, the more accurate the staging. High ligation of the IMA at its takeoff from the aorta used to be advocated to get the highest lymph nodes; however, subsequent studies have shown that the division of the IMA just below the left colic artery results in equivalent outcomes and decreases the risk of left colon ischemia.

For a sigmoid cancer without the evidence of distal spread, the resection should include the entire sigmoid colon to just above the descending colon–sigmoid junction proximally and to the true rectum where the taeniae coli spread out and become a full longitudinal coat of the rectum distally, plus at least 5 cm on either side of the tumor. If the tumor is at or adjacent to this distal level, a portion of the upper rectum should be removed as well (LAR). It is important to note that the point where the sigmoid becomes the rectum is defined by a complete longitudinal muscle layer and not by any extrinsic landmark such as the sacral promontory or the "peritoneal reflection," which are meaningless in this context.

Resection of the entire intraabdominal colon may be considered for patients with an obstructing cancer because resection of a dilated stool-laden colon may safely permit an ileorectostomy rather than a colostomy. Other indications for a total colectomy include synchronous cancers in separate segments of the colon cancer or in patients with known familial polyposis or Lynch syndrome because of the high risk of metachronous cancers.

Oophorectomy may be considered in postmenopausal women because approximately 6% of these patients have simultaneous drop metastases to the ovaries, and it removes the risk of ovarian cancer. Routine prophylactic oophorectomy does not improve survival in general. Isolated recurrence in an ovary is fairly uncommon, and less than 2% of women with CRC subsequently undergo ovarian resection. Additionally, spread to the ovaries is a sign of disseminated disease, and oophorectomy is not associated with increased survival.

Ref.: 3, 5, 9

23. Which of the following is true about HNPCC (Lynch syndrome)?

A. It is inherited as an autosomal recessive trait.

B. Most cancers in patients with HNPCC involve the right colon.

C. The average age at diagnosis is 62 years.

D. A segmental colectomy is frequently curative for these patients.

E. There is a high frequency of associated breast, brain, and lung cancers.

ANSWER: B

COMMENTS: HNPCC syndrome is categorized into two forms depending on whether it is isolated (Lynch syndrome I—colon cancer alone) or associated with extracolonic tumors (Lynch syndrome II—endometrial, ovarian, breast, urothelial, biliary, and gastric). HNPCC accounts for approximately 5% of all CRCs and is caused by mutations in one of the several mismatch repair genes, allowing the propagation of errors in DNA replication. These genes include *MSH2*, 60%; *MLH1*, 30%; *MSH6*, 7%–10%; and *PMS2*, <1%. Inheritance is autosomal dominant. Colon cancers are more common on the right colon (72%), are frequently synchronous (more than one at a time—18%), and are frequently metachronous after segmental colectomy (have a second colon cancer develop later—40% in 10 years). Therefore patients undergoing only segmental colectomy have a high rate of developing another colon cancer.

In HNPCC, the risk of developing colon cancer is over 80%, endometrial cancer 60%, stomach cancer 15%, ovarian cancer 10%, hepatobiliary cancer 5%, urinary tract cancer 5%, small bowel cancer 3%, and brain cancer 2%.

Although patients with HNPCC have a high rate of developing colon cancer, the overall survival is actually better in them than in patients with sporadic cancers.

Identifying patients and families with HNPCC requires vigilance but is quite important. The **Amsterdam Criteria**, developed in 1990, is the original method and uses the 3-2-1 rule:

- 3 successive generations affected by CRC,
- 2 first-degree relatives affected by CRC, and
- 1 affected person younger than 50 years.

This was fairly reliable in that people satisfying the criteria were highly likely to have HNPCC. However, there are many patients with HNPCC who do not quite satisfy these criteria, for example, small families with few siblings or cousins or spontaneous mutations. In addition, the presence of extraintestinal cancers was not included. Therefore, in 1998, the revised **Amsterdam II Clinical Criteria** were released:

- 3 or more relatives with an associated cancer (colorectal, endometrial, small intestine, ureter, or renal pelvis),
- 2 or more successive generations affected,
- 1 or more relatives diagnosed before the age of 50 years,
- 1 should be a first-degree relative of the other two,
- FAP should be excluded, and
- Tumors should be verified by pathologic examination.

The Amsterdam Criteria were developed before the genes responsible for HNPCC were known and before genetic testing was available. They are exclusionary with a high degree of specificity but low sensitivity (62%). Now, testing by immunohistochemical staining of tumor specimens and direct genomic characterization is possible and reasonably inexpensive. A new approach was needed. The National Cancer Institute developed the **Bethesda Guidelines** to identify patients who are candidates for genetic testing. These guidelines are much more inclusive and cast a wide net. Alone they are not terribly specific, but with appropriate testing, they are estimated to be 94% sensitive.

The current **Revised Bethesda Guidelines** from 2004 state that anyone who satisfies *any one* of the following criteria is a candidate for further testing:

- CRC diagnosed in a patient who is less than 50 years old
- Presence of synchronous or metachronous CRC or other Lynch syndrome–associated tumors, regardless of age
- CRC with high microsatellite instability histology diagnosed in a patient less than 60 years old
- CRC diagnosed in one or more first-degree relatives with a Lynch syndrome–associated tumor, with one of the cancers being diagnosed at less than 50 years of age
- CRC diagnosed in two or more first-degree or second-degree relatives with Lynch syndrome–associated tumors, regardless of age

Family members at risk should undergo biannual colonoscopy beginning at age 25 or 10 years younger than the age of the youngest affected family member. Women should have an annual pelvic examination and pelvic ultrasound to examine the ovaries and the thickness of the endometrial stripe. Serum markers for ovarian cancer should be checked, and mammograms should be obtained earlier than usually advised. Family members of an afflicted individual should be counseled and offered genetic screening.

Total colectomy with IRA should be recommended for HNPCC patients with a new colon cancer because of the high risk for metachronous tumors. If a woman has completed childbearing, hysterectomy and bilateral salpingo-oophorectomy should also be recommended at the time of colectomy.

Ref.: 9, 17

24. A 54-year-old patient presents with rectal bleeding and tenesmus. She has a history of cervical cancer and underwent a hysterectomy and radiation therapy 5 months ago. She has no personal or family history of cancer, abdominal problems, or rectal bleeding and has not traveled recently. A surveillance CT 1 month ago was negative. Which of the following is the most likely diagnosis?

A. Ulcerative colitis

B. Ischemic colitis

C. Radiation proctitis

D. Recurrent cervical cancer

E. Rectal cancer

ANSWER: C

COMMENTS: Radiation therapy is used in the treatment of cervical, uterine, anal, rectal, and prostate cancer. It is a very effective treatment but may result in severe side effects due to dose-dependent cell death in normal surrounding structures.

Injury from radiation therapy occurs via damage to DNA and production of oxygen free radicals. The maximum safe therapy is considered to be 6000 to 8000 cGy, depending on the tissue, but side effects can occur at much lower doses. The effects of acute radiation toxicity tend to manifest in the first 6 months as villous atrophy and degeneration of the mucosal lining. At 6 to 12 months following radiation, patients develop a progressive microvascular fibrosis (obliterative arteritis), causing thrombosis and ischemia.

Acute radiation proctitis typically manifests as diarrhea, mucous discharge, tenesmus, and bleeding. Chronic changes frequently present as nonhealing ulcerations and telangiectasia fistulas, thickening, and stricture. Symptoms differ between those induced with external beam radiation therapy and those induced with brachytherapy.

Most patients can be adequately treated with symptomatic control, antidiarrheals (after infectious causes are ruled out), and hydration. Sulfasalazine and sucralfate enemas can provide relief in some patients. Other modalities to control bleeding may include argon beam plasma (APC) coagulation, hydrocortisone enemas, and topical application of formaldehyde (4%–10%) under direct vision.

Although ulcerative colitis and new rectal primaries can present with tenesmus and bleeding, they are unlikely causes of new symptoms in this patient with prior radiation. Ischemic colitis must be ruled out but again is inconsistent with the clinical history. Recurrent cervical cancer is unlikely to cause these symptoms with normal imaging.

Ref.: 10

25. A 28-year-old patient with severe ulcerative colitis undergoes a total proctocolectomy with IPAA. Four days after the operation, she develops fever, anal pain, and tenesmus. Which of the following is the most likely diagnosis?

A. Small bowel obstruction

B. Pelvic sepsis

C. Ileoanal anastomotic stricture

D. Pouch–vaginal fistula

E. Pouchitis

ANSWER: B

COMMENTS: Creation of an IPAA is associated with low mortality but considerable morbidity. Small bowel obstruction can occur in up to 20% of patients; this high figure is expected given the extent of underlying inflammation as well as the colectomy and extensive mobilization of the small bowel.

Pelvic sepsis occurs in up to 5% of patients. It may present early or late, usually manifesting as an abscess or perineal fistula. The main symptoms are anal pain, tenesmus, fevers, and purulent discharge from the anus. The diagnosis is confirmed with CT imaging, which may show a discrete abscess or only soft tissue thickening. Antibiotics should be started immediately, and any fluid collections should be drained percutaneously or unroofed transanally if inaccessible. A return to the operating room for laparotomy is rarely necessary.

In the literature anastomotic stricture occurrence has been reported in a variable percentage of patients and is best avoided by a tension-free anastomosis and rapid control of any developing pelvic sepsis. The symptoms are generally more gradual, and the patient may have anal pain but generally no infectious symptoms. Prior to the closure of the temporary loop ileostomy, mild stenosis is expected, but it may be easily dilated at the closure operation. A pouch–vaginal fistula generally presents with isolated vaginal discharge or urinary tract infections.

Pouchitis is the most common long-term complication of IPAA. The symptoms are similar to pelvic sepsis and may include fevers, abdominal cramping, and diarrhea; however, this will occur much later in the clinical course. Pouchitis occurs in up to 25% of patients with an IPAA. It is usually treated with oral antibiotics and resolves quickly. Some patients have many recurrences or chronic inflammations. Crohn's disease in the pouch occurs about 4% of the time and should be ruled out as a cause of abscesses, fistulas, and pouchitis.

Ref.: 10

26. Which of the following neoplastic polyps is most likely to require surgical excision after a complete colonoscopic resection?

A. A 3-cm pedunculated carcinoma–containing adenomatous polyp with low-grade differentiation, no lymphovascular invasion, and no mucosal penetration that is resected piecemeal in five sessions

B. A 2-cm pedunculated carcinoma–containing adenomatous polyp with low-grade differentiation, positive lymphovascular invasion, and no mucosal penetration resected completely in one session

C. A 3-cm pedunculated hyperplastic polyp with no evidence of neoplasia

D. A 3-cm adenomatous noncancerous polyp with a 3-mm resection margin

E. A 1-cm hyperplastic polyp with a 1-mm resection margin

ANSWER: B

COMMENTS: Endoscopic polypectomy is an effective treatment that spares selected patients the morbidity of surgical resection in the treatment of advanced polyps. Most pedunculated polyps can be resected endoscopically. Large sessile polyps are more difficult to remove. Most can be safely removed in several pieces with no impact on recurrence, as long as the margins are clear.

All polyps undergo a complete pathologic examination after excision to determine not only whether the polyp is completely resected but also if high-risk factors are present that may indicate a higher likelihood of residual disease, lymphatic spread, or risk of recurrence.

Adenomas harbor a higher risk of malignancy than nonadenomatous polyps. Hyperplastic polyps harbor no risk, and serrated polyps are in between. Factors that predict focal carcinoma in an adenomatous polyp include increased size, high-grade dysplasia, and villous versus tubular structure.

Factors that are associated with an increased risk of spread when there is a focus of cancer are high tumor grade (poorly differentiated), penetration into the submucosa or deeper (T1 or greater vs. in situ location in the mucosa), lymphovascular invasion, and resection margin of less than 2 mm. Many of these patients will undergo surgical resection. In the absence of these factors, the metastatic spread would be exceedingly rare. Piecemeal removal of large polyps presents a problem since it may be impossible to determine if the resection margins are clear. Polyps of the rectum are considered more aggressive and require a more complete excision. A full-thickness transanal excision, with clear margins using either standard operating anal retractor for low lesions or TEM is recommended.

Ref.: 10

27. Which of the following is the best initial management for acute colonic pseudo-obstruction (Ogilvie's syndrome)?

A. Colonoscopy
B. Rectal tube decompression
C. Nasogastric tube decompression and correction of electrolytes
D. Neostigmine
E. Lower GI and gastrografin enema

ANSWER: C

COMMENTS: Ogilvie's syndrome was first described by Sir William Heneage Ogilvie in 1948. This is a syndrome of obstipation, acute distention, and dysmotility or ileus of the colon without evidence of a mechanical obstruction. It is associated with the use of opiates and neuroleptic medications, diabetes, myxedema, scleroderma, uremia, hyperparathyroidism, lupus, Parkinson's disease, retroperitoneal hematomas, and severe metabolic illnesses. It is commonly encountered in immobile hospitalized patients after orthopedic or neurosurgical procedures. Its pathophysiology is not clear but may involve an imbalance in autonomic neural function of the colon distal to the splenic flexure that results in a contraction of the distal part of the colon and functional obstruction. Frequently, the right and transverse sections of the colon are dilated compared with the distal colon. The risk of ischemia rises when the cecal diameter reaches 12 cm or more. If the patient is hemodynamically stable, without peritonitis, and without a known mechanical obstruction, initial management includes hydration, mobilization, correction of any electrolyte abnormalities, avoidance of offending drugs such as opiates, placement of a nasogastric tube if the stomach or small bowel is distended, tap water enemas, and serial abdominal examinations. Mechanical obstruction should be ruled out with a contrast enema or colonoscopy. Colonoscopy may be both diagnostic and therapeutic; it will rule out a mechanical problem such as carcinoma or volvulus, and decompression of the colon or reduction of a volvulus may be performed. Seventy percent of patients will improve with conservative treatment in the first 48 h. Neostigmine or colonoscopy should be considered if conservative treatment fails. Neostigmine is a cholinesterase inhibitor that produces colonic contraction; however, it can also cause bradycardia. All patients receiving neostigmine must be placed on a cardiac monitor, and atropine must be readily available to treat significant bradycardia. Placement of a rectal tube is rarely effective because the dilation is primarily in the proximal colon. Colonoscopy to the transverse colon is adequate for suction decompression. Colonoscopy may need to be repeated. Patients who fail nonoperative measures should be considered for surgical treatment such as cecostomy or resection if the cecum or right colon is compromised, ischemic, or perforated.

Ref.: 1, 10

28. Which of the following screening tests provides the greatest effectiveness (reduction in mortality) in detecting CRC?

A. Annual fecal occult blood test (FOBT)
B. Flexible sigmoidoscopy every 5 years
C. Colonoscopy every 10 years
D. Barium enema every 5 years
E. CT colonography

ANSWER: C

COMMENTS: Screening asymptomatic, average-risk patients for CRC with adenomatous polyp removal has been clearly shown to reduce the incidence of CRC and to increase the number of early cancers detected versus advanced cancers. However, screening must be accomplished in a cost-effective manner that encourages patient compliance. Screening tests mainly take the form of FOBT, flexible sigmoidoscopy, and colonoscopy.

The test that most easily accomplishes the goals of compliance and cost-efficacy is an annual examination of the stool for occult blood (FOBT). This test uses the peroxidase-like activity of hemoglobin. Three separate stool samples are collected on a guaiac paper, and hydrogen peroxide is added; if hemoglobin is present to catalyze the reaction, the colorless guaiac is oxidized to a blue-colored quinone. Normal blood loss in the stool is 2 mg of hemoglobin/g of stool; FOBT requires fecal blood loss of 10 mg of hemoglobin/g of stool to obtain a positive result. However, the sensitivity of FOBT is as low as 50%–85% in patients with known cancers. Mass screening programs with FOBT will yield positive results in 1%–8% of patients. The positive predictive value of a positive test result is 10% for cancer and 30% for adenoma. These programs diagnose a higher percentage of early localized cancers than may be expected otherwise, indicating the usefulness of such an approach. The risk reduction in CRC mortality ranges widely depending on the study and the type of FOBT used. Estimates range from 18% to 55%.

Combining annual FOBT with periodic flexible sigmoidoscopy every 5 years provides a greater risk reduction. Flexible sigmoidoscopy provides an effectiveness of approximately 34%–66%; effectiveness is increased in combination with annual FOBT. The benefits of this regimen above colonoscopy lie in a shorter, less costly procedure that does not require oral bowel preparation. Flexible sigmoidoscopy is estimated to detect 70% of lesions present.

When combined with FOBT, it provides reasonable sensitivity for the screening of a large population.

Double-contrast barium enema provides an alternate means of screening with an effectiveness of 33%–47%. It may provide improved visualization in colons with multiple strictures than flexible sigmoidoscopy or colonoscopy. It is generally used in conjunction with flexible sigmoidoscopy.

CT colonography (formerly called "virtual colonoscopy") was introduced in 1994. Like colonoscopy, it requires a bowel preparation. Air is insufflated into the colon followed by thin-cut images in a CT scanner in the prone and supine state. Three-dimensional reconstruction of the entire colon and the use of a "fly-through" view result in kinetic images that may allow better visualization behind the haustral folds than colonoscopy. However, only lesions greater than 1 cm are reliably seen, and residual stool may not be well differentiated from significant findings. Although CT colonography is effective as a screening tool versus no screening, it is not as effective as colonoscopy, it costs substantially more to achieve reasonable effectiveness, and it is not therapeutic since polypectomy and biopsies cannot be performed. Therefore it is primarily used in patients who cannot tolerate a colonoscopy or in patients with an incomplete colonoscopy because of difficult passage or obstruction.

Colonoscopy remains the screening test of choice since it is highly sensitive and specific as well as diagnostic and therapeutic. Colonoscopic screening has been shown to be the most effective method of risk reduction. Studies have shown 60%–90% reduction in the incidence of CRC in patients who are screened appropriately. Although complication rates are higher than other methods, the rate of perforation and significant bleeding is only 4 of 10,000 or 0.04%.

Current screening practices for asymptomatic patients endorsed by the American Cancer Society consist of the following:

- High-sensitivity FOBT with three consecutive stool samples yearly
- Flexible sigmoidoscopy every 5 years with FOBT every 3 years
- Colonoscopy every 10 years

Colonoscopy is also used as a diagnostic test when a person has symptoms, and as a follow-up test when the results of another screening test are unclear or abnormal.

Ref.: 10

29. Which of the following is true regarding rectal prolapse?

A. The extruded mucosa has radially orientated folds.

B. Rectal prolapse occurs mostly in men, with a male-to-female ratio of 6:1.

C. The Altemeier procedure involves a full-thickness resection of the prolapsed rectum through a perineal approach.

D. Fecal incontinence is not a predominant symptom in rectal prolapse.

E. Rectal prolapse is commonly attributed to intussusception of the rectum due to a neoplastic lead point.

ANSWER: C

COMMENTS: Rectal prolapse is a pelvic floor disorder that is most commonly found in women, with a 6:1 female-to-male ratio. This disorder has a bimodal distribution of incidence, with peak onsets within the first 3 years and after the seventh decade of life. There are varying degrees of prolapse—internal intussusception or occult rectal prolapse (or prolapse of the rectal wall without protrusion through the anus), procidentia (or complete protrusion of all layers of the rectum), and mucosal prolapse. Rectal prolapse is differentiated from incarcerated internal hemorrhoids by a close examination of the mucosal folds. Incarcerated internal hemorrhoids have a radially invaginated tissue, which distinguishes the hemorrhoidal cushion beds. Rectal prolapse has concentric (target) folds.

The pathophysiology of rectal prolapse is not clear, but several typical abnormalities have been identified. The normal rectal mesenteric attachments to the sacrum are lost, and the rectum sags down into the deep pelvis. Defecography studies have demonstrated that weakness of the pelvic floor allows full-thickness intussusception of the rectum through the anal canal and levator hiatus. Pudendal nerve injury due to stretching of the nerve in the ischiorectal fossa between its fixed exit from Alcock's canal and insertion into the sphincter muscles contributes to pelvic floor weakness. Direct trauma, obstetric injury, neuropathic diseases, such as diabetes, and neoplasms involving the sacral nerve root can all lead to pudendal nerve damage. Although neoplasm is a common cause of adult small bowel intussusception, it is not usually the cause of intussusception in rectal prolapse. The most common symptom is the sensation of an anal "mass" that reduces with manual pressure. Protrusion usually occurs with increased abdominal pressure such as during coughing or defecation. Fecal incontinence is a predominant symptom that is seen in 50%–75% of patients with rectal prolapse. Other symptoms include tenesmus and rectal pressure. Internal intussusception often presents with rectal pressure and obstructed defecation. It is best demonstrated by cine defecography.

Operative repairs for rectal prolapse can be done through either an abdominal or a perineal approach. The abdominal approach usually involves the resection of redundant sigmoid colon and rectopexy. This approach is generally reserved for healthier patients who can tolerate abdominal surgery. Either an open or minimally invasive approach can be used. The recurrence rate is low. The Altemeier procedure is a perineal approach that includes proctosigmoidectomy with a full-thickness resection of the redundant rectum and a variable amount of sigmoid while prolapsed. A levatorplasty is also often performed with this procedure to tighten the anal hiatus. Other repairs include the Delorme procedure (mucosal resection with plication of the rectal wall), rectopexy alone, rectopexy with mesh, and a Thiersch loop. Procedure selection is highly dependent on the extent of prolapse and the physiologic condition of the patient.

Ref.: 1, 11

30. Which of the following is the most common cause of massive colonic bleeding?

A. CRC

B. Ulcerative colitis

C. Diverticulosis

D. Ischemic colitis

E. Infectious colitis

ANSWER: C

COMMENTS: The causes of lower GI bleeding are many; it is accounted for predominantly by diverticular disease or angiodysplasia (60%), IBD (13%), anorectal disease such as hemorrhoids and fissures (11%), and neoplasia (9%). Few of these lead to massive bleeding. Frequently found to coexist, diverticulosis and angiodysplasia are responsible for most cases of massive colonic bleeding. The cause of angiodysplasia, or vascular ectasia, is unknown, but it may be related to degenerative vascular changes associated with aging and to colon wall muscular hypertrophy that obstructs the submucosal veins and leads to dilation and a propensity of these veins to bleed. Most cases of colonic angiodysplasia are located in the cecum and right colon. They may also be found in the small bowel, especially the terminal ileum. In contrast to diverticular disease, bleeding from angiodysplasia is venous and not as severe. Diverticulosis can also cause massive bleeding due to ruptured vasa recta in the neck of a diverticulum. Superficial mucosal ulceration in diverticula usually causes mild and self-limited bleeding. Ulcerative colitis is more likely to cause mild-to-moderate bleeding and is frequently associated with diarrhea and systemic signs of chronic illness such as weight loss and failure to thrive. Cancer of the colon generally causes occult rather than massive GI bleeding, with slow blood loss in stools rather than marked bright red blood or melena. Ischemic and infectious colitis may present with mild bleeding usually associated with abdominal pain and fevers, if infectious, or diffuse central or peripheral vascular disease, if ischemic.

Ref.: 3, 12, 13

31. An 18-year-old man with a 2-year history of ulcerative colitis is admitted for an acute exacerbation of his disease. He is febrile and tachycardic with a heart rate of 135 beats/min. His blood pressure is stable. Laboratories show a leukocytosis of 12.3 × 103/L, and plain radiographs show moderate colonic distention to 7 cm in the transverse colon. What is the next step in the treatment of toxic megacolon in this patient?

A. Nasoenteric decompression, broad-spectrum antibiotics, and intravenous steroids

B. Colonoscopic decompression

C. Emergency total abdominal colectomy with ileostomy

D. Nasoenteric decompression, broad-spectrum antibiotics, and infliximab

E. Diverting colostomy

ANSWER: A

COMMENTS: Toxic megacolon is most commonly seen in patients with IBD. Classically, it presents acutely in patients with ulcerative colitis (~5%) and less frequently in those with Crohn's colitis. Although the incidence of toxic megacolon is decreasing in IBD because of better medical management, it may also occur with severe *Clostridium difficile* colitis that is increasing. Toxic megacolon is a subset of toxic colitis. Both cause critical illness and can lead to perforation, peritonitis, and death.

The diagnosis of toxic megacolon is based on the clinical findings of fever, tachycardia, and abdominal distention, combined with radiographs showing colonic distention to 6 cm or greater and leukocytosis greater than 10.5 × 103/L. Successful management is predicated by early recognition and aggressive treatment. Immediate surgery is required for perforation and peritonitis. Otherwise, the patient is admitted to the intensive care unit for rapid fluid resuscitation, transfusion of blood products if needed, and nasogastric suction to minimize the accumulation of swallowed air in the colon. Air usually accumulates preferentially in the transverse colon as opposed to the cecum with distal colon obstruction, and this may be promoted by patients lying supine. Prompt administration of steroids is still felt to be an important component of therapy, and broad-spectrum antibiotics are routinely administered. Response to medical management is assessed with serial vital signs and abdominal radiographs.

Colonoscopy is not necessary in patients with known IBD since attempts at decompression are not helpful and intubation of the already tenuous and friable colon may cause perforation. In patients with no previous history of IBD, a careful proctoscopy to 10 to 15 cm with little insufflation is generally adequate to confirm IBD.

Infliximab is an anti-TNF-α antibody that blocks the TNF-α receptor, which in turns decreases inflammation. It is used to reduce the signs and symptoms of IBD and maintain remission. Infliximab is not used in the setting of acute toxic megacolon related to IBD.

Worsening colonic distention, fever, and leukocytosis are indications for urgent surgery. The operative procedure of choice is abdominal colectomy and ileostomy without proctectomy. The rectum or distal sigmoid may be closed as in a Hartmann's procedure. If the sigmoid is weak or thinned out, it may be exteriorized through the lower end of the midline incision, wrapped in wet gauze, and matured several days later at the bedside as a mucous fistula (Jones procedure). Total colostomy with preservation of the rectum allows a sphincter-preserving operation, usually an IPAA procedure, to take place once health has been restored.

Even when medical therapy of toxic colitis and megacolon is successful, most patients do not have a satisfactory long-term outcome and will require colectomy within the next 6 to 12 months for ongoing symptoms and even recurrent toxic colitis.

Ref.: 1, 6, 14, 15

32. In which of the following patients is colonoscopy indicated?

A. A patient with Crohn's colitis to monitor the efficacy of treatment

B. A patient currently admitted for his second attack of diverticulitis

C. A patient with multiple prior failed screening colonoscopies due to a tortuous colon

D. A 30-year-old patient (below screening age) with known hemorrhoids and rectal bleeding

E. A patient with a cecal volvulus and no peritoneal signs

ANSWER: D

COMMENTS: Different colonic diseases have different indications for and contraindications to colonoscopy.

Rectal bleeding: Patients with melena, hematochezia, other blood loss in the stool, and iron deficiency anemia of unknown etiology should always undergo evaluation of the entire colon, even if the patient is thought to have an anorectal source. Although bleeding from hemorrhoids, fissures, and other anorectal causes is quite common, it does not usually result in anemia, and a malignant source should always be ruled out.

IBD: Endoscopy aids in the diagnosis of IBD; however, it is not indicated for assessment of response to medical therapy, which can be done based on clinical findings alone. Patients with a history of ulcerative colitis for more than 8 to 10 years are at a higher risk for developing adenocarcinoma of the colon; their risk increases 1%–2% per year after 10 years. Therefore they should undergo regular surveillance colonoscopy with multiple biopsies to monitor for dysplasia, a known marker for increased cancer risk in IBD. This should be done even if the disease is in remission. The risk of cancer in patients with Crohn's disease is less well understood. It is likely that patients with pancolitis due to Crohn's disease probably have similar rates of cancer as do chronic ulcerative colitis patients. However, most Crohn's patients have segmental rather than diffuse colonic disease and so the risk may be relatively lower. Colonoscopy should not be performed during acute manifestations of IBD because of the potential for colonic perforation.

Ischemic colitis/diverticulitis: Colonoscopy is contraindicated in patients with acute peritoneal inflammation such as acute diverticulitis, peritonitis, or perforation. Colonoscopy may be performed after the acute inflammation has resolved to evaluate for cancer, polyps, or other causes of symptoms.

Volvulus/pseudo-obstruction: Colonoscopy is indicated for patients with sigmoid volvulus or pseudo-obstruction of the colon for decompression and to rule out other causes of symptoms, provided that there are no signs of peritoneal inflammation. Colonoscopic decompression of a cecal volvulus is usually not successful.

Routine screening: Screening begins at age 50 in the average-risk population and continues at 10-year intervals until age 75. Screening after this age is controversial. Colonoscopy is the gold standard since it is both diagnostic and therapeutic. Polyps may be removed and larger lesions may be biopsied. If polyps are found and removed, surveillance colonoscopy should be performed at more frequent intervals because of increased risk. CT colonography (formerly known as virtual colonoscopy) is useful in patients in whom colonoscopy was incomplete because of a tortuous sigmoid colon or pain. If there is any suspected lesion, a colonoscopy must be performed. If an adenomatous polyp or cancer is discovered during screening sigmoidoscopy, colonoscopy is indicated to exclude the possibility of proximal synchronous polyps (30%) or cancer (4%–8%).

Increased risk screening: Colonoscopy should be performed earlier and more frequently in patients with a known family history of cancer, such as HNPCC, FAP, and those having first-degree relatives with colon cancer. In general, patients with first-degree relatives with polyps or colon cancer should initiate screening at age 40 or 10 years younger than their relative's age of diagnosis; screening interval is dictated by the age of the affected relative, with younger age signifying increased family risk.

Ref.: 1, 5, 6, 15

33. Which of the following statements is correct?

A. Backwash ileitis is associated with ulcerative colitis.

B. Diversion colitis is associated with ulcerative colitis and Crohn's colitis.

C. Microscopic colitis is associated with *Campylobacter* infection.

D. Metronidazole is used to treat acute ileitis caused by *Yersinia* infection.

E. Pseudomembranous colitis is associated with amebiasis.

ANSWER: A

COMMENTS: Backwash ileitis consists of nonspecific inflammation and dilation of the ileum in patients with ulcerative colitis involving the entire colon. There is no thickening or narrowing as seen in Crohn's disease. Its presence does not imply a pre-Crohn's disease condition, nor does it imply a poor outcome after the IPAA procedure. It will resolve once the ulcerative colitis is treated.

Diversion colitis is found in segments of defunctionalized bowel, usually distal to a diverting ostomy or after a Hartmann's procedure. Colon epithelial cells seem to require nutrients from the luminal contents passing by, including short-chain fatty acids. Diversion colitis is thought to result when colonocytes are deprived of these compounds. This is supported by the observation that instillation of short-chain fatty acids ameliorates this condition. Preliminary trials on idiopathic ulcerative proctocolitis have shown a response to short-chain fatty acid enemas. Following reversal of the fecal diversion, the endoscopic findings of diversion colitis usually resolve.

Microscopic colitis (also known as lymphocytic colitis) is characterized by a history of watery diarrhea and microscopic inflammation of the colonic mucosa. The colitis often responds favorably to sulfasalazine. Collagenous colitis (which exhibits a collagenous band under the surface epithelium of the colon on a microscopic examination) may be a variant of this condition because patients have similar symptoms and also respond to sulfasalazine. Spontaneous remission of these two conditions is common. Most of these patients have been incorrectly labeled for years as having irritable bowel syndrome. Colonoscopy with biopsy may yield the correct diagnosis.

Campylobacter causes a diarrheal gastroenteritis that is often self-limited. However, it can cause severe dysentery, especially in a weakened host. It responds well to macrolide antibiotics including erythromycin, clarithromycin, or azithromycin.

Acute inflammatory ileitis causes right lower quadrant pain and is commonly confused with appendicitis or Crohn's disease. Acute ileitis may be due to infection with *Y. enterocolitica.* It is often self-limited but may be treated with antibiotics. It is often resistant to penicillin but is sensitive to aminoglycosides, sulfamethoxazole and trimethoprim (TMP-SMZ, Bactrim), ciprofloxacin, and doxycycline.

Antibiotic-induced colitis (also known as pseudomembranous colitis) is characterized by watery diarrhea, which is rarely bloody and is caused by the proliferation of *C. difficile*. The diagnosis is best made by detecting *C. difficile* toxin in the stool. Either oral vancomycin or metronidazole is used to treat this condition. The latter is less expensive and is therefore used more often.

Ref.: 15

34. With regard to the APC syndromes, which of the following statements is true?

A. Annual colonoscopic screening of family members should begin at the age of 25.

B. Twenty-five percent of the offspring of an afflicted individual will have the disease.

C. The risk for the development of colon cancer is approximately 50%.

D. Abdominal colectomy and ileoproctostomy eliminate the risk for carcinoma.

E. Periampullary tumors are an important cause of death.

ANSWER: E

COMMENTS: Most reports of FAP syndromes reflect experience in American and European populations, but these diseases have been identified in Africans and Asians as well. There is probably no race or geographic area that is exempt. These polyposis syndromes occur in approximately 1 in every 10,000 births. The disease is transmitted as an autosomal dominant trait, and therefore 50% of the offspring of an afflicted individual will have the disease. About 30%–40% of familial polyposis patients do not have a family history of polyposis, and these cases represent spontaneous mutations in the *APC* gene. FAP is the causative factor in about 1%–2% of all CRCs.

The polyps are not present at birth but usually first appear at puberty and gradually increase in number so that by the age of 21, the colon and rectum are carpeted by thousands of polyps. If left untreated, virtually all patients will develop CRC by 40 years of age. Some patients will also develop duodenal and jejunal polyps, which can be very difficult to manage. Periampullary cancer develops in about 5% of patients, primarily when they already have extensive duodenal polyps.

Surgical management is primarily aimed at reducing the risk of CRC. Since most patients will develop cancer by age 40, prophylactic colectomy is recommended in the teens to early 20s. The most common approach is proctocolectomy with anal mucosectomy to the dentate line and reconstruction with an IPAA. This procedure removes all of the at-risk colorectal mucosa while avoiding a permanent ileostomy.

Abdominal colectomy with IRA is still recommended occasionally since it is a relatively straightforward procedure and pelvic dissection is avoided. It is only appropriate if there are less than 20 polyps in the rectum and they can be cleared preoperatively. However, close surveillance of the rectal remnant by proctoscopy every 6 months is mandatory. The incidence of rectal cancer after IRA varies widely among series, probably because of variations in surveillance compliance. Rates of 10%–60% have been published from reputable institutions. In fact, patients are less likely to die of rectal cancer than of periampullary tumors or desmoids. Nevertheless, the importance of surveillance proctoscopy cannot be overemphasized. IRA should not be considered if there are large or dysplastic rectal polyps, or if the patient already has a colon cancer.

Attenuated FAP (aFAP), defined as between 20 and 100 polyps, is relatively uncommon. It seems to be due to mutations in a different part of the *APC* genome that is typical of FAP. Although there is a somewhat lower rate of cancer, it is still a high-risk mutation, and surgical management is usually recommended. An IRA procedure may be appropriate in many patients with aFAP.

Patients with a family history of FAP should be screened with flexible sigmoidoscopy starting at puberty. Annual sigmoidoscopy is recommended until age 20. Genetic screening is also available but is not 100% accurate, and therefore does not replace sigmoidoscopy. Colonoscopy is not necessary since all affected patients will have rectosigmoid polyps. Upper GI endoscopy screening should be performed to look for involvement of the stomach and duodenum every 1 to 3 years beginning at the age of 20 to 25. All polyps should be removed, if possible.

Ref.: 1, 3, 6, 16

35. Match the gene in the left column with the applicable statement in the right column:

A. *FAP*	a. Tumor-suppressor gene that regulates DNA transcription, common in many cancers, located on chromosome 17
B. *p53*	b. Late-occurring alteration resulting in the loss of cell-to-cell contact, thereby enhancing metastases
C. *hMSH2*	c. Tumor-suppressor gene (*APC*) located on chromosome 5
D. *DCC* (deleted in colorectal cancer)	d. Most common mutation found in patients with HNPCC
E. *K-ras*	e. Oncogene that produces a plasma membrane–based protein involved in the transduction of growth and differentiation signals. When mutated, the protein cannot regulate cell growth and differentiation

ANSWERS: A-c, B-a, C-d, D-b, E-e

COMMENTS: The *APC* gene is located on chromosome 5, is large (consisting of approximately 15 exons), and encodes for a cytoplasmic protein of 2843 amino acids. *APC* mutations occur in patients with both sporadic CRCs and familial polyposis, are frequent, are comparable in incidence with adenomas and carcinomas, and occur early in the development of cancer. The protein product of the *APC* gene is normally involved in maintaining cellular adhesion and suppressing neoplastic growth, but the mutant protein may not be capable of serving this function. The *APC* gene thereby acts as a tumor-suppressor gene. Approximately 35% of patients with sporadic cancers and up to 75% of those with polyposis cancers have *APC* mutations that can occur at variable points within the gene. This may explain the various phenotypes associated with the polyposis syndromes.

The *p53* gene is a tumor-suppressor gene located on chromosome 17. Mutations of this gene are the most common genetic abnormality found in various human cancers. The gene encodes for a nuclear phosphoprotein that regulates transcription and negatively influences cellular proliferation by binding at specific DNA sites. For example, cells damaged by ultraviolet light or radiation are kept from replicating by the wild-type (natural) p53 protein. Mutant *p53* binds to wild-type *p53*, thereby preventing specific binding to DNA and permitting tumor growth.

Mismatch repair genes correct errors of DNA replication. Alterations in these genes have been implicated in the pathogenesis of HNPCC. The genetic mutations identified are (1) *MSH2* on chromosome 2 (mutation of this gene may account for up to 60% of the genetic alterations seen in families with HNPCC); (2) *MLH1* on chromosome 3, which may act as a tumor-suppressor gene; (3) *MSH6* on chromosome 2; (4) *PMS1* on chromosome 2; and (5) *PMS2* on chromosome 7.

Mutations of the latter two genes account for only 10% of the mutations seen in families with HNPCC. Germline mutations of the *hMSH2* and *hMLH1* genes by themselves are not enough to produce the HNPCC phenotype. A somatic mutation of the remaining wild-type allele is also necessary.

The *DCC* gene is located on chromosome 18 and is one of the first mutations found to be associated with colon cancer. It encodes for a protein involved in cell-to-cell contact. Deletions of this gene have been found in 73% of patients with CRCs but in only 11% of those with adenomas, thus suggesting that gene loss occurred late during tumorigenesis. Cancers with the loss of the *DCC* gene are more likely to initially be seen as an advanced disease (in comparison with tumors maintaining this gene), and patient survival is consequently compromised.

The *K-ras* gene, an oncogene found on chromosome 12, encodes for a plasma membrane–based protein involved in the transduction of growth and differentiation signals. Approximately 50% of patients with CRC have *K-ras* mutations. Large adenomas and adenomas with small areas of invasive cancer have nearly the same incidence of *K-ras* mutations, thus suggesting that genetic alterations in the *K-ras* gene occur early (but not as early as *APC* mutations) during tumorigenesis. It has yet to be proved whether *K-ras* mutations have any prognostic significance.

Ref.: 17

36. A pedunculated 1.5-cm tubular adenoma is removed endoscopically from the sigmoid colon and found to contain well-differentiated adenocarcinoma extending to but not beyond the muscularis mucosae. The margin of resection is free of tumor. Select the best therapeutic option.

A. Observation only

B. Endoscopic fulguration of the polypectomy site

C. Operative colotomy and excision of the polypectomy site

D. Sigmoid colectomy

E. Laparoscopic segmental colectomy

ANSWER: A

COMMENTS: By definition, this lesion is classified as carcinoma in situ or intramucosal adenocarcinoma and is treated adequately by endoscopic polypectomy. Because a lymphatic plexus exists just below the muscularis mucosae, lymphatic dissemination is possible only when invasion deep to this level has occurred. The muscularis mucosae of the colon wall may extend for a variable distance into the stalk of the polyp and may not even reach the head. Pedunculated polyps consist of four anatomic levels: Haggitt's level 1 is the head itself, level 2 is the interface between the head and the stalk, level 3 is the stalk, and level 4 is the junction between the stalk and the colonic wall (Fig. 23A.2). Endoscopic polypectomy should be considered adequate treatment for a polyp containing invasive cancer at level 1, 2, or 3, if the carcinoma is well differentiated and does not exhibit invasion of the veins or lymphatics and the resection margins are free of cancer. For example, endoscopic polypectomy would be sufficient for a tubular adenoma with well-differentiated cancer extending to level 3 as long as there was no evidence of venous or lymphatic invasion and the margin of resection was free of disease. However, a poorly differentiated cancer extending to level 2 would require formal segmental resection either minimally invasive or by open means. Similarly, any polyp with cancer extending to level 4 requires segmental resection, regardless of differentiation or vascular invasion.

Laparoscopic colectomy is now widely accepted as equivalent to open operation for the cure of colon cancer when performed by experienced surgeons. The Clinical Outcomes of Surgical Therapy (COST) Study Group performed a randomized controlled trial comparing open colectomy with laparoscopically assisted colectomy and found no difference in intraoperative complications, reoperations, survival, and tumor recurrence. However, this patient does not need any further treatment other than observation and subsequent endoscopic surveillance.

Ref.: 1, 3, 18, 19

37. Which of the following is the most important prognostic determinant of survival after treatment of CRC?

A. Lymph node involvement

B. Transmural extension

C. Tumor size

D. Histologic differentiation

E. DNA content

ANSWER: A

COMMENTS: Of the many variables that affect the cure of patients with colon cancer, the status of the lymph nodes has consistently remained the most important. Even with modern aggressive therapy, the long-term survival of node-positive patients is approximately one-half that of node-negative patients. The extent of nodal disease also has an impact on the prognosis. Patients with four or more positive lymph nodes have a significantly lower 5-year survival rate than do patients with three or fewer positive nodes.

Tumor size in and of itself has no bearing on metastatic potential or prognosis. The DNA content of colorectal tumors has been studied extensively, and aneuploidy seems to correlate well with histologic differentiation, transmural penetration, and the presence of nodal metastases. However, the DNA content in general has not been shown conclusively to be an important independent prognostic indicator. Microsatellite instability is associated with inherited cancers but has also not been shown conclusively to be an independent prognostic indicator. A meta-analysis of 32 eligible studies involving 7642 patients noted that only about 15% of the CRC population had microsatellite instability reflecting inactivation of mismatch repair genes. In the remainder of the colorectal population (85%), colon cancer developed from other pathways and included aneuploidy, allelic losses, amplifications, and translocations. In this study and other studies, microsatellite instability was actually associated with a better prognosis in stage II cancers.

Ref.: 1, 3, 5, 20

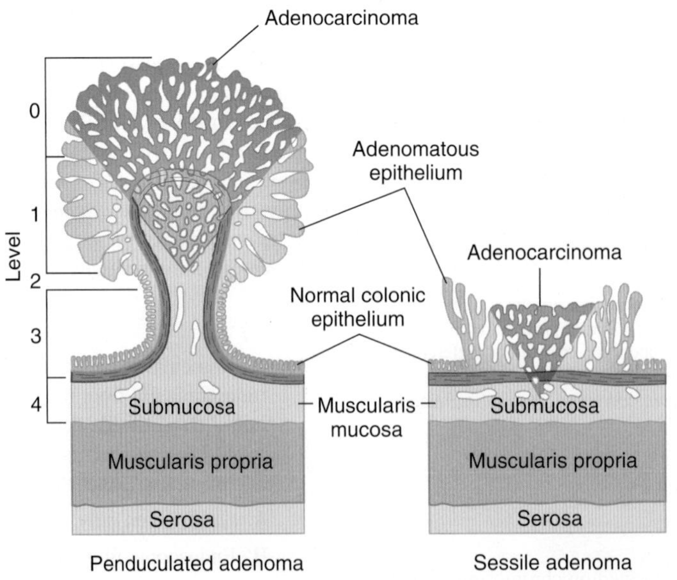

Fig. 23A.2 Haggitt level of malignant invasion in pedunculated and sessile adenomas. *(Source: Haggitt RC, Glotzbach RE, Soffer EE, et al. Prognostic factors in colorectal carcinoma arising in adenomas: implications for lesions removed by endoscopic polypectomy.* Gastroenterology. *1985;89:328–336.)*

38. Which of the following is true regarding EUS imaging?

A. Sedation is required.

B. The bowel must be prepared as for colonoscopy or colectomy.

C. Scanning is best performed with a 3.0-MHz crystal.

D. Imaging of lesions more than 10 cm from the anus is not possible.

E. Image-guided needle biopsy of extraluminal nodules is safe.

ANSWER: E

COMMENTS: Staging of rectal cancer has evolved over the past few years. Accurate staging helps determine appropriate treatment and predicts outcomes. EUS has been used for several decades and is generally performed as an office procedure without the need for sedation or formal bowel preparation. Both rigid probes and endoscopic mounted devices are available. A single enema is given 1 to 2 h before the examination to remove any stool from the rectal vault. Because only a minimal penetration of the rectal wall and perirectal tissues is required, a high-frequency ultrasound crystal is used (i.e., 7 or 10 MHz) to obtain a high resolution of the superficial structures. It is possible to image lesions in the mid and upper portions of the rectum, but to be certain that the ultrasound probe is in contact with neoplasms at this level, it is necessary to insert the probe under direct vision through a 2-cm-wide proctoscope.

EUS is used to stage rectal cancer. It is superior to CT for locoregional staging and has an overall accuracy for predicting tumor stage of up to 80%–95% as compared with CT, which is 65%–75% accurate. EUS also provides the benefit of guiding fine-needle aspiration biopsies to improve the accuracy of nodal staging. EUS demonstrates the depth of invasion of cancer (T stage) and nodal involvement (N stage). For endoscopic ultrasound to be accurate on staging lymph nodes, the nodes must be at least 5 mm. Interobserver variability in performing EUS can be a limitation. In addition, EUS is limited in restaging patients treated with neoadjuvant chemotherapy and radiation therapy because of the treatment-induced fibrosis. Therefore a complete staging with CT of the chest, abdomen, and pelvis; magnetic resonance imaging (MRI) of the pelvis; and examination under anesthesia (EUA) in earlier cases should be performed before initiating treatment. Ultrasound staging is as follows: uT1 is confined to the mucosa and submucosa, uT2 invades but does not penetrate through the muscularis propria, uT3 invades into the perirectal fat, uT4 invades into adjacent organs, uN0 has no lymph node enlargement, and uN1 has lymph node enlargement. Image-guided needle biopsy of extraluminal nodules is a safe procedure that can be performed under ultrasound guidance; suspicious perirectal nodules can also undergo a biopsy in this fashion. Only if the biopsy specimen contains benign lymphoid tissue can it be assumed that the nodule in question is truly free of cancer.

Pelvic MRI is now part of the recommended staging protocol. It is better at staging larger lesions, looking for extrarectal extension and venous, sacral, and pelvic side wall involvement. The likelihood of obtaining clear circumferential margins may also be predicted. EUS is more accurate for the staging of early lesions—T1 versus T2—and therefore it is very useful for deciding on local treatment for T0 and T1 lesions versus radical treatment for T2 and greater tumors.

Ref.: 23

39. A patient presents with a recently diagnosed 3-cm rectal cancer with its lower edge 4 cm from the anorectal ring. EUS shows a tumor extending through the muscularis propria with three adjacent lymph nodes measuring 1 cm each. CT scan does not show any evidence of distant spread to the liver or lungs. Which of the following is the most appropriate treatment for this patient?

A. APR with colostomy

B. LAR with total mesocolon excision and anastomosis

C. Chemotherapy and radiation followed by resection

D. Preoperative external beam radiation therapy

E. Preoperative chemotherapy

ANSWER: C

COMMENTS: Multiple studies have shown that radiation therapy to the pelvis decreases the rate of local and regional recurrence and that systemic chemotherapy reduces the rate of systemic progression. Preoperative combined chemotherapy as opposed to postoperative treatment is associated with lower complication rates and better clinical function. A variety of protocols have been studied globally. In the United States, a full-course radiation therapy consisting of about 5000 cGy to the pelvis and regional lymph node basins for over 6 weeks with a final boost to the primary tumor region with synchronous 5-fluorouracil (5FU)-based chemotherapy is standard. Radical resection of the rectum and mesentery with the lymph nodes by either APR with a permanent colostomy for low rectal lesions or LAR with anastomosis and temporary diverting loop ileostomy is performed 6 to 10 weeks following completion of the neoadjuvant therapy. After recovery from the operation, 6 to 12 months of chemotherapy are given, depending on the final pathology. Recent data show that up to 20% of patients will have a complete pathologic response to neoadjuvant treatment, meaning that no residual tumor is found in the resected specimen. However, a patient with a complete response cannot be reliably predicted based on current clinical evaluation or imaging. Therefore all patients proceed to resection unless they are medically unfit or refuse.

Short-course neoadjuvant therapy with 2500 cGy given for over 1 week followed by surgery 1 week later is used in some centers in Europe but is not standard in the United States. No trials have yet shown that the short-course therapy is as good as the long-course treatment.

This patient has stage III rectal cancer based on pretreatment clinical staging, which shows T3 invasion (through the muscularis propria), three enlarged perirectal lymph nodes (N1), and no evidence of distant spread (M0). Full neoadjuvant treatment with subsequent surgery is appropriate. LAR with a coloanal anastomosis is likely to be technically possible since a 2-cm margin from the anorectal ring should be achievable. Therefore APR is not necessary. In stage III patients, neoadjuvant therapy is associated with a significant increase in survival from 30% with surgery alone to 60%–70% with combined therapy.

Ref.: 9, 21, 23–25

40. A 62-year-old woman complains to her doctor of bright red blood per rectum, mixed with stool. On rectal examination, she is found to have a palpable mass at the tip of the finger. Proctoscopy shows the presence of a posterior 4-cm ulcerated mass that occupies 35% of the circumference beginning at 4 cm from the anorectal ring. A biopsy shows rectal adenocarcinoma, and a complete staging shows a T3 lesion and several enlarged lymph nodes, but no distant metastasis. Her carcinoembryonic antigen (CEA) level is normal. Select the most appropriate treatment for this patient.

A. Local excision
B. TEM excision
C. APR
D. Preoperative chemotherapy and radiation followed by resection
E. Fulguration

ANSWER: D

COMMENTS: The most common symptom of rectal cancer is hematochezia. Other symptoms include mucus discharge, tenesmus, and changes in bowel habits, often with a thin, pencil- or ribbon-like appearance. The workup for rectal cancer includes complete colonoscopy to exclude synchronous colon tumors, CT of the chest, abdomen, and pelvis, MRI of the pelvis, and EUA in selected patients who may be candidates for local treatment. The precise location is best determined by rigid proctosigmoidoscopy, which should be done even if the tumor has been diagnosed with colonoscopy to accurately assess orientation of the tumor and the level above the anal canal. The upper end of the anal canal is the anorectal ring that is typically 1 to 2 cm above the dentate line. This is the lowest level that resection may be performed without sacrificing the anal sphincters. A 2-cm margin is recommended since studies have shown that intramural spread of cancer below the visible and palpable margin is rarely beyond 1 cm.

Measurement of CEA levels is standard. Normal CEA levels are up to 5 μg/L. In smokers, they may be up to 7 μg/L. Although CEA levels are not useful for screening since only 70% of cancers express this antigen and levels are often normal in localized lesions, they are useful for follow-up. A baseline level is always drawn prior to initiating treatment. Very high levels, in the hundreds to thousands, are associated with metastatic disease. If the CEA is elevated and it normalizes after treatment, it may be useful for detecting recurrence. CEA levels are routinely checked every 3 months for several years.

Transanal excision is not part of the initial evaluation of rectal cancer and should be considered only after the evaluation is complete so that the appropriate treatment approach can be selected.

Preoperative clinical TNM staging (Table 23A.1) as well as the level of the lesion in the rectum guide therapeutic decisions. Stage I tumors do not require neoadjuvant therapy (preoperative radiation and chemotherapy). Ultrasound-staged T1 tumors can be treated with transanal local excision: either standard transanal excision with conventional operating anoscopes, TEM, or TAMIS using laparoscopic instruments. TEM uses carbon dioxide insufflation through a 40-mm operating rectoscope and a binocular magnifying visual system to create a better endoscopic visualization of the operative field. TEM is more likely to yield negative margins, an intact specimen, and lower recurrence than operations using conventional transanal instruments. The pitfall with any transanal approach is an inability to assess lymph node status. In T1 cancers, the incidence of lymphatic metastases is about 5%, and the outcomes of local excision versus radical excision are the same. Therefore they are considered safe for transanal excision. Ultrasound-staged T2 rectal cancers should undergo radical surgery because of the significant risk of lymph node metastases (25%–30%).

The ultrasound image of this patient showed penetration of the muscularis propria and possibly the mesorectal fat. Suspicious lymph nodes (spherical, hypoechoic) are seen as well. Therefore she is clinical stage III and should undergo neoadjuvant chemoradiation therapy before radical surgery.

APR involves a complete excision of the rectum and anus through a combined abdominal and perineal approach. APR leaves the patient with a permanent colostomy. Thus APR is indicated when the patient has poor preoperative sphincter control, the patient's body habitus is unfavorable, the tumor involves the anal sphincters, or part of the sphincter needs to be resected to obtain negative margins (as in a tumor less than 2 cm from the anorectal ring). LAR involves excision of the rectum and mesorectum through an abdominal approach and colorectal or coloanal anastomosis. A temporary loop ileostomy is often used to protect the low colorectal anastomosis, especially in radiated patients because of the higher risk of anastomotic leak.

In the United States, stages II and III rectal cancers are commonly treated with full-course neoadjuvant (preoperative) radiation therapy consisting of 5040 cGy and 5-FU-based chemotherapy. Fulguration is rarely used in current surgical practice because of the advances in transanal excision that provides a full-thickness specimen for pathology staging. It may be used in patients with small lesions below the peritoneal reflection that are poor surgical candidates or for small recurrences.

Ref.: 1, 22, 26

41. A 73-year-old man undergoes an exploratory laparotomy and small bowel resection for small bowel obstruction. During his postoperative course, the patient develops diarrhea, abdominal tenderness, and distention. He is diagnosed with a postoperative ileus. A stool specimen is sent that is positive for *C. difficile* toxin. He is developing a significant leukocytosis, fever, and elevated creatinine. What is the recommended treatment?

A. Metronidazole oral
B. IV vancomycin
C. Piperacillin-tazobactam
D. Vancomycin oral
E. IV metronidazole and vancomycin via a rectal tube

ANSWER: E

COMMENTS: Evidence shows that the incidence and virulence of *C. difficile* are increasing. Metronidazole and oral vancomycin have been known to be effective therapies for *C. difficile* since the late 1970s. IV vancomycin is ineffective in treating *C. difficile* colitis. A review conducted before 2000 showed that the failure rate of metronidazole for treatment of *C. difficile* colitis was 2.5% and the failure rate of treatment with oral vancomycin was 3.5%. Since 2000, there has been an increase in this failure rate, with recent data showing a metronidazole failure rate of 18.2%. Newer data also show that both agents still have similar efficacy in mild infection, but that vancomycin has superior efficacy in severe infection. Rectal administration of vancomycin may be employed as a treatment modality in severe infections and in patients who cannot tolerate oral administration as in the case of this patient with a postoperative ileus. Dual therapy of IV metronidazole and vancomycin may be employed in severe infections as well.

Ref.: 28, 29

42. Which of the following statistics are FALSE regarding CRC in the United States?

A. CRC rates are highest in black men and women.

B. CRC rates are lowest in Asian/Pacific Islander men and women.

C. Mortality rates are 30%–40% higher in women than in men.

D. Approximately 5% or 1 in 20 Americans will be diagnosed with a cancer of the colon or rectum in their lifetimes.

E. CRC is the third leading cause of cancer death in women.

ANSWER: C

COMMENTS: CRC is the third most commonly diagnosed cancer and the second leading cause of cancer death in men and women combined in the United States. Approximately 5% or 1 in 20 Americans will be diagnosed with a cancer of the colon or rectum in their lifetimes. There are approximately 150,000 new cases of CRC in the United States per year. CRC rates are highest in black men and women and lowest in Asian/Pacific Islander men and women. The incidence and death rates of CRC increase with age. Overall, 90% of new cases and 93% of deaths occur in people aged 50 years or older. Mortality rates are 30%–40% higher in men than in women. The median age of colon cancer diagnosis is 69 in men and 73 in women. The median age of rectal cancer diagnosis is 63 in men and 65 in women. CRC death rates have been declining since 1980 in men and since 1947 in women, and this can be attributable to improved screening, treatment, and decreases in exposure to risk factors.

Ref.: 30

43. A 32-year-old woman presents to the emergency department with abdominal pain that has gradually increased over the past week. The patient has a history of FAP and underwent a total proctocolectomy with IPAA at age 20. She has 5 to 6 soft to loose bowel movements per day, which is normal for her. A CT scan reveals a 10-cm soft tissue mass in the middle abdomen, displacing the loop of small bowel to either side. Upon review of a CT scan from several years prior, the mass was present but has grown from 7 cm. What is the next step in initial management?

A. External beam radiation

B. Surgical debulking

C. Chemotherapy

D. Daily tamoxifen

E. Core needle biopsy

ANSWER: D

COMMENTS: Extracolonic manifestations of FAP include adenomas of the upper GI tract, desmoid tumors, osteomas, pigmented lesions of the retina, and epidermoid cysts, as well as gastric, thyroid, suprarenal, and central nervous system cancers. The patient in this scenario has a desmoid tumor of the small bowel mesentery. This is a typical presentation of a patient with a history of FAP and the finding of an intraabdominal soft tissue mass. Desmoid tumors are benign growths that occur in 10%–20% of patients with FAP. They are a form of fibromatosis and are more common in patients with a family history of desmoids. Histologically, they consist of proliferating myofibroblasts. They have no malignant potential but often progress locally, infiltrating tissues and causing obstruction, vascular compromise, and pain. They are most commonly found in the abdomen, particularly in the small bowel mesentery, in the retroperitoneum, and in the abdominal wall. Occasionally they will develop in other sites. Desmoids are the second most common cause of death in patients with FAP, after GI malignancies.

Most desmoids grow slowly and may cause symptoms over time; some will grow faster. Some will grow, plateau, and then regress. There are no specific inciting factors, but the observation has been made that desmoids may grow more rapidly after abdominal surgery. They also have a high rate of recurrence after resection. Asymptomatic desmoid tumors demonstrating little or no growth can be observed. They should be followed with imaging to assess progression. Initial therapeutic measures are aimed at slowing growth. Several medications have been shown to be of benefit in some patients. Nonsteroidal antiinflammatory drugs (NSAIDs) such as sulindac and indomethacin have been used both to treat desmoids and to slow growth of polyps. Alone, they are not particularly effective. Antiestrogen agents such as tamoxifen and progesterone seem to have more effect. Tamoxifen is currently the mainstay of medical treatment. Combined therapy with an NSAID and tamoxifen may prove to be more effective. Overall, about 50% of patients have stabilization or reduction in tumor mass with medical therapy. Cytotoxic chemotherapy is rarely used but is an option when the tumor is growing rapidly and causing symptoms, does not respond to other medical therapy, is not resectable, or recurs rapidly after resection. Typical agents include doxorubicin and carboplatin.

Radiotherapy is rarely used for intraabdominal tumors because of the risks and side effects. These tumors are not particularly radiosensitive. Radiotherapy may be used for abdominal wall or extremity lesions. It also may be used as an adjuvant to surgery.

Surgical excision is the most effective means of eradicating these tumors; however, recurrence rates are over 60%, and clear margins may be difficult to achieve. There also may be significant morbidity with resection, including ischemia, short-bowel syndrome, and the loss of an ileoanal pouch, if present. The most problematic lesions are those in the base of the small bowel mesentery that surround major vessels such as the superior mesenteric artery and vein. If a large abdominal desmoid is causing obstruction, then a bypass is an alternative to resection.

Ref.: 31

44. Which of the following is NOT a principle of Enhanced Recovery After Surgery (ERAS) protocols in colorectal surgery?

A. Multimodal analgesia

B. Hypothermia

C. Minimizing perioperative starvation

D. Early postoperative ambulation

E. Avoiding aggressive perioperative fluid loading

ANSWER: B

COMMENTS: ERAS programs focus on many aspects of care of the surgical patient with the intent of decreasing pain and narcotic use, decreasing the length of stay, decreasing complication rates, reducing costs, and improving the overall experience. Many ERAS programs have risen in the setting of colorectal surgery. Due to the success of these programs, the concepts are being applied to other surgical specialties. Although there are variations in the details of the programs among institutions, there are well-established principles. The major elements within these enhanced recovery programs include preoperative education, multimodal analgesia (the use of epidural regional anesthesia, maximizing usage of nonopioid analgesic options, minimizing narcotic usage), limiting perioperative starvation (preoperative complex carbohydrate drinks, early refeeding), limiting intravenous fluids, maintaining normothermia, and early postoperative ambulation. Setting expectations and psychologically and emotionally supporting the patients by dedicated personnel helps. The average hospital stay after colectomy may be reduced from 5.5 to 3.5 days for laparoscopic surgery without an increase in readmission rates.

Ref.: 32, 33

45. A 58-year-old man had a left colectomy for a T2 N2 M0 colon cancer 4 years ago, followed by adjuvant chemotherapy. During a surveillance visit, his CEA is found to be elevated, and a CT scan revealed a large, 6-cm lesion in the liver. A subsequent biopsy is consistent with a metastatic recurrence. The positron emission tomography (PET) scan reveals no other extrahepatic lesions. What treatment should be offered to this patient with metastatic disease?

A. Systemic chemotherapy
B. Radiofrequency ablation plus systemic chemotherapy
C. Orthotopic liver transplant
D. Palliative care consult to discuss goals of care
E. Hepatic resection plus systemic chemotherapy

ANSWER: E

COMMENTS: Twenty percent of patients have metastasis at the time of diagnosis, with many more developing metastatic spread throughout the course of their disease. The most common site of metastasis is the liver; 80% of stage IV patients have hepatic spread, and 40% of these do not have the extrahepatic disease. Hepatic resection for isolated liver metastases has been clearly shown to be safe and efficacious in experienced hands. The traditional guidelines for recommending liver resection (metastasectomy) for patients with stage IV CRC are three or fewer lesions, disease limited to one side of the liver, no extrahepatic disease, and a willing patient who is a reasonable surgical candidate. The median survival for isolated liver metastases treated with only chemotherapy is 20 months. With hepatic resection, median survival is as much as 88% at 1 year and 43% at 5 years. The long-term survival is about 30%. Hepatic resections for colorectal hepatic metastases have become a much safer surgery over the years, with perioperative mortality of 1%–5%. The key to safety and efficacy in hepatic resections is the careful patient selection. Factors associated with poor survival include the presence of extrahepatic disease, inability to achieve a negative margin, short interval to recurrence, number and size of tumors, lymph node–positive primary, high preoperative CEA, advanced age, and significant comorbid disease. Other modalities available for treatment of hepatic metastases include radiofrequency ablation, staged resections for bilobar disease, and preoperative portal vein embolization or ligation to induce liver hypertrophy.

An evolving approach to bilobar disease is the two-step ALPPS (associating liver partition and portal vein ligation for staged hepatectomy) procedure. In the first operation, the liver is divided into two segments. The side to be retained (FLR, future liver remnant) is cleared of disease by limited resections with clear margins. The portal vein branch to the side to be removed is ligated. During the weeks following this, the FLR parenchyma undergoes remarkable hypertrophy. In the second operation a few weeks later, the planned resection is performed, leaving the hypertrophied side. This approach allows a much larger proportion of the liver to be resected, yet leaves enough for the patient to survive. Initial results are impressive, but a larger experience with longer follow-up is needed to assess its usefulness.

Ref.: 34–36

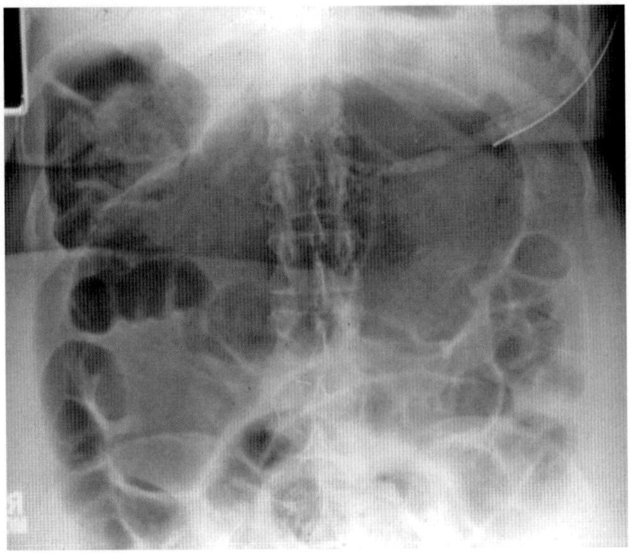

Fig. 23A.3 Plain abdominal radiograph. *(Source: BAOrkin.)*

46. A 60-year-old otherwise healthy woman presents to the emergency department for acute onset of lower abdominal pain with associated nausea and emesis. Her previous surgical history includes a total hysterectomy. On examination, she is distended and peritonitic. Her vitals show tachycardia and hypotension, and lab results show bicarb of 14 and lactic acid of 4.8. The emergency department orders a plain film (Fig. 23A.3). What is the optimal therapy for this patient?

A. Subtotal colectomy with end ileostomy
B. Endoscopic decompression, placement of a rectal tube, and sigmoid colectomy with primary anastomosis
C. Intraoperative decompression followed by subtotal colectomy
D. Laparotomy, detorsion, and cecostomy tube
E. Right hemicolectomy and primary anastomosis with or without diverting ileostomy

ANSWER: E

COMMENTS: Colonic volvulus refers to torsion of the bowel around its own mesentery. The word *volvulus* originates from the Latin word *volvere,* meaning “to twist.” Colonic volvulus is a rare cause of bowel obstruction, collectively accounting for only 2%–3% of cases of colonic obstruction in the United States. Sigmoid volvulus is the most common form and accounts for about two-thirds of cases. Cecal volvulus is present in almost one-third of cases, while volvulus of the transverse colon is extremely rare.

During intrauterine development of the fetus, the intestinal tract rotates counterclockwise and is drawn into the peritoneum and out of the yolk sac. The cecum normally fixes to the right retroperitoneum and posterolateral abdominal wall. Incomplete fixation with a mobile cecum puts patients at a risk for cecal volvulus. Other risk factors include previous surgery that may result in adhesions that create a point of fixation for twisting, chronic constipation with colon dilation, intestinal malformations including malrotation, excessive exercise, distal colon obstruction, very high fiber diets, and late pregnancy.

The patient in this scenario has a cecal volvulus as demonstrated by her radiograph. She has signs of ischemic bowel based on her physical examination, vitals, and acidotic state. She needs prompt surgical treatment. Mortality increases with both the presence of ischemic bowel and a delay in surgical treatment. Nonsurgical treatment has no role in a patient with evidence of bowel ischemia. Even if this patient was stable without any signs of bowel compromise, endoscopic decompression has been found to be ineffective in the majority of cases of cecal volvulus. A right hemicolectomy should be performed with a complete resection of all ischemic/gangrenous bowel and primary anastomosis if the margins appear healthy and well-perfused bowel. The decision to perform an end ileostomy is based on multiple factors including nutritional status, anemia, use of chronic steroids, other comorbidities, and the appearance of the tissues. In cases where there is no ischemic or gangrenous bowel, detorsion and cecopexy can be considered in the frail or elderly population where minimal surgery is preferred. This is reasonable although recurrence rates are higher. Detorsion and cecostomy tube are no longer performed because the complication and mortality rates are much higher than with cecopexy. Resection should always be performed in the case of ischemic bowel and should be attempted whenever possible, even in the cases of nonischemic bowel, when the patient can tolerate the operation because it is the definitive treatment and eliminates the risk of recurrence.

Ref.: 1, 37

47. Which statement is FALSE regarding sigmoid volvulus?

A. Sigmoid volvulus is commonly seen in patients who are elderly, debilitated, chronically constipated, or on psychotropic medications.

B. Mortality rates are lower when emergent decompression is performed before sigmoid resection.

C. Nonoperative reduction of sigmoid volvulus is successful in 70%–80% of cases.

D. If the gangrenous bowel is seen during decompression, a rectal tube should be placed to prevent recurrence.

E. Sigmoid resection within 2 to 3 days of decompression is the preferred definitive treatment.

ANSWER: D

COMMENTS: The prerequisite for the development of sigmoid or cecal volvulus is a mobile segment of bowel that can rotate around a mesentery whose points of fixation are in proximity. Typically, the cecum rotates around the ileocolic artery, while the sigmoid rotates around the IMA. Otherwise, there are surprisingly few similarities between sigmoid and cecal volvulus.

Volvulus of the cecum is found most frequently in persons 25 to 35 years of age, whereas it is unusual for sigmoid volvulus to occur in an active, otherwise healthy individual. Usually, it occurs in the elderly, debilitated persons, or those with psychiatric or neurologic disorders in which immobility, medications that impair bowel motility, and loss of accessory defecatory muscles may lead to constipation and elongation of the colon.

Both types of volvulus typically cause abdominal distention and pain. With cecal volvulus, plain abdominal films may show evidence of small bowel obstruction and a dilated colon segment extending into the left upper quadrant, whereas with sigmoid volvulus, the distended twisted loop has a fairly characteristic appearance of a "bent inner tube" extending into the right upper quadrant.

For sigmoid volvulus, endoscopic detorsion plus insertion of a rectal tube to evacuate the voluminous fecal contents is the preferred initial therapeutic approach but should be attempted only if the mucosa does not appear gangrenous. It should not be attempted if the patient has rebound abdominal tenderness or other signs of peritoneal inflammation. Evidence of gangrenous bowel mandates surgical management. Although nonoperative detorsion is successful approximately 70%–80% of the time, recurrence rates have been reported from 33% to as high as 90%, and therefore an elective resection of the elongated colon is recommended if the patient has an acceptable operative risk. Data from the Veterans Affairs (VA) Hospitals have reported mortality rates as high as 24% for patients undergoing initial emergency operations for sigmoid volvulus versus only 6% for patients initially treated with endoscopic decompression followed by scheduled sigmoid resection soon afterward.

Nonoperative colonoscopic reduction of cecal volvulus is difficult and usually ineffective. Prompt surgery is the mainstay of treatment for cecal volvulus. If gangrenous, the cecum must be resected. In the absence of vascular compromise, either resection or sutured cecopexy is a reasonable option. The most important determinant of a patient's outcome is whether bowel gangrene is present, with mortality being highest if surgery is performed for intestinal infarction or perforation. Mortality is also higher if operating for recurrent volvulus.

Ref.: 1, 3, 6, 37

48. Which of the following is not a type of cecal volvulus?

A. An axial volvulus from clockwise twisting where the torsed cecum remains in the right lower quadrant

B. Upward folding of the cecum

C. Downward folding of the cecum

D. A torsion of the cecum and a portion of the terminal ileum resulting in a displacement of the cecum out of the right lower quadrant

E. Bascule

ANSWER: C

COMMENTS: Sigmoid volvulus is the most common type of volvulus. Cecal volvulus accounts for approximately one-third of cases of colonic volvulus. The causes of cecal volvulus can be congenital or acquired. During embryological development, the cecum normally rotates into the right lower quadrant and becomes fixed to the retroperitoneal structures and right gutter. Incomplete fixation can put patients at a risk for cecal volvulus. Other risk factors include previous surgery (allowing adhesions to create a point of fixation for twisting), chronic constipation, intestinal malformation, excessive exercise, distal colon obstruction, very high fiber diets, and late pregnancy.

There are three types of cecal volvulus:

- Type I: Axial torsion—An axial volvulus from clockwise twisting of the cecum around the axis of the ileocolic artery. The cecum remains in the right lower quadrant.

- Type II: Loop torsion—A torsion of the cecum and a portion of the terminal ileum resulting in a displacement of the cecum out of the right lower quadrant into the left upper quadrant. This is the most common type.
- Type III: Cecal bascule type—The cecum flows upward into the midepigastrium or left upper quadrant on a tangential fold from the hepatic flexure in the right upper quadrant down toward the left lower quadrant.

Surgery is the mainstay of treatment for cecal volvulus. Right hemicolectomy is the procedure of choice since it eliminates the problem. If resection is not desired or the simplest procedure is preferred in a compromised patient, cecopexy by raising a flap of lateral peritoneum and fixing the cecum to the right gutter under this flap may be considered. However, recurrence rates are fairly high. If there is any compromise of the bowel such as gangrene or ischemia, resection is mandatory. In most circumstances, the primary ileocolic anastomosis is safe, although ileostomy and either distal closure or mucous fistula is an option.

Ref.: 38

49. A 56-year-old man is scheduled to undergo a laparoscopic segmental colectomy for a carcinoma of the descending colon. Which of the following statements is true concerning bowel preparation for colorectal operations?

A. Preoperative nonabsorbable oral antibiotics alone are effective in preventing postoperative wound infections.

B. Preoperative mechanical bowel cleansing alone is most effective in preventing postoperative wound infections.

C. A broad-spectrum antibiotic should be administered only once and just before surgery.

D. Mechanical cleansing with sodium phosphate is preferred in patients with renal insufficiency, cirrhosis, ascites, and congestive heart failure.

E. Mechanical cleansing should be used selectively in patients with a complete bowel obstruction or perforation.

ANSWER: C

COMMENTS: The colon contains a higher concentration of bacteria, both aerobic and anaerobic, than any other part of the body. Infectious complications constitute the major morbidity of colorectal operations and occur at higher rates than most other general surgery procedures. *Escherichia coli* is the most common aerobic organism and *Bacteroides* the most common anaerobic organism found in the colon. Mechanical cleansing of the colon has been a time-honored practice that can be achieved by the administration of a cathartic in combination with enemas or by peroral lavage with a nonabsorbable polyethylene glycol–electrolyte (PEG) solution administered the afternoon before surgery. Although there was a period when mechanical bowel preparation prior to colectomy was felt to be unnecessary, recent data have shown that the combination of mechanical preparation, oral antibiotics, and one preoperative dose of intravenous antibiotics within 30 min of the skin incision is the best approach to reduce colorectal surgical site infections.

Oral and rectal Fleet Phospho-Soda (sodium phosphate) was commonly used in the past because of its efficacy in mechanically cleansing the bowel with less volume. However, its use has been associated with significant electrolyte derangements causing compromise of patients with renal insufficiency, cirrhosis, ascites, and congestive heart failure. Therefore it was removed from the market. Polyethylene glycol is *not* contraindicated in patients with renal failure, cirrhosis, ascites, or congestive heart failure since it generally preserves electrolyte balance. Complete bowel obstruction and bowel perforation are absolute contraindications to mechanical bowel preparation.

Ref.: 1, 3, 9, 40

50. Which of the following is the *least* appropriate operative strategy for a patient presenting with sigmoid diverticulitis and localized peritonitis?

A. Sigmoid colectomy with primary anastomosis

B. Sigmoid colectomy with primary anastomosis and diverting ileostomy

C. Sigmoid colectomy with end colostomy and rectal stump

D. Drainage and ileostomy without resection

E. Total colectomy

ANSWER: E

COMMENTS: Diverticulitis is the inflammation caused by perforation of a colonic diverticulum. In many cases, the perforation is microscopic and results in local infection and inflammation in the bowel wall and adjacent mesentery. In complicated diverticulitis, a larger perforation may cause a phlegmon, abscess, fistula, or peritonitis. The severity of complicated acute diverticulitis is graded by the Hinchey classification:

- Stage I: Diverticulitis with a localized pericolic or mesocolic abscess
- Stage II: Diverticulitis with a pelvic abscess
- Stage III: Perforation with purulent peritonitis
- Stage IV: Perforation with fecal peritonitis

The Hinchey classification does not describe uncomplicated diverticulitis or late complications such as fistula or stenosis. It provides a loose guideline to the management of acute complicated disease. Historically, sigmoid colectomy with diverting colostomy and rectal stump—the Hartmann's procedure—was the primary treatment for acute diverticulitis. It is still the most common procedure performed in the acute setting. In recent years, primary anastomosis has been found to be reasonable for selected patients presenting with a walled off abscess or localized peritonitis. The anastomosis must be tension free, inflammation free, away from the inflammatory site or abscess cavity, and well vascularized. Tissues to be anastomosed must be healthy and not involved in the inflammatory process. The patient must be stable, and a complete washout should be performed.

A number of studies have been performed looking at the option of laparoscopic washout and drainage without resection. Although some surgeons have been enthusiastic, the studies are low powered and general consensus recommendations have not yet shifted to this approach. A recent multicenter, randomized trial from the Scandinavian countries showed that primary resection was superior to laparoscopic lavage. Mortality, quality of life, and hospital stay were not different; however, the reoperation rate was higher and several sigmoid cancers were missed.

Still, most cases of diverticulitis are managed nonoperatively with antibiotics. Radiologic drainage of localized abscesses is usually well tolerated. The general plan is for observation of uncomplicated patients. Interval resection is usually reserved for patients with a drained abscess, a fistula, or multiple episodes of diverticulitis. The need for resection after radiologic drain is now being questioned; this is currently being studied.

Ref.: 10, 27, 41

51. Which of the following is a known risk factor for the anastomotic leak?

A. Long rectal stump

B. Stapled anastomosis

C. Female gender

D. IRA

E. Prior operation

ANSWER: D

COMMENTS: Anastomotic leaks after a colorectal operation can present in a variety of ways, from isolated postoperative tachycardia to fulminant sepsis and peritonitis. Multiple factors have been implicated in the development of anastomotic leak, few of which are definitive. Implicated, or associated but not necessarily causal, are the use of drains, advanced malignancy, shock, malnutrition, emergent surgery, smoking, steroid use, male gender (related to a narrow pelvis), and technical reasons. The gut microbiome has recently been increasingly implicated in the development of leaks, independent of other predictors. Studies are in progress to evaluate this mechanism. Factors that have been definitively related are poor blood supply, tension on the suture line, use of radiated tissue, emergency operations, and contaminated fields. Anastomoses in the low rectum are more technically challenging and therefore at higher risk of a leak. Ileorectal anastomoses have the highest leak rate of any colonic anastomosis, although it is not clear why. Patients with Crohn's disease have a slightly higher incidence of anastomotic leaks. Extensive research has shown that there is no overall difference in the anastomotic leak rates of hand-sewn and stapled anastomoses. However, a deep pelvic colorectal anastomosis is much easier to construct with a stapler, while a hand-sewn anastomosis should be considered when the bowel is thick, edematous, or otherwise not suitable for stapling.

Ref.: 1, 41

52. Which of the following is true regarding ileostomy construction and management?

A. Approximately 95% of patients with an ostomy tolerate it well with the improved quality of life.

B. One-third of patients require revision of their ileostomy for parastomal hernias, prolapse, or wound care issues.

C. New-onset necrotic skin changes around an ostomy can always be attributed to poor wound care.

D. Ostomy retraction helps facilitate pouching.

E. The Brooke method of maturing an ileostomy prevents mucosal sloughing.

ANSWER: B

COMMENTS: When performed in low-risk patients with attention to good technique, the creation of a Brooke ileostomy is a safe and well-tolerated procedure with few postoperative complications. Originally described by Bryan Brooke in 1952, the everted and primarily matured ileostomy surmounted the problems of serositis, stenosis, and retraction, known as ileostomy dysfunction. The crucial elements of successful ostomy creation include preoperative site marking by a knowledgeable surgeon or enterostomal nurse, adequate mobilization of the mesentery to allow a tension-free ostomy, and primary maturation with eversion using tripartite sutures. Obese patients with a thick abdominal wall and deep skin folds present a challenge since site selection may be difficult and the mesentery may be thick and short. Inadequate maturation and excessive tension from the mesentery can cause retraction, which interferes with effective pouching, leading to wound care difficulties, skin rashes and breakdown, leakage, and occasional soft tissue infections. Finally, a poorly sized fascial aperture can lead to obstruction or ischemia if too small, or a parastomal or prolapse if too large. For these reasons, up to one-third of patients eventually require operative revision or reversal of their ostomy.

Peristomal rashes and skin breakdown are usually due to ineffective pouching because of poor patient education or compliance, or due to the ostomy problems such as retraction, prolapse, poor siting, or hernia. The services of a trained enterostomal nurse (WOCN, wound ostomy care nurse) are invaluable. Ideally, patients scheduled for surgery that will include an ostomy will have a preoperative WOCN consultation and organized postoperative training on ostomy care. WOCNs will also allow nonoperative management of many problems. Patients with Crohn's disease and, rarely, ulcerative colitis may develop pyoderma gangrenosum with serpiginous skin ulcers. Although pyoderma is typically developing in the pretibial skin, it can also develop around a stoma or in a skin incision. If pyoderma is suspected, the patient should be evaluated for Crohn's disease, if not already diagnosed. Treatment includes medical control of the IBD and local care with various immunosuppressive topical agents and ostomy appliances. Tacrolimus cream has been quite effective in many patients. The Brooke method of maturation refers to folding over the mucosa to hide the serosa, preventing serositis and ileitis. This method does not prevent mucosal sloughing, a complication related to ischemia.

Ref.: 39, 41

REFERENCES

1. Fry RD, Mahmoud N, Maron DJ, et al. Colon and rectum. In: Townsend CM, Beauchamp RD, Evers BM, et al., eds. *Sabiston Textbook of Surgery: The Biological Basis of Modern Surgical Practice*. 18th ed. Philadelphia: WB Saunders; 2008.
2. Pemberton JH, Phillips SF. Colonic absorption. *Perspect Colon Rectal Surg*. 1988;1:89–103.
3. Bullard KM, Rothenberger DA. Colon, rectum and anus. In: Brunicardi FC, Andersen DK, Billiar TR, et al., eds. *Schwartz's Principles of Surgery*. 9th ed. New York: McGraw-Hill; 2010.
4. Hookman P, Barkin JS. *Clostridium difficile* associated infection, diarrhea and colitis. *World J Gastroenterol*. 2009;15:1554–1580.
5. Corman ML. *Colon and Rectal Surgery*. 5th ed. Philadelphia: JB Lippincott; 2005.
6. Mazier WP, Levien DH, Luchtefeld MA, et al. *Surgery of the Colon, Rectum and Anus*. Philadelphia: WB Saunders; 1995.
7. Kaleya RN, Boley SJ. Colonic ischemia. *Perspect Colon Rectal Surg*. 1990;3:62–81.
8. Taylor I. Intestinal blood flow. *Perspect Colon Rectal Surg*. 1988;1:49–57.
9. Gordon PM, Nivatvongs S. *Principles and Practice of Surgery for the Colon, Rectum and Anus*. 2nd ed. St. Louis: Quality Medical; 1999.
10. Mulholland MW, Lillemoe KD, Doherty GM, Maier RV, Simeone DM, Upchurch GR, eds. *Greenfield's Surgery: Scientific Principles and Practice*. 5th ed. Philadelphia: Lippincott Williams & Wilkins; 2011.
11. Fischer JE, Bland KI, eds. *Mastery of Surgery*. 5th ed. Philadelphia: Lippincott Williams & Wilkins; 2007.
12. Boley SJ, Brandt LJ, Frank MS. Severe lower intestinal bleeding: diagnosis and treatment. *Clin Gastroenterol*. 1981;10:65–91.
13. Browder W, Cerise EJ, Litwin MS. Impact of emergency angiography in massive lower gastrointestinal bleeding. *Ann Surg*. 1986;204:530–536.
14. Wilhelm SM, McKenney KA, Rivait KN, et al. A review of infliximab use in ulcerative colitis. *Clin Ther*. 2008;30:223–230.
15. Sleisenger MH, Fordtran JS. *Gastrointestinal Disease: Pathophysiology, Diagnosis and Management*. 4th ed. Philadelphia: WB Saunders; 1989.

16. Fazio VW, ed. *Current Therapy in Colon and Rectal Surgery*. St. Louis: BC Decker; 1990.
17. Howe JR, Guillem JG. The genetics of colorectal cancer. *Surg Clin North Am*. 1997;77:175–196.
18. Gordon MS, Cohen AM. Management of invasive carcinoma in pedunculated colorectal polyps. *Oncology*. 1989;3:99–105.
19. Nelson H, Sargent DJ, Wieand HS, et al. A comparison of laparoscopically assisted and open colectomy for colon cancer. The Clinical Outcomes of Surgical Therapy Study Group. *N Engl J Med*. 2004;350:2050–2059.
20. Popat S, Hubner R, Houlston RS. Systematic review of microsatellite instability and colorectal cancer prognosis. *J Clin Oncol*. 2005;23:609–618.
21. Ahuja N. Rectal cancer. In: Cameron JL, ed. *Current Surgical Therapy*. 9th ed. Philadelphia: CV Mosby; 2008.
22. Kukreja SS, Agusti EE, Velasco JM, et al. Increased lymph node evaluation with colorectal cancer resection: does it improve detection of stage III disease? *Arch Surg*. 2009;144:612–617.
23. Saclarides TJ. Anorectal ultrasound. In: Machi J, Staren ED, eds. *Ultrasound for Surgeons*. 2nd ed. Philadelphia: Lippincott Williams & Wilkins; 2005.
24. Diaz-Canton EA, Pazdur R. Adjuvant therapy for colorectal cancer. *Surg Clin North Am*. 1997;77:211–228.
25. Fleshman JW, Myerson RJ. Adjuvant radiation therapy for adenocarcinoma of the rectum. *Surg Clin North Am*. 1997;77:15–26.
26. Turner J, Saclarides T. Transanal endoscopic microsurgery. *Minerva Chir*. 2008;63:401–412.
27. Haas EM, Bailey R, Farragher I. Application of 10 percent formalin for the treatment of radiation-induced hemorrhagic proctitis. *Dis Colon Rectum*. 2006;50:213–217.
28. Kelly CP, LaMont JT. *Clostridium difficile*—more difficult than ever. *N Engl J Med*. 2008;359:1932–1940.
29. Shen EP, Surawicz CM. Current treatment options for severe *Clostridium difficile*-associated disease. *Gastroenterol Hepatol*. 2008;4:134–139.
30. American Cancer Society. Colorectal cancer facts and figures 2014–2016. Available at: www.cancer.org.
31. Escobar C, Munker R, Thomas JO, Li BD, Burton GV. Update on desmoid tumors. *Ann Oncol*. 2012;23:562–569.
32. Abraham N, Albayati S. Enhanced recovery after surgery programs hasten recovery after colorectal resections. *World J Gastrointest Surg*. 2011;3(1):1–6.
33. Counihan TC, Favuzza J. Fast track colorectal surgery. *Clin Colon Rectal Surg*. 2009;22(1):60–72.
34. Frankel TL, D'Angelica MI. Hepatic resection for colorectal metastases. *J Surg Oncol*. 2014;109:2–7.
35. Shah SA, Bromberg R, Coates A, Rempel E, Simunovic M, Gallinger S. Survival after liver resection for metastatic colorectal carcinoma in a large population. *J Am Col Surg*. 2007;205(5):676–683.
36. Poston GJ, Adam R, Alberts S, et al. OncoSurge: a strategy for improving resectability with curative intent in metastatic colorectal cancer. *J Clin Oncol*. 2005;23(28):7125.
37. Gingold D, Murrell Z. Management of colonic volvulus. *Clin Colon Rectal Surg*. 2012;25:236.
38. Delabrousse E, Sarliève P, Sailley N, et al. Cecal volvulus: CT findings and correlation with pathophysiology. *Emerg Radiol*. 2007;14:411.
39. Murrell Z, Fleshner P. Ulcerative colitis: surgical management. In: Beck DE, Roberts PC, Saclarides TJ, et al. eds. *The ASCRS Textbook of Colon and Rectal Surgery*. 2nd ed. Springer Verlag, New York, NY.
40. Chen M, Song X, Chen LZ, Lin ZD, Zhang XL. Comparing mechanical bowel preparation with both oral and systemic antibiotics versus mechanical bowel preparation and systemic antibiotics alone for the prevention of surgical site infection after elective colorectal surgery: a meta-analysis of randomized controlled clinical trials. *Dis Colon Rectum*. 2016;59(1):70–78. PubMed PMID: 26651115.
41. Schultz JK, Yaqub S, Wallon C, et al. for SCANDIV Study Group. Laparoscopic lavage vs primary resection for acute perforated diverticulitis: the SCANDIV randomized clinical trial. *JAMA*. 2015;314(13):1364–1375. http://dx.doi.org/10.1001/jama.2015.12076. PubMed PMID: 26441181.

B. Anorectal Disease

John Kubasiak, M.D., and Marc Singer, M.D.

1. A 37-year-old man presents with a recurrent perianal abscess. The abscess was drained in the emergency department, and he is now being seen in the clinic for follow-up care. Which of the following is true about perirectal suppuration?

A. The pathophysiology of perirectal abscesses is related to infection of the perianal skin.

B. A horseshoe abscess is best drained at the bedside with the use of local anesthesia.

C. An intersphincteric abscess causes pain higher in the rectum, frequently without external manifestations.

D. Ischiorectal abscesses should be drained immediately under general anesthesia so that the fistula can be identified.

E. Perianal Crohn's disease is not a risk factor for recurrent disease.

ANSWER: C

COMMENTS: Most perirectal abscesses are the result of obstruction of the anal ducts and glands lying in the intersphincteric space. Horseshoe abscesses include bilateral ischiorectal, supralevator, or perianal abscesses that communicate. Horseshoe abscesses usually arise from infection of the posterior midline glands. A horseshoe ischiorectal abscess starts in the deep postanal space and extends bilaterally into each ischiorectal space. The patient is best treated in the operating room under regional or general anesthesia by incising the skin from the external sphincter to the coccyx. This exposes the superficial external sphincter, which is split longitudinally but not transected. The incision provides access to the deep postanal space. A probe is inserted into the posterior midline crypt and then into the deep postanal space. A seton is placed in this space and wrapped around the internal sphincter and superficial external sphincter. Counterincisions are made laterally along extensions of the abscess. An intersphincteric abscess is usually accompanied by pain and bulging inside the rectum but no external swelling. Treatment consists of transanally laying open the internal sphincter, beginning at the lower edge of the abscess and extending cephalad to the top of the abscess cavity. Most perianal abscesses can be drained with the use of local anesthesia, but if the patient has a high fever, significant leukocytosis, or extreme pain, treatment in the operating room under general anesthesia is preferable. Identification of a fistula may be deferred until there are clinical signs that a fistula is present, specifically, nonhealing of an abscess wound or recurrence of the abscess at the same location. Patients with anorectal Crohn's disease may experience recurrent abscesses despite maximal therapy. Anorectal abscesses may be the first manifestation of Crohn's disease in over 5% of patients, and up to 50% of patients with Crohn's disease will develop anorectal issues including abscesses, fistulas, anal ulcers, and large swollen skin tags at some point in their disease process.

Ref.: 1, 2, 4

2. All of the following are accepted applications of endorectal ultrasound except:

A. Assessing sphincter integrity in patients complaining of fecal incontinence

B. Determining whether a rectal cancer is suitable for local excision

C. Ruling out recurrent rectal cancer

D. Evaluating a transsphincteric anal fistula

E. Routine screening for rectal cancer

ANSWER: E

COMMENTS: Endorectal ultrasound imaging has had a significant impact on the diagnosis and management of a variety of anorectal diseases. The initial use of endoluminal ultrasound was for the staging of rectal cancers. The depth of penetration and the presence of abnormal lymph nodes were used to determine the stage of the cancer and its suitability for local excision. Generally, tumors that demonstrate deep penetration of the rectal wall have an increased likelihood of lymph node metastases and are not suitable candidates for transanal excision because of the unacceptably high recurrence rates associated with local excision of these advanced neoplasms. Most surgeons would restrict transanal excision to T1 tumors for curative intent. Recently, the use of ultrasound imaging for staging rectal cancers has been expanded to determine whether a lesion is advanced enough to warrant preoperative radiation therapy and chemotherapy. Ultrasound imaging can be used to assess the rectal wall and the extraluminal tissue for any sign of recurrent cancer following surgery. In this respect, it has distinct advantages over other imaging modalities, such as computed tomography, in that the probe is placed in direct contact with the operative site. Ultrasound has never been demonstrated to be beneficial for routine screening for rectal cancer. Ultrasound requires the application of the probe directly to the tissue of interest.

Endoscopic ultrasound (EUS) may be useful in several benign diseases of the anus and rectum. It may be used to image the sphincter mechanism in patients complaining of fecal incontinence. In fact, before a diagnosis of idiopathic or neurogenic incontinence is made, an ultrasound scan should be done to inspect the integrity of the sphincter. Ultrasound provides excellent diagnostic accuracy in determining disruptions of the internal and/or external sphincters. Although most anorectal abscesses and fistulas can be managed without imaging studies, ultrasound has proved useful for determining the extent of abscess collections laterally and in a cephalad direction. Furthermore, the relation of the tract of the fistula to the sphincter muscle can be assessed with ultrasound imaging. The internal opening can be identified as a hypoechoic disruption of the internal sphincter muscle. Hydrogen peroxide may be injected into the fistula tract during ultrasound scanning to further delineate the fistula tract.

Ref.: 3

3. A 36-year-old woman has prolapsing tissue and bleeding with bowel movements both in the toilet following forceful defecation and on the toilet paper. On examination, she has several large vascular lesions that are reducible with direct pressure. Which of the following statements regarding her most likely condition is true?

A. Internal hemorrhoids are vascular cushions arising proximal to the dentate line and are covered by anoderm.

B. Prolapsing hemorrhoids are external hemorrhoids covered by anoderm.

C. Bleeding internal hemorrhoids should be initially managed with surgical excision.

D. Thrombosed external hemorrhoids should be treated by hemorrhoidectomy with the patient under general anesthesia.

E. Recurrence is uncommon after surgical hemorrhoidectomy.

ANSWER: E

COMMENTS: Internal hemorrhoids are submucosal cushions normally located above the dentate line and are therefore covered by the transitional mucosa of the anal canal and not by anoderm. External hemorrhoids are the dilated veins of the inferior hemorrhoidal plexus located below the dentate line and are covered by anoderm. Prolapsing hemorrhoids are internal hemorrhoids that prolapse below the dentate line. Bleeding is the main manifestation of smaller internal hemorrhoids and is managed initially by rubber banding, infrared coagulation, or injection sclerotherapy. Surgery is reserved for internal hemorrhoids that do not respond to dietary measures and office procedures. Surgery may be the best initial therapy for large prolapsing internal hemorrhoids or for those that are acutely thrombosed and incarcerated. Thrombosed external hemorrhoids are most often treated by excision using local anesthesia in the office setting. General anesthesia is only required in the uncommon situation when they are quite large and circumferential. Internal hemorrhoidal recurrence is rare after formal surgical hemorrhoidectomy. When it does occur, it is usually related to inadequate removal of the rectal mucosa and hemorrhoidal tissue or inadequate management of chronic constipation.

Ref.: 1, 2, 5

4. A 40-year-old woman is evaluated for pain with defecation. The pain started acutely after a large bowel movement, is extremely intense following the passage of any stool, and persists for several hours. She is barely able to tolerate examination, which demonstrates a small defect in the anoderm located at the posterior midline. Which of the following statements regarding her condition is true?

A. Most lesions are located above the dentate line.

B. The lesions are always located at the posterior midline.

C. The operation of choice for this lesion is excision and posterior internal sphincterotomy.

D. Lateral partial subcutaneous sphincterotomy for lesions not in the midline is considered a definitive treatment.

E. Pharmacologic therapy with nitroglycerin, calcium channel blockers, or botulinum toxin may prove beneficial.

ANSWER: E

COMMENTS: An anal fissure is a tear of the skin-lined portion of the anal canal located below the dentate line. It is most commonly caused by hard bowel movements and straining. Occasionally, high internal anal sphincter tone is the cause. Gentle spreading of the buttocks is frequently all that is needed to reveal the fissure. Once the acute fissure is identified, digital examination and anoscopy may be deferred in the acute setting. About 90% of fissures (acute or chronic) are located in the posterior midline, an area where the anoderm is least supported by the sphincter and where blood flow is the poorest. The anterior midline is the second most common location and is involved in 10% of women. Fissures located laterally or multiple fissures should arouse suspicion for Crohn's disease, syphilis, tuberculosis, leukemia, or other causes, and therapy is directed toward the underlying disease. The initial treatment of a midline fissure is conservative and starts with a bowel management program including lubricants, fluids and fiber supplements, and warm baths. Over 90% of acute fissures will heal with this approach. Topical nitroglycerin or calcium channel blocking agents may help resolve chronic fissures in approximately 50% of patients; however, several weeks or months of treatment may be required. Botox injected directly into the internal sphincter on either side of the fissure may also produce healing in approximately 60% of patients. However, recurrence is common. Persistent chronic fissures are often used to high internal anal sphincter tension, which can be demonstrated on digital rectal examination or by anorectal manometry. Operative treatment consists of lateral partial internal sphincterotomy up to the dentate line to relax the internal sphincter. Posterior fissurectomy and sphincterotomy can lead to a keyhole defect and soiling. For this reason, lateral internal sphincterotomy has become the procedure of choice. Although mild incontinence to gas or diarrhea may be seen, it is infrequent enough to justify sphincterotomy in the small number of patients who do not respond to conservative therapies. External sphincterotomy should not be performed for anal fissure because it is not necessary and leads to unacceptably high rates of incontinence.

Ref.: 1, 2, 6

5. A 41-year-old patient with persistent pruritus ani is seen for further treatment after having undergone a biopsy. Which of the following statements is correct regarding possible causes of this problem?

A. Bowen's disease progresses rapidly to invasive cancer and requires urgent wide local excision.

B. Paget's disease of the perianal skin is often associated with breast cancer.

C. Basal cell carcinomas of the anal margin have an excellent prognosis.

D. Buschke-Löwenstein tumors are primarily treated by chemotherapy.

E. Surgical excision of Bowen's disease and Paget's disease requires 5-cm margins.

ANSWER: C

COMMENTS: Precursors to malignant disease are often found in the anal margin. Anal intraepithelial neoplasias, such as Bowen's or Paget's disease, can cause symptoms such as itching. Skin changes are usually present, and biopsy is indicated whenever the pruritus does not resolve with conservative measures. Bowen's disease represents high-grade dysplasia or squamous cell carcinoma in situ of the perianal skin. It is often associated with the human papillomavirus (HPV) (especially HPV types 16 and 18). It is usually indolent, and less than 5% progress to invasive cancer. Treatment consists of wide local excision with clear margins. Paget's disease is adenocarcinoma in situ of the perianal skin, usually from skin appendages such as ducts and glands. A lower gastrointestinal malignancy, usually a rectal or anal carcinoma, is found in 50%–70% of patients, but it is not associated with breast cancer. After evaluating the colon and anorectum for synchronous tumors, treatment is wide local excision. This disease may be multicentric, so circumferential mapping biopsies around the anal canal and perineum are part of the procedure. With HPV-related neoplasia, high-resolution anoscopy may be useful for targeting biopsies with excision or destruction of abnormal tissue, but this is primarily used in human immunodeficiency virus (HIV)–positive patients and men who have anoreceptive intercourse. Basal cell carcinoma of the perianal skin is rare and is associated with a 5-year survival rate of almost 100% following local surgical excision. Buschke-Löwenstein tumors, also called giant condylomas, are large verrucous squamous cell tumors of the anal canal and perineum due to HPV infection. Pathologically, they resemble condyloma and may have areas of invasive squamous cell carcinoma. They are rarely metastatic but may invade local structures around the anal canal or margin. Treatment consists of wide local excision or, rarely, abdominoperineal resection (APR) if the sphincter is invaded. Radiation therapy is occasionally used preoperatively to shrink large cancers or for patients with recurrent tumors.

Ref.: 1, 2, 7, 9

6. A 27-year-old man who engages in anal receptive intercourse has white, cauliflower-shaped masses throughout his perianal region and in the anal canal. Which of the following statements regarding his most likely condition is true?

A. The causative agent appears to be HPV.

B. Podophyllin, administered in a 25% solution, results in the resolution of the warts in 80% of patients, and recurrence rates are less than 10%.

C. Immunotherapy with vaccination is used as the initial treatment of small lesions.

D. Carcinoma frequently develops if the lesions are left untreated.

E. Surgical treatment involves excision and is not associated with any risk of transmission to health care providers.

ANSWER: A

COMMENTS: Anal infection with HPV is responsible for condyloma acuminatum, which appears as a group of cauliflower-shaped masses on the perianal skin and in the anal canal. The disease is transmitted by close contact and is seen in both genders regardless of whether anal intercourse is practiced. It is especially prevalent in anoreceptive men who have sex with men, and in this population, it is seen more often than genital warts. Another high-risk population consists of those receiving immunosuppression after organ transplantation. Podophyllin, a cytotoxic agent available in 10% and 25% solutions, must be applied by a physician. However, the results have been disappointing. Clearance of the warts has been noted in 22%–77% of patients, with recurrence rates being as high as 65%. Podophyllin may cause skin burns and cannot be used within the anal canal. Multiple treatments are usually necessary. Failure to treat intraanal lesions results in persistent disease. An autologous vaccine prepared from sampled condyloma can be injected weekly for 6 weeks. No adverse reactions have been seen, and resolution of lesions has been noted in up to 95% of patients. However, the process is not standardized, and so at present, such therapy is only considered for extensive, persistent, or recurrent cases of condyloma. Malignant transformation is a concern but occurs only rarely. Surgical treatment includes excision by one of three techniques (sharp excision with scissors, laser vaporization, or electrocautery excision and fulguration). Electrocautery is the preferred therapy and is associated with a recurrence rate of 10%–25%. With close follow-up and treatment of any recurrence, 95% of patients are rendered disease free. There is a risk of surgeon infection within the respiratory tract from the inhalation of vaporized viral particles. This risk can be minimized by using smoke evacuators and special masks during procedures.

Ref.: 7, 10

7. A 60-year-old woman complains of air and stool coming from her vagina. Digital rectal examination reveals an area of induration in the rectovaginal septum, although contrast barium enema does not demonstrate any abnormality. Which of the following statements regarding her probable condition is true?

A. Eighty-five percent of fistulas caused by obstetric trauma heal spontaneously.

B. Low rectovaginal fistulas may be treated effectively by primary fistulotomy.

C. Rectovaginal fistulas from Crohn's disease usually require proctectomy.

D. Repairs of radiation-induced rectovaginal fistulas generally include a stoma.

E. High rectovaginal fistulas respond well to fibrin glue.

ANSWER: D

COMMENTS: Rectovaginal fistulas are classified according to location and cause, which influences the type of corrective surgery required. High fistulas require an abdominal approach, whereas low fistulas can be repaired through a transanal, transperineal, or transvaginal approach. The common causes of these fistulas include obstetrical injuries, primary or recurrent cancer, radiation treatment of pelvic cancers, inflammatory bowel disease, trauma, or infection (e.g., cryptoglandular infection, tuberculosis, or lymphogranuloma venereum). Five percent of all vaginal deliveries are accompanied by third- or fourth-degree perineal lacerations. Approximately 10% of these repairs become disrupted and result in incontinence and/or a rectovaginal fistula. Approximately 50% of these obstetric fistulas heal spontaneously (not 85%); therefore if the patient's symptoms are not disabling, a 3- to 6-month waiting period is recommended. This waiting period also allows the tissue inflammation and edema to subside before surgical intervention. Repair of a fistula secondary to an obstetric injury can be performed transvaginally or transrectally. With the former, the tract is excised and the rectovaginal septum is inverted with serial purse-string sutures. With the latter, a flap consisting of mucosa, submucosa, and muscularis is advanced to cover the rectal side of the fistula. A diverting colostomy is not required unless previous surgical attempts have failed. A low anovaginal fistula may be treated by fistulotomy, but rectovaginal fistulas (even distal ones) should not be treated by this method. Partial or total incontinence may result if the fistula tract is divided.

High rectovaginal fistulas are best treated through a transabdominal approach so that coexisting pathologic conditions such as diverticulitis, cancer, or inflammatory bowel disease can be addressed. The rectovaginal septum is mobilized, the fistula is divided, the vagina is closed, and normal tissue (such as omentum or a muscle flap) is used to buttress the repair. Because the colon is not usually normal (inflammation or radiation injury), bowel resection is generally necessary.

Fistulas secondary to Crohn's disease do not always require proctectomy if the symptoms are minimal, the rectum is relatively healthy, and continence is normal. In such cases, an advancement flap can lead to healing. When there is refractory rectal Crohn's disease (especially the stricturing form) or incontinence, proctectomy with a colostomy is often ultimately needed. Radiation-induced fistulas may be very difficult to treat since the radiated tissue does not heal well. Repair requires use of nonradiated tissue, and so may include partial proctectomy with left colon-to-rectum anastomosis and/or use of an omental or gracilis muscle flap. A colostomy or ileostomy as sole therapy (e.g., a poor-risk patient with recurrent, unresectable cancer or multiple failed attempts at repair) or to divert stool from an anastomosis after resection of diseased bowel is often necessary.

Ref.: 8, 10

8. A 65-year-old woman presents to your office reporting 1 year of fecal incontinence. She states that she experiences the loss of loose stools twice per week. She typically passes five loose or watery stools daily. She has a history of four vaginal deliveries including at least one episiotomy. She had a normal screening colonoscopy 1 year ago. The most appropriate initial treatment for these symptoms is:

A. Colostomy

B. Bulk-forming agents and loperamide

C. Sacral nerve stimulation

D. Artificial bowel sphincter

E. Overlapping sphincteroplasty

ANSWER: B

COMMENTS: Fecal incontinence is commonly related to obstetric injuries, which result in a sphincter defect. However, the quality of the stool is also a common contributing cause of incontinence. A patient with marginal sphincter function may experience incontinence when the stool is loose or watery. Treatment with bulk-forming agents, such as psyllium husk, and/or loperamide will bulk the stool. Treatment of the diarrhea will cure the symptoms of incontinence in many patients. If unsuccessful, then physical therapy including biofeedback may be employed. Sphincter reconstruction and sacral nerve stimulation are well documented to improve symptoms; however, they should be reserved for patients who do not improve with medical therapy and bowel management.

Ref.: 10

9. A 47-year-old man presents with a 2.5-cm anal mass arising just proximal to the dentate line, involving > 1/2 of the circumference of the anal canal, and fixed to the internal sphincter muscle. Biopsies show squamous cell carcinoma. Metastatic evaluation is negative. What treatment would you recommend for this patient?

A. Low anterior resection with coloanal anastomosis

B. High-resolution anoscopy

C. 5-Flourouricil, mitomycin C, and radiation therapy

D. APR with colostomy

E. Wide local excision with clear margins and close surveillance

ANSWER: C

COMMENTS: This is a localized anal canal squamous cell carcinoma. TNM staging of anal carcinoma includes the size of the primary lesion. T1 lesions are 2 cm or less in diameter; T2 are > 2 cm to 5 cm, T3 are > 5 cm, and T4 are invading into an adjacent structure beyond the sphincter muscles. The lesion is staged as T2, N0, M0. Endorectal ultrasound or magnetic resonance imaging (MRI) may further define the depth of penetration, extension to other organs, and lymph node status. It is important to examine the inguinal lymph nodes since this is a common site of spread. The primary treatment of localized squamous cell carcinoma of the anal canal was defined by Norman Nigro, M.D. (the Nigro protocol), who demonstrated that combined chemoradiation therapy was much more effective than radical surgery (APR), with high rates of anal preservation. The modified Nigro protocol in use today includes a course of chemotherapy using 5-fluorouracil (5-FU) and mitomycin C and 6 weeks of radiation therapy to a dose of about 5400 cGy. Anal canal carcinoma must be differentiated from anal margin carcinoma. Any squamous cell carcinoma that has any part within the anal canal (from the anal verge to the anorectal ring) is considered an anal canal carcinoma, while anal margin lesions are entirely outside of the anal canal in the perineal skin. Anal margin carcinomas are treated by local excision with clear margins, which results in a high rate of cure. APR is reserved for persistent or recurrent cancer or if the patient has previously received radiation therapy for other indications. The modified Nigro protocol results in an initial complete response in 90% of patients. Salvage APR for persistence or recurrence results in a cure rate of 25%–50%. So, the overall 5-year disease-free survival for anal canal carcinoma is about 80%.

Ref.: 11

10. A 32-year-old male with third-degree internal hemorrhoids underwent an operative hemorrhoidectomy in the surgical center and was discharged home. What is the most common early postoperative complication after hemorrhoidectomy?

A. Urinary retention

B. Bleeding

C. Fecal Incontinence

D. Perirectal abscess

E. Anal fissure

ANSWER: A

COMMENTS: The most common early postoperative complication after hemorrhoid surgery is urinary retention. This typically occurs in 10% (2%–36%) of patients. The incidence of postoperative urinary retention is more common in men and is directly related to the volume of intravenous fluids administered. In addition, it may be related to narcotic administration and regional anesthesia. Other complications include bleeding (0.03%–6%), anal stenosis (0%–6%), infection (0.5%–5%), and incontinence (2%–12%). Bleeding is the next most common complication of stapled hemorrhoidopexy. Other complications unique to stapled hemorrhoidopexy include rectovaginal fistula, rectal perforation, rectal occlusion, and chronic pain related to an inappropriately distal staple line.

Ref.: 11, 12

11. A 47-year-old man with poorly controlled diabetes mellitus presents to your clinic complaining of anal bulging and bleeding with bowel movements. Anoscopy shows a single left lateral, second-degree internal hemorrhoid. You perform rubber band ligation without difficulty, and the patient is sent home. The following evening your answering service receives a call from the patient who is complaining of fever, anal pain, and difficulty urinating. What is your recommendation?

A. Encourage increased fluid intake, stool softeners, Sitz baths, and oral analgesics.

B. Tell the patient to call his primary care physician.

C. Ask the patient to return to the clinic in the morning.

D. Perform an examination under anesthesia urgently.

E. Remove the band in the office.

ANSWER: D

COMMENTS: Rubber band ligation is commonly performed for first- and second-degree hemorrhoids. The band is placed on the redundant mucosa a minimum of 2 cm proximal to the dentate line. This will slough off in 5-7 days and can be associated with light bleeding. Complications of banding include pain, thrombosis, bleeding, and perineal or pelvic sepsis. Placing the band too close to the dentate line will cause immediate pain and require removal. Thrombosis of the internal, external, or both complexes may be managed by observation and analgesics if mild or by operative hemorrhoidectomy if extensive. Significant bleeding is abnormal and may require control of the bleeding site in the office or the operating room (OR). Life-threatening sepsis due to necrotizing infection is rare but mandates immediate evaluation and treatment (fluid, antibiotics, and examination in the OR). This sepsis is associated with severe diabetes and states of immune suppression. Early recognition of this problem is critical, and treatment must be rapid.

Ref.: 12

12. A 45-year-old male with a 4-cm anal mass above the dentate line is found to have squamous cell carcinoma on biopsy. In this patient, which nodal basin is likely to be the initial site of spread?

A. Inferior mesenteric artery nodes

B. Internal iliac nodes

C. Inguinal nodes

D. Para-aortic nodes

E. Sister Mary Joseph node

ANSWER: B

COMMENTS: Lymphatic drainage of the upper and middle rectum includes the inferior mesenteric and para-aortic nodes. Drainage from the lower one-third of the rectum occurs partially in a cephalad direction toward the inferior mesenteric artery, but also laterally along the middle hemorrhoidal vessels to the internal iliac nodes. Anal canal lymphatic drainage is defined by the relationship of the lesion to the dentate line. Superior to the dentate line, drainage occurs to the inferior mesenteric and internal iliac nodes. Distal to or below the dentate line, drainage occurs along the inferior lymphatics to the superficial inguinal nodes. The Sister Mary Joseph node is a peri-umbilical nodule and often due to metastatic gastric or pancreatic cancer.

Ref.: 12

13. A 28-year-old Caucasian man presents with a 9-month history of anal pain during and after defecation with a trace of red blood on the toilet tissue. On anoscopy, there is an irregular fibrotic tear in the anoderm in the right lateral position. Further evaluation of this problem should include:

A. Colonoscopy

B. QuantiFERON gold test

C. Complete blood count

D. HIV testing

E. All of the above

ANSWER: E

COMMENTS: Chronic anal fissures in the lateral position are rare and should prompt consideration of alternative diagnoses. These include Crohn's disease, leukemia, tuberculosis, syphilis, HIV, or anal carcinoma. The QuantiFERON gold test is useful for diagnosing both active and latent *Mycobacterium tuberculosis* infection. Medical treatments such as bowel management, Sitz baths, topical lidocaine, topical nitroglycerin, or nifedipine may be initiated for pain relief and to promote healing. However, sphincterotomy should not be recommended until other causative disorders are identified and treated. Sphincterotomy in the setting of untreated Crohn's disease or HIV may result in nonhealing wounds and/or fecal incontinence.

Ref.: 12

14. An 89-year-old multiparous female with chronic obstructive pulmonary disease (COPD) presents with a 12-month history of a worsening anal bulge and fecal incontinence. On examination, she has a 5-cm full-thickness rectal prolapse. It is easily reduced but spontaneously reprolapses. What is the best surgical treatment for this patient?

A. Low anterior resection

B. Perineal rectosigmoidectomy

C. Transabdominal mesh rectopexy

D. Laparoscopic sigmoid resection

E. Robotic sigmoid resection and mesh rectopexy

ANSWER: B

COMMENTS: Full-thickness rectal prolapse involves all layers of the rectal wall. It is often associated with fecal incontinence, particularly in elderly multiparous patients. Initial treatment includes high-fiber diet and stool softeners to prevent straining. This may reduce the severity of the prolapse but will not cure it. In healthy patients with constipation, sigmoid resection with sutured rectopexy (Frykman procedure) can result in low rates of recurrence and improvement in constipation. Patients with fecal incontinence ideally should not undergo sigmoid resection, as this may worsen this symptom. Abdominal procedures should be avoided in older frail patients because of the risks. These patients are better suited for a perineal approach such as a perineal rectosigmoidectomy (Altemeier procedure). This is a low-risk operation that may be performed under regional anesthesia or even sedation with local anesthesia. The redundant rectum and colon are resected from the perineal approach with a coloanal anastomosis. A levateroplasty may be added to tighten up the levator hiatus and possibly improve incontinence. Although the loss of the rectal vault may worsen incontinence and frequency and the recurrence rate is higher than with abdominal procedures, the very low risk and rapid recovery make this the best operation in this group of patients.

Ref.: 12, 13

15. A 42-year-old previously healthy man has had a 4-day history of increasing rectal pain and difficulty sitting. Examination shows a 3-cm area of erythema and fluctuance consistent with a perianal abscess. Which of the following is true regarding the anatomic spaces in which this process may occur?

A. The supralevator space is situated above the levator ani muscles and is connected with the contralateral side anteriorly.

B. The retrorectal space lies between the rectum and the sacrum but below the rectosacral fascia.

C. The deep postanal space lies below the levator ani muscles and posterior to the external sphincter muscles.

D. The perianal space and the superficial postanal space lie deep to the superficial portion of the external anal sphincter.

E. The intersphincteric space lies just outside the conjoined longitudinal muscle.

ANSWER: C

COMMENTS: The supralevator space is bounded superiorly by the peritoneum, laterally by the pelvic walls, medially by the rectum, and inferiorly by the levator ani muscles (Figs. 23B.1 and 23B.2). It communicates with the contralateral side posteriorly. Infection in this space can arise from an abdominal or pelvic source (e.g., diverticulitis or pelvic inflammatory disease) or as an upward extension from an anorectal source. The retrorectal space lies above the rectosacral fascia between the upper two-thirds of the rectum and sacrum. The fascia runs downward and forward from the sacrum to the anorectal junction. The retrorectal space contains loose connective tissue and is a site for the formation of tumors arising from embryologic remnants (i.e., dermoids, teratomas, and chordomas). The retrorectal space is bounded anteriorly by the rectum, posteriorly by the presacral fascia, laterally by the pelvic side wall, superiorly by the peritoneal reflection, and inferiorly by the rectosacral fascia, below which is the supralevator space. The ischiorectal space lies below the levator muscle, above the transverse septum of the ischiorectal fossa, and between the external sphincter and the lateral pelvic wall. This space communicates posteriorly through the deep postanal space, which lies between the levator ani and the superficial external sphincter. The lower border of the deep postanal space is the anococcygeal ligament, which originates from the superficial portion of the external sphincter in the posterior midline. This communication allows an abscess in the deep postanal space to extend to both ischiorectal spaces (horseshoe abscess). The perianal space (the most common space involved in abscesses) lies superficial to the superficial external anal sphincter. The intersphincteric space lies within the conjoined longitudinal muscle, where the anal glands are also located. The perianal, ischiorectal, and supralevator spaces may connect posteriorly with their counterparts on the contralateral side to form a horseshoe connection in any of these spaces.

Ref.: 2, 4, 14

16. A 55-year-old man presents to the clinic with a long-standing anal fissure with pain on defecation and red streaking after bowel movements. He has failed conservative measures. On anoscopy you note a small posterior midline fissure with surrounding fibrosis, a skin tag, and a hypertrophied papilla. You plan a lateral internal sphincterotomy. In performing this procedure, you will divide a continuation of which muscle?

A. Puborectalis muscle

B. Muscularis propria of the rectum

C. Levator ani muscle

D. Conjoined longitudinal muscle

E. Subcutaneous external anal sphincter muscle

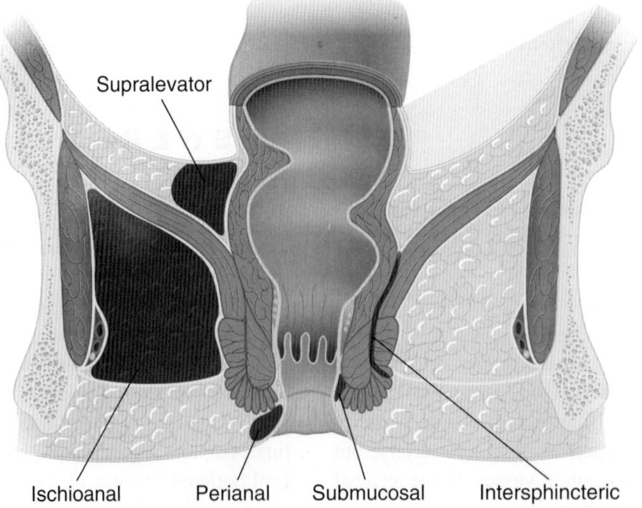

Fig. 23B.1 Coronal section diagram showing possible locations of perirectal abscesses and their relation to normal structures. *(From Vasilevsky CA, Gordon PH. Benign anorectal: abscess and stula. In: Wolff BG, Fleshman JW, Beck DE, eds.* The ASCRS Textbook of Colon and Rectal Surgery. *New York: Springer Science + Business Media, LLC; 2007:193, Fig. 13.1A and B.)*

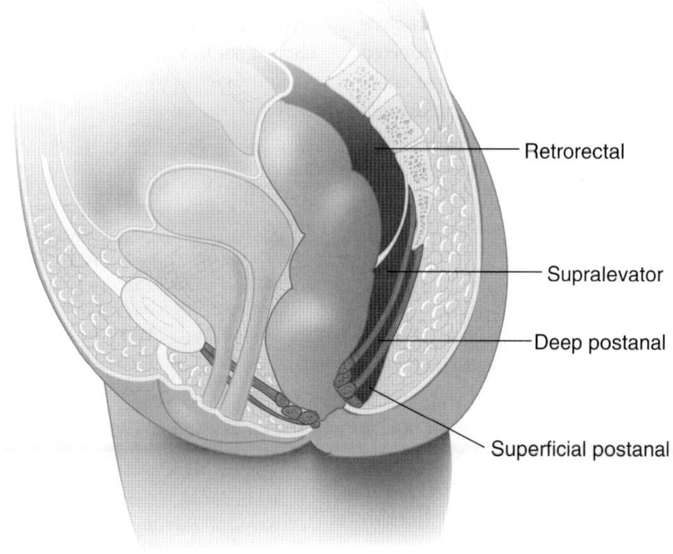

Fig. 23B.2 Sagittal section diagram showing possible locations of perirectal abscesses and their relation to normal structures. *(From Vasilevsky CA, Gordon PH. Benign anorectal: abscess and stula. In: Wolff BG, Fleshman JW, Beck DE, eds.* The ASCRS Textbook of Colon and Rectal Surgery. *New York: Springer Science + Business Media, LLC; 2007:193, Fig. 13.1A and B.)*

TABLE 23B.1 Classification of Internal Hemorrhoids

	First degree	Second degree	Third degree	Fourth degree
Finding	Bulge into the lumen of the anal canal ± painless bleeding	Protrude at the time of a bowel movement and reduce spontaneously	Protrude spontaneously or with bowel movement, require manual replacement	Permanently prolapsed and irreducible
Symptoms	Painless bleeding	Painless bleeding Anal mass with defecation Anal burning or pruritus Mucous leakage Fecal leakage	Painless bleeding Anal mass with defecation Feeling of incomplete evacuation Mucous leakage Fecal leakage Perianal burning or pruritus ani Difficulty with perianal hygiene	Painless or painful bleeding Irreducible anal mass Feeling of incomplete evacuation Perianal burning or pruritus ani Difficulty with perianal hygiene
Signs	Bright red bleeding Bleeding at end of defecation Blood drips or squirts into toilet Bleeding may be occult	Bright red bleeding Prolapse with defecation Anemia extremely rate	Bright red bleeding Blood drips or squirts into toilet Prolapsed hemorrhoids reduce manually Perianal stool or mucus Anemia extremely rare	Bright red bleeding Blood drips or squirts into toilet Prolapsed hemorrhoids always out Perianal stool or mucus

From Cintron JR, Abcarian H. Benign anorectal: hemorrhoids. In: Wexner SD, ed. *The ASCRS Textbook of Colon and Rectal Surgery*. New York: Springer Science + Business Media, LLC; 2009:229, Table 23B.1.

ANSWER: B

COMMENTS: The internal anal sphincter represents the distal 2.5 to 4.0 cm of the circular muscle layer (muscularis propria) of the rectum. This sphincter is therefore smooth muscle and under autonomic control. In its basal state, it is contracted, creating a natural barrier to the loss of stool and gas. The external anal sphincter is a continuation of the puborectalis muscle. This sphincter is a striated muscle, and like the other pelvic floor muscles, it is maintained by an unconscious resting tone at the level of the cauda equine but can be voluntarily relaxed and contracted. The conjoined longitudinal muscle combines with fibers of the levator ani and then descends and crosses the external anal sphincter to insert into the perianal skin.

Ref.: 15

17. A 33-year-old woman with a history of multiple pregnancies and irritable bowel syndrome (IBS) presents to the clinic with an anal bulge. She has a history of bulging with bowel movements, fecal leakage, and occasional bright red bleeding on the toilet paper. On anoscopy, you note two enlarged hemorrhoid plexuses: one left lateral and one right posterior. Both prolapse with Valsalva and reduce spontaneously. What degree do these represent?

A. First-degree hemorrhoids

B. Second-degree hemorrhoids

C. Third-degree hemorrhoids

D. Fourth-degree hemorrhoids

E. Rectal prolapse

ANSWER: B

COMMENTS: The internal hemorrhoidal tissues originate proximal to the dentate line and are vascular structures that are covered by mucosa (transitional and columnar epithelium). The anal canal from 1 to 2 cm above the dentate line is viscerally innervated and is insensitive to pain, touch, or temperature, and therefore amenable to office procedures without the need for anesthetics. Internal hemorrhoids are classified by 4 degrees depending on the amount of prolapse. Table 23B.1 reviews the differences in internal hemorrhoids by degree.

Ref.: 16

18. An 18-year-old otherwise healthy college student presents to your office complaining of chronic, recurrent pain, and drainage from a wound at the superior aspect of his gluteal cleft. On examination, he has a single midline pit with minimal serous drainage and no surrounding erythema. There are no surrounding sinus tracts. He has never received medical attention for this issue. The most appropriate management is:

A. A cleft lift procedure

B. Observation

C. Topical clindamycin

D. Excision with off-midline closure

E. Incision and drainage

ANSWER: D

COMMENTS: This patient suffers from pilonidal disease. This is mostly likely due to hair follicles that become distended with keratin and then subsequently infected, rupturing into the subcutaneous tissue. This is most likely due to micro-trauma related to the weight of the buttocks having its greatest support (and effect) at the midline skin of the gluteal cleft. The patient does not have an abscess or cellulitis. Therefore drainage or antibiotics are not indicated. Pilonidal disease will cause recurrent symptoms unless definitively treated with excision closure of the midline pit(s) and elimination of the associated epithelialized sinus tract extending from the pit to the abscess cavity. This may be accomplished by excision removing the midline pit, epithelialized tract, and abscess cavity. Excision may be accompanied by leaving the wound open. This is an acceptable treatment option; however, it requires dressing changes that are difficult for patients to perform themselves. The cleft lift procedure has been demonstrated to achieve high rates of cure, with few wound complications; however, as the initial procedure for uncomplicated disease is not indicated, it may be overly aggressive. As the pilonidal is not infected, incision and drainage is not indicated. Simple excision and closure of the wound is indicated. Off-midline closure has been established as the preferred technique compared with midline closure, as this reduces the tension on the wound caused by the weight of the buttocks.

Ref.: 17

REFERENCES

1. Bullard KM, Rothenberger DA. Colon, rectum and anus. In: Brunicardi FC, Andersen DK, Billiar TR, et al., eds. *Schwartz's Principles of Surgery*. 9th ed. New York: McGraw-Hill; 2010.
2. Nelson H, Cima RR. Anus. In: Townsend CM, Beauchamp RD, Evers BM, et al., eds. *Sabiston Textbook of Surgery: The Biological Basis of Modern Surgical Practice*. 18th ed. Philadelphia: WB Saunders; 2008.
3. Saclarides TJ. Anorectal ultrasound. In: Machi J, Staren ED, eds. *Ultrasound for Surgeons*. 2nd ed. Philadelphia: Lippincott Williams & Wilkins; 2005.
4. Glasgow SC, Dietz DW. Anorectal abscess and fistula. In: Cameron JL, ed. *Current Surgical Therapy*. 9th ed. Philadelphia: Mosby; 2008.
5. Gregorcyk SG, Huber Jr PJ. Hemorrhoids. In: Cameron JL, ed. *Current Surgical Therapy*. 9th ed. Philadelphia: Mosby; 2008.
6. Costedio M, Cataldo PA. Anal fissures. In: Cameron JL, ed. *Current Surgical Therapy*. 9th ed. Philadelphia: Mosby; 2008.
7. Ayscue JM, Smith LE. Tumors of the anal region. In: Cameron JL, ed. *Current Surgical Therapy*. 9th ed. Philadelphia: Mosby; 2008.
8. Tran NA, Thorson AG. Rectovaginal fistula. In: Cameron JL, ed. *Current Surgical Therapy*. 9th ed. Philadelphia: Mosby; 2008.
9. Corman M. *Colon and Rectal Surgery*. Philadelphia: JB Lippincott; 2005.
10. Gordon PH, Nivatvongs S. *Principles and Practice of Surgery of the Colon, Rectum and Anus*. St. Louis: Quality Medical; 1999.
11. Senagore AJ, Singer M, Abcarian H, et al. A prospective, randomized, controlled multicenter trial comparing stapled hemorrhoidopexy and Ferguson hemorrhoidectomy: perioperative and one-year results. *Dis Rectum*. 2004;47(11):1824–1836.
12. Beck DE, Roberts PL, Saclarides TJ, et al. In: *The ASCRS Textbook of Colon and Rectal Surgery*. New York: Springer Science & Business Media; 2011.
13. Nelson RL, Thomas K, Morgan J, et al. Nonsurgical therapy for anal fissure. *Cochrane Database Syst Rev*. 2012;2:CD003431.
14. Vasilevsky CA, Gordon PH. Benign anorectal: abscess and stula. In: Wolff BG, Fleshman JW, Beck DE, eds. *The ASCRS Textbook of Colon and Rectal Surgery*. New York: Springer Science + Business Media, LLC; 2007:192–193.
15. Cintron JR, Abcarian H. Benign anorectal: hemorrhoids. In: Wexner SD, ed. *The ASCRS Textbook of Colon and Rectal Surgery*. New York: Springer Science + Business Media, LLC; 2009:225–254.
16. Cintron JR, Abcarian H. Benign anorectal: hemorrhoids. In: Wexner SD, ed. *The ASCRS Textbook of Colon and Rectal Surgery*. New York: Springer Science + Business Media, LLC; 2009:229.
17. Nelson JM, Billingham RP. Pilonidal disease and hidradenitis suppurativa. In: Wolff BG, Fleshman JW, Beck DE, eds. *The ASCRS Textbook of Colon and Rectal Surgery*. New York: Springer Science + Business Media, LLC; 2007:228–239.

SECTION VI

LIVER, BILIARY TRACT, PANCREAS, AND SPLEEN

CHAPTER 24

LIVER AND PORTAL VENOUS SYSTEM

Nasim T. Babazadeh, M.D., and Edie Y. Chan, M.D.

1. Which of the following statements about the anatomy of the liver is true?

A. The right and left lobe are divided by the falciform ligament.

B. The portal triad consists of the hepatic artery, hepatic vein, and bile duct.

C. The caudate lobe has its own separate arterial supply.

D. The right lobe contains anterior and posterior segments.

E. The American system describes eight segments.

ANSWER: D

COMMENTS: The surgical anatomy of the liver is based on the distribution of the hepatic veins and portal structures, and it has been modified several times. There are two main anatomic classification systems for the liver: the American system and the French system. In both these systems, the liver is divided into right and left lobes by the Cantlie line, a longitudinal plane that extends from the gallbladder fossa to the inferior vena cava. This plane, also called the portal fissure, contains the middle hepatic vein and the bifurcation of the portal vein. In the American system, the liver is further broken down into four segments, with each lobe containing two segments. The right lobe of the liver consists of posterior and anterior segments. The left lobe consists of a medial segment (quadrate lobe) and a lateral segment divided by the falciform ligament. The caudate lobe can be considered anatomically independent of the right and left lobes because it receives portal and arterial blood supply from both sides and has venous drainage directly into the inferior vena cava.

In the French system, developed by C. Couinaud, the two lobes of the liver are broken down into eight segments. These eight segments are formed by three vertical planes (scissurae) created by the right, middle, and left hepatic veins, which results in four sectors. These four sectors are further divided by a plane created by the branching portal system. Therefore the left lobe, according to the French system, is divided into medial and lateral segments by the left hepatic vein. The lateral sector of the left lobe consists of a superior segment (II) and an inferior segment (III). The medial sector of the left lobe is segment IV. The right lobe consists of anteromedial and posterolateral sectors divided by a vertical plane containing the right hepatic vein. The anteromedial sector is made up of segment V (inferior) and segment VIII (superior), and the posterolateral sector is made up of segment VI (inferior) and segment VII (superior).

Ref.: 1–3

2. Which of the following statements is true about the hepatic arterial supply?

A. Aberrant hepatic arterial anatomy is present in less than 5% of all patients.

B. The cystic artery is usually a branch off the proper hepatic artery.

C. A "replaced" right hepatic artery arises from the superior mesenteric artery.

D. The hepatic artery provides 75% of the blood flow to the liver.

E. The hepatic artery lies dorsal to the portal vein within the hepatic hilum.

ANSWER: C

COMMENTS: The hepatic arterial supply is normally derived from the celiac axis by way of the common hepatic artery, which becomes the proper hepatic artery after giving off the gastroduodenal branch and subsequently bifurcates into right and left hepatic branches. The hepatic artery lies ventral to the portal vein. The middle hepatic artery is usually a branch off the left hepatic artery, and the cystic artery is generally a branch off the right hepatic artery. There is, however, significant variability in hepatic arterial anatomy in up to 50% of patients. In approximately 15% of individuals, the right hepatic artery arises from the superior mesenteric artery (replaced right hepatic artery) and is found in the right dorsal border of the hepatoduodenal ligament. In roughly 10% of individuals, the left hepatic artery originates from the left gastric artery and is located in the gastrohepatic ligament. These commonly encountered variants can have important surgical implications during upper abdominal operations. The arterial blood supply accounts for only 25% of hepatic blood flow, with the remainder being supplied by the portal vein.

Ref.: 1–3

3. Which of the following statements about the anatomy of the hepatic veins is true?

A. The left hepatic vein drains the entire left lobe.

B. Veins from the caudate lobe enter both the left and middle hepatic veins.

C. The middle hepatic vein usually joins the left hepatic vein.

D. There are valves in the hepatic venous system.

E. Hepatic veins have prominent hyperechoic walls on ultrasound imaging.

ANSWER: C

COMMENTS: The hepatic veins begin in the liver lobules as the central veins and coalesce to form the right, left, and middle hepatic veins, which drain into the inferior vena cava and are of considerable surgical importance because they define the three vertical scissurae of the liver. The right vein, which is generally the largest, drains most of the right lobe. The left vein drains the lateral segment of the left lobe and a portion of the medial segment as well. The middle vein drains the inferoanterior portion of the right lobe and the inferomedial segment of the left lobe. This vein joins the left hepatic vein in 80% of individuals and enters the inferior vena cava directly in the remainder. There are also smaller veins, particularly those draining the caudate lobe dorsally, that enter directly into the inferior vena cava. The human hepatic venous system has no valves. The portal veins and hepatic veins can readily be differentiated from each other on the basis of their distinctive sonographic features. The portal veins (not the hepatic veins) have prominent hyperechoic walls.

Ref.: 1–4

4. Which of the following statements is true about the portal vein?
   A. It is formed by the junction of the inferior mesenteric vein and splenic vein.
   B. It is the most dorsal structure in the hepatoduodenal ligament.
   C. It contains the valves of Mirizzi.
   D. The right portal vein typically branches later than the left portal vein.
   E. It carries deoxygenated blood and provides only 10% of the liver's oxygenation.

ANSWER: B

COMMENTS: The portal vein is usually formed dorsal to the neck of the pancreas by the junction of the superior mesenteric vein and splenic veins. It ascends posterior to the common bile duct and hepatic artery in the hepatoduodenal ligament. These three structures make up the portal triad. There are no valves in the portal venous system (Pablo Mirizzi described valves in the common hepatic duct that do not exist). The portal vein bifurcates just outside the liver. The right portal vein has anterior and posterior branches that typically diverge only a short distance from the bifurcation and then quickly dive into the liver parenchyma. The left portal vein has a longer transverse portion (pars transversus) and then angulates anteriorly in the umbilical fissure (pars umbilicus), where it gives off medial branches to segment IV and lateral branches to segments II and III. The portal vein provides approximately 75% of the hepatic blood flow, and although the blood is largely deoxygenated, it provides up to 50%–70% of the liver's oxygenation secondary to the portal system's large volume flow rate.

Ref.: 1–3

5. Which of the following characteristics is typically seen on ultrasound imaging of the hepatic portal vein branches?
   A. Hyperechoic vessel walls
   B. Hepatofugal blood flow
   C. Diastolic reversal of blood flow
   D. Location between hepatic segments
   E. Vertical orientation

ANSWER: A

COMMENTS: The portal veins and hepatic veins can readily be differentiated from each other on the basis of their distinctive sonographic features. The portal vein and its branches have prominent hyperechoic walls. This appearance has been attributed to the accompanying intrahepatic branches of the hepatic artery and bile duct, which are not generally seen individually on external ultrasound imaging. In contrast, the hepatic veins appear to be essentially "wall less." They are anechoic or hypoechoic tubular structures that are vertically oriented and increase in caliber as they course toward the inferior vena cava. The portal veins are more transversely oriented and of larger caliber centrally. The portal vein branches are located within the anatomic liver segments, and the hepatic veins are found between the segments. Doppler ultrasound permits characterization of flow patterns in the hepatic vessels. Under normal circumstances, portal vein flow is toward the liver (hepatopedal). Flow in the portal vein is usually of fairly low velocity, with minor undulations and continued forward flow during diastole. Flow in the hepatic veins is hepatofugal and varies according to the cardiorespiratory cycle. The portal veins are horizontally oriented, whereas the hepatic veins are vertically oriented.

Ref.: 4

6. Which of the following is true regarding the hepatic functional unit?
   A. The center of the hepatic lobule is the hepatic venule.
   B. Blood flows from the hepatic vein to the portal triad.
   C. Zone I is the most susceptible to hypoxic injury.
   D. Hepatocytes in zone I have the lowest oxygen tension.
   E. Bile flows toward the centrilobular hepatic venule.

ANSWER: A

COMMENTS: The functional histologic unit of the liver is the acinus. At the center of the acinus is the portal triad, which consists of a terminal branch of the portal vein (portal venule) along with a hepatic arteriole and bile ductule. Blood from the terminal portal venule goes into the hepatic sinusoids, around which hepatocytes are located. Eventually, blood returns to the central vein leading to the terminal hepatic venules at the periphery of the acinar unit. The hepatocytes of the acinus are divided into three zones, with zone I being closest to the afferent portal venule and zone III being nearest the efferent central hepatic venule. Zone II is between these two points. Within the acinus, there is a gradient of solute concentration and oxygen tension that is greatest near the portal venules at the center of the acinus. The hepatocytes in zone I are therefore exposed to more oxygen and are less subject to hypoxia compared with the hepatocytes near the periphery of the acinus (zone III). This explains the histologic pattern of centrilobular necrosis that occurs following ischemia. The hepatic venule is at the center of the histologic hepatic lobule. Each hepatic lobule is thus surrounded by several peripheral acini. Bile is formed within the hepatocytes and empties into terminal canaliculi, which coalesce into bile ducts. The bile then flows toward the portal triad.

Ref.: 1, 3

7. What is the pathologic feature of cirrhosis?
   A. Apoptosis of hepatocytes, involving lobules and portal tracts
   B. Fat accumulation in hepatocytes

C. Brown pigment in hepatocytes

D. Periductal fibrosis with an onion-skin appearance

E. Dense matrix material deposition in the perisinusoidal space

ANSWER: E

COMMENTS: Cirrhosis may be due to many processes. It is defined as end-stage liver damage with hepatocyte death and disruption of hepatic parenchyma by diffuse fibrosis (dense matrix material deposition) and abnormal nodular architecture. Pathologic characteristics include fibrous septa around regenerative nodules of hepatocytes. The bands of fibrosis originate from stellate cells located beneath endothelial cells that line the sinusoids, in the space of Disse (perisinusoidal space).

Clinical manifestations include increased hepatic pressure, portal venous congestion and portal hypertension, ascites, coagulopathy, steroid hormone imbalances, encephalopathy, hepatorenal syndrome, and hepatopulmonary syndrome. Despite historical schools of thought, it is now known that even in late-stage disease, some regression of cirrhosis is possible.

Apoptosis of hepatocytes involving lobules and portal tracts is seen in hepatitis. Fat accumulation in hepatocytes is seen in the alcoholic fatty liver disease. Brown pigment in hepatocytes, or hemosiderosis, is due to iron deposition in hepatocytes in hemochromatosis. Periductal fibrosis with an onion-skin appearance is seen in primary biliary cirrhosis.

Ref.: 5–7

8. Which of the following statements related to liver embryology is true?

A. The liver is derived from the hindgut.

B. Two umbilical veins carry placental blood to the liver.

C. One umbilical artery carries placental blood to the placenta.

D. The ductus venosus shunts blood from the portal vein to the systemic circulation.

E. The falciform ligament is the obliterated ductus arteriosus.

ANSWER: D

COMMENTS: The liver, gallbladder, and biliary tree are derived from a ventral diverticulum of the junction of the foregut and midgut.

In fetal circulation, one umbilical vein carries oxygenated blood from the placenta to the ductus venosus, which shunts blood from the portal vein to the inferior vena cava. The result is that the maternal blood, which has already undergone hepatic metabolism in the mother, largely bypasses the fetal liver. Two umbilical arteries carry deoxygenated blood back to the placenta. In the transition to extrauterine circulation, the umbilical vein degenerates as flow ceases, and stasis and thrombosis cause ductus venosus closure.

In the adult, the falciform ligament carries the umbilical vein remnant from the umbilicus. The ligamentum teres extends from the falciform ligament and carries the obliterated umbilical vein to the undersurface of the liver. The ligamentum venosum derives from the ductus venosus.

Ref.: 7–8

9. During fasting, the liver provides energy substrates by all but which of the following mechanisms?

A. Glycogenolysis

B. Glycolysis

C. Gluconeogenesis from alanine

D. Gluconeogenesis from lactate

E. Formation of ketone bodies from fatty acids

ANSWER: B

COMMENTS: The liver plays a pivotal role in energy metabolism. In the fed state, glucose is converted to glycogen for storage. The liver itself obtains its energy primarily from ketoacids rather than glucose, although it can use glycolysis during periods of glucose excess (fed state). During fasting, the liver provides glucose by the breakdown of the stored glycogen (glycogenolysis). Glucose is a critical energy source for red blood cells, the central nervous system, and the kidneys. Because glycogen stores are depleted after about 48 h, the liver generates glucose from other sources. Alanine, other amino acids, lactate, and glycerol can serve as carbon sources for gluconeogenesis. Lipolysis occurs during prolonged fasting, and the fatty acids released from adipose stores are oxidized in hepatocytes to form ketone bodies. Ketone bodies are an important alternative fuel source for brain and muscle.

Ref.: 1, 3, 9

10. The cytochrome P-450 system transforms compounds by all except which of the following mechanisms?

A. Oxidation

B. Hydrolysis

C. Conjugation

D. Reduction

E. Hydrogenation

ANSWER: C

COMMENTS: The liver is responsible for the biotransformation of many endogenous and exogenous substances. For the most part, this process detoxifies potentially injurious substances and facilitates their elimination. In some instances, however, hepatic biotransformation produces more toxic metabolites. There are two general mechanisms by which the liver accomplishes biotransformation: oxidation, reduction, and hydrolysis (phase I reactions) and conjugation (phase II reactions). The cytochrome P-450 enzyme system catalyzes phase I reactions. The second mechanism involves an array of enzymes that conjugate substances with other endogenous molecules. These reactions are referred to as phase II reactions, and their purpose is to convert hydrophobic compounds to hydrophilic ones that are water soluble and can thus be eliminated in bile or urine. The liver is also the principal site of conversion of ammonia to urea via the urea cycle, which is a separate process.

Ref.: 1, 3, 9

11. A 63-year-old woman with unresectable cholangiocarcinoma undergoing palliative therapy presents with fever, right upper quadrant pain, jaundice, and cough for 1 day. Temperature was 101.7°F, pulse 93 beats/min, blood pressure 112/65 mmHg, respiratory rate 20 breaths/min, and saturation 98% on room air. Physical examination shows a soft and nondistended abdomen with tenderness in the right upper quadrant and hepatomegaly. Lab results include a white blood cell count of 14,000/mm^3 and alkaline phosphatase level of 215 IU/L. Chest x-ray shows an elevated right hemidiaphragm and right lower lobe atelectasis. Ultrasound is performed showing a round hypoechoic lesion within the liver, with well-defined borders and several internal echoes, mildly dilated intrahepatic bile ducts, and no cholelithiasis or pericholecystic fluid. In addition to further imaging, what is the most appropriate management?

A. Antibiotics for 10 to 14 days

B. Percutaneous drainage and intravenous (IV) antibiotics

C. Endoscopic retrograde cholangiopancreatography

D. Laparoscopic cholecystectomy

E. Emergent exploratory laparotomy

ANSWER: B

COMMENTS: Liver abscesses classically present as fever, right upper quadrant pain, nausea, pleuritic chest pain, cough or dyspnea, and sometimes with sepsis. They may be pyogenic (bacterial), amebic, or fungal. Pyogenic abscess is usually polymicrobial, although common microbes include *Escherichia coli* or other gram-negative bacteria, *Streptococcus* species, and anaerobes such as *Bacteroides*.

Patient risk factors include underlying biliary cancer, recent ablative liver therapy, or liver transplantation. Today, the most frequent source of pyogenic abscess is a contiguous infection in the biliary tract, such as cholangitis. Other sources include infectious foci within the portal venous drainage system, direct extension from perihepatic sites, and hematogenous spread. The right lobe is the most commonly involved, which has been attributed to a streaming effect on the portal vein. Approximately 20% of pyogenic abscesses are cryptogenic.

The diagnosis is based on the clinical findings and hepatic imaging and may be confirmed by fine-needle aspiration. While ultrasound is a good modality to visualize the liver abscess, gallbladder, and intrahepatic bile ducts, computed tomography (CT) is more sensitive and further allows for evaluation of another underlying cause such as a biliary tree cancer.

Treatment of pyogenic abscess requires eradication of both the abscess and the source. Treatment of the abscess usually requires drainage by operative or percutaneous approaches. Antibiotic therapy alone may suffice for the treatment of multiple small abscesses.

Ref.: 1–2

12. A 30-year-old man visiting from Mexico comes to the emergency department with a history of 2 weeks of right upper quadrant pain and tenderness, fevers, chills, and diarrhea. He is febrile to 102.9°F. His heart rate and blood pressure are 120 beats/min and 100/75 mmHg, respectively. Laboratory results include a white blood cell count of 16,000/mm^3, aspartate aminotransferase (AST) level of 50 IU/L, and alanine aminotransferase (ALT) level of 93 IU/L. Ultrasound of the abdomen shows a 4 × 7-cm^2 round, hypoechoic, nonhomogeneous lesion abutting the liver capsule without rim echoes. Subsequent CT also demonstrates a non–rim-enhancing hypoechoic lesion with a smaller adjacent lesion measuring 2 × 2 cm^2. Which of the following is the most appropriate course of action?

A. Observation

B. Open surgical drainage

C. Broad-spectrum antibiotics and percutaneous drainage

D. Serologic testing for *Entamoeba histolytica* and oral metronidazole

E. Therapeutic fine-needle aspiration

ANSWER: D

COMMENTS: Amebic abscesses are caused by the protozoan *E. histolytica*, which is spread through the fecal–oral route. Once ingested, the cysts pass into the intestines, where the trophozoite is released and transmitted to the colon. These trophozoites can then invade the colonic mucosa and subsequently reach the liver via the portal vein. In the liver, these trophozoites produce a liquefaction necrosis responsible for the classic "anchovy paste" appearance. Protozoa are not usually isolated from the abscess because they are located in the peripheral rim of tissue.

Diagnosis requires hepatic imaging (usually ultrasound or CT) and serologic testing for the presence of *E. histolytica* antibodies as well as a thorough history and physical examination. The patient in this question is a young man from an endemic region who has signs and symptoms similar to those of a pyogenic liver abscess; however, his classic history and the lack of rim enhancement on imaging suggest the diagnosis of amebic abscess rather than a pyogenic abscess. Hepatic amebiasis is treated primarily by the administration of amebicidal drugs, with metronidazole being the drug of choice. Percutaneous aspiration may be indicated if the patient does not respond to medical management or the diagnosis is in question. Percutaneous or operative drainage is also indicated in the presence of secondary bacterial infection, which occurs in about 10% of amebic abscesses.

Ref.: 1, 2

13. A 50-year-old woman complains of a 4-month history of right-sided abdominal pain and nausea. Her vital signs are stable, and she is afebrile. Her physical examination is unremarkable except for hepatomegaly. Ultrasound of the abdomen shows an 8-cm well-circumscribed cyst with a rosette appearance. What is the preferred treatment of this patient?

A. Pericystectomy

B. Percutaneous catheter drainage

C. Transperitoneal surgical drainage

D. Metronidazole

E. Albendazole

ANSWER: A

COMMENTS: The helminth *Echinococcus granulosus* is responsible for most hydatid diseases of the liver. It is usually a unilocular process involving the right lobe, although it may be manifested as multiple cysts. Complications include intrabiliary, intraperitoneal, or intrapleural rupture; secondary infection; anaphylaxis; and mass replacement of the liver. These lesions often have a calcified wall and can be diagnosed serologically by indirect hemagglutination tests, complement fixation tests, serum immunoelectrophoresis, and, formerly, the Casoni skin test. CT and ultrasound may demonstrate characteristic daughter cysts (hydatid sand) or granddaughter cysts (rosette appearance) within the cyst. Treatment is primarily surgical. Percutaneous aspiration or drainage is generally contraindicated because of the risk for intraperitoneal dissemination; however, since the advent of chemotherapeutic agents such as albendazole, some clinicians have proposed percutaneous drainage. The principles of surgical therapy are to avoid spillage and remove the entire germinal layer. The cyst consists of an inner germinal layer (endocyst) and an outer fibrous membrane layer (pericyst). Resection is usually accomplished by pericystectomy. Anatomic hepatic resection is not generally required but may be used. Surgery, in addition to preoperative and postoperative benzimidazole compounds, has been shown to be very effective. Metronidazole is used for the treatment of amebic liver abscesses. Because 20% of echinococcal cysts exhibit biliary communication, assessment by preoperative ERCP or intraoperative cholangiography is important in any patient with jaundice, cholangitis, elevated liver enzyme levels, or bile noted during resection. Scolicidal agents should be used with caution because of the risk of sclerosing the bile ducts in the event that the agent finds its way into the ductal system.

Ref.: 1

14. A 28-year-old asymptomatic white woman is incidentally found to have a 3.5-cm hypervascular lesion with a central scar in the right lobe of her liver. On delayed images, there is increased uptake of contrast material in the scar in comparison with the surrounding liver parenchyma. She is otherwise healthy and takes no medications. Liver enzyme and α-fetoprotein levels are within normal limits. Which of the following is the most appropriate management of this patient?

A. Open liver resection
B. Open surgical biopsy
C. Observation
D. Chemoembolization
E. Hepatic artery embolization

ANSWER: C

COMMENTS: This patient has focal nodular hyperplasia (FNH), which is often found incidentally on imaging or during laparotomy. FNH is a benign liver tumor that predominantly occurs in women in the third to fifth decades of life. It is similar to hepatic adenoma (HA) but with important differentiating clinical and histologic features and therapeutic implications. Both occur most commonly in women of childbearing age; however, HA is associated with the use of oral contraceptives and anabolic steroids and is also seen in certain glycogen storage diseases. HA is usually symptomatic (80% of cases) and is associated with rupture and bleeding in a substantial proportion of patients, whereas FNH is usually asymptomatic and found incidentally. Furthermore, HA has the potential for malignant transformation, whereas the risk for malignancy in FNH is unlikely but uncertain. Histologically, HA consists of hepatocytes without bile ducts or Kupffer cells. FNH contains Kupffer cells along with a central stellate scar surrounded by fibrous tissue. Scanning for Kupffer cell activity with technetium-99m (99mTc)-labeled sulfur colloid is thus useful in differentiating the lesions. Because of the asymptomatic nature of this patient, small size of the lesion, and negligible risk for malignant transformation, observation is appropriate. Surgical resection is reserved for symptomatic patients or when the diagnosis is uncertain.

Ref.: 1–3, 9

15. Right upper quadrant abdominal pain develops in a 25-year-old woman taking oral contraceptives. CT demonstrates a hypodense, 6-cm mass in the right lobe of the liver. A 99mTc-labeled scan reveals a defect in the area of the mass. Angiography reveals a hypervascular tumor with a peripheral blood supply. Which of the following is the appropriate management?

A. Discontinuation of oral contraceptives and observation with serial CT
B. Percutaneous needle biopsy
C. Hepatic resection
D. Arterial embolization
E. Radiation therapy

ANSWER: C

COMMENTS: The imaging characteristics described are typical of HA. Because HA does not contain Kupffer cells, it does not take up radioisotope. This point may be useful for differentiating HA from FNH but not necessarily from other mass lesions of the liver. Percutaneous biopsy of suspected HA is not advisable because of the risk for hemorrhage. HAs associated with oral contraceptives tend to be larger and have a higher risk for bleeding. Regression does not reliably occur with cessation of oral contraceptives. However, for lesions smaller than 4 cm, a trial of cessation of contraceptives or steroids with observation may be attempted. Resection is indicated for most suspected HAs, particularly for symptomatic lesions, for patients not taking oral contraceptives, and if the diagnosis is uncertain. Embolization may be useful for treating hemorrhage in a patient whose HA is inoperable. Radiation has no role in the management of HA.

Ref.: 1–3, 9

16. A 75-year-old woman with recurrent breast cancer undergoes CT of the chest, abdomen, and pelvis for metastatic workup. She is found to have a 7-cm liver mass. Follow up triple-phase CT shows a hypervascular lesion with peripheral to central enhancement. It is thought to be a hemangioma. She denies abdominal pain or any episodes of jaundice. What would be a reasonable indication for operative intervention?

A. Pain, shortness of breath, early satiety
B. Hemorrhage
C. High-output cardiac failure
D. Disseminated intravascular coagulation (DIC)
E. All of the above

ANSWER: E

COMMENTS: Hepatic hemangiomas are the most common benign hepatic tumor. They have no risk of malignant degeneration and are often found incidentally. They typically appear as hypervascular lesions with initial peripheral enhancement followed by late central enhancement, which follows the direction of blood flow into the lesion. Biopsy is not necessary and furthermore carries the risk of hemorrhage.

Asymptomatic uncomplicated hemangiomas are simply observed. Indications for surgical resection include symptoms from mass effect, consumptive coagulopathy manifesting as DIC (seen in Kasabach-Merritt syndrome), high-output cardiac failure from arteriovenous shunting, or rupture and hemorrhage. Enucleation can generally be performed, without formal liver resection being necessary.

Ref.: 1–3, 7, 9–11

17. A 50-year-old woman with hypertension presents to her primary care physician (PCP) with right upper quadrant pain and jaundice. There is a palpable soft mass along her liver edge. Workup is negative for viral hepatitis, and liver enzymes are mildly elevated. Right upper quadrant ultrasound shows a 4-cm cystic structure that is extrahepatic and separate from the gallbladder. ERCP is performed and demonstrates a biliary diverticulum obstructing the common bile duct. What is the most appropriate next step in management?

A. Observation
B. Percutaneous drainage
C. Cholecystectomy
D. Resection
E. Hepaticojejunostomy

ANSWER: D

COMMENTS: When a cyst is an incidental finding with no symptoms and the diagnosis is secure, no further intervention is indicated. In larger cysts, there is a risk of biliary obstruction leading to pancreatitis, cholangitis, and obstructive jaundice, and symptomatic patients should undergo resection. Percutaneous drainage or injection of alcohol or other sclerosing agents does not suffice and is not recommended. If a cyst is found to communicate with the bile ducts, either excision or Roux-en-Y cystojejunostomy may be performed.

Choledochal cysts are classified into five types. Type I cysts are saccular dilatations of the entire common bile duct, and treatment is Roux-en-Y hepaticojejunostomy. Type II cysts, like in this case, are true diverticula of the common bile duct, and treatment is simple excision. Type III cysts, also called choledochodeles, are local dilations of the distal common bile duct extending into the duodenal wall, and treatment is marsupialization or excision.

Type IV cysts are multiple and involve both intra- and extrahepatic ducts. Type V cysts are intrahepatic cysts and the rarest type. They are sometimes associated with congenital hepatic fibrosis and medullary sponge kidney. Treatment of type IV and V cysts depends on the extent of liver tissue involved. Excision, often requiring Roux-en-Y jejunostomy, is preferred over drainage. However, resection may not be an option at all, such as in the case of multifocal cysts involving both lobes with background hepatic fibrosis.

Ref.: 1, 3, 7, 9, 12

18. Which of the following statements is true regarding intrahepatic cholangiocarcinoma?

A. Survival following resection is generally lower than that for distal bile duct cancer.
B. Resection is contraindicated unless histologically negative margins can be obtained.
C. The best survival is achieved with liver transplantation.
D. Adjuvant chemotherapy improves survival following resection.
E. None of the above.

ANSWER: A

COMMENTS: Cholangiocarcinoma arises from the bile duct epithelium and can occur anywhere along the biliary tract. It constitutes 5%–20% of primary liver cancers. Tumors arising from the extrahepatic bile ducts differ from those located intrahepatically in terms of their clinical findings, therapy, and prognosis. Tumors of the extrahepatic bile ducts are typically manifested as biliary obstruction. Intrahepatic tumors appear similar to hepatocellular cancer, a liver mass with absent or vague symptoms such as pain, weight loss, nausea, and anorexia. The treatment of choice is surgical excision, which is associated with a 15%–20% 5-year survival rate. The prognosis is best for tumors of the distal bile ducts that can be resected by a pancreaticoduodenectomy. Tumors involving the bifurcation of the bile duct (Klatskin tumor) are less often resectable. Tumor size and the presence of satellite nodules are correlated with outcome. Histologically negative margins are always desirable, but prolonged survival can be attained even with microscopically involved margins. If the tumor cannot be resected, improved survival has been noted with bypass or stenting procedures. Liver transplantation for cholangiocarcinoma has been associated with frequent recurrence and has not generally been encouraging. Adjuvant chemotherapy has not typically been useful for bile duct cancer.

Ref.: 1, 13–14

19. A 75-year-old man with hepatitis C cirrhosis presents for an annual checkup. He denies any new complaints, including jaundice, abdominal pain, ascites, gastrointestinal bleeding, or encephalopathy. Temperature is 99.1°F, pulse 85 beats/min, blood pressure 109/78 mmHg, respiratory rate 18 breaths/min, and saturation 98% on room air. What studies should be ordered?

A. None
B. Ultrasound
C. α-Fetoprotein (AFP) level
D. Esophagogastroduodenoscopy (EGD)
E. CT scan

ANSWER: B

COMMENTS: Hepatocellular carcinoma (HCC) is among the most common cancers worldwide. Anyone with cirrhosis is at risk, and some etiologies of cirrhosis are independent risk factors separate from cirrhosis. For example, in hepatitis B infection, HCC can develop without underlying cirrhosis. Other populations at risk include patients with hepatitis C, alcoholic liver disease, hemochromatosis, alpha-1-antitrypsin deficiency, primary sclerosing cholangitis, aflatoxins, HA, anabolic steroid use, and pesticides.

HCC screening is therefore recommended in all individuals with cirrhosis. The recommended screening method is ultrasonography every 6 months. Ultrasonography is 60%–90% sensitive, depending on the size of the lesions. Adding AFP testing is no longer recommended due to its cost and false-positive rates.

Ref.: 1, 3, 7, 15

20. A 69-year-old woman with Child's C cirrhosis has an elevated AFP and a new liver mass on ultrasound. Triple-phase contrast CT confirms a 3.5 ×4-cm^2 mass with arterial enhancement and venous washout. She is otherwise healthy with no cardiopulmonary disease. What is the next most appropriate step in workup and treatment?

A. Interventional radiology (IR) biopsy and pathology
B. Neoadjuvant chemotherapy
C. Liver resection
D. Liver transplant
E. Assess portal vein pressures

ANSWER: D

COMMENTS: In a patient with positive HCC screening, diagnosis is generally made by imaging. Triple-phase magnetic resonance imaging (MRI) is more sensitive and specific than triple-phase CT, but the latter is more often used. The characteristic description of HCC is a lesion with arterial enhancement and venous washout. Biopsy is usually not necessary, except for unusual cases in which the clinical diagnosis is still in doubt.

Management of HCC is resection, and the most important factor in assessing candidacy for liver resection is a hepatic reserve. In general, a patient with Child's A cirrhosis can tolerate up to 50% liver resection, and Child's B up to 25% liver resection. Liver resection is contraindicated in Child's C cirrhosis, and transplant has better survival than resection in these patients. Portal vein hypertension must also be taken into account, as liver resection may not be tolerated if portal vein pressures are above 10 mmHg. The Barcelona Clinic Liver Cancer (BCLC) staging system is often used to guide HCC treatment based on patient and tumor factors.

Liver transplantation is indicated in Child's C cirrhosis as long as the patient is thought to be able to tolerate this. The Milan criteria have been proposed to define HCC tumors in Child's C cirrhosis that would benefit from transplantation. These are tumors in which there is no extrahepatic disease, no macrovascular invasion, and either one tumor up to 5.0 cm in size, or up to three tumors and each up to 3.0 cm in size. Patients with a new HCC diagnosis are awarded additional model for end-stage liver disease (MELD) exception points to minimize waiting list dropout due to disease progression.

Ref.: 3

21. Appropriate use of locoregional therapies in patients with HCC includes all of the following except:

A. An attempt at down-staging tumors initially regarded as unresectable

B. To maintain a patient within transplant listing criteria

C. Treatment of multiple small tumors that are multifocal

D. Treatment of tumors that are in locations of anatomic constraint

E. An alternative to resection in patients with good hepatic reserve

ANSWER: E

COMMENTS: Locoregional therapies, such as radiofrequency ablation, transarterial chemoembolization (TACE), and radiation, have been used with the aim of down-staging tumors initially regarded as unresectable. The resectability of a tumor is determined by a number of factors including hepatic reserve, patient functional status, and tumor size. Resection is still preferred over locoregional therapy and should be performed in patients without contraindication.

Additionally, locoregional therapies have been used in patients with cirrhosis who do not qualify for liver transplantation based on the Milan criteria, in efforts to bring or maintain them within transplant listing criteria. Other uses include treatment of multiple bilobar tumors unresectable due to distribution and tumors in locations that are difficult to access surgically. Finally, another role for these modalities is in the treatment of liver metastases from colorectal cancer.

Ref.: 13, 16

22. A 55-year-old woman with a history of colorectal cancer 10 years ago, treated with right hemicolectomy and chemotherapy and with no evidence of disease since then, presents with vague abdominal pain. Temperature is 98.7°F, pulse 67 beats/min, blood pressure 132/78 mmHg, and saturation 99% on room air. Labs are remarkable for AST 67 IU/L, ALT 83 IU/L, and carcinoembryonic antigen (CEA)-27 ng/mL. Triple-phase contrast CT shows a new peripheral liver mass that slightly enhances on arterial phase. She has hypertension that is well controlled with medications. What are the most likely diagnosis and most appropriate management of her liver lesion?

A. FNH; observation

B. Primary liver cancer; resection

C. Primary liver cancer; chemotherapy

D. Metastatic colorectal cancer; resection

E. Metastatic colorectal cancer; palliation

ANSWER: D

COMMENTS: Metastatic liver tumors are much more common than primary liver tumors. The liver is the most common site of colorectal cancer metastasis, followed by the lung. Other common sources of liver metastases include pancreas, lung, and breast carcinomas. A new hepatic lesion with a known history of one of these carcinomas is generally sufficient for diagnosis, without a need for biopsy. CEA is usually elevated as well if colorectal cancer is the primary.

Characteristics that further support metastasis over primary liver cancer include a history of primary cancer, peripheral residing lesions, multiple lesions, and mass hypovascularity (hence only slightly enhancing compared with adjacent liver parenchyma).

Resection of hepatic metastases from colorectal cancer provides a clear survival advantage over any other treatment and should be performed whenever possible. Over the past two decades, improvements in intraoperative techniques have afforded improved outcomes in liver surgery. Experienced centers demonstrate 5-year survival rates of 25%–40% with mortality rates of less than 5%.

Candidacy for resection is similar to that in HCC and, in other words, depends highly on hepatic reserve. In general, an isolated liver and/or lung metastasis in a patient with colorectal carcinoma should be resected unless contraindicated. This patient should also undergo surveillance colonoscopy to evaluate for local recurrence.

Ref.: 3

23. Which of the following is the most accurate method for identifying hepatic metastases?

A. Transabdominal ultrasound

B. CT

C. Laparoscopy

D. Intraoperative palpation

E. Intraoperative ultrasound imaging

ANSWER: E

COMMENTS: Transabdominal ultrasound is as accurate as CT for detecting liver tumors that are 2 cm in size or larger. For smaller lesions, CT is more accurate, although it can miss the smallest lesions (<1 cm). Laparoscopy is useful for identifying small metastases on the liver or peritoneal surfaces that escape discovery by noninvasive preoperative imaging modalities. Laparoscopy has been incorporated into the staging workup of a variety of intraabdominal malignancies, including those of the liver. However, one of its limitations is its ability to assess the interior structure of solid organs. It is now well recognized that intraoperative ultrasound is the most accurate method for detecting and assessing hepatic tumors. Not only does intraoperative ultrasound discover more lesions than any other modality (including palpation), but it also clearly demonstrates the anatomic relationship of tumors to important vascular structures, which is a critical determinant of resectability and the extent of resection necessary. Intraoperative ultrasound can be performed with handheld or laparoscopic transducers. Experience with intraoperative ultrasound for liver tumors has shown that the sonographic findings affect the surgical management of one-third to one-half of patients. Intraoperative ultrasound imaging has become an indispensable component of hepatic surgery.

Ref.: 4

24. A 56-year-old woman with hepatitis C cirrhosis has had a worsening mental status that has now progressed to hepatic coma. Which of the following can be used for initial treatment of a patient in a hepatic coma?

A. Reduction of dietary protein to 50 g/day or less
B. Control of active bleeding
C. Lactulose
D. Neomycin
E. All of the above

ANSWER: E

COMMENTS: Treatment of hepatic encephalopathy and coma is aimed at limiting the nitrogen that the liver must metabolize by eliminating nitrogenous material from the gastrointestinal tract and by inhibiting its absorption. At the same time, precipitating causes are sought and treated. Nutritional support is important and can be initiated with standard amino acids and restriction of dietary protein. Cessation of any gastrointestinal bleeding from varices is an important step in reducing the conversion of intraluminal blood to ammonia. Lactulose acts as a cathartic and also inhibits the absorption of ammonia by acidifying the colon. Nonabsorbable antibiotics, such as neomycin and kanamycin, reduce colonic flora and the production of ammonia. Systemic antibiotics may be useful for treating specific infections that precipitate encephalopathy but are not indicated empirically. Because the colon is the major site of ammonia absorption, colon resection or exclusion has been suggested to improve encephalopathy but is not a widely used therapeutic measure.

Ref.: 1–3

25. A 43-year-old man with alcoholic cirrhosis has had increasing abdominal distention over the last month. His vital signs are stable, and he is afebrile. Physical examination reveals a distended abdomen with a fluid wave. The initial management of the patient's ascites should include all of the following except:

A. Transjugular intrahepatic portosystemic shunt (TIPS)
B. Sodium restriction
C. Diuretic administration
D. Fluid restriction
E. Diagnostic paracentesis

ANSWER: A

COMMENTS: Ascites is the most common major complication of hepatic cirrhosis. It is associated with a 2-year survival rate of 50%, and its onset in a cirrhotic patient should prompt an evaluation for liver transplantation. Treatment of ascites depends on its cause, and therefore diagnostic paracentesis is required after a history and physical examination. Abdominal ultrasound can confirm the presence of ascites if it is not certain by examination. The serum-ascites albumin gradient is useful diagnostically. A high gradient (1.1 g/dL) indicates portal hypertension and suggests that the patient will be responsive to medical management consisting of sodium restriction (2000 mg/day) and oral diuretics. Usually, both spironolactone and furosemide are administered to produce fluid loss and natriuresis. Spironolactone alone may cause hyperkalemia, and furosemide alone is less effective. Medical therapy controls ascites in about 90% of patients. When the ascites is refractory, serial therapeutic paracenteses (with or without the administration of albumin or other plasma volume expanders) are indicated. Liver transplantation is the ultimate treatment. A peritoneovenous shunt is an option for patients with refractory ascites who are not transplantation candidates or who cannot undergo repeated paracenteses. These shunts are fraught with potential complications, however, and do not prolong survival in comparison with medical management. TIPSs or operative side-to-side–type portosystemic shunts may control the ascites in select patients.

Ref.: 17

26. What is the preferred site for needle entry in paracentesis?

A. 3 cm medial and 3 cm superior to the anterior superior iliac supine (ASIS) on either side
B. 3 cm medial and 3 cm superior to the ASIS in the right lower quadrant (RLQ)
C. 3 cm medial and 3 cm superior to the ASIS in the left lower quadrant (LLQ)
D. 3 cm medial to and at the level of the ASIS on either side
E. Midline at linea alba, inferior to arcuate line

ANSWER: C

COMMENTS: The mechanism of ascites in cirrhosis is thought to be a result of the local release of vasodilators, such as nitric oxide. This causes splanchnic arterial vasodilation, leading to a reduction in effective arterial blood volume. The impending result is systemic vasoconstriction and renal sodium-retention, leading to total body fluid retention.

The serum-ascites albumin gradient (SAAG) is used to help determine the etiology of ascites. SAAG-serum albumin – ascitic albumin. SAAG $\geq$ 1.1 is consistent with portal hypertension, such as from cirrhosis, Budd-Chiari syndrome, portal vein thrombosis, congestive heart failure, liver lesion, and alcoholic hepatitis. SAAG $<$ 1.1 points to other nonhepatic etiologies, such as peritoneal carcinomatosis, nephrotic syndrome, and pancreatitis. Diagnostic paracentesis should be performed on all patients with new-onset ascites, as the etiology of the ascites will guide treatment.

The management of ascites due to portal hypertension includes dietary sodium restriction, fluid restriction, and diuretics. For ascites refractory to medical therapy, treatment options include large-volume paracentesis, TIPS, and peritoneovenous shunt. Liver transplantation is the definitive treatment, and ascites in a patient with cirrhosis should prompt an evaluation for liver transplantation.

In paracentesis, the generally accepted site for needle entry is 3 cm medial and 3 cm superior to the ASIS in the LLQ. Although controversial, a common practice is to follow paracentesis with albumin 1-g infusion for every 100 cc removed, in an attempt to maintain plasma oncotic pressure.

Ref.: 7, 17–18

27. A 43-year-old woman with primary biliary cirrhosis complicated by massive ascites, hepatic encephalopathy, and multiple episodes of upper gastrointestinal bleed requiring endoscopic management presents with hematemesis. Temperature is 98.7°F, pulse 109 beats/min, blood pressure 103/77 mmHg, respiratory rate 20 breaths/min, and saturation 97% on 2 L of nasal cannula oxygen. After acute resuscitation with intravenous fluids and blood products, EGD is performed showing multiple bleeding esophageal varices, which undergo endoscopic band ligation. When the patient is stabilized, TIPS is considered. Further workup including chest radiography shows a large right pleural effusion. What is the most important relative contraindication for portovenous shunting?

A. Hepatic encephalopathy
B. Concern for continued active hemorrhage
C. Massive ascites
D. Pleural effusion
E. No contraindications to TIPS

ANSWER: A

COMMENTS: Portal hypertension is responsible for the majority of the morbidity and mortality associated with cirrhosis, such as variceal bleeding, refractory ascites, and hepatic hydrothorax. First-line therapy for patients with primary variceal bleeding is endoscopic therapy with variceal band ligation or sclerotherapy. However, there is a high risk for rebleeding not amenable to endoscopic techniques (refractory bleeding) or continuation of bleeding (recurrent bleeding).

This patient has failed medical and endoscopic management of variceal bleeding. TIPS is very effective at reducing or normalizing portal pressure, the underlying cause of variceal bleeding. Other indications for TIPS include refractory ascites, hepatic hydrothorax, and Budd-Chiari syndrome refractory to anticoagulation. The mechanism is via diverting blood into systemic circulation and decompressing the portal system. Because hepatic metabolism is bypassed, hyperammonemia may occur manifesting clinically as worsening hepatic encephalopathy. Hepatic encephalopathy is therefore a relative contraindication to TIPS.

Ref.: 1, 3, 13, 19

28. A 57-year-old man with alcoholic cirrhosis presents with abdominal pain and a large umbilical hernia. Temperature is 97.8°F, pulse 78 beats/min, blood pressure 105/63 mmHg, respiratory rate 16 breaths/min, and saturation 98% on room air. Exam shows a large, dull to percussion abdomen with flank fullness, a fluid shift, and a reducible umbilical hernia. What is the most appropriate management?

A. Observation
B. Diuresis and paracentesis
C. Elective surgical repair
D. Emergent surgical repair
E. Liver transplantation

ANSWER: C

COMMENTS: Umbilical hernias are common in patients with ascites, occurring in up to 20% of these patients. They develop as a result of increased intraabdominal pressure, muscle wasting, fascial thinning, and nutritional deficits. Ascites management should be optimized prior to repair in order to decrease intraabdominal pressure and minimize recurrence. Ascites management should be optimized prior to repair to minimize recurrence.

Asymptomatic hernias should be observed. Indications for repair include symptoms, leakage of ascitic fluid, incarceration, and strangulation. Spontaneous rupture and massive leakage of ascitic fluid is a surgical emergency due to the risk of peritonitis and death. Unfortunately, the recurrence rate following repair in patients with ascites is as high as 73%.

Ref.: 1–2, 20

29. Which of the following statements is true regarding spontaneous bacterial peritonitis (SBP)?

A. The diagnosis can be made clinically without paracentesis.
B. Infection is most commonly polymicrobial.
C. Antibiotic therapy is reserved for patients with positive findings on ascitic fluid culture.
D. Gram-negative enteric bacteria are often present.
E. None of the above.

ANSWER: D

COMMENTS: SBP is a potentially lethal complication of ascites that affects about 10% of patients with cirrhotic ascites. Fever and abdominal pain are common manifestations, but the signs and symptoms may be subtle. Diagnosis requires paracentesis with a demonstration of an elevated ascitic fluid polymorphonuclear neutrophil (PMN) count (>250 cells/mm^3) or, eventually, positive findings on culture. Antibiotic therapy should be instituted promptly based on an elevated ascitic fluid PMN count or on symptoms even if the PMN count is lower. Infection is usually from one organism, most commonly *E. coli*, *Klebsiella*, or pneumococcus. A third-generation cephalosporin is typically the preferred antibiotic. Differentiation from bacterial peritonitis secondary to a surgical condition is critical. Patients with SBP typically respond to appropriate antibiotics within 48 h, and ascitic PMN counts decrease. Failure to improve, the presence of polymicrobial infection, or ascitic fluid with a total protein level greater than 1 g/dL, a lactate dehydrogenase (LDH) level greater than the serum level, or a glucose level less than 50 mg/dL suggests secondary peritonitis. Risk factors for SBP include previous SBP, variceal hemorrhage, and low-protein ascites (<1.0 g/dL). Short- or long-term prophylactic antibiotics may be appropriate for high-risk patients.

Ref.: 3, 17

30. Eight weeks after open heart surgery with transfusions, a 56-year-old man notes dark urine, fatigue, and anorexia. Physical examination discloses only mild, tender hepatomegaly. Laboratory investigations reveal a bilirubin level of 2 mg/dL; an AST level of 540 IU/L; an ALT level of 620 IU/L; an alkaline phosphatase level of 1120 IU/L; and negative assay results for hepatitis B surface antigen (HBsAg), hepatitis B core antibody (anti-HBc), immunoglobulin M anti-hepatitis A virus (HAV) antibody (IgM anti-HAV), and anti-hepatitis C virus (HCV) antibody (anti-HCV). Which of the following is the most likely explanation for the patient's clinical condition?

A. Acute viral hepatitis A
B. Acute viral hepatitis B
C. Acute viral hepatitis C
D. Acute viral hepatitis D
E. Acute viral hepatitis E

ANSWER: C

COMMENTS: Posttransfusion non-A, non-B hepatitis is mostly the result of HCV infection. The incubation period is usually 5 to 10 weeks, and the mean peak aminotransferase levels are 500 to 1000 IU/L. Anti-HCV antibody is commonly not detectable until 18 weeks after onset of the illness. Approximately 70% of patients with acute hepatitis C progress to chronic hepatitis and potentially cirrhosis. The negative serologic study results exclude acute infection with HAV and HBV. Hepatitis D (delta) virus (HDV) is capable of infecting only patients who also have HBsAg because HDV is an incomplete RNA virus. Hepatitis E (epidemic) virus is rare, except in association with water-borne epidemics in India, the Middle East, and South America.

Ref.: 1, 3

31. Which of the following clinical conditions is indicated by the presence of serum antibodies against hepatitis B surface antigen (anti-HBs) and absence of serum anti-HBc?

A. Active, acute infection with HBV
B. Normal response to vaccination with the hepatitis B vaccine
C. Chronic active hepatitis secondary to HBV
D. Recovery with subsequent immunity following acute hepatitis B
E. Asymptomatic chronic carrier of HBV

ANSWER: B

COMMENTS: The pattern of negative HBsAg, positive anti-HBs, and positive anti-HBc assays is seen during the recovery phase following acute hepatitis B and clearance of HBsAg from the liver. This antibody pattern may persist for years and is not associated with liver disease or infectivity. Vaccination with the hepatitis B vaccine (genetically manufactured HBsAg particles without HBcAg or HBV DNA) is associated with the development of anti-HBs antibody alone. Active, ongoing infection with HBV, whether acute hepatitis, chronic active hepatitis, or an asymptomatic chronic carrier state, is manifested by the presence of HBsAg and anti-HBc in serum.

Ref.: 1, 3

32. A 32-year-old man with no past medical history is brought to the emergency room with altered mental status. Temperature is 100.4°F, pulse 89 beats/min, blood pressure 101/70 mmHg, respiratory rate 19 breaths/min, and saturation 97% on room air. The examination is notable for being awake but not oriented, inconsistently following commands, jaundice, and scleral icterus. Labs are remarkable for sodium 127 mEq/L, AST 2100 IU/L, ALT 2399 IU/L, and international normalized ratio (INR) 1.6. The next most important step in management is:

A. Broad-spectrum antibiotics and percutaneous drainage
B. IV fluid resuscitation and copper chelation
C. Calculate MELD for transplant candidacy
D. Emergent TIPS
E. Transfer to a liver transplant center for emergent evaluation

ANSWER: E

COMMENTS: Acute liver failure (ALF) is a rare but serious emergency, with mortality approaching 60%–80%. It is defined as a new-onset liver disease with no preexisting cirrhosis, occurring over a span of less than 26 weeks, with an INR ≥ 1.5 and hepatic encephalopathy. Complications include multiorgan system failure, intracranial hypertension, and rapid death. Therefore timely transfer to a liver transplant center intensive care unit is important. Outcomes following liver transplantation in these patients are poor compared with patients with elective transplants after being on the transplant waiting list.

The MELD scoring system is not applicable in ALF. Instead, the King's College Criteria is the algorithm aimed at identifying patients that would benefit from liver transplantation versus those in whom it would likely be futile.

The most common cause is acetaminophen overdose, but other causes include other drugs, hepatitis B infection, autoimmune hepatitis, Wilson disease, acute Budd-Chiari syndrome, and HELLP (hemolysis, elevated liver enzymes, low platelet count) syndrome. Wilson disease is an autosomal recessive disorder of adenosine triphosphate (ATP)-mediated hepatocyte copper transport, causing copper buildup in tissues, with resultant cirrhosis and neurologic manifestations. Half of the patients have Kayser-Fleischer rings in the cornea. Even if this patient's ALF is due to Wilson disease, in the fulminant presentation of this disease, chelator treatment is ineffective, and liver transplantation is still indicated.

Ref.: 3

33. During liver resection, where is the most common site of life-threatening hemorrhage?

A. Main hepatic arteries
B. Portal vein branches
C. Intrahepatic vena cava
D. Hepatic vein branches
E. Hepatic artery variants

ANSWER: D

COMMENTS: The crucial steps in a liver resection involve inflow occlusion at the porta hepatis, followed by parenchymal transection, and finally outflow control of the hepatic veins. A thorough exploration of the abdomen must take place at the beginning because findings may affect management and lead one to abort surgery, such as in the case of diffuse peritoneal implants. Additionally, vascular variants such as a replaced right hepatic artery would affect subsequent steps. Intraoperative ultrasound (IOUS) is an important technique for surveying the liver and delineating intrahepatic vasculature and tumor location. IOUS should be repeated throughout the operation.

Hemorrhage is one of the major hazards during liver resection. Troublesome bleeding is most likely to occur during the division of the hepatic parenchyma, and life-threatening hemorrhage is most commonly from the hepatic veins and their branches.

A variety of intraoperative techniques have been used in an effort to minimize the risk of hemorrhage. Note that inflow occlusion at the porta hepatis (Pringle maneuver) would not occlude hepatic vein hemorrhage. Total hepatic vascular isolation requires occlusion of the inferior vena cava above and below the liver, in addition to the Pringle maneuver.

A disadvantage of any vascular occlusion, however, is the potential for ischemic injury to the liver. This may be particularly hazardous in patients with underlying hepatocellular disease to begin with. Additional techniques that have been employed to help limit blood loss often involve interventions by anesthesia to achieve low central venous pressure, head-down positioning, and vasodilator effects.

Ref.: 3, 13, 21–22

34. What is the difference between a standard right hepatectomy and extended right hepatectomy?

A. Extended includes left lobe segments III and IV

B. Extended includes the middle hepatic vein and its parenchymal counterparts

C. Extended includes segment IV and includes the middle hepatic vein

D. Extended includes everything until the line transecting the gallbladder and inferior vena cava (IVC)

E. Extended includes dissection in the plane of the falciform ligament

ANSWER: C

COMMENTS: Extended right hepatectomy includes not only the anatomic right lobe (segments V through VIII), but also segment IV. Additionally, the plane of transection is carried over to the left of the middle hepatic vein. Therefore inflow control is not adequately obtained by ligating the right portal vein and right hepatic artery at the porta hepatis. Smaller inflow vessels need to be ligated within the umbilical fissure.

Left lobectomy includes segments II, III, and IV. Left lateral segmentectomy includes only segments II and III. The umbilical fissure is the segmental plane between the medial and lateral segments of the left lobe of the liver.

A portion of the left branch of the portal vein, known as the pars umbilicus, runs in the inferior portion of the falciform ligament. Dissection is therefore never carried out directly in the segmental fissure. During left lateral segmentectomy, the plane of the parenchymal dissection is to the left of the fissure, whereas with right trisegmentectomy, the parenchyma is divided to the right of the fissure. Both right and left lobectomies involve dissection well to the right of this plane.

Ref.: 1–3, 22

REFERENCES

1. Sicklick JK, D'Angelica M, Fong Y. The liver. In: Townsend CM, Beauchamp RD, Evers BM, et al., eds. *Sabiston Textbook of Surgery: The Biological Basis of Modern Surgical Practice*. 19th ed. Philadelphia: Elsevier Saunders; 2012.
2. Cheng EY, Zarrinpar A, Geller DA, Goss JA, Busuttil RW. Liver. In: Brunicardi FC, Anderson DK, Billar TR, et al., eds. *Schwartz's Principles of Surgery*. 10th ed. New York: McGraw-Hill; 2015.
3. Greenfield LJ, Mulholland MW. Hepatobiliary and portal venous system section. In: Mulholland MW, Lillemoe KD, Doherty GM, et al., eds. *Greenfield's Surgery: Scientific Principles and Practice*. 5th ed. Philadelphia: Lippincott Williams & Wilkins; 2011.
4. Deziel DJ. Hepatobiliary ultrasound. *Probl Gen Surg*. 1997;14:13–24.
5. Theise ND. Liver, gallbladder, and biliary tract. In: Kumar V, Abbas AK, Aster JC, eds. *Robbins Basic Pathology*. 9th ed. Philadelphia: Elsevier Saunders; 2013.
6. Sattar HA. *Fundamentals of Pathology*. 1st ed. Chicago: Pathoma LLC; 2011.
7. Fiser SM. *The ABSITE Review*. 4th ed. Philadelphia: Lippincott Williams & Wilkins; 2014.
8. Goldberg S, Ouellette H. *Clinical Anatomy Made Ridiculously Simple*. 4th ed. Miami: MedMaster, Inc; 2011.
9. Mulvihill SJ. Liver, biliary tract and pancreas. In: O'Leary JP, Tabuenca A, eds. *The Physiologic Basis of Surgery*. 4th ed. Philadelphia: Lippincott Williams & Wilkins; 2008.
10. Sachs TE, Choti MA. Cavernous hepatic hemangioma. In: Cameron JL, Cameron AM, eds. *Current Surgical Therapy*. 11th ed. Philadelphia: Elsevier Saunders; 2014.
11. Hirose K. The management of benign liver lesions. In: Cameron JL, Cameron AM, eds. *Current Surgical Therapy*. 11th ed. Philadelphia: Elsevier Saunders; 2014.
12. Mequid RA, Van Arendonk KJ, Lipsett PA. *The Johns Hopkins ABSITE Review Manual*. 2nd ed. Philadelphia: Lippincott Williams & Wilkins; 2014.
13. Blumgart LH. *Surgery of the Liver, Biliary Tract and Pancreas*. 4th ed. Edinburgh: Churchill-Livingstone; 2006.
14. Roayaie S, Guarrera JV, Ye MQ, et al. Aggressive surgical treatment of intrahepatic cholangiocarcinoma: predictors or outcome. *J Am Coll Surg*. 1998;187:365–372.
15. AASLD Practice Guideline, Management of Hepatocellular Carcinoma: An Update. Bruix J, Sherman M. http://www.aasld.org/practice guidelines/Documents/Bookmarked%20Practice%20Guidelines/HCC Update2010.pdf
16. Locke JE, Cameron AM. Treatment for hepatocellular carcinoma. In: Cameron JL, Cameron AM, eds. *Current Surgical Therapy*. 11th ed. Philadelphia: Elsevier Saunders; 2014.
17. Runyon BA. Management of adult patients with ascites caused by cirrhosis. *Hepatology*. 1998;27:264–272.
18. Latt NL, Gurakar A. The management of refractory ascites. In: Cameron JL, Cameron AM, eds. *Current Surgical Therapy*. 11th ed. Philadelphia: Elsevier Saunders; 2014.
19. Azene EM, Hong K. Transjugular intrahepatic portosystemic shunt. In: Cameron JL, Cameron AM, eds. *Current Surgical Therapy*. 11th ed. Philadelphia: Elsevier Saunders; 2014.
20. Rosemurgy AS, Statman RC, Murphy CG, et al. Postoperative ascitic leaks: the ongoing challenge. *Surgery*. 1992;111:623–625.
21. Melendez JA, Arslan V, Fischer ME, et al. Perioperative outcomes of major hepatic resections under low central venous pressure anesthesia: blood loss, blood transfusion and the risk of postoperative renal dysfunction. *J Am Coll Surg*. 1998;187:620–625.
22. Melstrom LG, Fong Y. The management of malignant liver tumors. In: Cameron JL, Cameron AM, eds. *Current Surgical Therapy*. 11th ed. Philadelphia: Elsevier Saunders; 2014.

CHAPTER 25

GALLBLADDER AND BILIARY TRACT

Scott Schimpke, M.D., Benjamin R. Veenstra, M.D., and Keith Millikan, M.D., F.A.C.S.

1. Which surgeon performed the world's first laparoscopic cholecystectomy?

A. Karl Langenbuch

B. Phillipe Mouret

C. J. Barry McKernan

D. William B. Saye

E. Eric Mühe

ANSWER: E

COMMENTS: Karl Langenbuch performed the very first operation to remove the gallbladder on July 15, 1882. The **first "laparoscopic" cholecystectomy** was performed by Eric Mühe in Germany in 1985. Although technically different from modern laparoscopic cholecystectomy, it was a landmark contribution. Mühe was severely criticized and, in fact, vilified by the surgical community at the time. Only years later was the significance of his accomplishment recognized. Phillip Mouret, a French surgeon from Lyons, performed the procedure in 1987. This was after Mühe had already performed 94 such "laparoscopic" cholecystectomies. J. Barry McKernan and William B. Saye are credited with performing the first laparoscopic cholecystectomy in the United States on June 22, 1988 in Marietta, Georgia.

Ref.: 1

2. During palpation of the hepatoduodenal ligament, a pulsation is felt dorsal and slightly to the right of the common bile duct (CBD). Which of the following does this pulsation most likely represent?

A. A normal common hepatic artery

B. A normal right hepatic artery

C. A replaced right hepatic artery

D. A gastroduodenal artery

E. A right renal artery

ANSWER: C

COMMENTS: The most common variation in **hepatic arterial anatomy** is origination of the right hepatic artery from the superior mesenteric artery. This is a replaced hepatic artery and not simply an accessory vessel that can be sacrificed with impunity. When an operation is performed in the right upper part of the abdomen, the pulsations encountered in the porta hepatis and gastrohepatic ligaments should be assessed. If the hepatic artery is absent or small, the surgeon must be alert to the possibility of a replaced hepatic vessel. When the right hepatic artery originates from the superior mesenteric artery, it courses dorsal to the head of the pancreas and the portal vein and is usually identified dorsolateral to the CBD. This vessel and its origin can readily be identified with intraoperative ultrasonography. Only rarely does a replaced right hepatic artery course through the pancreas. A replaced left hepatic artery originates from the left gastric artery and is located in the gastrohepatic ligament, where it is frequently encountered during operations on the stomach and gastroesophageal junction.

Ref.: 2, 3

3. Which of the following anatomic features may contribute to stricture formation after injury to the CBD?

A. The blood supply to the supraduodenal bile duct has a longitudinal pattern.

B. The blood supply to the supraduodenal bile duct has a lateral pattern.

C. The blood supply to the supraduodenal bile duct has a segmental end-artery arrangement.

D. The blood supply to the CBD is derived primarily from the common hepatic artery.

E. The blood supply to the CBD has a fragile anastomotic network.

ANSWER: A

COMMENTS: Ischemia is an important contributing factor to the development of postoperative **bile duct stricture**. The blood supply to the area of the bile duct bifurcation and the distal retropancreatic duct is primarily lateral in arrangement, whereas the blood supply to the supraduodenal portion of the bile duct has a primarily axial or longitudinal pattern. The so-called 3- and 9-o'clock arteries and other small vessels arise from the right hepatic artery and the retroduodenal artery, which is a branch of the gastroduodenal artery, and form the skeleton of a pericholedochal plexus of vessels. An additional source of blood supply to the CBD can be the retroportal artery. This vessel arises from the celiac axis or the superior mesenteric artery and generally joins the retroduodenal artery; however, in approximately one-third of individuals it ascends the back of the CBD to the right hepatic artery. The portion of the bile duct supplied by the longitudinal vessels receives most of its arterial blood supply from below, thus rendering the proximal portion of the duct subject to ischemia after injury or transection.

Ref.: 2–4

4. In this intraoperative cholangiogram (Fig. 25.1), a separately inserting right sectional duct would insert into which labeled structure?

A. 3

B. 5

C. 6

D. 7

E. 2

ANSWER: B

COMMENTS: Variations in the **anatomy of the extrahepatic bile ducts** are common. The surgeon must be cognizant of these variations and learn to recognize and identify them to prevent inadvertent injury to the bile ducts during cholecystectomy. Approximately two-thirds of individuals have the "textbook" anatomy, with the anterior (segments V and VIII) and posterior (segments VI and VII) sectional ducts from the right joining to form the main right hepatic duct, which then joins the main left hepatic duct to form the common hepatic duct.

In 15%–25% of individuals, the anterior or posterior sectional duct from the right lobe inserts separately **into the common hepatic duct** (labeled 5 in the above image). This duct is therefore at risk for injury during cholecystectomy if the anatomy is not recognized. One of the most common variations in cystic duct anatomy is direct insertion into one of these separately inserting right hepatic ducts. The structures labeled in the above image are as follows: 1, right hepatic duct; 2, left hepatic duct; 3, cystic duct; 4, two surgical clips securing cholangio catheter; 5, common hepatic duct; 6, CBD; 7, pancreatic duct; 8, ampulla of Vater; 9, duodenum.

Ref.: 2, 4–6

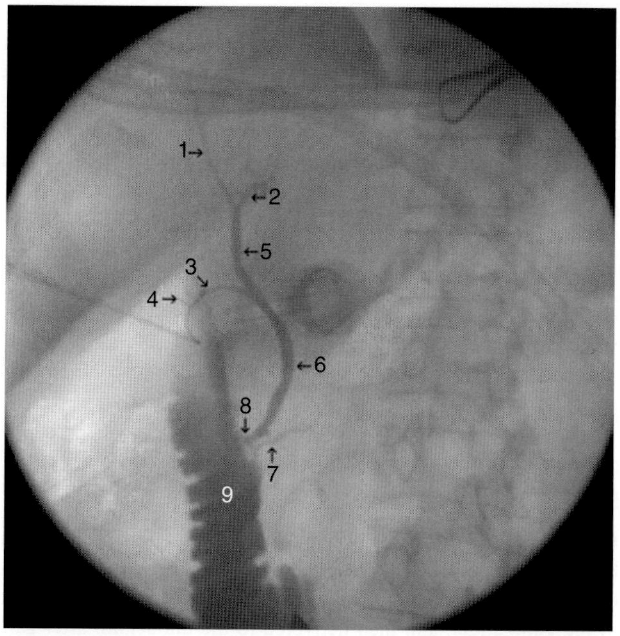

Fig. 25.1 (Question 4). *(Source: Massearweg NN, Flum DR. Role of intraoperative cholangiography in avoiding bile duct injury.* J Am Coll Surg. *2007;204(4):656–664. Copyright © 2007 American College of Surgeons.)*

5. In this transverse laparoscopic ultrasound scan of the hepatoduodenal ligament (Fig. 25.2), what structure is labeled by the straight black arrow?

A. CBD

B. Cystic duct

C. Common hepatic artery

D. Right hepatic artery

E. Right hepatic duct

ANSWER: C

COMMENTS: See Question 6.

Ref.: 7

6. In this transverse laparoscopic ultrasound scan of the hepatoduodenal ligament (Fig. 25.3), which structure is labeled by the thick black arrow?

A. Portal vein

B. Common hepatic artery

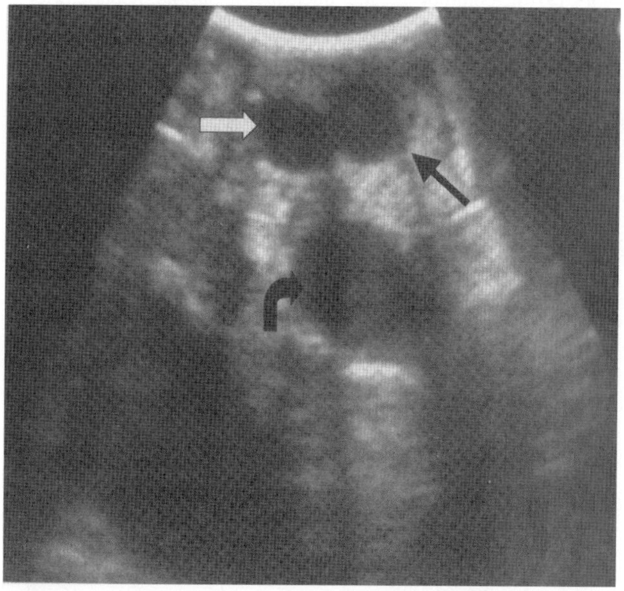

Fig. 25.2 (Question 5). *(Source: Machi J, Staren ED.* Ultrasound for Surgeons. *Philadelphia: Lippincott Williams & Wilkins; 2005; image is Fig. 6, page 292.)*

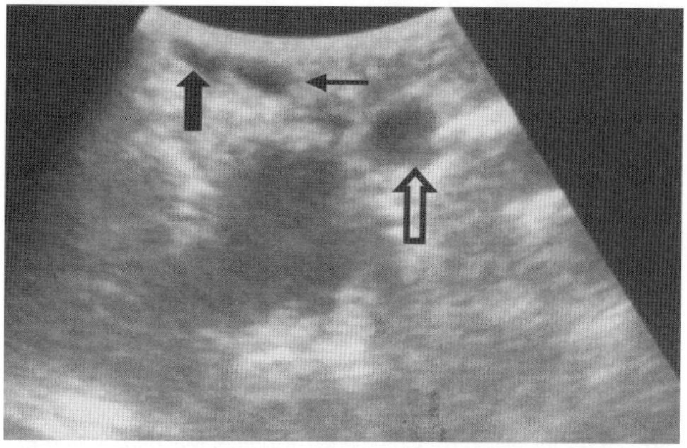

Fig. 25.3 (Question 6 - Stem). *(Source: Machi J, Staren ED.* Ultrasound for Surgeons. *Philadelphia: Lippincott Williams & Wilkins; 2005; image from Fig. 9, page 294.)*

C. Cystic duct
D. CBD
E. Common hepatic duct

ANSWER: C

COMMENTS: Intraoperative ultrasound imaging, whether laparoscopic or open, is an accurate method for identifying bile duct anatomy and assessing the bile duct for stones during cholecystectomy. The transverse scans of the hepatoduodenal ligament in Questions 5 and 6 depict typical anatomy. In the transverse plane, the structures of the hepatoduodenal ligament have a "**Mickey Mouse**" configuration. The cross-sections of the bile duct and common hepatic artery appear as smaller hypoechoic circles anterior to the larger portal vein. This configuration changes as one scans more proximal or distal along the hepatoduodenal ligament (Fig. 25.4). The structures labeled in the scan from Question 5 are as follows: *white arrow*, CBD; *straight black arrow*, common hepatic artery; *curved black arrow*, portal vein. The structures labeled in the scan from Question 6 are as follows: *thick black arrow*, cystic duct (just superior to junction with hepatic duct); *thin black arrow*, common hepatic duct; *arrow outline*, hepatic artery.

Ref.: 7

7. If a patient has complete bile duct obstruction, which of the following does not occur?
   A. Triglyceride absorption
   B. Vitamin K absorption
   C. Cholesterol synthesis
   D. Bilirubin conjugation
   E. All of the above

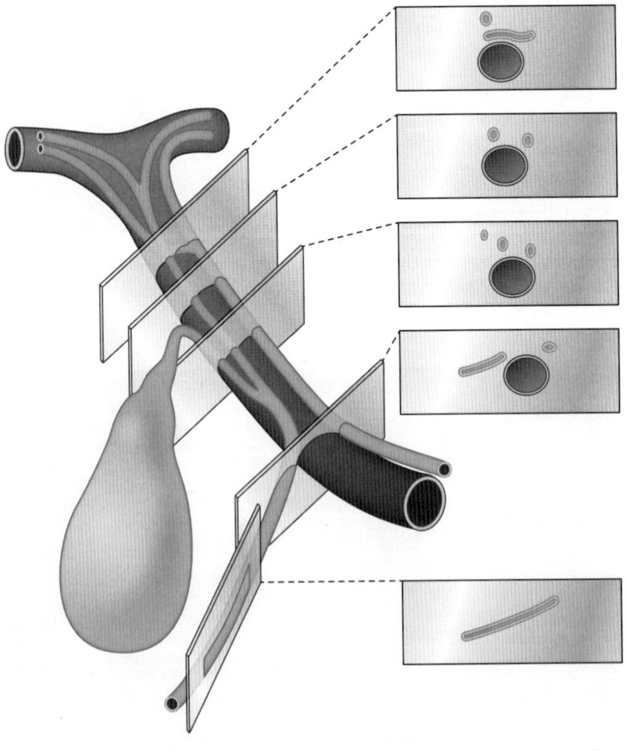

Fig. 25.4 (Question 6 - Comments). *(Source: Machi J, Staren ED. Ultrasound for Surgeons. Philadelphia: Lippincott Williams & Wilkins; 2005; image from Fig. 8, page 294.)*

ANSWER: B

COMMENTS: Bile has a number of critical functions related to the digestion and absorption of fats and the elimination of various endogenous and exogenous substances. Bile interacts with pancreatic lipase and colipase in the intraluminal hydrolysis of dietary triglycerides. It subsequently solubilizes the monoglycerides and fatty acids produced by triglyceride metabolism by forming mixed micelles. The micelles facilitate mucosal uptake of triglycerides by permitting transport across the water barrier adjacent to the enterocyte membrane. Although bile therefore plays an important role in triglyceride absorption, a substantial amount of triglycerides can be absorbed, even in the absence of bile, because of the long length of the intestine. The same is not true for the fat-soluble vitamins A, D, E, and K, which are minimally water soluble and are not absorbed in any substantial amount in the absence of micelles. Patients with longstanding **cholestasis** generally require supplementation of these fat-soluble vitamins to prevent the clinical effects of deficiency. Bile is the sole pathway for elimination of bilirubin and cholesterol from the body. Bilirubin is secreted into hepatic bile by an active transport mechanism following hepatic uptake and conjugation. Cholesterol is eliminated both by synthesis of bile acids from cholesterol and by solubilization of cholesterol in bile during secretion.

Ref.: 4

8. Cholic acid is converted by bacteria to which of the following secondary bile acids?
   A. Deoxycholic acid
   B. Chenodeoxycholic acid
   C. Lithocholic acid
   D. Ursodeoxycholic acid
   E. None of the above

ANSWER: A

COMMENTS: The primary human **bile acids** cholic acid and chenodeoxycholic acid are synthesized from cholesterol in the liver. The secondary bile acids deoxycholic acid and lithocholic acid are formed in the intestine as the result of bacterial enzyme activity. 7-Ketolithocholic acid is also a secondary bile acid. It is converted to the tertiary bile acid ursodeoxycholic acid in the liver.

Ref.: 2–4, 8

9. Conjugated bile acids are primarily absorbed in the intestine by which of the following mechanisms?
   A. Active transport in the colon
   B. Passive transport in the colon
   C. Active transport in the ileum
   D. Passive transport in the ileum
   E. Bacterial translocation

ANSWER: C

COMMENTS: Enterohepatic cycling of bile acids begins at the hepatocyte level. Bile acids are conjugated in the liver with glycine or taurine, secreted into the biliary system, concentrated and stored in the gallbladder, and then delivered to the duodenum after gallbladder contraction. Most bile acids are efficiently resorbed in the intestine. The site and mechanism of intestinal absorption differ according to the form of the bile acid and its corresponding lipid solubility. Conjugated bile acids are predominantly ionized in the intestinal pH range and are relatively lipid insoluble. Conjugated forms are therefore absorbed by an active transport mechanism in the terminal ileum. This mechanism accounts for approximately 70%–80% of the enterohepatic circulation. Bacterial deconjugation of bile acids occurs in the colon and small intestine, as does conversion of primary bile acids to secondary forms. Deconjugation raises the pK_a of bile acids and enables resorption by passive nonionic diffusion, which occurs predominantly in the colon but to some extent in the small intestine as well. Both primary and secondary bile acids are resorbed and taken back to the liver. Unconjugated forms are then reconjugated and resecreted. Hepatic bile therefore contains both primary and secondary bile acids, with the primary bile acids normally constituting 60%–90% of the total bile pool. Hepatic synthesis of new bile acids approximates fecal losses of 300 to 600 mg/day.

The bile acid pool cycles four to eight times per day, and hepatic secretion is dependent on enteral return. Disruption of this cycle therefore diminishes bile acid secretion. Clinical conditions that may be associated with bile acid malabsorption include ileal disease or resection, small bowel dysmotility or obstruction, and blind loop syndrome. Clinical consequences of this disordered physiology may include fat malabsorption, deficiencies of fat-soluble vitamins (A, D, E, and K), choleretic diarrhea caused by impaired colonic water absorption by bile acids, and formation of gallstones.

Ref.: 2–4, 8

10. Which of the following usually produces gallbladder contraction?

A. Adrenergic stimulation
B. Vasoactive intestinal peptide (VIP)
C. Somatostatin
D. Cholecystokinin (CCK)
E. Secretin

ANSWER: D

COMMENTS: Gallbladder function is subject to many neurohormonal influences. Generally, stimulation of parasympathetic vagal nerves causes gallbladder contraction, and stimulation of sympathetic nerves from the celiac ganglion causes gallbladder relaxation. Regulation of gallbladder function is actually a complex process that involves the interaction of various neural, hormonal, and peptidergic stimuli on various receptors located on the gallbladder muscle, blood vessels, and nerves. Cholinergic stimuli (including vagal) and CCK cause contraction. CCK receptors can be found on both gallbladder smooth muscle cells and intrinsic cholinergic nerves. Adrenergic stimulation (sympathetic) usually causes relaxation, but selective stimulation of certain adrenergic receptors can cause contraction. VIP and somatostatin inhibit gallbladder contraction, which can account for clinical biliary manifestations in patients with tumors that secrete those substances or in patients being administered somatostatin agonists. Many other peptides, hormones, and neurotransmitters may also affect gallbladder function, although their clinical significance is not completely known.

Ref.: 3

11. Which of the following is true regarding gallbladder volume during the interdigestive period?

A. It correlates with CCK plasma levels.
B. It depends on peristalsis of the CBD.
C. Volume is constant.
D. The gallbladder gradually fills, with cyclic periods of emptying.
E. The gallbladder gradually fills, uninterrupted.

ANSWER: D

COMMENTS: Bile flow in the biliary tract varies according to the fasting or fed state of the individual. **CCK**, which is released by the duodenum in response to the ingestion of food substances, facilitates delivery of bile to the intestine by stimulating contraction of the gallbladder and relaxation of the sphincter of Oddi. Normal contraction of the gallbladder in response to meals results in approximately 80% emptying in 2 h. CCK has no role in the interdigestive or fasting period. The CBD is for the most part a passive conduit in humans and does not play an active role in biliary motility.

Filling of the gallbladder after it has emptied (i.e., **the fasting state**) depends on neural and hormonal factors that relax the gallbladder and increase resistance of the sphincter of Oddi. During this fasting state, the gallbladder **gradually fills**, but this filling is **interrupted by cyclic periods of emptying**, during which time approximately one-third of the gallbladder volume is dispensed. This cyclic pattern during fasting correlates with the interdigestive myoelectric migratory complex of the intestine and is related to increased levels of plasma motilin. Motilin is a 21–amino acid peptide, and plasma motilin levels vary cyclically during the fasting period.

Ref.: 3, 8

12. Which of the following is decreased after cholecystectomy?

A. Size of the bile acid pool
B. Rate of enterohepatic recycling
C. Rate of bile acid secretion
D. Cholesterol solubility in bile
E. Rate of bilirubin conjugation

ANSWER: A

COMMENTS: The total size of the **bile acid pool** is diminished after **cholecystectomy** as a result of loss of the gallbladder reservoir. However, cholecystectomy produces a more continuous flow of bile into the intestine, which increases the frequency of enterohepatic cycling and stimulates bile acid secretion. For these reasons, even though the size of the bile acid pool is diminished, cholecystectomy improves cholesterol solubility in bile. The solubility of cholesterol in bile depends on the relative molar concentration of cholesterol in relation to the concentration of bile acids and the phospholipid lecithin.

Ref.: 2

13. Which of the following is not a part of the process of cholesterol gallstone formation?

A. Supersaturation of bile with cholesterol
B. Bilirubin deconjugation
C. Crystal nucleation

D. Aggregation of cholesterol monomers

E. Stone growth

ANSWER: B

COMMENTS: Cholesterol gallstone formation is a complex physicochemical process. The requisite steps in the genesis of cholesterol stones can be conceptually simplified as cholesterol saturation, nucleation, and stone growth. The cholesterol content of bile must exceed the capacity of bile to solubilize cholesterol in vesicles and micelles. Cholesterol supersaturation alone, however, is not sufficient to cause stones because this process can occur in normal individuals. Nucleation must also take place; that is, cholesterol monohydrate crystals must form and aggregate. Finally, the crystals must enlarge by fusion or continued solid deposition to produce a stone large enough to be clinically relevant. Bacterial infection is thought to be an important pathogenic factor in the development of some pigment stones but not generally cholesterol stones. Bacterial infection is associated with deconjugation of bilirubin and subsequent formation of insoluble calcium bilirubinate complexes. Bacterial infection can also result in the production of glycocalyx, an adhesive glycoprotein that plays a role in pigment stone formation.

Ref.: 2, 3, 8

14. In which of the following patients with symptomatic cholelithiasis would pigment gallstones be expected?

A. A 45-year-old (y/o) male with a body mass index (BMI) of 49

B. A 27-y/o female status post ileal resection

C. A-38 y/o female with rapid weight loss after a sleeve gastrectomy

D. A 65-y/o female on estrogen therapy

E. A 30-y/o male who is a competitive eater (high-calorie diet)

ANSWER: B

COMMENTS: Changes in bile composition that either increase the relative concentration of cholesterol or decrease the relative concentration of bile acids favor **cholesterol gallstone formation**. Situations that lead to increased hepatocyte cholesterol secretion include obesity, rapid weight loss, diets high in calories and polyunsaturated fats, and estrogen therapy (Choices A, C, D, and E). Theoretically, a relative decrease in the size of the bile acid pool would predispose a person to cholesterol gallstone formation in situations where there is excessive bile acid loss (e.g., ileal disease or resection). However, stones associated with ileal disease or resection are of the **pigment type**. Additionally, total parenteral nutrition (TPN) is associated with pigment gallstones in a high proportion of patients, depending on the duration of therapy.

Ref.: 2, 3

15. Which of the following is the main chemical component of pigment gallstones?

A. Cholesterol

B. Calcium bilirubinate

C. Calcium carbonate

D. Calcium phosphate

E. Calcium oxalate

ANSWER: B

COMMENTS: Pigment gallstones are composed primarily of calcium precipitated with bilirubin, carbonate, phosphate, or palmitate anions. Two relatively distinct types of pigment gallstones are recognized: *black* pigment gallstones and *brown* pigment gallstones. There are differences between black and brown pigment gallstones in terms of gross appearance, chemical composition, pathogenesis, and clinical implications. Black pigment gallstones are small and spiculated. They contain calcium bilirubinate primarily in polymerized form, as well as calcium carbonate or phosphate. Brown pigment gallstones are soft and yellow-brown and are also composed primarily of calcium bilirubinate, but they contain more calcium palmitate (fatty acid derived from lecithin) and cholesterol than do black stones. The oxalate salts of calcium play no role in gallstone disease.

Ref.: 2, 8

16. Which of the following features is more characteristic of black pigment gallstones than brown pigment gallstones?

A. Association with hepatic cirrhosis

B. Association with bacterial infection

C. Location in the CBD

D. Treatment requiring bile duct drainage

E. Higher risk for cholangitis

ANSWER: A

COMMENTS: There are some important clinical differences between patients with **black pigment gallstones** and those with **brown pigment gallstones**. It is postulated that these stones form by different pathogenic mechanisms. Stasis and infection are critical factors in the formation of brown pigment gallstones. Bile culture results are positive in most patients with brown pigment gallstones, and scanning electron microscopy demonstrates bacterial colonies or casts within the stones. Brown pigment gallstones are found more frequently in the CBD than in the gallbladder. They occur in older patients with stasis and in postcholecystectomy patients.

Black pigment gallstones are thought to have a metabolic cause. They often occur in patients with cirrhosis or hemolysis. The precise role of stasis and infection in black stone formation remains unclear, however. Approximately 20% of patients with black pigment gallstones have positive bile culture results, and some investigators have demonstrated bacteria in black stones. A subset of patients with gallstones have combined features of both black and brown pigment gallstones. The important therapeutic implication in differentiating black from brown pigment gallstones is that patients with brown pigment gallstones may require a definitive biliary drainage procedure to prevent recurrence, whereas patients with black pigment gallstones may be treated successfully by cholecystectomy alone.

Ref.: 2, 3, 8

17. A 22-y/o female presents to your office with postprandial epigastric pain. Which of the following sonographic findings is not a feature of gallstone disease?

A. Hyperechoic intraluminal structure

B. Mobility of the intraluminal structure

C. Shadowing posterior to the structure

D. Acoustic enhancement posterior to the structure

E. Sonographic Murphy's sign in acute cholecystitis

ANSWER: D

COMMENTS: External ultrasound (US) imaging has a sensitivity of about 95% for the diagnosis of gallstones. The three **sonographic criteria for gallstones** are (1) the presence of a hyperechoic intraluminal focus, (2) shadowing posterior to that focus, and (3) movement of the focus with changes in position of the patient. Problems in interpretation arise when all of these criteria are not fulfilled. For example, small stones may not shadow well, and impacted stones do not move. Ultrasound imaging may also fail to diagnose stones if the gallbladder cannot be visualized well because it is contracted or close to excessive bowel gas. For an optimal elective ultrasound scan, the gallbladder should be examined after the patient has fasted for about 6 h. Posterior acoustic enhancement is a sonographic feature of hypodense structures such as cysts. The signals behind the structure are "whiter" because the sound wave energy is less attenuated as it passes through. Additionally, a cholesterol polyp on US is seen with a nonmobile, hyperechoic focus with associated "comet tail" artifact. A sonographic Murphy's sign refers to tenderness when the ultrasound transducer is placed over the gallbladder. This is a typical finding in a patient with gallstones and acute cholecystitis.

Ref.: 7

18. Ultrasound imaging reveals gallstones in an asymptomatic 50-y/o woman. Which of the following is the recommended treatment?

A. Observation

B. Laparoscopic cholecystectomy

C. Open cholecystectomy

D. Ursodeoxycholic acid

E. Extracorporeal shock wave lithotripsy (ESWL)

ANSWER: A

COMMENTS: The appropriate management of **asymptomatic cholelithiasis** is sometimes controversial. First, the physician must determine whether the patient is in fact asymptomatic because gastrointestinal (GI) complaints other than pain may be attributable to biliary tract disease. It was formerly thought that symptoms would eventually develop in most patients with silent gallstones and that the risk for subsequent complications was high. Subsequent studies suggested that symptoms develop in about 1%–2% of patients each year and that serious complications are relatively infrequent. The morbidity, mortality, and cost of intervention in these patients may exceed those of expectant therapy. The availability of laparoscopic cholecystectomy has not changed the basic indications for surgery, although it has probably altered the symptomatic threshold for surgical referral. Nonoperative pharmacologic dissolution and ESWL are neither definitive nor cost effective.

Therefore the current incidental finding of asymptomatic cholelithiasis is not an indication for therapy in most situations. Circumstances that may be exceptions and that merit consideration on an individual basis include (1) a transplant patient with anticipated immunosuppression because of the risk for sepsis, (2) anticipated long-term parenteral nutrition because of associated stasis and sludge formation, (3) anticipated pregnancy because of the possibility of becoming symptomatic as gallbladder emptying is impaired and because of the potential risk imposed on both the mother and fetus if complicated cholelithiasis occurs, (4) concurrent abdominal surgery for an unrelated problem because of the relative ease and safety of incidental cholecystectomy in most situations and in consideration of the potential for postoperative cholecystitis otherwise, and (5) bariatric operations because of the high incidence of gallstones associated with obesity and during rapid weight loss. In patients requiring massive intestinal resection, concomitant cholecystectomy has been recommended even when the gallbladder is normal because disease will probably develop during parenteral nutrition.

Ref.: 2, 3, 8

19. In a patient with which of the following conditions is early elective cholecystectomy for symptomatic gallstones *not* indicated?

A. Elderly status

B. Diabetes mellitus

C. Child class C cirrhosis

D. TPN-induced gallstones

E. Chronic renal failure

ANSWER: C

COMMENTS: Patients with certain medical conditions are often considered to be at higher risk for morbidity and mortality from gallstone disease. Complications of cholelithiasis, such as sepsis, perforation, and choledocholithiasis, more frequently develop in elderly patients. They also have a higher mortality rate during emergency operations. Elective cholecystectomy can usually be performed safely in the elderly and is recommended for symptomatic patients. Although the supportive evidence has not always been conclusive, diabetic patients may also be at increased risk, particularly if emergency intervention is required, and should therefore be considered for early elective cholecystectomy. Gallstones develop in a high proportion of patients maintained on long-term TPN, and reports suggest that complications, emergency operations, and mortality are more frequent in this population as well. Early cholecystectomy is therefore indicated. **Cholecystectomy** is also indicated for patients with chronic renal failure, particularly if they are candidates for renal transplantation. Patients with hepatic cirrhosis, however, have high morbidity and mortality rates related to cholecystectomy, especially those with hepatocellular dysfunction and portal hypertension. In selected patients, with Child-Pugh A and B cirrhosis, laparoscopic cholecystectomy can be performed safely with acceptable morbidity. However, patients with Child-Pugh class C have an unacceptably high risk of morbidity and mortality and therefore cholecystectomy is not advised.

Ref.: 3, 9

20. A patient with abdominal pain has a normal ultrasound of the gallbladder, followed by a CCK-stimulated cholescintigraphy (CS) scan that demonstrates an ejection fraction (EF) of 14% with reproduction of symptoms. Which of the following is true regarding biliary dyskinesia?

A. Cholecystectomy is not indicated because persistent or recurrent symptoms are likely.

B. Cholecystectomy is successful (resolution or improvement of symptoms) 50% of the time.

C. Reproduction of symptoms during CCK-stimulated CS scan is the most accurate predictor of success after laparoscopic cholecystectomy.

D. In patients diagnosed with biliary dyskinesia, improved outcomes postlaparoscopic cholecystectomy are noted in those with an EF closer to zero.

E. The technique used for CCK-stimulated CS in the diagnosis of biliary dyskinesia is important.

ANSWER: E

COMMENTS: Biliary dyskinesia is a subsegment of Functional Disorders of the Gallbladder as defined by the Rome III criteria. Diagnosis is suspected when both typical and atypical biliary symptoms are found in the absence of stones or sludge on ultrasonography. **CCK-stimulated CS** has been useful for identifying patients who may have symptoms as a result of motility disorders of the gallbladder, specifically biliary dyskinesia. The technique used is important as multiple studies have examined the optimal approach and have found this to be an infusion of 0.02 µg/kg of sincalide in infused over 30 min in patients who have been fasting for 3 to 4 h. In general, laparoscopic cholecystectomy is recommended for patients with typical symptoms and an EF of less than 35%–40% on CCK-CS, with success rates between 85% and 90%. Although initially thought to be a predictor of success, CCK provocation tests (reproduction of pain with CCK-CS) are not believed to be accurate as CCK stimulates other organs that also can contribute to the pain. No studies to date have found a concrete correlation between decreasing EF and improved outcome.

Ref.: 3, 10

21. Laparoscopic cholecystectomy is most strongly contraindicated in which of the following situations?

A. Pregnancy

B. Previous upper abdominal surgery

C. Known CBD stones

D. Recent myocardial infarction (MI) with severe coronary artery disease noted on cardiac catheterization, requiring full anticoagulation

E. Gallbladder cancer

ANSWER: D

COMMENTS: When **laparoscopic cholecystectomy** was first introduced worldwide during the late 1980s, there were a number of circumstances in which it was more or less strongly contraindicated. Today, most contraindications are relative, and in fact the laparoscopic approach is preferred when possible in certain situations that were initially considered contraindications (e.g., acute cholecystitis, choledocholithiasis, and obesity). Basically, the surgeon must be adequately trained and the patient must be reasonably fit for an operation and give informed consent that includes the possibility of laparotomy. It must be recognized that there are patients for whom the potential physiologic consequences of CO_2 pneumoperitoneum are more important, but the presence of underlying disease itself does not prohibit a laparoscopic approach. In fact, laparoscopic cholecystectomy may be more beneficial to the postoperative course of a compromised patient. Pregnancy is not a contraindication with appropriate precautions, although the physiologic effects on the fetus are not completely known. Originally deemed a contraindication to laparoscopic cholecystectomy because of risk for dissemination, gallbladder cancer is being reevaluated. Recent literature shows favorable long-term oncologic results in appropriately selected patients (those with early-stage gallbladder cancer with no evidence of liver invasion). Any contraindication to open surgery remains a contraindication to laparoscopic surgery, as illustrated by the individual with recent MI and severe cardiac disease.

Ref.: 3, 11

22. Most major bile duct injuries during laparoscopic cholecystectomy occur in patients under which of the following circumstances?

A. Acute cholecystitis

B. Gallstone pancreatitis

C. Choledocholithiasis

D. Elective cholecystectomy

E. Conversion of a laparoscopic procedure to an open procedure

ANSWER: D

COMMENTS: There are several **risk factors** for **bile duct injury** during **laparoscopic cholecystectomy**. Pathologic risk factors include severe acute or chronic inflammation. Several studies have found a statistical correlation between the rate of duct injury and the presence of acute cholecystitis. Bleeding has long been implicated as a factor predisposing to duct injury during open or laparoscopic cholecystectomy. Injuries are sometimes attributed to the "anomalous" anatomy of the bile ducts. More often than not, however, such "anomalies" are simply common anatomic variations that the surgeon must recognize to prevent injury (see Question 27). The surgeon's experience, or the "learning curve," is clearly a risk factor because higher rates of duct injury have been well documented in less experienced surgeons. It is interesting to note that there is no convincing evidence that duct injury is more frequent during cases involving laparoscopic management of CBD stones, possibly because these procedures are performed by more experienced surgeons. Unfortunately, most major bile duct injuries during laparoscopic cholecystectomy have occurred in elective and otherwise uncomplicated cases. Despite the presence or absence of risk factors, the primary problem resulting in duct injury is misidentification of the anatomy. The most frequent mechanism of injury is mistaking a major bile duct for the cystic duct and clipping and cutting it. This pitfall is best avoided by correct operative strategy, which means appropriate retraction and adequate dissection to obtain the "critical view of safety." The **critical view** is achieved by dissecting the base of the gallbladder off the liver for an adequate distance to visualize the cystic plate and to verify that the only structures entering the gallbladder are the true cystic duct and the cystic artery. Intraoperative bile duct imaging with cholangiography or laparoscopic ultrasonography can also aid in discerning the anatomy. If the cystic duct cannot be conclusively identified, the surgeon must resort to alternative approaches such as laparoscopic subtotal cholecystectomy, conversion to an open operation, or termination of the procedure.

Ref.: 12

23. Which of the following statements regarding the critical view of safety is ***true***?

A. It helps to recognize a bile duct injury, but does not prevent it.

B. It can be achieved in every laparoscopic cholecystectomy.

C. It does not apply if the patient has aberrant anatomy.

D. It was first described in 1995 in response to increasing bile duct injury rates with the advent of the laparoscopic cholecystectomy.

E. Interest in the critical view of safety has dwindled in recent years due to improved technology.

ANSWER: D

COMMENTS: See Question 24.

Ref: 12

24. Which of the following statements about "infundibular technique" is **true**?

A. The CBD can be mistaken for the cystic duct when obtaining this view.

B. It requires dissection of the cystic plate over the bottom third of the gallbladder.

C. It has been shown to prevent bile duct injuries.

D. It facilitates identification of the anatomy in the hepatocystic triangle.

E. It requires clearance of the hepatocystic triangle.

ANSWER: A

COMMENTS: Drs. Strasberg, Hertl, and Soper first described the critical view of safety in 1995 in response to an increasing bile duct injury rate with the advent of the laparoscopic cholecystectomy. It has been shown to prevent bile duct injuries and is internationally accepted as a standard practice. In 2014, Dr. Brunt made it the central focus of the SAGES safe cholecystectomy program, which was formed to further propagate a "universal culture of safety in cholecystectomy." The three criteria to fulfill the critical view of safety are (1) clearance of tissue from the hepatocystic triangle, (2) complete dissection of the bottom one-third of the cystic plate, and (3) two and only two structures are seen entering the gallbladder. If these criteria cannot be achieved, it should alert the surgeon that the anatomy is not clearly defined, it is not safe to proceed, and an alternate strategy should be employed. Adjunct measures that can assist with identifying the biliary anatomy include intraoperative ultrasound or cholangiogram. Otherwise, another operative strategy should be to perform a subtotal cholecystectomy (see Question 39). The infundibular technique involves encircling the cystic duct and tracing it up to the characteristic funnel-shaped junction with the gallbladder. It does not require further clearance of the hepatocystic triangle, identification of the cystic artery, or cystic plate dissection. The CBD can be mistaken for the cystic duct using this technique, resulting in a bile duct injury. Therefore it is an unreliable method of ductal identification and should be abandoned.

Ref.: 12, 13

25. A surgeon encounters difficulty during an elective laparoscopic cholecystectomy in a healthy 25-y/o woman and converts to an open procedure. The 4-mm common hepatic duct has been transected 1 cm below the bifurcation. Which of the following procedures is the most appropriate?

A. Duct-to-duct repair over a T-tube

B. Duct-to-duct repair without a stent

C. Roux-en-Y hepaticojejunostomy

D. Hepaticoduodenostomy

E. Ligation of the duct and placement of a drain

ANSWER: C

COMMENTS: When a transection or resection **injury of the extrahepatic biliary tree** is discovered at the time of cholecystectomy, the surgeon must make some careful decisions. Repair at the time is preferable, provided that the surgeon is adequately experienced in performing such a repair so that a successful outcome is likely. Unfortunately, the weight of evidence indicates that most primary repairs by the initial operating surgeon have failed, thus necessitating repeated operations and other interventions. The initial repair of a major duct injury has the best chance for long-term success. A less experienced surgeon should not attempt anastomosis of a small bile duct but seek the help of an experienced colleague if available. Otherwise, drains should be placed and transfer to an experienced hepatobiliary surgeon arranged. If repair at the time is appropriate, the standard reconstruction for this type of injury is a Roux-en-Y hepaticojejunostomy. Duct-to-duct repairs usually fail in this situation. Hepaticoduodenostomy is not recommended for an injury at this level.

Ref.: 14

26. How would the bile duct injury described in Question 25 be classified?

A. Bismuth type 1

B. Bismuth type 2

C. Bismuth type 3

D. Bismuth type 4

E. Bismuth type 5

ANSWER: B

COMMENTS: The **Bismuth classification of bile duct injuries** and strictures describes the level of injury in relation to the bifurcation of the main right and left hepatic ducts. Higher injuries are more difficult. They require a greater degree of technical skill and expertise to reconstruct, and reconstructions may have a lower long-term success rate. Many of the injuries resulting from laparoscopic cholecystectomy have been higher than those seen with open cholecystectomy. Moreover, many injuries, initially lower, end up being higher when repaired because of the need to debride unhealthy ductal tissue as a result of ischemia or inflammation and infection caused by bile leakage. With a type 1 injury, 2 cm or more of the common hepatic duct is preserved below the bifurcation. With a type 2 injury, less than 2 cm remains. A type 3 injury reaches the bifurcation with preservation of continuity between the right and left ducts. A type 4 injury involves destruction of the hepatic duct confluence with separation of the right and left hepatic ducts. A type 5 injury involves a separate inserting right sectoral duct with or without injury to the common hepatic duct.

Ref.: 4

27. What is the most common anatomic reason for a type B (Strasberg classification) bile duct injury during a laparoscopic cholecystectomy?

A. A short cystic duct

B. An aberrant right hepatic duct

C. A replaced right hepatic artery

D. A replaced left hepatic artery

E. An aberrant left hepatic duct

ANSWER: B

COMMENTS: A type B iatrogenic injury is an occlusion of part of the biliary tree, which is usually caused by an aberrant right hepatic duct. Normal variants include the cystic duct emptying into a right hepatic duct, which then drains into the CBD, or a low-entering right hepatic duct on the CBD. In both scenarios a surgeon can falsely identify the aberrant right duct as the cystic duct. The

Strasberg classification is generally the easiest to follow and is more applicable in the days of laparoscopy (see Fig. 25.5 below).

Ref.: 12, 15

28. On the second postoperative day following an elective laparoscopic cholecystectomy, a 40-y/o woman complains of nausea and abdominal pain. Examination shows a temperature of 100°F (37.8°C), a pulse of 100 beats/min, mild abdominal distention, and moderate right upper quadrant (RUQ) tenderness. Which of the following would be the most appropriate *initial* step?

A. Administration of intravenous (IV) antibiotics
B. Magnetic resonance cholangiopancreatography (MRCP)
C. Hepatobiliary iminodiacetic acid (HIDA) scan
D. Endoscopic retrograde cholangiopancreatography (ERCP)
E. Percutaneous transhepatic cholangiography (PTC)

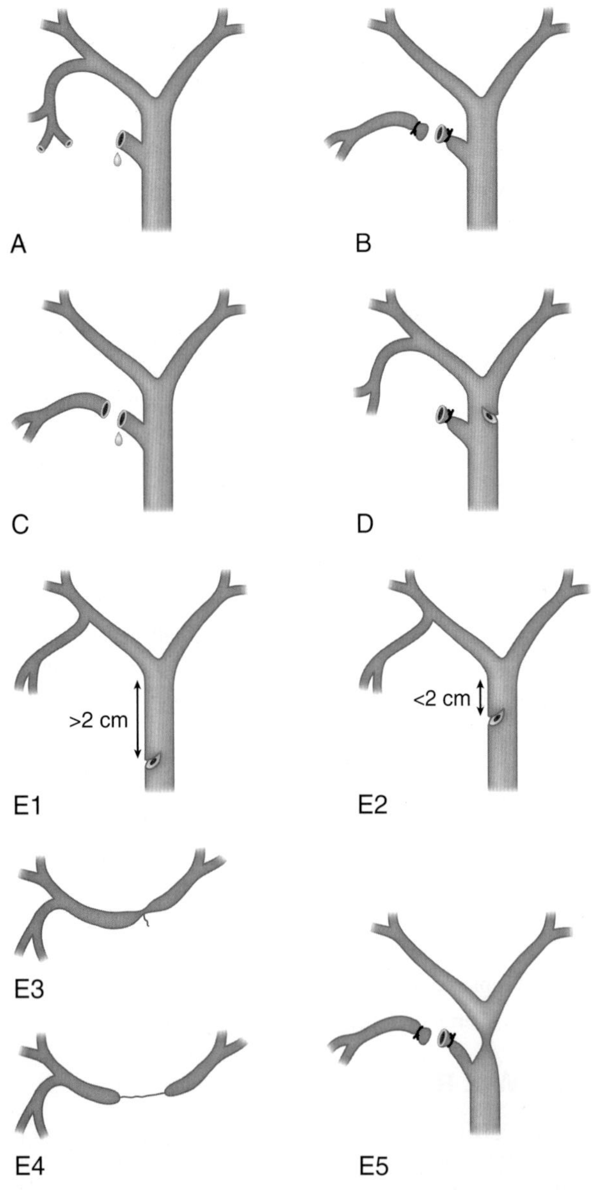

Fig. 25.5 (Question 27 - Comments). *(Source: Chari RS, Shah SA. Biliary system. In: Townsend CM, Beauchamp RD, Evers BM, et al., eds.* Sabiston Textbook of Surgery. *20th edition. Elsevier; 2017: Philadelphia, PA. chapter 54, Fig. 54.39.)*

ANSWER: C

COMMENTS: A bile leak should be highly suspect in the above patient, as it occurs in 1%–2% of patients after elective cholecystectomy. Other problems such as retained bile duct stones or intestinal injury can occur as well, although they are less frequent.

A HIDA scan is often the most reasonable initial investigation as it can demonstrate whether the leak is ongoing, unlike ultrasound or computed tomography (CT). These two imaging studies can demonstrate fluid collections or intrahepatic bile duct dilation and would be reasonable after a HIDA is obtained. If a fluid collection is seen, percutaneous aspiration can determine whether the fluid is bile. If a bile leak is confirmed, cholangiography is necessary to establish the site of leakage and help determine further therapy. **Endoscopic cholangiography** is generally the first choice and may be all that is necessary for bile leaks that originate from lateral injuries, the cystic duct stump, or the gallbladder fossa. **PTC** is necessary for complete anatomic definition in patients with transection or resection injuries or injuries to sectoral hepatic ducts that may not be in continuity with the rest of the extrahepatic bile ducts. MRCP is not an initial diagnostic examination but can be useful for delineation of bile duct anatomy in complex situations.

Ref.: 14, 16

29. Which of the following is true regarding the use of intraoperative cholangiography (IOC) and bile duct injury during laparoscopic cholecystectomy?

A. Selective use of IOC effectively prevents bile duct injury.
B. Routine use of IOC effectively prevents bile duct injury.
C. Selective use of IOC is associated with a higher rate of bile duct injury.
D. The severity of bile duct injury is independent of the use of IOC.
E. Use of IOC increases the intraoperative diagnosis of injury.

ANSWER: E

COMMENTS: As long as there are imaging studies to assess the bile ducts intraoperatively, the debate between proponents of routine versus selective use of such studies will continue. Proponents of IOC argue that its routine or liberal use can be advantageous in terms of bile duct injury and that there is an association between routine IOC and lower rates of duct injury. **Cholangiograms** can be incomplete or misinterpreted, however, and injuries can occur after IOC has been done. Properly performed IOC does not prevent **duct injury**. There is a compelling argument that IOC may limit the severity of duct injury. For example, IOC may allow a surgeon to recognize that the cholangiogram catheter has been placed in the common duct and not in the cystic duct before transection of the common duct. Some evidence suggests that the number of high duct injuries and anastomotic repairs required to remedy duct injuries has been lower when IOC was performed. The use of IOC increases the intraoperative recognition of any injury that has occurred. About 70%–90% of injuries have been identified intraoperatively when IOC has been performed compared with only 15%–25% of injuries when IOC has not been performed. Failure to interpret the results of IOC correctly can account for missed injuries. The two primary reasons for misinterpreting the results of IOC are failure to completely visualize the proximal ducts (including both the right anterior and posterior ducts) and extravasation of dye of uncertain origin.

Ref.: 17

30. A ^{99m}Tc-iminodiacetic acid scan in a fasting patient demonstrates the following: normal liver activity, no gallbladder visualization at 60 min, intestinal activity present at 60 min, and gallbladder visualization at 120 min. These findings are most consistent with which of the following situations?

A. Normal study results
B. Acute calculous cholecystitis
C. Acute acalculous cholecystitis
D. Chronic cholecystitis
E. Partial bile duct obstruction

ANSWER: D

COMMENTS: Since the mid-1970s, technetium-labeled derivatives of iminodiacetic acid (i.e., **HIDA**, para-isopropylacetanilido-iminodiacetic acid (PIPIDA), and diisopropyl iminodiacetic acid (DISIDA) have been important in the evaluation of **biliary tract disease.** After IV injection, these radioisotopes are taken up by the liver and excreted into the biliary tract. The characteristics of a normal study include visualization of the gallbladder within 60 min in fasting patients and the appearance of radioisotope in the duodenum by about the same time. In nonfasting patients, visualization of the gallbladder may be delayed. The hepatic phase of the study may demonstrate mass lesions or diminished uptake in patients with hepatic dysfunction. Such results are similar to those of a liver scan. With both calculous and acalculous acute cholecystitis, the gallbladder is not visualized because of cystic duct obstruction. No visualization or delayed visualization is common with chronic cholecystitis. The distinction between acute and chronic cholecystitis therefore depends on the clinical findings, not simply on abnormal scan results. Bile duct obstruction may cause delayed or absent clearance of isotope from the liver or delayed hepatic uptake. Radioisotope scans can be useful in the clinical assessment of disorders other than cholecystitis, including biliary motility, biliary-enteric anastomosis, bile fistulas or leaks, and enterogastric reflux.

Ref.: 2, 3

31. A 65-y/o female presents with RUQ pain, nausea, and vomiting. Her temperature is 38°C, heart rate (HR) is 115 beats/min, and blood pressure is (BP) 88/62 mmHg; she is saturating 92% on 2-L nasal cannula. Her abdominal examination is significant for a positive Murphy's sign. Laboratory values are significant for a white blood cell (WBC) count of 19,000/mm^3 and a normal total bilirubin. Ultrasound shows a gallbladder wall of 5 mm, pericholecystic fluid, gallstones, and a CBD diameter of 4 mm. She is admitted to the surgical intensive care unit (SICU), IV fluids and vasopressors are started, and antibiotics are administered. Which is the most appropriate surgical management?

A. Percutaneous cholecystestomy tube placement followed by cholecystectomy before hospital discharge
B. Emergent cholecystectomy
C. Percutaneous cholecystostomy tube placement followed by cholecystectomy in 3 months
D. Percutaneous cholecystostomy tube placement and cholecystectomy only if her symptoms recur
E. Percutaneous cholecystostomy tube placement only

ANSWER: C

COMMENTS: See Question 33.

Ref: 18–22

32. A 27-y/o female presents with RUQ pain, which started 12 h ago. Her vitals are normal, and her examination is significant for RUQ tenderness without peritonitis. Laboratory values are significant for a WBC count of 12,000/mm^3 and normal total bilirubin. Ultrasound shows a gallbladder wall of 4 mm, pericholecystic fluid, gallstones, and a CBD diameter of 3 mm. Which is the most appropriate surgical treatment?

A. IV fluids, antibiotics, and interval elective cholecystectomy in 1 month after her symptoms resolve
B. ERCP with sphincterotomy for biliary decompression
C. Cholecystectomy within 72 h of onset of symptoms
D. Biliary drainage followed by interval cholecystectomy within 72 h of onset of symptoms
E. Percutaneous cholecystostomy tube placement

ANSWER: C

COMMENTS: See Question 33.

Ref: 18–22

33. A 36-y/o male presents with RUQ pain, nausea, and vomiting, which started 5 days ago. His vitals are significant for a HR of 106 beats/min and BP 126/75 mmHg. His examination is significant for RUQ tenderness and positive Murphy's sign, but no peritonitis. Laboratory values are significant for a WBC count of 19,000/mm^3 and normal total bilirubin. Ultrasound shows a gallbladder wall of 5 mm, pericholecystic fluid, gallstones, and a CBD diameter of 3 mm. Which is the most appropriate surgical treatment?

A. Percutaneous cholecystostomy tube placement
B. Immediate cholecystectomy
C. Cholecystectomy within 72 h of admission
D. IV fluids, antibiotics, and interval elective cholecystectomy in 3 months after his symptoms resolve
E. ERCP with sphincterotomy for biliary decompression

ANSWER: B

COMMENTS: The Tokyo Guidelines, originally published in 2007 with revision in 2013, are the expert consensus on the diagnosis and management of both cholangitis and cholecystitis. The three diagnostic criteria for acute cholecystitis are (A) local signs of inflammation (e.g., Murphy's sign, RUQ mass/pain/tenderness), (B) systemic signs of inflammation [e.g., fever, elevated C-reactive protein (CRP), or elevated WBC count], and (C) imaging characteristic of acute cholecystitis (e.g., wall thickening, pericholecystic fluid). For a suspected diagnosis of acute cholecystitis, one item in A and one item in B must be present. For a definite diagnosis, one item must be present from (A), (B), *and* (C). Grade III (severe) acute cholecystitis is associated with organ dysfunction with any of the following signs: hypotension, altered mental status, $PaO_2/FiO_2 < 300$, oliguria or serum creatinine > 2 mg/dL, INR > 1.5, or platelet count < 100,000/mm^3. Grade II (moderate) acute cholecystitis is associated with any one of the following conditions: elevated WBC count (>18,000/mm^3), palpable tender mass in the RUQ, duration of complaints > 72 h, or marked local inflammation (gangrenous cholecystitis, pericholecystic abscess, hepatic abscess, biliary peritonitis, or emphysematous cholecystitis). Grade I (mild) acute cholecystitis does not meet the criteria of grade II or III. Initial treatment for all grades includes IV fluid resuscitation and initiation of antimicrobials. For grade I (mild) acute cholecystitis, cholecystectomy within 72 h of onset of symptoms or if no response to medical treatment within 24 h AND still within the 72 h since the onset of symptoms is recommended. For grade II (moderate) acute cholecystitis, immediate cholecystectomy or biliary drainage if the patient is at high surgical risk is recommended. For grade III (severe) acute cholecystitis, antibiotics and supportive measures are recommended. Performing an emergent biliary drainage as soon as the patient is stable is then recommended. For patients who undergo biliary drainage and have gallbladder stones, an elective cholecystectomy should be performed 3 months after the patient's condition improves. The patient in Question 31 presents with grade III (severe) cholecystitis as evidence by organ dysfunction (hypotension). The recommended initial treatment is percutaneous cholecystostomy tube placement. The patient in Question 32 presents with grade I (mild) cholecystitis, and cholecystectomy is recommended within 72 h since the onset of symptoms. The patient in Question 33 presents with grade II (moderate) cholecystitis; the recommended treatment is immediate cholecystectomy or biliary drainage if the patient is at a high surgical risk.

Ref.: 18–22

34. A 46-y/o male presents with 2 days of RUQ pain. His labs are significant for a WBC count of 15,000/mm^3. His ultrasound notes numerous gallstones with wall thickening and pericholecystic fluid. On examination, his temperature is 99.5°F, and he has a positive Murphy's sign. What is the best management for this individual?

A. Early laparoscopic cholecystectomy

B. Delayed cholecystectomy after "cool-down" period

C. IV antibiotics

D. Percutaneous cholecystostomy tube

E. Early open cholecystectomy

ANSWER: A

COMMENTS: The former debate over early versus late **cholecystectomy** for **acute cholecystitis** has been put to rest. Prospective studies have demonstrated that early cholecystectomy within the first few days is not associated with higher morbidity or mortality and that delayed surgery requires longer hospitalization, is more expensive, and risks recurrent biliary problems before definitive therapy. Most patients are treated effectively by stabilization and prompt surgery. From a technical standpoint, cholecystectomy is often easier during the first day or two of the patient's illness when the inflammation tends to be more edematous rather than necrotic and hyperemic, as it becomes when the process progresses. Most advocate cholecystectomy within the first 72 h, while others push this to within the first 96 h. Laparoscopic cholecystectomy is the preferred treatment in most circumstances, with decreased length of stay and morbidity compared with open cholecystectomy. However, conversion to an open procedure is required more often than when the procedure is performed electively for nonacute symptoms.

Ref.: 2, 3

35. With regard to acalculous cholecystitis, which of the following statements is true?

A. It most commonly affects elderly patients in an outpatient setting.

B. The primary pathophysiologic feature involves gallbladder stasis.

C. HIDA scan results are usually normal.

D. Ultrasound imaging of the gallbladder is usually normal.

E. Treatment requires cholecystectomy.

ANSWER: B

COMMENTS: Approximately 5%–10% of acute cholecystitis cases occur in patients without gallstones. The primary predisposing factor is gallbladder stasis with subsequent distention and ischemia. **Acalculous cholecystitis** typically develops in hospitalized patients, often after trauma, unrelated surgery, or other critical illnesses. Factors present in these patients that may contribute to biliary stasis include hypovolemia, intestinal ileus, absence of oral nutrition, multiple blood transfusions, narcotic use, and positive pressure ventilation. Because of the clinical situation in which acute acalculous cholecystitis occurs, the diagnosis may not be readily apparent. The patient may have fever or unexplained sepsis, and abdominal signs may not be initially appreciated. The results of imaging studies are generally abnormal. Because of stasis and functional obstruction of the cystic duct, HIDA scanning fails to allow visualization of the gallbladder, and ultrasonography may demonstrate sludge, thickening of the gallbladder wall, or pericholecystic fluid. None of these findings are specific for the presence of acute acalculous cholecystitis, however, and the diagnosis must rely on clinical suspicion.

Standard surgical treatment consists of cholecystectomy (or cholecystostomy for patients who are too infirm to withstand general anesthesia). Percutaneous cholecystostomy can be a valuable technique for establishing gallbladder decompression in these critically ill patients. Later cholecystectomy may not be required if stones are not present and subsequent cholangiography demonstrates a patent cystic duct. Cholecystectomy is the only effective treatment if the gallbladder is necrotic or gangrenous.

Ref.: 2, 3

36. The pertinent area of a plain x-ray film of the abdomen of a 78-y/o diabetic man with RUQ pain is shown in Fig. 25.6. Which of the following is the appropriate next step?

A. Ultrasound imaging of the gallbladder

B. CT

C. HIDA scan

D. Cholecystectomy

E. ERCP

ANSWER: D

COMMENTS: Emphysematous cholecystitis occurs most typically in elderly diabetic men. Curvilinear radiolucencies in the RUQ have the configuration of the gallbladder, are in the location of the gallbladder, and are diagnostic of gas in the gallbladder wall. In their totality, they are pathognomonic of emphysematous cholecystitis. Gas may also be seen in the gallbladder lumen. This condition is associated with a high incidence of gallbladder necrosis, perforation, and sepsis. Unnecessary diagnostic examinations would only delay prompt surgical therapy and possibly affect the outcome adversely. Urgent surgery is needed. An ultrasound study of an emphysematous gallbladder would show highly reflective shadows as a result of the gas. Differentiation from bowel gas

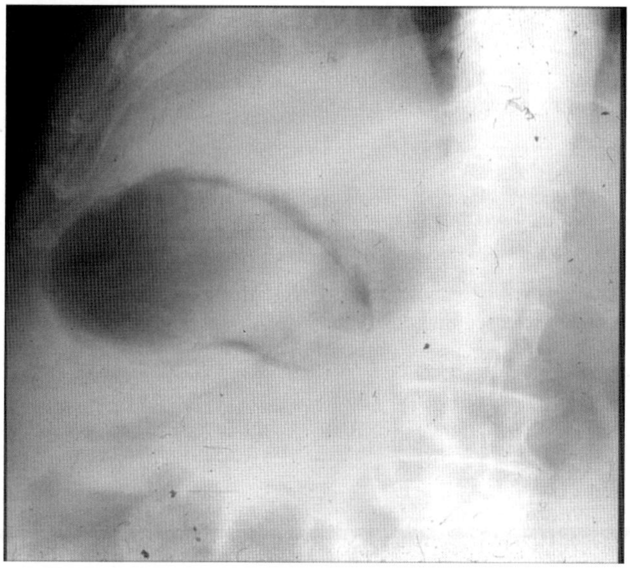

Fig. 25.6 (Question 36 - Stem). *(Source: Ash-Miles J, Roach H, Virjee J, Callaway M. More than just stones: a pictorial review of common and less common gallbladder pathologies.* Curr Probl Diagn Radiol. *2008;37(5):189–202, Fig. 21.)*

may be difficult, although the diagnosis is usually evident. About one-third of patients do not have stones. CT would show the abnormal gas in the gallbladder wall, lumen, or both. HIDA scans would fail to allow visualization of the gallbladder. ERCP is unnecessary.

Ref.: 2, 3

37. A 26-y/o female who is 10 weeks pregnant presents to your office with symptomatic cholelithiasis. She has had two recent trips to the emergency room for significant pain. Her ultrasound from her most recent visit demonstrates a wall of 3 mm, no pericholecystic fluid, an impacted stone in the neck of the gallbladder, and a CBD of 4 mm. On examination, she has mild RUQ pain but no Murphy's sign. The most appropriate management is:

A. Urgent laparoscopic cholecystectomy

B. Percutaneous cholecystostomy tube

C. Laparoscopic cholecystectomy in 4 weeks

D. Open cholecystectomy in 4 weeks

E. Nonoperative management until term and postpartum laparoscopic cholecystectomy

ANSWER: C

COMMENTS: While elective operations during pregnancy have traditionally been avoided for fear of miscarriage/fetal loss and birth defects secondary to anesthetic effect, the data supporting this are mostly theoretical. The largest study following the outcomes of women undergoing nonobstetric surgery was based on the Swedish Birth Registry. They found no increased risk for congenital malformations or stillbirth when compared with the control population. However, the rates of low birth weight were significantly higher in the surgical group. Additionally, the authors noted an increased incidence of preterm birth and an increased rate of neonatal death within 7 days in the surgery group. However, the authors did note that it was difficult to separate the many possible confounding factors (operation type, surgical indication, and type of anesthesia used) that could contribute to the aforementioned adverse outcomes.

In the case of semielective surgery, as illustrated in the above question, the risks and benefits must be carefully weighed. Symptomatic **gallstone disease** is second to appendicitis as the most common nonobstetric surgical problem that affects **pregnant women**. The overwhelming majority of women who become symptomatic during the first trimester of pregnancy will have continuing or recurrent symptoms before delivery. Without definitive treatment, rehospitalizations are frequent and there is an ongoing risk to both the mother and the fetus. Most propose that the second trimester is the ideal time to operate. This avoids the risk of spontaneous miscarriage and the theoretic concern of teratogenicity in the first trimester, while also avoiding the risk of preterm birth in the third trimester. That being said, **laparoscopic cholecystectomy** has been performed successfully during all stages of pregnancy. In late term, however, the size of the gravid uterus interferes with trocar placement. For this reason, many surgeons prefer an open approach if surgery is necessary during the third trimester.

Ref.: 11, 23, 24

38. A 35-y/o female with a BMI of 42 presents for evaluation for bariatric surgery. After discussion, you decide to proceed with a laparoscopic Roux-en-Y gastric bypass procedure. You notice in her chart that a previous RUQ ultrasound shows that she has gallstones, but she denies any symptoms. Which is the most appropriate management of this patient?

A. Perform Roux-en-Y bypass with concomitant cholecystectomy.

B. Perform Roux-en-Y bypass followed by interval cholecystectomy in 1 month.

C. Recommend a gastric band to prevent complications from her cholelithiasis.

D. Proceed with Roux-en-Y bypass and only perform a cholecystectomy in the future if she becomes symptomatic.

E. Recommend a sleeve gastrectomy to prevent complications from her cholelithiasis.

ANSWER: D

COMMENTS: Rapid weight loss (>25% of original weight) is the most significant risk factor for gallstone formation after bariatric surgery. The caloric restriction reduces bile acid secretion, which, combined with excess cholesterol, results in supersaturated bile and stone formation. In addition, for Roux en y gastric bypass (RYGBP), the decreased CCK secretion and (potential) inadvertent injury to the hepatic branch of the vagus nerve during gastric pouch formation may lead to delayed gallbladder emptying and stone formation. Prophylactic cholecystectomy during a bariatric operation was once a routine procedure, but now is no longer recommended. It increases intraoperative time and hospital length of stay. Recent studies have shown the postoperative symptomatic cholelithiasis rate for both Roux-en-Y gastric bypass and sleeve gastrectomy is similar and low at 6%–8%. It is even lower for laparoscopic adjustable gastric band likely due to the decreased postoperative weight loss. Therefore the most appropriate management is selective cholecystectomy in patients who become symptomatic.

Ref: 25–27

39. A 68-y/o male presented to the hospital with chronic cholecystitis. He was taken to the operating room for a laparoscopic cholecystectomy. Intraoperatively, the critical view of safety could not be obtained due to dense adhesions in the hepatocystic triangle. Which is the most reasonable next operative step?

A. Obtain the infundibular view and then proceed with cholecystectomy.

B. Abort the operation.

C. Proceed with subtotal fenestrating cholecystectomy.

D. Proceed with subtotal reconstituting cholecystectomy.

E. Both C and D.

ANSWER: E

COMMENTS: Safe management of a patient with a difficult laparoscopic cholecystectomy requires technical skill, considerable judgment, and familiarity with a spectrum of operative options. Such options include open cholecystectomy, "fundus first" cholecystectomy, laparoscopic or open cholecystostomy, and laparoscopic or open subtotal cholecystectomy. Alternatives to total cholecystectomy can help avoid major bile duct or vascular injury under difficult circumstances. Cholecystostomy tube placement can be lifesaving; potential disadvantages include tube complications, the possible need for a reoperation later, and possible inability to place a tube if the gallbladder is necrotic or gangrenous. Subtotal cholecystectomy can help avoid a bile duct injury and bleeding and reduce the need for cholecystostomy and reoperation. The ability to safely perform subtotal excision of the gallbladder laparoscopically can decrease the rate of conversion to an open operation and potential morbidity in critically ill patients. Two types of subtotal cholecystectomy have been described. A subtotal fenestrating cholecystectomy does not leave a remnant gallbladder, whereas a subtotal reconstituting cholecystectomy does. There are no long-term data as to which is superior. The goal for both is to resolve the patient's symptoms and avoid a second operation/procedure. Aborting the operation is a very reasonable and safe option if the surgeon does not feel comfortable proceeding, but would not be ideal, as it would require an additional intervention.

Ref.: 28

40. A 71-y/o female presents to your office for a persistent high-output biliary fistula 3 weeks after you performed a subtotal fenestrating cholecystectomy with subhepatic Jackson Pratt (JP) drain placement for acute cholecystitis. She is asymptomatic. What is the next step in management?

A. ERCP

B. Observation as a persistent fistula is expected after a subtotal fenestrating cholecystectomy

C. Reoperation to close the fistula

D. Make her nil per os and start TPN

E. Octreotide infusion

ANSWER: A

COMMENTS: A bile leak is not uncommon following subtotal cholecystectomy, especially of the fenestrated type, but most is self-limited and will close without any intervention. A persistent bile leak after a subtotal fenestrating cholecystectomy should raise concern for a distal biliary obstruction. In this case, the most likely etiology would be a retained stone. Therefore an ERCP would be both diagnostic and therapeutic. There is no role for TPN or octreotide or reoperation in this patient.

Ref.: 28

41. When compared with standard three-or four-port laparoscopic cholecystectomy, single-incision laparoscopic surgery (SILS) is associated with which of the following?

A. Decreased rate of trocar site hernias

B. Increased bile duct injuries

C. Decreased pain

D. Decreased hospital stay

E. Increased operative time

ANSWER: E

COMMENTS: There has been substantial interest in the development of single-incision laparoscopic approaches for many operations, including cholecystectomy, colectomy, fundoplication, and appendectomy. Proponents of **SILS** cite the potential advantages of decreased pain and improved cosmesis in comparison with laparoscopic operations using multiple trocar sites. So far, for most surgeons, SILS has been more difficult and time-consuming than standard laparoscopic approaches.

Two recent meta-analyses have examined postoperative outcomes between single-incision and multiport cholecystectomy. In the first meta-analysis, seven randomized controlled studies were included. The primary outcomes measured were postoperative complications and postoperative pain score, while secondary outcomes measured were operating time and length of hospital stay. The only difference found between the two was operative time, being longer in the SILS group. In the second meta-analysis, nine randomized controlled trials were included. They found significantly improved cosmesis postoperatively, with no difference in pain score or hospital stay. Postoperative complications, while higher in the SILS group, were not statistically significant.

Ref.: 29–31

42. With regard to choledocholithiasis, which of the following statements is true?

A. Common-duct stones are present in one-third of patients undergoing cholecystectomy.

B. The incidence of common-duct stones is highest in elderly patients.

C. Most common-duct stones are composed of calcium bilirubinate.

D. Common-duct stones are found more frequently when cholecystectomy is performed for chronic cholecystitis than for acute cholecystitis.

E. Laparoscopic cholecystectomy is contraindicated if choledocholithiasis is suspected.

ANSWER: B

COMMENTS: About 8%–18% of patients with symptomatic gallstones have **choledocholithiasis**, which has a spectrum of clinical manifestations. Approximately 6% of patients undergoing cholecystectomy have CBD stones that were completely unsuspected. Proper recognition of common-duct stones is important because of the associated risk for biliary tract obstruction and cholangitis. The incidence of choledocholithiasis increases with each decade over the age of 60 years. Most common-duct calculi originate in the gallbladder and are therefore of the cholesterol variety. Friable "earthy" stones (brown-colored gallstones) contain calcium complexed with bilirubinate and other anions and arise de novo in the common duct in association with biliary stasis and infection. Choledocholithiasis occurs as often with acute cholecystitis as with chronic cholecystitis. Therefore appropriate evaluation of the patient for potential choledocholithiasis is mandatory. Laparoscopic cholecystectomy is the preferred approach for patients with choledocholithiasis. This can be accomplished in conjunction with preoperative ERCP for patients with a high likelihood of common-duct stones. For those at intermediate or low risk for common-duct stones, intraoperative duct imaging (cholangiography, laparoscopic ultrasound) is performed. If stones are found in the common duct, most can then be cleared with laparoscopic techniques.

Ref.: 2, 3

43. Which of the following is the best indication for preoperative ERCP in a patient with gallstones?

A. Obstructive jaundice

B. Gallstone pancreatitis

C. History of jaundice

D. Alkaline phosphatase levels elevated to twice the normal

E. Ultrasound demonstrating numerous small calculi within the gallbladder

ANSWER: A

COMMENTS: The rationale for **preoperative ERCP** is to identify and remove CBD stones so that patients may subsequently undergo laparoscopic cholecystectomy and, it is hoped, avoid the potential need for an open operation or for operative treatment of the CBD. However, because endoscopic evaluation of the bile duct entails its own risks, it should be selected for patients at the highest risk for choledocholithiasis. Unfortunately, there are no absolute predictors of CBD stones. The yield of ERCP in identifying CBD stones is highest in patients with obstructive jaundice or clinical cholangitis or when a duct stone is actually seen on ultrasound. In all other circumstances, most patients have negative endoscopic cholangiograms, and the examination was not necessary for most of these patients. As the number of parameters suggestive of CBD stones increases, however, so does the likelihood of finding stones. There is no substitute for good clinical judgment in the use of preoperative ERCP. It is an unquestionably valuable tool for diagnosing and removing CBD stones, but its overuse is dangerous and must be discouraged. **Magnetic resonance cholangiopancreatography** can be a useful noninvasive screening tool for choledocholithiasis that allows ERCP to be reserved for those with positive studies. Another option for the diagnosis of bile duct stones is an endoscopic ultrasound, which has a specificity and sensitivity of 95% and 98%, respectively. It is less invasive than an ERCP and uses no contrast or radiation.

Ref.: 32, 33

44. An intraoperative cholangiogram obtained during laparoscopic cholecystectomy shows several 2- to 3-mm filling defects in the distal common duct. What should be done next?

A. Complete the laparoscopic cholecystectomy and perform ERCP postoperatively.

B. Perform open surgical CBD exploration.

C. Administer glucagon, and flush the CBD through the cystic duct.

D. Laparoscopically dilate the cystic duct, and perform transcystic choledochoscopy.

E. Perform laparoscopic choledochotomy.

ANSWER: C

COMMENTS: Choledocholithiasis discovered **intraoperatively** can often be managed laparoscopically, depending on a number of considerations, such as the size, number, and location of the stones and the size and anatomy of the bile ducts. When approaching common bile stones laparoscopically, one should start with simple techniques and progress to more complex maneuvers as necessary. Small stones can often be cleared by flushing the common duct through a transcystic catheter after glucagon has been administered to relax the choledochoduodenal sphincter. Other transcystic manipulations can be used if the cystic duct is dilated or dilatable (with hydrostatic balloons) and provided that there is a relatively direct course between the cystic duct and the CBD. Such techniques include retrieval with balloon catheters or stone baskets under fluoroscopic or choledochoscopic visualization. Experienced laparoscopic surgeons can perform choledochotomy when the CBD is sufficiently large and simpler efforts have failed. In general, the surgeon should not leave common-duct stones untreated but may elect to terminate the procedure when (1) the stones are very small or questionable, (2) the CBD is narrow, (3) laparoscopic clearance is not feasible, and (4) the morbidity of an open CBD exploration is judged to be too high for a particular patient. Intraoperative endoscopic retrieval of CBD stones has been successful but may be logistically impractical. Relying on postoperative endoscopy for intentionally neglected stones carries the risk that endoscopic removal may fail. A traditional open CBD exploration is a safe, reliable fallback for most patients when laparoscopic methods are unsuccessful and the duct is not too small.

Ref.: 34

45. A 35-y/o female presents with choledocholithiasis. A laparoscopic cholecystectomy with biliary clearance is recommended. Which of the following is ***FALSE*** regarding laparoscopic CBD exploration (LCBDE) versus preoperative ERCP followed by laparoscopic cholecystectomy?

A. Morbidity and mortality are equivalent.

B. Hospital stay is shorter for the LCBDE group.

C. Cost is greater for the ERCP followed by the LC group.

D. There are fewer retained stones after the laparoscopic common bile duct exploration (LCBDE) group.

E. Successful CBD clearance is equivalent between the two.

ANSWER: D

COMMENTS: The ideal method of treating choledocholithiasis is controversial. The two-stage approach involves a preoperative ERCP for the CBD clearance followed by laparoscopic cholecystectomy. The alternative one-stage procedure is laparoscopic cholecystectomy with LCBDE. The morbidity and mortality rates are equivalent between the two groups. The CBD clearance rates are also equivalent, both around 90%. The one-stage approach is more cost effective, and the overall hospital stay for the patient is shorter. However, the operative time is longer for the one-stage approach. There is no significant difference in rates of retained stones between the two groups (both 8%–15%).

Ref.: 35, 36

46. When compared with IOC, laparoscopic ultrasound for evaluation of the CBD during cholecystectomy is most associated with each of the following *except*:

A. Better sensitivity for detecting common-duct stones
B. Less time requirement
C. Less need for dissection of cystic structures
D. More accurate identification of the proximal bile ducts
E. Better identification of vascular variations

ANSWER: D

COMMENTS: IOC and **intraoperative ultrasonography** are the most commonly used methods for evaluating the bile ducts during cholecystectomy. Some of the advantages of sonography are that it is relatively quick, it can be performed without the need for dissection of the cystic duct, and it can easily be repeated. Intraoperative ultrasound is more sensitive than IOC for the detection of small stones or sludge in the CBD, although these findings may not necessarily be clinically relevant. Sonography can also demonstrate the vascular anatomy of the hepatoduodenal region. Ultrasound is less reliable than cholangiography for delineation of the anatomy of the proximal bile ducts, such as the presence of separately inserting segmental hepatic ducts. Both imaging methods can be useful in the avoidance of bile duct injury.

Ref.: 37

47. Which of the following is the best treatment for a patient with choledocholithiasis 3 years after cholecystectomy?

A. Administration of ursodeoxycholic acid
B. Percutaneous transhepatic stone extraction
C. Endoscopic sphincterotomy and stone extraction
D. LCBDE and T-tube placement
E. Open CBD exploration and choledochoduodenostomy

ANSWER: C

COMMENTS: Most **CBD stones** found in patients after cholecystectomy can be treated successfully by nonoperative methods. **Stone extraction** through a T-tube or endoscopically after endoscopic sphincterotomy if the patient does not have a T-tube in place results in successful duct clearance with a low complication rate in more than 90% of patients. By definition, bile duct stones occurring more than 2 years after cholecystectomy are considered primary common-duct stones. These are pigment gallstones related to biliary stasis and infection rather than the typical cholesterol stones found in the gallbladder. In addition to stone removal, some type of ductal drainage procedure is therefore also indicated in most of these patients to prevent stone recurrence.

When performed by experienced clinicians, endoscopic sphincterotomy is successful in more than 90% of patients, and when combined with endoscopic extraction with the use of balloon catheters or baskets, results in stone clearance in 85%–90% of patients. Duct stones have been removed successfully via the percutaneous transhepatic route when endoscopic approaches are not successful.

A number of situations may make endoscopic clearance of bile duct stones difficult or unsuccessful, including large impacted stones, the presence of a distal bile duct stricture, previous gastrectomy with gastroenterostomy or Roux-en-Y anastomosis, complications of endoscopic sphincterotomy before stone extraction, or the presence of a duodenal diverticulum. For patients with an altered GI tract, as is the case in those with a Roux-en-Y reconstruction, there are specialized endoscopic or combined endoscopic and laparoscopic approaches available to access the biliary tree. If access to the bile duct can be achieved endoscopically, adjuvant modalities, such as **intracorporeal fragmentation techniques** (i.e., mechanical, electrohydraulic, or laser lithotripsy) or ESWL, may allow successful removal of even difficult stones. Reoperation on the biliary tract for clearance of duct stones is reserved for physiologically fit patients in whom other extraction techniques are unsuccessful. Ursodeoxycholic acid does not dissolve pigment stones.

Ref.: 2, 3

48. Which of the following is the most appropriate initial test for the evaluation of obstructive jaundice?

A. HIDA scan
B. Ultrasound imaging
C. CT
D. PTC
E. ERCP

ANSWER: B

COMMENTS: All of the aforementioned **imaging** modalities may be useful for evaluating a patient with **obstructive jaundice**. Overall, ultrasound is the most cost-effective initial examination. It permits identification or visualization of ductal dilation, suggests the level of obstruction, and provides information about the liver, the pancreas, and the presence or absence of calculous disease. CT or magnetic resonance imaging may best delineate the anatomy of mass lesions in the hepatobiliary and pancreatic region and assist in the preoperative assessment of resectability. **Magnetic resonance cholangiography** can provide precise delineation of ductal anatomy and is increasingly important in the evaluation of malignant disease. PTC can demonstrate the proximal extent of obstruction and is useful for assessing the suitability of the proximal hepatic ducts for anastomosis. **ERCP** is particularly useful in cases of distal biliary tract obstruction and allows evaluation of the ampullary region. Both PTC and ERCP allow cytologic or histologic sampling, and both can be used to place catheters for decompression of the obstructed biliary tract. Although ^{99m}Tc-iminodiacetic acid scans can demonstrate ductal obstruction, they do not provide sufficient anatomic definition to determine cause or assist in making therapeutic decisions.

Ref.: 2, 3

49. Two weeks following hepaticojejunostomy for the treatment of a benign bile duct stricture, a patient has a serum bilirubin level of 6 mg/dL. The patient was jaundiced for 4 weeks before the operation and had a preoperative serum bilirubin level of 12 mg/dL. Which of the following is the most likely explanation for this current serum bilirubin level?

A. Anastomotic stricture
B. Persistent delta-bilirubinemia
C. Postoperative hepatitis
D. Normal expected decline after relief of any obstructive jaundice
E. Renal failure

ANSWER: B

COMMENTS: After relief of biliary obstruction, there is a prompt increase in bile flow, and normal bile acid secretion resumes within several days. Serum bilirubin levels decline approximately 50% by 36 to 48 h after surgery and 8% per day thereafter. This rate varies depending on the duration of the jaundice. **Delta-bilirubin** is a form of bilirubin that is covalently bonded to albumin and is measured as part of the direct bilirubin fraction. As such, it is not filtered by the kidneys and has the same serum half-life as albumin, approximately 18 days, which accounts for the slow decline in serum bilirubin levels observed in patients following relief of longstanding jaundice. Although 90% of patients who had jaundice for 1 week or less have a normal serum bilirubin level 3 to 4 weeks postoperatively, only one-third of patients who had jaundice for 4 weeks or longer obtain normal levels by the same time. Anastomotic stenosis does not usually develop early during the postoperative period. Postoperative hepatocellular dysfunction as a result of hepatitis or other causes can occur early in the postoperative period, but it is a less likely cause of hyperbilirubinemia in a patient whose serum bilirubin levels are gradually declining and who would be anticipated to have persistent delta-bilirubinemia.

Ref.: 4

50. Which of the following is the most likely explanation for a serum bilirubin level of 40 mg/dL in a patient with obstructive jaundice?

A. The patient has complete biliary obstruction.
B. The duration of obstruction has exceeded 2 weeks.
C. The patient has associated renal dysfunction.
D. The patient has malignant biliary obstruction.
E. The patient also has Gilbert disease.

ANSWER: C

COMMENTS: In the presence of **complete biliary obstruction**, **serum bilirubin** levels generally plateau at 25 to 30 mg/dL. At this point, the daily bilirubin load equals that excreted by the kidneys. Situations in which even higher bilirubin levels can be found include renal insufficiency, hemolysis, hepatocellular disease, and, rarely, a bile duct–hepatic vein fistula. Hyperbilirubinemia tends to be more pronounced in patients with obstruction caused by malignant disease than with obstruction resulting from benign causes. However, malignant obstruction in the absence of the previously enumerated factors does not produce this degree of hyperbilirubinemia.

Ref.: 4

51. Which of the following conditions is usually associated with the highest incidence of positive bile culture results?

A. Acute cholecystitis
B. Chronic cholecystitis
C. Choledocholithiasis
D. Postoperative bile duct stricture
E. Bile duct malignancy

ANSWER: D

COMMENTS: Recognition of clinical situations in which bacteria are likely to be present in bile is important because the presence of bacteria in bile is correlated with the risk for postoperative infectious complications. Prophylactic antibiotics have decreased infectious morbidity in patients older than 50 years and in those with jaundice, acute cholecystitis, or choledocholithiasis and **cholangitis**. Bile cultures are positive in approximately 5%–40% of patients with chronic cholecystitis, 29%–54% of patients with acute cholecystitis, 60%–80% of patients with choledocholithiasis, 59%–93% of patients with cholangitis, and nearly all patients with bile duct stricture. Bacterial infection of bile occurs in 25%–50% of patients with malignant obstruction. Bile culture results are expected to be positive in any patient with an indwelling biliary tube.

Ref.: 2, 4, 38

52. Which of the following organisms is most commonly isolated from bile?

A. *Escherichia coli*
B. *Clostridium* spp.
C. *Bacteroides fragilis*
D. *Pseudomonas* spp.
E. *Enterococcus* spp.

ANSWER: A

COMMENTS: All of the aforementioned organisms are found in the biliary tract, but gram-negative aerobic organisms, particularly *E. coli* and *Klebsiella*, are found most frequently. Other gram-negative aerobic bacteria that can be cultured are *Pseudomonas* and *Enterobacter* spp. Gram-positive organisms, especially *Enterococcus* spp. and *Streptococcus faecalis*, are also frequently observed. Anaerobes are now recognized in 4%–20% of cases, most commonly *B. fragilis*, followed by *Clostridium* spp. Polymicrobial infection occurs in approximately 60% of cases. Prophylactic or therapeutic antibiotic therapy must be effective against the anticipated organisms and tailored according to the local antibiogram. Specific antibiotic administration and duration also depend on whether it is community-acquired or health care–associated and the severity grade of the biliary tract infection. For community-acquired grade III and health care–associated biliary infections, consider adding coverage for extended-spectrum beta-lactamase (ESBL)-producing organisms, *Pseudomonas and Enterococcus* spp. Data available on the duration of therapy are scarce, and so the following is based on expert opinion. For grade I cholecystitis, antibiotic therapy can be stopped within 24 h after cholecystectomy or continued for 4 to 7 days if there are emphysematous changes, necrosis, or perforation of the gallbladder. For cholangitis (any grade), grade II/III cholecystitis, and health care–associated biliary infections, antibiotic therapy should continue for 4 to 7 days after source control is achieved. Certain clinical scenarios, such as bacteremia, may require a prolonged antibiotic course.

Ref.: 2, 4, 8, 38

53. Which of the following is the most common mechanism leading to bacteria in bile:

A. Ascending infection from the duodenum
B. Hematogenous portal venous spread
C. Hematogenous arterial spread
D. Lymphatic spread
E. Systemic immunosuppression

ANSWER: B

COMMENTS: Bile is usually sterile. There are various routes by which bacteria can reach the biliary tract, and although not proved, dissemination from the portal venous system via the liver is favored as the most common mechanism. Ascending infection from the duodenum does not occur to a significant extent. In addition, evidence suggests that the direction of lymphatic flow is from the liver downward rather than in the reverse direction. Hematogenous dissemination via hepatic arterial flow is a mechanism of hepatic abscess formation and may lead to bactibilia but is thought to be less common than portal venous spread.

Ref.: 2, 4

54. Which of the following conditions is sufficient to cause cholangitis with bacteremia?

A. Bacteria in bile
B. Complete duct obstruction
C. Bacteria in bile with bile duct obstruction
D. None of the above
E. Any of the above

ANSWER: C

COMMENTS: The pathophysiology of **cholangitis** requires *both* bacterial infection of bile and bile duct obstruction with elevated intraductal pressure. Neither the presence of bacteria in bile nor biliary obstruction alone is sufficient to produce bacteremia. When bacteria are present in bile and common-duct pressures exceed 20 cm H_2O, cholangiovenous and cholangiolymphatic reflux occurs and results in systemic bacteremia. Partial or complete bile duct obstruction may produce cholangitis if bacteria are present. In fact, cholangitis occurs more commonly with partial obstruction because it is more frequently associated with stone disease, whereas complete obstruction is more often found with malignancy. Calculous disease is the most common cause of cholangitis, which is understandable because it is associated with both bile duct obstruction and bacterial infection.

Ref.: 2, 8

55. If an antibiotic is effective against the bacteria present in bile, which of the following is the most important consideration for effective treatment of biliary tract infection?

A. Serum concentration of the antibiotic
B. Bile concentration of the antibiotic in an unobstructed biliary tract
C. Bile concentration of the antibiotic in an obstructed biliary tract
D. Potential renal toxicity of the antibiotic
E. Potential hepatic toxicity of the antibiotic

ANSWER: A

COMMENTS: The most important pharmacologic considerations pertaining to selection of **antimicrobial agents** for the treatment of **biliary sepsis** are the spectrum of antibacterial activity of the agent and achievement of adequate serum levels of the drug. Therapy cannot be adequate if the agents selected are not effective against the anticipated organisms (i.e., gram-negative Enterobacteriaceae, enterococci, and anaerobes) or if dosing does not produce sufficient serum levels. The significance of biliary levels of antibiotics is often discussed, but they are of little clinical importance. High bile levels of an antibiotic are meaningless if the agent is not effective against the bacteria present. Moreover, agents that achieve high concentrations in the normal biliary tract may not reach such levels in the presence of biliary obstruction. Aminoglycosides, for example, have traditionally been effective agents against the gram-negative organisms that cause biliary sepsis, but they are not concentrated in bile. The potential nephrotoxicity of an antibiotic is an important consideration because the risk for renal compromise already exists in a patient with sepsis and biliary obstruction. This has encouraged the use of nonaminoglycoside drugs for gram-negative coverage, but this consideration is not as important as the activity spectrum and adequate serum levels of the drugs.

Ref.: 2, 4

56. All of the following are poor prognostic factors in a patient with cholangitis except:

A. Renal failure
B. Liver abscess
C. Cirrhosis
D. Cholangiocarcinoma
E. Ileus

ANSWER: E

COMMENTS: Charcot's triad, which consists of fever, jaundice, and upper abdominal pain, is the clinical hallmark of acute cholangitis. When accompanied by shock and changes in mental status, it is referred to as **Reynold's pentad**. The current mortality rate in patients with acute cholangitis is approximately 5%. *Poor prognostic factors* include renal failure, liver abscess, cirrhosis, and proximal malignant obstruction. Cholangitis varies widely in severity, and treatment must be individualized according to the patient's condition. Initial therapy consists of fluid resuscitation and antibiotics that are effective against gram-negative organisms, enterococci, and anaerobes. Approximately 5%–10% of patients initially have severe toxic cholangitis and manifestations of the Reynold's pentad. Patients who fail to improve or who deteriorate despite antibiotic and fluid support require urgent biliary decompression. This can generally be accomplished nonoperatively by percutaneous transhepatic or endoscopic approaches depending on the suspected location of the obstruction based on ultrasonographic findings and on the availability of local expertise in these procedures. The ability to decompress the biliary tract nonoperatively in these cases has been advantageous because it not only allows stabilization of a high percentage of patients but also permits diagnostic cholangiography to be performed when the patient is stabilized. When initial operative decompression of the biliary tract was the only approach for these critically ill patients, the mortality rate was high, and there was a frequent need for subsequent reoperation on the biliary tract because of the inability to identify or deal with the underlying pathologic condition at the time of the initial operation. If effective nonoperative drainage of the biliary tract is not possible, surgery should not be delayed in these critically ill patients. T-tube decompression of the CBD is performed. Choledochoduodenostomy is not performed in critically ill patients, but it can be considered if the CBD is dilated to 15 mm or greater, the patient is physiologically stable, and other conditions permit safe performance of an anastomosis.

Ref.: 2, 8

57. A 46-y/o female presents with fevers to 38°C and jaundice for 5 days after an uneventful laparoscopic cholecystectomy for symptomatic cholelithiasis. Her HR is 105, but otherwise her vitals are normal. An ultrasound reveals no fluid collections but shows a CBD diameter of 9 mm. Laboratory values include a WBC count of 10,000/mm³ and a total bilirubin of 3 mg/dL. What is the most appropriate management?

A. IV fluid resuscitation and antibiotics only
B. Emergent endoscopic biliary drainage
C. Emergent bile duct exploration
D. Percutaneous cholecystostomy tube placement
E. IV fluids resuscitation and antibiotics, and biliary drainage if no response to treatment in 24 h

ANSWER: E

COMMENTS: See Question 58.

Ref: 18, 39–40

58. A 38-y/o male presents to the emergency department with fevers and RUQ pain. His temperature is 39°C, he is tachycardic to 110, and the remainder of his vitals are normal. On abdominal examination, he has a positive Murphy's sign. Laboratory values are significant for a WBC count of 15,000/mm³ and a total bilirubin of 5.5 mg/dL. Ultrasound shows a thickened gallbladder wall, stones, pericholecystic fluid, and a CBD diameter of 8 mm. What is the most appropriate ***initial*** management?

A. IV fluids resuscitation and antibiotics, and biliary drainage if no response to treatment in 24 h
B. IV fluids resuscitation, antibiotics, and urgent biliary drainage
C. Cholecystectomy
D. Percutaneous cholecystostomy tube placement
E. IV fluid resuscitation and antibiotics only

ANSWER: B

COMMENTS: As discussed in Question 33, the Tokyo Guidelines also provide diagnostic criteria and a management algorithm for the treatment of acute cholangitis. The three diagnostic criteria for acute cholangitis are (A) signs of systemic inflammation (e.g., fever, abnormal WBC, increased CRP), (B) cholestasis, and (C) imaging suggestive of biliary dilatation and/or etiology of obstruction (stricture, stone, etc.). A patient has a suspected diagnosis of cholangitis if he or she has one item in A and one item in either B or C. A patient has a definite diagnosis of cholangitis if he or she has one item from A, B, *AND* C. The guidelines stratify patients into severity grades, which allow recommendations for management. Grade III (severe) acute cholangitis is associated with organ dysfunction with any of the following signs: hypotension, altered mental status, $PaO_2/FiO_2 < 300$, oliguria or serum creatinine > 2 mg/dL, INR > 1.5, or platelet count < 100,000/mm³. Grade II (moderate) acute cholangitis is associated with any two of the following conditions: abnormal WBC count (>12,000/mm³, <4000/mm³), fever ≥ 39°C, age ≥ 75 years old, total bilirubin ≥ 5 mg/dL, or hypoalbuminemia (lower limit of normal × 0.7). Grade I (mild) acute cholangitis does not meet the criteria of grade II or III. Initial treatment for all grades includes IV fluid resuscitation and initiation of antimicrobials. For grade I (mild), when no response to the initial treatment is observed within 24 h, biliary tract drainage is recommended. For grade II (moderate), biliary tract drainage is immediately performed, in conjunction with IV fluids and antibiotics. For grade III (severe), after IV fluid resuscitation with antibiotics, organ system supportive care takes priority (positive pressure ventilation, vasopressors, etc.) and biliary tract drainage is recommended when safe to do so. Treatment for the etiology of acute cholangitis (e.g., cholecystectomy for gallstones) is considered once acute illness has resolved. The patient in Question 57 presents with grade I (mild) cholangitis after a laparoscopic cholecystectomy, likely from a retained stone. The recommended treatment is IV fluids and antibiotics with biliary drainage reserved for patients who do not improve within 24 h. The patient in Question 58 presents with grade II (moderate) cholangitis. The recommended treatment is IV fluids, antibiotics, and urgent biliary drainage.

Ref.: 18, 39–40

59. Ultrasound of the gallbladder demonstrates a 5-mm hyperechoic focus along the gallbladder wall that does not move or produce shadowing and that has a "comet tail" echo pattern behind it. What is the most likely diagnosis?

A. Adenomatous polyp
B. Cholesterol polyp
C. Gallstone
D. Adenomyomatosis
E. Xanthogranulomatous inflammation

ANSWER: B

COMMENTS: The term ***hyperplastic cholecystosis*** describes a group of benign proliferative conditions of the gallbladder, including cholesterolosis and adenomyomatosis, or adenomatous hyperplasia. These conditions can be symptomatic and are often diagnosed on the basis of their sonographic features. **Cholesterolosis** consists of deposits of cholesterol in foamy histiocytes in the gallbladder wall. A localized collection of such cholesterol-laden cells covered by a normal layer of epithelium and connected to the mucosa by a small pedicle is known as a cholesterol polyp. Ultrasound imaging shows hyperechoic foci with a "comet tail" artifact. Unlike gallstones, the foci do not move or produce acoustic shadowing. **Adenomatous hyperplasia** is a proliferative lesion characterized by increased thickness of the mucosa and muscle along with mucosal diverticula known as Rokitansky-Aschoff sinuses. Segmental, diffuse, and localized forms of adenomyomatous hyperplasia have been described. Of these, a localized form involving the fundus of the gallbladder is most frequently encountered. Ultrasound demonstrates a mass lesion or "pseudotumor." **Adenomatous polyps** are true neoplasms derived from the glandular epithelium of the gallbladder. **Xanthogranulomatous inflammation** is a condition in which foamy histiocytes are found in conjunction with inflammatory cells and a fibroblastic vascular reaction, often with mucosal ulceration.

Ref.: 7

60. With regard to adenomyomatosis of the gallbladder, which of the following statements is true?

A. It is a premalignant lesion.
B. It results from chronic inflammation.
C. It may cause RUQ pain in the absence of gallstones.
D. It is rarely associated with cholelithiasis and cholecystitis.
E. It is not an indication for cholecystectomy in asymptomatic patients.

ANSWER: C

COMMENTS: Adenomyomatosis is a hyperplastic abnormality of the gallbladder that is not related to inflammation or neoplasia.

Approximately one-half or more of patients with adenomyomatosis also have cholelithiasis and cholecystitis, but the relationship is not causal. Adenomyomatosis is not a premalignant lesion. The hyperplastic conditions of adenomyomatosis and cholesterolosis may be associated with functional abnormalities of the gallbladder, as evidenced by disturbances in motility or hyperconcentration during oral cholecystography. These abnormalities may be the cause of biliary tract symptoms in patients with hyperplastic cholecystosis in the absence of cholelithiasis. Cholecystectomy can relieve the symptoms in these patients.

Ref.: 1, 2

61. Which of the following is the *second most common* type of biliary-enteric fistula?

A. Cholecystocolic

B. Cholecystoduodenal

C. Cholecystoduodenocolic

D. Choledochoduodenal

E. Choledochogastric

ANSWER: A

COMMENTS: Almost all **internal biliary fistulas** are acquired communications between the extrahepatic biliary tree and the intestinal tract. In rare instances, acquired or congenital bronchobiliary or acquired pleurobiliary fistulas occur. Biliary-enteric fistulas most commonly involve the gallbladder and the duodenum (70%–80% of cases) and are the result of chronic inflammation caused by gallstone disease. The second most common fistula occurs between the gallbladder and colon; infrequently, the stomach or multiple sites (cholecystoduodenocolic) are involved. Occasionally, the biliary site of the fistula is the CBD. Choledochoduodenal fistulas are most frequently caused by penetrating peptic ulcers, but they might occur in patients with choledocholithiasis and previous cholecystectomy. Other, less common causes of biliary-enteric fistulas are malignancy and penetrating trauma.

Ref.: 2, 4

62. A 73-y/o female presents with acute onset of abdominal distention, pain, nausea and vomiting. She has no previous surgeries. She has no abdominal or inguinal hernias on examination. Abdominal x-ray shows dilated small bowel with air-fluid levels and pneumobilia (Fig. 25.7). The obstruction is most likely at which site?

A. Pylorus

B. Duodenum

C. Jejunum

D. Ileocecal valve

E. Colon

ANSWER: D

COMMENTS: Gallstone ileus is a rare cause of intestinal obstruction. It is a misnomer because it is a mechanical obstruction and not an ileus. The most common etiology is erosion of a large gallstone into the duodenum via a cholecystoduodenal fistula, where the stone passes in the GI tract until it obstructs at the ileocecal valve. Other, less common, locations of fistulas include cholecystogastric and cholecystocolic, which can cause gastric outlet obstruction and colonic obstruction, respectively. After resuscitation, the priority is relieving the obstruction by removing the stone.

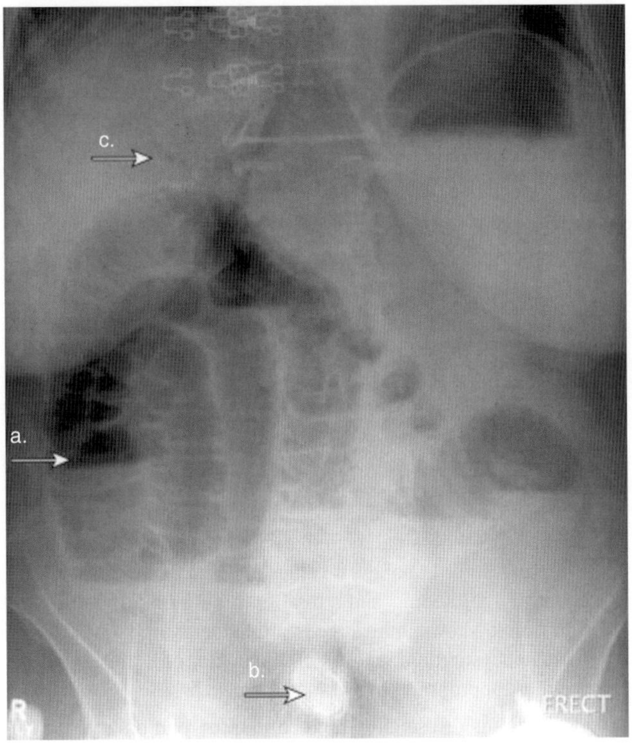

Fig. 25.7 (Question 62 - Stem). *(Source: Cameron JL, Cameron AM. Management of Gallstone Ileus.* Current Surgical Therapy. Cameron JL, Cameron AM, eds. *12th Edition. Elsevier; Philadelphia, PA. 2017, Fig. 2.)*

The biliary management is controversial, as many of the fistulas close spontaneously. Concomitant cholecystectomy and closure of the fistula during the index operation or a two-step staged operation are described in the literature.

Ref.: 41

63. With regard to the management of a patient with gallstone ileus, which of the following statements is true?

A. Initial tube decompression and nonoperative management allow spontaneous stone passage in one-third of patients.

B. Operative treatment attempts to displace the stone into the colon without enterotomy.

C. Operative treatment involves enterotomy proximal to the site of obstruction.

D. Cholecystectomy and fistula repair at the time of stone removal are contraindicated.

E. Standard treatment is initial laparotomy for stone removal and reoperation for cholecystectomy when the patient is stable.

ANSWER: C

COMMENTS: **Gallstone ileus** is mechanical obstruction of the GI tract caused by a gallstone that has entered the intestine via an acquired biliary-enteric fistula. Although gallstone ileus accounts for only 1%–3% of all small bowel obstructions, it is associated with a higher mortality rate than other nonmalignant causes of bowel obstruction because it tends to occur in the elderly population and typical cases are characterized by diagnostic delay as a result of waxing and waning of symptoms ("tumbling obstruction"). Pathognomonic radiologic features include a gas pattern of small bowel obstruction with pneumobilia and an opaque stone outside the expected location of the gallbladder. Not all of these radiologic features are usually present, however. The most common site of obstruction is the terminal ileum. Infrequently, sigmoid obstruction occurs in an area narrowed by intrinsic colonic disease.

Initial therapy is appropriate resuscitation followed by surgery. Spontaneous passage is a rare phenomenon, and nonoperative management is associated with a prohibitive mortality rate. Stone removal is best accomplished with an enterotomy placed proximal to the site of obstruction. Care must be taken to search for additional intestinal stones, which are present in 10% of patients. Attempts to crush the stone extraluminally or to milk it distally are contraindicated because they may cause bowel injury. In rare instances, small bowel resection is necessary if there is ischemic compromise or bleeding at the site of impaction.

The main controversy regarding surgical treatment of gallstone ileus is whether a definitive biliary tract operation with **cholecystectomy**, **fistula repair**, and possible common-duct exploration should be performed at the time of stone removal. This decision must be based on sound surgical judgment and consideration of the underlying physiologic status of the patient and the anatomic status of the RUQ. Up to one-third of patients who do not undergo definitive biliary surgery experience recurrent biliary symptoms, including cholecystitis, cholangitis, and recurrent gallstone ileus. Furthermore, the rate of spontaneous fistula closure is open to question. For these reasons, a definitive one-stage procedure should be considered in physiologically fit patients if RUQ dissection does not prove unduly hazardous from a technical standpoint, particularly if residual stones can be demonstrated in the RUQ. In properly selected patients, a definitive one-stage procedure is not associated with higher operative morbidity or mortality rates. However, because most of these patients are elderly and have a high incidence of comorbid disease, surgical therapy has been limited to stone removal in most instances. **Interval cholecystectomy** should be considered for patients with postoperative biliary symptoms and for those with residual RUQ stones, provided that they are physiologically fit. In reality, because of the compromised underlying status of many of these patients, interval elective procedures are not commonly performed.

Ref.: 2, 4

64. Which clinical scenario is not an indication for early (within 48 to 72 h) ERCP in a patient with proven gallstone pancreatitis?

A. Cholecystitis

B. Severe pancreatitis as measured by the Ranson score

C. Concomitant cholangitis

D. Choledocholithiasis

E. Both A and B

ANSWER: E

COMMENTS: Gallstone disease is the most common cause of acute pancreatitis in the United States. Early studies have shown that patients with acute pancreatitis have a much higher rate of gallstones in their stool (85%–95%) compared with patients who only have symptomatic cholelithiasis (10%). In addition, these series showed a high prevalence of impacted ampullary stones in patients who underwent surgery within 48 h after admission for acute pancreatitis. Today, the debate of which patients benefit from a preoperative ERCP and the timing of this continues to be controversial. Agreed-upon indications for an ERCP include cholangitis, evidence of choledocholithiasis (visualized CBD stones or dilated CBD), persistent biliary obstruction (bilirubin level > 4 mg/dL), or clinical deterioration with the biliary system as the suspected source. Intermediate risk factors for CBD stones include age > 55 years, cholecystitis, a dilated CBD > 6 mm without visualized stones, bilirubin level 1.8 to 4 mg/dL, or other abnormal liver function tests. First-line endoscopic ultrasound or MRCP should be considered for these patients. Patients with none of these sequelae of gallstone pancreatitis require no further intervention. Ultimately, cholecystectomy is advised during the hospital admission as the rate of recurrent pancreatitis or biliary complications is unacceptably high after hospital discharge.

Ref.: 42–44

65. A 22-y/o female presents to the emergency room with RUQ pain and jaundice. Ultrasound shows a normal-appearing gallbladder without stones, but a diffusely dilated CBD. Follow-up ERCP confirms a diffusely dilated fusiform extrahepatic bile duct without filling defects, and normal-appearing intrahepatic biliary anatomy. What is the most appropriate management of this patient?

A. Observation, since there is no evidence of choledocholithiasis

B. Cholecystectomy

C. Hepaticoduodenostomy

D. Complete surgical excision of the dilated bile duct segment and reconstruction with a hepaticojejunostomy

E. Transduodenal excision of the dilated intramural segment within the duodenal wall

ANSWER: D

COMMENTS: Choledochal cysts are a rare cause of RUQ pain and jaundice. They are more common in women of Asian descent and are usually diagnosed in infants, but may present in adults as well. They are premalignant lesions, carrying a 10%–30% risk of carcinoma, so observation is not appropriate. The most accepted theory of their pathogenesis is related to an anomalous pancreaticobiliary junction, which allows pancreatic fluid to reflux up into the biliary tract. This results in chronic inflammation and cystic degeneration of the bile duct. This patient has a type I cyst, which involves fusiform dilatation of the extrahepatic biliary tree and is treated by complete excision and hepaticojejunostomy reconstruction. Type II cysts appear as a diverticulum off the CBD and are treated by excision, as well as biliary-enteric drainage if an anomalous pancreaticobiliary junction is present. Type III cysts, also known as choledochoceles, appear as intramural CBD cystic dilatation within the duodenal wall. Their pathogenesis is not clear and so treatment is directed at relieving the biliary or duodenal obstruction (if present). This can be approached via a transduodenal excision or endoscopic sphincteroplasty. Type IV disease involves both the intra- and extrahepatic biliary trees. Treatment depends on the anatomic pattern of disease. Type V disease, also known as Caroli disease, involves only the intrahepatic bile ducts. Surgical treatment ranges from liver resection to transplantation depending on the extent of ductal involvement.

Ref.: 15

66. With regard to balloon dilation of benign biliary strictures, which of the following statements is true?

A. Dilation can be performed via the transhepatic or endoscopic route.

B. Repeated dilations are not often required.

C. Perforation of the bile duct is the most frequent complication.

D. Better success is obtained with anastomotic strictures than with primary duct strictures.

E. The long-term success rate is better than that achieved with surgical repair.

ANSWER: A

COMMENTS: Nonoperative **dilation of benign biliary strictures** via endoscopic or percutaneous transhepatic access is an alternative to surgery that may be appropriate for some patients. Repeated dilations are often required, but overall success rates of 70%–80% at 2 to 3 years of follow-up have been reported. Success has generally been somewhat higher in patients with primary ductal strictures than in those with strictures of biliary-enteric anastomoses. Bleeding and sepsis have been the most frequent complications and can be life-threatening. Data on long-term results are limited. Comparison between balloon dilation and surgery has demonstrated better long-term results (approximate mean follow-up at 5 years) with surgery, but no difference in overall morbidity, hospitalization, or cost between the two therapies. It cannot be ensured that the treatment groups are comparable, however. Nonoperative dilation of biliary strictures may be appropriate as initial treatment of a strictured biliary anastomosis or for patients in whom surgical repair is deemed excessively difficult or dangerous. The decision about how a biliary stricture is initially treated and when nonoperative maneuvers are abandoned in favor of surgery should be made in consultation with a skilled endoscopist, an interventional radiologist, and an experienced hepatobiliary surgeon.

Ref.: 2, 3

67. A 40-y/o man is evaluated for fluctuating jaundice, pruritus, and fatigue. Liver enzyme levels demonstrate cholestasis. Ultrasound imaging does not show gallstones or bile duct dilation. What diagnostic test should be obtained next?

A. Measurement of serum antimitochondrial antibodies

B. CT

C. HIDA scan

D. ERCP

E. Liver biopsy

ANSWER: D

COMMENTS: The findings described are fairly typical of **sclerosing cholangitis**, which can also be discovered in asymptomatic patients based on a cholestatic liver enzyme pattern. Sclerosing cholangitis is a disease of undetermined cause characterized by inflammatory fibrosis and stenosis of the bile ducts. The process can be considered primary when no specific etiologic factor is identified or secondary when associated with specific causes, such as bile duct stones, operative trauma, hepatic arterial infusion of chemotherapeutic agents, or intraductal instillation of various irritants for the treatment of echinococcal disease. Primary sclerosing cholangitis may be an isolated finding or may occur in conjunction with a variety of other disease processes, most commonly ulcerative colitis and pancreatitis. Although the cause of primary sclerosing cholangitis is unknown, most attention has focused on an autoimmune or infectious cause. Evidence of an autoimmune cause is largely inferential and based on the association of sclerosing cholangitis with a variety of autoimmune diseases. Abnormal immunologic parameters can be found in the serum of some patients with sclerosing cholangitis, but there are no specific serologic markers for the disease. Antimitochondrial antibodies are generally associated with primary biliary cirrhosis. The diagnosis is usually made following ERCP showing multiple strictures and dilations, which give a “beaded” appearance to the ducts. Magnetic resonance imaging of the bile ducts may also show abnormalities. Typically, sclerosing cholangitis is a diffuse process that affects both the intrahepatic and extrahepatic bile ducts. In some cases, more limited involvement of the distal bile duct, the intrahepatic ducts, or the area of the bifurcation can be seen. Liver biopsy may show fibro-obliterative cholangitis or cirrhosis as the disease progresses.

Ref.: 2–4

68. Definitive treatment of a patient with sclerosing cholangitis and biliary cirrhosis involves which of the following?

A. Ursodeoxycholic acid

B. Corticosteroids

C. Endoscopic balloon dilation and stenting

D. Extrahepatic bile duct resection and transhepatic stenting

E. Hepatic transplantation

ANSWER: E

COMMENTS: Once **sclerosing cholangitis** has progressed to cirrhosis, the only definitive treatment is **hepatic transplantation**. The results of transplantation are generally similar to those obtained when it is performed for other indications. Before the development of cirrhosis, a number of medical and surgical therapies may be useful. Pharmacologic approaches have included the use of immunosuppressants, bile acid–binding agents, and antifibrotic and antimicrobial drugs. Unfortunately, there is little evidence that any medical therapy has been effective in slowing progression. Some hopeful results have been reported with ursodeoxycholic acid, which may improve liver enzyme test results and liver histologic study results. Dominant strictures can be treated operatively or by nonoperative dilation via endoscopic or percutaneous transhepatic approaches. The long-term efficacy of nonoperative approaches has often been limited, however. Select patients with predominantly extrahepatic or bifurcation strictures have been treated successfully with bile duct resection followed by Roux-en-Y reconstruction and long-term anastomotic stenting.

Ref.: 2–4

69. A 63-y/o female undergoes a laparoscopic cholecystectomy for symptomatic cholelithiasis. The pathology report states that there is a foci of carcinoma which invades, but does not penetrate through, the lamina propria. What is the most appropriate management?

A. Laparoscopic resection of the gallbladder fossa

B. Open extended cholecystectomy including segment 4b and 5 liver resection as well as removal of porta hepatis lymph nodes

C. Cholecystectomy is sufficient

D. CBD excision to achieve negative margins with Roux-en-Y hepaticojejunostomy reconstruction
E. Radiation and chemotherapy

ANSWER: C

COMMENTS: Gallbladder cancer is an aggressive malignancy that is often asymptomatic until it reaches an advanced stage. This is an early-stage T1a tumor that was found incidentally. The treatment is cholecystectomy alone because the tumor is limited to the lamina propria and the chance of lymph node disease is less than 3%. A more advanced T1b tumor, which presents with invasion of the muscularis proper with evidence of lymphovascular invasion, requires an open extended cholecystectomy. Resection includes a 2-cm rim of liver parenchyma from the gallbladder fossa (segments 4b and 5) as well as removal of pericholedochal, periportal, hepatoduodenal, right celiac, and posterior pancreaticoduodenal lymph nodes. Prognosis is substantially improved if an R0 resection can be obtained. Therefore a CBD resection with a Roux-en-Y hepaticojejunostomy reconstruction may be necessary to achieve a negative cyst duct margin. Radiation therapy and chemotherapy have generally been ineffective for the treatment of gallbladder cancer.

Ref: 15

70. Ultrasound imaging demonstrates a 15-mm polypoid lesion in the gallbladder of an asymptomatic 60-y/o patient. Which of the following best describes the recommended treatment?

A. Observation with repeated ultrasound studies in 6 months
B. Cholecystectomy
C. Cholecystectomy if the patient is female
D. Cholecystectomy only if symptoms develop
E. Cholecystectomy only if the patient also has gallstones

ANSWER: B

COMMENTS: Polypoid lesions of the gallbladder may be benign, premalignant, or malignant. Inflammatory polyps and cholesterol polyps are benign, nonneoplastic lesions. Benign adenomas are neoplasms that have a malignant potential similar to that of adenomas arising in other areas of the GI tract. Polypoid lesions are typically diagnosed by ultrasound imaging and occasionally by other imaging modalities, such as CT. The indications for cholecystectomy for the treatment of a polypoid lesion are (1) symptoms and (2) possible malignancy.

The **risk for malignancy** is related to the size of the lesion; it is higher for lesions that are 10 mm or larger and is quite substantial for lesions measuring 15 mm. Therefore cholecystectomy is performed if the patient has biliary tract symptoms—regardless of polyp size or the presence or absence of gallstones—or if the lesion is larger than 10 mm. Polypoid lesions in patients 60 years or older are also more frequently malignant. The use of **laparoscopic cholecystectomy** for polypoid lesions is controversial. Proponents argue that the laparoscopic approach is appropriate because most polyps are benign and even limited cancers may be cured by cholecystectomy alone. However, gallbladder leakage is not infrequent during laparoscopic cholecystectomy, and consequent dissemination of otherwise "curable" early cancers has been reported. It is generally advised that "**open cholecystectomy**" be performed for patients considered at risk for gallbladder cancer.

Ref.: 45

71. Which of the following is a contraindication to resection of an adenocarcinoma of the bile duct?

A. Tumor location in the distal CBD
B. Tumor location at the bifurcation of the bile duct
C. Invasion of the right and left portal vein
D. Invasion of the right portal vein and right hepatic artery
E. None of the above

ANSWER: C

COMMENTS: Cancers of the extrahepatic bile ducts usually carry a poor prognosis because these tumors are frequently beyond the confines of surgical resection at the time of diagnosis. Substantial palliation can often be achieved with therapy directed at the relief of biliary obstruction. The prognosis is related to tumor location, resectability, and histologic pattern. Proximal lesions at or near the hepatic bifurcation are most common but are also least often resectable and therefore have a less favorable prognosis. Aggressive resection of proximal lesions, usually including hepatic resection, can improve survival. Hilar cholangiocarcinoma (Klatskin tumor) is considered unresectable if there is metastatic disease, bilateral involvement of the portal vein or hepatic artery, or bilateral extension of the tumor to second-order biliary radicles. **Hepatic transplantation** for otherwise unresectable tumors is performed at highly specialized centers, but is not the standard of care. Distal lesions resectable by pancreaticoduodenectomy have the best prognosis, with a 5-year survival rate of approximately 30%–50%. Palliative decompression can be achieved by surgical anastomosis, surgical intubation, or endoscopic or percutaneous catheter placement. The most appropriate method of palliative decompression for a particular patient depends on tumor location and extent, the patient's underlying condition, the expertise of the surgeon, and the anticipated complications associated with each technique. Nonoperative decompression is preferred for patients who are demonstrated to have metastasis or otherwise unresectable disease before surgery.

Ref.: 3, 4

REFERENCES

1. Reynolds W. The first laparoscopic cholecystectomy. *JSLS*. 2001; 5(1):89–94.
2. Chari RS, Shah SA. Biliary system. In: Townsend CM, Beauchamp RD, Evers BM, et al., eds. *Sabiston Textbook of Surgery: The Biological Basis of Modern Surgical Practice*. 18th ed. Philadelphia: WB Saunders; 2008.
3. Mullholland MW, Lillemoe KD, Doherty GM, et al., eds. *Greenfield's Surgery: Scientific Principles and Practice, Hepatobiliary and Portal Venous System Section*. 4th ed. Philadelphia: Lippincott Williams & Wilkins; 2006.
4. Blumgart LH. *Surgery of the Liver, Biliary Tract and Pancreas*. 4th ed. Edinburgh: Churchill-Livingstone; 2006.
5. Yoshida J, Chijiwa K, Yamaguchi K, et al. Practical classification of the branching types of the biliary tree: an analysis of 1,094 consecutive direct cholangiograms. *J Am Coll Surg*. 1996;82:37–40.
6. Massearweg NN, Flum DR. Role of intraoperative cholangiography in avoiding bile duct injury. *J Am Coll Surg*. 2007;204(4):656–664.
7. Machi J, Staren ED. *Ultrasound for Surgeons*. Philadelphia: Lippincott Williams & Wilkins; 2005.
8. Mulvihill SJ. Liver, biliary tract, and pancreas. In: O'Leary JP, Tabuenca A, eds. *The Physiologic Basis of Surgery*. 4th ed. Philadelphia: Lippincott Williams & Wilkins; 2008.
9. Delis S, Bakoyiannis A, Madariaga J, Bramis J, Tassopoulos N, Dervenis C. Laparoscopic cholecystectomy in cirrhotic patients: the value of MELD score and Child-Pugh classification in predicting outcome. *Surg Endosc*. 2010;24(2):407–412.

10. Vassiliou MC, Laycock WS. Biliary dyskinesia. *Surg Clin N Am.* 2008;88(6):1253–1272.
11. Yoon YS, Han HS, Cho JY, et al. Is laparoscopy contraindicated for gallbladder cancer? A 10-year prospective cohort study. *J Am Coll Surg.* 2015;221(4):847–853.
12. Strasberg SM, Hertl M, Soper NJ. An analysis of the problem of biliary injury during laparoscopic cholecystectomy. *J Am Coll Surg.* 1995;180: 101–125.
13. Strasberg SM, Eagon CJ, Drebin JA. The "hidden cystic duct" syndrome and the infundibular technique of laparoscopic cholecystectomy—the danger of the false infundibulum. *J Am Coll Surg.* 2000;191(6):661–667.
14. Lillemoe KD. Current management of bile duct injury. *Br J Surg.* 2008;95:403–405.
15. Jackson PG, Evans SRT, eds. *Sabitston Textbook of Surgery: Biliary System.* 20th ed. Philadelphia: Elsevier, Inc; 2017.
16. Deziel DJ. Complications of cholecystectomy. *Surg Clin North Am.* 1994;74:809–823.
17. Woods MS, Traverso LW, Kozarek RA, et al. Biliary tract complications of laparoscopic cholecystectomy are detected more frequently with routine intraoperative cholangiography. *Surg Endosc.* 1995;9: 1076–1080.
18. Okamoto K, Takada T, Strasberg SM, et al. TG13 management bundles for acute cholangitis and cholecystitis. *J Hepatobiliary Pancreat Sci.* 2013;20(1):55–59.
19. Yamashita Y, Takada T, Strasberg SM, et al. TG13 surgical management of acute cholecystitis. *J Hepatobiliary Pancreat Sci.* 2013;20(1):89–96.
20. Tsuyuguchi T, Itoi T, Takada T, et al. TG13 indications and techniques for gallbladder drainage in acute cholecystitis (with videos). *J Hepatobiliary Pancreat Sci.* 2013;20(1):81–88.
21. Kimura Y, Takada T, Strasberg SM, et al. TG13 current terminology, etiology, and epidemiology of acute cholangitis and cholecystitis. *J Hepatobiliary Pancreat Sci.* 2013;20(1):8–23.
22. Yokoe M, Takada T, Strasberg SM, et al. TG13 diagnostic criteria and severity grading of acute cholecystitis (with videos). *J Hepatobiliary Pancreat Sci.* 2013;20(1):35–46.
23. Date RS, Kaushal M, Ramesh A. A review of the management of gallstone disease and its complications during pregnancy. *Am J Surg.* 2008;196:599–608.
24. Schwartz N, Adamczak J, Ludmir J. Surgery during pregnancy. In: Gabbe SG, Niebyl JR, Galan HL, et al., eds. *Obstetrics: Normal and Problem Pregnancies.* 6th ed. St Louis: Saunders; 2012.
25. Villegas L, Schneider B, Provost D, et al. Is routine cholecystectomy required during laparoscopic gastric bypass? *Obesity Surg.* 2004; 14(2):206–211.
26. Li VK, Pulido N, Fajnwaks P, Szomstein S, Rosenthal R, Martinez-Duartez P. Predictors of gallstone formation after bariatric surgery: a multivariate analysis of risk factors comparing gastric bypass, gastric banding, and sleeve gastrectomy. *Surg Endosc.* 2009;23(7):1640–1644.
27. Moon RC, Teixeira AF, DuCoin C, Varnadore S, Jawad MA. Comparison of cholecystectomy cases after Roux-en-Y gastric bypass, sleeve gastrectomy, and gastric banding. *Surg Obes Relat Dis.* 2014;10(1):64–68.
28. Strasberg SM, Pucci MJ, Brunt ML, Deziel DJ. Subtotal cholecystectomy: "fenestrating" vs "reconstituting" subtypes and the prevention of bile duct injury: definition of the optimal procedure in difficult operative conditions. *J Am Coll Surg.* 2016;222(1):89–96.
29. Podolsky ER, Curcillo II PG. Single port access (SPA) surgery: a 24-month experience. *J Gastrointest Surg.* 2010;14:759–767.
30. Markar SR, Karthikesalingam A, Thrumurthy S, Muirhead L, Kinross J, Paraskeva P. Single-incision laparoscopic surgery (SILS) vs. conventional multiport cholecystectomy: systematic review and meta-analysis. *Surg Endosc.* 2012;26(5):1205–1213.
31. Garg P, Thakur JD, Garg M, Menon GR. Single-incision laparoscopic cholecystectomy vs. conventional laparoscopic cholecystectomy: a meta-analysis of randomized controlled trials. 2012;16(8):1618–1628.
32. Barkun AN, Barkun JS, Fried GM, et al. Useful predictors of bile duct stones in patients undergoing laparoscopic cholecystectomy. *Ann Surg.* 1994;220:32–39.
33. Tse F, Barkun J, Romagnuolo J, et al. Non-operative imaging techniques in suspected biliary tract obstruction. *HPB (Oxford).* 2006;(8):409–425.
34. Petelin J. Laparoscopic approach to common duct pathology. *Am J Surg.* 1993;165:487–491.
35. Bansal VK, Misra MC, Rajan K, et al. Single-stage laparoscopic common bile duct exploration and cholecystectomy versus two-stage endoscopic stone extraction followed by laparoscopic cholecystectomy for patients with concomitant gallbladder stones and common bile duct stones: a randomized controlled trial. *Surg Endosc.* 2014;28(3):875–885.
36. Dasari BV, Tan CJ, Gurusamy KS, et al. Surgical versus endoscopic treatment of bile duct stones. *Cochrane Database Syst Rev.* 2013;(9): CD003327.
37. Perry KA, Myers JA, Deziel DJ. Laparoscopic ultrasound as the primary modality for bile duct imaging during cholecystectomy. *Surg Endosc.* 2008;22:208–213.
38. Gomi H, Solomkin JS, Takada T, et al. TG13 antimicrobial therapy for acute cholangitis and cholecystitis. *J Hepatobiliary Pancreat Sci.* 2013;20(1):60–70.
39. Kiriyama S, Takada T, Strasberg SM, et al. TG13 guidelines for diagnosis and severity grading of acute cholangitis (with videos). *J Hepatobiliary Pancreat Sci.* 2013;20(1):24–34.
40. Miura F, Takeda T, Strasberg SM, et al. TG13 flowchart for the management of acute cholangitis and cholecystitis. *J Hepatobiliary Pancreat Sci.* 2013;20(1):47–54.
41. Bailey EH, Sharp KW, eds. *Current Surgical Therapy: Gallstone Ileus.* 11th ed. Philadelphia: Elsevier, Inc; 2014.
42. Frossard JL, Spahr L. ERCP for gallstone pancreatitis. *NEJM.* 2014;370(20):1954–1955.
43. Fogel EL, Sherman S. ERCP for gallstone pancreatitis. *NEJM.* 2014;370(2):150–157.
44. Acosta JM, Ledesma CL. Gallstone migration as a cause of acute pancreatitis. *NEJM.* 1974;290:484–487.
45. D'Angelica M, Dalal KM, DeMatteo RP, et al. Analysis of the extent of resection for adenocarcinoma of the gallbladder. *Ann Surg Oncol.* 2009;16:806–816.

CHAPTER 26

PANCREAS

Joseph Broucek, M.D., Benjamin R. Veenstra, M.D., and Keith Millikan, M.D., F.A.C.S.

1. A 58-year-old woman with jaundice underwent endoscopic retrograde cholangiopancreatography (ERCP) (see Fig. 26.1) as a part of her diagnostic workup. On the basis of this radiograph, what is the most likely diagnosis?

A. Chronic pancreatitis

B. Pancreatic cancer

C. Cholangiocarcinoma

D. Pancreas divisum

E. Ectopic pancreas

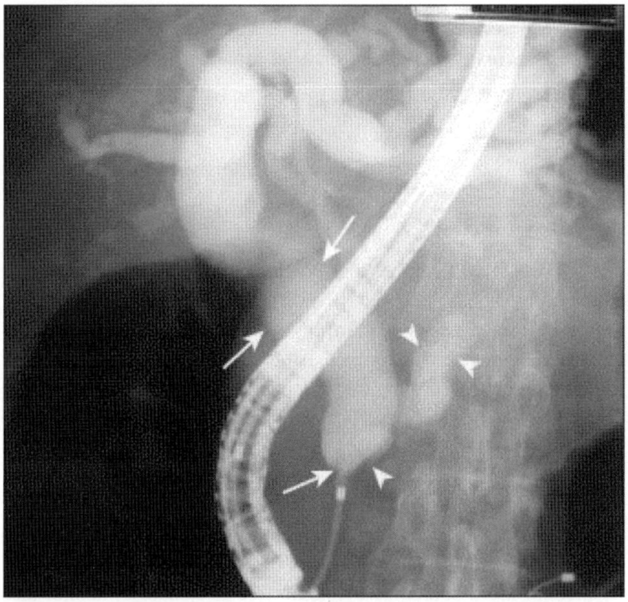

Fig. 26.1 ERCP demonstration of a "double-duct" sign in pancreatic carcinoma with proximal biliary dilation (arrows) and dilated pancreatic duct (arrowheads). *From Shah P, Spencer G, Kochman ML. ERCP. In: Baron TH, Kozarek R, Carr-Locke DL, eds.,* Approach to the Dilated Bile Duct and Pneumobilia. *2nd ed. Philadelphia: Elsevier Saunders; 2013:313–322.e2. Chapter 33.*

ANSWER: B

COMMENTS: This ERCP study shows the classic "double-duct sign:" dilation of the biliary system above an area of abrupt narrowing and abrupt termination of the main pancreatic duct. These findings place the primary abnormality in the geographic location of the pancreatic head, and it is not uncommon for a pancreatic neoplasm to involve both ducts. Chronic pancreatitis may cause biliary obstruction, but the obstruction in the biliary systems is usually more distal. Likewise, there are no coexistent changes in this patient, such as irregular beading of the pancreatic duct, to suggest that chronic pancreatitis is present. Cholangiocarcinoma may be responsible for the stenosis in the biliary system, but cholangiocarcinomas rarely become large enough to involve the pancreatic duct. With pancreas divisum, injection of the major papilla opacifies only a short, tapering ventral duct draining the caudal portion of the pancreatic head and uncinate process. Injection of the minor papilla demonstrates the dorsal duct draining the major portion of the gland.

Ref.: 1, 2

2. You diagnose the patient in Question 46 with an insulinoma. Magnetic resonance imaging (MRI) shows a lesion in the body of the pancreas. Which of the following statements is true regarding the preferred treatment?

A. Diazoxide is the preferred initial method of management.

B. Enucleation is acceptable for localized pancreatic lesions.

C. Because most lesions are multiple or diffuse, total or nearly total pancreatectomy is generally necessary.

D. Because most lesions are malignant, adjuvant streptozocin is usually indicated.

E. Parathyroid adenoma should be excluded or treated before pancreatic resection.

ANSWER: B

COMMENTS: Insulinomas are usually single and benign and are rarely ectopic. Localization of an insulinoma can be difficult, and preoperative imaging along with thorough mobilization and exploration of the pancreas is mandatory. Intraoperative ultrasonography is indispensable. For localized lesions, simple enucleation is the preferred treatment, but the integrity of the pancreatic duct must be ascertained. If the lesion cannot be identified and the biochemical basis of the diagnosis is firm, blind distal pancreatic resection with a careful histologic examination of the specimen may be necessary. Intraoperative monitoring of serum glucose levels has also been used. Diazoxide inhibits insulin release from beta cells and is occasionally used for preoperative control or for patients with recurrent postoperative hypoglycemia. For patients with metastatic malignant insulinoma, tumor debulking may be beneficial, as is the use of streptozocin and 5-fluorouracil. Gastrinoma, not insulinoma, is the most common pancreatic adenoma associated with multiple endocrine adenomatosis type I syndrome. Parathyroid disease should be excluded or treated before surgical intervention for gastrinoma.

Ref.: 1–3

3. Which of the following features is characteristic of Zollinger-Ellison syndrome but not of Verner-Morrison syndrome?
   A. Diarrhea
   B. Hypercalcemia
   C. Hypocalcemia
   D. Increased gastric acid secretion
   E. Malignancy

ANSWER: D

COMMENTS: Zollinger-Ellison syndrome is caused by a gastrin-producing islet cell tumor. Verner-Morrison syndrome is caused by an islet cell tumor that produces vasoactive intestinal peptide. Zollinger-Ellison syndrome is associated with a marked increase in gastric acid secretion and with diarrhea. Hypercalcemia may occur because of associated parathyroid abnormalities. Verner-Morrison syndrome is characterized by watery diarrhea, hypokalemia, and achlorhydria. Hypercalcemia may occur, but the parathyroids are usually normal. Both syndromes are frequently the result of malignant islet cell tumors.

Ref.: 1–3

4. Which of the following is not a feature of the clinical syndrome associated with a glucagon-producing islet cell tumor?
   A. Rash
   B. Diabetes
   C. Seizures
   D. Glossitis
   E. Anemia

ANSWER: C

COMMENTS: Patients with **glucagon-secreting tumors** have diabetes, anemia, weight loss, venous thrombosis, glossitis, and a characteristic cutaneous lesion known as necrolytic migratory erythema. The lesion is rare and often metastatic at the time of diagnosis. Treatment is directed at achieving as complete a resection as possible. Postoperatively, chemotherapy with dacarbazine or streptozocin may be useful for a residual or recurrent disease.

Ref.: 1–3

5. A 27-year-old male presents to the trauma bay after being hit in the mid-abdomen with a large steel post at the construction site where he works. Focused assessment with sonography for trauma scan of the abdomen shows free fluid, and the patient is becoming more tachycardic in the trauma bay despite fluids and pain control. He is taken to the operating room, and complete transection of the pancreatic neck is identified. There are no associated organ injuries. Which of the following treatments is most appropriate?
   A. Placement of drains and closure of the abdomen
   B. Distal pancreatectomy with ligation of the proximal duct
   C. Roux-en-Y pancreaticojejunostomy to the distal pancreas with ligation of the proximal duct
   D. Roux-en-Y pancreaticojejunostomy to both the proximal and distal segments of the pancreas
   E. Pancreaticoduodenectomy with Roux-en-Y pancreaticojejunostomy to the distal duct

ANSWER: B

COMMENTS: Pancreatic contusions or lacerations without ductal disruption are managed by drainage alone. The pancreatic neck is a frequent site of pancreatic injury when it occurs with blunt trauma. Distal pancreatectomy with identification and closure of the proximal duct and drainage is safe, and resections involving up to 80% of an otherwise normal gland can be accomplished without subsequent endocrine insufficiency. In theory, Roux-en-Y pancreaticojejunostomy may be desirable to preserve pancreatic tissue, but it is not recommended for the management of acute injuries because of the risk associated with a pancreatic anastomosis and the need to open the gut. Pancreaticoduodenectomy is indicated for patients with severe combined duodenal, pancreatic, and bile duct injuries. Most **pancreatic injuries** are the result of penetrating trauma, although the gland is vulnerable to blunt trauma because of its fixed position anteriorly over the vertebral column. The presence of significant pancreatic injury following blunt trauma is often not initially apparent. Hyperamylasemia in serum or peritoneal fluid suggests the diagnosis, but a negative peritoneal tap or lavage does not exclude retroperitoneal injury. Retroperitoneal hematomas in the upper part of the abdomen should be explored to exclude pancreatic ductal injury. Pancreatitis is the most common cause of pseudocyst, although about 25% occur as a result of trauma.

Ref.: 1–3

6. The mechanism of alcohol-induced acute pancreatitis is thought to involve all of the following except:
   A. Pancreatic ductal obstruction
   B. Pancreatic exocrine hypersecretion
   C. Hypertriglyceridemia
   D. Acetaldehyde toxicity
   E. Genetic defect in lysosomal membranes

ANSWER: E

COMMENTS: Ethanol is the prevalent etiologic factor in acute pancreatitis. There are several contributory mechanisms by which **alcohol-induced pancreatic injury** occurs. Ethanol causes pancreatic ductal hypertension by increasing ampullary resistance and by intraductal deposition of stone proteins. Concomitantly, ethanol stimulates gastric acid secretion and increases pancreatic exocrine secretion via the release of secretin. The combination of ductal obstruction with stimulated secretion may result in enzyme extravasation. Acetaldehyde, the metabolic product of ethanol, injures acinar cells by increasing membrane permeability and disrupting the microtubule structure. The elevated levels of serum triglycerides induced by alcohol are a source of cytotoxic free fatty acids. Alcohol also impairs normal trypsin inhibition and reduces pancreatic blood flow. All of these effects may contribute to intraglandular enzyme activation and the development of acute alcoholic pancreatitis.

Ref.: 1, 3

7. In North America, chronic pancreatitis is most commonly related to chronic alcohol ingestion. Which of the following is the second most common cause?
   A. Gallstones
   B. Drugs
   C. Infection
   D. Malnutrition
   E. Idiopathic

ANSWER: E

COMMENTS: In the Western world, **alcohol** use accounts for about 75% of cases of **chronic pancreatitis**. Approximately 20% of cases are considered idiopathic. In parts of Africa and Asia, protein malnutrition is an important etiologic factor. Other, less common causes of chronic pancreatitis include pancreatic duct obstruction (secondary to stenosis or pancreas divisum), hyperparathyroidism, trauma, cystic fibrosis (CF), and hereditary causes. Unlike acute pancreatitis, calculous biliary disease is not a typical cause of chronic pancreatitis. Certain infections (particularly viral) and drugs are among the many factors that can produce acute, rather than chronic, pancreatitis.

Ref.: 3

8. Endoscopy demonstrates a 1-cm submucosal nodule with central umbilication in the second portion of the duodenum. This finding is usually associated with which of the following?

A. Peptic ulceration
B. Increased risk for pancreatic cancer
C. Islet cell hyperplasia
D. Absence of symptoms
E. Intussusception

ANSWER: D

COMMENTS: A **heterotopic pancreas** is a pancreatic tissue located at sites other than the normal location of the gland. Ectopic pancreatic tissue has been described at many anatomic locations but is typically found in the stomach, the duodenum, or a Meckel's diverticulum. Theories of origin include metaplasia (the favored theory) and transplantation. Histologic findings range from those of a rudimentary structure to a fully formed gland. Most heterotopic rests contain ducts, and both endocrine and exocrine elements may be present. This entity is not uncommon, being described in 1%–2% of autopsies. It is usually asymptomatic. When symptoms occur, they are related to the location of the ectopic site and include obstruction (as a result of intussusception), ulceration, and bleeding. Although malignancy has been reported, there is no evidence that heterotopic pancreatic tissue is predisposed to cancer. The typical gross appearance is a submucosal nodule, often with central umbilication. Resection is indicated for symptomatic lesions and is appropriate diagnostically for incidental lesions discovered during operations for other reasons.

Ref.: 1, 2, 4

9. What is the recommended treatment of duodenal obstruction caused by an annular pancreas?

A. Endoscopic division of the associated duodenal web
B. Gastrojejunostomy
C. Duodenoduodenostomy
D. Surgical division of the annular tissue
E. Pancreaticoduodenectomy

ANSWER: C

COMMENTS: An **annular pancreas** is a congenital anomaly involving a band of pancreatic tissue encircling the second portion of the duodenum. The annular tissue appears to originate from the embryologic ventral pancreas. Causal theories include abnormal fixation of the ventral pancreatic primordium before gut rotation, failure of involution of part of the ventral pancreas, and the development of heterotopic pancreatic tissue in the duodenum. Approximately one-half of these cases are diagnosed in infants and the remainder in adults, with a peak during the fourth decade of life. Most patients are asymptomatic. Clinical findings are obstruction in infants and children and obstruction, ulceration, or pancreatitis in adults. Associated anomalies include duodenal stenosis or atresia and Down syndrome. Treatment of symptomatic patients consists of surgical bypass by duodenoduodenostomy or duodenojejunostomy. Gastrojejunostomy can also alleviate obstruction but risks marginal ulceration. Resection or division of the annular band is not advised because it risks the development of a pancreatic fistula and may fail to relieve the obstruction.

Ref.: 1, 2, 4

10. The embryologic ventral pancreas forms which area of the fully developed gland?

A. Superior head
B. Uncinate process
C. Neck
D. Body
E. None of the above because it regresses

ANSWER: B

COMMENTS: The pancreas is formed from two outpouchings of the primitive gut. The **dorsal pancreas** originates from the duodenum, and the **ventral pancreas** begins as a bud from the hepatic diverticulum, which itself is an outpouching of the duodenum. Other outgrowths from the hepatic diverticulum mature into the liver, gallbladder, and bile ducts. During normal fetal development, the ventral pancreas rotates along with the primitive gut and fuses with the dorsal component. The ventral pancreas constitutes the uncinate process and the inferior portion of the head of the gland in the fully developed state, and the dorsal pancreas forms the remainder of the gland. Abnormalities in this developmental process result in recognized congenital anomalies that can be clinically important. An understanding of this embryologic development is also important for recognizing the relationship of the pancreas to adjacent vascular structures during pancreatic operations.

Ref.: 1, 3, 4

11. A 68-year-old man presents with painless jaundice. He has a history of diabetes, hypertension, and alcohol abuse. He has a 40-pack-year tobacco history. He has been hospitalized for pancreatitis three times in the past. Computed tomography (CT) scan shows a 2-cm lesion in the head of the pancreas. Endoscopic ultrasound (EUS) and biopsy confirm pancreatic adenocarcinoma. He asks you what most likely would have contributed to this diagnosis of ductal adenocarcinoma of the pancreas.

A. Chronic pancreatitis
B. Diabetes mellitus
C. Cigarette smoking
D. Coffee consumption
E. Alcohol consumption

ANSWER: C

COMMENTS: Epidemiologic studies have identified various demographic, medical, environmental, and dietary factors that have some relationship to **pancreatic cancer**. The most firmly established risk factor is cigarette smoking. Experimentally, nitrosamines have been found to be carcinogenic. In addition, the carcinogens in cigarettes have been related to *K-ras* oncogene mutations, which are frequent in pancreatic cancer. Alcohol has not been demonstrated conclusively to be a risk factor independent of cigarettes. The previously reported association of pancreatic cancer with coffee consumption is questionable. Diets high in fats and meat may be associated with pancreatic cancer, whereas diets high in fruits and vegetables may be protective. Certain occupational and industrial exposures have an increased risk. There may be some association with diabetes mellitus and certain forms of chronic pancreatitis, but the relationship is not considered causal. Previous gastrectomy has been associated with increased risk, whereas tonsillectomy has been observed to be protective.

Ref.: 1, 3, 4

12. The medical intensive care unit service consults you on hospital day 2 for a 57-year-old male being treated for alcoholic pancreatitis. At admission, his white blood cell (WBC) count was 17,000, glucose was 100 mg/dL, aspartate aminotransferase (AST) was 400 IU/L, alanine aminotransferase (ALT) was 150 IU/L, and lactate dehydrogenase (LDH) was 200 IU/L. Today his creatinine is 2.1 mg/dL with a stable blood urea nitrogen (BUN), his base deficit is 7 mEq/L, pO_2 is 72 mmHg, calcium is 7.5 mg/dL, and base deficit is 8 mEq/L. He does not appear to be heavily third spaced. What is his likelihood of mortality?

A. 0%

B. 10%

C. 20%

D. 40%

E. 80%

ANSWER: D

COMMENTS: Several systems have been devised to gauge the severity of acute pancreatitis. These systems involve multiple clinical, biochemical, and, sometimes, radiologic criteria. The most widely used system in the United States, developed by Ranson, was based on retrospective analysis and subsequent prospective verification. The **Ranson criteria** include 11 parameters determined at the time of admission or during the subsequent 48 h. Patients with three or more criteria have more severe disease and are at increased risk for septic complications and death. The criteria reflect the patient's underlying status, the severity of the retroperitoneal inflammatory process, and the effects on renal and respiratory function. The Ranson criteria were originally developed for alcoholic pancreatitis and have been modified somewhat for gallstone pancreatitis. For example, a rise in the serum BUN level of more than 2 mg/dL is 1 of the 10 criteria for gallstone pancreatitis, but the rise must be more than 5 mg/dL to meet the criteria for alcoholic pancreatitis (a subtle point). The criteria include the following at admission: age > 55 years, WBC > 16 cells per MCL, blood glucose > 200 mg/dL, AST > 250 IU/L, and LDH > 350 IU/L. At 48 h from admission, the additional criteria include the following: calcium < 8 mg/dL, hematocrit fall > 10%, hypoxemia (pO_2 < 60 mmHg), BUN increased by 5 mg/dL or more, base deficit > 4, and sequestration of fluid > 6 L. A score of 0 to 2 assigns a 2% mortality, 3 to 4: 15%, 5 to 6: 40%, and greater than 7: 100%. Other physiologic scoring systems, such as the Acute Physiology, Age, and Chronic Health Evaluation II, are also useful prognostically, although they are not designed specifically for acute pancreatitis.

Ref.: 1, 3, 4

13. Hyperamylasemia is diagnostic of acute pancreatitis when associated with which of the following laboratory findings?

A. Hyperlipasemia

B. Increased urinary amylase levels

C. Amylase-creatinine clearance ratio (ACCR) greater than 5%

D. Hypocalcemia

E. None of the above

ANSWER: E

COMMENTS: The **diagnosis of acute pancreatitis** is based on signs and symptoms, supported by biochemical findings and morphologic abnormalities seen on imaging studies such as CT. No biochemical feature is pathognomonic of acute pancreatitis. Hyperamylasemia, hyperlipasemia, and elevations in urinary amylase levels and the **ACCR** are typical of acute pancreatitis but are not specific or sensitive, and they can occur with other abdominal and extraabdominal disorders. Hypocalcemia may occur as a consequence of pancreatitis, but it is also nonspecific. There is no absolute level of serum amylase or lipase that is diagnostic of acute pancreatitis. Marked elevations are more indicative of pancreatitis but are not themselves diagnostic. Both amylase and lipase levels may be elevated in a number of conditions that can be confused with acute pancreatitis, such as acute cholecystitis, perforated peptic ulcer, and intestinal infarction. Moreover, severe pancreatitis can occur without substantial elevations in these serum enzymes. Elevations in serum and urinary **amylase** levels and in the ACCR, as determined by the following equation, are typical of acute pancreatitis.

$$ACCR = U_{amy}/S_{amy} \times S_{cr}/U_{cr} \times 100$$

where U = urine, S = serum, amy = amylase, and cr = creatinine. Elevation of the ACCR above the normal 2%–5% range is not specific for pancreatitis, but a normal ratio in the presence of hyperamylasemia suggests that the hyperamylasemia is the result of something other than pancreatitis. Serum and urinary amylase levels and the ACCR may be normal in patients with chronic pancreatitis or elevated during an acute exacerbation. Renal disease may be associated with low urinary amylase levels and an elevated ACCR. Common duct stones may produce hyperamylasemia without true pancreatitis. The urinary amylase level is elevated, although the ACCR may be normal. With macroamylasemia, amylase forms complexes with serum proteins too large for glomerular filtration. The serum amylase level is therefore elevated, but urinary amylase levels and the ACCR are low. The diagnosis can be confirmed by electrophoresis. Abdominal pain has been reported in more than one-half of patients with macroamylasemia, although the biochemical abnormality is probably not etiologically related to the pain. Hyperamylasemia predominantly caused by salivary amylase may also be associated with a low urinary amylase level and ACCR because compared with the pancreatic isoenzyme, the salivary isoenzyme is cleared more slowly by the kidneys.

Ref.: 1–4

14. At the time of laparotomy for a patient presenting with a known diagnosis of pancreatic cancer, the patient is found to have an unresectable pancreatic cancer locally invading the antrum of the stomach and retroperitoneum. There are no lesions identified elsewhere in the abdomen. Which of the following statements regarding management is correct?

A. The preferred management is to close the patient and place an endoscopic stent postoperatively.

B. Proceed with pancreaticoduodenectomy.

C. Choledochoduodenostomy is preferred.

D. Gastrojejunostomy should be performed.

E. Gastrojejunostomy should not be performed.

ANSWER: D

COMMENTS: Most patients with **pancreatic cancer** do not have resectable disease. **Palliative treatment** is directed to relieve obstruction of the bile duct and duodenum and to alleviate pain. For lesions demonstrated to be unresectable before laparotomy, nonoperative relief of biliary obstruction can be achieved by the endoscopic (preferred) or transhepatic route. Surgical bypass generally provides more durable relief with less need for further intervention. It is preferred for patients when unresectability is determined at the time of laparotomy.

Pancreatic cancers can obstruct the duodenum or the proximal jejunum near the ligament of Treitz. Traditionally, many surgeons have favored routine "double bypass" (biliary and duodenal) for operated patients because the rate of duodenal obstruction that develops later in patients treated by biliary bypass alone has been cited to be 5%–30%. However, duodenal obstruction does not develop in most patients, and gastrojejunostomy is sometimes associated with problems such as bleeding or delayed gastric emptying. The selective approach is therefore appropriate. Patients with obstructive symptoms or impending obstruction as a result of tumor location should undergo gastrojejunostomy. **Gastrojejunostomy** is also advisable for patients with an anticipated longer survival, such as those whose lesions are not resected because of local tumor invasion but because of hepatic or peritoneal metastases. Endoscopic placement of a **duodenal stent** is another option, but the results are not always satisfactory.

Additionally, choledochojejunostomy, cholecystojejunostomy, **hepaticojejunostomy**, and choledochoduodenostomy are each appropriate for the management of distal bile duct obstruction. A Roux-en-Y configuration is preferred by many surgeons for choledochojejunostomy reconstruction, although a simple loop (with or without distal enteroenterostomy) also suffices. Cholecystojejunostomy is relatively simple but should be avoided if the gallbladder is diseased or when cystic duct patency cannot be demonstrated or may be jeopardized by tumor proximity. It is sometimes taught that choledochoduodenostomy should be avoided with malignant obstruction because of possible tumor growth and eventual reobstruction. In reality, choledochoduodenostomy can be an effective solution provided that the common bile duct is sufficiently dilated and the duodenum is pliable and unobstructed.

Ref.: 1–4

15. A 45-year-old woman was seen at an outside hospital with abdominal pain, and a CT scan was performed showing a pancreatic cyst. The interventional radiologist drained the cyst during that admission, and the patient was sent home. She presents now to your hospital, and a CT scan again shows a septated, 10-cm cystic mass in the head of the pancreas. Which of the following statements constitutes appropriate advice?

A. The lesion is benign and requires no intervention.

B. The lesion is malignant and probably incurable.

C. Pancreaticoduodenectomy is indicated.

D. Percutaneous needle biopsy is indicated.

E. Drainage by Roux-en-Y cyst jejunostomy is indicated.

ANSWER: C

COMMENTS: Cystadenoma and **cystadenocarcinoma** are **cystic neoplasms of the pancreas** that are most commonly manifested as mass lesions in middle-aged women. Serous and mucinous types are recognized, and the risk for malignancy is significant with the mucinous variety. Cystadenoma is more common than its malignant counterpart, but malignant transformation may occur. EUS with sampling for cytology, mucin, and carcinoembryonic antigen can be useful for gauging the likelihood of cancer. Without resection, however, exclusion of malignancy can be difficult. Internal drainage of cystic neoplasms is not an appropriate therapy. Complete excision should be carried out whenever possible. The 5-year survival rate after resection of cystadenocarcinoma is approximately 50%. Occasionally, islet cell tumors, ductal adenocarcinomas, or other unusual tumors (e.g., papillary and cystic pancreatic neoplasms) have cystic components.

Ref.: 1–4

16. The uncinate process of the pancreas is directly adjacent and ventral to which of the following?

A. Splenic vein

B. Inferior vena cava

C. Superior mesenteric artery

D. Left renal vein

E. Fourth portion of the duodenum

ANSWER: B

COMMENTS: The pancreas can be divided into various parts: head, uncinate, neck, body, and tail. The uncinate process is the portion of the gland that extends to the left, dorsal to the portal vein and superior mesenteric artery and ventral to the aorta and inferior vena cava. The uncinate process is located caudad and ventral to the left renal vein and cephalad to the distal duodenum. Understanding the extent and location of the uncinate is important during resection of the head of the pancreas. The blood supply of the uncinate is derived from numerous short branches of the superior mesenteric artery and portal vein. When performing pancreaticoduodenectomy, these branches must be carefully controlled to prevent bleeding and avoid injury to the superior mesenteric artery or portal vein.

Ref.: 1–4

17. Which of the following vascular relationships is not an important consideration during resection of the head of the pancreas?

A. Arterial supply of the pancreatic head from the splenic artery

B. Confluence of the splenic vein and superior mesenteric vein dorsal to the pancreatic neck

C. Absence of ventral portal vein branches dorsal to the pancreatic neck
D. Origin of the right hepatic artery from the superior mesenteric artery
E. Origin of the middle colic artery from the superior mesenteric artery

ANSWER: A

COMMENTS: The relationship of the pancreas to neighboring organs and to critical vascular structures is of great surgical significance. The **arterial supply** to the head of the gland is derived from both the gastroduodenal and the superior mesenteric arteries via the anterior and posterior pancreaticoduodenal arcades. For the most part, the head of the pancreas and the duodenum have a shared blood supply, so they must generally be resected together. However, techniques for "duodenal-sparing" resection of the pancreatic head or "pancreatic-sparing" duodenectomy are appropriate in selected circumstances.

The body and tail of the **pancreas** receive their blood supply mainly from multiple branches of the splenic artery, which also connect with superior mesenteric sources. Variations in major arteries—such as the origin of the right hepatic artery from the superior mesenteric artery and the origin of the middle colic artery from the superior mesenteric artery or dorsal pancreatic artery—place these vessels in close proximity to the head and neck of the pancreas, where they are subject to injury during pancreatectomy. The junction of the splenic vein and superior mesenteric vein to form the portal vein lies behind the neck of the pancreas. Usually, these vessels do not have large anterior tributaries in this area, but appropriate caution must nonetheless be exercised when developing this plane during pancreatic operations.

Ref.: 1–4

18. A jaundiced, otherwise healthy patient is noted to have a 3-cm mass in the head of the pancreas on CT. EUS-guided fine-needle aspiration shows cancer. The mass abuts the portal vein, but there is no clear evidence of vessel involvement or metastatic disease. You proceed to the operating room. Intraoperatively, you are concerned about the resectability of the tumor. In which of the following situations is resection contraindicated?

A. 70% abutment of the superior mesenteric artery
B. Tumor located in the neck of the pancreas
C. Inability to verify malignancy histologically before resection
D. 40% abutment of the superior mesenteric vein
E. Tumor invading the portal vein

ANSWER: A

COMMENTS: When the clinical situation suggests a resectable **pancreatic neoplasm** in a good-risk patient with biliary obstruction, surgery for potential resection is generally indicated without additional tests. Routine **preoperative biliary decompression** is not advantageous in this setting because it does not improve operative outcomes and may increase the morbidity associated with resection. Endoscopic biliary decompression is invaluable, of course, for palliation of obstruction in patients deemed inoperable or if operation is to be delayed. CT or MRI is usually adequate in assessing the extent of disease and resectability preoperatively. EUS is extremely useful for identifying small tumors that are inapparent on CT, for obtaining cytologic material, and somewhat for assessing vascular invasion. Imaging criteria for what constitutes a borderline case vary but would commonly include tumors that abut a substantial (half or greater) circumference of adjacent vessels (hepatic artery, superior mesenteric artery, portal vein) or that narrow the portal-splenic vein confluence. **Resection of a pancreatic malignancy** offers the only chance for cure. Most commonly, resection of ductal carcinomas involves pancreaticoduodenectomy because most potentially resectable tumors are located in the head or uncinate process of the gland. Tumors originating in the body or tail of the pancreas are often not diagnosed until they are beyond the confines of surgical resection. However, location alone does not contraindicate resection because, stage for stage, tumors in the body have the same survival as tumors in the head of the pancreas. Resection is indicated for physiologically fit patients (age alone is not a contraindication) who do not have metastases beyond the field of resection. Histologic or cytologic confirmation of malignancy can often be obtained intraoperatively but is not necessary before resection if the clinical circumstances suggest cancer and the surgeon is appropriately experienced. For some tumors with local vascular invasion, en bloc resection with reconstruction of the involved vessels is appropriate if a tumor-free resection can be accomplished. **Positive lymph nodes** outside the resection field, peritoneal metastases, and liver metastases generally contraindicate resection for adenocarcinoma of the exocrine pancreas. However, tumor "debulking" and resection of liver metastases can be beneficial in patients with functioning tumors of the endocrine pancreas.

Ref.: 1–4

19. Which of the following would not be appropriate for the management of steatorrhea in a patient with chronic pancreatitis?

A. Restriction of fat to 75 g/day
B. Encapsulated pancreatic enzymes
C. Encapsulated pancreatic enzymes and a proton pump inhibitor
D. Nonencapsulated pancreatic enzymes
E. Nonencapsulated pancreatic enzymes and a proton pump inhibitor

ANSWER: C

COMMENTS: Gross **steatorrhea** and diarrhea occur when pancreatic exocrine function is reduced to about 10% of normal. Therapy involves limitation of fat intake and administration of adequate amounts of exogenous pancreatic enzyme preparations to provide at least 10% of the normal lipolytic activity in the duodenum at the time when the food substrate is present. Various commercial formulations of pancreatic enzymes are available. Nonencapsulated forms may improve the malabsorption but can be ineffective because of inactivation in the stomach when the pH falls below 4. The addition of H_2 blockers may then be useful. Enteric-coated preparations release their enzymes at a pH above 5. Therefore they are useful for patients whose gastric pH remains low to ensure that the enzyme is not released until it reaches the duodenum. The use of encapsulated forms with H_2 blockers is counterproductive because the enzyme is released in the stomach and is then inactivated if the pH falls. In addition, enteric-coated preparations are microspheres of varying sizes, and the larger ones do not empty into the duodenum until after the food substrate does.

Ref.: 3, 4

20. A 42-year-old female presents to the emergency department (ED) with nausea, vomiting, and pain in the epigastrium and right upper quadrant (RUQ). She is afebrile and hemodynamically stable. Her WBC is 10,000 cells per MCL without a left shift, and total bilirubin is 2.5 mg/dL. The common bile duct was not identified on subsequent ultrasound due to overlying bowel gas. Magnetic resonance cholangiopancreatography (MRCP) confirms a gallstone in the common bile duct with proximal dilation. **Incidentally**, she is found to have pancreatic divisum. What is the etiology of this?

A. Aplasia of the dorsal pancreatic anlage
B. Aplasia of the ventral pancreatic anlage
C. Incomplete rotation of the ventral pancreatic anlage
D. Failed fusion of the ventral and dorsal pancreatic parenchyma
E. Failed fusion of the ventral and dorsal pancreatic ducts

ANSWER: E

COMMENTS: Pancreas divisum currently refers to congenital variations of the pancreatic ducts that result from failed or incomplete fusion of the embryologic ventral and dorsal ductal systems. (Historically, the term may also refer to the rare failure of parenchymal fusion.) There may be complete separation of the ducts, an absent or minimal ventral duct, or only a few meager connections between the systems. As a consequence, most of the pancreatic duct drainage is through the dorsal duct joining the duodenum at the minor papilla. Any existing ventral ducts (Wirsung's) drain only the uncinate process and the caudal head of the gland rather than the bulk of the gland at the major papilla, as when normally developed. Some variation of pancreas divisum is present in about 10% of the population. In some individuals, it is clinically significant if the relatively stenotic minor papilla imposes an obstruction to ductal flow. This can potentially result in recurrent abdominal pain, acute pancreatitis, or even chronic pancreatitis. The diagnosis is usually made by ERCP, and cannulation of the minor papilla may be required to image the dorsal duct. MRCP might also demonstrate this ductal anatomy. The vast majority (95%) of individuals with **pancreas divisum** are asymptomatic.

Ref.: 1–5

21. The bicarbonate concentration of pancreatic secretions is:

A. Primarily increased by cholecystokinin (CCK)
B. Primarily decreased by secretin
C. Independent of acinar cell secretion
D. Reciprocally related to the chloride concentration
E. Reciprocally related to the sodium concentration

ANSWER: D

COMMENTS: The **centroacinar cells** secrete a bicarbonate-rich solution by an active transport mechanism, primarily in response to secretin. **Cholecystokinin** is the primary stimulant of enzyme secretion from the acinar cells. The bicarbonate and chloride contents of pancreatic juice are reciprocally related. As ductal flow rates increase, the bicarbonate concentration increases and the chloride concentration decreases. This is the result of two processes: (1) changes in passive exchange of intraductal bicarbonate for intracellular chloride and (2) changes in the relative contribution of acinar cell secretion. Acinar cells secrete fluid high in chloride in addition to digestive enzymes. In contradistinction to anion concentrations, the concentrations of sodium and potassium in pancreatic duct secretions remain relatively constant despite the flow rate and are similar to their concentrations in plasma.

Ref.: 1, 3, 5

22. Which pancreatic islet cell type produces a hormonal peptide to stimulate glycogenolysis and gluconeogenesis?

A. Alpha cell
B. Beta cell
C. Delta cell
D. F cell
E. Pancreatic polypeptide (PP) cell

ANSWER: A

COMMENTS: See Question 23.

Ref.: 1–3, 5

23. Pancreatic delta cells secrete which inhibitory peptide?

A. Bombesin
B. Glucagon
C. Somatostatin
D. Insulin
E. Pancreatic polypeptide

ANSWER: C

COMMENTS: The **endocrine pancreas** is composed of various cells located in the islets of Langerhans, approximately 1 million of which are interspersed with the acinar and ductal elements throughout the gland. The hormonal peptides produced by the islets affect a wide range of metabolic and physiologic actions. The primary function of the endocrine pancreas is to regulate glucose homeostasis. Beta cells, which are the most numerous, produce insulin. Insulin promotes glucose transport, stimulates protein synthesis, and inhibits glycogenolysis and lipolysis. Alpha cells secrete glucagon, which counterbalances insulin by stimulating hepatic glycogenolysis, gluconeogenesis, ketogenesis, and lipolysis. Glucagon also inhibits intestinal motility and gastric acid and pancreatic exocrine secretion. Somatostatin, produced by delta cells, has a broad range of inhibitory effects on the gastrointestinal tract, including inhibition of secretion of other pancreatic peptides; inhibition of gastric, biliary, intestinal, and pancreatic exocrine secretions; and inhibition of gastrointestinal motility. PP cells are the source of pancreatic polypeptide. Pancreatic polypeptide inhibits pancreatic exocrine secretion and biliary and gut motility. Clinically, deficiency of pancreatic polypeptide has been linked to diabetes following resection of the pancreatic head or chronic pancreatitis. Because postprandial secretion of pancreatic polypeptide is dependent on vagal innervation, it has been used to assess the completeness of vagotomy.

Ref.: 1–3, 5

24. Which of the following statements is true regarding blood flow to the pancreas?

A. Islet cells receive a greater proportion of pancreatic blood flow than do the exocrine elements.
B. CCK and secretin regulate secretion by altering the blood flow.
C. Fragile anastomotic networks predispose the gland to ischemia.

D. The blood supply to the islet cells is independent of the acinar supply.

E. Pancreatic blood flow is highly sensitive to changes in systemic blood pressure.

ANSWER: A

COMMENTS: The microcirculation of the pancreas is complex and has important correlations with the endocrine and exocrine functions of the gland. The rich anastomotic supply from various sources makes pancreatic ischemia unusual. The islets receive a disproportionately large amount of total **pancreatic blood flow** (10%–25%) relative to their mass (1%–2%). Both the islets and exocrine tissue have an arteriolar blood supply. The acinar tissue is also perfused by blood that drains from the islets, a mechanism referred to as the islet–acinar or insuloacinar portal system. This system is the structural basis for endocrine regulation of exocrine function. Insulin receptors are present on acinar cells, and the density of receptors is higher on acini located near the islets. Because the islets themselves often have a central-to-peripheral pattern of perfusion, insulin from the centrally located beta cells can influence the other peripheral islet cell types. In addition, some islets are apparently perfused in a peripheral-to-central pattern. CCK and secretin have relatively little effect on the blood flow and thus exert their stimulatory effects independently. Pancreatic blood flow is maintained relatively constant despite changes in arterial pressure.

Ref.: 3–5

25. What is the leading cause of death from acute pancreatitis?

A. Hemorrhage

B. Pseudocyst rupture

C. Secondary pancreatic infection

D. Biliary sepsis

E. Renal failure

ANSWER: C

COMMENTS: Formerly, death from acute pancreatitis often occurred early in the course of the disease as a result of the acute effects of hypovolemia and inadequate resuscitation. In the current era, about 80% of deaths are attributed to secondary pancreatic infection, which develops in approximately 10% of patients with acute pancreatitis. Fatal pancreatic sepsis typically progresses to multisystem organ failure, and deaths occur later in the course of the disease. To have an impact on this disease, therapeutic efforts have therefore focused on the prevention and early diagnosis of pancreatic infection and on more effective methods of surgical therapy.

Ref.: 6

26. A 58-year-old man with recurrent alcoholic pancreatitis presents to the ED with 3 days of worsening abdominal pain, nausea, and vomiting. Further questioning elicits symptoms including rigors and subjective fevers. His temperature is 102.5°F, WBC is 23,000 cells per MCL, heart rate is 105 beats/min, and blood pressure is 118/64 mmHg. CT scan is obtained, which shows a hypoenhancing pancreas with necrosis and air bubbles, a small pseudocyst, and a second peripancreatic fluid collection. Which of the following complications of acute pancreatitis is associated with the highest mortality rate?

A. Peripancreatic abscess

B. Infected pancreatic pseudocyst

C. Infected pancreatic necrosis

D. Sterile pancreatic necrosis

E. Bile duct obstruction

ANSWER: C

COMMENTS: **Retroperitoneal infection** is a serious, often fatal, complication of **acute pancreatitis**. The early literature pertaining to the local infectious sequelae of pancreatitis may be confusing because of nonselective use of the term "pancreatic abscess" to describe infectious complications, which vary in severity. Pancreatic abscess best describes a localized collection of drainable pus in or around the pancreas. Pancreatic abscess and infected pseudocyst can be treated effectively by external drainage, and the anticipated mortality rate for each is about 5%. Pancreatic necrosis is a manifestation of severe pancreatitis. When accompanied by infection, it has been associated with a mortality rate that may exceed 40%, which is higher than that for noninfected necrosis. Infected pancreatic necrosis is treated by operative debridement and open or closed retroperitoneal drainage. Patients with sterile necrosis may require operative intervention as well but are generally treated nonoperatively with intensive support as long as their condition permits.

Ref.: 4, 6

27. An alcoholic patient has acute pancreatitis with five of the Ranson criteria. He gradually improves over a 14-day hospitalization, but then a pulse of 120 beats/min, a temperature of 39°C, and abdominal distention develop. CT is performed, and the results are shown below (Fig. 26.2). The next most appropriate therapy is which of the following measures?

A. Antibiotics

B. Percutaneous catheter drainage

C. Peritoneal lavage

D. Endoscopic cyst gastrostomy

E. Operative drainage

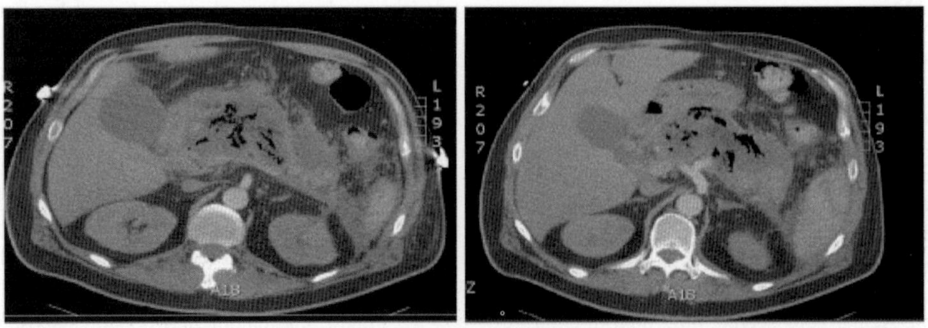

Fig. 26.2 *From Jeyarajah DR, Osman HG, Patel S. Advances in management of pancreatic necrosis.* Curr Probl Surg. *2014;51(9):374–408.*

ANSWER: E

COMMENTS: Pancreatic infection complicating acute pancreatitis should be suspected in any patient who fails to improve following supportive medical therapy or improves but then demonstrates deterioration. Pancreatic infection occasionally occurs early during the chronologic course of the disease, typically occurring later, as in the patient described. CT is the best method for imaging the pancreas. The results of CT in this patient demonstrate air in the pancreas, which is characteristic of a pancreatic infection. The technique of dynamic pancreatography can identify ischemic areas of pancreas and is useful for evaluating patients who may have pancreatic necrosis. **Dynamic pancreatography** is performed by serially imaging the pancreas after bolus injection of an intravenous contrast agent. Percutaneous needle aspiration of fluid collections or necrotic areas found on CT can be performed to identify the presence of infection and guide therapeutic decisions about the need for drainage. When pancreatic infection is present, operative drainage and debridement are indicated. Interest has been focused on the selection of closed or open methods of operative drainage. Minimal-access operative approaches are also used to drain and debride pancreatic necrosis in the hope of lowering morbidity in these ill patients. Percutaneous catheters can drain thin fluid but are usually inadequate for the management of infected pancreatic necrosis. Peritoneal lavage has been used early in the course of patients with severe acute pancreatitis. Endoscopic cyst gastrostomy may be appropriate for some patients with pancreatic pseudocysts. These latter two modalities have no role in the management of infected pancreatic necrosis.

Ref.: 4, 6

28. A 45-year-old man is admitted with severe alcoholic pancreatitis. CT scan shows 20% pancreatic sterile necrosis. Which of the following statements best describes the current use of antibiotics for this patient?

A. Systemic antibiotics are not indicated unless his condition deteriorates.

B. Systemic antibiotics are indicated for coverage of gut-derived bacteria.

C. Systemic antibiotics are indicated for coverage of gut-derived bacteria and fungal organisms.

D. Nonabsorbable antibiotics are indicated for gut decontamination.

E. Systemic antibiotics are not indicated if enteric antibiotics can be tolerated.

ANSWER: A

COMMENTS: The risk for **infected pancreatic necrosis** is related to the clinical severity and duration of disease and to the extent of necrosis. Strategies to decrease secondary pancreatic infection focus on patients at higher risk. Unfortunately, controlled trials of systemic antibiotics for prophylaxis against secondary infection have yielded conflicting results. These differences are probably because of numerous factors, including heterogeneity in the severity of disease, patient characteristics, and concomitant therapy among those studied, as well as differences in study methodologies. Current practice favors systemic antibiotics for patients with severe disease and more extensive (>30%) necrosis based on studies demonstrating fewer septic complications and perhaps decreased mortality. However, not all studies have shown benefit, and the risk for subsequent infection with multiresistant bacterial or fungal organisms may be increased, particularly if prophylactic antibiotic use is prolonged. Because the gut is typically the source of the offending organisms, the use of nonabsorbable enteral antibiotics for selective gut decontamination has had some appeal. The effect of this measure remains unclear, and it is not typically used. Enteric feedings are beneficial to maintain the gut mucosal barrier to bacterial translocation. However, the efficacy of enteric feeding alone for prevention of secondary pancreatic infection has not been demonstrated.

Ref.: 7, 8

29. A 54-year-old male presents to the ED with RUQ pain and epigastric pain and associated emesis. Lab results are significant for a total bilirubin of 1.9 g/dL, WBC of 11,500 cells per MCL, and lipase level of 300 U/L, and AST/ALT are mildly elevated. An US is performed showing a duct of 6 mm and numerous mobile stones in the gallbladder. Acute gallstone pancreatitis is diagnosed. Which of the following is considered standard treatment?

A. Urgent (within 24 h) cholecystectomy and common bile duct exploration

B. Urgent ERCP and subsequent laparoscopic cholecystectomy

C. Initial supportive therapy with cholecystectomy performed during the same admission

D. Initial supportive therapy with cholecystectomy performed in 6 to 8 weeks

E. Initial supportive therapy with cholecystectomy performed only if symptoms recur

ANSWER: C

COMMENTS: Gallstone pancreatitis is related to the passage of stones through the ampulla of Vater. Patients with smaller gallstones have an increased risk for the development of this manifestation. **Cholecystectomy** is indicated because gallstone pancreatitis is a recurrent problem in 30%–50% of patients if surgery is not performed. The traditional controversy has involved the timing of surgery. Proponents of immediate intervention have found a higher incidence of choledocholithiasis but have not demonstrated that this approach is safer than delayed surgery or that it is necessary for most patients. Most surgeons advise initial nonoperative therapy until the patient's signs and symptoms subside (most do within 2 to 3 days), followed by elective cholecystectomy with intraoperative imaging of the common bile duct by cholangiography or intraoperative ultrasonography during the same hospitalization.

The role of urgent **endoscopic retrograde cholangiopancreatography** and **endoscopic sphincterotomy** for the **management of biliary pancreatitis** has been controversial. The vast majority (97%) of patients with gallstone pancreatitis have mild pancreatitis that improves rapidly. ERCP finds common duct stones in only a small percentage of patients and is not indicated routinely. Some trials comparing urgent ERCP and sphincterotomy with traditional treatment have suggested benefit in patients with severe pancreatitis, but this has not been consistently observed. ERCP is indicated for patients with concomitant obstructive jaundice and biliary sepsis. Less invasive methods of duct imaging, such as **MRCP** or EUS, might be useful in patients at an intermediate risk for choledocholithiasis but are not necessary for most with biliary pancreatitis. For the small proportion of patients with severe biliary pancreatitis, early cholecystectomy should be avoided. Treatment in this group is directed at resolution of the pancreatitis and its complications. When the pancreatitis has subsided, delayed cholecystectomy is indicated.

Ref.: 9

30. Which of the following is the preferred nutritional support for a patient with severe pancreatitis?

A. Nasogastric feeding

B. Feeding via percutaneous endoscopic gastrostomy

C. Nasojejunal feeding

D. Parenteral amino acids and glucose

E. Parenteral amino acids, glucose, and lipids

ANSWER: A

COMMENTS: Nutritional support is a critical component of the successful management of patients with severe **pancreatitis**. Mortality is reduced by positive nitrogen balance. Direct delivery of nutrients into the jejunum is the preferred route. **Enteral feeding** helps maintain the intestinal mucosal barrier and prevent infection from early bacterial translocation. Enteral feeding is associated with a lower risk for infection and shorter hospital stay than is parenteral nutrition. Moreover, enteric feeding helps avoid catheter-related sepsis and other complications of central venous lines. Recent studies have shown feeding into the stomach to be at least equal to nasojejunal feedings. Oral feeding is cheaper and easier to manage than jejunal feedings. Nasojejunal tubes may require radiologically guided or endoscopic placement.

If nutritional goals cannot be met within a few days of initiation, parenteral nutritional support may also be necessary. Intravenous lipids are not detrimental and prevent essential fatty acid deficiency.

Ref.: 10, 30, 31

31. A 45-year-old nondiabetic patient with chronic alcoholic pancreatitis and intractable abdominal pain has extensive fibrosis of the intrapancreatic duct and distal common bile duct. The pancreatic duct measures 8 mm. Which of the following choices constitutes the best treatment?

A. Sphincteroplasty

B. Lateral pancreaticojejunostomy

C. Whipple procedure

D. Total pancreatectomy

E. Continued nonoperative therapy

ANSWER: C

COMMENTS: Pain is the primary indication for surgery in patients with chronic pancreatitis. Selection of the best **operation** for a particular patient must include consideration of the anatomy of the gland, preexisting endocrine or exocrine dysfunction, compliance and the rehabilitative capacity of the patient, postoperative endocrine or exocrine deficiency, and the likelihood of postoperative pain relief. Patients with small ducts disease are treated by resection if surgery is necessary. Resection of the pancreatic head in properly selected patients has generally yielded better long-term results for pain relief than those yielded by tail resection. The head of the pancreas is often enlarged and bulky in chronic pancreatitis and has been considered to be the "pacemaker" of the disease. A number of operative techniques are available for resection of the pancreatic head including Whipple procedure. This strategy is best employed in patients with calcified obstructive fibrosis of the bile duct, pancreatic duct, and/or duodenum.

Other patients with a dilated duct (>6 mm) and without focal findings restricted to the head of the pancreas are candidates for ductal drainage, with lateral pancreaticojejunostomy being the best choice for these procedures. It is important to achieve adequate decompression of the enlarged pancreatic head and uncinate process during drainage procedures. Variations such as the **Frey or Beger procedure** are intended to accomplish this. The Frey procedure involves patients with increased disease in the head of the pancreas where portions of the head are cored out, and a lateral pancreaticojejunostomy is performed along the opened pancreatic duct.

The Beger procedure involves total excision of the head and neck of the pancreas, with a residual edge of pancreas preserving the duodenum and bile duct remains. A loop of jejunum is then brought up, and distal pancreaticojejunostomy as well as a pancreaticojejunostomy to the residual edge of the pancreas is performed. Further, a jejunojejunostomy is performed for duodenal drainage. Sphincteroplasty does not play a role in the management of patients with established chronic pancreatitis.

Total or nearly total (95%) resections have higher long-term morbidity and mortality rates related to postoperative endocrine insufficiency. Although endocrine and exocrine function tends to deteriorate over time in patients with chronic pancreatitis, some evidence suggests that pancreaticojejunostomy halts or delays this decline better than does nonoperative therapy.

Ref.: 1, 4, 11, 32

32. CT demonstrates a 5-cm peripancreatic fluid collection in a patient 3 weeks after an episode of acute pancreatitis. The patient is eating and does not have clinical signs of infection. What is the recommended treatment?

A. Expectant management without intervention

B. Nothing by mouth and total parenteral nutrition

C. Percutaneous catheter drainage of the fluid collection

D. Endoscopic drainage

E. Reimaging in 3 to 6 weeks and surgery for internal drainage if the collection persists

ANSWER: A

COMMENTS: Peripancreatic fluid collections can be found in about 20% of patients with acute pancreatitis. Many of them resolve spontaneously and should not be mistaken for pancreatic pseudocysts. If the patient is stable, can eat, and does not have clinical evidence of infection or other complications, expectant management is indicated. The fluid collection can be monitored with ultrasonography or CT in 1 to 3 months. If the patient has persistent pain and is unable to eat, nutrition by postpyloric enteral feeding, or parenteral nutrition if necessary, may be instituted for several weeks to allow resolution or maturation of the collection into a pseudocyst. If the patient has a symptomatic or complicated fluid collection that requires early intervention, some method of external drainage must be used. If the fluid is thin, endoscopic or percutaneous catheter drainage may suffice. Operative drainage is preferred if there is substantial necrotic debris, as there often is, or if there is concern about infection. Operative drainage might be accomplished with minimal-access approaches.

Ref.: 1, 4, 12

33. Which of the following is the most important determinant of the need for drainage of a pancreatic pseudocyst?

A. Pseudocyst symptoms

B. Pseudocyst size

C. Pseudocyst duration

D. Associated chronic pancreatitis

E. Patient age

ANSWER: A

COMMENTS: Historically, **pancreatic pseudocysts** larger than 5 to 6 cm and present for longer than 6 weeks were thought to have a low rate of spontaneous resolution and a high rate of complications. They were therefore treated by operative drainage. Current understanding of the natural history of pseudocysts is that the rate of spontaneous resolution is higher and the rate of complications is lower than previously thought. Pseudocyst size and duration are therefore no longer absolute criteria for intervention. Rather, pseudocyst-related symptoms are the primary indication for treatment. Large pseudocysts are more likely to be symptomatic and less likely to resolve spontaneously compared with small pseudocysts. In addition, pseudocysts in patients with chronic pancreatitis are unlikely to resolve but may not require intervention if they are stable, asymptomatic, and uncomplicated.

Ref.: 1, 4, 12

34. A patient with chronic pancreatitis is unable to eat because of persistent postprandial pain. CT is performed (shown below). What is the recommended treatment?

A. Nothing by mouth and total parenteral nutrition for 4 to 6 weeks

B. Percutaneous catheter drainage

C. Endoscopic drainage

D. Operative internal drainage

E. Operative external drainage

ANSWER: D

COMMENTS: **Pseudocysts** that develop in patients with **chronic pancreatitis** can be considered mature when they are discovered unless there has also been a recent episode of acute pancreatitis. The indications for treatment of a pancreatic pseudocyst are (1) persistent symptoms (pain, inability to eat, or biliary or gastrointestinal obstruction), (2) enlargement, or (3) the onset of a pseudocyst-related complication (infection, hemorrhage, or rupture). Operative internal pseudocyst drainage into the stomach, jejunum, or duodenum is generally the preferred treatment, depending on the location of the pseudocyst. For patients with chronic pancreatitis, it is critical to evaluate the pancreatic duct to determine whether a concomitant duct drainage procedure is necessary. **Pseudocyst drainage** can be accomplished laparoscopically in some situations. Pseudocysts in the tail of the gland are sometimes best treated by distal pancreatectomy. Percutaneous or endoscopic drainage of established pseudocysts is still being debated. These techniques can successfully treat pseudocysts in some circumstances but have definite limitations and potential complications.

Ref.: 1, 4, 12

35. A 64-year-old man is evaluated for abdominal pain. CT shows segmental dilation of the main pancreatic duct to greater than 10 mm in the head of the gland with mural nodules. Which of the following is the next most appropriate recommendation?

A. EUS

B. ERCP

C. Serum cancer antigen 19-9

D. Total pancreatectomy

E. Abstinence from alcohol and CT repeated in 3 months

ANSWER: A

COMMENTS: An **intraductal papillary mucinous neoplasm (IPMN)** of the pancreas is a premalignant condition characterized by papillary projections of mucin-secreting epithelial cells, excessive mucin production, and cystic dilation of the pancreatic duct. The patient may already have cancer when initially seen or may be at some other stage along the process of malignant transformation, which occurs relatively slowly. IPMNs are divided into a main duct type and a branch duct type depending on the areas of the pancreatic ducts that are involved. The goals of evaluation are to identify factors associated with a higher risk for malignancy and to determine the anatomic extent of the disease. EUS is usually the next step in evaluation when IPMN is suspected. EUS can identify diffuse or segmental dilation of the pancreatic duct and the size of cystic lesions or mural nodules and can guide fine-needle aspiration to assess cytology and molecular tumor markers. ERCP shows duct dilation without strictures, filling defects from mucus or nodules, and commonly a patulous papillary orifice with mucus. ERCP also permits sampling of mucus and therapeutic clearance if mucus obstruction is a problem. If available, direct pancreatoscopy and intraductal ultrasound can be adjuncts to ERCP for determining the extent of an IPMN.

Ref.: 13

36. A 68-year-old male presents to his primary care physician (PCP) with abdominal pain in the epigastrium and associated nausea. No other significant findings are observed. The patient denies any alcohol or tobacco use. The PCP sends him to the ED for a CT scan, which shows a lesion in the pancreas. The patient subsequently undergoes an EUS/ERCP, which shows mucin at the ampulla. MRI and biopsy results confirm a main duct–type IPMN. Which of the following features of IPMN of the pancreas is associated with the lowest risk for cancer?

A. Branch duct type with mural nodularity

B. Branch duct type smaller than 3 cm

C. Main duct type with diffuse dilation to greater than 10 mm

D. Main duct type with segmental dilation

E. Multifocal IPMN

ANSWER: B

COMMENTS: Progression of IPMN through the adenoma cancer sequence is considered a slow process that requires perhaps 10 to 20 years. Main duct–type tumors have a greater risk for malignancy than the branch duct type. The Sendai Consensus Guidelines identified the following features as risk factors for cancer and as general indicators for resection: main pancreatic duct dilation to greater than 10 mm, cyst size larger than 3 cm, presence of mural nodules, and atypical cytology. Additional risk factors include high-grade dysplasia, multifocal or synchronous tumors, and increasing cyst size during follow-up. In branch duct–type tumors, mural nodularity or atypical cytology may be more important determinants than size.

Ref.: 14, 15, 16

37. A 58-year-old male is referred to you by his PCP for evaluation of pancreatic exocrine insufficiency. Upon evaluation of the patient, you suspect insufficiency due to malnutrition. You perform a standard secretin test. Which of the following test findings correlate with this diagnosis?

	Total Secretion Volume	Bicarbonate Secretion	Enzyme Secretion
A.	Normal	Normal	Decreased
B.	Decreased	Decreased	Decreased
C.	Increased	Normal	Normal
D.	Decreased	Normal	Normal
E.	Normal	Normal	Normal

ANSWER: A

COMMENTS: The secretin test of pancreatic exocrine insufficiency is considered the classic testing method. The patient fasts overnight, and the next day, a double-lumen tube is placed into the duodenum through which basal secretion levels are collected for reference. Next, an intravenous bolus of two units of secretin/kg is administered, followed by four 20-min collection periods. Normal levels include 2 mL/kg of pancreatic fluid per hour, bicarbonate concentration of 80 mmol/L, bicarbonate output of 10 mmol/L/h, and amylase of 6 to 18 IU/kg. Bicarbonate is the biggest discriminator between normal patients and dysfunction. "A" represents malnutrition. "B" represents end-stage pancreatitis or advanced pancreatic cancer. "C" is hemochromatosis (associated Zollinger-Ellison syndrome or cirrhosis). "D" is early pancreatic cancer. Other tests that could be performed include 5,5-dimethyl-2,4-oxazolidinedione (DMO), Lundh, or the noninvasive triolein breath test.

Ref.: 17

38. Which of the following statements is true regarding acute pancreatitis?

A. Twenty-five percent of patients with the diagnosis of idiopathic acute pancreatitis (IAP) will have a recurrence in their lifetime.

B. The diagnosis of IAP is made in up to 30% of cases of acute pancreatitis.

C. Pancreatic divisum is the most common congenital abnormality of the pancreas occurring in 15% of the general population and is a potential contributor to IAP.

D. Patients with CF have a 10%–15% incidence of pancreatitis during their lifetime, secondary to their disease.

E. None of the above.

ANSWER: B

COMMENTS: The etiology for acute pancreatitis is determined in 70%–90% of cases, and thus up to 30% of cases are deemed idiopathic. Further extensive investigation is warranted as over 50% of IAP will recur, increasing a person's risk of developing chronic pancreatitis. Entities such as biliary sludge/microlithiasis, sphincter of Oddi dysfunction, pancreatic divisum, hereditary pancreatitis, CF, choledochocele, anomalous pancreaticobiliary junction, annular pancreas, and tumors can all be less obvious causes of acute pancreatitis in cases deemed "idiopathic." Pancreatic divisum is the most common congenital malformation of the pancreas in 5%–8% of the general population. CF is an autosomal recessive disease where a mutation in a regulator gene encoding cyclic adenosine monophosphate regulates chloride ion channels. This disease leads to pancreatitis by diminished pancreatic enzyme secretion in 2% of CF patients.

Ref.: 18

39. Which of the following statements is true regarding chronic pancreatitis?

A. Patients with chronic pancreatitis tend to die from complications of smoking, diabetes, and chronic alcohol use.

B. There is no difference in the rate of pancreatic carcinoma between patients with chronic pancreatitis and the general population.

C. Pancreatic cancer in patients with chronic pancreatitis is the leading cause of mortality.

D. There is no difference in the rate of extrapancreatic malignancies between patients with chronic pancreatitis and the general population.

E. None of the above.

ANSWER: A

COMMENTS: Patients with chronic pancreatitis have an overall higher rate of mortality compared with that of the general population. The 20-year survival after diagnosis is approximately 69%–80% (three- to fourfold higher mortality than general population). Interestingly, the mortality is usually not due to the progression of their pancreatitis to carcinoma, but due to the comorbidities that often go along with patients who suffer from pancreatitis, including alcoholic cirrhosis, diabetes, and smoking-related cardiovascular disease. Of note, patients with chronic pancreatitis have an elevated risk of extrapancreatic malignancy (10%–15%) affecting mostly the upper and lower airways as well as the gastrointestinal tract. The rate of pancreatic cancer is noted to be 1.8% at 10 years postdiagnosis and 4% at 20 years, which is higher than that of the general population (approximately 1.5% lifetime risk).

Ref.: 19–22

40. A 55-year-old woman with a history of ulcerative colitis presents to your office with a new onset of vague epigastric pain and jaundice. She denies any weight loss. To her knowledge, this has not happened before. Lab results are significant for a WBC of 12,000 cells per MCL and a total bilirubin of 2.0 mg/dL. You send her to the emergency room for a CT scan (see Fig. 26.3). Subsequent ERCP

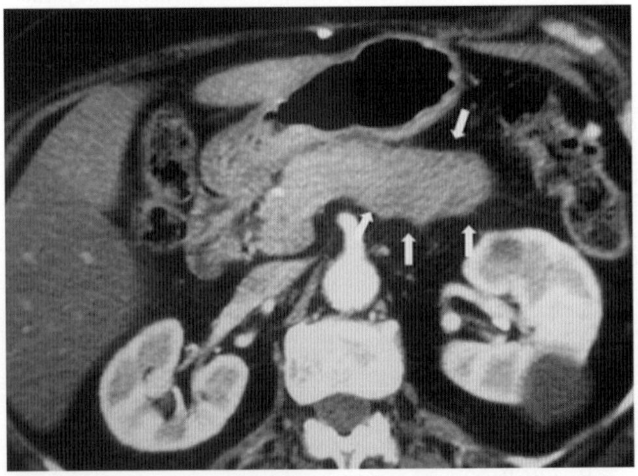

Fig. 26.3 Contrast-enhanced CT shows an enlarged pancreatic body and tail (arrows). *From Buscarini E, Frulloni L, De Lisi S, Falconi M, Testoni PA, Zambelli A. Autoimmune pancreatitis: a challenging diagnostic puzzle for clinicians.* Dig Liver Dis. *2010;42(2):92–98.*

showed areas of irregular narrowing throughout the intrapancreatic common bile duct. No masses are identified on EUS. What is the initial treatment of choice for this patient?

A. Puestow procedure
B. Total pancreatectomy
C. Whipple procedure
D. Steroids
E. Frey procedure

ANSWER: D

COMMENTS: Autoimmune pancreatitis can be very difficult to diagnose and is the cause of acute pancreatitis in 4%–6% of cases. Patient age varies between 30 and 70 years, and it affects men more often than women. The majority (70%–80%) present with painless jaundice. Acute pain, typical of classic pancreatitis, is rare. Additionally, one may see associated symptoms of pancreatic insufficiency, as this disease may have been ongoing without notice. Systemic inflammation/inflammatory reactions may be associated affecting kidney, lung, biliary tree, salivary glands, and gastrointestinal (GI) tract. Ulcerative colitis is observed in 30% of cases of associated systemic disease. On CT or US, a boggy, thick, "sausage-shaped" pancreas can be seen often with a rim of hypo- or hyperattenuation (early versus late). Irregularities in the intrapancreatic portion of the common bile duct can also be seen. Immunoglobulin G4 levels are thought to be associated with autoimmune pancreatitis, but using levels as a diagnostic marker is highly debated. Antinuclear antibody levels may also be elevated, indicating an autoimmune process. Steroids are considered as standard therapy for this etiology of pancreatitis (typically 30 to 40 mg of prednisone for 1 week).

Ref.: 23, 24

41. A 62-year-old male with an extensive history of recurrent alcoholic pancreatitis presents to the ED with progressively worsening shortness of breath. His last attack of pancreatitis was 9 months ago. At that time, a new fluid collection around the pancreas and extensive calcifications throughout the pancreas were noted. On examination, he is saturating 94% on room air. Auscultation of the lungs reveals absent breath sounds two-thirds of the way up his left lung fields. The right chest has breath sounds throughout. X-ray shows a large left pleural effusion. WBC count is 6,000 cells per MCL, and the patient is afebrile and hemodynamically stable. He has vague abdominal pain and had one episode of emesis in the ED. The ED resident orders a CT chest/abdomen displayed below (Fig. 26.4).

What is the most likely diagnosis?

A. Pneumonia
B. Sympathetic effusion
C. Pancreatic fistula
D. Reactive effusion
E. Diaphragmatic hernia

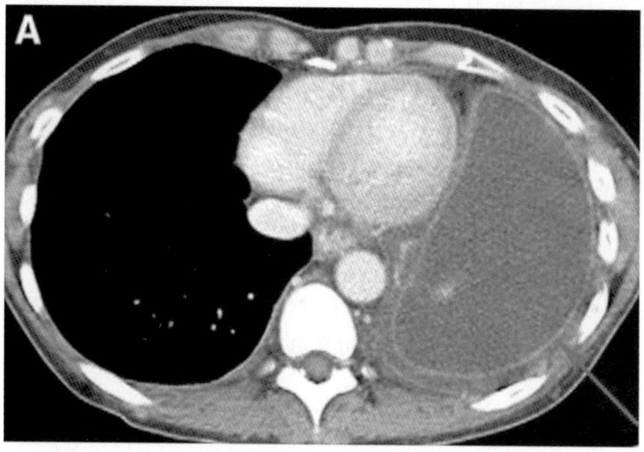

Fig. 26.4 *From King JC, Reber HA, Shiraga S, Hines OJ. Pancreatic–pleural fistula is best managed by early operative intervention.* Surgery. *2010;147(1):154–159.*

ANSWER: C

COMMENTS: Pancreatic–pleural fistula is a very rare entity and complication of chronic/recurrent pancreatitis. This usually evolves from a disruption in the pancreatic duct (often posterior), followed by fluid tracking in the retroperitoneum and up along the aorta or esophagus into the pleural space. Initial nonoperative therapy can include nil per os status, total parenteral nutrition, repeat thoracentesis, and octreotide. Interventional therapy utilizing ERCP to stent the ductal defect (if present) may also be attempted. Conservative treatment has an efficacy of 30%–60% and a recurrence rate of 15%. Operative therapy for failed conservative therapy, including duct ligation and resection or Roux-en-Y reconstruction, has an efficacy of 90% with an 18% recurrence. Regardless of treatment modality, patients often require prolonged hospitalization. Currently, treatment consists of several weeks of conservative management before progressing to surgical intervention.

Ref.: 25, 26

42. A 65-year-old male presents to the ED with two episodes of bloody emesis. His vitals are within normal limits other than mild tachycardia up to 110 beats/min. His hemoglobin is 9 g/dL (on prior lab testing, his baseline was 11 g/dL). His medical history is significant for hypertension, diabetes, 40-pack-year smoking history, alcohol abuse, and chronic pancreatitis. A nasogastric tube is placed, and some bright blood-tinged fluid is aspirated. No further episodes of emesis

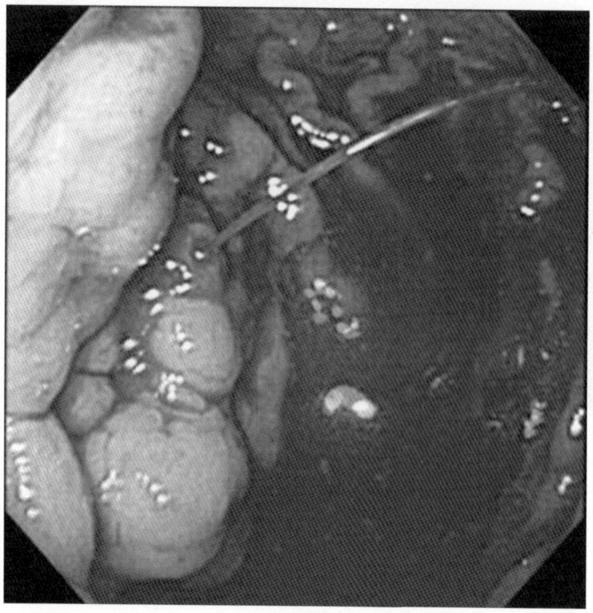

Fig. 26.5 *From Liang TJ, Chen YC, Liang HL, Liu SI, Chang PM. Balloon-occluded retrograde transvenous obliteration for intractable gastric variceal bleeding.* J Formos Med Assoc. *2013;112(7):426–429. © 2012.*

occur. A CT scan is obtained and shows a hypoechoic focus within the splenic vein and a calcified pancreas. He is sent for esophagogastroduodenoscopy, which is shown below (Fig. 26.5).
Which is the most definitive management?

A. Splenectomy
B. Gastric variceal banding
C. Propranolol
D. Porto-caval shunt
E. Spleno-renal shunt

ANSWER: A

COMMENTS: Discussions over the role of splenectomy have evolved as the quality and frequency of CT scans have risen. Splenic vein thrombosis is thought to occur in 7%–20% of patients with recurrent pancreatitis. This can lead to left-sided portal hypertension and subsequent development of gastric varices. Clinically significant hemorrhage secondary to variceal bleeding occurs in only 4% of those with pancreatitis-induced splenic vein thrombosis. Since not all patients who have splenic vein thrombosis will present with GI hemorrhage, prophylactic splenectomy has fallen out of favor. Splenectomy is now reserved for those who present with hemorrhagic complications of splenic vein thrombosis.

Ref.: 27–29

43. A 57-year-old male presents to the ED with complaints of epigastric abdominal fullness and occasional pain over the past 8 months with associated nausea. He confirms a long-standing history of acute on chronic pancreatitis secondary to alcohol abuse. A CT scan from a prior admission 10 months ago showed a large pancreatic pseudocyst. In the ED, he has one episode of blood-tinged emesis. He remains hemodynamically stable, with a hemoglobin of 10 g/dL. A CT scan is obtained (see Fig. 26.6).

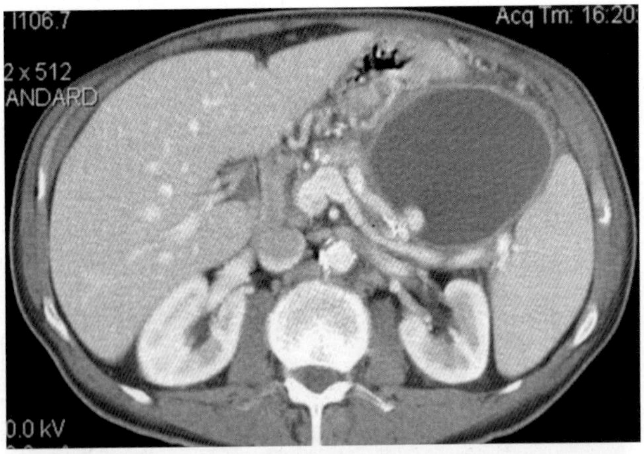

Fig. 26.6 *From Donatini G, Iacconi P, De Bartolomeis C, et al. Massive upper gastrointestinal bleeding from a pancreatic pseudocyst rupture: a case report.* Cases J. *2009;2(1):6793.*

What is the appropriate next step in management?

A. Exploratory laparotomy
B. Interventional radiology (IR) angiography and embolization
C. Laparoscopic cystogastrostomy
D. Endoscopic cystogastrostomy
E. IR percutaneous drainage

ANSWER: B

COMMENTS: This patient has a diagnosis of splenic artery pseudoaneurysm with a likely fistulous connection to a pancreatic pseudocyst. His nausea is likely due to gastric compression from this pseudocyst. As the patient is hemodynamically stable, IR embolization of the aneurysm to prevent further bleeding is the most appropriate next step in management, followed by surgical cystogastrostomy once his bleeding risk is controlled. Rupture is associated with 50% mortality. Planning a cystogastrostomy without management of an associated pseudoaneurysm can lead to intraoperative hemorrhage, delayed hemorrhage, and an increased risk to the patient. Pseudoaneurysms are rare complications (3%–10% incidence) caused by pancreatic enzymes eroding into the surrounding vasculature. The splenic artery is most frequently involved, but reports of involvement of gastroduodenal, pancreaticoduodenal, gastric, and hepatic arteries exist.

Ref.: 33, 34

44. Of the following listed genetic mutations, which occurs least frequently in the pathway of pancreatic carcinogenesis?

A. *p16* oncogene mutation
B. *p53* oncogene mutation
C. *DPC4* tumor suppressor gene deletion
D. *DNA* mismatch repair gene deletion
E. *BRCA1*

ANSWER: D

COMMENTS: Several mutations are considered significant and contributory to the development and progression of pancreatic cancer. The aforementioned mutations have all been shown to be involved in this process. Of the mutations mentioned, deletion of the DNA mismatch repair gene occurs least frequently at a rate of 4% in pancreatic cancer. When mutations in DNA mismatch repair genes occur, errors in DNA coding are unable to be repaired. Oncogene p16 is involved in phosphorylation of growth factors and regulatory proteins, and thus loss of this gene leads to unchecked cellular checkpoints. The p53 gene is well studied and involved in a variety of cancers. Its gene product includes a DNA-binding protein that induces apoptosis, thus functioning as a cellular checkpoint. This is inactivated in up to 75% of pancreatic neoplasms. DPC4 is located on chromosome 18q, and this chromosome is missing in 90% of pancreatic cancers. This gene product functions as a tumor suppressor and is specifically mutated in 50% of pancreatic cancers. Of note, BRCA2, well known for its involvement in ovarian and breast cancers, has shown increased risk of pancreatic cancer in those with this mutation.

Ref.: 35, 36

45. Which of the following familial genetic syndromes is not associated with pancreatic cancer?

A. Familial atypical multiple mole melanoma syndrome (FAMMM)
B. Familial adenomatous polyposis (FAP)
C. Hereditary nonpolyposis colorectal cancer (HNPCC)
D. Autosomal dominant polycystic kidney disease (ADPKD)
E. All of the above

ANSWER: D

COMMENTS: One in 71 people in the United States will develop pancreatic cancer in their lifetime; 5%–10% of these cancer occurrences can be associated with another well-known inherited disorder. FAMMM is an autosomal dominant disorder associated with an increased risk of melanoma and dysplastic nevi. It involves alteration in the gene encoding for p16 protein on chromosome 9p (involved in phosphorylation of growth factors and regulatory proteins, and thus loss of this gene leads to unchecked cellular checkpoints). There is an associated 58% risk of developing pancreatic cancer by age 80 in those affected. FAP is another autosomal dominant gene mutation involving the *APC* gene, with primary risk involving colon cancer. Associated extracolonic malignancies involve duodenal, thyroid, hepatic, and pancreatic cancers. HNPCC is again primarily associated with colon cancer, with lifetime risk ranging from 52%–82%. The defect involves a mutation in DNA mismatch repair. Extracolonic malignancies include endometrial, ovarian, gastric, and pancreatic cancers (1%–4%, associated medullary histology). ADPKD has not been reliably shown to be associated with pancreatic cancer.

Ref.: 37, 38

46. A 52-year-old male and his family are referred to you for evaluation after the diagnosis of pancreatic adenocarcinoma. After a review of his imaging, the patient is observed to have a resectable disease and is a candidate for a Whipple procedure. They read on a website that the procedure can be performed in two ways. When discussing pylorus-preserving versus pylorus-resecting (standard) pancreaticoduodenectomy, which of the following statements is true?

A. On average, there is no difference in operative time between the two procedures.

B. Patients who undergo pylorus-preserving pancreaticoduodenectomy have a lower rate of pancreatic leak and fistula development.

C. Patients undergoing pylorus-resecting pancreaticoduodenectomy have less blood loss and less need for blood transfusions.

D. Patients with pylorus-preserving pancreaticoduodenectomy have a higher rate of delayed gastric emptying.

E. None of the above.

ANSWER: D

COMMENTS: Pancreatic cancer is the fourth leading cause of cancer deaths in men and fifth leading cause in women. The classic Whipple procedure (involving antrectomy) is associated with operative mortality rates of 5% in expert hands at high-volume centers. However, it is also associated with morbidity as high as 30%–40% including fistulas, early and late dumping, weight loss, and reflux. An extensive Cochrane review and a meta-analysis of approximately eight randomized clinical trials both support that there is no difference in overall operative morbidity including fistulas, wound infection, postoperative bleeding, biliary leak, or pancreatic leak between the two techniques. There is no difference in operative mortality or oncologic outcome based on procedure type as well. Pylorus-preserving Whipple procedure seems to have lower operative time, less intraoperative blood loss, and decreased need for transfusions compared with pylorus-resecting Whipple procedure, but it does have a higher rate of delayed gastric emptying.

Ref.: 39, 40

47. Which of the following is true regarding neoadjuvant treatment for resectable pancreatic cancer?

A. It is associated with increased morbidity and mortality at 30 days postoperatively.

B. Radiation alone is considered as the optimal neoadjuvant therapy in this disease.

C. It is associated with a lower rate of pancreatic fistula and deep space infection postoperatively.

D. It is the standard of care.

E. None of the above.

ANSWER: C

COMMENTS: Often a debated topic, neoadjuvant versus surgery as the first strategy has been an issue of much interest in the pancreatic surgery community. Some surgeons advocate surgery first in order to attack the disease process early, prevent spread, and work with virgin tissue planes. Others advocate for a neoadjuvant approach for several reasons. One is a possibly improved management of micrometastatic disease. Another reason is to see which patients progress early versus those who would likely benefit from surgery without delaying time to chemotherapy for those who progress aggressively. Clinical trials regarding the neoadjuvant approach boast improved overall survival; however, there is no true randomized trial comparing neoadjuvant to surgery first, as it is difficult to accrue patients when the two treatment arms are so drastically different. A recent review of the American College of Surgeons-National Surgical Quality Improvement Program (ACS-NSQIP) data of over 1500 patients with pancreatic cancer does show that patients who underwent neoadjuvant therapy prior to surgical resection had a lower rate of pancreatic fistula (7.3% vs. 15.4%) and deep space infection (3% vs. 10.3%) compared with the surgery-first patients. Also, overall 30-day postoperative morbidity and mortality are reported to be no different in the ACS-NSQIP data set. There is no clear national consensus at this time as to which approach should be the standard of care.

Ref.: 41–43

48. A 60-year-old female is referred to your junior partner for the diagnosis of IPMN. She asks you for advice regarding any other workup that she may have missed. You recommend a colonoscopy. A stage II colon cancer in the sigmoid colon is diagnosed. How should you proceed?

A. Colon resection followed by pancreas resection at a second surgery

B. Pancreas resection followed by colon resection at a second surgery

C. Neoadjuvant chemoradiation

D. Simultaneous resection of both the IPMN and colon cancer

ANSWER: D

COMMENTS: Extrapancreatic malignancies have been observed more commonly in patients with IPMN than in those with ductal cancer of the pancreas or other cystic pancreatic neoplasms. The reason for this is not known. No particular genetic predisposition for IPMN has been identified. Extrapancreatic cancer has been reported in approximately one-third of patients with IPMN. Gastric cancer and colon cancer have been the most frequent. No specific guidelines exist, but based on these findings, screening upper gastrointestinal endoscopy and colonoscopy would be appropriate recommendations in these patients. Should an extrapancreatic malignancy be identified, simultaneous resection is often indicated.

Ref.: 16, 44

49. Which of the following studies is the most effective in identifying and localizing pancreatic neuroendocrine neoplasms?

A. MRI

B. Positron emission tomography/CT

C. Octreotide scan

D. Endoscopy with EUS

E. Ultrasound

ANSWER: D

COMMENTS: EUS, in experienced hands, is associated with up to 93% sensitivity and 95% specificity when localizing a suspected neuroendocrine tumor of the pancreas, particularly in the head. Another highly regarded imaging modality with high accuracy (>75%) is somatostatin receptor scintigraphy (SRS; octreotide scan). The accuracy of CT scan alone ranges from 64% to 82%, and MRI is slightly better at above 74% sensitivity, similar to SRS. Limits of EUS include the inability to evaluate the liver for disease. Thus when using EUS to localize neuroendocrine tumors of the pancreas, SRS or another imaging modality would be needed to evaluate for metastatic disease.

Ref.: 45–47

50. A 48-year-old female presents to the ED with her third episode of blurred vision, palpitations, and weakness. Glucose level is 38 mg/dL. Her symptoms resolve with the administration of glucose. On her prior two presentations, her glucose levels were 35 and 42 mg/dL, respectively, and she was responsive to glucose administration. She is referred to you by the hospitalist for concerns of an insulinoma. Which is the first best diagnostic test?

A. Check proinsulin levels

B. Oral glucose tolerance test

C. Monitored fast

D. Check C-peptide levels

E. Hemoglobin A1c

ANSWER: C

COMMENTS: Insulinoma is the most common functional neoplasm of the endocrine pancreas and is evenly distributed throughout the pancreas; 10% of insulinomas are associated with MEN-1, 10% are malignant, and 90% are sporadic and solitary. Patients present with symptoms of hypoglycemia during fasting, low levels of glucose less than 50 mg/dL, and relief of symptoms with exogenous glucose (referred to as "Whipple triad"). Symptoms can include findings associated with catecholamine surge including palpitations, diaphoresis, and tachycardia. Also, neurologic symptoms such as confusion, seizures, and irritability may be observed.

Differential diagnosis can include tumors, such as mesothelioma and sarcoma, adrenal insufficiency, and self-administration of insulin. In order to make the diagnosis of insulinoma, first a 24-h monitored fast should be performed. This includes glucose and insulin samples every 4 to 6 h in addition to samples at any time that symptoms appear during this period. Insulin-to-glucose ratios greater than 0.4 (normal are less than 0.3) after a prolonged fast are highly sensitive for the diagnosis. Levels of C-peptide and proinsulin are elevated often in these patients as well but are not so in patients who self-administer insulin.

The absolute diagnosis is made with these six key features: (1) displayed blood glucose levels ≤ 40 mg/dL, (2) concomitant insulin levels ≥ 3 U/L, (3) C-peptide levels ≥ 200 pmol/L, (4) proinsulin levels ≥ 5 pmol/L, (5) β-hydroxybutyrate levels ≤ 2.7 mmol/L, and (6) absence of sulfonylurea (metabolites) in the plasma or urine.

Ref.: 48, 49

REFERENCES

1. Steer ML. Exocrine pancreas. In: Townsend CM, Beauchamp RD, Evers BM, et al., eds. *Sabiston Textbook of Surgery: The Biological Basis of Modern Surgical Practice*. 18th ed. Philadelphia: WB Saunders; 2008.
2. Fisher WE, Andersen DK, Bell RH, et al. Pancreas. In: Brunicardi FC, Andersen DK, Billar TR, et al., eds. *Schwartz's Principles of Surgery*. 9th ed. New York: McGraw-Hill; 2010.
3. Mulholland MW, Lilleomoe KD, Doherty GM, et al., eds. *Greenfield's Surgery: Scientific Principles and Practice*. 4th ed. Philadelphia: JB Lippincott; 2006.
4. Howard J, Idezuki Y, Ihse I, et al., eds. *Surgical Diseases of the Pancreas*. 3rd ed. Baltimore: Williams & Wilkins; 1998.
5. Mulvihill SJ. Liver, biliary tract, and pancreas. In: O'Leary JP, Tabuenca A, eds. *The Physiologic Basis of Surgery*. 4th ed. Philadelphia: JB Lippincott; 2008.
6. Deziel DJ, Prinz RA. Bacteriology of necrotizing pancreatitis. *Probl Gen Surg*. 1996;13:22–28.
7. Villatoro E, Bassi C, Larvin M. Antibiotic therapy for prophylaxis against infection of pancreatic necrosis in acute pancreatitis. *Cochrane Database Syst Rev*. 2006;4:CD002941.
8. Buchler M, Malfertheiner P, Freiss H, et al. Human pancreatic tissue concentration of bactericidal antibiotics. *Gastroenterology*. 1992;103:1902–1908.
9. Sharma VK, Howden CW. Meta-analysis of randomized controlled trials of endoscopic retrograde cholangiography and endoscopic sphincterotomy for the treatment of acute biliary pancreatitis. *Am J Gastroenterol*. 1999;94:3211–3214.
10. McClave SA, Chang WK, Dhaliwal R, et al. Nutrition support in acute pancreatitis: a systematic review of the literature. *J Parenter Enteral Nutr*. 2006;30:143–156.
11. Prinz RA, Deziel DJ, eds. Chronic pancreatitis. *Problems in General Surgery*. 1998;15(1):80–89.
12. Deziel DJ, Prinz RA. Drainage of pancreatic pseudocysts: indications and long term results. *Dig Surg*. 1996;13:101–108.
13. Pais SA, Attasaranya S, Leblanc JK, et al. Role of endoscopic ultrasound in the diagnosis of intraductal papillary mucinous neoplasms: correlation with surgical histopathology. *Clin Gastroenterol Hepatol*. 2007;5:489–495.
14. Tanaka M, Chari S, Adsay V, et al. International consensus guidelines for management of intraductal papillary mucinous neoplasms and mucinous cystic neoplasms of the pancreas. *Pancreatology*. 2006;6:17–32.
15. Schmidt CM, White PB, Waters JA, et al. Intraductal papillary mucinous neoplasms: predictors of malignant and invasive pathology. *Ann Surg*. 2007;246:644–651.
16. Yoon WJ, Ryu JK, Lee JK, et al. Extrapancreatic malignancies in patients with intraductal papillary mucinous neoplasm of the pancreas: prevalence, associated factors, and comparison with patients with other pancreatic cystic neoplasms. *Ann Surg Oncol*. 2008;15:3193–3198.
17. Riall TS. Pancreas anatomy and physiology. In: Mulholland MW, Lillemoe KD, Doherty GM, Maier RV, Simenone DM, Upchurch GR, eds. *Greenfield's Surgery: Scientific Principles and Practice*. 5th ed. Lippincott, Williams & Wilkins; 2011. Chapter 51.
18. Levy M. Idiopathic acute recurrent pancreatitis. *Am J Gastroenterol*. 2001;96(9):2540–2555.
19. Zyromski NJ, Howard TJ. Chronic pancreatitis. In: Mulholland MW, Lillemoe KD, Doherty GM, Maier RV, Simenone DM, Upchurch GR, eds. *Greenfield's Surgery: Scientific Principles and Practice*. 5th ed. Lippincott, Williams & Wilkins; 2011.

20. Nøjgaard C, Bendtsen F, Becker U, Andersen JR, Holst C, Matzen P. M1383 mortality and prognostic factors in chronic pancreatitis—a long-term follow-up study of a Danish cohort. *Gastroenterology*. 2010;138(5):5–393.
21. Pedrazzoli S, Pasquali C, Guzzinati S, Berselli M, Sperti C. Survival rates and cause of death in 174 patients with chronic pancreatitis. *J Gastrointest Surg*. 2008;12(11):1930–1937.
22. Seicean A, Tantau M, Grigorescu M, et al. Mortality risk factors in chronic pancreatitis. *J Gastrointest Liver Dis*. 2006;15(1):21–26.
23. Buscarini E, Frulloni L, De Lisi S, Falconi M, Testoni PA, Zambelli A. Autoimmune pancreatitis: a challenging diagnostic puzzle for clinicians. *Dig Liver Dis*. 2010;42(2):92–98.
24. Hart PA, Zen Y, Chari ST. Recent advances in autoimmune pancreatitis. *Gastroenterology*. 2015;149(1):39–51.
25. King JC, Reber HA, Shiraga S, Joe Hines O. Pancreatic–pleural fistula is best managed by early operative intervention. *Surgery*. 2010;147(1): 154–159. Web.
26. Virgilio E, Mercantini P, Catta F, Grieco M, Cavallini M, Ferri M. Pancreaticopleural fistula. *Surg Infect*. 2016;17(2):266–267.
27. Chen BC. Isolated gastric variceal bleeding caused by splenic lymphoma-associated splenic vein occlusion. *World J Gastroenterol*. 2013;19(40):6939.
28. Gotto A, Lieberman M, Pochapin M. Gastric variceal bleeding due to pancreatitis-induced splenic vein thrombosis. *BMJ Case Rep*. 2014 Mar 24; 2014. pii: bcr2013201359 http://dx.doi.org/101136/bcr-2013-201359.
29. Heider TR, Azeem S, Galanko JA, Behrns KE. The natural history of pancreatitis-induced splenic vein thrombosis. *Ann Surg*. 2004;239(6): 876–882.
30. Eatock FC, Chong P, Menezes N, et al. A randomized study of early nasogastric versus nasojejunal feeding in severe acute pancreatitis. *Am J Gastroenterol*. 2005;100(2):432–439.
31. Oláh A, Romics Jr L. Enteral nutrition in acute pancreatitis: a review of the current evidence. *World J Gastroenterol*. 2014;20(43):16123.
32. Traverso LW. The Whipple procedure for severe complications of chronic pancreatitis. *Arch Surg*. 1993;128(9):1047.
33. Donatini G, Iacconi P, Bartolomeis CD, et al. Massive upper gastrointestinal bleeding from a pancreatic pseudocyst rupture: a case report. *Cases J*. 2009;2(1):6793.
34. Son C, Liu C, Wang X-M. Pancreatitis associated with splenic artery pseudoaneurysms. *J App Radiol*. 18 June 2016;2013(1 Feb). Web.
35. Nakeeb A, Lillemoe KD. Neoplasms of the exocrine pancreas. In: Mulholland MW, Lillemoe KD, Doherty GM, Maier RV, Simenone DM, Upchurch GR, eds. *Greenfield's Surgery: Scientific Principles and Practice*. 5th ed. Lippincott, Williams & Wilkins; 2011. Chapter 54.
36. Winter JM, Maitra A, Yeo CJ. Genetics and pathology of pancreatic cancer. *HPB*. 2006;8(5):324–336.
37. Solomon S, Das S, Brand R, Whitcomb DC. Inherited pancreatic cancer syndromes. *Cancer J*. 2012;18(6):485–491.
38. Hruban R, Kern S. *Hereditary pancreatic cancer. Atlas Gene & Cytogenet Oncol Haematol*. 2001;5(1):72–75.
39. Diener MK, Fitzmaurice C, Schwarzer G, et al. Pylorus-preserving pancreaticoduodenectomy (pp Whipple) versus pancreaticoduodenectomy (classic Whipple) for surgical treatment of periampullary and pancreatic carcinoma. *Cochrane Database Syst Rev*. 2014;2:CD006053.
40. Yang C, Wu H-S, Chen X-L, et al. Pylorus-preserving versus pylorus-resecting pancreaticoduodenectomy for periampullary and pancreatic carcinoma: a meta-analysis. *PLoS ONE*. 2014;9(3):e90316.
41. Asare EA, Evans DB, Erickson BA, Aburajab M, Tolat P, Tsai S. Neoadjuvant treatment sequencing adds value to the care of patients with operable pancreatic cancer. *J Surg Oncol*. 2016;114(3):291–295.
42. Cooper AB, Parmar AD, Riall TS, et al. Does the use of neoadjuvant therapy for pancreatic adenocarcinoma increase postoperative morbidity and mortality rates? *J Gastrointest Surg*. 2014;19(1):80–87.
43. Tsai S, Evans DB. Therapeutic advances in localized pancreatic cancer. *JAMA Surg*. 2016;151(9):862–868.
44. Sparr JA, Bandipalliam P, Redston MS, Syngal S. Intraductal papillary mucinous neoplasm of the pancreas with loss of mismatch repair in a patient with Lynch syndrome. *Am J Surg Pathol*. 2009;33(2): 309–312.
45. Anderson M. Endoscopic ultrasound is highly accurate and directs management in patients with neuroendocrine tumors of the pancreas. *Am J Gastroenterol*. 2000;95(9):2271–2277.
46. Kennedy EP, Brody JR, Yeo CJ. Neoplasms of the endocrine pancreas. In: Mulholland MW, Lillemoe KD, Doherty GM, Maier RV, Simenone DM, Upchurch GR, eds. *Greenfield's Surgery: Scientific Principles and Practice*. 5th ed. Lippincott, Williams & Wilkins; 2011.
47. Oberg K. Diagnostic work-up of gastroenteropancreatic neuroendocrine tumors. *Clinics*. 2012;67(S1):109–112.
48. Anderson CW, Bennett JJ. Clinical presentation and diagnosis of pancreatic neuroendocrine tumors. *Surg Oncol Clin N Am*. 2016;25(2): 363–374.
49. Kennedy EP, Brody JR, Yeo CJ. Neoplasms of the endocrine pancreas. In: Mulholland MW, Lillemoe KD, Doherty GM, Maier RV, Simenone DM, Upchurch GR, eds. *Greenfield's Surgery: Scientific Principles and Practice*. 5th ed. Lippincott, Williams & Wilkins; 2011. Chapter 55.

CHAPTER 27

SPLEEN AND LYMPHATIC SYSTEM

Gillian Alex, M.D., and Edie Chan, M.D.

1. Which of the following statements regarding splenic anatomy is true?
   A. The splenic ligaments are all avascular.
   B. The tail of the pancreas is often contained in the splenorenal ligament.
   C. The average weight of the adult spleen is 300 g.
   D. The first branches of the splenic artery are the short gastric arteries.
   E. The accessory spleens are most commonly found in the greater omentum.

ANSWER: B

COMMENTS: Although the majority of the splenic ligaments are in fact avascular, the gastrosplenic ligament contains the short gastric vessels. Additionally, in the case of portal hypertension, other splenic ligaments may become vascularized. The tail of the pancreas may be injured during splenectomy because it often lies within the splenorenal ligament. The average weight of the adult spleen is 150 g (range, 75 to 300 g). The first branches of the splenic artery are the pancreatic branches and then the short gastric, the left gastroepiploic (which may also give rise to the short gastric arteries), and the terminal splenic branches. The splenic artery divides into segmental branches that enter the trabeculae of the spleen. There are two types of anatomy of the splenic artery: the distributive and magistral. The distributive subtype is much more common (70% of individuals) and is characterized by a short splenic artery trunk and multiple long branches entering the spleen. Conversely, the magistral type has a long main trunk that divides relatively near the hilum. Accessory spleens are common, especially in patients with hematologic disorders, and are found in 15%–35% of patients. In decreasing order of frequency, they are found in the splenic hilum, gastrosplenic ligament, splenocolic ligament, splenorenal ligament, greater omentum and mesentery, and the left pelvis along the left ureter or by the left testis or ovary, but they have been identified anywhere within the peritoneal cavity.

Ref.: 1, 2

2. Which statement regarding the segments and function of the spleen is true?
   A. The white pulp consists of lymphatic sheaths surrounding vessels and is where B-lymphocyte precursors mature before migrating to the red pulp.
   B. The white pulp usually constitutes 50% of a normal spleen.
   C. The major function of the red pulp is to store old or defective erythrocytes for future use.
   D. The marginal zone is the zone usually absent except in the presence of lymphoma.
   E. The spleen can act as a large reservoir of platelets, erythrocytes, and other lymphatic cells.

ANSWER: E

COMMENTS: The white pulp of the spleen consists of lymphatic sheaths that usually surround splenic blood vessels. The white pulp contains plasma cells and lymphocytes and functions as the immune center of the spleen. The lymphatic sheaths contain mostly T cells, as well as some B-cell follicles that can be either primary or secondary (after stimulation by antigen). The white pulp makes up approximately 25% of a normal spleen. The red pulp is the largest component of the spleen and represents a network of sinuses that filter the blood. Here, red cells are removed from the circulation and destroyed. The junction between the red pulp and white pulp is the marginal zone, which allows additional antigen presentation and contributes further to the lymphatic functions of the spleen. The spleen serves as a large reservoir. As much as 30% of an individual's platelets reside in the normal spleen. In disease states such as portal hypertension, splenic sequestration can trap an even larger proportion of the body's circulating cells, including as much as 90% of the total number of platelets.

Ref.: 1, 2

3. A 49-year-old woman with Felty's syndrome undergoes successful splenectomy. Several years after surgery, examination of her peripheral blood smear would reveal which one of the following to be true?
   A. Howell-Jolly bodies, which are suggestive of the presence of an accessory spleen
   B. Stippling, spur cells, and target cells because of the lack of filtration
   C. High levels of properdin and tuftsin
   D. No change in the level of antibodies needed to clear organisms as in the presplenectomy state
   E. Red blood cells undergoing maturation more quickly

ANSWER: B

COMMENTS: Howell-Jolly bodies are abnormal cytoplasmic inclusions within red blood cells. They are seen in individuals who have undergone splenectomy because normally they are removed by a functioning spleen, and thus their absence would suggest the presence of an accessory spleen. Stippling, spur cells, and target cells are all functionally altered erythrocytes that are normally cleared from the circulation by the spleen and thus are commonly seen following splenectomy. Properdin and tuftsin are important opsonins manufactured in the spleen. Properdin helps initiate the alternative pathway of complement activation, which is particularly useful for fighting encapsulated organisms. Tuftsin enhances the phagocytic activity of granulocytes. Asplenic individuals lack the ability to produce these substances. The spleen is the initial site of immunoglobulin (Ig) M synthesis in response to bacteria. Without this primary defense mechanism, asplenic individuals require increased levels of antibodies to clear organisms relative to the presplenectomy state. Erythrocytes do not undergo maturation more quickly after splenectomy. As part of its "pitting" function, the spleen removes cytoplasmic inclusions [particles such as nuclear remnants (Howell-Jolly bodies), insoluble globin precipitates (Heinz bodies), and endocytic vacuoles] from within circulating red blood cells. Felty's syndrome is an uncommon disorder marked by splenomegaly, neutropenia, and rheumatoid arthritis. Patients may have thrombocytopenia and anemia, with a predisposition to infections. Splenectomy in patients with Felty's syndrome is beneficial in correcting the anemia and neutropenia associated with this syndrome.

Ref.: 1, 2

4. A 39-year-old male comes to you with easing bruising and mucosal bleeding. His complete blood count (CBC) shows a hemoglobin level of 8.2 g/dL and platelet count of 56,000/mm^3. You obtain a peripheral smear that shows increased megakaryocytes and reticulocytes. Which of the following is associated with this condition?

A. Splenomegaly must exist for this condition to occur.
B. All patients with this condition will have reticulocytosis.
C. Early satiety is an important symptom that may suggest splenomegaly.
D. Left upper quadrant pain is the most common symptom in this process.
E. The disease will not correct with splenectomy.

ANSWER: C

COMMENTS: The criteria for the diagnosis of hypersplenism are (1) documented anemia, thrombocytopenia, or leukopenia; (2) normal compensatory response from the bone marrow to correct the cytopenia; and (3) correction of the cytopenia by splenectomy. In patients with splenomegaly, all activities of the spleen are thought to be markedly accentuated. Although splenomegaly is almost always associated with hypersplenism, not all cases of hypersplenism are associated with splenomegaly. Patients may have an anatomically normal spleen with abnormal function. The most frequently reported symptom of splenomegaly is early satiety from the mass effect of the enlarging spleen on the stomach. The left upper quadrant pain is more frequently associated with conditions that cause an acute distension of the splenic capsule such as abscess or hematoma formation after trauma.

Ref.: 1

5. A 24-year-old female is to undergo an elective splenectomy for β-thalassemia. Which of the following recommendations should you make to her regarding vaccinations?

A. She should be vaccinated against *Streptococcus pneumoniae*, *Neisseria meningitidis*, and *Haemophilus influenzae* 14 days before splenectomy.
B. She should be vaccinated against *S. pneumoniae, N. meningitidis*, and *H. influenzae* at the time of splenectomy.
C. She should be vaccinated against *S. pneumoniae*, *N. meningitidis*, and *H. influenzae* 1 year after splenectomy.
D. She should be vaccinated against *S. pneumoniae* alone 14 days after splenectomy and given a booster dose of *N. meningitidis* vaccine.
E. She should be vaccinated against *S. pneumoniae* alone 14 days before splenectomy and given a booster dose of *N. meningitidis* vaccine.

ANSWER: E

COMMENTS: Asplenic patients are at an increased risk of severe sepsis following splenectomy. A series of case reports in the 1980s and 1990s reports about a 3.2% incidence of postsplenectomy sepsis. Patients are at the highest risk in the first year after splenectomy. Since the spleen has an important immunologic role in the opsonization of encapsulated organisms, asplenic patients are at an increased susceptibility to these bacteria—*S. pneumoniae*, *H. influenzae*, and *N. meningitidis*. The most common organism that causes postsplenectomy sepsis is *S. pneumoniae*. The current guidelines recommend that all patients receive the *S. pneumoniae* vaccine 14 days prior to surgery. The ideal timing for vaccination after trauma splenectomy or unanticipated splenectomy during surgery for other reasons should be 14 days postoperatively. The patient in this question is 24 years old and has already presumably received her Haemophilus influenza type B (HiB) vaccine and therefore does not need to be redosed. If she had not been vaccinated against HiB, the vaccination would be indicated. She has also most likely received an *N. meningitidis* vaccine as well and therefore only needs a booster dose.

Ref.: 3

6. A 4-year-old male with sickle cell anemia undergoes splenectomy for sequestration crisis. His mother wants to know if he is now at an increased risk for infection and would like to know if he is going to require lifelong antibiotics. How do you advise her?

A. He needs to take lifelong daily prophylaxis with amoxicillin.
B. He needs daily prophylaxis with amoxicillin until age 5 and 1 year after splenectomy.
C. Antibiotics prophylaxis is not indicated.
D. Antibiotic prophylaxis is not indicated unless he becomes immunocompromised.
E. He only needs to take antibiotics if he develops a fever.

ANSWER: B

COMMENTS: Patients and families need to be educated that the asplenic state carries a small risk of overwhelming and life-threatening infection. Sepsis in this population carries a 50% mortality risk. It is crucial that asplenic patients adhere to vaccination and antibiotic prevention guidelines and inform all caregivers of their asplenic state. It is recommended that all asplenic children under age 5 receive daily oral antibiotic prophylaxis with a penicillin derivative or antibiotic with similar coverage. If children receive a splenectomy at age 4, it is recommended that they continue prophylaxis for 1 year following splenectomy when the rate of infection is the highest.

Ref.: 1, 3

7. A 43-year-old man has thrombocytopenia, ecchymosis, and a history of melena. His primary doctor suspects that he might have idiopathic thrombocytopenia purpura (ITP). Which of the following is true about this condition?

A. It is characterized by a low platelet count, mucosal hemorrhage, normal bone marrow, and an enlarged spleen.
B. It is caused by a splenic overproduction of IgM, which attacks the platelet membrane and causes platelet destruction.
C. The bone marrow often hypertrophies to counteract the increased platelet destruction.
D. It affects young men more commonly than women.
E. Diagnosis requires exclusion of other causes of thrombocytopenia.

ANSWER: E

COMMENTS: ITP is a disorder of increased platelet destruction caused by autoantibodies to platelet membrane components. This results in platelet phagocytosis in the spleen, and the bone marrow does not adequately compensate for this increased destruction. Although ITP is characterized by a low platelet count, mucosal hemorrhage, and relatively normal bone marrow (not hyperactive), the spleen is not enlarged. The autoantibodies are IgG antibodies, not IgM, directed against the platelet fibrinogen receptor. The mechanism underlying the use of intravenous (IV) IgG for the treatment of ITP is that IgG saturates the fibrinogen receptors so that they will not bind and thus destroy platelets. This autoimmune disorder affects women more commonly than men. A diagnosis of ITP requires exclusion of other potential causes of thrombocytopenia such as drugs, myelodysplasia, thrombotic thrombocytopenia purpura (TTP), systemic lupus erythematosus, lymphoma, and chronic disseminated intravascular coagulation.

Ref.: 1, 2

8. A 37-year-old female has just completed treatment with steroids for ITP. Her platelet count is currently 37,000/mm^3. She is asymptomatic. Which of the following is the next step in her management?

A. Splenectomy
B. Rituximab
C. Intravenous immunoglobulin (IVIG)
D. Observation
E. Eltrombopag

ANSWER: D

COMMENTS: The initial treatment for ITP is high-dose steroids, usually 1 mg/kg of prednisone a day. The goal of therapy is to induce remission and increase platelet counts to >100,000/mm^3. This is effective in roughly 75% of patients. Treatment is initiated when platelet counts fall to less than 20,000/mm^3 or less than 50,000/mm^3 in patients who are symptomatic. Although the initial response to steroid therapy is good, it only persists in 15%–25% of patients. Patients who are symptomatic and fail steroid therapy should then progress to receiving IVIG; if this fails at correction of thrombocytopenia, then elective splenectomy is the next step in management. Not all patients respond to splenectomy. For these patients, rituximab (a monoclonal antibody against CD20 on B cells) and eltrombopag (thrombopoietin receptor agonist) are fourth-line options. The patient in this question is asymptomatic and therefore can be managed with observation.

Ref.: 1, 2, 4

9. Which of the following is true of thrombocytopenic purpura?

A. It is characterized by widespread occlusion of arterioles and capillaries by hyaline membranes composed of platelets and fibrinogen.
B. Splenectomy is curative and is the first line for treatment.
C. Central nervous system manifestations such as intracerebral hemorrhage are exceedingly rare.
D. The pathogenesis is well understood and is marked by antibodies to vessel wall antigen.
E. Plasmapheresis is only used as a salvage therapy in the treatment of TTP.

ANSWER: A

COMMENTS: This patient has thrombotic thrombocytopenic purpura. The disease is characterized by occlusion of arterioles and capillaries by hyaline deposits of aggregated platelets and fibrin. The pathogenesis is not well understood or described; the most accepted theory is that it is an autoimmune disease that causes there to be antibodies to small vessel antigens. The success of plasmapheresis as a treatment supports this idea, but a signal antibody has not been identified. The first-line therapy is plasmapheresis. Fresh-frozen plasma and high-dose corticosteroids may be used to control bleeding. Splenectomy is not curative and is considered only for salvage therapy. Mortality rates in patients with TTP can approach 50%, mostly from intracranial hemorrhage or renal failure. The disease can have a rapidly fulminant course. Most long-term survivors of TTP have undergone splenectomy. Platelet transfusion does not control the bleeding, and therapy should be focused on high-volume plasmapheresis.

Ref.: 1

10. A 17-year-old male is being worked up for jaundice and anemia. His peripheral smear shows spherocytes. His Coomb's test is negative, and an osmotic fragility test is positive. Other than his jaundice, he denies any other symptoms. Right upper quadrant ultrasound shows a normal gallbladder without stones. What is the best surgical option to offer this patient?

A. Surgery is not indicated
B. Splenectomy
C. Cholecystectomy
D. Splenectomy and cholecystectomy
E. Bone marrow biopsy

ANSWER: B

COMMENTS: Hereditary spherocytosis (HS) is inherited in an autosomal dominant fashion and is the most common of the congenital hemolytic anemias. It affects around 1/5000 individuals. There are numerous genetic defects responsible for this disease that affect proteins on the cytoskeleton of red blood cells—spectrin and ankyrin. This causes loss of flexibility and makes them more susceptible to destruction in the spleen. Diagnosis is made by peripheral smear, which will exhibit spherocytes. Spherocytes can also be seen in other hemolytic anemias, but a Coomb's test will be negative only with HS. The osmotic fragility test is diagnostic. Treatment is splenectomy, which should be delayed until children are at least 4 to 6 years of age. Moreover, 30%–60% of patients with HS will develop gallstones. Concomitant splenectomy and cholecystectomy is recommended in patients with gallstones. The patient in this question is symptomatic from his HS and requires splenectomy; he does not have gallstones on ultrasound and therefore does not need his gallbladder removed at this time.

Ref.: 1

11. Which of the following hematologic disorders is unlikely to respond to splenectomy?

A. Idiopathic thrombocytopenic purpura
B. Autoimmune hemolytic anemia secondary to warm antibodies
C. Autoimmune hemolytic anemia secondary to cold antibodies
D. HS
E. Thalassemia

ANSWER: C

COMMENTS: Hematologic disorders that respond to splenectomy are conditions of cells that are destroyed in the spleen. The spleen contains macrophages with Fc fragments that bind to IgG. ITP is caused by IgG antibodies to platelets; autoimmune hemolytic anemias are either caused by IgG (warm) or IgM (cold) antibodies. IgM is not cleared in the spleen but in the liver. Therefore splenectomy is not helpful in patients with an autoimmune hemolytic anemia due to cold antibodies. Patients with HS and thalassemia do benefit from splenectomy.

Ref.: 1, 2

12. A 47-year-old woman with a history of a radical mastectomy 20 years previously has had a long-standing lymphedema of her upper extremity on the treated side. She is now complaining of a reddish blue nodule on her arm and dyspnea on exertion. Which one of the following is not true regarding her condition?

A. The lymphatic system is a collection of small lymphatic vessels that parallel the major blood vessels and may contain red blood cells, bacteria, and proteins.
B. The lymphatic system has valves.
C. Her reddish blue nodule probably represents a benign condition related to a long-standing lymphedema.
D. Extrinsic factors such as muscle contraction, arterial pulsation, and respiratory movement aid in the movement of lymph flow.
E. Measurement of the protein content of edema fluid can be used to assess the lymphatic function of her arm.

ANSWER: C

COMMENTS: This patient has a lymphangiosarcoma following mastectomy complicated by untreated chronic lymphedema, or Stewart-Treves syndrome. This malignant tumor is rare and typically occurs in patients with long-standing lymphedema. It is characterized by a rapid and aggressive course and a tendency to metastasize to the lungs early, as suggested by her history of dyspnea. Treatment often involves multimodality therapy, and amputation of the limb may be necessary. The lymphatic system begins as a network of valveless capillaries in the superficial dermis that drain into a secondary system of valved vessels in the deep or subdermal layer, which then drain into major lymphatic channels that parallel the major blood vessels. Intradermal lymphatics can be evaluated by the intradermal injection of blue dye. Lymphangiography is rarely done as a mapping technique for patients with lymphedema because it may worsen the symptoms. Proteins, red blood cells, and lymphocytes that make their way into the extracellular fluid readily enter the lymphatic vessels. Measurement of the protein content of edema fluid in an extremity can be used to assess the status of lymphatic function. The protein content should be less than 1.5 mg/dL; higher values suggest declining lymphatic return.

Ref.: 5

13. A 61-year-old heavy smoker undergoes computed tomography (CT) of the abdomen after a motor vehicle accident. The scan reveals a 4-cm irregular hypodensity in the spleen without other associated lymphadenopathy or masses. Which of the following statements is true regarding primary and metastatic tumors of the spleen?

A. Vascular neoplasms, including hemangiomas and angiosarcomas, are the most common primary tumors of the spleen.
B. With the exception of lymphomas, the spleen is rarely a site of metastatic involvement from primary tumors.
C. Splenectomy is often curative for primary tumors of the spleen.
D. A laparoscopic approach to splenectomy for malignancy is associated with inferior outcomes.
E. Most splenic metastases are symptomatic.

ANSWER: A

COMMENTS: Not infrequently, lung cancer metastasizes to the spleen. Other common primary tumors that may metastasize to the spleen include breast cancer and melanoma, as well as ovarian, gastric, and colon cancers. The most common primary splenic tumors are vascular in origin and include hemangiomas (benign) and angiosarcomas (malignant). They later may be associated with environmental exposure to vinyl chloride or thorium dioxide. Most splenic metastases are asymptomatic and are found at autopsy in about 7% of cancer patients. Occasionally, secondary tumors in the spleen may cause symptomatic splenomegaly or splenic rupture. By the time that metastases are detected, splenectomy is rarely curative, but it may be palliative in appropriately selected symptomatic patients or be a reasonable therapy for isolated splenic metastases. The laparoscopic approach to splenectomy is appropriate for most splenic tumors.

Ref.: 1

14. A 32-year-old woman comes to the emergency department complaining of pain in her foot and calf. She reports that her left leg has been swollen for the last 15 years. She has a temperature of 101.5°F and reports that she had a splinter removed from her leg 1 week earlier. Her left lower extremity is swollen from the foot to the inguinal ligament, and she has erythema of the foot and calf. In addition to cellulitis, what is the most likely underlying diagnosis?

A. Chronic venous insufficiency
B. Deep venous thrombosis
C. Lymphedema praecox
D. Meige's disease
E. Milroy's disease

ANSWER: C

COMMENTS: Chronic venous insufficiency is usually bilateral and marked by signs of venous stasis such as hemosiderin deposits and possibly ulceration. Deep venous thrombosis would be manifested acutely and would be unlikely to have such a long-standing history. Swelling of an extremity from a pathologic condition of the lymphatic system is classified as primary or secondary lymphedema. Primary lymphedema is an uncommon condition and is not related to any extrinsic process. Primary lymphedema is divided into three groups, depending on age at diagnosis. With an onset before completion of the first year of life, it is called congenital lymphedema (or Milroy's disease if associated with a family history). Lymphedema praecox refers to the onset of primary lymphedema before the age of 35. It is the most common form of primary lymphedema and affects women four times more commonly than men. Onset is usually during puberty, and 70% of cases are unilateral, with the left side more commonly affected than the right. Lymphedema tarda (or Meige's disease) refers to swelling of the legs that occurs after the age of 35. It is the least common form of primary lymphedema. Secondary lymphedema can be the result of multiple disease processes, including but not limited to infection, trauma, filariasis, lymph node dissection, and exposure to radiation. The mainstay of lymphedema treatment is conservative and nonoperative. The goals of therapy are the prevention of infection and reduction of subcutaneous fluid volume with the use of decongestive massage therapy, pneumatic compression devices, and fitted elastic stockings. Diuretics are not used routinely but may be useful in women with premenstrual fluid retention. Recurrent lymphangitis is common following injury, and streptococci are the usual offending organisms. Penicillin is an appropriate therapy. Rarely, a protein-losing enteropathy attributed to lymphatic obstruction of the small bowel develops in patients with lymphedema. Various surgical procedures have been described for the treatment of lymphedema, including removal of skin, subcutaneous tissue, and fascia, followed by split-thickness skin graft reconstruction (the Charles operation); excision of strips of skin and subcutaneous tissue, followed by primary closure; and the creation of buried dermal flaps. All these procedures are associated with significant failure rates.

Ref.: 6, 7

15. A 64-year-old female presents to you with a palpable lymph node in her right axilla. Her family history is positive for a maternal aunt with breast cancer diagnosed at age 78 and a paternal grandmother who died from breast cancer at 42. What is the most likely etiology of this mass?

A. Breast cancer
B. Melanoma
C. Lymphoma
D. Reactive lymphadenopathy
E. Lung cancer

ANSWER: D

COMMENTS: Unilateral lymphadenopathy is a physical finding that should prompt a thorough evaluation, because a minority of patients (~25%) will have an underlying malignancy. The most common diagnosis in the setting of this presentation is reactive lymphadenopathy. Of those that do have an underlying malignancy, lymphoma is the most common followed by a carcinoma. Women with this presentation should have a formal breast examination and examination of the contralateral axilla. Women over the age of 35 should also undergo a mammography. The best imaging modality for the axilla is ultrasound, which can reliably predict lymph nodes suspicious for malignancy. A biopsy is warranted in patients with lymph nodes concerning for malignancy. For patients with a non-concerning history and physical examination and ultrasound showing benign-appearing lymph nodes, observation is appropriate.

Ref.: 8, 9

16. What is the next step in the management of the patient in Question 15?

A. Excisional biopsy
B. Breast examination and mammogram
C. Fine-needle aspiration (FNA)
D. Ultrasound
E. Observation

ANSWER: B

COMMENTS: Unilateral lymphadenopathy is a physical finding that should prompt a thorough evaluation, because a minority of patients will have an underlying malignancy. The most common diagnosis in the setting of this presentation is reactive lymphadenopathy. Of those that do have an underlying malignancy, lymphoma is the most common followed by a carcinoma; only about 1% of women with breast cancer will present this way. Women with this presentation should have a formal breast examination and examination of the contralateral axilla. Women over the age of 35 should also undergo a mammography. The best imaging modality for the axilla is ultrasound, which can reliably predict lymph nodes suspicious for malignancy. A biopsy is warranted in patients with lymph nodes concerning for malignancy. The patient in this question is a 64-year-old female with a positive family history of breast cancer; while the most likely diagnosis is reactive lymphadenopathy, an occult breast cancer must be excluded. This patient should undergo a thorough breast examination and mammogram.

Ref.: 8, 9

17. Regarding lymphedema after breast cancer surgery, which of the following is true?

A. It can occur after sentinel lymph node biopsy.
B. Exercise worsens lymphedema.
C. Weight loss does not have an effect on lymphedema.
D. Any therapy to reduce lymphedema should be delayed until the patient has completely healed from surgery.
E. Laser therapy has not been shown to decrease rates of lymphedema.

ANSWER: A

COMMENTS: Lymphedema is the accumulation of protein-rich fluid in tissue with inadequate lymphatic drainage. Lymphedema occurs at rates reported from 20% to 30% after mastectomy and up to as high as 7% after sentinel lymph node biopsy. Patients at risk of lymphedema should maintain a normal body weight, as obesity is a known risk factor for lymphedema. Additionally, exercises specifically aimed at improving lymphedema have been developed and have been shown to be beneficial in the treatment and prevention of lymphedema. Many institutions have initiated specific exercise regimens as soon as 48 h after surgery.

Ref.: 6, 7

18. A 56-year-old male presents to the emergency department complaining of nonspecific abdominal pain. A CT scan is ordered that shows a hypoattenuating well-defined intrasplenic lesion, with a thin wall and no peripheral enhancement. How would you manage this patient?

A. Splenectomy

B. Magnetic resonance imaging (MRI) of the abdomen

C. Angioembolization

D. Observation

E. Aspirate contents and then replace with hypertonic saline

ANSWER: D

COMMENTS: Splenic cysts are common lesions seen across all age groups and are often multifocal. The diagnosis is usually made incidentally on ultrasound or CT scan. Splenic cysts usually have no clinical significance unless they reach a large size and cause expansion of the splenic capsule. Elective splenectomy has been performed for large symptomatic cysts. Additional benign lesions of the spleen include hemangiomas, lymphangiomas, pseudotumors, hamartomas, and echinococcal cysts. All of these lesions, except echinococcal cysts, can be managed expectantly until symptomatic from mass effect. The echinococcal cyst is the only parasitic cyst involving the spleen. The incidence of echinococcal cyst in the spleen compared with the liver is a ratio of approximately 30:1. However, the spleen is the third most common site of echinococcal cysts behind the liver and the lung. The treatment for echinococcal cysts can include splenectomy. However, if there is a high risk of rupture, contents can be aspirated and replaced with hypertonic saline. Angioembolization is not used for the treatment of splenic lesions; its use is reserved for cases of splenic bleeding.

Ref.: 1, 2

19. You are consulted on a 29-year-old male admitted to the medical intensive care unit (MICU) with a past medical history of IV drug abuse but otherwise healthy. He is febrile with a temperature of 102.3°F, heart rate of 117 beats/min, and blood pressure of 94/62 mmHg. A CT scan was obtained that shows a lesion with a peripherally enhancing rim. After a 2-L resuscitation, his heart rate decreases to 102 beats/min, and his blood pressure improves to 108/70 mmHg. How would you manage this patient?

A. IV antibiotics and observation

B. IV antibiotics alone

C. IV antibiotics and percutaneous drainage

D. IV antibiotics and splenectomy

E. Observation alone

ANSWER: D

COMMENTS: Splenic abscess is associated with significant mortality, which in most series ranges between 40% and 100%. Typically, pathogenesis is caused by seeding of the spleen by bacteria from endocarditis or IV drug abuse. There have been some instances where the abscess is spread by a direct contamination of an intraperitoneal source. In 80% of cases additional sources of infection are identified, but in 20% of cases only the spleen is identified as an infectious source. Enteric organisms account for two-thirds of splenic abscesses, and *Staphylococcus* and *Streptococcus* cause the remainder of the cases. Presenting symptoms are generally fever and leukocytosis, with possible left upper quadrant tenderness. Plain abdominal films may show gas in the left upper quadrant. Otherwise ultrasound or CT scan can be diagnostic. Splenectomy is the treatment of choice if the patient is stable enough to undergo laparotomy. If patients are too unstable to undergo laparotomy or have multiple sources of infection, then percutaneous drainage is an option. The patient in this question stabilized with fluids and had the spleen as his sole source of infection; therefore laparotomy with splenectomy would be an appropriate approach to management.

Ref.: 1

20. After failing medical therapy, a 46-year-old woman with ITP is referred to you for splenectomy. She is very interested in a laparoscopic procedure. Review of her CT scan shows a normal-sized spleen and normal splenic vascular anatomy. Which of the following is true about laparoscopic splenectomy?

A. Operative mortality rates are the same regardless of the underlying disease type.

B. Laparoscopic splenectomy has similar success rates as open splenectomy, except when performed for ITP.

C. The rate of conversion from laparoscopic to open splenectomy is 0%–20%.

D. Laparoscopic splenectomy can be considered for spleen sizes up to 35 cm.

E. Laparoscopic splenectomy results in a higher incidence of splenosis than does the open approach.

ANSWER: C

COMMENTS: Laparoscopic splenectomy is increasingly being selected as a technique when elective splenectomy is indicated. The operative morbidity and mortality rates after splenectomy are higher for patients with the malignant hematologic disease than for those with benign disease. The risk of postoperative portal venous thrombosis is greatest for patients with myeloproliferative disorders. For idiopathic thrombocytopenic purpura, laparoscopic splenectomy has success rates similar to those of open splenectomy. Regardless of the surgical approach, when splenectomy is performed for hematologic disease, a careful search for accessory spleens must be performed. Their appearance may mimic that of a lymph node, and they may more easily be palpated than visualized, thus giving rise to concern that the laparoscopic approach may overlook some accessory spleens. The conversion rate in an open procedure is reported to range from 0% to 20%. Conversion is usually secondary to bleeding, but extensive adhesions, obesity, and splenomegaly may also be factors. Spleens up to 20 to 25 cm in size are amenable to laparoscopic splenectomy. A splenic size of 35 cm is generally too large for a laparoscopic approach. The laparoscopic approach does not result in a higher incidence of splenosis (autotransplantation and subsequent growth of splenic fragments from an injured spleen that may remain functional and occasionally cause pain or symptoms related to a mass effect).

Ref.: 1, 2

21. A 14-year-old girl is involved in a high-speed car accident and has a mildly distended abdomen, a seatbelt sign, and a positive focused abdominal sonography for trauma (FAST) examination. She is tachycardic and found to have a splenic injury on CT. She fails the nonoperative management over the next day because of transfusion requirements. At the time of exploration, which of the following is most correct?

A. Eighty percent of the spleen can be sacrificed at splenorrhaphy before total splenectomy should be performed.

B. Although available techniques for splenorrhaphy include argon beam coagulation, fibrin glue, and mattress suturing with pledgets, mesh wrap should not be done because of the increased risk for infection.

C. Splenorrhaphy is especially advantageous in the setting of pancreatic or hollow viscus injury because it decreases the occurrence of subphrenic abscess.

D. Splenorrhaphy may be attempted safely in patients with severe head injuries.

E. Splenorrhaphy is best used only for grades I and II injuries.

ANSWER: C

COMMENTS: Splenorrhaphy is a useful tool to allow preservation of the spleen. Only one-third of the spleen is required for retention of its immunologic benefit; injuries requiring the sacrifice of more than two-thirds of the spleen are best treated by splenectomy. Available tools for splenorrhaphy include all those listed in choice B. The use of a mesh wrap has not contributed to an increased incidence of infection following splenorrhaphy, even in the setting of associated hollow viscus injury. It is true that splenorrhaphy decreases the incidence of abscess formation following pancreatic or hollow viscus injury. In unstable patients or those with severe head injuries, expeditious splenectomy should be performed if needed instead of a partial splenectomy or splenorrhaphy because the latter tends to be more time-consuming. There is no grade restriction for performing splenorrhaphy after injury, and it may be done as long as one-third of the spleen remains viable for continued immunologic function.

Ref.: 2

22. A 23-year-old sustains blunt force trauma in a high-speed motor vehicle accident. Abdominal CT demonstrates a subcapsular hematoma involving 60% of the surface area of the spleen without obvious injury to the hilum. The patient has a heart rate of 110 beats/min and blood pressure of 105/60 mm Hg. Correct statements regarding the management of this patient include which of the following?

A. A Kehr's sign is a contraindication to nonoperative management given the high associated severity of injury.

B. Diagnostic peritoneal lavage is not sensitive for the detection of splenic injury.

C. For patients with moderate to severe splenic injuries managed nonoperatively, follow-up abdominal CT is indicated in 2 to 3 days.

D. Angiography is required in all patients with splenic injury to exclude unsuspected areas of active hemorrhage not seen on CT.

E. Nonoperative management may be pursued, provided that the patient is hemodynamically stable; the injury can be clearly classified by imaging, and transfusion requirements remain less than six units of packed red blood cells.

ANSWER: C

COMMENTS: This patient has a grade III splenic injury. Kehr's sign (pain referred to the left shoulder) does correlate highly with splenic injury but does not mandate operative management. Diagnostic peritoneal lavage is perhaps too sensitive in detecting significant splenic injury and has largely been replaced by ultrasound. Follow-up scans are recommended to exclude any vascular blush not seen on initial imaging because of sampling error with larger cuts or subsequent lysis of clot. Angiography, with possible angioembolization, should be pursued if a vascular blush appears on CT in patients with grade III and higher injuries or in patients with any grade of injury if frank hemorrhage from the splenic artery is seen. It is not required for all patients. Criteria for nonoperative management include hemodynamic stability, documented CT classification of injury, absence of additional injuries necessitating surgery, and transfusion of two or fewer units of red blood cells (not six units). The success of nonoperative management is reported to be 70%–90% for children and 40%–50% for adults treated in trauma centers. The differing success rates may be related to both anatomic considerations and mechanisms of injury.

Ref.: 1

REFERENCES

1. Fracker M. The spleen. In: Mulholland MW, Greenfield LJ, eds. *Greenfield's Surgery: Scientific Principles & Practice*. 5th ed. Philadelphia, PA: Wolters Kluwer/Lippincott Williams & Wilkins; 2011.
2. Demetriades D, Lam L. Splenectomy and splenorrhaphy. In: Fisher JE, Bland KE, eds. *Mastery of Surgery*. 6th ed. Philadelphia: Lippincott Williams & Wilkins; 2012.
3. Solomon CG, Rubin LG, Schaffner W. Care of the asplenic patient. *N Engl J Med*. 2014;371:349–356.
4. American Society of Hematology. Guidelines for the investigation and management of idiopathic thrombocytopenic purpura in adults, children and in pregnancy. *Br J Haematol*. 2003;120(4):574–596. Available at http://doi.org/4131. [pii].
5. Wong S. Sarcomas of soft tissue and bone. In: Mulholland MW, Greenfield LJ, eds. *Greenfield's Surgery: Scientific Principles & Practice*. 5th ed. Philadelphia, PA: Wolters Kluwer/Lippincott Williams & Wilkins; 2011.
6. Pippins B, Baxter T. The lymphatics. In: Iraklis I, ed. *Sabiston Textbook of Surgery: The Biological Basis of Modern Surgical Practice*. 19th ed. Philadelphia: Elsevier; 2012.
7. Cormier JN, Rourke L, Crosby M, Chang D, Armer J. The surgical treatment of lymphedema: a systematic review of the contemporary literature (2004-2010). *Ann Surg Oncol*. 2012;19(2):642–651. Available at http://doi.org/10.1245/s10434-011-2017-4.
8. King T, Morrow M. Breast disease. In: Mulholland MW, Greenfield LJ, eds. *Greenfield's Surgery: Scientific Principles & Practice*. 5th ed. Philadelphia, PA: Wolters Kluwer/Lippincott Williams & Wilkins; 2011.
9. Schwab FD, Burger H, Isenschmid M, Kuhn A, Mueller MD, Gunthert AR. Suspicious axillary lymph nodes in patients with unremarkable imaging of the breast. *Eur J Obstet Gynecol Reproduct Biol*. 2010;150(1):88–91. Available at http://doi.org/10.1016/j.ejogrb.2010.02.011.

SECTION VII

VASCULAR AND THORACIC

CHAPTER 28

VASCULAR SURGERY

A. Vascular Surgery Principles

John Kubasiak, M.D., and Richard Keen, M.D.

1. A patient with severe peripheral vascular disease underwent aortobiliac bypass grafting 9 months ago and now presents with hematochezia and a syncopal episode. Along with the administration of intravenous antibiotics, reasonable treatment or diagnostic modalities include which of the following?
   A. Magnetic resonance imaging (MRI)
   B. Tagged red blood cell scanning
   C. Bilateral axillofemoral bypass
   D. Unilateral axillofemoral and femorofemoral bypass followed by removal of the graft
   E. Colonoscopy

ANSWER: D

COMMENTS: The general approach to the treatment of **aortoenteric fistulas (AEFs)** and infections involves prompt diagnosis, antibiotics, removal of the entire prosthesis, and reestablishment of vascular continuity through noncontaminated fields. MRI has the highest sensitivity for graft infections but is ill suited to unstable patients. Computed tomography (CT) scans can be obtained rapidly and are abnormal 91% of the time in patients with an AEF. Abnormal CT findings include perigraft fluid, gas, and tissue inflammation. They actually demonstrate the AEF in only 33% of cases. Although arteriography may help in planning the site of distal anastomosis, it rarely demonstrates the fistula and can take considerably longer. Colonic ischemia is more common in the immediate postoperative period.

In hemodynamically unstable patients, esophagogastroduodenoscopy of the third and fourth portion of the duodenum should be performed first, with aggressive resuscitation and rapid transfer to the operating room (OR). Extraanatomic axillofemoral and femorofemoral grafts permit revascularization through a clean field distal to the original site. In situations requiring revascularization through a contaminated area, autologous tissue such as a femoral vein graft can be used. Bilateral axillofemoral grafts should be used as a secondary option because of the diminished outflow compared with unilateral axillofemoral and femorofemoral grafts. Delayed excision of the graft is recommended only in patients who are hemodynamically stable and do not demonstrate a false aneurysm at the site of the fistula.

Ref.: 1, 2

2. Fasciotomy should be performed in patients with which of the following signs or symptoms?
   A. Tense fullness of the compartment in an otherwise asymptomatic patient
   B. Extremity ischemia for greater than 2 h
   C. Swollen leg following revascularization, with progressively worsening neurologic signs
   D. Traumatic injuries of the popliteal artery
   E. Compartmental pressure higher than 15 mmHg and unreliable findings on physical examination

ANSWER: C

COMMENTS: Compartment syndromes occur whenever tissue pressure within a confined anatomic space becomes sufficiently elevated to impair venous return. It can be due to bleeding within a compartment or to reperfusion edema. There is no absolute pressure above which the syndrome invariably occurs, but nutrient blood flow in the muscle ceases between 30 and 40 mmHg. In addition, a difference between the diastolic blood pressure and intercompartmental pressure greater than 30 mmHg is indicative of impaired blood flow. At minimum, such elevated pressures mandate close follow-up neurovascular examinations in reliable patients. Successful treatment is based on early, accurate diagnosis. Prolonged ischemia is associated with compartment syndrome due to the reperfusion injury and release of free radicals. Diminished or absent pulses are a late finding; by the time this is appreciated, irreversible neurologic damage may have occurred. Compartmental syndromes are best diagnosed by having a high index of suspicion. A tense compartment alone in the absence of elevated pressures or physical findings is not an absolute indication for fasciotomy. Traumatic injury to the popliteal artery is not an absolute indication for fasciotomy unless the repair/revascularization occurred more than 4 to 6 h from the time of injury.

Ref.: 1–3

3. Which of the following is not an independent risk factor for the development of coronary and peripheral atherosclerosis?
   A. Cigarette smoking
   B. Hypercholesterolemia
   C. Diabetes mellitus
   D. Hypertension
   E. Hypercoagulable conditions

ANSWER: E

COMMENTS: Hypercoagulable conditions are associated with an increased risk of thrombosis, but they are not an independent **risk factor for atherosclerosis**. Smoking is a risk factor owing to the release of oxidative free radicals, which damage the vascular endothelium. Hypercholesterolemia with total serum levels greater than 200 mg/dL and elevated low-density lipoprotein fractions are also associated with an increased risk. Diabetes mellitus and hypertension are independent risk factors in proportion to their severity.

Ref.: 1–3

4. Which of the following statements about leg swelling due to venous insufficiency or lymphedema is true?

A. Edema forms when the hydrostatic pressure in the interstitium is higher than that in the lymphatics or venules.

B. Venous insufficiency causes pigmentation and hypertrophic changes in the skin over the ankle and subsequent lymphedema with fibrosis.

C. Lymphedema can be diagnosed by ultrasound imaging.

D. Operative intervention is commonly used for lymphedema.

E. Late sequelae of lymphedema include thinned skin and pitting edema.

ANSWER: B

COMMENTS: Edema formation is governed by the balance between hydrostatic and oncotic pressures in the interstitium versus the lymphatics and venules. Hyperpigmentation and cicatrix formation in the gaiter region (legs from ankle to knees) is pathognomonic of venous insufficiency and is caused by the breakdown of extravascular red blood cells and subcutaneous scar tissue (liposclerosis). In severe cases of untreated chronic venous insufficiency, scar tissue formation can cause local destruction of leg lymphatics and secondary formation of lymphedema. Any severe hypoproteinemia can also cause lymphedema. Early lymphedema may present with pitting, but after subsequent protein deposition in the extremity and damage to the lymphatics, the adipose tissue fibroses and the skin thickens. **Venous insufficiency** can be recognized clinically by filling of varices and also on color Doppler imaging. Due to the size of the lymphatics, they are not visible on ultrasound imaging, and only nonspecific subcutaneous edema may be visible. Operations for lymphedema are generally not performed. Operations for venous insufficiency include perforator vein ligation, varicose vein ligation and stripping, deep vein valve plasty, and laser and radiofrequency ablations of greater and lesser saphenous veins.

Ref.: 1–3

5. A 45-year-old woman was hit by a car. On arrival to the trauma bay, she is protecting her airway with rapid breaths, and she has sinus tachycardia. Focused assessment with sonography for trauma (FAST) examination is positive for free intraabdominal fluid. She is taken to the OR for exploration. Which of the following correctly describes the zone and contents of the retroperitoneum?

A. Zone 3: Kidneys

B. Zone 1: Rectum and anus

C. Zone 1: Inferior vena cava (IVC)/Aorta

D. Zone 2: Iliac artery

E. Zone 3: Duodenum

ANSWER: C

COMMENTS: Zone 1 of the retroperitoneum contains the IVC, aorta to the bifurcation of the iliac, and the pancreas and duodenum. All hematomas in zone 1 require exploration. Zone 2 has two sections, each comprising the area around a kidney. Penetrating wounds to this zone are typically explored, while blunt injuries are typically observed unless there is an expanding hematoma or injury to the hilum. Zone 3 includes the contents of the pelvis including the iliac and femoral arteries. Blunt injuries to this region are likely venous and should prompt interventional radiology evaluation and treatment. Penetrating injuries to zone 3 should be explored.

Ref.: 4

6. A 70-year-old male who had undergone endovascular abdominal aneurysm repair 1 year ago complains of back and abdominal pain and then collapses. His blood pressure is 90/40 mmHg. The patient denies a history of peptic ulcer or alcohol abuse. What is the most likely diagnosis?

A. AEF

B. Bleeding duodenal ulcer

C. Ruptured abdominal aortic aneurysm (AAA)

D. Pancreatitis

E. Diverticulitis

ANSWER: C

COMMENTS: The diagnosis of **ruptured AAA** must be considered in a patient with abdominal pain, back pain, and hypotension. Up to 1% of patients with stent graft repair of AAAs have a late rupture. After **endovascular repair**, up to 50% of patients develop an **endoleak** (persistent flow within an aneurysm sac despite an excluded aneurysm). Type 1 endoleak occurs when a persistent channel of blood flow develops owing to inadequate or ineffective seal at the graft ends. Type 2 endoleak occurs when there is persistent collateral blood flow into the aneurysm sac, usually retrograde from lumbar arteries or the inferior mesenteric artery. Type 3 is a graft defect endoleak, such as when the sections pull apart. Type 4 is a graft-fabric porosity endoleak.

Ref.: 4

7. Which of the following statements concerning fibromuscular dysplasia of the carotid arteries is true?

A. The incidence in males and females is approximately equal.

B. Atherosclerosis is common when fibromuscular dysplasia is present.

C. The patient should undergo operative dilatation before transient ischemic attacks (TIAs) or stroke occurs.

D. The process can also occur in the subclavian, internal iliac, and mesenteric vessels.

E. Approximately 25% of patients have associated intracranial aneurysms.

ANSWER: E

COMMENTS: Fibromuscular dysplasia occurs predominantly in females and can also involve the renal, external iliac carotid, and vertebral arteries. The subclavian and mesenteric vessels are not involved. Symptomatic patients may undergo graded intraluminal dilatation through an arteriotomy in the common carotid artery or percutaneous treatment with balloon angioplasty. Asymptomatic patients may be followed.

Approximately 13%–35% of patients have atherosclerosis of the carotid bifurcation. The incidence of intracranial aneurysms is 23%.

Ref.: 4

8. An 18-year-old male sustains a gunshot wound (GSW) to the right chest just below the clavicle. A chest tube is placed, and 2000 mL of blood is evacuated. On the way to the OR, you rehearse the exposure of the axillary artery with the intern. What muscle needs to be divided to expose the entire length of the axillary artery?

A. Pectoralis major

B. Pectoralis minor

C. Deltoid

D. Sternocleidomastoid

E. None of the above

ANSWER: B

COMMENTS: The subclavian artery becomes the axillary artery as it passes beyond the lateral margin of the first rib. The artery is divided into three sections defined by the pectoralis minor muscle. The medial aspect is the first section, the portion deep to the pectoralis minor is the second section, and the aspect lateral to the pectoralis minor is the third portion. Exposure of the axillary artery can be achieved by a subclavicular incision; the pectoralis major fibers are spread, and the pectoralis minor is then encountered and divided. The axillary vein typically runs superior to the artery. The brachial plexus is intimately involved at this level, so care must be taken not to injure the nerve fibers.

Ref.: 4, 5

9. A 35-year-old male is brought to the trauma bay by police officers after a domestic disturbance call. The patient had punched through a fish tank and, despite a tourniquet, is still slowly bleeding from the wound. You clean the wound and take him to the OR for exploration. The radial artery is completely transected, but a Doppler signal can be heard in the palmar arch and at the base of the thumb when the tourniquet is released. Which is the appropriate treatment for this injury?

A. Ligation of the radial artery

B. Reverse saphenous vein interposition

C. Expanded polytetrafluoroethylene (ePTFE) graft

D. Endovascular stenting

E. None of the above

ANSWER: A

COMMENTS: Laceration to the distal forearm can injure the radial or ulnar arteries. The ulnar artery is deeper and less commonly injured. The radial and ulnar arteries connect via the palmar arch. The dominant perfusion to the hand is delivered via the ulnar artery. In a patient with an intact palmar arch, one of the arteries may be safely ligated. In a dirty wound with no evidence of acute hand ischemia, simple ligation is the appropriate treatment. Patency rates following repair of the ulnar or radial artery are around 50%–60%, likely due to the small caliber of the vessel and the collaterals at that level. Following ligation, the majority of patient symptoms are related to nerve or tendon injury. In patients without an intact arch who present with hand ischemia, primary repair or repair with saphenous vein interposition is required.

Ref.: 6, 7

10. Which of the following is characteristic of ischemic extremity rest pain?

A. Initially occurs mostly in the morning

B. Can be relieved by placing the involved extremity in the supine position

C. Is usually located at the toes

D. Can be relieved by intravenous heparin

E. Can be relieved with cilostazol (Pletal)

ANSWER: D

COMMENTS: Extremity angina occurs most commonly at night because when patients with severe lower-extremity arterial insufficiency lie supine, they lose the added benefit of gravity for perfusing the lower extremity. Patients with nocturnal **ischemic rest pain** quickly discover that walking, standing, or sleeping in a chair relieves this pain, which is centered over the metatarsal heads, not the toes. Pain in the toes suggests gout or infection. Intravenous heparin causes vasodilation by promoting the release of nitric oxide, thereby improving extremity arterial circulation. Intravenous heparin can reduce rest pain until the arterial circulation can be improved with a bypass operation or angioplasty. Cilostazol improves claudication-impaired distance walking but has not been shown to be effective for treating ischemic rest pain.

Ref.: 1–3, 8

11. Which of the following statements regarding claudication is true?

A. The term claudication originated from the Latin root word meaning "to shuffle."

B. Without intervention, the risk of limb loss approaches 15% at 5 years.

C. It is not alleviated significantly with cilostazol.

D. It can be managed successfully without arteriography, balloon angioplasty, or operation in most cases.

E. Optimal treatment includes limits on exercise and walking.

ANSWER: D

COMMENTS: Claudication is derived from the Latin verb meaning "to limp." The risk of limb loss for all claudicant patients is 5% over 5 years. Over the long term, the risk of limb loss drops substantially, from 12% to 2%, if a patient successfully stops smoking. Claudication usually can be treated safely with medication. Several medications, including cilostazol and pentoxifylline, have been shown to improve walking distance. "Stop smoking and keep walking" summarizes the treatment strategy for most patients. A regular, organized walking program generally doubles the walking distance.

Ref.: 1–3, 8, 9

12. A 19-year-old male is stabbed anterior to the sternocleidomastoid muscle. He has an expanding hematoma and develops hoarseness and stridor. After intubation, he is brought to the OR and the wound explored via an incision anterior to the sternocleidomastoid muscle. An injury 2 cm distal to the bifurcation of the common carotid artery is seen. While trying to gain control of the distal internal carotid artery, what structure is at risk for injury?

A. Vagus nerve

B. Recurrent laryngeal nerve

C. Hypoglossal nerve

D. Inferior root of ansa cervicalis

E. None of the above

ANSWER: C

COMMENTS: The neck is divided into three zones: zone 1 is from the inferior cricoid cartilage to the thoracic outlet; zone 2 extends from the superior to the cricoid cartilage to the angle of the mandible; AND zone 3 extends from the angle of the mandible to the skull base. Vascular injuries in zone 1 will typically require thoracic exposure to gain proximal control. Injuries in zone 3 are protected by the bone of the mandible and the skull base; therefore interventional radiology is the mainstay of treatment. In experienced hands, some zone 3 injuries can be accessed with adjunct maneuvers including subluxation of the mandible or partial craniotomy for access to the skull base. Zone 2 of the neck is accessed via an incision along the anterior border of the sternocleidomastoid muscle. The vascular sheath is then opened; division of the facial vein and sometimes the omohyoid muscle allows for access to the carotid artery. Injury to the hypoglossal nerve will lead to ipsilateral deviation of the tongue toward the side of the injury on protrusion.

Ref.: 10

13. A 23-year-old male with a gunshot wound just superior to the clavicle presents to the emergency room (ER) with an expanding hematoma. Exposure of the first section of the vertebral artery involves:

A. Interventional radiology

B. Unroofing the transverse foramen

C. Neurosurgical consultation

D. Division of the distal sternocleidomastoid muscle

E. Division of the skull base

ANSWER: D

COMMENTS: The vertebral artery is divided into four segments: the first segment is preforaminal (V1) from the origin of the artery to the transverse process of the sixth cervical vertebra. V2 (foraminal) is the segment that runs from C6 to C2 within the transverse process. V3 is the segment before the skull base as it exits the transverse process. Distal to the foramen magnum, the vessel is intracranial/intradural (V4). Injuries to V1 can be approached surgically; those in the further segments require special expertise and consultation with neurosurgery and neurointerventional radiology. The supraclavicular approach can provide excellent exposure to V1. This incision is made parallel to the clavicle, and the distal sternocleidomastoid muscle is divided. The carotid sheath and contents are retracted medially, and the anterior scalene muscle is retracted laterally to expose the vertebral artery. This exposure also gives access to the origin of the carotid artery.

Ref.: 11

14. A 21-year-old male sustains a gunshot wound to the right abdomen just lateral to and below the umbilicus. His abdomen is distended, and a FAST examination is positive. In the OR you identify a right iliac vein injury. What maneuver might be required to access the right iliac vein?

A. Division of the right iliac artery

B. Transection of the right ureter

C. Hip disarticulation

D. Tamponade with Foley catheter

E. None of the above

ANSWER: A

COMMENTS: The distal aorta and the iliac vessels are contained within zone 3 of the abdomen. Iliac vein injuries can result in large-volume blood loss. The iliac arteries overlie the iliac veins; therefore injury to the vein in this location may require division of the common iliac artery with primary repair after the vein injury is addressed. The iliac vein may be ligated if necessary. If the vein is ligated distal to the bifurcation, there is an increased risk for developing deep vein thrombosis; therefore postoperative anticoagulation versus IVC filter should be considered. Concomitant injury to the ureters is common and should be addressed after vascular control has been obtained.

Ref.: 12

15. In a low-resistance arterial vascular system, at which percent diameter reduction does a stenosis become flow limiting?

A. 10%

B. 20%

C. 40%

D. 50%

E. 80%

ANSWER: D

COMMENTS: In low-resistance arterial systems, such as the internal carotid artery, the total blood flow across a stenosis does not decrease until the diameter is reduced by approximately 50%. This corresponds to a 75% reduction in the cross-sectional area. The total blood flow is maintained by increasing the velocity. Shear stress (drag along the wall) and viscosity limit further increase in velocity once the stenosis exceeds 50%. Short stenosis of less than 50% does not usually require intervention since the total blood flow is not altered. A longer stenosis increases the shear stress, so a lesser degree of stenosis over a longer length can be flow limiting.

Ref.: 8, 13

16. Which of the following characterize duplex ultrasound imaging?

A. It is a combination of Doppler and D-mode ultrasound imaging.

B. Lower frequencies (e.g., 3 MHz) are better suited for deep abdominal imaging, and higher frequencies (e.g., 7 MHz) are better for more superficial structures such as in situ vein grafts.

C. High-frequency ultrasound waves have higher energy than do low-frequency ultrasound waves.

D. Diagnosis of deep venous thrombosis (DVT) is made by the absence of color flow imaging alone.

E. Calcification within a diseased artery is usually severe enough to prevent an adequate vascular ultrasound examination.

ANSWER: B

COMMENTS: Duplex ultrasound imaging consists of the B-mode image (picture) and Doppler shift, which measures the velocity of the flowing blood. High-frequency transducers (7 to 10 MHz) are used for superficial structures, with applications such as saphenous vein mapping and in situ vein bypasses or pedal bypasses. These higher-frequency transducers have a greater resolution but lower energy and cannot penetrate as deeply as can lower-frequency, higher-energy transducers (3 or 5 MHz). Since venous flow velocity is slower than arterial flow, artifacts such as those due to transducer movement are more common. When evaluating for a DVT, it is helpful to use B-mode imaging to show a dilated noncompressible vein. B-mode imaging (rather than color Doppler) allows better assessment of vein compressibility and is not confused by an artifact introduced by transducer movement. The absence of flow in that segment of vein with augmentation and lack of respiratory variation confirm the diagnosis. Arterial wall calcium occasionally interferes with vascular ultrasound scans by blocking ultrasound wave transmission, but it is unusual that an adequate vascular examination of the carotid or other structure cannot be performed because of severe calcifications.

Ref.: 8, 9, 13

17. The advantages of lower-extremity arterial Doppler examinations performed with waveform analysis compared with the ankle-brachial index (ABI) alone include which of the following?

A. Calcification of the artery by diseases such as diabetes mellitus and chronic renal failure make the arterial wall incompressible, causing the ABI to be artificially decreased and unreliable.

B. Inflow disease can be recognized by the delay in the downstroke of the waveform.

C. The loss of reversal of flow when the arterial waveform transforms from triphasic to biphasic is observed with exercise or with moderate atherosclerosis.

D. The ABI can be used to diagnose an arteriovenous fistula.

E. The ABI can be used to diagnose a DVT.

ANSWER: C

COMMENTS: The ABI is a measurement for quantifying extremity ischemia, based on the assumption that the flow in the limb is proportional to the blood pressure in the limb. The ABI is obtained with a blood pressure cuff and a handheld Doppler instrument. The cuff is applied at the point at which the pressure measurement is desired. The Doppler device is placed over any vessel distal to the cuff, but routinely it is the radial artery in the upper extremity or the posterior tibial or dorsal pedal artery in the lower extremity. The cuff is inflated to a pressure greater than the systolic pressure. The pressure at which the arterial Doppler signal returns as the cuff is deflated is the pressure used to calculate the ABI. Diabetes and renal failure cause calcification of the axial extremity arteries, making the arteries noncompressible. The ABI is artificially elevated with these conditions.

When the ABI is falsely elevated (ABI > 1.2), one must depend on the Doppler waveform to assess the degree of extremity ischemia. Waveforms become monophasic in diseased arteries regardless of whether the vessels are compressible. The degree of arterial inflow disease (above the inguinal ligament) can be assessed by examining the femoral artery waveform. Prolongation of the arterial upstroke to more than 180 ms is suggestive of the significant iliac disease. Digital artery pressures are useful for quantifying ischemia in patients with diabetes and renal failure, since these vessels are usually compressible even under such conditions. Pressures less than 30 mmHg are consistent with severe ischemia in nondiabetic patients, and those less than 50 mmHg are consistent with severe ischemia in diabetic patients.

Reversal of blood flow direction is caused by vascular resistance. Exercise causes vasodilation in the muscular beds and decreases resistance. The first change one observes in the waveform morphology due to mild atherosclerotic disease is the loss of flow reversal when the waveform changes from triphasic to biphasic. Duplex imaging is required to diagnose arteriovenous fistulas and DVTs. The ABI alone is inadequate for diagnosing these conditions.

Ref.: 8, 9, 13

18. What is the most common cause of a congenital hypercoagulable disorder?

A. Protein S deficiency

B. Protein C deficiency

C. Antithrombin III deficiency

D. Activated protein C resistance (APC-R; factor V Leiden mutation)

E. Homocysteinemia

ANSWER: D

COMMENTS: Hemostasis is a finely tuned balance between coagulation and fibrinolysis. The existence of a congenital defect in the procoagulant or anticoagulant proteins can shift this balance and cause increased bleeding or increased thrombotic tendencies, respectively. **Hypercoagulable states** are the most common cause of early bypass graft failure in young adults who require vascular interventions for limb salvage. More than half of patients under the age of 50 who require a lower-extremity bypass and experience early graft thrombosis have a hypercoagulable state.

The existence of **protein C, protein S, and antithrombin III deficiencies** has been known for some time, but until recently a specific inherited hypercoagulable state could not be identified in as many as 80% of patients. It is now known that APC-R is the most common inherited hypercoagulable state, existing in more than 50% of patients with inherited thrombosis tendencies. The cause of APC-R is an amino acid substitution of glutamine for arginine in the encoding for factor V. Patients with APC-R have a poor anticoagulant response to activated protein C, a vitamin K–dependent anticoagulant protein. When protein C is activated, it normally degrades activated clotting factors Va and VIIa. The altered factor V, or Leiden mutation (named after the Dutch city where it was first found), is resistant to the degrading action of APC. The altered, activated factor V retains its procoagulant activity, and the hemostatic balance is shifted toward thrombosis.

Antithrombin III is the major plasma inhibitor of thrombin. Heparin performs its anticoagulant function by forming a trivalent molecule of heparin–antithrombin III–thrombin to inactivate thrombin. Antithrombin III deficiency is rare, with an incidence of only 1:5000. Thrombotic events are usually triggered by trauma, operation, or pregnancy.

Proteins C and S are both vitamin K–dependent anticoagulant proteins synthesized by the liver. The incidence of congenital protein C deficiency is 1:200. Protein C and S deficiencies are found in 20% of patients under the age of 50 with arterial thrombosis, but the combined incidence is much less than the incidence of APC-R.

The treatment for antithrombin III, protein C, and protein S deficiencies is lifelong warfarin anticoagulation. Heparin must be given before initiating warfarin anticoagulation in these patients to protect against warfarin-induced skin necrosis. All patients with thrombosis who are to receive warfarin therapy should receive heparin during the first 3 to 4 days of warfarin therapy because the half-life of the anticoagulation protein C is much less, since it is degraded much faster than the procoagulant vitamin K–dependent factors II, IX, and X.

Mild homocysteinemia exists in 5%–7% of the population. Elevated levels of homocysteine occur because of a defect in the pathway that metabolizes methionine. The treatment for homocysteinemia is the B vitamin folate 1 to 5 mg/day.

Ref.: 8, 9, 13

19. What is the most common cause of an acquired hypercoagulable state?

A. Smoking

B. Heparin-induced thrombocytopenia (HIT)

C. Antiphospholipid antibody (e.g., lupus anticoagulant)

D. Warfarin

E. Oral contraceptives

ANSWER: A

COMMENTS: Smoking is the most common cause of **acquired hypercoagulability**. It is the most important factor that determines the short- and long-term results of any vascular intervention. The mechanisms of action of smoking are multiple and include both vasoconstriction and a measurable elevation of plasma fibrinogen levels, which itself is a risk factor for thrombosis.

The next most common cause of acquired hypercoagulability is **HIT**. HIT affects 2%–3% of all patients who receive heparin. Antibodies to heparin form because it is obtained from bovine or porcine sources. The clinical manifestations are a falling platelet count, increasing resistance to anticoagulation with heparin, and new paradoxical thrombotic events while receiving heparin treatment. Although low-molecular-weight heparin has a lower incidence of HIT than the standard heparin, 25% of patients with HIT who receive low-molecular-weight heparin manifest heparin allergy. The treatment for HIT is cessation of all heparin. Warfarin-induced skin necrosis is unusual when heparin is given for the first 3 days of warfarin therapy.

Antiphospholipid syndrome (APS) is common, affecting 1%–5% of the population. Specific types are lupus anticoagulant and anticardiolipin antibodies. Since the incidence of APS increases with age, 50% of patients over the age of 80 have APS. This syndrome is recognized by prolongation of the baseline partial thromboplastin time (PTT). Brain thromboplastin is the reagent used for triggering the intrinsic clotting system when the PTT is measured. Patients with APS have serum antibodies that consume this reagent, resulting in a prolonged PTT. This is an unforgiving hypercoagulable state with an incidence of thrombotic complications approaching 50%.

Warfarin and oral contraceptives are less common causes of hypercoagulability.

Ref.: 8, 9, 13

REFERENCES

1. Ernst CB, Stanley JC. *Current Therapy in Vascular Surgery*. 4th ed. St. Louis: CV Mosby; 2001.
2. Sabiston DC, Townsend CM. Vascular section. In: Townsend CM, Beauchamp RD, Evers BM, et al., eds. *Sabiston Textbook of Surgery: The Biological Basis of Modern Surgical Practice*. Philadelphia: Saunders/Elsevier; 2008.
3. Schwartz SI, Brunicardi FC. Arterial disease. In: Brunicardi FC, Andersen DK, Billiar TR, et al., eds. *Schwartz's Principles of Surgery*. New York: McGraw-Hill; 2010.
4. Cronenwett JL, Johnston KW. *Rutherford's Vascular Surgery*. 7th ed. Philadelphia: Saunders; 2010.
5. Mattox KL, Moore EE, Feliciano DV. *Trauma*. 7th ed. New York: McGraw-Hill Medical; 2013.
6. Aftabuddin M, Islam N, Jafar MA, Haque E, Alimuzzaman M. Management of isolated radial or ulnar arteries at the forearm. *J Trauma*. 1995;38(1):149–151.
7. Franz RW, Skytta CK, Shah KJ, Hartman JF, Wright ML. A five-year review of management of upper-extremity arterial injuries at an urban level I trauma center. *Ann Vasc Surg*. 2012;26(5):655–664.
8. Moore WS. *Vascular and Endovascular Surgery: A Comprehensive Review*. 7th ed. Philadelphia, PA: Saunders Elsevier; 2006. xviii, 972.
9. Yao STJ, Pierce WH. *Practical Vascular Surgery*. Stamford, CT: Appleton & Lange; 1999.
10. Kim T, Chung S, Lanzino G. Carotid artery-hypoglossal nerve relationships in the neck: an anatomical work. *Neurol Res*. 2009;31(9):895–899.
11. Hatzitheofilou C, Demetriades D, Melissas J, Stewart M, Franklin J. Surgical approaches to vertebral artery injuries. *Br J Surg*. 1988;75(3):234–247.
12. Haan J, Rodriguez A, Chiu W, Boswell S, Scott J, Scalea T. Operative management and outcome of iliac vessel injury: a ten-year experience. *Am Surg*. 2003;69(7):581–586.
13. Porter JM, Taylor LM. *Basic Data Underlying Clinical Decision Making in Vascular Surgery*. St. Louis: Quality Medical Publishing; 1994.

B. Cerebrovascular Disease

Elizabeth Aitcheson, M.D.

1. A 70-year-old woman with 90% stenosis of her right internal carotid artery (ICA) undergoes carotid endarterectomy (CEA). Postoperatively, she complains of right-sided headache. The evening of postoperative day 1 she has a seizure. A computed tomography (CT) shows acute cerebral hemorrhage. What measures might have prevented this?

A. Aspirin therapy
B. Preoperative cerebral imaging
C. Better postoperative blood pressure control
D. Therapeutic anticoagulation
E. Intraoperative shunting

ANSWER: C

COMMENTS: This woman's symptoms are consistent with **hyperperfusion syndrome** after CEA. With a chronic carotid stenosis, cerebral vessels in turn remain dilated to maintain cerebral blood flow. Restoration of blood flow through the carotid by endarterectomy can therefore lead to increase in pressure of cerebral vessels resulting in cerebral edema. Most commonly, the syndrome presents with ipsilateral headache and can progress to seizures and even intracerebral hemorrhage. Strict blood pressure control is required to decrease the risk for hyperperfusion syndrome in the perioperative period.

Ref.: 1

2. For patients with carotid stenosis, preoperative medication regimen consists of:

A. Antiplatelet therapy
B. Warfarin
C. Antiplatelet therapy and statin
D. Lovenox
E. No medication therapy needed preoperatively

ANSWER: C

COMMENTS: Antiplatelet therapy should be initiated preoperatively in all patients if possible. The regimen should include aspirin 81 or 325 mg daily or clopidogrel. Perioperative clopidogrel has resulted in decreased observed embolic events, correlating with decreased stroke risk when started in the perioperative period. Dual antiplatelet therapy may also be associated with decreased stroke risk compared with single-agent therapy. Statins should also be initiated as statin therapy decreases 30-day risk for transient ischemic attack (TIA), stroke, and mortality. The effect of statins is thought to be related to pleiotropic arterial effects.

Ref.: 1, 2

3. A 65-year-old female with diabetes and hypertension presents after an episode of transient left arm weakness. Duplex ultrasound (US) demonstrated a 70% stenosis of her right ICA. What treatment is recommended?

A. CEA within 6 months of symptoms
B. CEA after 6 months
C. No treatment
D. Carotid artery stenting (CAS) within 6 months
E. CAS after 6 months

ANSWER: A

COMMENTS: Currently, **CEA** is recommended in symptomatic patients with >70% stenosis or >50% stenosis with an irregular plaque. CEA decreases the stroke rate from 26% to 9% over 2 years in the >70% stenosis group, according to the North American Symptomatic Carotid Endarterectomy Trial (NASCET). Looking specifically at the moderate stenosis group (classified as patients with 50%–60% stenosis), the risk was reduced from 22.2% to 15.7% (5 year). Similar results were also obtained in the European Carotid Surgery Trial. CEA performed within 6 months of TIA was associated with a perioperative mortality less of than 6%. For TIA or nondisabling stroke, CEA should be performed >48 h after an event, but <2 weeks, as the benefit of CEA is highest given the risk for recurrent stroke during the first 6 weeks. For disabling stroke, timing is more controversial. CAS is usually reserved for patients at higher surgical risk during CEA, although recent trials have shown noninferiority of CAS compared with CEA for many patients.

Ref.: 1–3

4. The risk for perioperative stroke among symptomatic patients undergoing CEA is:

A. Between 5% and 10%
B. <1%
C. Between 10% and 15%
D. <5%
E. >15%

ANSWER: D

COMMENTS: Predicting **perioperative stroke rates** is important in evaluating candidacy for intervention for carotid stenosis. Trials have shown a rate of 3.2% in symptomatic patients compared with a rate of 1.4% in asymptomatic patients. These strokes are usually ipsilateral to the lesion, but patients have demonstrated contralateral stroke as well, believed to be from emboli into cerebral circulation during surgery. The highest risk time for emboli is believed to be during carotid artery clamp placement and removal.

Ref.: 1–3

5. A 65-year-old man undergoes CEA for 75% stenosis of his left ICA. On arrival at the intensive care unit, he develops aphasia. What is the next step in management?

A. Serial neurologic examinations
B. Anticoagulation
C. CT head

D. No intervention required

E. Return to the operating room (OR)

ANSWER: E

COMMENTS: Perioperative stroke is a feared complication after CEA. Aphasia immediately after surgery may indicate occlusion of the repaired carotid that necessitates immediate return to the OR. Frank carotid occlusion can be quickly diagnosed with bedside US; however, acute ipsilateral stroke may result from occlusion of the artery, emboli originating from the arteriotomy closure, intimal flap, or distal dissection. Direct and immediate evaluation is necessary in the setting of postoperative stroke.

Ref.: 1–3

6. A 72-year-old male undergoes duplex US that shows a 55% stenosis of his right ICA. What additional factor would be an indication for right-sided CEA?

A. Transient loss of vision in the right eye

B. Transient right-arm and -leg weakness

C. Transient aphasia

D. Multiple major medical comorbidities, high risk for anesthesia

E. Prolonged right-leg weakness

ANSWER: A

COMMENTS: The NASCET recommends intervention in symptomatic patients with stenosis greater than 50%. In asymptomatic patients, intervention would be indicated if stenosis was greater than 60%. Symptoms for a right-sided lesion would include ipsilateral amaurosis fugax, which involves transient loss of vision. Transient aphasia would be more consistent with a left-sided lesion. Motor symptoms resulting from a right-sided lesion would more involve the contralateral extremity; therefore weakness on the right side would also be more consistent with a left-sided lesion. Patients with complicated medical comorbidities who represent higher operative risks may be more appropriate for CAS rather than endarterectomy.

Ref.: 3

7. A 68-year-old male underwent right CEA for a symptomatic 70% ICA stenosis. Surveillance duplex US at 6 months showed increased velocities and concern for 50% restenosis. What therapy should be offered?

A. Carotid stent

B. Reoperation endarterectomy

C. Repeat duplex US at 1 year

D. Therapeutic anticoagulation

E. No further treatment or surveillance necessary

ANSWER: C

COMMENTS: Recurrent stenosis after endarterectomy is most commonly caused by neointimal hyperplasia. If found on duplex examination within the first 6 months, the area should be followed with serial duplex US because one-third of these lesions will spontaneously regress. Operation intervention may be appropriate for a persistent restenosis after 1 to 2 years. Restenosis rates range from 5% to 22%, with females; smokers; and patients with hypertension, diabetes, or hyperlipidemia at the highest risk.

Ref.: 3

8. A 55-year-old woman undergoes duplex US of her carotids; it demonstrates an increased velocity but no identifiable atherosclerosis. Follow-up magnetic resonance angiogram (MRA) demonstrates a "string-of-beads" pattern. She is asymptomatic, with no prior TIA or stroke. What is the next step in management?

A. Coumadin therapy

B. CEA

C. Carotid artery stent

D. No further treatment

E. Aspirin

ANSWER: E

COMMENTS: Imaging findings mentioned above are consistent with fibromuscular dysplasia. **Fibromuscular dysplasia** usually affects women in their 40s or 50s and can affect the carotid, vertebral, renal, or iliac arteries. For carotid arteries, changes are usually bilateral and involve the "string-of-beads" appearance on imaging, consistent with the sequence of stenosis and dilation. There are several different types, the most common being medial fibrodysplasia, where smooth muscle is replaced by fibroconnective tissue. Stroke risk is reported at 8% in women and 4% in men, but surgery is rarely indicated. Because the patient in this question is asymptomatic, antiplatelet therapy is the recommended treatment. If she were to develop symptoms such as TIA or stroke, endovascular treatment is an option.

Ref.: 3

9. Stroke is the third leading cause of death in the United States. Which list accurately reflects the causes of stroke from most to least common?

A. Atherothrombotic, cardiac, intraparenchymal hemorrhage

B. Cardiac, intraparenchymal hemorrhage, atherothrombotic

C. Atherothrombotic, intraparenchymal hemorrhage, cardiac

D. Intraparenchymal hemorrhage, cardiac, atherothrombotic

E. Intraparenchymal hemorrhage, atherothrombotic, cardiac

ANSWER: A

COMMENTS: The most common cause of stroke is from **atherothrombotic** events, accounting for 50%–66% of strokes. Cardiac sources represent 20% of cerebrovascular accidents (CVAs), while 15% result from intraparenchymal and subarachnoid hemorrhage. Risk factors for stroke include age, hypertension, diabetes, hyperlipidemia, smoking, and male gender. Specifically, in patients with carotid disease, stroke is usually due to turbulent flow across atherosclerotic plaque leading to atheroembolization.

Ref.: 3

10. Duplex evaluation of a 70-year-old female shows a 35% stenosis of her right ICA. She is otherwise healthy with no prior symptoms, prior TIAs, or stroke. What treatment would you recommend?

A. CEA

B. Carotid stenting

C. Carotid artery bypass

D. Aspirin therapy

E. No intervention

ANSWER: D

COMMENTS: For **asymptomatic patients**, CEA is recommended when a stenosis is greater than 60%. Given that the aforementioned patient shows a 35% stenosis and no symptoms, CEA and CAS would not be recommended as risks outweigh potential benefits. She should be managed medically with antiplatelet and statin therapy. Management is based on findings of the Asymptomatic Carotid Atherosclerosis Study and Asymptomatic Carotid Surgery Trial, where stroke risk over 5 years was reduced significantly compared with medical management for a stenosis greater than 60%. This recommendation may change given the overall reduction in the annual stroke rate in asymptomatic patients with increased use of optimal medical therapy (aspirin and statin, blood pressure and diabetes management, smoking cessation) since these studies were published.

Ref.: 1, 4

11. Amaurosis fugax is brought about by occlusion of which of the following arteries?

A. Facial artery
B. Occipital artery
C. Retinal artery
D. Posterior auricular artery
E. Ophthalmic artery

ANSWER: C

COMMENTS: About 75% of patients who suffer a stroke have had a previous TIA. **Amaurosis fugax**, one type of TIA (lasting minutes to hours), is manifested as ipsilateral blindness, described by the patient as a window shade pulled across the eye. It is caused by emboli traveling via the ophthalmic artery—the first intracerebral branch of the ICA—and lodging in the retinal artery. These emboli may be seen on fundoscopic examination and are called Hollenhorst plaques. The other arteries listed are branches of the external carotid artery. There are eight branches of the external carotid artery: superior thyroid, lingual, facial, ascending pharyngeal, occipital, posterior auricular, superficial temporal, and maxillary.

Ref.: 5, 6

12. Carotid body tumors are most commonly manifested by which of the following?

A. Hypertension
B. Painless neck mass
C. Cranial nerve deficit
D. Horner syndrome
E. Cerebral ischemia

ANSWER: B

COMMENTS: The carotid body is 3 to 4 mm in size and located within the adventitial tissue of the carotid bifurcation. It arises from paraganglionic cells of neural crest origin. **Carotid body tumors (chemodectomas)** are uncommon, slow growing (they may even remain stationary for long periods), and usually manifested as a painless mass. There are two types of carotid body tumors: sporadic (5% of which are bilateral) and autosomal-dominant familial (32% of which are bilateral). The criteria for malignancy are controversial and influenced by the tumor's location, its biologic behavior, or evidence of local invasion or distal spread. Most are benign. Definitive treatment is excision.

Ref.: 5, 6

13. Most patients with "subclavian steal" syndrome have which of the following conditions?

A. Reversal of flow in the ipsilateral vertebral artery
B. Disabling neurologic symptoms
C. Upper extremity claudication
D. Equal systolic blood pressure in both arms
E. Require operative intervention

ANSWER: A

COMMENTS: "Subclavian steal" syndrome results from a high-grade stenosis or occlusion of the subclavian artery causing decreased systolic pressure distal to the obstruction. This causes blood to flow from the brain and basilar artery in a retrograde manner through the vertebral artery to provide perfusion to the arm. Most patients with this phenomenon are asymptomatic and do not require intervention; however, symptoms such as arm and hand pain and weakness, paresthesias, and vertebral artery insufficiency (often presenting with dizziness or syncope) may require carotid-subclavian artery bypass or transposition.

Ref.: 5, 6

14. With regard to symptoms of ischemia secondary to vertebral-basilar insufficiency, which of the following statements is correct?

A. They include diplopia, ataxia, vertigo, and tinnitus.
B. They are usually indistinguishable from those of carotid insufficiency.
C. They usually reflect unilateral vertebral disease.
D. They are most commonly caused by emboli.
E. They are caused by a diffuse, ulcerated stenosis of the artery.

ANSWER: A

COMMENTS: Stenosis of the vertebral artery usually involves a localized segment near its origin from the subclavian artery. Unlike carotid plaques, the stenotic lesions are usually smooth and nonulcerated, and the ischemia is generally attributed to decreased flow rather than an embolic phenomenon. Although one vertebral artery is usually dominant, a unilateral vertebral stenosis rarely produces symptoms. Associated atherosclerotic involvement of the basilar artery is also common. Symptoms of ischemia caused by vertebral-basilar insufficiency are the same as those of brainstem ischemia and produce a characteristic clinical syndrome (diplopia, dysarthria, vertigo, and tinnitus) quite distinct from the cerebral hemispheric ischemia produced by carotid disease.

Ref.: 6

15. A patient with a symptomatic 85% carotid stenosis is found to have a 50% stenosis of the contralateral carotid artery that is not symptomatic. Appropriate initial treatment includes which of the following?

A. Simultaneous bilateral CEA

B. Staged bilateral CEA with a 1-week interval between stages

C. CEA on the symptomatic side only

D. CEA on the side with the greatest stenosis, regardless of symptoms

E. Antiplatelet therapy and follow-up with duplex scans

ANSWER: C

COMMENTS: Evaluation of patients with a symptomatic disease who are found to have an **asymptomatic stenosis on the contralateral side** suggests that TIAs related to the asymptomatic lesion may develop in 10%–15% of patients. For patients with 50%–75% asymptomatic lesions, the rate of CVA is approximately 1%, although the risk in patients with more significant narrowing is not known and may be higher. For this patient, the asymptomatic contralateral disease can be managed expectantly because cerebral ischemic symptoms, if they do develop, will most likely present as TIAs and can prompt intervention at that time.

Ref.: 7

REFERENCES

1. Beaulieu RJ, Abularrage CJ. Carotid endarterectomy. In: Cameron JL, Cameron AM, eds. *Current Surgical Therapy*. 11th ed. Philadelphia: Elsevier; 2014.
2. Lin PH, Huynh TT. Cerebrovascular occlusive disease. In: Mullholland MW, Lillemoe KD, Doherty GM, et al., eds. *Greenfield's Surgery: Scientific Principles and Practice*. 5th ed. Philadelphia: Lippincott Williams & Wilkins; 2011.
3. Fisher JE. *Mastery of Surgery*. 6th ed. Philadelphia: Lippincott Williams & Wilkins; 2012.
4. Gupta K, Shah Z. What is the future of asymptomatic carotid artery disease? *Am Coll Cardiol*. Available at: http://www.acc.org/latest-in-cardiology/articles/2015/06/16/10/57/what-is-the-future-of-asymptomatic-carotid-artery-disease#sthash.lCl0YaYM.dpuf]%5C. Accessed June 16, 2015.
5. Riles TS, Rockman CB. Cerebrovascular disease. In: Townsend Jr CM, Beauchamp RD, Evers BM, et al., eds. *Sabiston Textbook of Surgery: The Biological Basis of Modern Surgical Practice*. 18th ed. Philadelphia: WB Saunders; 2008.
6. Lin PH, Kougias P, Bechara C, et al. Arterial disease. In: Brunicardi FC, Andersen DK, Billiar TR, et al., eds. *Schwartz's Principles of Surgery*. 9th ed. New York: McGraw-Hill; 2010.
7. Ernst CB, Stanley JC. *Current Therapy in Vascular Surgery*. 4th ed. St. Louis: CV Mosby; 2001.

C. Thoracic Aorta

Elizabeth Aitcheson, M.D.

1. All of the following are risk factors for thoracic aortic aneurysm (TAA) rupture except:
   A. Symptomatic aneurysm
   B. Concurrent dissection
   C. Increased patient age
   D. Anticoagulation use
   E. Rapidly increasing size

ANSWER: D

COMMENTS: TAAs are those occurring distal to the left subclavian vein. They are thought to result from degeneration of the media of the aortic wall combined with local hemodynamic forces. In the thorax, an aortic diameter greater than 3.5 cm is usually considered dilated and greater than 4.5 cm is considered aneurysmal. TAAs are significantly less common than infrarenal abdominal aortic aneurysms (AAAs), although as many as 25% patients with TAA may also have an abdominal aneurysm. The risk for rupture is increased with increasing aneurysm size, advanced age, history of chronic obstructive pulmonary disease (COPD), and concurrent dissection. Pain or symptoms that can be attributed to the aneurysm (usually caused by the compression of nearby structures) are also associated with an increased risk for rupture. The 5-year rupture risk is approximately 20% and incidence is 3.5/100,000 patient-years. Anticoagulation is not a risk factor for rupture.

Ref.: 1, 2

2. Which of the following patients has an indication for descending TAA repair?
   A. A 55-year-old man with a 4-cm TAA
   B. A 65-year-old woman with a 7-cm TAA
   C. A 50-year-old woman with TAA growing at the rate of 5 mm in a year
   D. A 90-year-old man with a 5.5-cm TAA with ejection fraction (EF) < 30%
   E. A 35-year-old man with Marfan syndrome with a 1.5-cm TAA

ANSWER: B

COMMENTS: Size and growth rate classically are used to determine when to surgically intervene on patients with aortic aneurysms. Both larger size and fast growth rate put patients at an increased risk for rupture. Patients with aneurysms smaller than 6 cm are at low-enough risk for rupture to be observed rather than intervened. This threshold may be lower in patients with chronic dissection or Marfan syndrome (usually 5 cm). Growth rates of greater than 1 cm per year are also considered an indication for intervention due to increased rupture risk, especially in larger aneurysms. Patient comorbidities, including reduced EF heart failure, must also be considered in the decision-making process for operative intervention.

Ref.: 1, 2

3. Which of the following is associated with descending TAAs?
   A. 10% of patients have synchronous ascending aortic aneurysms.
   B. 50% of patients have a concomitant AAA.
   C. 75% of patients also have COPD.
   D. 3% of patients also have renal insufficiency (elevated creatinine).
   E. 60% of patients also have reduced EF heart failure.

ANSWER: A

COMMENTS: Descending TAAs are associated with concomitant AAA or ascending thoracic aneurysms in 25% and 10% of cases, respectively. A history of COPD is considered as a risk factor for rupture of thoracic aneurysms, but it is not present in such a large majority of patients with TAA. About 15% of patients with TAA have preoperative renal insufficiency, which puts them at a higher risk for perioperative renal failure. Patients are also at a higher risk for perioperative complications with EF < 30%, but this level of heart failure is not seen in a majority of patients.

Ref.: 1, 2

4. Which of the following is not used as an adjunct for organ protection in open repair of TAAs?
   A. Preoperative clopidogrel
   B. Instillation of cooled lactated Ringer's, mannitol, and methylprednisolone solution into the renal artery
   C. Cerebrospinal fluid (CSF) drainage
   D. Minimizing visceral ischemic time with inline mesenteric shunting
   E. Reconstruction of renal arteries

ANSWER: A

COMMENTS: Ischemia during an aortic repair represents an important operative concern during open thoracic aneurysm repair. Several adjuncts have been developed to minimize ischemia time to certain organs in order to limit the postoperative organ dysfunction. The main areas of concern are the spinal cord, kidneys, and bowel. CSF drainage has been shown to help with spinal cord perfusion during surgery. Shunting of mesenteric vessels (celiac and superior mesenteric arteries) can decrease bowel ischemic time without interfering in the operative field. Finally, cooling of the kidneys and reconstruction of the renal arteries (either because of location or stenosis) are renal protective strategies. Preoperative clopidogrel therapy is not used for organ protection.

Ref.: 1, 2

5. Which statement is true concerning thoracic endovascular aorta repair (TEVAR) in comparison with open repair and endovascular aortic repair (EVAR)?
   A. TEVAR has been used for only degenerative causes of aneurysms, while EVAR is used for a variety of aortic pathologies.
   B. TEVAR has a higher complication rate compared with the open repair of TAAs.
   C. TEVAR devices require smaller-bore delivery devices compared with EVAR.
   D. Proximal and distal seal zones should be at least 15 mm in length.
   E. Open TAA repair has a lower associated morbidity than open AAA repair.

ANSWER: D

COMMENTS: Open repair of TAAs carries the morbidity of a thoracotomy as well as complications associated with cross-clamping of the proximal aorta. Given this risk TEVAR represents a less-morbid alternative repair option. TEVAR does have certain anatomic requirements, especially the proximal seal zone, which ideally should be at least 15 mm in length to allow for an adequate seal. Compared with EVAR, TEVAR requires larger-bore delivery devices, and special consideration may be needed in case of narrowing of calcified iliac arteries. Finally, compared with EVAR, TEVAR has been used for a wider range of aortic pathologies including traumatic aortic rupture.

Ref.: 1, 2

6. What is the appropriate Crawford classification for a descending thoracic aneurysm beginning in the distal aorta above the diaphragm and extending to the infrarenal aorta?
   A. Crawford I
   B. Crawford II
   C. Crawford III
   D. Crawford IV
   E. Undefined category

ANSWER: C

COMMENTS: The Crawford classification of descending TAAs was developed to help define the portion of the aorta that would require resection in open repair. Crawford I involves the aorta from the left subclavian takeoff to the renal arteries. Crawford II involves the aorta from the left subclavian takeoff to the aorta distal to the renal arteries. Crawford III involves the aorta distal to the subclavian takeoff but above the diaphragm, to the infrarenal aorta. Crawford IV involves the aorta below the diaphragm to below the renal arteries.

Ref.: 1, 2

7. Which is a true statement about the DeBakey and Stanford classifications of aortic dissection?
   A. A dissection can be both Stanford class A and DeBakey type II.
   B. Stanford class A dissections are treated with aggressive medical management of blood pressure.
   C. DeBakey type III dissections are proximal to the left subclavian artery.
   D. Stanford class B dissections are always considered surgical emergencies.
   E. Chronic Stanford A dissections account for 60% of all dissections.

ANSWER: A

COMMENTS: The Stanford classification divides aortic dissections into those that involve the ascending aorta and those that do not. Aortic dissections can either be acute or chronic (greater or less than 2-week duration). Acute Stanford class A dissections, representing 60% of all dissections, are considered surgical emergencies. Stanford class B dissections are further divided into complicated (which may require intervention) and uncomplicated (asymptomatic, which can be treated with aggressive medical management) dissections. The DeBakey classification is determined by proximal and distal extent of dissection. Type I involves the ascending and descending aorta, type II only the ascending aorta, and type III only distal to the left subclavian artery takeoff. Therefore Stanford class A dissections include DeBakey type I and II dissections.

Ref.: 1, 2

8. A 55-year-old female is brought in after a high-speed motor vehicle collision. She is initially hypotensive with a blood pressure of 80/40 mmHg, which responds to resuscitation. Chest radiograph shows a widened mediastinum, and on physical examination, she is tender in the right upper quadrant with a positive focused assessment with sonography for trauma examination. She only transiently responds to resuscitation and again becomes hypotensive. Which statement is true concerning appropriate initial management?
   A. She should be taken immediately for computed tomography (CT) angiography of the chest to evaluate the widened mediastinum.
   B. The most likely site of traumatic aortic rupture is the ascending aortic arch.
   C. Initial treatment should focus on the intraabdominal source of hemorrhage as the likely cause of hypotension.
   D. She should be taken emergently for TEVAR for suspected traumatic rupture of the aorta.
   E. Traumatic aortic ruptures are more likely to result in mortality after initial presentation to the emergency room rather than in the field.

ANSWER: C

COMMENTS: Patients with multiple injuries that include suspected aortic injury should have other sources of hemorrhage addressed first (e.g., extensive pelvic fractures or intraabdominal injuries). Further evaluation of aortic injury/widened mediastinum with CT angiography may be delayed in the setting of hemodynamic instability and alternate source of hemorrhage (in this patient, the likely source is intraabdominal). TEVAR may be appropriate for this injury, but it is not the first intervention that should be considered. The most common site for blunt aortic injury is just distal to the left subclavian artery origin.

Ref.: 1, 2

9. Regarding TAAs in patients with Marfan syndrome, which of the following statements is true?

A. Less than 50% of patients with Marfan syndrome survive past the age of 45 years.

B. The descending aorta is always affected.

C. All aneurysmal dilations greater than 4 cm should be treated with prophylactic replacement of the aortic root.

D. Surgical repair of an ascending aortic aneurysm usually requires aortic repair only.

E. The perioperative mortality rate exceeds 15%.

ANSWER: A

COMMENTS: The severely diminished longevity of patients with the Marfan syndrome has been well-documented. Less than 50% of patients with the syndrome survive past the age of 45 years. Cardiac deaths account for more than 90% of early deaths of a known cause, and 75% of these deaths are secondary to complications from aortic root dilation or aortic dissections. Prophylactic aortic root replacement is recommended for all aneurysms larger than 6 cm in diameter. In contrast to the atherosclerotic aneurysmal disease, aneurysmal dilations in patients with Marfan syndrome involve not only the entire aorta, including the coronary sinuses, but also the cardiac valvular tissues. Therefore replacement of the entire aortic root, including the aortic valve, with a composite valve graft is required in the majority of patients. Improved techniques of myocardial protection have resulted in perioperative mortality rates of less than 5% in the most recent series.

Ref.: 2

10. With regard to ascending aortic aneurysms, which of the following statements is true?

A. They are most often caused by connective tissue abnormalities.

B. They are not related to earlier venereal disease.

C. Primary tumors of the aorta are common.

D. They are usually associated with aortic insufficiency.

E. Death is generally caused by a rupture with resulting hemothorax.

ANSWER: A

COMMENTS: Etiologic factors involved in aortic aneurysms vary according to the location of an aneurysm. In the ascending aorta, a connective tissue abnormality recognized histologically as cystic medial necrosis is the most common underlying abnormality. This is the defect seen in aneurysms associated with Marfan syndrome. Other known causes, such as syphilitic aneurysms, are steadily decreasing in frequency, and atherosclerotic aneurysms of the ascending aorta are relatively uncommon. Primary tumors originating from the aorta (most commonly sarcomas) are extremely rare. Aortic insufficiency occurs only when there is associated annular dilation or when one or more aortic cusps are sheared off by an acute dissection. Death from an ascending aortic aneurysm is usually caused by cardiac failure secondary to chronic untreated aortic insufficiency or rupture into the pericardium with pericardial tamponade.

Ref.: 3, 4

11. With regard to the clinical characteristics and management of ascending aortic aneurysms, which of the following statements is true?

A. Most ascending aortic aneurysms are symptomatic.

B. Valvular murmurs are rare.

C. Aortography is contraindicated because of the risk for causing dissection of an aneurysm with the catheter.

D. Operative management with the placement of a composite graft of aortic conduit and aortic valve is the treatment of choice for all ascending aortic aneurysms.

E. CT with contrast is a good noninvasive modality with which to delineate the size and extent of an aortic aneurysm.

ANSWER: E

COMMENTS: Although relatively uncommon, an ascending aortic aneurysm may be manifested as a mass in the anterior aspect of the chest. Patients are usually asymptomatic, with aneurysms discovered on routine chest radiographs. Aneurysms can be localized (saccular) or more generalized (fusiform). When symptoms are present, they are commonly related to congestive heart failure caused by the dilation of the aortic annulus, which results in aortic insufficiency and its characteristic murmur (an early diastolic murmur at the second interspace along the right sternal border). This murmur is often present even in asymptomatic patients.

Aortography confirms the diagnosis and is important for defining the dimensional extent of an aneurysm and its relationship to the rest of the aorta, its major branches, and the coronary ostia.

Surgical correction is clearly the treatment of choice, with surgical options determined by the presence of valve pathology. Valve-sparing operations are carried out in patients with preserved valve function. If aneurysms are associated with the massive dilation of the aortic root, aortic annulus, and aortic leaflets, a composite graft is used (Bentall operation).

CT with intravenous contrast enhancement and magnetic resonance imaging (MRI) are excellent noninvasive modalities that can delineate the extent and size of an aneurysmal aorta.

Ref.: 3, 4

12. Which of the following is correct about the superior vena cava syndrome (SVCS)?

A. Bronchogenic carcinoma with invasion into the mediastinum is the leading cause of SVCS.

B. Venous pressure in the superior vena cava (SVC) rarely exceeds 15 mmHg.

C. Acute obstruction of the SVC is seldom clinically significant because of the large number of collateral vessels available.

D. Occlusion of the SVC between the azygos vein and the right atrium is more symptomatic than an occlusion above the azygos vein.

E. Surgical correction is usually indicated.

ANSWER: A

COMMENTS: SVCS results when blood flow through the SVC becomes obstructed. More than 70% of SVC obstructions are caused by malignant tumors, most often mediastinal invasion by bronchogenic carcinoma. When obstruction occurs, venous pressures rise to 20 to 50 mmHg.

Acute complete obstruction allows little time for the formation of collateral vessels and can therefore produce significant edematous laryngeal obstruction and even fatal cerebral edema. A more gradual onset of obstruction results in the characteristic clinical picture of facial swelling and dilation of the collateral veins of the head and neck, arms, and upper thoracic areas. Obstruction between the azygos vein and the right atrium is less disabling because the azygos vein provides a large collateral venous channel for drainage of the SVC system into the inferior vena cava (IVC) system. Obstruction above the azygos vein eliminates this collateral channel and is not as well tolerated.

The treatment of choice for obstruction caused by associated malignancy is prompt radiation therapy, often in association with diuretics and chemotherapy. An operation is rarely indicated for the management of SVC obstruction because of the technical difficulties associated with vena cava grafts, the underlying poor prognosis in patients with malignant conditions, and the usual adequacy of collateral venous circulation in the rare instances of slowly developing obstruction caused by benign conditions. The only indication for surgery is the unusual instance of a benign problem in which the collateral circulation does not relieve the symptoms. Management may include angioplasty, stenting, anatomic bypass, or non-anatomic bypass. In general, autologous grafts have performed better than prosthetic grafts.

Ref.: 3, 4

13. With regard to transverse aortic arch aneurysms, which of the following statements is true?

A. Cystic medial necrosis is a major cause.

B. Repair is associated with the highest operative mortality rate of any of the aortic aneurysms.

C. Differentiation from mediastinal tumors is usually possible on standard chest radiographs.

D. Deep hypothermia with circulatory arrest and cardiopulmonary bypass is rarely used.

E. All of the above.

ANSWER: B

COMMENTS: Transverse aortic arch aneurysms almost always are the result of atherosclerosis. In asymptomatic individuals, they are most often detected on routine chest radiographs. However, aortography and CT are required to differentiate them from mediastinal tumors and to define the vascular anatomy before repair. Concomitant association with coronary and cerebrovascular disease, together with the need to disrupt flow to the brain temporarily during repair, has resulted in an operative mortality rate exceeding that for repair of other aortic aneurysms. The introduction of cardiopulmonary bypass and hypothermic circulatory arrest has significantly reduced this operative mortality rate. Spiral CT is used rather than aortography in some centers.

Ref.: 3, 4

14. Radiographic signs of aortic injury secondary to blunt chest trauma include all of the following except:

A. Widening of the mediastinum

B. Blunting of the aortic knob

C. Right apical capping

D. Depression of the left main bronchus

E. Deviation of the trachea to the right

ANSWER: C

COMMENTS: Blunt injury to the thoracic aorta may occur without clinical signs or symptoms. Frequently, the mechanism of injury (sudden deceleration from vehicular accidents or falls) and a high index of suspicion obligate the examining physician to rule out aortic trauma by aortography or CT angiography. Radiographic signs of aortic injury, when present, include blunting of the aortic knob, widening of the mediastinum (to 7.0 cm), deviation of the trachea to the right, blunting of the left apex, and depression of the left main bronchus. Even when these radiographic signs are present, CT angiogram or aortography is required to precisely define the anatomy and the extent of the vascular injury.

Ref.: 3–5

REFERENCES

1. Beaulieu RJ, Abularrage CJ. Carotid endarterectomy. In: Cameron JL, Cameron AM, eds. *Current Surgical Therapy*. 11th ed. Philadelphia: Elsevier; 2014.
2. Mullholland MW, Lillemoe KD, Doherty GM, et al., eds. *Greenfield's Surgery: Scientific Principles and Practice*. 5th ed. Philadelphia: Lippincott Williams & Wilkins; 2011.
3. LeMaire SA, Sharma K, Coselli JS. Thoracic aneurysms and aortic dissection. In: Brunicardi FC, Andersen DK, Billiar TR, et al., eds. *Schwartz's Principles of Surgery*. 9th ed. New York: McGraw-Hill; 2010.
4. Safi HJ, Estrera AL, Miller CC, et al. Thoracic vasculature with emphasis on the thoracic aorta. In: Townsend Jr CM, Beauchamp RD, Evers BM, et al., eds. *Sabiston Textbook of Surgery: The Biological Basis of Modern Surgical Practice*. 18th ed. Philadelphia: WB Saunders; 2008.
5. LeMaire SA, Sharma K, Coselli JS. Thoracic aneurysms and aortic dissection. In: Brunicardi FC, Andersen DK, Billiar TR, et al., eds. *Schwartz's Principles of Surgery*. 9th ed. New York: McGraw-Hill; 2010.

D. Abdominal Aorta

M. Caroline Nally, M.D.

1. What is the most common organism that causes infected abdominal aortic aneurysms (AAAs)?
   A. *Escherichia coli*
   B. *Bacteroides*
   C. *Salmonella*
   D. *Pseudomonas aeruginosa*
   E. *Streptococcus*

ANSWER: C

COMMENTS: Infected AAAs account for less than 1% of all repairs. There are four different causes of an infected aneurysm. (1) Mycotic aneurysms involve a septic embolus from the heart infecting an artery. (2) Microbial arteritis involves bacteria infecting an atherosclerotic artery to cause aneurysmal degeneration (80% of infected aneurysms). (3) Existing aneurysms that become infected. (4) Traumatic pseudoaneurysm that has concomitant bacterial inoculation. Salmonella causes 40% of all aneurysmal infections, with most others being caused by *Streptococcus*, *Staphylococcus*, *Bacteroides*, *Arizona hinshawii*, *E. coli*, and *P. aeruginosa*. Blood cultures are positive in only 50% of cases. Computed tomography (CT) is the most useful diagnostic study, with images showing periaortic mass, aneurysm at an atypical location, periaortic fluid or gas, retroperitoneal inflammation, or frank rupture. The aneurysm is usually saccular or eccentric. Treatment involves the removal of all infected tissue and restoration of distal flow.

Ref.: 1

2. What is the best way to perform an endovascular repair of a juxtarenal aortic aneurysm?
   A. Using a standard endograft
   B. Using an individually designed fenestrated endograft that contains orifices for the renal and visceral vessels
   C. Using a covered stent
   D. Only via a hybrid endovascular and an open approach
   E. Only via an open approach

ANSWER: B

COMMENTS: Aneurysms that extend to the level of the renal arteries present increased difficulty in management and, ultimately, lead to increased morbidity and mortality rates. Renal and visceral ischemia associated with aortic occlusion during the proximal anastomosis leads to 15%–20% of patients having complications. Therefore it is not recommended that patients undergo elective operative repair until the aneurysm is greater than 6 cm in diameter. Open approaches to juxtarenal aortic aneurysms include retroperitoneal and transperitoneal approaches. The availability of individually customized fenestrated endografts has made endovascular repair a viable option for these difficult aneurysms. Endografts that can be placed in a short infrarenal neck and have fenestrations for the renal and visceral vessels are now available. The endovascular technique has been proven to be safe, feasible, and successful in preventing aneurysm rupture. If the patients have an extensive disease and are not candidates for an individualized fenestrated endograft, they may benefit from a hybrid operation incorporating endovascular and open techniques.

Ref.: 1

3. What is the best treatment for inflammatory aortic aneurysms?
   A. Systemic corticosteroids
   B. Systemic antibiotics
   C. No treatment is needed
   D. Open repair
   E. Endovascular repair

ANSWER: E

COMMENTS: About 5% of AAAs are considered inflammatory. They have a dense inflammatory response encasing the anterior and lateral walls of the infrarenal aorta with sparing of the posterior aspect. The inflammatory response consists of a dense cellular infiltrate with a white, glistening appearance. The cause is unknown, but 20% of patients with inflammatory aneurysms have some other autoimmune disorder. Patients are usually male and often have the triad of a pulsatile abdominal mass, abdominal pain, and elevated erythrocyte sedimentation rate. Imaging [CT or ultrasound (US)] shows the thickened aortic walls and can be confused with a ruptured AAA. Treatment is essentially the same as for other aneurysms. Nonoperative treatment with corticosteroids has been deemed ineffective and largely abandoned. There is no role for antibiotics. Despite the thickening of the walls, these patients still have a risk for rupture similar to aneurysms of similar etiology and therefore should undergo repair. The open repair is complicated by the dense adhesions created by the aneurysm to surrounding structures such as ureters, duodenum, and colon. This makes the endovascular approach the optimal treatment as there is no extensive dissection, and reviews have shown that the inflammatory process resolves spontaneously in 50% of patients after endovascular repair.

Ref.: 2

4. Which of the following is the most common graft-related late complication of aortic bypass grafts?
   A. Graft occlusion caused by progressive atherosclerosis
   B. Suture line pseudoaneurysm
   C. Aortoenteric fistula
   D. Distal embolization
   E. Infection caused by transient bacteremia

ANSWER: A

COMMENTS: The most common graft-related late complication is graft occlusion, which develops in 10%–35% of patients. The most frequent cause of graft occlusion is progressive atherosclerosis, which usually occurs at or just beyond the distal anastomosis. Other late complications include anastomotic pseudoaneurysm (1%–5%) and graft infection (1%), both of which occur more often when a femoral anastomosis is involved. An aortoenteric fistula is rare but carries a high mortality rate (50%).

Ref.: 2

5. Which of the following is not an acceptable treatment option for a patient with late aortic graft limb occlusion?
   A. Percutaneous atherectomy
   B. Thrombolytic therapy
   C. Graft limb thrombectomy
   D. Femorofemoral bypass
   E. Aortofemoral bypass reoperation

ANSWER: A

COMMENTS: The most common graft-related complication following aortofemoral bypass is thrombosis of one limb. Graft limb occlusion occurs in 10%–20% of patients, depending on the duration of follow-up. Late graft limb occlusion is most commonly caused by progressive atherosclerotic disease at or just beyond the distal anastomosis. Other causes include worsening disease of the outflow vessels (commonly the proximal profunda femoris), thrombosis of an anastomotic aneurysm, arterial embolism from a cardiac source, low-output states, hypercoagulable states, and iatrogenic injury to the graft or native vessels following cardiac catheterization or diagnostic angiography. Preoperative angiography should be performed in all patients with late aortic graft limb occlusion, except in those with profound limb ischemia. In high-risk or inactive patients without evidence of limb-threatening ischemia, a nonoperative approach may be the most prudent course. Thrombolytic therapy has been used in patients with acute graft thrombosis. It can be performed in patients without profound lower extremity ischemia as it requires an extended amount of time to dissolve the thrombus. Complications such as bleeding, distal embolization, and worsening ischemia may occur. Surgical revision of the graft is often required following successful thrombolysis. Most patients with graft limb occlusion are treated via an operative approach. In patients with short duration, unilateral occlusion and absence of proximal aortic disease, a graft limb thrombectomy has been shown to be 90% successful. To prevent recurrent thrombosis, revision of the anastomosis is often required. If the graft limb cannot be opened, femorofemoral bypass can be performed quickly, under limited anesthesia and with a lower risk than recurrent aortic surgery. In patients with proximal aortic disease, anastomotic complications, or significant degeneration or dilation of the original prosthesis, redo aortofemoral or thoracofemoral bypass may be considered; however, in high-risk patients or those with a hostile abdomen, the axillofemoral bypass may be preferred. Regardless of the technique, revision of the outflow tract may be necessary. It may require profundaplasty, graft limb extension, and bypass to the popliteal or tibial level. Distal grafts are required in 25%–50% of all procedures for graft limb occlusion. Percutaneous artherectomy involves the use of a catheter with a sharp rotating blade to remove plaque and debris in small, native vessels; therefore it is not appropriate for the treatment of aortic graft limb occlusion.

Ref.: 1, 3

6. With regard to the approach for an open repair of AAAs, which of the following statements is true?
   A. There is no true indication for a retroperitoneal approach.
   B. Extension of the aneurysm to the right common iliac artery is a contraindication to a retroperitoneal approach.
   C. The retroperitoneal approach is associated with a higher incidence of paralytic ileus.
   D. The midline transperitoneal approach is associated with a higher incidence of pulmonary complications.
   E. The retroperitoneal approach can be used for the repair of ruptured AAAs.

ANSWER: E

COMMENTS: There are many reported indications for the retroperitoneal approach to the infrarenal aorta. A "hostile abdomen," usually resulting from multiple transabdominal procedures, irradiation, or the presence of enteric or urinary stomas, is the most common. The retroperitoneal approach is also useful for patients with ascites, peritoneal dialysis catheters, morbid obesity, inflammatory aneurysms, or a horseshoe kidney. Relative contraindications to use of the retroperitoneal approach include the presence of right renal artery stenosis, ruptured AAA, and an AAA with a left-sided inferior vena cava. The presence of a right common iliac artery aneurysm is not an absolute contraindication to the retroperitoneal approach. In these cases, the right iliac aneurysm is excluded by oversewing the ostium of the right common iliac artery through the open aorta, making a right lower quadrant transplant incision, ligating the distal neck of the iliac aneurysm, and extending the right limb of the bifurcated aortic graft to the right external iliac or right common femoral artery. Alternatively, the distal neck of the aneurysm is not ligated, but the distal right external iliac or the proximal right common femoral artery is ligated, followed by extension of the right limb of the graft to the right common femoral artery. The latter approach has the disadvantage of allowing backflow to the iliac aneurysm via the right internal iliac artery, which may result (on rare occasion) in enlargement and rupture of the iliac aneurysm. Although most surgeons avoid the retroperitoneal approach for ruptured AAAs, several centers with extensive experience have reported the successful use of this approach in select cases of ruptured AAAs.

At least four prospective randomized studies have confirmed that the retroperitoneal approach is associated with a decreased incidence of postoperative ileus and a shorter hospital stay. There was no significant difference in the incidence of pulmonary complications, perhaps because of the increasing use of epidural analgesia in the postoperative period for patients undergoing an AAA repair.

Ref.: 3

7. With regard to the operative technique of AAA repair, which of the following statements is true?
   A. Bifurcation grafts are preferable to straight grafts, even if the iliac vessels are not involved.
   B. An endovascular approach is most commonly used today.
   C. Bleeding lumbar vessels are routinely ligated from outside the aneurysm sac.
   D. The inferior mesenteric artery (IMA) is routinely reimplanted in elderly patients to prevent ischemia of the left colon.
   E. Flow should be restored first to the external iliac vessels when the cross-clamps are removed.

ANSWER: B

COMMENTS: Details of the operative technique for the repair of AAAs vary somewhat, depending on individual circumstances, but several general principles should apply. Proximal control is established distal to the renal vessels with left renal vein preservation when there is adequate normal aorta below the renal arteries for clamping and sewing; however, with improved endovascular treatment options, open operations require suprarenal clamping. Manipulation of the aorta is kept to a minimum to prevent embolization of the contents of the aneurysm. After the proximal and distal clamps are applied, the aneurysm is opened and the thrombus is evacuated. The lumbar vessels are ligated from within the aneurysm sac. The IMA can usually be safely ligated at its origin, thereby avoiding damage to collateral vessels within the mesentery of the left colon. If backflow from the IMA is poor, consideration should be given to reimplanting the artery to the side of the prosthesis. Prior to ligation, some surgeons evaluate IMA flow by viewing backflow or measuring stump pressure. Pressure lower than 40 mmHg is a reason for reimplantation.

Flow to at least one hypogastric artery should be preserved to maintain collateral flow to the colon via the middle hemorrhoidal arteries. If the ischemic injury to the left colon is suspected, a flexible sigmoidoscopy should be performed.

A tube graft is preferable to a bifurcated graft when the common iliac arteries are uninvolved. Tube grafts obviate the need for an additional anastomosis and decrease the dissection around the parasympathetic nerves and iliac veins and arteries.

Extensive aneurysms involving the celiac, superior mesenteric, or renal artery require more complex revascularization procedures, including mesenteric vessel reimplantation.

After graft placement, proper techniques of aortic flushing and sequential unclamping are important to minimize the risk for hypotension and distal embolization. The latter is accomplished by adequate flushing before completing the distal anastomosis and opening the circulation first into the internal iliac and then into the external iliac arteries.

Hypotension after the removal of the aortic cross-clamp is believed to occur as a result of washout of acidic metabolites and vasoactive substances from the ischemic lower extremities, third-space loss into permeable distal tissues, and sudden flow into vasodilated beds, as well as vascular steal secondary to reactive hyperemia in the lower extremities.

The aneurysm sac should be closed over the prosthetic graft to isolate the graft from the duodenum and to minimize the risk for erosion and fistulization.

Ref.: 1, 2, 4

8. Which one of the following complications occurs most commonly after successful repair of an open AAA in a 58-year-old man?

A. Sexual dysfunction

B. Ischemic colitis

C. Renal failure

D. Peripheral embolization

E. Leg paralysis

ANSWER: A

COMMENTS: All of these complications may occur after repair of an AAA, but with appropriate operative technique, most are uncommon. Changes in sexual function, however, are common. Retrograde ejaculation has been reported in as many as two-thirds and loss of potency in as many as one-third of such patients. These changes may result from an injury to the autonomic nerve fibers overlying the anterior aorta near the origin of the IMA or from an injury to fibers overlying the proximal left common iliac artery and aortic bifurcation. Avoiding excessive aortic dissection in this region can help minimize this complication. Documentation that sexual dysfunction existed preoperatively is of obvious importance in aortoiliac surgery because the incidence of impotence in men of this age with no aortoiliac occlusive disease is considerable. Revascularization of the internal iliacs at the time of aortoiliac reconstruction for occlusive disease may reverse vasculogenic impotence in patients with distal obstructive disease.

Ref.: 1, 2, 4

9. Which of the following is the most common manifestation of an AAA?

A. Incidental finding on physical examination or CT performed for unrelated disease

B. Back or abdominal pain

C. Acute rupture

D. Spontaneous thrombosis with peripheral ischemia

E. Peripheral embolization

ANSWER: A

COMMENTS: Approximately three-fourths of all AAAs are discovered incidentally and are asymptomatic. The most common complaint in patients with symptoms is a vague abdominal pain. Patients may also note back or flank pain. AAAs may expand without symptoms, rupture, embolize, thrombose, erode into the adjacent vertebral bodies, or partially obstruct the duodenum or ureters (inflammatory aneurysms). Rare manifestations include aortoenteric fistula and aortocaval fistula. The latter are accompanied by an abdominal bruit, venous hypertension, and high-output cardiac failure. Rupture may mimic other acute intraabdominal emergencies, such as diverticulitis and renal colic, and may be manifested as acute abdominal pain followed by transient hypotension and eventually vascular collapse. Signs and symptoms of acute ischemia in the lower extremities may follow thrombosis or embolization from an abdominal aneurysm.

Ref.: 1, 2, 4

10. What is the blood supply to the aorta?

A. Vasa vasorum

B. Vasa recta

C. Arteriocapillaries

D. Vasa previa

E. Vasa vena

ANSWER: A

COMMENTS: Arteries are composed of three layers. The intima is the innermost layer that contains the endothelial cells. The internal elastic membrane separates the intima from the media. The media is the major structural component of the artery containing smooth muscle cells, elastin, proteoglycans, and collagen. The external elastic membrane separates the media from the adventitia. The adventitia provides 60% of the strength of the blood vessel and contains elastic tissue, fibroblasts, and collagen. During an endarterectomy, the cleavage plane is just superficial to the external elastic membrane. The blood supply to the inner media comes from the direct diffusion from the blood within the lumen. The outer media is supplied by small penetrating arteries called vasa vasorum. Hypertrophy of the vasa vasorum on the thoracic and abdominal aorta can be a sign of severe underlying atherosclerosis.

Ref.: 5

11. Where does an aortoenteric fistula usually form?

A. Stomach

B. Third portion of the duodenum

C. Fourth portion of the duodenum

D. Sigmoid

E. Rectum

ANSWER: B

COMMENTS: Aortoenteric fistula is the most severe manifestation of an aortic graft infection. It has a reported incidence of 0.04%–0.07% in autopsy series. It usually presents as a herald upper or lower gastrointestinal bleed, but can then turn into massive exsanguination if left untreated. This should be suspected in all patients with a history of abdominal aortic surgery who present with a gastrointestinal bleed. Although the diagnosis can at times be made with endoscopy, CT is a more sensitive study to demonstrate erosion or frank graft exposure. This usually occurs at the third portion of the duodenum as there is a point of contact with the proximal graft anastomosis. An endovascular graft can be placed across the aortoenteric fistula as a temporizing measure, but it has a high rate of reintervention, making definitive surgical repair necessary.

Ref.: 1, 6

12. Which of the following is not a risk factor for developing an AAA?

A. Hypertension

B. Diabetes

C. Tobacco use

D. Male gender

E. Hyperlipidemia

ANSWER: B

COMMENTS: Risk factors for developing an AAA include age, male gender, family history, tobacco use, hypertension, hyperlipidemia, and height. Connective tissue disorders, such as Marfan syndrome, and concurrent aneurysmal or atherosclerotic disease are also associated with aneurysm development. Aneurysmal enlargement is associated with factors that result in the weakening of the arterial wall and increased local hemodynamic factors including heritable conditions like Marfan syndrome, familial thoracic aortic aneurysm and dissection, and vascular-type Ehlers-Danlos syndrome. Other factors that lead to AAA expansion include advanced age, severe cardiac disease, previous stroke, tobacco use, and cardiac or renal transplant. AAA rupture is associated with female gender, large initial diameter of AAA, higher mean blood pressure, length of time smoking, cardiac or renal transplantation, chronic obstructive pulmonary disease (COPD), and critical wall stress–wall strength relationship. Cross-sectional aneurysm diameter is the most widely accepted surrogate for rupture risk.

AAA Diameter (cm)	Rupture Risk (%/year)
<4	0
4 to 5	0.5 to 5
5 to 6	3 to 15
6 to 7	10 to 20
7 to 8	20 to 40
>8	30 to 50

Ref.: 6

13. What is an indication for the surgical repair of an aortic abdominal aneurysm?

A. Size larger than 4.5 cm

B. Growth of more than 5 mm in 1 year

C. Growth of more than 5 mm in 6 months

D. Fusiform anatomy

E. An aneurysm of any size in a patient with hypertension

ANSWER: C

COMMENTS: Size is predominantly used to determine the need for an operative repair of an AAA. Surgical treatment is recommended for aneurysms that are larger than 5.5 cm in maximal diameter or those that grow more than 5 mm in 6 months or more than 1 cm in 1 year. Although this remains the standard, there is evidence to suggest that smaller aneurysms (especially in women) can exhibit more rapid growth that can increase the risk for rupture at smaller sizes. Autopsy studies have shown evidence of rupture in up to 12% of aneurysms less than 5 cm in diameter. Finally, aneurysms with saccular anatomy are more likely to rupture. Saccular aneurysms appear as an outpouching of the aorta compared with fusiform aneurysms that appear spindle-shaped.

Ref.: 6

14. Who should be screened for AAAs?

A. Men over the age of 55 years with a personal history of smoking

B. Women over the age of 55 years with a personal history of smoking

C. Men over the age of 55 years with a family history of AAA

D. Men over the age of 55 years with no family history of AAA

E. Women over the age of 55 years with a family history of AAA

ANSWER: C

COMMENTS: The Clinical Practice Council of the Society for Vascular Surgery reviewed available evidence-based data to make recommendations for the screening of AAAs. One-time screening should be performed for all men 65 years or older with greater than 100 pack-year cigarette smoking history and men 55 years or older with a family history of AAA. Screening for women is recommended for those over the age of 65 years with a family history of AAA or a personal history of smoking. After an aneurysm has been detected, additional screening is recommended based on size.

Size (cm)	Recommended Timing of Repeat Screening
<2.6	No further screening
2.6 to 2.9	5 years
3 to 3.4	3 years
3.5 to 4.4	12 months
4.5 to 5.4	6 months

Ref.: 6

15. Which is the least appropriate conduit for the replacement of an infected arterial graft?

A. Polytetrafluoroethylene (PTFE)
B. Rifampin-soaked graft
C. Silver-coated polyester graft
D. Cryopreserved arterial allograft
E. Saphenous or femoral vein allograft

ANSWER: A

COMMENTS: Extensive infection of previously placed arterial graft resulting in anastomotic pseudoaneurysm requires a complete removal of the graft and debridement of all infected or devitalized tissue and restoration of flow. This can be done as a single or staged procedure. Reconstruction can occur in situ or via an extraanatomic bypass. Complications of this procedure include recurrent graft infection, graft thrombosis, and aortic stump disruption and can cause serious morbidity and mortality. These are prevented through debridement, layered closure, flap coverage when needed, and appropriate selection of new conduit material. Appropriate options include rifampin-soaked or silver-coated polyester graft, cryopreserved arterial allograft, or vein allograft. Prosthetic graft is discouraged in grossly purulent operative fields due to its likelihood of reinfection. Endovascular repair is not recommended in infected fields because it does not include debridement of the infected tissue.

Ref.: 6

16. What is the treatment for uncomplicated Stanford type B aortic dissections?

A. Aggressive medical management
B. Open operative replacement of the ascending and descending aorta
C. Open operative replacement of the ascending aorta
D. Endovascular stent graft placement
E. Open operative replacement of the descending aorta

ANSWER: A

COMMENTS: Aortic dissection occurs when a tear in the intimal layer of the vessel permits blood to create a false channel within the wall, causing the aorta to be divided into a true and a false lumen. There are two different classification systems, Debakey and Stanford, based on the anatomic location of the dissection. Debakey type I involves the ascending and thoracoabdominal aorta. Debakey type II is limited to the ascending aorta. Debakey type IIIa is limited to the descending thoracic aorta. Debakey type IIIb involves the descending thoracic and abdominal aorta. Stanford type A involves the ascending aorta, while Stanford type B does not. Diagnosis can be made with CT and echocardiogram to assess the proximal aorta and heart. Acute type A dissection is considered a surgical emergency. Treatment often includes replacement of the aortic valve and the ascending aorta. Type B is characterized as acute (presentation within 14 days of symptoms) or chronic and complicated or uncomplicated. Type B dissections usually begin from a primary tear in the proximal descending thoracic aorta just distal to the origin of the left subclavian artery and usually extend antegrade (but can extend retrograde). Traditionally, aggressive medical management has been the treatment for uncomplicated type B dissections. With advances in endovascular treatments, this management paradigm has started to shift. Specifically, 91% of patients who undergo stent graft placement have been found to have aortic remodeling, which decreases the risk for aneurysmal degeneration in future years. Only 19% of those who undergo medical management have aortic remodeling. The potential for survival benefit following endovascular stenting may increase the use of this technique. Complications of type B dissections include rupture, aneurysmal degeneration, intractable pain, and evidence of malperfusion. Malperfusion to the lower extremities, viscera, or spine can be caused as a result of the dynamic compression of the true lumen by the false thrombosis of either lumen or by the extension of the dissection onto the branch vessels. Signs of malperfusion include renal insufficiency, abdominal pain, mesenteric ischemia, lower extremity ischemia, paresthesia, or paraplegia. Surgical treatment includes replacement of the descending aorta or fenestration of the abdominal aorta to address visceral or limb malperfusion. Endovascular stent grafts can be used to cover the entry tear, therefore depressurizing the false lumen, expanding the true lumen, and allowing for thrombosis of the false lumen and aortic remodeling.

Ref.: 6

17. What is a type III endoleak?

A. Failure to seal between components of a modular graft system
B. Continued filling of the aneurysm sac by the hypogastric, inferior mesenteric, or lumbar arteries
C. Seepage through a porous graft material
D. Failure to seal the proximal seal zone
E. Failure to seal the distal seal zone

ANSWER: A

COMMENTS: Endovascular repair of AAAs was first described by Parodi et al. in 1991. When compared with an open repair of AAA, it is associated with a shorter length of stay and a lower 30-day morbidity and mortality, but it does not improve the quality of life beyond 3 months or survival beyond 2 years. These advantages have made endovascular repair the preferred treatment for patients with suitable anatomy. However, the implementation of endovascular repair has brought in a different set of complications called endoleaks: continued blood flow into the aneurysm sac. Type I endoleak is the failure to seal the proximal (type Ia) or distal (type Ib) seal zones. These are usually detected at the time of the procedure and should be immediately corrected with more aggressive balloon inflation within the seal zone, placement of additional graft components, or placement of balloon expandable stents. Type II endoleak is the most common type and involves the continued filling of the aneurysm sac by the inferior mesenteric or lumbar arteries. Treatment of type II endoleak is indicated if the size of the sac increases. Treatment options include embolization of the feeding vessels, laparoscopic ligation of the feeding vessels, or sac puncture and embolization. Type III endoleaks represent a failure of the seal between components of a modular graft system. All type III endoleaks should be treated with angioplasty or relining the area of separation with new graft components. Type IV endoleaks involve the seepage of blood through the porous graft material. These are usually self-limiting and resolve after procedural anticoagulation is reversed. Other complications of endovascular AAA repair include device migration, iliac limb thrombosis, or occlusion or graft breakdown. CT surveillance is recommended at 1, 6, and 12 months postoperatively and annually thereafter. If no endoleaks are detected, patients can be transitioned to longer interval screening times and/or the use of ultrasound instead of CT.

Ref.: 6

18. Which of the following is not a noted complication that occurs after an open aortic surgery?

A. Cardiac ischemia

B. Limb ischemia

C. Cerebral ischemia

D. Renal insufficiency

E. Anastomotic pseudoaneurysms

ANSWER: C

COMMENTS: Cardiac ischemia is the most frequent complication after an open aortic surgery, causing 50% of deaths associated with aortic reconstruction. Nearly all patients with occlusive aortic disease also have some degree of coronary pathology. Stress testing, cardiac angiography, and coronary intervention can help to identify and treat patients at the highest risk for postoperative cardiac event. Limb ischemia due to thrombosis occurs in 5%–10% of patients. Renal insufficiency is another common complication and can be caused by embolization from clamping, prolonged suprarenal clamp time, intrinsic renal artery disease, hypovolemia, or hypoperfusion. It directly relates to a patient's preoperative renal and cardiac function. It can be minimized by having a precise plan for clamping sites and sequence based on preoperative imaging studies. Anastomotic pseudoaneurysms can be sterile or caused by infection. They usually occur at the femoral anastomosis opposed to the aortic or iliac anastomoses. This is thought to be secondary to the higher rate of infection and wound breakdown in the femoral area. The diagnosis of postoperative pseudoaneurysms in the iliac or aortic position is based on imaging. There is a higher rate of detection of pseudoaneurysms on imaging than on clinical exam. As pseudoaneurysms are often caused by infection, a full infectious workup should be performed once one is found. This includes history, physical examination, cultures, laboratories, and imaging (including nuclear medicine–tagged white blood cell scans).

Ref.: 6

REFERENCES

1. Reddy DJ, Shepard AD. Aortoiliac disease. In: Mullholland MW, Lillemoe KD, Doherty GM, et al., eds. *Greenfield's Surgery: Scientific Principles and Practice*. 4th ed. Philadelphia: Lippincott Williams & Wilkins; 2006.
2. Lin PH, Kougias P, Bechara C, et al. Arterial disease. In: Brunicardi FC, Andersen DK, Billiar TR, et al., eds. *Schwartz's Principles of Surgery*. 9th ed. New York: McGraw-Hill; 2010.
3. Ernst CB, Stanley JC. *Current Therapy in Vascular Surgery*. 4th ed. St. Louis: CV Mosby; 2001.
4. Cronenwett J, Johnston W, eds. *Rutherford's Vascular Surgery*. 7th ed. Philadelphia: WB Saunders; 2010.
5. Beckles DL, Wait MA. The cardiovascular system. In: O'Leary JP, Tabuenca A, eds. *The Physiologic Basis of Surgery*. 4th ed. Philadelphia: Lippincott Williams & Wilkins; 2008.
6. Tracci MC, Cherry KJ. The aorta. In: Townsend CM, Beauchamp RD, Evers BM, et al., eds. *Sabiston Textbook of Surgery: The Biological Basis of Modern Surgical Practice*. 19th ed. Philadelphia: Elsevier Inc; 2012.

E. Peripheral Vascular—Lower Extremity

Vidyaratna Fleetwood, M.D., and Neha Sheng, M.D.

1. After undergoing femoral embolectomy and fasciotomy, a patient becomes oliguric, and his urine is brownish red in color. Immediate treatment includes which of the following?

A. Cessation of intravenous administration of heparin

B. Restoration of the serum potassium level

C. Intravenous administration of sodium bicarbonate and mannitol

D. Renal arteriography

E. Intraarterial vasodilators

ANSWER: C

COMMENTS: When an extremity has been subjected to ischemia and muscular necrosis occurs, reperfusion can result in metabolic acidosis and profound hyperkalemia. Rhabdomyolysis releases myoglobulin, which precipitates in acidic urine and produces brownish red urine that is free of red blood cells. Treatment of patients in this situation requires prompt reversal of hyperkalemia to prevent cardiac arrest (intravenous insulin and glucose), administration of sodium bicarbonate to alkalinize the urine and to treat the systemic metabolic acidosis, and osmotic diuresis with mannitol to prevent renal tubular obstruction. Fasciotomy is indicated if it has not already been performed. Continuation of anticoagulation therapy is critical because the patient remains at a significant risk for recurrent embolism from the underlying cardiac disease. Less than 10% of arterial emboli involve the renal vessels, and renal arteriography is not indicated in this case.

Ref.: 1

2. After undergoing brachial artery catheterization for coronary angiography, a patient complains of hand numbness, and the previously present radial pulse is noted to be absent. Which of the following is the appropriate treatment?

A. Administration of systemic vasodilators

B. Surgical exploration and topical application of papaverine

C. Percutaneous balloon dilation of the brachial artery

D. Brachial artery exposure with direct repair of the injured segment

E. Arteriography to determine the presence of thrombus at the catheterization site

ANSWER: D

COMMENTS: Iatrogenic arterial injuries may result from the placement of needles and catheters for radiographic studies or monitoring purposes. Arterial occlusion usually occurs because of thrombosis in association with intimal injury. Treatment consists of prompt exploration with arteriotomy and thrombectomy. Intimal damage may be treated by segmental excision with direct anastomosis or by placing a short vein patch. Surgery should not be delayed by attributing the ischemia associated with arterial injury to arterial "spasm." Arteriography to confirm what is already clinically apparent delays the required surgical exploration and is not usually indicated.

Ref.: 1

3. Which of the following is the most common site of atherosclerotic occlusion in the lower extremities?

A. Aortic bifurcation

B. Common femoral artery

C. Profunda femoris artery

D. Proximal superficial femoral artery

E. Distal superficial femoral artery

ANSWER: E

COMMENTS: Although atherosclerotic disease frequently involves the area of arterial bifurcations, such as the aortic, iliac, and common femoral bifurcations, the most common site of occlusion in the lower extremities is the distal superficial femoral artery. The occlusion occurs in the adductor canal proximal to the popliteal fossa and is related to the anatomic relationship of the artery to the adductor magnus tendon at this site. However, affected patients frequently have disease at several levels, which emphasizes the need for accurate angiographic assessment before revascularization procedures. Occlusive disease of the superficial femoral artery alone is generally associated with intermittent claudication but not with tissue loss or pain during rest. The profunda femoris artery usually remains patent and serves as an important source of collateral blood flow.

Ref.: 2

4. Most arterial emboli originate from which one of the following sites?

A. Cardiac valves

B. Left atrium

C. Left ventricle

D. Thoracic aorta

E. Abdominal aorta

ANSWER: B

COMMENTS: Most arterial emboli originate in the heart. Less than 10% arise from ulcerated plaques in the aorta, carotid arteries, or subclavian arteries. The most common intracardiac site is the left atrium, in which thrombi form because of stasis in patients with atrial fibrillation, mitral valvular disease, or both. A rare source of left atrial emboli is a left atrial myxoma. Left ventricular thrombi are a potential source of embolism in patients with myocardial infarction, left ventricular aneurysm, congestive heart failure, or cardiomyopathy. Valvular sources of emboli include vegetative endocarditis and thrombi formed on mechanical prosthetic heart valves. Paradoxical emboli arising from the venous system may reach the arterial circulation through a patent foramen ovale.

Ref.: 1, 2

5. Which of the following statements is true regarding arterial occlusive disease of the lower extremities?

A. Intermittent claudication is a symptom of acute arterial occlusion.

B. Rest pain usually occurs in the same muscle groups affected by claudication and is often relieved by the dependent positioning of the affected extremity.

C. Changes such as hair loss, brittle nails, and muscle atrophy generally precede symptoms of claudication.

D. Tissue necrosis is more likely in the presence of multilevel distal arterial disease.

E. Arterial ulcerations, such as those of venous insufficiency, characteristically begin near the malleoli.

ANSWER: D

COMMENTS: Chronic arterial occlusion of the lower extremities is a result of atherosclerotic disease of the aorta and its branches. It can be diagnosed by the presence of characteristic signs and symptoms. The classic symptom, intermittent claudication, is cramping pain in specific muscle groups that occurs when blood flow is inadequate for meeting the demands of exercise. The pain usually occurs below the level of occlusion. Hence, claudication of the buttock and thigh muscles is suggestive of aortoiliac obstruction, and calf claudication is suggestive of femoral artery obstruction. As the chronic ischemia progresses, trophic changes such as hair loss, nail brittleness, and muscular atrophy occur. Ischemic pain during rest is a manifestation of the end-stage disease and characteristically involves the more distal aspects of the arterial circulation, such as the toes and feet. Pain is typically felt across the metatarsal heads. Associated physical findings include exacerbation of pain with elevation of the extremity, relief of pain by the dependent positioning of the extremity, and dependent rubor (redness of the feet) caused by reactive hyperemia. Tissue necrosis usually signifies a multilevel disease of the distal arterial tree since chronic proximal occlusion alone is associated with the development of collateral circulation, which is normally adequate for preventing necrosis and gangrene. Most ulcers resulting from arterial insufficiency involve the toes or plantar surface of the foot and are painful, whereas venous ulcers are less painful and typically occur near the malleoli.

Ref.: 1, 2

6. Regarding Buerger's disease, which of the following statements is correct?

A. It is most frequently found in African-American men aged 20 to 40 years.

B. Recurrent migratory superficial phlebitis often follows arterial involvement.

C. Sympathectomy is effective in 50% of patients, but arterial reconstruction offers better long-term results.

D. Cessation of cigarette smoking is the primary therapy.

E. It can be treated successfully with anticoagulants, vasodilators, and steroids.

ANSWER: D

COMMENTS: Buerger's disease (thromboangiitis obliterans) is an inflammatory process of uncertain etiology that produces thrombosis of medium-sized and small arteries and veins. The disease typically affects young men who are heavy smokers. It is rare in African-Americans. Recurrent migratory superficial thrombophlebitis involving the pedal veins often predates arterial involvement by several years. Both the upper and lower extremities can be affected, and ischemic gangrene frequently results. Complete cessation of tobacco use is the most important aspect of treatment and may produce remission. Simply decreasing the frequency of tobacco use is ineffective. Arterial reconstruction is not usually possible because distal small vessels are frequently involved. Cervical or lumbar sympathectomy is useful in 50% of patients. No pharmacologic treatment has proved widely successful.

Ref.: 1, 2

7. Regarding the appropriate management of popliteal aneurysms, which of the following statements is true?

A. A popliteal artery aneurysm should be managed conservatively if it is 3 cm in diameter and if the patient is asymptomatic.

B. Popliteal aneurysms are bilateral in up to 25% of patients.

C. Excision with end-to-end anastomosis is the procedure of choice for popliteal artery aneurysms.

D. The presence of a popliteal aneurysm should heighten suspicion for arterial aneurysms in the abdomen and thorax.

E. Rupture is the most common complication of a popliteal aneurysm.

ANSWER: D

COMMENTS: Peripheral aneurysms are primarily atherosclerotic in origin, associated with hypertension, and frequently multiple. Popliteal artery aneurysms are the most common; they are bilateral in 50%–70% of patients and approximately 50% are associated with femoral or aortic aneurysms. Patients with bilateral popliteal artery aneurysms have a 70% chance of having an AAA. Patients with popliteal aneurysms therefore require a thorough assessment to rule out other associated aneurysms. Popliteal aneurysms present a high risk for limb loss because of thrombosis or embolism, and rupture is very rare. Popliteal aneurysms should be operated on if mural thrombus is identified in the vessel and if the patient has symptoms of ischemia or mass effect. There is a debate about the size at which popliteal aneurysms should be repaired, with some advocating a criterion of 2 cm, others advocating 3 cm, and still others recommending that the decision be based upon the presence of symptoms and mural thrombus. Proximal and distal ligation with interposition grafting is the procedure of choice. Occasionally, if the aneurysm is small and the artery is tortuous, excision with end-to-end anastomosis is feasible.

Ref.: 2

8. Regarding Raynaud disease or phenomenon, which of the following statements is correct?

A. It is characterized by sequential phases of pallor, cyanosis, and rubor in the upper extremities that are initiated by exposure to heat or emotional stress.

B. It is seen most frequently in elderly women.

C. It is characterized by a pathologic mechanism that involves vasospasm with a reduction in dermal circulation.

D. β-Blockers often yield symptomatic control.

E. Cervical sympathectomy is usually the primary therapy.

ANSWER: C

COMMENTS: Raynaud disease or phenomenon is the most common vasospastic disorder, and it most frequently affects young women (90% of patients are younger than 40 years). It may exist as a primary disorder (Raynaud disease) or as a secondary manifestation (Raynaud phenomenon) of disorders such as scleroderma, Buerger's disease, or thoracic outlet syndrome. The classic pattern of pallor, cyanosis, and rubor occurs after exposure to cold or stress. Vasospasm with a decrease in dermal circulation results in pallor. Cyanosis occurs because of sluggish flow of blood. Reactive hyperemia then develops as the vasospasm subsides. Avoidance of initiating factors is often adequate. Calcium channel blockers are the initial drug of choice.

Ref.: 2

9. A 61-year-old male smoker presents to your clinic with complaints of posterior calf pain consistently appearing after walking two blocks. This prevents him from performing many of his activities of daily living, as walking is his primary form of transport. Ankle-brachial indices (ABIs) were obtained and were found to be greater than 0.9 bilaterally. What is the most appropriate next step?

A. Reassurance and 1-year follow-up
B. Repeat ABIs
C. Exercise ABIs
D. Imaging of the lumbar spine
E. Catheter-directed angiography

ANSWER: C

COMMENTS: The ABI is a simple, informative, noninvasive method of evaluating lower extremity perfusion. The test is generally performed at rest, with the patient positioned supine. A pneumatic pressure cuff is placed just above the elbow and ankle on each side. The cuff is then inflated to suprasystolic pressure; as the cuff is deflated, the pressure reading when the Doppler signal returns is recorded. The pressure in the bilateral brachial arteries, dorsalis pedis arteries, and posterior tibial arteries is recorded. The higher brachial artery systolic pressure serves as the denominator for the ABI on both lower extremities. The numerator is determined by the higher value between the dorsalis pedis and posterior tibial arteries on each side. A normal ABI is 0.9 to 1.2; claudication usually occurs between 0.4 and 0.8; ischemic rest pain usually arises at 0.2 to 0.4; and gangrene can develop at less than 0.2.

There are two main limitations to ABIs. In diabetic patients, medial calcinosis of the vessels limits compressibility, preventing accurate measurement and manifesting as false elevation of the ABI, often greater than 1.2. These patients can be evaluated with digital pressures in the toes. Alternate modalities include computed tomography (CT) angiography, magnetic resonance angiography (MRA), and catheter-directed angiography. The second limitation is the measurement of pressures at rest. For some patients, the ABIs may be normal at rest and may diminish with exercise. For these patients, ABI measured after exercise may reveal the underlying arterial occlusive disease.

Further evaluation is necessary before providing reassurance only in a patient with significant lifestyle handicap due to symptoms. Repeat measurement of ABI at rest would be of low yield. The presenting symptoms of the patient in this vignette are highly consistent with vascular claudication. In the event that exercise ABI is normal, spinal stenosis should be considered and imaging of the lumbar spine would be indicated.

Both CT angiography and catheter-directed angiography are indicated for surgical planning in patients with an established diagnosis of arterial occlusive disease and an indication for surgery. Exercise ABI can help establish the diagnosis in this patient. Prior to establishing the diagnosis, angiography would be an unnecessarily invasive modality and should be deferred.

Ref.: 1, 2

10. A 64-year-old male with a history of ischemic rest pain for which he underwent a prosthetic femoral–popliteal artery bypass 5 months ago presents in the emergency department with groin pain, erythema, tenderness, and mass. He is afebrile and normotensive. Laboratory results show a leukocyte count of 9000 per uL and an erythrocyte sedimentation rate of 150 mm/hr. An ultrasound of the groin demonstrates an echolucent rim, or "halo sign," around the anastomosis. What is the most likely diagnosis?

A. Inguinal hernia
B. Lymphatic leak
C. Wound infection
D. Lymphadenopathy
E. Graft infection

ANSWER: E

COMMENTS: See Question 11 for comments.

Ref.: 1, 2

11. For the patient in the prior problem, what is the most likely organism?

A. *Staphylococcus aureus*
B. *S. epidermidis*
C. *Pseudomonas aeruginosa*
D. *Escherichia coli*
E. *Mycoplasma*

ANSWER: B

COMMENTS: Vascular prostheses are sometimes necessary in the absence of a suitable vein autograft. These have multiple limitations including cost, lower patency rate than autogenous conduit, and increased risk for infection. The overall risk for infection varies by graft site but ranges from 2% to 6% at the femoral level. Infection can be acquired by local contamination from skin or lymph or from hematogenous seeding from any source. Most prosthetic graft infections are thought to be initiated at the time of implantation and are frequently acquired from the skin.

The presentation of graft infection varies by organism. The most common organism found in late graft infections is *S. epidermidis*. This is a low-virulence organism and usually presents late, sometimes months to years postoperatively. This organism does not usually produce systemic symptoms or leukocytosis, although the erythrocyte sedimentation rate is frequently elevated. The patients often present with local manifestations, such as chronically draining purulent groin sinuses, chronic wound infection with exposed graft, anastomotic pseudoaneurysm, or thrombosis. High-virulence organisms such as *S. aureus*, *P. aeruginosa*, and *E. coli* frequently present in the earlier postoperative phase, with systemic symptoms and sepsis. *S. aureus* is the second most common organism isolated after *S. epidermidis*. *Mycoplasma* is an uncommon isolate.

The diagnosis of a graft infection can be made on clinical examination or with imaging. CT scans are frequently the first images obtained and can show gas, fluid around the graft, and false aneurysm. Ultrasound is a sensitive and noninvasive adjunct. The findings mostly associated with graft infection are an echolucent rim, or halo sign, around the graft, signifying perigraft fluid, as well as anastomotic pseudoaneurysms. The gold standard treatment for graft infection is complete excision of the prosthetic graft.

Ref.: 1, 2

12. A patient undergoes femoral artery bypass for a traumatic injury to the lower extremity incurred 6 h prior to the operative repair. He later develops increasing pain, pallor, and coolness in his calf. He becomes oliguric, and his urine changes color to brownish red. Which of the following findings is not consistent with his pathology?

A. Pain out of proportion to physical examination

B. Urinalysis with large amounts of blood noted on dipstick but few red blood cells on microscopic analysis

C. Creatinine phosphokinase (CPK) deposition in the renal tubules

D. Numbness in the web space between the first two toes

E. Compartment pressure greater than 30 mmHg

ANSWER: C

COMMENTS: See Question 13.

Ref.: 2

13. For the patient in Question 12, what is the next step?

A. Placement of Foley urinary catheter

B. CT angiography

C. Measurement of compartment pressures

D. Fasciotomy of the affected extremity

E. Serial examinations

ANSWER: D

COMMENTS: Compartment syndrome of the extremity results from an increased pressure within a volume-limited, closed space. The pressure results from edema of the compartment musculature secondary to reperfusion injury. The investing fascia creates a barrier to the expansion of the tissues and compresses the vasculature, causing ischemia. An early sign of compartment syndrome is a loss of sensation in the first interdigital space. Other classic signs of compartment syndrome include paresthesia, pallor, poikilothermia, pain out of proportion to examination, and motor weakness, and a late sign is pulselessness. A direct measurement of the compartment pressure greater than 30 mmHg is pathognomonic.

The muscle necrosis of compartment syndrome causes myoglobin and CPK to be released. Myoglobin deposits in the renal tubules, causing tubular injury and acute renal failure if untreated. Myoglobin registers on urinalysis as hemoglobin, leading to the classic findings of bloody urine—in appearance and on dipstick test—with few blood cells detected under microscopy. The treatment of renal failure due to compartment syndrome includes alkalinization of the urine and mannitol infusion.

Hyperkalemia is a common complication of myonecrosis and can cause arrhythmias if not treated aggressively.

Compartment syndrome is ultimately a clinical diagnosis. Increased serum CPK levels and compartment pressures and myoglobinuria can provide a clue to diagnosis, but any patient with clinical risk factors—prolonged leg ischemia for greater than 4 h—and new findings consistent with compartment syndrome should be taken immediately to the operating room for fasciotomy. A delay in treatment, whether by the lack of recognition or pursuing further unnecessary imaging, can lead to further ischemia and ultimate loss of limb.

Ref.: 1, 2

14. For an acute arterial embolus to the lower extremity with limb-threatening ischemia, appropriate initial treatment includes which of the following?

A. Intravenous heparin bolus (80 units/kg) followed by continuous infusion (18 units/kg per hour)

B. Delay in heparinization until anesthesia is administered because heparinization precludes spinal anesthesia

C. Routine preoperative trial of vasodilators

D. Attempt at thrombolytic therapy with drugs such as tissue plasminogen activator (0.5 mg/h)

E. Immediate angiography before an operation

ANSWER: A

COMMENTS: Treatment of arterial embolism must be initiated promptly to prevent irreversible ischemic damage. Intravenous heparin should be administered to prevent the formation and propagation of thrombosis distal to the embolus and is the most important first step. Heparinization should not be delayed, particularly because most embolectomies can be performed with the use of local anesthesia. Furthermore, the degree of distal thrombosis is an important determinant of surgical success and limb salvage. Although arterial spasm accompanies acute arterial occlusion, the routine use of vasodilators is not advocated. Fibrinolytic agents have an important role in the treatment of patients with acute thrombosis superimposed on chronic ischemia. However, their routine use in the treatment of acute arterial embolism with limb-threatening ischemia is not advocated. Because patients with arterial embolism often have associated cardiac disease and may be compromised further by the metabolic effects of ischemic tissue, preoperative attention must be given to careful physiologic monitoring and to the fluid balance, electrolyte balance, and arterial blood gas status of the patient.

Ref.: 1, 2

15. Regarding aortoiliac atherosclerotic occlusive disease, which of the following statements is correct?

A. Impotence is a common finding that results from decreased blood flow through the external iliac vessels.

B. Thigh or buttock claudication (or both) is typical, and toe ulceration or gangrene secondary to atherosclerotic emboli is occasionally present.

C. Lower extremity hair loss and nail brittleness occur in 60% of patients.

D. Hemorrhage and sepsis are the principal causes of death after aortoiliac reconstruction.

E. Percutaneous angioplasty with stenting of iliac lesions only occasionally relieves symptoms.

ANSWER: B

COMMENTS: An accurate history and physical examination can help establish the diagnosis of aortoiliac atherosclerotic occlusive disease. The classic clinical presentation, Leriche syndrome, includes intermittent claudication of the thighs or buttocks, impotence, and diminished or absent femoral pulses. Impotence is caused by internal iliac arterial occlusion, which reduces blood flow through the internal pudendal artery and the corpora cavernosa. However, with aortoiliac involvement alone, trophic changes are rarely present because collateral flow originating from the lumbar and epigastric arteries is preserved. Nutritional changes, such as hair loss and brittle nails, when present, are indicative of additional distal arterial occlusive disease. Although distal tissue necrosis is often suggestive of more distal occlusive disease, the possibility of emboli from atherosclerotic plaque in the aortoiliac vessels must always be considered. This has been referred to as the "blue toe syndrome" and can occur even in the absence of occluding lesions. The principal cause of death in this group of patients is coronary artery disease. Iliac angioplasty with stenting is particularly successful in treating short-segment iliac disease. When a multilevel disease necessitates conventional distal bypass techniques, adequate inflow may be established with balloon angioplasty of the iliac arteries.

Ref.: 1–3

16. Any patient with intermittent calf claudication should be advised of which of the following?

A. Angiography should be performed early to determine the extent of the arterial disease.

B. Surgical reconstruction should be performed to prevent the progression of disease and the development of pain at rest with gangrene.

C. Nonoperative treatment is sufficient for 50% of patients.

D. There are no indications for arterial revascularization in patients with claudication.

E. Claudication progresses to gangrene in 2%–3% of patients per year.

ANSWER: E

COMMENTS: The goals of **therapy for the occlusive arterial disease** of the lower extremities are to relieve pain, prevent limb loss, and maintain bipedal gait. Most patients with intermittent claudication alone remain stable or even improve with appropriate conservative management. Such management includes a formal exercise program, smoking cessation, and risk reduction and may include medications such as cilostazol (Pletal). Daily aspirin therapy has been shown to be beneficial for such patients by reducing the risk for morbidity from concomitant atherosclerotic disease, such as stroke and myocardial infarction. Prophylactic surgical intervention is not indicated. Patients with claudication have a low rate of progression to gangrene. In fact, more than 75% of these patients remain stable, and the amputation rate is less than 7% in patients treated nonoperatively and observed for up to 8 years. In patients with severe claudication and marked involvement of the tibial vessels, the disease progresses to gangrene in 2%–3% of patients annually. This contrasts with patients having pain at rest, ulceration, or gangrene, who are at risk for limb loss and should be evaluated for revascularization. Surgical intervention is reserved for patients whose lifestyle or livelihood is impaired by their symptoms and who do not otherwise have a limiting cardiac disease. Arteriography is indicated for patients who are considered candidates for surgery or angioplasty, but it should be preceded by less invasive testing, such as arterial blood flow studies.

Ref.: 1–3

17. Occlusive tibioperoneal disease does not occur commonly in patients with which of the following entities?

A. Buerger's disease

B. Raynaud phenomenon

C. Diabetes mellitus

D. Arterial emboli

E. Tobacco use

ANSWER: B

COMMENTS: Although common patterns of atherosclerotic occlusive disease involve the femoral artery or the more proximal aortoiliac system, diabetic patients characteristically acquire a pattern of distal occlusive disease involving the distal popliteal artery and the tibial and metatarsal vessels. Buerger's disease, or thromboangiitis obliterans, is associated with tobacco use; it results in inflammatory thrombosis of the small and medium sized vessels of the upper and lower extremities. This type of distal involvement may also be seen in patients with an arterial embolism. Patients with tibioperoneal involvement are often initially found to have advanced ischemia rather than simple claudication, and arterial reconstruction may necessitate bypass grafting to target vessels at the ankle or proximal part of the foot. Raynaud syndrome is characterized by vasospasm of the small arteries and arterioles of the most distal portions of the extremities, such as in the hands, feet, and digits.

Ref.: 2, 3

18. A patient with atrial fibrillation arrives at the emergency room with a cold, pulseless leg and undergoes femoral embolectomy. His pedal pulses are palpable. He subsequently develops compartment syndrome. A single-incision decompressive fasciotomy is performed. After the procedure, his CPK levels continues to rise rapidly. What is the most likely diagnosis?

A. Inadequate fasciotomy

B. Missed arterial injury

C. New embolus at an alternate site

D. Crush injury from prolonged immobility

E. Myocardial infarction

ANSWER: A

COMMENTS: Treatment for compartment syndrome of the lower extremity involves a four-compartment fasciotomy. The fasciotomy can be performed using a single- or double-incision technique; two-incision fasciotomy is standard.

In the single-incision approach, the skin is incised at a point 1 cm anterior to the fibular head and carried down to just superior to the lateral malleolus. From this incision, the fascia of the anterior, lateral, and superficial posterior compartments can be accessed and opened. The deep posterior compartment can be accessed by dissecting the soleus off of the fibula.

In the double-incision approach, the soleus is left in place and a second incision is made 1 cm posterior to the medial border of the tibia in order to access the deep compartment.

Incomplete fasciotomy with inadequate release of the posterior compartment is a risk for the fasciotomy procedure, and meticulous surgical technique should be used to prevent this technical error. A generous length of fasciotomy of each compartment should be performed to prevent inadequate fasciotomy.

Missed arterial injury after embolectomy and new embolus are unlikely and would clinically manifest in other ways.

New crush injury is not likely.

Myocardial infarction, while less likely than incomplete fasciotomy in this case, is certainly a concern in the high-risk vascular patient population and should be ruled out if any clinical suspicion exists.

Ref.: 2, 3

19. Which of the following statements is NOT true regarding endovascular management of lower extremity ischemia?

A. Iliac stenosis may be treated with endovascular techniques, but occlusions must be addressed surgically.

B. Superficial femoral artery stenosis greater than 10 cm in length has much-reduced patency after endovascular therapy than an open surgical therapy.

C. If percutaneous balloon angioplasty results in the flow-limiting dissection of the target artery, placement of a stent is indicated.

D. Endovascular stents can be placed primarily to treat severe arterial occlusions or recurrent stenosis.

E. Infrapopliteal angioplasty results in a 2-year limb salvage rate of 50%–80% despite much lower patency rates.

ANSWER: A

COMMENTS: Endovascular techniques play an integral role in the management of peripheral arterial occlusive disease. Long-term patency following angioplasty depends largely on the site being treated and the severity of the stenosis. Proximal, larger-caliber arteries have the best initial and long-term results, whereas distal sites have lower patency rates. Results are better for the treatment of short, focal stenosis rather than long stenosis in diffusely diseased arteries. Stenoses less than 2 cm are considered ideal lesions for percutaneous treatment, whereas those longer than 10 cm have poor patency with endovascular repair. Iliac stenosis and occlusions may both be treated with percutaneous endovascular technique. Although initial success rates in treating occlusions are somewhat lower, some series have shown similar long-term patency rates for both stenosis and occlusions of the iliac artery. This may be due partly to increased use of intravascular stents when treating occlusions. Although stents certainly have a role in treating postangioplasty dissections or residual stenosis, primary stent placement may be considered for treating longer, more complex lesions, recurrent lesions, lesions likely to embolize (e.g., arteries with ulcerated plaque), and occlusions. In poor operative candidates with limb-threatening ischemia, infrapopliteal angioplasty may be considered. Although the 2-year limb salvage rate for such procedures has been reported to be 50%–80%, patency rates are significantly lower at 30%–40%.

Ref.: 3

20. Regarding atheroembolic disease of the lower extremities, which of the following is true?

A. Atheroemboli commonly cause acute occlusion of the common femoral bifurcation.

B. Normal pedal pulses are commonly found in patients with atheroembolic disease.

C. The most common source of atheroemboli is superficial femoral artery atherosclerotic disease.

D. Medical therapy is associated with a low rate of recurrence.

E. Aortofemoral bypass, femoropopliteal bypass, extraanatomic bypass with aortic exclusion, and localized endarterectomy are not indicated for the management of atheroembolic disease.

ANSWER: B

COMMENTS: The term *atheroemboli* describes cholesterol or atherothrombotic microemboli. Both aneurysms and atherosclerotic plaque may be the sources of microemboli. The aortoiliac atherosclerotic disease is the most common source of lower extremity microemboli. Although macroemboli from cardiac sources tend to lodge at the bifurcations of large vessels, microemboli commonly lodge in the distal small vessels, such as the digital arteries of the toes. Cholesterol debris is often found on pathologic review of patients with atheroemboli. Patients typically have a sudden appearance of painful, mottled areas on their toes. Microemboli may lodge in the capillaries of the skin and lead to livedo reticularis of the knees, thighs, and buttocks. Typically, patients have palpable pedal pulses. Duplex scans may help define atherosclerotic lesions, but CT angiography and conventional angiography are more sensitive diagnostic methods for determining the source of emboli.

Medical management alone (e.g., with antiplatelet agents, steroids, aspirin, or warfarin) is associated with a high rate of recurrence. Warfarin may lead to exacerbation of the condition because of plaque destabilization. Surgical intervention is indicated to remove the embolic source and reconstruct the arterial tree if necessary. Aortofemoral bypass, femoropopliteal bypass, extraanatomic bypass with aortic exclusion, and localized endarterectomy may all be indicated, depending on the location and extent of disease. Endovascular therapy with covered stents may also treat this condition, depending on the anatomy of the embolic source.

Ref.: 1–4

21. Regarding popliteal entrapment syndrome, which of the following is true?

A. The syndrome commonly affects men before the age of 40.

B. Limb-threatening ischemia is the most common manifestation.

C. Fibrous bands of the popliteus muscle most commonly cause arterial impingement.

D. CT is the diagnostic procedure of choice.

E. Symptoms are usually treated by exercise and antiplatelet medications.

ANSWER: A

COMMENTS: The popliteal artery entrapment syndrome most commonly affects men before the age of 40. The most common finding is mild, intermittent claudication. Arterial thrombosis or occlusion is rare. Other, less common causes of claudication in young adults include premature atherosclerosis caused by malignant hyperlipidemia, adventitial cystic disease, chronic exertional compartment syndrome, and vasculitis secondary to collagen vascular disorders. Physical examination typically reveals a loss of tibial pulses with active plantar flexion or passive dorsiflexion to tighten the gastrocnemius muscle. Noninvasive blood flow studies and duplex scanning may also reveal the abnormality when done in conjunction with these flexion maneuvers. The most sensitive diagnostic study is MR imaging, which can delineate the musculotendinous structures of the popliteal fossa and document their dynamic relationship with the popliteal vessels. The most common abnormality encountered is medial deviation of the popliteal artery around the medial head of the gastrocnemius muscle. Five other anatomic variants have been described. Surgical repair is the only effective treatment for symptomatic patients. Resection or release of the variant musculotendinous structures is performed. Arterial reconstruction is necessary when stenotic or aneurysmal lesions are present. Surgical repair is also recommended for asymptomatic patients who are noted to have anatomic variants on the opposite side to prevent the development of secondary vascular complications.

Ref.: 3, 4

22. A 50-year-old male patient presents to the emergency room with complaints of acute right lower extremity pain and pallor. On examination, the dorsalis pedal and posterior tibial arterial pulses are absent and no pedal arterial signal is audible to Doppler examination, but a venous signal can be obtained. He has decreased sensation and range of motion in his right foot but is still able to walk with it with some support; he is complaining of profound pain. Which of the following is the most appropriate definitive treatment?

A. Systemic heparinization alone

B. Heparinization and thrombolysis

C. Thrombolysis alone

D. Systemic heparinization and surgical thromboembolectomy

E. Amputation

ANSWER: D

COMMENTS: This patient is presenting with acute limb ischemia (ALI), one of the most common vascular emergencies. This is most commonly caused by cardiac emboli, but may occur in the setting of acute thrombosis of chronic arterial occlusive disease. The treatment depends on the severity of ischemia and viability of the foot.

ALI is staged as follows: I, viable; IIa, threatened marginally; IIb, threatened immediately; and III, irreversible.

Grade	Category	Sensorimotor	Doppler
I	Viable	No sensorimotor deficits	+ Arterial signal + Venous signal
IIa	Marginally threatened	Minimal deficits	± Arterial signal + Venous signal
IIb	Immediately threatened	Mild-to-moderate deficits	− Arterial signal + Venous signal
III	Irreversible	Profound deficit	Absent signals

An accurate grading of injury is crucial, especially when differentiating between marginally and immediately threatened. Grade I ischemia can often be safely treated with heparin infusion alone if there are no sensory or motor deficits and serial history and physical examination reveal improvement. Grade III ischemia is irreversible and is best treated with amputation prior to the onset of gangrene or myonecrosis.

Grade IIa injury can be treated with either surgical revascularization or catheter-directed thrombolysis. The latter often requires multiple returns to the procedure suite for reimaging and adjustment of the catheter. However, grade IIb injury—with marked sensorimotor deficits and pain—is more safely treated with an urgent surgical embolectomy or emergent bypass.

An important point is that all patients with acute limb injury should receive heparin infusion regardless of other treatments, immediately upon diagnosis, unless there is any contraindication to anticoagulation.

Ref.: 2, 5

23. The patient in Question 22 returns to the clinic after catheter-directed angiography. The images demonstrate mild, nonocclusive stenosis along the length of the superficial femoral artery with less than 30% luminal narrowing. He has extensive infrapopliteal disease beginning at the origin of the anterior tibial artery, with multiple tandem stenosis along his anterior tibial, peroneal, and posterior tibial arteries. All arteries are observed to disappear midway down his calf with no detectable runoff to the foot. During his stay in your clinic, the patient mentions increasing pain. On examination of his foot, his ulcer is now erythematous and foul-smelling with purulent exudate. Red streaks extend along the dorsum of his foot. What is the next step in management?

A. Trial of broad-spectrum antibiotics alone

B. Transmetatarsal amputation

C. Guillotine amputation at the ankle

D. Below-knee amputation

E. Femoral–popliteal bypass

ANSWER: C

COMMENTS: This patient has progressed to wet gangrene. Only single-vessel runoff to the foot is needed to heal wounds, but absent runoff is a poor prognostic factor for healing. With wet gangrene, intravenous antibiotics will not be sufficient; debridement is necessary, and amputation is often indicated. Guillotine amputation above the level of infection should be the first step. Revision to a formal amputation should be planned several days later, should no further debridement be necessary.

However, the imaging in this patient indicates extensive infrapopliteal disease with no apparent targets for bypass placement; therefore definitive amputation will be required at the transtibial level. The presence of a palpable popliteal pulse indicates that he is likely to heal at this level of amputation.

Ref.: 2, 5

24. A 24-year-old male presents in your trauma bay with a gunshot wound to his right arm. He has a decreased right radial pulse and a nonexpanding hematoma in his forearm but no hard signs of arterial injury; he therefore undergoes CT angiography. The images demonstrate contrast extravasation from the radial artery. On examination, he has no sensory or motor deficits and his palmar arch is intact. Which of the following is true?

A. The ulnar artery is the dominant circulation to the hand in 60% of people.

B. The radial artery may be safely ligated in this patient.

C. Arterial reconstruction is mandatory in this patient.

D. An interposition graft using the ipsilateral cephalic vein is necessary to prevent neurologic sequelae.

E. Selective angiography and coiling should be performed.

ANSWER: B

COMMENTS: Expedient diagnosis and management of extremity injuries are essential to reduce the risk for limb loss. Hard signs indicate a very high probability of vascular injury and require immediate operative exploration; these include absent distal pulses, palpable thrill or audible bruit, an actively expanding hematoma, and active pulsatile bleeding. Soft signs suggest an injury, but additional workup is indicated to confirm the diagnosis. Soft signs of vascular injury include diminished but distal pulses, history of significant hemorrhage prior to arrival in the trauma bay, neurologic deficits, and proximity of the injury to the vessel.

Further imaging may be obtained with CT angiography or invasive arteriography. CT angiography has the advantage of being quicker and less invasive and has been found to be equally reliable at diagnosing the arterial injury.

If only one of the forearm arteries is injured and an Allen test reveals a patent palmar arch, the injury can be safely ligated. If an Allen test reveals that the palmar arch is not intact or neurovascular symptoms are present, hand perfusion is likely dependent on the injured vessel and arterial reconstruction is indicated.

If both forearm arteries are injured, the ulnar artery should be preferentially repaired as it is the dominant circulation to the hand in 95% of patients. Like the brachial, the forearm arteries are most commonly amenable to mobilization and end-to-end repair.

In this case, bleeding is evident on imaging and the patient must undergo surgical exploration for control of hemorrhage. Since the patient has a patent palmar arch, the radial artery may be ligated.

Ref.: 2, 5

25. A patient sustains a penetrating injury to his radial artery, causing an expanding hematoma in his forearm. As the operating room is being prepared, you attempt to obtain a baseline neurologic examination. Which of the following motor deficits appears first?

A. Inability to oppose thumb and index finger

B. Inability to oppose the thumb and fifth finger

C. Inability to adduct and abduct the fingers

D. Inability to flex wrist

E. Inability to extend elbow

ANSWER: C

COMMENTS: Patients with compromised extremities of any etiology should undergo a full neurologic examination prior to an operation to allow full assessment of postoperative recovery and any inadvertent intraoperative nerve injury. In the upper extremity, the brachial plexus forms three separate nerve trunks that divide to form the radial, median, and ulnar sensorimotor nerves and the musculocutaneous sensory nerve.

The ulnar nerve provides sensory input to the medial palm and fourth and fifth fingers as well as controls finger abduction and adduction via the interossei. The functions of the interossei are the first to be lost in an ischemic insult.

The radial nerve carries sensory information from the upper arm proximal to the elbow and controls elbow flexion and extension and wrist extension.

The median nerve is sensory to the lateral palm and first three fingers and controls thumb movements other than adduction (ulnar) and extension (radial). Apposition, or using the index finger and thumb for a pincer-like movement, and opposition of the thumb to the fifth finger are controlled by the median nerve.

Nerve deficits in vascular trauma patients can be secondary to the initial ischemic insult, compression, traction injury of the nerves, or cautery damage intraoperatively. Occupational therapy consultation is recommended for persistent postoperative neurapraxias. Any progressive nerve deficit after an adequate repair should prompt evaluation for a postoperative hematoma or compartment syndrome.

Ref.: 3, 5

26. A 65-year-old diabetic patient with a history of smoking presents to your clinic with an ulcer of the foot. He has never been evaluated by a vascular surgeon but has undergone an ABI measurement, ordered by his primary care physician. The results revealed elevated indices of 1.8 bilaterally. He denies fevers or other systemic symptoms and has not noticed ascending foot pain, but he does note an occasional "pins and needles" sensation in both feet. On examination, he has a painless ulcer present on the plantar surface of the left foot, underlying the second metatarsal head. There is black eschar at the edges of the ulcer. The ulcer is deep to the subcutaneous tissue, but no bone is exposed. There is no significant surrounding erythema; minimal granulation tissue is present. His left dorsalis pedis and posterior tibial arterial pulses are absent, but a weak popliteal pulse is present. What is the next step in management?

A. Leg elevation and reassurance

B. A course of broad-spectrum antibiotics

C. Wide debridement of the wound

D. Second ray amputation

E. CT or catheter-directed angiography

ANSWER: E

COMMENTS: This patient is presenting with a diabetic foot ulcer, likely due to repeated foot trauma. He has diminished protective sensation on his foot due to diabetic neuropathy. The wound has no clinical signs of infection in this vignette and should be treated with local wound care and pressure offloading with orthotics.

However, given his concomitant arterial disease, the patient requires further evaluation of his arterial perfusion and revascularization if indicated. His elevated ABIs provide a clue to the extensive degree of calcifications in his vessels.

Further imaging is indicated by CT angiography, catheter-directed angiography, or MRA. In patients with extensive calcification, CT imaging may be of limited utility, as the calcifications obscure adequate evaluation of the infrapopliteal arteries. Furthermore, the contrast load can be hazardous to patients with preexisting renal compromise. Catheter-directed angiography is a highly sensitive and specific modality. It can be performed using a lower contrast dose, but this imaging modality does require invasive arterial access. MRA is highly sensitive and specific for arterial disease; however, arterial calcifications are not well detected.

Leg elevation is a useful adjunct in an edematous leg but should be avoided in patients with suspected ischemic disease, as it reduces flow to the foot. Antibiotics and wide debridement are not necessary in this patient who does not have signs of active infection. Second ray amputation would be premature without evaluation for adequate perfusion for wound healing.

Ref.: 5

27. A 75-year-old woman, who had for dry gangrene of the left third toe, underwent a femoral to popliteal bypass with synthetic graft 3 weeks ago. She now presents with groin edema and drainage of copious serosanguinous fluid from her incision. She has no systemic symptoms of infection. Her leukocyte count and erythrocyte sedimentation rate are normal. Compression dressings are applied and the patient is placed on bed rest, but the drainage worsens. Which of the following is the most definitive step in management?

A. A brief course of antibiotics

B. Opening of the wound at bedside for drainage

C. Operative reexploration

D. Graft excision

E. Upper extremity musculocutaneous free flap

ANSWER: C

COMMENTS: Lymphatic complications occur in up to 6% of groin operations. Lymphatic complications can be prevented by minimizing dissection medial to the femoral vessels and by meticulously ligating all lymphatics and closing the wound in multiple layers. Extensive dissection in the groin, presence of prosthetic material, and reoperation are risk factors for lymphocele or lymphorrhea. These complications occur more commonly in older patients, diabetics, and smokers. The diagnosis of lymphorrhea is usually made clinically, by persistent leakage of clear or yellow fluid from the groin incision. Patients generally present without infectious symptoms or leukocytosis, which can help differentiate a wound infection. Secondary graft infection is unusual but can occur.

The initial treatment is conservative management, including compression wraps of the extremity, local wound care, and bed rest with leg elevation. If large volume output continues after several days, surgical closure with lymphatic ligation should be pursued. Leaking lymphatics can be identified intraoperatively with the aid of isosulfan blue administration.

In this case, the patient has failed conservative management and must undergo reexploration for ligation of the lymphatic leak. Antibiotics are often used as an adjunct to prevent graft infection but are not definitive treatment. Opening the wound at the bedside can expose an underlying graft or femoral vessels under nonsterile conditions and should be avoided. A flap may be considered but a musculocutaneous free flap is unnecessary. In severe cases, especially if prosthetic graft is present, a sartorius muscle rotational flap may be considered to decrease the rate of recurrence. Graft excision is required if the graft is demonstrated to be infected.

Ref.: 5

28. Which of the following is true regarding the thoracic outlet syndrome (TOS)?

A. Venous TOS is the most prevalent subtype.

B. Subclavian stents are the most effective treatment for venous TOS.

C. Arterial TOS is most commonly caused by bony abnormalities, such as a cervical rib.

D. Venous TOS is most commonly caused by bony abnormalities, such as a cervical rib.

E. Neurogenic TOS is an operative emergency to prevent progressive neurapraxia.

ANSWER: C

COMMENTS: TOS is a general term for many symptoms and signs resulting from compression of the neurovascular bundle in the thoracic outlet. The neurovascular bundle consists of the brachial plexus, subclavian vein, and subclavian artery; therefore there are three types of TOS: neurogenic, venous, and arterial.

The neurogenic subtype is most common at 95% of TOS cases; venous is 3%, and arterial is 1%. Neurogenic is most commonly caused by neck trauma or falls. Predisposing factors are a cervical rib or scalene muscle fibrosis. The symptoms are extremity pain, paresthesias, and weakness; patients can also present with neck pain and headaches. Diagnosis is made with electromyography (EMG) and appropriate imaging. The initial treatment is physical therapy, to which 20%–30% of patients respond; the rest can be considered for first rib resection.

Venous TOS, or Paget-Schrotter syndrome, results from axillary-subclavian vein thrombosis due to compression. It is more common in patients with an occupational need for repetitive upper arm and shoulder movements. The symptoms are upper extremity edema, pain and sometimes cyanosis of the extremity, and dilated veins with collateralization. Pain is common. The initial diagnostic workup consists of duplex ultrasound; venography can be used if ultrasonography is equivocal. The treatment is surgical relief of compression via rib resection, with or without thrombus removal (via thrombolysis and/or thrombectomy) and vein reconstruction for any stenosis. The patient should still undergo 3 to 6 months of therapeutic anticoagulation for complete treatment of the deep venous thrombosis. Stents are likely to occlude due to compressive forces and have no role in the treatment.

Arterial TOS is most commonly caused by a cervical rib. These patients most commonly present with hand ischemia due to microembolization but may also have mild exertional arm pain or unilateral Raynaud syndrome. CT or MRA may aid in the diagnosis. There is no role for medical therapy of arterial TOS. Surgical treatment involves resecting the cervical rib, first rib, and scalenus muscle.

Ref.: 5

29. A 70-year-old man with ischemic rest pain of the right foot undergoes a femoral to popliteal bypass with a reversed saphenous vein graft. He continues to smoke. At his 6-month surveillance visit, a routine duplex ultrasound demonstrates suspicion for graft stenosis. Which of the following is true?

A. Either increased blood flow velocities at the level of the stenosis or decreased velocities in the distal graft on ultrasound can indicate graft stenosis.

B. Focal, mildly stenotic lesions are best addressed with reoperation and short-segment bypass.

C. Long-segment stenosis is most amenable to endovascular intervention such as balloon angioplasty.

D. Late graft failure is usually due to a technical error.

E. Infrapopliteal grafts have the lowest incidence of failure.

ANSWER: A

COMMENTS: The life span of a bypass is limited largely by the conduit. Autogenous vein grafts are preferentially used due to a higher patency rate than synthetic grafts. When an adequately sized autogenous conduit is unavailable, a graft must be used. Patency is adversely affected by grafts performed below the knee, continued tobacco use, poor distal runoff, and small vein size (<4 mm). The primary patency rate for femoral to suprageniculate popliteal artery bypass with saphenous vein conduit is 80%–90% at 1 year; synthetic grafts have been shown to have a 1-year patency approaching that of saphenous vein grafts. Infrapopliteal grafts with saphenous vein conduit have patency rates of 75%–80% at 1 year. With prosthetic conduit, that patency is reduced to less than 50%.

Graft stenosis or occlusion can occur at any time in the postoperative period. Early graft thrombosis, occurring within 30 days of surgery, is generally thought to be technical in nature or due to an insufficient conduit (e.g., small-diameter autogenous vein conduit). Graft failures occurring within the first 2 years, but after the initial postoperative period, are usually due to neointimal hyperplasia at the anastomoses or prior valve sites within vein grafts. Late graft failures occurring beyond 2 years are typically a result of the progression of atherosclerotic occlusive disease within the inflow or outflow arteries.

Surveillance is generally performed with a combination of clinical examination and ultrasound, followed by angiography if stenosis is suspected. Absolute velocities greater than 300 cm/s or a 3.5:1 velocity ratio (the ratio of a segment with increased velocity compared with that of proximal segment), along with a reduction in the ABI (by 0.15 or more), are indicative of severe graft stenosis. There is an intermediate risk for stenosis with peak systolic velocities less than 180 cm/s or less than 45 cm/s, or velocity ratios greater than 2:1.

Stenosis can be treated by percutaneous balloon angioplasty, operative patch angioplasty, or revision. Focal stenosis developing after the initial perioperative period may be treated with endovascular techniques. However, long-segment stenosis, early graft stenosis, and anastomotic stenosis are best treated with surgical revision.

Ref.: 3, 5, 6

REFERENCES

1. Belkin M, Owens CD, Whittemore AD, et al. Peripheral arterial occlusive disease. In: Townsend Jr CM, Beauchamp RD, Evers BM, et al., eds. *Sabiston Textbook of Surgery: The Biological Basis of Modern Surgical Practice*. 18th ed. Philadelphia: WB Saunders; 2008.
2. Lin PH, Kougias P, Bechara C, et al. Arterial disease. In: Brunicardi FC, Andersen DK, Billiar TR, et al., eds. *Schwartz's Principles of Surgery*. 9th ed. New York: McGraw-Hill; 2010.
3. Cronenwett J, Johnston W, eds. *Rutherford's Vascular Surgery*. 7th ed. Philadelphia: WB Saunders; 2010.
4. Ernst EB, Stanley JE. In: *Current Therapy in Vascular Surgery*. 4th ed. St. Louis: CV Mosby; 2001.
5. Fischer JE. *Mastery of Surgery*. 6th ed. Philadelphia: Lippincott Williams and Wilkins; 2011.
6. Zwiebel WJ, Pellerito JS. *Introduction to Vascular Ultrasonography*. 5th ed. Philadelphia: Elsevier Saunders; 2005.

F. Venous

MacKenzie Landin, M.D., and Joseph Durham, M.D.

1. A patient presents with superficial thrombophlebitis associated with varicose veins; the treatment plan may include which of the following measures?
   A. Excision of the entire vein and administration of intravenous antibiotics
   B. Iodine-125 (^{125}I)–labeled fibrinogen scan, hospitalization, and heparinization
   C. Ligation of the vein proximal and distal to the thrombosis, bed rest, and intravenous antibiotics
   D. Bed rest, elastic support hose, leg elevation, and antibiotics
   E. Warm packs, elastic support hose, nonsteroidal antiinflammatory drugs, and ambulation with limited sitting or standing

ANSWER: E

COMMENTS: The usual aim when treating **superficial thrombophlebitis** is to relieve the symptoms. The inflammation is nonbacterial, and antibiotics are not necessary unless there is evidence of secondary infection. These thrombi almost never embolize to the lungs unless they have propagated to the deep venous system. Fortunately, superficial venous thrombosis rarely progresses to deep vein thrombosis (DVT), making anticoagulation unnecessary.

Superficial phlebitis in these locations is best evaluated with duplex ultrasound scanning. Unlike the recommendations made for DVT, the goal for superficial thrombosis is to prevent venous stasis to lessen thrombus propagation risk. This is accomplished by frequent walking, using elastic stocking support, and keeping the leg elevated above the level of the heart when in the supine position. In other words, the patient should either walk or lie down with the leg elevated. Sitting and standing still for extended periods should be avoided whenever possible. Superficial thrombophlebitis is an acute problem, and symptoms from it usually resolve in 6 to 8 weeks. Antiinflammatory drugs are of variable effectiveness. Aspirin usually suffices. Recurrent superficial thrombophlebitis may respond to proximal ligation followed by vein stripping.

Ref.: 1, 2

2. Which of the following is true regarding ileofemoral venous thrombosis?
   A. Edema is rarely present.
   B. The left side is more frequently involved.
   C. It commonly results from an indwelling catheter.
   D. It is the most common site of lower-extremity DVT.
   E. It rarely results in elevated venous pressure.

ANSWER: B

COMMENTS: The signs and symptoms of **DVT** vary according to the vein involved. The most frequent site of thrombosis is the calf, with the lesion generally arising in the sinuses of the soleus muscle. Calf vein thrombi usually produce pain and localized tenderness. Little swelling occurs (typically less than a 1.5-cm difference in diameter between the calves, although it is entirely absent in 30% of patients), and venous pressure is normal. **Femoral vein thrombi** produce pain in the calf, popliteal region, or adductor canal. Swelling is generally present up to the mid-calf, and venous pressure is elevated. Ileofemoral thrombi are often localized but may extend to the calf. The left leg is involved twice as often as the right, probably because of the longer course of the left iliac vein and its compression by the right iliac artery. As venous pressure becomes elevated, the leg becomes painful, edematous, swollen, and pale (phlegmasia alba dolens). In this condition, the blanched appearance of the limb is the result of edema and not arterial spasm, as previously thought. More extensive ileofemoral venous thrombosis, in which a clot is propagated distally and into the ileofemoral venous tributaries, can obstruct all venous drainage, impair arterial inflow, and produce ischemia and threatened loss of the limb. This condition, phlegmasia cerulea dolens, is a surgical emergency.

Ref.: 1, 2

3. A 28-year-old overweight woman comes to the emergency department with a reddened, painful "knot" 8 cm above the medial malleolus. Examination in the standing position demonstrates a palpable vein above and below a tender nonfluctuant 2-cm mass. The patient is afebrile and has no other abnormalities on physical examination. Which of the following is the most likely diagnosis?
   A. Early DVT
   B. Superficial venous thrombosis
   C. Suppurative thrombophlebitis
   D. Cellulitis
   E. Insect bite

ANSWER: B

COMMENTS: **Superficial venous thrombi** may be associated with thrombophlebitis, which is an acute, nonbacterial inflammation that produces pain, redness, and swelling. Thrombi, however, may form without producing any signs or symptoms. Superficial thrombophlebitis usually appears as a localized process over the course of a superficial vein. It occurs in association with intravenous catheters in the upper extremity and within varicosities in the lower extremity. The presence of distended varicosities above and below the lesion aids in the diagnosis. The diagnosis is usually readily made from the history and findings on physical examination. Lack of blood flow through the vein can be confirmed with Doppler ultrasound imaging, but this test is usually an unnecessary clinical examination, is unclear, or there is a concern for extension into the deep venous system.

The diagnoses of cellulitis, insect bite, subcutaneous hematoma, and traumatic ecchymosis must be considered when evaluating these lesions. An insect bite is frequently associated with itching. The presence of hematoma or ecchymosis may indicate trauma as the cause. Suppurative thrombophlebitis must also be considered, especially in patients with fever and leukocytosis. Suppurative thrombophlebitis is characterized by purulence within the vein and is generally a complication of intravenous cannulation. The presence of increased redness, pain, fluctuance, fever, and leukocytosis is more typical of bacterial infection than of superficial thrombophlebitis.

Ref.: 1–3

4. Regarding the workup of patients with DVT, which of the following statements is true?

A. Ascending venography has high specificity for the diagnosis of DVT.

B. Magnetic resonance imaging (MRI) can detect central but not iliac venous thrombi.

C. Doppler ultrasound imaging and impedance plethysmography are equally useful in diagnosing femoral, popliteal, and major calf vein thromboses.

D. Doppler ultrasound and impedance plethysmography are equally sensitive in diagnosing ileofemoral venous occlusion.

E. Isotope scanning differentiates between active thrombosis and inflammatory fibrous exudate.

ANSWER: A

COMMENTS: **Isotope scans** with ^{125}I-labeled human fibrinogen are used to detect clot formation or thrombus propagation. Studies of even the sickest patient are possible with portable instrumentation. Isotope scanning is not useful in patients with superficial **thrombophlebitis**, overlying recent incisions, traumatic injuries, hematomas, cellulitis, active arthritis, or primary lymphedema because it cannot differentiate between active inflammatory fibrous exudate and thrombus formation. Upper thigh and pelvic lesions are often confounded by high background counts of the isotope within the pelvic organs. An isotope scan can be 90% accurate in detecting the onset of thrombosis when performed serially (daily) in high-risk patients. Isotope scanning is now almost never used for clinical diagnosis and is reserved for research studies. **Doppler ultrasound imaging** is useful for detecting occlusions of major veins. It can also detect incompetence of the deep and perforator veins, but it cannot differentiate between old and new thrombi nor can it help diagnose small, nonobstructing thrombi. Duplex scanning with B-mode ultrasound imaging is the best noninvasive study for DVT. This test can reliably differentiate extrinsic venous compression from DVT and new thrombi from old, and it can determine valvular competence. Superficial and deep veins of the calf and thigh, as well as the iliac veins and inferior vena cava (IVC), can also be visualized. These tests are viewed as the preferred initial tests for DVT. Impedance plethysmography is more accurate than Doppler ultrasound for diagnosing femoral, popliteal, and major calf vein thrombosis but less accurate than duplex scanning. Venography is still considered the definitive test for the diagnosis of DVT and is used to resolve equivocal results obtained by the noninvasive techniques but is rarely necessary.

Ref.: 1–3

5. Which of the following is true?

A. The calf muscle pump has minimal importance in regard to the venous flow rate.

B. Postthrombotic syndrome may occur in more than one-half of patients after an episode of DVT.

C. Veins are less stiff than arteries per unit of cross-sectional area.

D. Valvular incompetence contributes to the development of varicose veins but not to the development of venous stasis ulcers.

E. Venous pressure at the foot is greatly increased while walking.

ANSWER: B

COMMENTS: The **calf muscle pump** is the most important mechanism for preventing the accumulation of interstitial fluid. While standing, **venous pressure** may exceed 100 mmHg. This pressure is greatly reduced while walking. Postthrombotic syndrome occurs in up to 60% of patients following DVT. It is caused by valvular incompetence in deep veins below the knee and in perforating veins. Venous hypertension results in brawny discoloration and venous stasis disease. Varicose veins result when incompetent valves allow reflux of blood proximally to distally. Veins have less elastic tissue than arteries and are stiffer per unit of cross-sectional area.

Ref.: 3

6. Which of the following statements is true?

A. The major indication for deep venous thrombectomy is recurrent pulmonary embolism (PE).

B. Open thrombectomy for ileofemoral DVT rarely results in less swelling, pain, and venous stasis than conservative therapy does.

C. Thrombectomy is contraindicated in patients with phlegmasia cerulea dolens.

D. Ileofemoral thrombosis from a pelvic infection is best treated by thrombectomy.

E. Caval interruption should always precede ileofemoral thrombectomy.

ANSWER: B

COMMENTS: The role of surgery in the treatment of **acute DVT** is limited because of the effectiveness of medical management, the high incidence of residual or recurrent venous obstruction, and the valvular incompetence that occurs after operative correction. Surgery is usually reserved for major obstruction of the subclavian, iliac, or femoral vein and when the immediate- or long-term function of the limb is in jeopardy. Clinical studies have not demonstrated that thrombectomy leads to less swelling, pain, and venostasis than does nonoperative therapy. The progression of ileofemoral thrombosis to the stage of near total occlusion, with tenderness, massive edema, and cyanosis (phlegmasia cerulea dolens), may lead to venous gangrene. When it occurs, failure of the patient to respond promptly to treatment consisting of leg elevation and heparinization or thrombolytic therapy (or both) is an indication for thrombectomy.

Although there is a theoretical advantage to caval interruption before thrombectomy, ileofemoral thrombectomy can be performed safely without caval interruption.

Septic ileofemoral thrombi (usually as a result of pelvic infection) are a contraindication to thrombectomy.

Operations for subclavian vein thrombosis should include resection of the first rib or cervical rib (or both) because most thrombi originate at the point where the clavicle crosses the first rib. Failure to resect these structures is associated with a high rate of postoperative recurrence.

The success of venous thrombectomy depends on early surgery, good technique, and complete removal of the thrombus. Surgery is not as useful after 7 to 10 days, and the best results are obtained when thrombectomy is performed within 48 h of the appearance of symptoms.

PE that recurs despite proper medical therapy is best treated with a caval filter.

Ref.: 1, 2

7. A 56-year-old man has had heaviness, tiredness, and aching of the lower part of his left leg for the past several months. The symptoms are relieved by leg elevation. He mentions that he is awakened from sleep because of calf and foot cramping but that walking or massage relieves it. On physical examination, he has thick, darkly pigmented skin; nonpitting edema bilaterally; and a superficial ulcer 2 cm in diameter and 5 cm above and behind the medial malleolus, which is slightly painful. The most likely diagnosis is which of the following?

A. Arterial insufficiency with ulceration

B. Isolated symptomatic varicose veins

C. Diabetic neuropathy with ulceration

D. Deep venous insufficiency with incompetent perforator veins

E. Diabetic ulcer

ANSWER: D

COMMENTS: The most common symptoms associated with **venous insufficiency** are aching, swelling, and night cramps of the involved leg. The symptoms often occur after periods of sitting or inactive standing. Elevation of the leg frequently provides relief. Although the edema of venous insufficiency can occur with varicose veins alone, it is usually associated with deep venous abnormalities and incompetent perforating veins. Night cramps are the result of sustained contractions of the calf and foot muscles and are relieved by massage, ambulation, and proper management of the underlying venous insufficiency. Brawny, nonpitting edema is the result of increased connective tissue in the subcutaneous tissue. Brown discoloration is the result of hemosiderin deposition. **Ulceration** is most common in patients with deep venous abnormalities and incompetent perforators. In such cases, the ulcers are usually located above and posterior to the malleoli (medial more than lateral), thus reinforcing their relationship with perforator abnormalities. When patients with a history of DVT are monitored beyond 10 years, ulcers ultimately develop in up to 20%.

In contrast to arterial ulcers, **venous ulcers** are superficial and rarely penetrate the fascia. The pain of arterial insufficiency is often increased with leg elevation. Ulcers associated with arterial insufficiency may occur anywhere on the lower part of the leg but usually occur distally, with the toe often being involved first. Arterial ulcers have an associated blue erythematous border and are more painful than venous ulcers. Shallow ulcers of the ankle that closely resemble venous stasis ulcers may develop in patients with diabetes mellitus. Treating them as venous stasis ulcers (i.e., with leg elevation, an Unna boot, and other measures) may be disastrous because of the associated arterial insufficiency. Patients with diabetes often have decreased vibration and position sense and decreased reflexes due to peripheral neuropathy. Ulcers associated with neuropathy can be found on weight-bearing areas and are not usually associated with pain.

Ref.: 1, 2

8. The therapeutic plan for the patient in Question 7 should include which of the following measures?

A. Varicose vein ligation and stripping as soon as possible

B. Ligation of the medial perforating veins as soon as possible

C. Initial treatment consisting of appropriate leg wraps, leg elevation, and ambulation with avoidance of prolonged sitting or standing

D. Ulcer debridement, vein stripping, and skin grafting

E. Laser ablation

ANSWER: C

COMMENTS: Operative treatment of venous insufficiency in most instances is an adjunct to aggressive conservative management. Leg elevation, active exercise, and elastic compression form the cornerstone of nonoperative management. The goals of compression are to relieve symptoms and reduce swelling. When ulcers are present, local medications should be avoided unless evidence of infection exists. Ulcers smaller than 3 cm in diameter often heal with the aforementioned treatment.

The indications for superficial vein ligation, endovenous ablation, and stripping are moderate to severe symptoms without other signs of venous insufficiency, venous insufficiency with recurrent ulceration despite aggressive medical management, and occasionally, severe varicosities without symptoms. **Ligation of incompetent perforating veins** can be an important addition to the treatment of venous insufficiency, particularly if done before development of ulceration. Ligation was once often performed through a longitudinal incision placed posterior and superior to the malleoli, as first described by Robert Linton. Subfascial endoscopic techniques have reduced the morbidity associated with this technique. When present, incompetent superficial veins should be stripped as part of the procedure. Postoperatively, conservative measures must be continued aggressively. Obstructions of the ileofemoral or femoropopliteal veins have been bypassed with the use of ipsilateral (femoropopliteal occlusions) or contralateral (ileofemoral occlusions) saphenous veins.

Ref.: 1, 2

9. Which is true regarding lymphatic anatomy?

A. The limb lymphatic vessels are valveless.

B. The lymphatic system begins just below the dermis as a network of fine capillaries.

C. Red blood cells and bacteria do not enter lymphatic capillaries.

D. Extrinsic factors (e.g., muscle contraction, arterial pulsations, respiratory movement, and massage) aid in the movement of lymph flow.

E. All of the above.

ANSWER: D

COMMENTS: The **lymphatic system** begins as a network of valveless capillaries in the superficial dermis. There is a second valved plexus in the deep or subdermal layer that joins with the first to form the lymphatic vessels, and their course parallels that of the major blood vessels. Lymph flow toward the heart is aided by massage, arterial pulsations, respiratory movement, and muscle contraction. Intradermal lymphatics can be evaluated by the intradermal injection of patent blue dye. The capillaries normally become visible as a fine network 30 to 60 s after the injection. Lymphangiography is rarely used to visualize the lymphatic vessels because it may make the lymphedema worse. Unlike veins, these vessels appear to be of uniform caliber throughout their course.

Lymphatic vessels are readily entered by the proteins present in the extracellular fluid. Red blood cells and lymphocytes enter lymphatic vessels by separating the endothelial cells at their junctions.

Lymphedema occurs when the lymphatics are obstructed, too few in number, or nonfunctional, which results in the retention of interstitial fluid with a high protein concentration. Tissue oncotic pressure increases, and fluid is drawn into the interstitium. Measurement of the protein content of the edema fluid (normally <1.5 mg/dL) can be used to assess the status of lymphatic function in the edematous extremity.

Ref.: 1, 2, 4

10. Which statement is true regarding the cause and complications of lymphedema?

A. Primary lymphedema appears at birth, is more common in females, and occurs in the right leg more often than in the left.

B. Milroy disease is a form of primary lymphedema that is gender linked.

C. A lymphangiogram usually demonstrates a point of obstruction of the lymphatics in primary lymphedema.

D. Primary lymphedema almost always progresses to involve both lower extremities.

E. The major complication of lymphedema is the later development of lymphangiosarcoma.

ANSWER: B

COMMENTS: Primary lymphedema is caused by an abnormal development resulting in aplasia, hypoplasia, or varicosities of the lymphatic vessels. Congenital lymphedema (Milroy disease) is present at birth and is a familial, gender-linked condition, but a family history is present in less than 5% of patients. Primary lymphedema usually appears in individuals during their teens, more commonly in females, and it often develops insidiously. The left limb is more frequently involved than the right (3:1), and often only one limb is involved.

Secondary lymphedema is the result of an obstruction to or destruction of normal lymphatic channels and can be caused by a tumor, repeated infection, or parasitic infection (particularly filariasis), or it can occur following radiation treatment or lymph node dissection. Lymphangiography often demonstrates a discrete obstruction. Recurrent infections of venous stasis ulcers can destroy lymphatic vessels and lead to lymphedema.

The inability to clear proteins leads to edema formation, which gradually increases over time and becomes woody because of the presence of fibrous tissue in the subcutaneous region. Repeated infection hastens the accumulation of this fibrous tissue. In some patients, blisters develop that contain edema fluid, or chyle. The major complication of lymphedema is recurrent attacks of cellulitis or lymphangitis, often following a minor injury. β-Hemolytic streptococci are the organisms responsible, and the infection spreads rapidly because the protein-containing edema fluid is an excellent culture medium.

Lymphangiosarcoma is a rare complication of a long-standing lymphedema that is most frequently described in patients following radical mastectomy (Stewart-Treves syndrome). It appears as a blue or purple nodule with a satellite lesion. Metastases develop early, primarily to the lungs.

Rarely, a protein-losing enteropathy that has been attributed to lymphatic obstruction of the small bowel develops in patients with lymphedema.

Ref.: 1, 2, 4

11. Regarding the treatment of lymphedema, which of the following statements is true?

A. More than 50% of patients ultimately require an operation.

B. Diuretics have a crucial role in the conservative management of early lymphedema.

C. Pneumatic compression devices can damage the remaining lymphatics and should not be used.

D. Microsurgically constructed lymphovenous shunts are far more effective than excisional procedures.

E. All surgical procedures for lymphedema have significant failure rates.

ANSWER: E

COMMENTS: The mainstay of **management of lymphedema** is conservative and nonoperative. Less than 5% of patients require an operation. The goals of the therapy are prevention of infection and reduction of subcutaneous fluid volume. Fluid volume is reduced by elevating the extremity during sleep and using pneumatic compression devices and carefully fitted elastic support stockings. Diuretics are not used routinely but may be useful in women who retain fluid during the premenstrual period. Patients prone to recurrent lymphangitis require intermittent long-term antibiotic therapy at the first sign of infection. The drug of choice is penicillin because streptococci are the usual infecting organisms. Secondary lymphedema requires treatment of the underlying cause, such as giving diethylcarbamazine for filariasis and appropriate antibiotics for tuberculosis or lymphogranuloma venereum.

Edema that is excessive and interferes with normal activity and the presence of severe recurrent cellulitis are indications for surgery. Patients with minimal edema, gross obesity, and progressing disease are not candidates for surgery. Excisional procedures include removal of the skin, subcutaneous tissue, and fascia, followed by split-thickness skin graft reconstruction (the Charles operation); excision of strips of the skin and subcutaneous tissue, followed by primary closure; and creation of buried dermal flaps. Physiologic procedures to restore or enhance lymphatic drainage include insertion of silk, Teflon, or polystyrene threads into the subcutaneous tissue; construction of pedicle grafts from the involved limb to the trunk; and microsurgical lymphovenous shunts using dilated lymphatics or the capsule and efferent channels of isolated lymph nodes anastomosed to neighboring veins. All procedures are associated with significant failure rates.

Ref.: 1, 2, 4

12. Which of the following is least likely to occur with acquired peripheral arteriovenous fistulas (AVFs)?

A. Bacterial endocarditis

B. Distal embolization

C. Peripheral arterial insufficiency

D. Congestive heart failure

E. Venous aneurysm formation

ANSWER: B

COMMENTS: Acquired peripheral AVFs are most commonly the result of a penetrating trauma, which causes injury to an adjacent artery and vein. The upper and lower extremities are the most frequent sites. Other causes include suture ligation of adjacent vessels, vessel catheterization for diagnostic or therapeutic study, erosion of an adjacent vein by an atherosclerotic aneurysm, periarterial abscess, or neoplasm. Another cause is a remnant fistula following in situ peripheral artery bypass. Small fistulas may close spontaneously. Fistulas that persist lead to dilation and ectasia of the proximal artery, and the adjacent vein becomes thick walled, dilated, and aneurysmal. The intimal damage that occurs leads to increased risks for infection and bacterial endocarditis. Depending on the size and location of the fistula, the significant flow may lead to arterial insufficiency distal to the fistula ("steal phenomenon"). Venous congestion, chronic venous stasis changes, edema, and venous varicosities may also occur. In young children, a peripheral fistula may lead to limb length inequality if it is present before the closure of the epiphyseal plate. If the fistula is large, signs and symptoms of high-output congestive heart failure may develop. Temporary compression of the fistula may elicit a Branham-Nicoladoni sign, with a rise in the diastolic blood pressure and a decrease in the heart rate. Peripheral AVFs do not cause thrombosis or distal embolization.

Ref.: 2, 3, 5

13. A 17-year-old boy comes to the emergency department complaining of swelling of his left arm and cyanosis 1 h after strenuous weight lifting. Venography demonstrates subclavian-axillary vein thrombosis. Which treatment is most appropriate?

A. All patients can expect an asymptomatic recovery if treated promptly with anticoagulants only.

B. The patient may be treated effectively with acetylsalicylic acid only.

C. The patient will need lifelong anticoagulation with Coumadin.

D. The patient requires catheter-directed thrombolysis and resection of the first rib if patency is restored and venous narrowing is demonstrated.

E. The patient requires first rib resection only.

ANSWER: D

COMMENTS: Primary DVT of the upper extremity is a rare entity that accounts for 2%–3% of all patients with thoracic outlet syndrome. A young healthy athlete is a typical patient. Males are affected twice as often as females. Almost all have a history of strenuous or repetitive physical activity 24 to 48 h earlier. During hyperabduction of the arm, the subclavian vein is compressed at the costoclavicular space, which is the most medial aspect of the thoracic outlet. Trauma at this location causes intimal injury, followed by thrombus formation in the axillary and subclavian veins. All patients complain of swelling and cyanosis of the affected extremity when initially seen, and pain develops in the majority of patients.

Catheter-directed thrombolysis is the first line of treatment. If the resolution of thrombus is documented after thrombolysis and extrinsic compression is identified at the level of the costoclavicular space, resection of the first rib is recommended. It is performed through the axillary, infraclavicular, or supraclavicular approach during the same hospitalization or later. Additional treatment options include anticoagulation and delayed outlet decompression, outlet decompression with external venolysis, outlet decompression followed by angioplasty, and outlet decompression with venous reconstruction. The decision regarding which option to use is based on the level of the patient's discomfort and findings on venography.

Ref.: 3

14. A 67-year-old man is in the hospital for the treatment of bilateral PE and DVT. Heparin was started with transition to Coumadin. On day 5, the patient's platelet count was 75,000/mm^3, a decrease from an original level of 250,000/mm^3. On physical examination, he was noted to have ischemic changes in the right upper extremity and right lower extremity. Which of the following statements is true?

A. Low-molecular-weight heparin (LMWH) can be used safely as a substitute for unfractionated heparin.

B. Venous thrombosis is the most likely cause of this patient's problem.

C. Subcutaneous administration of heparin is not associated with this problem.

D. Direct thrombin inhibitors are used as the first line of treatment.

E. Antiplatelet agents are not necessary as an additional treatment.

ANSWER: D

COMMENTS: Heparin-induced thrombocytopenia (HIT) is an immune-mediated adverse drug reaction that can occur in up to 5% of patients undergoing treatment with unfractionated heparin. The initial diagnosis of this condition is clinical. The occurrence of HIT is independent of the route of administration. Two forms of acute HIT have been reported. Mild (type 1) thrombocytopenia occurs 2 to 7 days after the initiation of full-dose heparin therapy. It is nonimmune in nature. Platelet counts usually remain above 100,000/mm^3, and treatment can be continued without any risk for complications. Severe (type 2) thrombocytopenia occurs much less frequently, 5 to 10 days after the initiation of full-dose or low-dose heparin therapy. It is an immune-mediated syndrome. Platelet counts drop below 100,000/mm^3, or there is a more than 50% drop from baseline. Laboratory confirmation of the presence of heparin-induced antibodies is available, but not always in a timely fashion for decision-making. Platelet-associated immunoglobulin G (IgG) levels are almost always elevated, but testing for them is not very specific. The C-serotonin platelet release assay, heparin-induced platelet aggregation assay, and flow cytometric studies are very sensitive and specific. Paradoxically, severe HIT is associated with thrombotic complications, including arterial thrombosis with a platelet-fibrin clot (so-called white clot), which may cause myocardial infarction or stroke or necessitate amputation of a limb. Arterial or venous thrombosis may develop in up to 75% of patients, and the mortality rate is 25%–30%. Direct thrombin inhibitors, such as lepirudin and argatroban, are the first line of treatment, with the choice of agent depending on the patient's comorbid conditions (lepirudin depends on renal clearance, and argatroban depends on hepatic functional status). Each agent has a relatively short half-life. Antiplatelet medications (e.g., aspirin and clopidogrel [Plavix]) should be used for all patients with HIT.

Ref.: 3

15. Which of the following regarding treatment of DVT is true?

A. Thrombus removal is associated with high morbidity and is rarely indicated.

B. Catheter-based thrombolysis has complication rates equivalent to those of systemic thrombolysis.

C. LMWH and unfractionated heparin are associated with equivalent rates of HIT.

D. Intracranial bleeding, reported in 5% of patients, is the most common major complication of catheter-based thrombolysis.

E. Early thrombus resolution is associated with improved long-term outcomes.

ANSWER: E

COMMENTS: Postthrombotic syndrome results in venous valvular incompetence and subsequent venous hypertension. Clinically, this is manifested as a lower-extremity edema, cutaneous stasis changes, venous varicosities, and venous stasis ulceration. These sequelae are termed *postthrombotic syndrome*. Early clot thrombolysis is associated with a reduced incidence of postthrombotic syndrome. Substantial evidence suggests that patients with extensive clot burden (i.e., iliac vein clot) have improved outcomes with thrombus removal versus anticoagulation alone. Data regarding thrombus removal for infrainguinal DVT are lacking. Catheter-based delivery of thrombolytic agents is associated with fewer complications than the systemic thrombolytic therapy. The most common complication is major bleeding, seen in 5%–10% of patients; it is usually located at the puncture site. Intracranial bleeding was reported in less than 1% of patients in multiple studies.

Ref.: 3

16. Which of the following is true?

A. An extended indication for a vena cava filter is in low-risk trauma patients.

B. A relative indication for a filter is a small adherent thrombus within the iliac vein.

C. Vena cava filters should not be placed after pulmonary thromboembolectomy.

D. Vena cava filters can be placed in pregnant women.

E. None of the above.

ANSWER: D

COMMENTS: Vena cava filters are medical devices used to prevent lower-extremity venous thrombi from embolizing into the pulmonary system. The ideal filter is one that does not stimulate clot formation and has the ability to filter blood effectively, but does not hinder flow. The filter itself should be easy to insert, deploy, and reposition. Ideal filters can be visualized on MRI and have low-risk for complications like migrating, fracture, occlusion, perforation, and insertion-site thrombosis. There are several absolute and relative indications for vena cava filter insertion. Absolute indications for insertion include contraindication to anticoagulation, recurrent disease despite adequate anticoagulation, and significant bleeding that prevents anticoagulation. Relative indications include clots with a large free-floating iliocaval thrombus, pre- or postpulmonary thromboembolectomy, thromboembolic disease with limited cardiopulmonary reserve, poor compliance with medications, thrombolysis of iliocaval thrombus, and ataxia or significant fall risk. Extended indications for filter insertion include high-risk trauma patients with head or spine injury; patients with spine, pelvis, or long-bone fractures; patients with a history of bariatric surgery; preoperative patients with multiple risk factors for venous thromboembolism; and high-risk immobilized patients. Contraindications to a vena cava filter include complete thrombosis of the IVC; an inability to gain access to the IVC secondary to severe venous obstruction; and uncorrectable severe coagulopathy or thrombocytopenia. Special situations requiring caution include pediatric patients and patients with uncontrolled bacteremia. Pregnant women can have filters placed, usually suprarenal in location, when they develop a clot and cannot be given anticoagulation.

Ref: 6

17. The CEAP classification is a formal system for classifying venous disease based on the **C**linical picture, **E**tiology of the disease, **A**natomic distribution, and **P**athophysiology of venous disease. A patient with telangiectasias on physical examination of the lower extremity would be classified with which clinical stage?

A. 0

B. 1

C. 3

D. 5

E. 4

ANSWER: B

COMMENTS: Classification systems help to standardize diagnosis and treatment. The CEAP classification system was created to aid in diagnosing the severity of a disease and to improve the care of patients with venous disease. According to this system, a patient with C0 has no visible or palpable signs of venous disease. C1 is someone who has telangiectasias or reticular veins on examination. A telangiectasia is a "spider" vein that is a collection of smaller veins, each less than 1 mm in size. A reticular vein is a vein below the dermis that is between 1 and 3 mm and usually tortuous. C2 patients have varicose veins, and C3 patients have significant edema. C4 is divided into 4a, those with skin changes including pigmentation and/or eczema, and 4b, skin changes of lipodermatosclerosis and or atrophie blanche. C5 includes healed venous ulcers, and C6 has active ulceration. An "S" designation is for patients with symptoms of aching pain, tightness, skin irritation, heaviness, and muscle cramps. An "A" designation is for patients who are asymptomatic. The **E**tiology of a disease can be congenital, primary, or secondary. The pathophysiology for the venous problem can be due to reflux, obstruction, or both. Generally, patients with C3 or C4 usually have nonoperative management. Their treatment includes compression stockings and skin lubricants. C5 and C6 can undergo operative intervention depending on the etiology and anatomy of the disease to prevent a long-term ulcer recurrence.

Ref.: 7, 8

18. Your patient is a 34-year-old female who participates in triathlons in the summertime. She notices her legs have become tender to touch, and they are affecting her ability to exercise. On examination, you appreciate hyperpigmented lower extremities, bilaterally, with a prior ulcer, which has now healed. What treatment is offered to patients of any stage of venous disease?

A. Compression stockings

B. Sclerotherapy

C. Vein stripping
D. Powered phlebectomy
E. Keep extremity dependent

ANSWER: A

COMMENTS: All patients with venous complaints are recommended to wear compression stockings. Stockings can either be elastic or inelastic. Inelastic stockings can come in the form of Unna boots, Velcro bandages, etc. The benefit of compression stockings depends on the level the compression is applied to, the type of compression applied, and the underlying venous problem. When inelastic bandages are used and the patient is standing, 30 mmHg is applied, which causes a decrease in the venous filling index and the residual venous volume. The goal of compression stockings is to improve the venous pump and decrease the venous volume in the lower extremity. Evidence has shown that compression stockings reduce the incidence of postthrombotic syndrome and increase ulcer healing rates.

Surgical treatment of varicose veins can be done with sclerotherapy, stab phlebectomy, or powered phlebectomy. Sclerotherapy entails injection of a sclerosing agent (like hypertonic saline, polidocanol, or sodium tetradecyl) into the vein causing obliteration of the lumen. Stab phlebectomy is performed when a small incision is made overlying the varicosity, and then it is avulsed and the limb is compressed to tamponade any bleeding and prevent hematoma formation. Powered phlebectomy involves injecting the area surrounding the veins, which prevents bleeding. The vein is then emulsified by a device that combines a rotating ablator with a suction component. Powered phlebectomy is faster than stab phlebectomy as it treats a larger area and offers the same cosmesis.

Ref.: 7

19. There is a 61-year-old female with duplex proven saphenous insufficiency. She has failed conservative management with compression and leg elevation. Which of the following are options to treat her disease?

A. Percutaneous laser ablation
B. Powered phlebectomy
C. Sclerotherapy
D. Vein stripping
E. All of the above

ANSWER: E

COMMENTS: Varicose veins are irregular superficial veins that are sometimes associated with chronic disease of deep veins. Patients who experience local trauma, prolonged sitting or standing, pregnancy, or have a family history are at risk for developing varicose veins. Treatment may be offered to patients as the varicosities can cause pain, cramping, or be cosmetically unappealing. There are a variety of methods used for treatment. Percutaneous laser therapy can be used for telangiectasias, reticular veins, and branch varicose veins. Laser therapy of various wavelengths has been used for a saphenous application; 90%–100% of patients do not develop recurrent varicosities. A complication of laser therapy is thermal damage to surrounding structures. Sclerotherapy has been used to treat varicosities that remain following a saphenous ablation or small isolated varicosities, telangiectasias, and reticular veins. The concentration of a sclerosant, liquid or foam, depends on the vein size and the agent used. Side effects of sclerotherapy include burning, itching, and muscle spasm. If the sclerosant extravasates from the vein, the surrounding fat becomes necrotic, ulcerations can form, and the surrounding skin can become hyperpigmented. Ultrasound-directed foam sclerotherapy has been shown to be 84% effective in eliminating reflux for 1 year. It has been shown that more veins are present at 10-year follow-up when foam is used alone, compared with foam plus surgery. Phlebectomy is the sharp dissection and resection of the offending vein. Small incisions are made, and the vein is removed from its bed. Tumescent anesthesia, or field anesthesia, can be applied to a larger area allowing for powered phlebectomy to be used. Powered phlebectomy is the method of illuminating the vein, morcellizing it, and aspirating it from the field. There is no difference in cosmetic outcome compared with sclerotherapy, and powered phlebectomy has an associated higher cost. Vein stripping is when a refluxing vein is removed after high ligation. The saphenous vein is stripped after ligation of the saphenous at the saphenofemoral junction. It is usually removed from the groin to the knee, but if there is disease past the knee, the vein can be taken down to the level of the ankle. Complications of great saphenous vein surgery include DVT, wound infection, nerve damage, and development of a hematoma.

Ref.: 7, 8

20. A 58-year-old male develops unilateral leg swelling that worsens with exercise. He notes that when his symptoms are severe, his toes turn blue. What is the likely diagnosis?

A. Superficial vein thrombus
B. Venous claudication
C. Arterial claudication
D. Deep vein thrombus
E. PE

ANSWER: B

COMMENTS: Venous claudication occurs with exercise. Patients can develop cyanosis of the affected extremity, increased swelling, and increased prominence of the superficial veins that are relieved by rest and elevation of the extremity. This disease process is the most debilitating when there is a proximal obstruction of venous outflow.

Ref: 7

21. Which of the following tests will determine the venous filling index?

A. CT angiography
B. Duplex ultrasound
C. Air plethysmography
D. Venogram
E. MRI

ANSWER: C

COMMENTS: To determine how severe a patient's venous disease is, one can perform air plethysmography. The extremity to be evaluated is fitted in a plastic cylinder filled with air over the calf and foot. There is a change in volume of the canister during exercise or change in position. The change in volume is used to calculate the venous filling index. The venous filling index is 90% of resting standing venous volume divided by the time it takes to reach 90% of venous volume as the patient shifts from the supine to the standing position (mL/s). A venous filling index of 2 mL/s or less is consistent with a competent venous system. If the venous filling index (VFI) is greater than 2 mL/s, this finding suggests venous insufficiency. Plethysmography can be used to differentiate between patients with and without disease, but it cannot stratify patients by symptom severity.

Ref: 7

22. Which is the correct statement?

A. Reteplase converts plasminogen to plasmin; plasmin then degrades clots.

B. Urokinase is derived from bacteria.

C. Tissue plasminogen activator is an enzyme made by the kidney that converts plasminogen to plasmin.

D. Anistreplase is a combination of streptokinase and plasminogen.

E. Streptokinase is a recombinant human tissue plasminogen activator.

ANSWER: D

COMMENTS: There are several pharmaceutical agents that can be used to lyse clots. Patients who undergo catheter-directed thrombolysis for iliofemoral venous thrombosis have been shown to improve physical functioning and have less health distress and fewer postthrombotic syndromes. Thrombolytic agents lyse fibrin clots by catalyzing the formation of plasmin, which attacks and degrades fibrin, fibrinogen, and other proteins. Tissue plasminogen activator converts plasminogen to plasmin; plasmin then degrades clots. Streptokinase is derived from streptococci bacteria. It combines with plasminogen and forms a complex that catalyzes the plasminogen-to-plasmin reaction of other precursor molecules. However, as it is derived from bacteria, it has a high immunogenicity preventing it from being used repeatedly by the same subject. Urokinase is generated by the human kidney and acts in a similar fashion. Reteplase is a recombinant human tissue plasminogen activator, which is used for coronary reperfusion in patients with acute myocardial infarction, catheter-directed thrombolysis in DVT, and arterial occlusion. Anistreplase is another second-generation thrombolytic agent, which combines human plasminogen with bacterial-derived streptokinase. It has a long half-life, but like streptokinase, has antigenic properties.

Ref.: 9, 10

23. What is the least appropriate therapy for a patient affected by phlegmasia cerulea dolens?

A. Systemic anticoagulation

B. Targeted thrombolysis

C. Thrombectomy

D. Observation

E. Combination therapy of A, B, and C

ANSWER: D

COMMENTS: Damage to distal valves following the development of a DVT can result in venous reflux and postthrombotic sequelae. Phlegmasia cerulea dolens is the disease process characterized by a DVT, which extends and causes massive thrombosis compromising venous outflow and as a result causes ischemia. When treating this disease, the goal is to prevent progression to venous gangrene, shock, or death. Risk factors for this disease are malignancy, femoral vein catheterization, HIT, antiphospholipid syndrome, surgery, heart failure, and pregnancy. Observation in this case is not appropriate. Systemic anticoagulation may not be enough therapy to prevent the development of phlegmasia cerulea dolens after DVT. When primary ciliary dyskinesia (PCD) is diagnosed, it should be treated with targeted thrombolysis, thrombectomy, or systemic anticoagulation or a combination.

Ref.: 11, 12

24. A 64-year-old male undergoes a penectomy and lymphadenectomy for penile cancer and develops significant scrotal and bilateral lower-extremity swelling for 5 years. What intervention is the least appropriate at this time?

A. Microsurgery

B. Decongestive physiotherapy

C. Benzopyrone trial

D. Reductive surgery

E. Compression therapy

ANSWER: A

COMMENTS: Lymphedema occurs because of increased flow of fluid out of the capillary and into the interstitium as well as decreased flow out of the interstitium. Possible causes of lymphedema include increased capillary permeability, venous hypertension, and decreased oncotic pressure within the capillary. There are congenital causes of lymphedema; however, acquired causes are more common. Malignancy and its treatment (surgery and radiation) are the most common acquired causes of lymphedema in the United States. When lymphedema persists for longer periods, the subcutaneous tissue becomes thickened and fibrotic allowing for increased deposition of adipose tissue. When the lymphedema is severe, it is known as elephantiasis. Nonoperative strategies like compression therapy, decongestive physiotherapy, and elevation are attempted first as surgical therapy has a high associated morbidity with complications including recurrence, infection, and difficulty with wound healing. Benzopyrone has been used with mixed results. It works to decrease vascular permeability and increase macrophage activity. When nonoperative therapies fail, microsurgery can be considered only for early disease. Microsurgery involves either lymph node transfer or lymphaticolymphatic anastomoses to increase the absorption of lymph from the interstitium. However, when the disease is chronic, there is irreversible damage to the lymphatics, and attempts to restore flow will fail. Therefore for patients who fail nonoperative therapies and have a debilitating disease, reductive surgery or excisional surgery can be attempted. Reductive surgery is the debulking of affected tissue followed by skin grafting of the remaining wounds. This procedure was described by surgeon Sir Richard Henry Havelock Charles in 1912, who performed the procedure for an incapacitating disease.

Ref.: 13

25. A 71-year-old female presents with bilateral lower-extremity edema. Her right leg has a large ulceration over the medial thigh. Which intervention has the greatest chance for cure?

A. Wide local excision with lymphadenectomy

B. Wide local excision

C. Amputation of the right lower extremity

D. Amputation of the right lower extremity with lymphadenectomy

E. None of the above

ANSWER: C

COMMENTS: The patient described has bilateral lower-extremity lymphedema with the development of an ulcerating skin lesion concerning for lymphangiosarcoma. First described by Fred Stewart and Norman Treves in 1948, it is classically seen in patients after surgery in the upper extremity who developed chronic lymphedema. Lymphangiosarcoma can also develop in the lower extremity. On physical examination, there can be hyperkeratotic nodules, fissures, and papules among lymphedematous skin. Large lymphangiosarcomas are typically treated with amputation. Smaller disease may be treated with wide local excision if 2- to 3-cm margins can be obtained. Patients who undergo wide local excision may need formal amputation if there is a local recurrence. Chemotherapy is available for patients with inoperable disease, recurrent disease not amenable to surgery, or those unwilling to undergo amputation. Median survival is 19 months, and 5-year survival is 8.5%–13.6%.

Ref.: 14, 15

26. Match the mechanism of action to the corresponding drug.

A. Argatroban is a direct thrombin inhibitor.

B. Rivaroxaban (Xarelto) and fondaparinux prevent activation of factors II, VII, and IX.

C. Enoxaparin (Lovenox) inhibits vitamin K epoxide reductase.

D. Coumadin (warfarin) is a factor Xa inhibitor.

E. Heparin has a long half-life.

ANSWER: A

COMMENTS: Heparin was discovered in 1916 and was first used in 1935. It activates antithrombin III, inhibiting thrombin and Xa activity. It has a short half-life and therefore is given parenterally. In long-term users, side effects like osteoporosis, HIT, and bleeding can occur. LMWH, enoxaparin, is an alternative to heparin. It can be given subcutaneously, allowing for in-home application. LMWH is efficacious in treating DVT and has decreased bleeding risk compared with heparin. Argatroban is a direct thrombin inhibitor of both free thrombin and fibrin-bound thrombin and does not require a cofactor. Fondaparinux and rivaroxaban are both factor Xa inhibitors. Finally, Coumadin (warfarin) irreversibly inhibits vitamin K epoxide reductase, which prevents factors II, VII, IX, and X from being active.

Ref.: 7, 16, 17

27. An 85-year-old female with a medical history of atrial fibrillation has her home Coumadin held during her hospital admission. Which of the following is true?

A. Coumadin should not be held.

B. The patient can only be bridged with heparin, and once the partial thromboplastin times (PTTs) are therapeutic, the Coumadin can be restarted.

C. LMWH can be given as a weight-based dose, and after it has circulated, Coumadin can be restarted.

D. The patient's Coumadin can be restarted without bridging therapy.

E. The patient is at a decreased risk for forming a venous clot.

ANSWER: D

COMMENTS: The Bridging Anticoagulation in Patients who Require Temporary Interruption of Warfarin Therapy for an Elective Invasive Procedure or Surgery (BRIDGE) trial was a randomized, double-blind, placebo-controlled trial to determine the need for bridging anticoagulation after Coumadin had been held for an elective procedure in patients with atrial fibrillation. The trial showed that discontinuing warfarin treatment without a bridge was not inferior to discontinuing with a bridge (LMWH) in relation to the development of arterial thromboembolism. A safety outcome measured in this study was the risk for major bleeding. Bridging therapy was associated with a three-time greater risk. There were no significant differences between groups in regard to myocardial infarction, venous thromboembolism, or death.

Ref: 7, 16, 18

REFERENCES

1. Freischlag JA, Heller JA. Venous disease. In: Townsend Jr CM, Beauchamp RD, Evers BM, et al., eds. *Sabiston Textbook of Surgery: The Biological Basis of Modern Surgical Practice*. 18th ed. Philadelphia: WB Saunders; 2008.
2. Liem TK, Moneta GL. Venous and lymphatic disease. In: Brunicardi FC, Andersen DK, Billiar TR, et al., eds. *Schwartz's Principles of Surgery*. 9th ed. New York: McGraw-Hill; 2010.
3. Cronenwett J, Johnston W, eds. *Rutherford's Vascular Surgery*. 7th ed. Philadelphia: WB Saunders; 2010.
4. Pipinos II , Baxter BT. The lymphatics. In: Townsend Jr CM, Beauchamp RD, Evers BM, et al., eds. *Sabiston Textbook of Surgery: The Biological Basis of Modern Surgical Practice*. 18th ed. Philadelphia: WB Saunders; 2008.
5. Ernst EB, Stanley JE, eds. *Current Therapy in Vascular Surgery*. 3rd ed. St. Louis: CV Mosby; 1995.
6. Rectemwald J, Krishnamurthy V. Vena cava filter placement. In: *Fisher's Mastery of Surgery*. Philadelphia: Lippincott Williams & Wilkins; 2012:2408–2413.
7. Wakefield T, Dalsing M. Venous disease. In: *Greenfield's Surgery: Scientific Principles and Practice*. 5th ed. Philadelphia: Lippincott Williams & Wilkins; 2010.
8. Marston W. Surgical treatment of varicose veins. In: *Fisher's Mastery of Surgery*. Philadelphia: Lippincott Williams & Wilkins; 2012:2414–2421.
9. Axelrod D, Wakefield T. Future directions in antithrombotic therapy: emphasis on venous thromboembolism. New antithrombotic therapy. *J Am Coll Surg*. 2001;192(5):642–651.
10. Frangos SG, Chen AH, Sumpio B. Vascular drugs in the new millennium. *J Am Coll Surg*. 2000;191(1):76–92.
11. Barham K, Shah T. Phlegmasia cerulea dolens. *N Eng J Med*. 2007;356(3):e3.
12. Mumoli N, Invernizzi C, Luschi R, et al. Images in cardiovascular medicine phlegmasia cerulea dolens, AHA. *Circulation*. 2012;125:1056–1057.
13. Doscher ME, Herman S, Garfein ES. Surgical management of inoperable lymphedema: the re-emergence of abandoned techniques. *J Am Coll Surg*. 2012;215(2):278–283.
14. Wysocki WM, Komorowski A. Stewart-Treves syndrome. *J Am Coll Surg*. 2007;205(1):195.
15. Schiffman S, Berger A. Stewart-Treves syndrome. *J Am Coll Surg*. 2006;204(2):238.
16. Guyatt GH, Akl EA, Crowther M, et al. Antithrombotic therapy and prevention of thrombosis, 9th edition: American College of Chest Physicians Evidence-Based Clinical Practice Guidelines. *Chest*. 2012;141(2 Suppl):7s–47s.
17. Axelrod D, Wakefield T. Future directions in antithrombotic therapy: Emphasis on venous thromboembolism. *J Am Coll Surg*. 2001;192(5): 641–651.
18. Douketis D, Spyropoulos AC, Kaatz S, et al. Perioperative bridging anticoagulation in patients with atrial fibrillation. *N Engl J Med*. 2015;373(9):823–833.

G. Amputations

Jennifer Son, M.D., and Erin Farlow, M.D.

1. For recurrent melanoma confined to an extremity, which of these does not confer an increase in survival?
   A. Simple excision
   B. Isolated limb perfusion (ILP) with hyperthermia and chemotherapeutic agent
   C. Amputation
   D. Wide local excision
   E. Immunotherapy

ANSWER: C

COMMENTS: For recurrent melanoma confined to an extremity, simple excision can usually eradicate the disease. Simple excision is sufficient, and a wide local excision is not necessary because it does not improve the recurrence rate. For larger numbers of lesions, simple excision becomes technically prohibitive. For these patients, ILP is the treatment of choice. ILP involves surgical isolation of an extremity's circulation and placing that circulation into an extracorporeal circulation, which is separated from the systemic circulation. After creating the new circuit, the isolated limb is perfused with high doses of heated chemotherapy.

In the era of ILP and immunotherapy to treat melanoma, amputation is performed rarely to treat locoregionally intractable extremity melanoma. Kapma and colleagues presented a series of 451 patients who underwent 501 ILPs over a 23-year period, with only 11 patients (2.4%) who needed to undergo an amputation for locoregionally intractable melanoma. Amputation for melanoma confers no increase in survival and should be performed only for palliation.

Ref.: 1–3

2. Which type of traumatic amputation is least favorable for replanting?
   A. Crush amputation
   B. Guillotine amputation
   C. Avulsion amputation
   D. None of the above can be replanted
   E. All are equally favorable for replanting

ANSWER: C

COMMENTS: Replantation is the reattachment of the part that has been completely amputated. A guillotine amputation is when the tissue is cut with a sharp object and is minimally damaged. Crush amputations have a local injury, which can often be converted into a guillotine amputation by debriding the edges of the wound. Finally, an avulsion amputation is the most unfavorable type as the extensor tendons are shredded or avulsed at their musculotendinous junctions and nerves are stretched or ripped.

Ref.: 4

3. All are indications for replantation of amputated parts except:
   A. Thumb amputations
   B. Multiple injured digits or digits amputated distal to the flexor digitorum superficialis (FDS) insertion
   C. Guillotine amputations at the hand, wrist, and forearm
   D. Amputations in children
   E. A psychotic patient who has willfully self-amputated the part

ANSWER: E

COMMENTS: There are general indications for the replantation of amputated parts, but the overriding decision is still to save life before limb. Although patients and family members may desire replantation, it is not performed in patients with severe associated medical problems or injuries. Replantation is also generally not considered under the following circumstances:

1. Severe crush or multilevel injury of the amputated part
2. A psychotic patient who has willfully self-amputated the part
3. Amputation of a single digit proximal to the FDS distal insertion (zone 2), except for single-digit amputations in children or those with a demanding profession (e.g., a musician)
4. Amputation in patients with severely atherosclerotic arteries (sometimes this can only be determined when exploring the vessels in the operating room)

Indications for replantation of amputated parts are as follows:

1. Whenever possible for a thumb amputation (it provides > 40% of the overall hand function)
2. Single digits that have been amputated distal to the FDS insertion (e.g., a manual worker may likely desire revision of amputation and to return to work quickly)
3. Multiple injured digits
4. Most amputations in children, including single-digit amputations
5. Guillotine-sharp clean amputations at the hand, wrist, or distal forearm

Ref.: 4–6

4. Select the correct timing for reattaching the structure during a replantation:
   A. Veins are attached first to decrease the incidence of venous congestion.
   B. Arteries are attached before veins in order to clear lactic acid and decrease ischemic time.
   C. Nerves are attached first to prevent further injury and restore function to the digits.
   D. Bone is attached last to prevent bone shortening and to prevent a tension-free closure.
   E. Muscles and tendons are attached last to avoid obscuring the operative field.

ANSWER: B

COMMENTS: With only a few minor variations, the sequence of replantation has been standardized. Preliminary exploration of the distal amputated part under a microscope by an initial surgical team determines whether a replantation is technically possible. Bone shortening allows the skin to be debrided back to where it is free of contusion, and direct tension-free closure can be achieved. This is the reason why bone is usually attached first. The order of repair is usually bone, tendons, muscle units, arteries, nerves, and finally veins. The establishment of arterial flow before venous flow clears lactic acid from the replanted part. The functional veins can now also be detected by spurting bleeding. However, blood loss must be closely monitored. For major replantations, reestablishing arterial circulation as rapidly as possible is crucial to limiting the ischemia time.

Ref.: 4

5. In bed-ridden patients who are unable to care for themselves, which type of amputation is best for dry gangrene of the foot?

A. Syme's amputation

B. Below-knee amputation

C. Above-knee amputation

D. Autoamputation with revascularization for optimal healing

E. Any of the above

ANSWER: C

COMMENTS: During the selection of amputation levels, one should consider the objectives of removing all nonviable tissue while ensuring primary wound healing and an acceptable functional result. The outcome following a below-knee amputation is far better than that following amputation at the ankle despite the higher level. In cases where the patient has severe depression of mental status such that he or she is unable to ambulate, communicate, or provide self-care, an above-knee primary amputation should be considered. Severe, long-standing contractures can occur with below-knee amputations in this bed-ridden patient group, leading to pressure ulceration of the stump and further surgery. It is also less likely to heal than the above-knee amputation.

The Syme's amputation involves disarticulation at the ankle. It has fallen into disfavor because it is technically demanding and, more importantly, it is more difficult to create a well-fitting prosthetic for a Syme's amputation than for a below-knee amputation.

Autoamputation of a foot rarely occurs, and revascularization to a leg with a nonsalvageable foot is rarely indicated.

Ref.: 6

6. In trauma patients with mangled extremity injuries:

A. Amputation constitutes a treatment failure

B. Clinical testing such as skin color, temperatures, capillary refill, ankle-brachial indices, and angiographic studies should always be performed to test perfusion of a traumatized limb and determine salvagability

C. Limb salvage often is technically possible but at the cost of multiple surgeries and possible long-term functional deficits

D. Tourniquets should always be applied to prevent massive hemorrhage

E. None of the above

ANSWER: C

COMMENTS: When an extremity in injured, limb salvage is the primary objective so as to give the patient the maximum benefit of a full recovery to be able to perform activities of daily living. In evaluating an extremity, skin color, temperature, and capillary refill as well as other studies such as ankle-brachial indices (ABIs) and angiography may be performed to assess the viability of that extremity. At times when limb salvage is not possible due to hemodynamic instability or severity of injury, amputation must be performed. This does not constitute treatment failure if it saves the patient's life. Mangled extremities frequently require multiple surgical interventions including arterial and venous repair, bony fixation, and soft tissue fixation. The patient should be assessed for adequate health and mental capacity to tolerate repeated surgery and prolonged recovery. Finally, tourniquets are not always applied to an extremity in the field unless there is torrential hemorrhage in the field.

Ref.: 6, 7

7. What is not a contraindication to a below-knee amputation?

A. Absence of popliteal pulse

B. Presence of gangrene that would involve the posterior flap

C. Flexion contracture of the knee greater than 20 degrees

D. Patient's inability to ambulate, communicate, and provide self-care

E. Presence of paresthesia

ANSWER: A

COMMENTS: In cases where the patient has severe depression of mental status such that he or she is unable to ambulate, communicate, or provide self-care, an above-knee primary amputation should be considered. Severe, long-standing contractures can occur with below-knee amputations in this bed-ridden patient group.

A useful algorithm is described by Dwars and colleagues. The authors analyzed a series of 85 lower-extremity amputations and determined that the presence of a palpable pulse immediately above the level of amputation correlated well with primary wound healing and a 100% negative predictive value. The absence of palpable pulses was of no use in selecting an amputation level. Contraindications to a below-knee amputation include situations wherein the gangrenous or infectious process extends to involve the anterior portion of the lower extremity within 4 or 5 cm of the tibial tuberosity or would involve the posterior skin flap, a flexion contracture greater than 20 degrees, or neurologic dysfunction creating muscle spasticity or rigidity on the affected side.

Ref.: 7

8. Primary amputation should be strongly considered in a mangled lower extremity when popliteal artery transection and tibia and fibula fractures are combined with:

A. Popliteal vein transection

B. Tibial nerve transection

C. Deep peroneal nerve transection

D. Extensive skin loss

E. Inability to dorsiflex the foot

ANSWER: B

COMMENTS: The decision to perform a primary amputation or attempt reconstruction is based on hemodynamic stability, soft and bony tissue injury, severity of ischemia (based on clinical or other studies as mentioned in Question 7), duration of ischemia, and the mechanism of injury. The Mangled Extremity Severity Score is a commonly used scoring system that is based on (1) the degree of energy of injury, (2) the degree of limb ischemia, (3) patient age, and (4) the presence and degree of shock. High scores predict limb salvage. However, attempting limb salvage does not mean that the patient will be without complications such as osteomyelitis, non-union, having a nonfunction limb, and undergoing other surgeries. In general, primary amputation should be considered for patients who are hemodynamically unstable, have profound ischemia of greater than 6 h, have a complete amputation, and have a tibia/fibula fracture with a transection of the tibial nerve. A tibial nerve transection leads to paralysis of muscles in the superficial and deep posterior compartments. Patients with inability to dorsiflex the foot usually have an injury to the deep peroneal nerve that leads to a loss of function in the muscles in the anterior compartment, leading to foot drop. This is usually managed with an ankle-foot orthotic.

Ref.: 8, 9

9. Which of the following best predicts healing of a below-knee amputation?

A. Warm skin over the ankle

B. Presence of a popliteal pulse

C. Trancutaneous oximetry reading of 25 mmHg of calf

D. Absence of gangrene above the ankle

E. Popliteal systolic pressure of greater than 50 mmHg

ANSWER: B

COMMENTS: In general, the presence of pulses above the site of amputation predicts healing of an amputation. For example, a palpable femoral pulse predicts the healing of an above-knee amputation, and a popliteal pulse predicts the healing of a below-knee amputation. A dorsalis pedis (DP) pulse predicts the healing of a transmetatarsal amputation (TMA). There are noninvasive tests that predict the healing, such as transcutaneous oximetry readings >40 mmHg (<20 mmHg predict the nonhealing). Further tests may be needed for those that fall in between 20 and 40 mmHg. A popliteal pressure >70 mmHg measured with Doppler and blood pressure cuff predicts healing. One study showed that a palpable popliteal pulse, in addition to using Doppler studies, was associated with a 97% healing rate.

Ref.: 9, 10

REFERENCES

1. Blansfield JA, Pingpank JF. Isolated limb perfusion and extremity amputations. In: Evans SRT, ed. *Surgical Pitfalls*. Philadelphia, PA: Elsevier; 2009:497–501.
2. Kapma MR, Vrouenraets BC, Nieweg OE, et al. Major amputation for intractable extremity melanoma after failure of isolated limb perfusion. *Eur J Surg Oncol*. 2005;31:95–99.
3. Fraker DL. Hyperthermic regional perfusion for melanoma and sarcoma of the limbs. *Curr Probl Surg*. 1999;36:841–907.
4. Netscheer D, Murphy K, Fiore NA. Hand surgery. In: Townsend CM, Beauchamp RD, Evers BM, et al., eds. *Sabiston Textbook of Surgery: The Biological Basis of Modern Surgical Practice*. 19th ed. Philadelphia: Saunders/Elsevier; 2012.
5. Soucacos PN. Indications and selection for digital amputation and replantation. *J Hand Surg Br*. 2001;26:572–581.
6. Neschis DG, Golden M. Arterial disease of the lower extremity. In: Norton JA, Bollinger J, Chang RR, Lowry AE, eds. *Surgery: Basic Science and Clinic Evidence*. 2nd ed. New York: Springer-Verlag; 2001.
7. Dwars BJ, van den Broek TA, Rauwerda JA, Bakker FC. Criteria for reliable selection of the lowest level of amputation in peripheral vascular disease. *J Vasc Surg*. 1992;15:536–542.
8. Quirke T, Sharma P, Boss W, et al. Are type IIIC lower extremity injuries an indication for primary amputation? *J Trauma*. 1996;40:992–996.
9. Mulholland M, Greenfield LJ. Orthopaedic trauma. In: Mullholland MW, Lillemoe KD, Doherty GM, et al., eds. *Greenfield's Surgery: Scientific Principles and Practice*. 5th ed. Philadelphia: Lippincott Williams & Wilkins; 2011.
10. Malone J, Anderson G, Lalka S, et al. Prospective comparison of noninvasive techniques for amputation level selection. *Am J Surg*. 1987;154:179–184.

CHAPTER 29

THORACIC SURGERY

Justin M. Karush, D.O., and Andrew T. Arndt, M.D.

A. Lung and Airway

1. A patient who has remained intubated endotracheally for a prolonged period (>4 weeks) is at risk for the development of tracheal injury. All of the following are true of postintubation tracheal injury except:

   A. Symptoms usually appear many months after extubation.

   B. Dyspnea on exertion is the primary symptom.

   C. It is often misdiagnosed as asthma or bronchitis.

   D. Bronchoscopy is the best mode of evaluation.

   E. Treatment options include tracheal dilation, laser resection, internal stent placement, and staged reconstruction.

ANSWER: A

COMMENTS: Tracheal injury after endotracheal intubation can occur at the cuff level, as a result of stomal injury, or can occur in the glottic and subglottic areas. It is typically caused by scarring at the site of compression of the tracheal mucosa by the balloon from the endotracheal tube. Symptoms usually appear within 1 to 6 weeks of intubation. Dyspnea on exertion is the primary symptom. The severity usually correlates with the degree of tracheal stenosis. Dilation, laser treatment, and stent placement are most often used as temporizing measures to allow inflammation or to allow the patient's overall condition to improve. Most functionally significant strictures are best treated by segmental resection and primary anastomosis.

Ref.: 1, 2

2. Approximately 2 weeks after placement of a tracheostomy tube, copious bleeding from within and around the tracheostomy tube develops in a 65-year-old man. Which of the following choices is the best management for this problem?

   A. Removal of the tracheostomy tube at the bedside

   B. Right posterolateral thoracotomy to access trachea and innominate artery

   C. Tracheal stent placement

   D. Resection of the innominate artery

   E. Arterial wall repair of the innominate artery

ANSWER: D

COMMENTS: A **tracheoinnominate artery fistula** is a rare, but often fatal, complication of intubation or tracheostomy. It has a reported mortality rate of 86%. The most common cause is the placement of the tracheostomy tube too low, with subsequent erosion of the anterior tracheal wall into the innominate artery. Massive hemoptysis and episodic hemoptysis are the most common symptoms. Management includes hyperinflation of the tracheal tube cuff, finger compression of the innominate artery, and emergency return to the operating room (OR) for control of the airway and operative repair. Following orotracheal intubation, exposure is initially achieved via a collar incision at the stoma, with extension into the midline for a sternotomy. The tracheal defect may be closed primarily and covered with soft tissue or be left open to heal by secondary intention if grossly infected. Repair of the innominate artery is associated with a high incidence of failure. Once the vascular defect is identified, the artery is divided proximal and distal to the defect and the divided edges are oversewn. The stumps are then buried under healthy tissue.

Ref.: 1, 2

3. A 53-year-old woman is evaluated for worsening stridor. She also complains of worsening dyspnea. Imaging studies demonstrate no lung pathology but are suggestive of an endotracheal lesion. Bronchoscopy confirms the presence of a primary tracheal tumor. Which of the following statements is true?

   A. It occurs more frequently in women.

   B. A tracheal tumor is best treated with radiation therapy to provide the optimal chance for long-term survival.

   C. The most common histologies are adenoid cystic carcinoma and squamous cell carcinoma.

   D. It is usually found incidentally.

   E. Imaging studies allow adequate characterization of tracheal tumors.

ANSWER: C

COMMENTS: Primary tumors of the trachea are rare and account for less than 0.2% of all respiratory tract malignancies in the United States. A male-to-female ratio of 7:3 is reported. Patients typically have progressive respiratory symptoms, including cough and hemoptysis. Hoarseness and dysphagia are less common. Although endoscopic resection, radiotherapy, and tracheal resection are all available treatment modalities, surgical resection with airway reconstruction provides the best chance for long-term survival in appropriately selected patients. Despite imaging studies visualizing these tumors, bronchoscopic evaluation is extremely important in planning resection.

Ref.: 1, 2

4. A stage I thymoma has been diagnosed in a 41-year-old woman. Through which of the following surgical approaches should a thymectomy not be performed?

A. Transcervical collar incision

B. Median sternotomy

C. Partial sternal split

D. Video-assisted thoracoscopy (VATS)

E. Posterolateral thoracotomy through the sixth intercostal space

ANSWER: E

COMMENTS: Thymectomy is performed most commonly for patients with myasthenia gravis. Indications for thymectomy include the presence of **thymoma** and a diagnosis of myasthenia without thymoma in patients whose disease is refractory to medical therapy or who cannot tolerate or are noncompliant with medical treatment. Thymectomy is also indicated for patients with other less common thymic neoplasms such as thymic carcinoma and thymic carcinoid tumors. Various surgical techniques for thymectomy have been advocated and include all of the approaches listed. The debate regarding which technique has the best results has not been resolved. A posterolateral thoracotomy through the sixth intercostal space would be too low and would provide suboptimal exposure.

Ref.: 1, 2

5. All of the following mediastinal tumors are found in the anterior mediastinum except:

A. Thymoma

B. Thyroid mass

C. Lymphoma

D. Teratoma

E. Ganglioneuroma

ANSWER: E

COMMENTS: Mediastinal masses are characterized by their location in the three compartments of the mediastinum: anterior, middle, and posterior. The **anterior mediastinum** extends vertically from the thoracic inlet to the diaphragm and is bounded anteriorly by the sternum and posteriorly by the brachiocephalic vessels, aorta, and pericardium. The **middle mediastinum** is defined as the space that contains the heart and pericardium. The posterior mediastinal compartment is defined anteriorly by the heart and trachea, laterally by the mediastinal pleura, and posteriorly by the vertebrae. The differential diagnosis of an anterior mediastinal mass includes thymoma, thyroid, lymphoma, and teratoma as the most common tumors. Neurogenic tumors such as ganglioneuromas are most often located in the **posterior mediastinum**.

Ref.: 1, 2

6. A 58-year-old smoker with a history of ethanol abuse was found unconscious after multiple episodes of vomiting. Shortly after this episode, he was noted to have pneumomediastinum and a left pleural effusion on chest radiograph.

In this case, which of the following is most likely the cause of the pneumomediastinum?

A. Esophageal perforation

B. Tracheobronchial injury

C. Rupture of terminal alveoli from pressure generated by coughing or straining against a closed glottis

D. Extension of a pneumothorax

E. Penetrating trauma

ANSWER: A

COMMENTS: Pneumomediastinum refers to the presence of air in the mediastinal space. The most common source is rupture of terminal alveoli caused by coughing or straining against a closed glottis. The air escapes the distal lung tissue, but the visceral pleura remains intact. The air then courses along the perivascular or peribronchial space into the mediastinum. This process is rarely clinically significant and almost always requires no intervention except reassurance and a brief period of observation. Pneumomediastinum may also arise from more significant injury to the tracheobronchial tree or from esophageal perforation. Tracheobronchial injuries should be evaluated with bronchoscopy. An esophagogram with or without esophagoscopy can be performed to evaluate for esophageal injury. The history of recent vomiting and left pleural effusion suggest esophageal perforation in this patient. Rarely, gas extension from the neck, usually secondary to trauma or surgical procedures, or from the abdominal cavity, usually after perforation of retroperitoneal hollow viscera, may result in pneumomediastinum.

Ref.: 1, 2

7. As part of a lung cancer screening protocol, a 62-year-old male with a 30-pack-year smoking history undergoes low-dose computed tomography (CT) of the chest. A 6-cm mass is identified invading the chest wall. Which of the following statements is correct?

A. Pain is an uncommon finding with tumors invading the chest wall.

B. Two uninvolved ribs above and below the site of invasion are required to obtain negative margins.

C. Anterior chest wall resections are more likely to require reconstruction than are posterior chest wall resections.

D. Postoperative radiation is beneficial even if negative margins are obtained.

E. Preoperative radiation is warranted for all tumors invading the chest wall.

ANSWER: C

COMMENTS: Chest wall invasion is identified in approximately 5%–8% of patients undergoing resection for non–small-cell lung cancer (NSCLC). Localized chest wall pain is a very common finding in patients with chest wall invasion; however, the absence of pain does not conclusively rule out invasion. Aside from Pancoast tumors (which benefit from neoadjuvant chemoradiation), tumors invading the chest wall can proceed directly to the lung and en bloc chest wall resection should be performed if N2 disease is not present; preoperative radiation is not indicated. The goal of surgery is to perform a complete (R0) resection, and adjuvant radiation is not indicated if surgical margins are negative. The chest wall resection should incorporate one uninvolved rib above and below the site of invasion to ensure a negative margin. Generally speaking, defects ≥5 cm or involving three or more ribs require chest wall reconstruction with prosthetic and/or muscle flap coverage. However, posteriorly based defects are often covered by the scapula and its associated musculature, and posterior defects of up to 10 cm or those comprising up to ribs 1 to 4 do not typically warrant reconstruction.

Ref.: 4

8. A 76-year-old cachectic-appearing male presents 4 weeks after a right pneumonectomy for stage IIb NSCLC with a cough productive of foul-smelling sputum. He is febrile to 102°F and has a leukocytosis of 15,000 uL. Chest x-ray (CXR) demonstrates a right-sided air-fluid level approximately half way up his thorax. What is true about his current condition?

A. It is best treated with a chest tube inserted, with the patient in the right lateral decubitus position.

B. It is more common after right pneumonectomy.

C. The first step in the management is to place the patient supine and emergently intubate to protect his airway.

D. CXR represents normal findings 4 weeks after a pneumonectomy, and other sources of infection should be sought.

E. Intravenous (IV) antibiotics and CT of the chest are the first steps in managing this patient.

ANSWER: B

COMMENTS: Bronchopleural fistula (BPF) refers to a communication between the bronchial tree and pleural space. It can develop from a variety of causes, including infectious, malignant, and traumatic, but the majority of cases occur following lung resection, particularly pneumonectomy (incidence of 1.5%–11.1%). BPF after pneumonectomy results in prolonged hospital courses and mortality rates of up to 71%. Most postpneumonectomy BPFs present within the first 3 months after surgery. Risk factors for BPF after pneumonectomy include anatomic, technical, and patient factors. Right pneumonectomy has a four- to five-fold higher incidence of BPF than does left pneumonectomy, and the reason for this is multifactorial. Anatomically, compared with the left, the right mainstem bronchus has less natural mediastinal tissue coverage, a more vertical orientation (allows pooling of secretions and pressure on the stump), and a poorer blood supply (one bronchial artery versus two and fewer direct branches from the aorta). Technical factors associated with an increased risk for BPF include devascularization of the bronchial stump, a long bronchial stump, and residual disease at the stump. Patient factors are numerable but principally include the need for postoperative mechanical ventilation as well as preoperative radiation, poor respiratory function, poor nutritional status, chronic steroid use, and surgery for infection. Initial diagnosis of BPF is based on clinical findings (fever, excessively productive cough) and CXR findings of new or dropping air-fluid level in the pneumonectomy space. Principles of BPF management include drainage of the pleural space (tube or open-window thoracostomy), debridement and reinforced closure of the bronchial stump (if nutritional status and overall condition allow), and obliteration of the pleural space (muscle flap, thoracoplasty, etc.). It is absolutely critical in the initial management of these patients to protect the remaining lung. Until the infection is adequately drained, the patient must not be placed supine, not for CT scan, chest tube placement, bronchoscopy, or intubation.

Ref.: 5

9. Which of the following statements about the National Lung Screening Trial (NLST) is true?

A. Patients with a minimum of 40 pack-years of smoking were included in this trial.

B. Patients aged 45 to 80 years were eligible for screening.

C. The NLST demonstrated a 20% reduction in lung cancer mortality in those screened with CT.

D. A CXR or low-dose CT scan annually for 10 years was required for screening.

E. CXR was found to be equivalent to CT scan in screening for lung cancer.

ANSWER: C

COMMENTS: The **NLST** was a multicenter randomized study comparing low-dose helical CT with chest radiograph in the screening of lung cancer in a high-risk population. Eligible participants were aged between 55 and 74 years, had at least a 30-pack-year history of smoking, and were either active smokers or had quit within the past 15 years. Participants underwent three screenings at 1-year intervals. The principal findings of the study included a 20% relative reduction in the rate of death from lung cancer and a 6.7% relative reduction in all-cause mortality in the CT group versus the chest radiograph group.

Ref.: 6

10. A 55-year-old male presents with a clinically staged IIIa (T2N2M0) right upper lobe (RUL) NSCLC. Which of the following statements is true?

A. Endobronchial ultrasound (EBUS) should be performed to establish pathologic diagnosis, followed by mediastinoscopy if negative.

B. Mediastinal sampling is not required as the patient should be referred to oncology for definitive chemotherapy.

C. Mediastinal lymph nodes should be sampled at the time of resection of the primary tumor.

D. Mediastinoscopy should be performed to establish pathologic diagnosis, followed by EBUS if negative.

E. Compared with EBUS, mediastinoscopy has better sensitivity, negative predictive value (NPV), and diagnostic accuracy in sampling mediastinal lymph nodes.

ANSWER: A

COMMENTS: The American College of Chest Physicians (ACCP) published its third edition for the diagnosis and management of lung cancer in 2013. With regard to the **methods of staging NSCLC**, the ACCP offers a grade 1B recommendation that "in patients with a high suspicion of N2,3 involvement ... a needle technique ... is recommended over surgical staging as a best first test." The ACCP subsequently offers that surgical staging (such as mediastinoscopy or VATS) should be performed if the clinical suspicion of mediastinal node involvement remains high after a negative needle biopsy. Needle techniques include endobronchial ultrasound-needle aspiration (EBUS-NA), endoscopic ultrasound-needle aspiration (EUS-NA), and combined EUS/EBUS-NA. Prospective studies have demonstrated that the diagnostic sensitivity, accuracy, and NPV of EBUS-NA are *higher* than those of mediastinoscopy for cN1-3 NSCLC. In one study, EBUS was found to have a sensitivity of 88.0%, specificity of 100%, accuracy of 92.9%, positive predictive value of 100%, and NPV of 85.2%.

However, given the operator dependence of EBUS, mediastinoscopy is still largely considered the gold standard for invasive mediastinal staging, and it is appropriate to perform mediastinoscopy after a negative EBUS if clinical suspicion for positive mediastinal lymph nodes is high.

Ref.: 7, 8

11. A 74-year-old male presents with biopsy-proven lung adenocarcinoma, but no mediastinal disease is found on positron emission tomography (PET)/CT. Which of the following characteristics does not require mediastinal lymph node sampling prior to definitive treatment?

A. Peripherally located T2 tumor

B. Centrally located T1 tumor

C. Clinically positive N1 disease

D. CT-positive mediastinal lymph nodes that have no PET avidity

E. None of the above

ANSWER: E

COMMENTS: Lymph node status has key prognostic and therapeutic indications for patients with clinically resectable NSCLC; **invasive mediastinal staging** is therefore a component of the workup of most NSCLCs. However, it is reasonable to omit invasive mediastinal staging in selected patients. The ACCP gives a grade 2B recommendation that "for patients with a peripheral clinical stage IA tumor (negative nodal involvement by CT and PET), it is suggested that invasive preoperative evaluation of the mediastinal nodes is not required." The rationale for this guideline is that T1-2N0 tumors have a false-negative mediastinal assessment of ~10% by CT and ~4% by PET. Furthermore, this false-negative rate is lower for T1 than for T2 lesions when additional subgroup analysis is performed. Therefore given the likelihood of radiographically occult N2 disease being <4% for peripheral T1 lesions, preoperative invasive mediastinal staging is not absolutely required. Patients undergoing surgery for peripheral T1N0 tumors must still undergo mediastinal lymph node dissection or systematic sampling at the time of resection of the primary tumor.

Ref.: 7, 9

12. A 66-year-old female with a clinically staged T1N0 squamous cell lung carcinoma undergoes a thoracentesis for a moderate pleural effusion. Pleural fluid analysis reveals an exudative effusion, and cytology is positive for malignant cells. What is the correct stage of this patient?

A. Stage I

B. Stage II

C. Stage IIIa

D. Stage IIIb

E. Stage IV

ANSWER: E

COMMENTS: As with other cancers, lung cancer is staged according to the TNM staging system, in which T refers to size, location, and invasiveness of the primary tumor; N refers to the extent of nodal involvement; and M refers to the presence of metastatic disease. Accurate staging of lung cancer is critical to optimize treatment planning and also provides significant prognostic information. According to the 7th edition of the International **Staging System for NSCLC**, a malignant pleural effusion represents M1a disease and makes this a stage IV cancer. The full TNM descriptors and stage groupings are depicted in Table 29.1.

Ref.: 3, 10

TABLE 29.1 TNM Staging System for Lung Cancer (Seventh Edition)

Primary tumor (T)	
T1	Tumor ≤3 cm diameter, surrounded by lung or visceral pleura, without invasion more proximal than lobar bronchus[a]
T1a	Tumor ≤2 cm in diameter
T1b	Tumor >2 cm but ≤3 cm in diameter
T2	Tumor >3 cm but ≤7 cm, or tumor with any of the following features: • Involves main bronchus, ≥2 cm distal to carina • Invades visceral pleura • Associated with atelectasis or obstructive pneumonitis that extends to the hilar region but does not involve the entire lung
T2a	Tumor >3 cm but ≤5 cm
T2b	Tumor >5 cm but ≤7 cm
T3	Tumor >7 cm or any of the following: • Directly invades any of the following: chest wall, diaphragm, phrenic nerve, mediastinal pleura, parietal pericardium, or main bronchus <2 cm from carina (without involvement of carina) • Atelectasis obstructive pneumonitis of the entire lung • Separate tumor nodules in the same lobe
T4	Tumor of any size that invades the mediastinum, heart, great vessels, trachea, recurrent laryngeal nerve, esophagus, vertebral body, carina, or with separate tumor nodules in a different ipsilateral lobe
Regional lymph nodes (N)	
N0	No regional lymph node metastases
N1	Metastasis in ipsilateral peribronchial and/or ipsilateral hilar lymph nodes and intrapulmonary nodes, including involvement by direct extension
N2	Metastasis in ipsilateral mediastinal and/or subcarinal lymph node(s)
N3	Metastasis in contralateral mediastinal, contralateral hilar, ipsilateral or contralateral scalene, or supraclavicular lymph node(s)
Distant metastasis (M)	
M0	No distant metastasis
M1	Distant metastasis
M1a	Separate tumor nodule(s) in a contralateral lobe; tumor with pleural nodules or malignant pleural or pericardial effusion
M1b	Distant metastasis (in extrathoracic organs)

TABLE 29.1 TNM Staging System for Lung Cancer (Seventh Edition)—Cont'd

Stage groupings			
Stage IA	T1a–T1b	N0	M0
Stage IB	T2a	N0	M0
State IIA	T1a, T1b, T2a	N1	M0
	T2b	N0	M0
Stage IIB	T2b	N1	M0
	T3	N0	M0
Stage IIIA	T1a, T1b, T2a, T2b	N2	M0
	T3	N1, N2	M0
	T4	N0, N1	M0
Stage IIIB	T4	N2	M0
	Any T	N3	M0
Stage IV	Any T	Any N	M1a or M1b

[a]The uncommon superficial spreading tumor of any size with its invasive component limited to the bronchial wall, which may extend proximal to the main bronchus, is also classified as T1a.

Adapted from Goldstraw P, Crowley J, Chansky K, et al. The IASLC Lung Cancer Staging Project: proposals for the revision of the TNM stage groups in the forthcoming (seventh) edition of the TNM classification of malignant tumours. *J Thorac Oncol.* 2007;2:706.

B. Mediastinum

1. The correct T stage for a patient with a 6-cm peripheral lung adenocarcinoma is:

A. T1a

B. T1b

C. T2a

D. T2b

E. T3

ANSWER: D

COMMENTS: As with other cancers, lung cancer is staged according to the TNM staging system, in which T refers to size, location, and invasiveness of the primary tumor; N refers to the extent of nodal involvement; and M refers to the presence of metastatic disease. Accurate staging of lung cancer assists with treatment planning and provides important prognostic information. According to the 7th edition of the International **Staging System for NSCLC**, a 6-cm peripheral NSCLC falls into the T2b category based on size criteria (tumor >5 but ≤7 cm). The full TNM descriptors and stage groupings can be found in Table 29.1.

Ref.: 10

2. During a right upper lobectomy, frozen section analysis of the bronchial margin is positive for malignant disease. What is the next most appropriate step?

A. Perform a right pneumonectomy

B. No further management is required

C. Refer the patient for radiation therapy of the bronchial stump

D. Place a well-vascularized autologous tissue flap on the bronchial stump

E. Perform a sleeve lobectomy

ANSWER: E

COMMENTS: The goal of a curative resection for NSCLC is to achieve an R0 resection—that is, to remove all macroscopic and microscopic disease—as the residual disease is known to adversely affect survival. To that end, the intraoperative frozen section is a frequently used tool to assess the bronchial margin during lung cancer operations. The utility in studying the bronchial margin via frozen section is to allow reexcision of the bronchial stump if needed. The first approach to reexcision of a positive bronchial stump is to perform a parenchymal-sparing resection—either a **bronchoplastic or sleeve resection**—if possible. If that is not feasible, additional parenchymal resection should be performed (bilobectomy, pneumonectomy) if the patient can tolerate it. Adjuvant radiation to the stump is an option in patients with residual disease, but its availability does not obviate the need for an appropriate oncologic (R0) resection. Covering a stump that was previously radiated or is likely to be radiated with autologous tissue should be considered, but this step alone is an inappropriate oncologic management of the residual disease. Clearly, offering no additional management is not an appropriate strategy.

Ref.: 11, 12

3. When a level 4R lymph node is biopsied during mediastinoscopy, an immediate rush of dark blood is obtained. Which of the following statements is correct?

A. The complication rate for mediastinoscopy is approximately 10%.

B. The first step is to remove the mediastinoscope and apply pressure to the wound.

C. Perform an emergent right thoracotomy.

D. Perform an emergent sternotomy.

E. The most common vessel injured during mediastinoscopy is the azygous vein.

ANSWER: E

COMMENTS: The complication rate for **mediastinoscopy** is reported as anywhere from 1% to 3.7% in several large publications. Although major bleeding has lethal potential, it represents only 0.3% of all complications. Major bleeding is defined as any bleeding that requires an additional incision for control. The most common vessel injured is the azygous vein given its proximity to the R4 nodal station. This is followed by the right main pulmonary artery and the innominate artery. The first step when bleeding occurs is to pack through the mediastinoscope, not to remove it. If the bleeding does not resolve with this maneuver, the surgeon must communicate with the OR team to ensure that all elements of resuscitation are available and the operative plan is clearly understood. The standard approach to mediastinal hemorrhage is median sternotomy; however, if the surgeon is certain that the bleeding is from the azygous vein, better exposure is achieved through a right thoracotomy.

Ref.: 13

4. A 76-year-old man with stage III chronic obstructive pulmonary disease (COPD) presents to the emergency department (ED) with shortness of breath. Evaluation reveals a 3-cm right middle squamous cell carcinoma. After negative EBUS evaluation of his mediastinum, he is referred for right middle lobectomy. Preoperative evaluation of his lung function reveals a forced expiratory volume 1.0 (FEV_1) of 35% and a diffusion capacity for carbon monoxide (DLCO) of 35%. What is the next most appropriate step in his evaluation?

A. Cardiopulmonary exercise testing (CPET)

B. No further testing required; he is not a surgical candidate based on his pulmonary function tests (PFTs)

C. Referral for lung-volume–reduction surgery

D. No further testing required; he should be offered surgical resection

E. Perform 6-min walk test

ANSWER: A

COMMENTS: A careful **preoperative assessment of lung function** is critical for every patient being evaluated for lung resection. Specifically, PFTs allows prediction of morbidity and mortality after thoracic surgery. Postoperative predicted FEV_1 and DLCO, which are calculated solely on the number of remaining lung segments after resection, are critical determinants of postoperative risk. Although based on historical data, a predicted postoperative FEV_1 or DLCO of 40% is still considered the cutoff for high risk. For patients with values in this range, a quantitative ventilation/perfusion (VQ) scan is performed to assess regional perfusion. Additionally, high-risk patients should be further evaluated with CPET, which assesses oxygen consumption (VO_2) and is a measure of functional capacity. A VO_2max greater than 15 represents an average risk, and a VO_2max less than 10 indicates high risk. More recent data from the National Emphysema Treatment Trial (NETT) Research Group suggests that selected patients with severe emphysema and otherwise poor candidates for lung resection by PFTs alone may even improve after resection. Additionally, significant improvements in postoperative care, including management of pain with epidurals, intensive pulmonary toilet exercises, and early ambulation, improve outcomes in higher-risk patients and have made determination of resectability a case-by-case decision.

Ref.: 1, 14

5. Which of the following histologic subtypes of lung adenocarcinoma is associated with the lowest risk for recurrence?

A. Lepidic
B. Acinar
C. Papillary
D. Micropapillary
E. Solid

ANSWER: A

COMMENTS: Lung adenocarcinoma demonstrates great histologic variability, and in 2011, a **new histologic classification for lung adenocarcinoma** was adopted by the World Health Organization (WHO). This was based on prognostic data that were validated in multiple large, independent, and international analyses. In the previous revision published by the WHO (2004), the majority were classified as mixed type despite tremendous variability in clinical outcome. Overwhelming evidence supports that specific histologic patterns have significant prognostic value. For example, adenocarcinoma in situ [formerly bronchioloalveolar carcinoma (BAC)] and minimally invasive adenocarcinoma are small (less than 3 cm) lepidic predominant tumors that have a nearly 100% 5-year survival with no recurrences. Among invasive adenocarcinoma, five subtypes have been identified. Lepidic predominant tumors have the lowest risk for recurrence. Acinar and papillary tumors are classified as associated with intermediate risk for recurrence. Micropapillary or solid predominant tumors are classified as associated with high risk for recurrence or cancer-related death.

Ref.: 15, 16

6. A 55-year-old male with significant history of alcohol abuse presents with fevers, cough, and chest pain. CT scan is performed, and it demonstrates a 4-cm RUL cavitary lesion consistent with lung abscess. Which of the following is an indication for continued nonoperative management?

A. Development of BPF
B. Massive hemoptysis
C. Suspicion of underlying malignancy
D. Lack of clinical improvement after 4 weeks of appropriate antibiotics
E. Empyema

ANSWER: D

COMMENTS: A **lung abscess** is a cavity within the lung parenchyma, which is filled with varying degrees of pus and air. Most commonly these abscesses result from aspiration, although previous cavitation resulting from neoplasm, infarct, or structural lung disease can lead to secondary infection and abscess formation. Typically, they develop in the dependent segments of the lung (posterior segment of the RUL and superior segment of the lower lobes). Patients with lung abscesses usually present with cough, fever, dyspnea, chest pain, and malaise. If the cavity drains into the tracheobronchial tree, patients will complain of foul-smelling sputum. The mainstay of successful treatment of lung abscesses is prolonged antibiotic therapy. The course of antibiotics is typically 6 to 8 weeks, and radiographic resolution usually lags behind by 4 to 5 months. Indications for surgical intervention include persistence of abscess despite adequate medical therapy, empyema, BPF, massive hemoptysis, and suspicion of malignancy.

Ref.: 2

7. Which of the following is the most common benign lung tumor?

A. Leiomyoma
B. Hamartoma
C. Myoepithelioma
D. Mucinous cystadenoma
E. Mucous gland adenoma

ANSWER: B

COMMENTS: **Benign lung lesions** are rare. In some reports, they comprise less than 1% of all resected lung masses. They can arise from any of the various cell types that are present in the lung. In the workup of a lung mass, numerous characteristics are used to evaluate the probability of malignancy, including standardized uptake value (SUV) avidity, growth rate, and radiographic appearance. However, none of these modalities allows for certain determination, and resection is frequently required to delineate benign from malignant lesions. Hamartomas are the most common benign lung lesions and account for more than 70% of nonmalignant tumors of the lung. They typically present as parenchymal lesions but can also be endobronchial and may require resection even if proven benign as they can cause obstructive symptoms (pneumonia, hemoptysis, and cough). The presence of cartilage is diagnostic of a hamartoma. In many cases calcification is seen, and it gives rise to the bosselated or "popcorn" shape classically attributed to hamartomas.

Ref.: 2

8. A 25-year-old man undergoes a CXR to evaluate a shoulder injury that he sustained during a tennis match. A 4-cm anterior mediastinal mass is found and confirmed by CT scan. Tumor markers show an elevated beta-human chorionic gonadotropin (β-hCG) and alpha-fetoprotein. What is the most likely diagnosis?

A. Thymoma
B. Teratoma
C. Nonseminomatous germ cell tumor
D. Seminoma
E. Lymphoma

ANSWER: C

COMMENTS: Although **germ cell tumors** usually arise in gonadal tissue, the anterior mediastinum is the most common site of extragonadal disease. Germ cell tumors account for 15%–20% of anterior mediastinal masses and are divided into benign and malignant lesions. Mediastinal teratoma is a benign mass that accounts for 60% of all germ cell tumors. On CT, these are well-circumscribed masses that may contain calcification and have variable enhancement owing to the frequent presence of different tissue types (muscle, bone, fat). As these tumors can grow very large and compress surrounding mediastinal structures, the treatment is complete excision. Malignant mediastinal germ cell tumors are divided into seminomatous and nonseminomatous tumors, and differentiation is crucial because treatment is widely different. Pure seminomas have no elevation in tumor markers (alpha-fetoprotein and β-hCG) and are treated with radiation alone. Nonseminomatous tumors are defined by elevations in both tumor markers and are usually treated with chemotherapy alone. In both cases surgery is reserved for residual masses after treatment.

Ref.: 2

C. Chest Wall

1. Which of the following tumor markers is not indicated in the workup of an anterior mediastinal mass?
   A. Antiacetylcholine receptor antibody
   B. Lactate dehydrogenase (LDH)
   C. Alpha-fetoprotein
   D. Carcinoembryonic antigen (CEA)
   E. Beta-HCG

ANSWER: D

COMMENTS: The differential diagnosis of an **anterior mediastinal mass** includes thymoma, lymphoma, germ cell tumors, and thyroid goiter. As management of these tumors varies significantly, accurate diagnosis is paramount. Mediastinal masses are typically identified on routine CXR or found incidentally on CT scan. However, imaging alone is generally nondiagnostic, and other factors must be considered in order to make appropriate recommendations. These include the patient's demographics, medical history, physical examination, symptoms, and blood work. Tumor markers should be obtained on all patients presenting with anterior mediastinal masses. Antiacetylcholine receptor antibody is indicated in patients with either a history or physical examination consistent with myasthenia gravis. LDH should be obtained for suspicion of lymphoma, especially in young women with B-symptoms who present with adenopathy and a mediastinal mass. Lastly, β-hCG and alpha-fetoprotein are diagnostic of nonseminomatous germ cell tumors, which typically present in young men.

Ref.: 2

2. A 14-year-old boy has an anterior chest wall deformity that includes a depression in the body of the sternum, as well as in the lower costal cartilage. Which of the following statements regarding his chest wall deformity is accurate?
   A. There is a 4:1 male-to-female preponderance.
   B. Occurrence is more common on the left side than on the right side.
   C. There is a high incidence of spontaneous resolution.
   D. There is an association with Marfan syndrome in more than 10% of patients.
   E. It is frequently associated with syndactyly.

ANSWER: A

COMMENTS: **Pectus excavatum** and **pectus carinatum** are the most common chest wall deformities. Carinatum is anterior angulation of the sternum, whereas excavatum is posterior angulation. Asymmetry of the depression can occur, such as the right side being more involved than the left side. It is usually present at birth but may worsen significantly during adolescence because of the rapid growth of the individual. Pectus excavatum occurs four times more commonly in males than in females and is rarely seen in the African-American or Hispanic population. Although rare cases of spontaneous resolution occur, the majority of children have deformities that persist or worsen with time, especially during rapid growth periods. Approximately 65% of patients with Marfan syndrome have chest wall deformities, with pectus excavatum being the most common. However, only 2% of all patients with pectus excavatum have Marfan syndrome. **Poland's syndrome** is a congenital anomaly characterized by the absence of the sternal head of the pectoralis major and minor muscles. It is associated with anomalies, including hypoplasia of the breast/nipple complex, rib aplasia, lung hernia, small and elevated scapula (Sprengel deformity), cervical vertebral fusion (Klippel-Feil syndrome), syndactyly, and renal anomalies. Malignancies such as leukemia, lymphoma, cervical cancer, and lung cancer have also been associated.

Ref.: 1, 2

3. A 45-year-old man is being evaluated for a painful right chest wall mass emanating from the ribs. Workup suggests that this is a primary lesion of the chest wall. What is the most common primary malignant chest wall neoplasm in an adult?
   A. Osteosarcoma
   B. Soft tissue sarcoma
   C. Ewing sarcoma
   D. Chondrosarcoma
   E. Plasmacytoma

ANSWER: D

COMMENTS: Most **primary chest wall tumors** are benign, whereas most malignant chest wall neoplasms are metastatic. The most common primary malignant chest wall mass in adults is **chondrosarcoma**. It accounts for 50% of malignant chest wall tumors and 25% of all primary chest wall masses. Eighty percent of chondrosarcomas occur in the ribs and 20% in the sternum. Surgical resection is the best treatment of chondrosarcoma because these tumors are extremely resistant to radiation therapy and chemotherapy. Wide resection is typically curative. If left untreated, metastases typically occur late. Ewing sarcoma and primitive neuroectodermal tumors are the most common primary chest mall malignancies in children. These tumors are best treated by resection and radiation therapy. Chemotherapy can be used to control distant disease. Plasmacytoma is a local manifestation of multiple myeloma that is often manifested as a rib lesion in older men. Osteosarcomas have a bimodal distribution; they occur between the ages of 10 and 25 years and then again after the age of 40 years, often in association with many other diseases. Primary soft tissue sarcomas of the chest wall are uncommon.

Ref.: 1, 2

4. Regarding the diagnosis and management of thoracic outlet syndrome:
   A. An operation is the primary treatment.
   B. It is recognized in approximately 2% of the population.

C. Neurogenic symptoms primarily result from compression of the phrenic nerve between the anterior and middle scalene muscles.

D. Patients may have primarily neurogenic symptoms, vascular symptoms, or a combination of both.

E. Decreased nerve conduction velocity of the median nerve at the elbow is strongly suggestive.

ANSWER: D

COMMENTS: Thoracic outlet syndrome is compression of the subclavian vessels or the brachial plexus (or both) as these structures exit the chest at the junction of the scalene muscles and the bony thorax. Most of the compression occurs at the first rib. It is present in approximately 8% of the population. Patients may have neurologic symptoms, signs of vascular compression, or a combination of both. Although the phrenic nerve lies on the anterior scalene muscle, neurogenic symptoms occur from compression of the brachial plexus between the scalene triangle and the bony thorax. Pain and paresthesia symptoms predominate, particularly in the ulnar nerve distribution. The initial treatment of most patients with thoracic outlet syndrome is nonoperative and consists of patient education on positioning, behavior modification, and physical therapy. Surgery is usually reserved for the 5% of patients with persistent symptoms despite nonoperative treatment. **Delayed nerve conduction velocity** across the thoracic outlet is consistent with thoracic outlet syndrome, and decreased velocity around the elbow is indicative of ulnar nerve entrapment or neuropathy.

Ref.: 1, 2

5. A 31-year-old man is brought to the trauma department 10 min after a gunshot wound to the left side of his chest. On arrival, he loses his vital signs. He is already intubated with endotracheal tube placement confirmed, and an ongoing resuscitation effort is maintained. In preparing for emergency thoracotomy, which of the following best characterizes the necessary incision and position of the patient?

A. Posterolateral incision through the fourth intercostal space and the patient in the lateral decubitus position

B. Anterior incision through the second intercostal space and the patient in the supine position

C. Anterolateral incision through the fourth or fifth intercostal space and the patient in the supine position

D. Vertical incision along the anterior axillary line through the sixth intercostal space and the patient in the supine position

E. Anterolateral incision through the sixth intercostal space and the patient in the lateral decubitus position

ANSWER: C

COMMENTS: The most common **emergency thoracotomy incision** is an anterolateral incision. It allows quick access to the thoracic cavity for control of life-threatening hemorrhage. This is performed with the patient supine and begins along the inframammary fold. The incision is turned superiorly along the medial aspect after crossing the midclavicular line so that if extension across the sternum is required, the incision is not too low. The pericardium, lungs, pulmonary hilum, and descending thoracic aorta from the left side are readily accessible through this incision. If on entering the chest, high apical bleeding is encountered consistently with injury to a great vessel, the apex of the chest should be packed and the appropriate counterincision made. All of the other incisions listed are used in thoracic surgery for various exposures but are not generally indicated for trauma.

Ref.: 1, 2

6. A healthy 45-year-old female, with normal pulmonary function, presents with left arm pain. CT scan shows a 3.4-cm irregular mass at the apex of the right lung involving the first and second ribs anteriorly. Transthoracic needle biopsy demonstrates primary lung adenocarcinoma. PET scan and mediastinoscopy demonstrate no metastatic disease. What is the best initial treatment for this patient?

A. Right upper lobectomy with en bloc chest wall resection

B. Induction chemotherapy and radiation

C. Right VATS lobectomy

D. Definitive chemotherapy and radiation

E. Right pneumonectomy, mediastinal lymph node dissection, and adjuvant chest wall radiation

ANSWER: B

COMMENTS: Pancoast tumors, also called *superior sulcus tumors*, are (typically) NSCLCs that arise in the extreme apex of the lung, occupying the superior sulcus—the uppermost portion of the costovertebral gutter. They can directly invade adjacent structures, including the first and second ribs, vertebral bodies, subclavian vessels, and brachial plexus. The most common presenting symptom is shoulder pain that often radiates down the arm in the ulnar distribution, caused by the invasion of the lower trunk of the brachial plexus as well as of the parietal pleura, ribs, or vertebral bodies. Intrinsic hand muscle wasting and Horner syndrome are also classically present. Because the tumors are peripherally located, respiratory symptoms tend to be uncommon until late in the disease. Unlike other NSCLCs that invade the chest wall more inferiorly and can proceed directly to resection, Pancoast tumors are best treated with neoadjuvant chemoradiation followed by en bloc resection of the tumor and involved chest wall structures. Some centers resect even in the face of vertebral body or subclavian artery invasion. Contraindications to surgery include motor loss to arm, N2 or M1 disease, disease progression with neoadjuvant therapy, and invasion of the trachea, esophagus, or mediastinum.

Ref.: 5

7. A 46-year-old woman with a history of previously treated breast cancer presents with pain over her left fourth and fifth ribs posteriorly. CT scan reveals a mass in the posterior paravertebral chest wall. What is the most common radiation-induced chest wall tumor?

A. Primitive neuroectodermal tumor

B. Malignant fibrous histiocytoma

C. Osteochondroma

D. Chondroma

E. Osteosarcoma

ANSWER: E

COMMENTS: Radiation-induced malignancies are rare, comprising about 3%–6% of all sarcomas. Most commonly, osteosarcoma arises in the chest wall, status post radiation therapy for breast cancer. Like all sarcomas, the most important prognostic factors are tumor size and grade. Most radiation-induced sarcomas are high grade. These tumors are typically symptomatic. Biopsy sites, either incisional or needle, need to be carefully planned as to be resectable along with the primary tumor. Complete surgical resection with adjuvant chemotherapy is the mainstay of treatment. No study has demonstrated a survival benefit of preoperative versus postoperative chemotherapy, and this practice is institution dependent. Chondroma and osteochondroma are the most common benign chest wall tumors in children and adults, respectively. Primitive neuroectodermal and malignant fibrous histiocytomas are the most common malignant chest wall tumors in children and adults, respectively.

Ref.: 2

D. Pleura

1. A 20-year-old tall, thin man experiences spontaneous right-sided pneumothorax. On further questioning and examination, it is revealed that approximately 1 year earlier he was hospitalized and had a right chest tube placed for a similar problem. What is the optimal treatment option for this patient at this time?

A. Observation and discharge

B. Repeated tube thoracostomy maintained until resolution

C. Needle aspiration and discharge

D. Lobectomy and hospitalization

E. Thoracoscopic pleurodesis and apical wedge resection

ANSWER: E

COMMENTS: Primary spontaneous pneumothorax occurs in young patients without significant lung disease, whereas secondary spontaneous pneumothorax occurs in patients with COPD. The most common cause of primary spontaneous pneumothorax is rupture of small apical blebs. In the United States, tube thoracostomy with water seal drainage is the usual first-line treatment of a moderate-to-large pneumothorax in a patient with a first-time occurrence. Needle aspiration of air from the pleural space is more commonly done in Europe. Patients with small, first-time pneumothoraces can be safely observed. Approximately 20%–30% of patients have a recurrence within 2 years of the first episode. After three or more episodes of spontaneous pneumothorax, the rate of recurrence rises to 50%–70% in the following 2 years. It is for this reason that surgery is indicated if there is a recurrence. Operative intervention may be considered after a first episode of spontaneous pneumothorax in patients with previous pneumonectomy, a history of untreated bilateral pneumothorax, or an occupation that poses an elevated risk for the development of pneumothorax, such as an airline pilot or underwater diver.

Ref.: 1, 2

2. Management of chylothorax includes all of the following except:

A. Drainage of the pleural space

B. Fluid, electrolyte, and nutritional support

C. External beam radiation therapy

D. Surgical ligation of the thoracic duct

E. Octreotide

ANSWER: C

COMMENTS: Chylothorax is the accumulation of excess lymphatic fluid in the pleural space. It is usually a result of injury to the **thoracic duct** or one of its major branches and occasionally results from obstruction of the duct. The thoracic duct at the level of the diaphragm runs extrapleurally along the left anterior surface of the vertebral bodies, posterior to the esophagus, between the aorta and azygous vein. A triglyceride level of 110 mg/dL has a 99% likelihood of being chylous versus 5% when the drainage is 50 mg/dL. The most common causes are trauma, neoplasms, tuberculosis, and venous thrombosis. Treatment options are divided into operative and nonoperative categories. Drainage of the pleural space is the basic treatment of any significant accumulation of fluid. Prevention of dehydration and malnutrition and correction of electrolyte imbalance are important for higher-output chyle leaks. The most effective means of reducing chyle production is limitation or elimination of oral intake and institution of total parenteral nutrition. Somatostatin, octreotide, etilefrine, mechanical ventilation with positive end-expiratory pressure, and embolization of the thoracic duct have been used with variable success. In general, 25%–50% of chyle leaks close spontaneously within 2 weeks of nonoperative treatment. Surgical treatment is recommended for persistent leaks and can be performed with a variety of described techniques. Successful operative management relies on an anatomic understanding of the course of the thoracic duct. Prolonged drainage only results in dehydration, malnutrition, and immunologic compromise secondary to the loss of fluid, fats, proteins, and T lymphocytes.

Ref.: 1, 2

3. A 60-year-old former smoker is being evaluated for progressive dyspnea and is found to have a large left-sided effusion. Workup reveals that his effusion is secondary to a malignant pleural mesothelioma of sarcomatoid histology. Which of the following is true regarding his diagnosis?

A. Only approximately 20% of malignant pleural mesotheliomas are not asbestos related.

B. It is related to infection with *Histoplasma.*

C. Its incidence is decreasing.

D. Malignant pleural mesothelioma cannot be treated with surgery.

E. It has a 5- to 10-year latency period after exposure to asbestos.

ANSWER: A

COMMENTS: Malignant mesothelioma is a rare tumor of the pleura. It is classified histologically into three subtypes: epithelioid, sarcomatoid, and mixed. The incidence is believed to be related to the industrial use of asbestos, particularly in occupations that expose individuals to the amphibole fibers of asbestos. Approximately 80% of malignant pleural mesotheliomas are secondary to asbestos exposure. Other factors that may contribute to the development of malignant pleural mesothelioma include radiation, non–asbestos-containing mineral fibers, organic chemicals, viruses, genetic predisposition, pleural scarring, and chronic inflammation. Despite governmental regulations on asbestos exposure in the second half of the 20th century, the incidence of malignant pleural mesothelioma has been rising in the United States since 1980. The latency period between exposure to asbestos and disease is 20 to 50 years. Twenty percent of cases are not related to **asbestos exposure**. Overall survival is grim. The best overall survival appears to be achieved with multimodality therapy consisting of combinations of surgery, chemotherapy, and radiation therapy. In appropriately selected patients, surgical treatment options include pleurectomy with decortication and extrapleural pneumonectomy. Controversy exists regarding which procedure is best.

Ref.: 1, 2

4. A 24-year-old woman is a passenger in a motor vehicle collision. On arrival to the trauma bay, a chest radiograph is suggestive of a left hemothorax. A tube thoracostomy is performed, and a copious amount of bloody effusion is evacuated. Blood continues to be drained from her chest. In blunt chest trauma with hemothorax, which of the following is an indication for surgical exploration?

   A. Initial chest tube output exceeding 1500 mL
   B. Hourly chest tube output of up to 100 mL for three consecutive hours
   C. Declining hemoglobin or hematocrit
   D. Increasing opacities on chest radiography
   E. Presence of pneumothorax

ANSWER: A

COMMENTS: Blunt injury to the thorax often results in varying degrees of hemothorax, pneumothorax, or both. Tube thoracostomy is the initial management of all injuries, both blunt and penetrating, to the thoracic cavity that result in **hemothorax** or **pneumothorax**. Many such injuries can be managed with tube thoracostomy alone. With regard to hemothorax, two metrics are generally accepted as indications for thoracotomy: (1) volume of initial drainage after tube thoracostomy of 1500 mL or more or (2) ongoing bloody chest tube output of greater than 200 mL/h. A drop in hemoglobin or hematocrit is often associated with a multiply injured trauma victim and is not by itself an indication for thoracotomy. Opacities on a chest radiograph in trauma patients are relatively nonspecific and may represent lung contusion, atelectasis, pneumonia, pleural effusion, or retained hemothorax. Their presence, although important to ongoing care of the patient, is not an indication for surgical exploration. Most pneumothoraces from trauma will resolve with tube thoracostomy.

Ref.: 1, 2

5. Two months following right-sided pneumonectomy, a right-sided empyema develops in a 60-year-old man. Conservative measures followed by lesser invasive measures to address this problem are not successful. Therefore the patient is scheduled for open drainage of his empyema. Which of the following is true?

   A. It is typically used in any patient able to tolerate general anesthesia.
   B. It is best suited if the underlying lung reexpands after drainage and is not well adherent to the surrounding chest wall.
   C. It is particularly useful if a BPF is present.
   D. It cannot be used in the setting of a BPF.
   E. It can be considered as an alternative first-line therapy in lieu of a chest tube.

ANSWER: C

COMMENTS: Empyema is defined as a purulent pleural effusion. The most common source of infection is the lung, but bacteria may enter the pleural space through the chest wall, from below the diaphragm, or through the mediastinum. The mainstays of treatment are antibiotics and drainage of the pleural space. Diagnostic thoracentesis is often performed, but definitive pleural drainage must be undertaken to control the infection. This can be performed by closed tube thoracostomy, pigtail catheter, VATS, or open thoracotomy. Open drainage of an empyema is best suited for chronic empyema with fixed underlying lung parenchyma that does not reexpand. Open drainage is particularly useful if a **BPF** is present. The drainage technique of open-window thoracostomy is credited to Dr. Leo Eloesser. In 1935 he described an open thoracic window for tuberculous empyemas in which a U-shaped flap of skin and subcutaneous tissue was created and sewn to the most dependent portion of the empyema cavity after removing two to three underlying ribs and intercostal muscles. The **Eloesser flap** is performed with a thoracotomy incision over the empyema, rib resection, and marsupialization of the skin edges to the parietal pleura to prevent closure of the incision. The **Clagett procedure** can be used if a BPF is not present and consists of open pleural drainage, serial operative debridement, and eventual chest closure after filling the chest cavity with antibiotic solution. It is most often used for an infected pneumonectomy space.

Ref.: 1, 2

6. A 55-year-old male with a 25-pack-year history of smoking is 6 months status post-coronary artery bypass grafting (CABG) and presents to the emergency room (ER) with shortness of breath and fever. A CXR is performed, which demonstrates a large left pleural effusion. Thoracentesis is performed, and 2 L of serous fluid is obtained. Pleural fluid analysis is pending. Which of the following statements is correct?

   A. Congestive heart failure is the most likely cause of an exudative effusion.
   B. Repeat imaging is unnecessary if the patient's symptoms resolve after thoracentesis.
   C. A chest tube should always be inserted to ensure complete drainage.
   D. Cytology is a necessary part of this patient's pleural fluid analysis.
   E. The patient should be taken to the OR for placement of a PleurX catheter.

ANSWER: D

COMMENTS: Pleural effusion is one of the most common pathologies faced by thoracic surgeons. With a broad differential, they frequently present both diagnostic and therapeutic dilemmas. Thoracentesis with the pleural fluid analysis is the mainstay of diagnosis and can also be definitively therapeutic. The initial analysis of an effusion focuses on the ratio and absolute value of protein and LDH (**Light's criteria**). This allows us to classify an effusion as exudative (high protein and LDH ratio) or transudative (low protein and LDH ratio). The most common causes of an exudative pleural effusion are infection (parapneumonic), inflammation [acute respiratory distress syndrome (ARDS)], and malignancy. The most common cause of a transudative pleural effusion is heart failure. Drainage of the effusion and treatment of its underlying cause is the mainstay of management (i.e., diuresis for heart failure or antibiotics for parapneumonic effusions). However, there are several other characteristics that predict failure of conservative management and may require more aggressive intervention. It is critically important to identify the presence of a loculated pleural effusion, which is unlikely to allow complete drainage with tube thoracostomy alone.

Although a loculated effusion in general can be appreciated on recumbent CXR, this is best evaluated with CT scan. Furthermore, imaging must be obtained to evaluate for adequate lung expansion after any initial drainage procedure, as trapped lung is a common complication of chronic effusions and may require decortication to manage properly. Cytology has a notoriously high false-negative rate, but is a critical component of the workup of a pleural effusion, especially in patients with risk factors for lung cancer. In the case of recurrent malignant effusions, one therapeutic option is to place a tunneled chest tube (PleurX catheter) that allows the patient to drain his or her own effusion at home.

Ref.: 4

E. Diaphragm

1. During the performance of trisegmentectomy in a patient with colorectal metastasis to the right lobe of the liver, a brisk venous-like type of bleeding arises posterior to the liver. The surgeon decides to extend the incision through a median sternotomy. What is the best location to take down and repair the diaphragm so that the phrenic nerve is not injured?
   A. Centrally along the middle of the diaphragm, beginning medially at the central tendon and moving laterally toward the chest wall
   B. Along the posterior third between the aorta and the esophagus
   C. Circumferentially at the periphery of the diaphragm
   D. Centrally along the middle of the diaphragm in a vertical line from anterior to posterior
   E. Medially in a linear fashion at the junction of the diaphragm and the mediastinal pleura

ANSWER: C

COMMENTS: The **diaphragm** is innervated by the **phrenic nerves**. Arising from cervical roots C3, C4, and C5, the nerves originate at the superior border of the thyroid cartilage, pass along the anterior scalene muscles bilaterally, and descend through the mediastinum along the middle of the pericardium anterior to the hilum of the lungs. The right phrenic nerve reaches the diaphragm just lateral to the inferior vena cava. The left phrenic nerve enters the diaphragm lateral to the left border of the heart. Both nerves divide at the level of the diaphragm or just above it into several branches. There are three main muscular branches on the surface of the diaphragm. One is directed anteromedially toward the sternum, another is directed anterolaterally toward the central tendon, and the third is directed posteriorly. When taking down the diaphragm for surgical exposure, it is of paramount importance to avoid injury to these branches. The best approach to divide the diaphragm is along the peripheral circumference with just enough muscle left on the chest wall for sturdy reapproximation. Generally, it is advised that one stay at least 5 cm lateral to the edge of the central tendon to avoid the posterolateral and anterolateral branches of the phrenic nerve.

Ref.: 1, 2

2. A Bochdalek congenital diaphragmatic hernia:
   A. Is right sided 90% of the time
   B. Is located anteriorly at the sternocostal junction
   C. Usually has a hernia sac with associated abdominal contents
   D. Is related to failure of development or fusion of the pleuroperitoneal membranes
   E. Is associated with other congenital anomalies in less than 10% of patients

ANSWER: D

COMMENTS: Congenital diaphragmatic hernias are divided into two subtypes: Bochdalek and Morgagni. Both types occur as a result of abnormalities during embryogenesis, specifically failure of development or fusion of the pleuroperitoneal membranes that usually make up the diaphragm between the fourth and eighth weeks of gestation. In **Morgagni hernias**, the defect occurs at the sternocostal hiatus through which the superior epigastric vessels pass from the abdomen to the retrosternal area. **Bochdalek hernias** occur in the posterolateral portion of the diaphragm and are left sided in 90% of cases. Most are found incidentally or are recognized after organ incarceration or volvulus. All Morgagni hernias have a sac that usually contains omentum and may also contain stomach, small bowel, or colon. Most (90%) Bochdalek hernias do not have a sac. Congenital diaphragmatic hernia (CDH) is associated with other congenital abnormalities in 45%–50% of live births.

Ref.: 1, 2

3. A newborn infant begins to experience respiratory distress approximately 4 h after delivery. On examination, the newborn is tachypneic, with sternal, subcostal, and supraclavicular retractions. Decreased breath sounds are noted, and bowel sounds are present on the left side of the chest. The abdomen is scaphoid. Which of the following is not part of the management of this newborn?
   A. Immediate operative repair
   B. Extracorporeal membrane oxygenation (ECMO)
   C. High-frequency oscillatory ventilation
   D. Inhaled nitric oxide
   E. Inotropic and vasopressor support

ANSWER: A

COMMENTS: Treatment of **CDH** often begins with a prenatal diagnosis via ultrasound. If a prenatal diagnosis is made, delivery should take place in a center capable of delivering advanced neonatal and pediatric surgical care with reasonable experience in dealing with CDH. Stabilization of the patient and delayed surgical repair are the standard of care for newborns with CDH. Stabilization begins with respiratory support, including immediate intubation. Additional measures of support, including ECMO, oscillatory ventilation, inhaled nitric oxide, and hemodynamic support, can be used as the clinical condition warrants. Immediate surgical repair before stabilization and support is associated with significant morbidity and mortality. Tube thoracostomy is not routinely described as an adjunct in the preoperative care of patients with CDH, presumably because of the presence of herniated abdominal contents on the ipsilateral side of the chest and the absence of a true pneumothorax. The respiratory distress and hypoxia that are present are usually secondary to pulmonary hypoplasia. Finally, a tube thoracostomy is not typically used after repair because of concern for negative intrapleural pressure causing barotrauma and alveolocapillary membrane damage.

Ref.: 1, 2

4. A 26-year-old man was the driver in a high-speed motor vehicle collision in which the side of his car was hit in a lateral fashion ("T-boned"), and he sustained left-sided blunt chest wall injury. On evaluation, his primary survey is intact.

He does have some left lateral rib fractures on the lower aspect of the left side of his chest. His chest radiograph shows an elevation in the costophrenic angle with air-fluid levels in the chest. Before undergoing chest CT, a nasogastric tube is placed, and during confirmatory radiographs, diagnosis of the injury is made. Which of the following is true regarding this patient's injury?

A. It must be repaired with a patch.

B. It can be readily identified on radiographs or CT.

C. It heals spontaneously.

D. It is best identified and repaired via laparotomy.

E. It requires full excision of the diaphragm with prosthetic repair.

ANSWER: D

COMMENTS: Injury to the diaphragm accounts for only 3% of all trauma-related injuries, with the majority occurring on the left side rather than on the right side. Blunt injuries usually occur secondary to high-speed motor vehicle crashes. A lateral impact is more likely to cause the injury than a frontal impact. Initial chest radiographic findings are normal in 50% of patients, and pneumothorax or hemothorax is seen in the remaining 50% of patients with a **diaphragmatic injury**. CT, though helpful in the evaluation of other injuries to the thorax and abdomen, aids in the diagnosis of a diaphragm injury only if abdominal viscera herniate into the pleural space. This is less common in the acute setting. The diagnosis of a diaphragm injury is best made with a high index of clinical suspicion based on the mechanism of injury and an injury pattern that is confirmed by thorough exploration via laparotomy. Recently, **laparoscopic exploration** of the abdomen has been used in the diagnosis of diaphragmatic injuries. Almost all trauma-related diaphragm injuries in the acute setting can be repaired primarily with a continuous monofilament suture 1-0 or larger in size. In general, in the acute setting a transabdominal approach is preferred, although some have advocated a right thoracic approach for right-sided injuries regardless of the time from injury. Classically, a thoracic approach is reserved for injuries seen in a delayed fashion.

Ref.: 1, 2

5. Regarding the management of diaphragmatic eventration, which of the following statements is correct?

A. Most blunt diaphragmatic injuries occur on the right.

B. Plication results in substantial and durable improvements in spirometry.

C. Diaphragmatic pacing is only effective when the phrenic nerve is damaged.

D. Diaphragmatic eventration is better tolerated in neonates than in adults.

E. Traumatic diaphragmatic injuries that are diagnosed promptly should always be explored from the chest.

ANSWER: B

COMMENTS: Diaphragmatic eventration refers to the elevation of the diaphragm, usually affecting one hemidiaphragm or the other. In adults, the most common causes include spinal cord disease, trauma, infiltration of the phrenic nerve by tumor, or iatrogenic injury. Patients present with restrictive lung disease, which may ultimately progress to respiratory failure. In neonates, diaphragmatic eventration is poorly tolerated, and surgical intervention is nearly always required. In adults, surgical indications are less well defined, but surgery is generally reserved for patients with progressive symptoms. The most common procedure performed is plication of the diaphragm where several rows of imbricating sutures are used to gather excess tissue and displace the diaphragm caudally. This procedure, which may be performed thoracoscopically, results in significant and durable improvements in spirometry. Diaphragmatic pacing is a therapy considered for patients with diaphragmatic paralysis. The ideal patient for this has central nervous system or upper motor neuron disease and requires an intact phrenic nerve. Traumatic injuries to the diaphragm are rare, but occur more commonly on the left where the diaphragm is not protected by the liver. Such an injury identified promptly should be explored from the abdomen due to the association with other intraabdominal injuries.

Ref.: 2

REFERENCES

1. Patterson GA, Cooper JD, Deslauriers J, et al., eds. *Pearson's Thoracic and Esophageal Surgery*. 3rd ed. Philadelphia: Churchill Livingstone; 2008.
2. Sellke FW, del Nido PJ, Swanson SJ, eds. *Sabiston and Spencer Surgery of the Chest*. 7th ed. Philadelphia: WB Saunders; 2005.
3. Detterbeck FC, Boffa DJ, Tanoue LT. The new lung cancer staging system. *Chest*. 2009;136:260–271.
4. Shields TW, Locicero J, Reed CE, et al., eds. *General Thoracic Surgery*. 7th ed. Philadelphia: Lippincott Williams & Wilkins; 2009.
5. Sugarbaker D, Bueno R, Colson YL, et al., eds. *Adult Chest Surgery*. 2nd ed. New York: McGraw-Hill Education; 2015.
6. National Lung Screening Trial Research Team, Aberle DR, Adams AM, et al. Reduced lung-cancer mortality with low-dose computed tomographic screening. *N Engl J Med*. 2011;365(5):395–409.
7. Silvestri GA, Gonzalez AV, Jantz MA, et al. Methods for staging non-small cell lung cancer: diagnosis and management of lung cancer, 3rd ed: American College of Chest Physicians evidence-based clinical practice guidelines. *Chest*. 2013;143(5S):e211S–e250S.
8. Um SW, Kim HK, Jung SH, et al. Endobronchial ultrasound versus mediastinoscopy for mediastinal nodal staging of non-small-cell lung cancer. *J Thorac Oncol*. 2015;10(2):331–337.
9. Cho S, Song IH, Yang HC, et al. Predictive factors for node metastasis in patients with clinical stage I non-small cell lung cancer. *Ann Thorac Surg*. 2013;96(1):239–245.
10. Goldstraw P, Crowley J, Chansky K, et al. The IASLC Lung Cancer Staging Project: proposals for the revision of the TNM stage groups in the forthcoming (seventh) edition of the TNM classification of malignant tumors. *J Thorac Oncol*. 2007;2:706–714.
11. Maygarden SJ, Detterbeck FC, Funkhouser WK. Bronchial margins in lung cancer resection specimens: utility of frozen section and gross evaluation. *Modern Pathol*. 2004;17:1080–1086.
12. Owen RM, Force SD, Gal AA, et al. Routine intraoperative frozen section analysis of bronchial margins is of limited utility in lung cancer resection. *Ann Thorac Surg*. 2013;95(6):1859–1866.
13. Park BJ, Flores R, Rusch V, et al. Management of major hemorrhage during mediastinoscopy. *J Thorac Cardiovasc Surg*. 2003;126(3):726–731.
14. National Emphysema Treatment Trial Research Group. A randomized trial comparing lung-volume–reduction surgery with medical therapy for severe emphysema. *N Engl J Med*. 2003;348:2059–2073.
15. Travis WD, Brambilla E, Noguchi M, et al. International Association for the Study of Lung Cancer/American Thoracic Society/European Respiratory Society international multidisciplinary classification of lung adenocarcinoma. *J Thorac Oncol*. 2011;6:244–285.
16. Kadota K, Lee M, Adusumilli P. The new international multidisciplinary histological classification of lung adenocarcinoma and clinical implications for Indian physicians. *Biomed Res J*. 2014;1(1):6–22.

SECTION VIII

SUBSPECIALTIES FOR THE GENERAL SURGEON

CHAPTER 30

HEAD AND NECK

Peter Papagiannopoulos, M.D., and Samer Al-Khudari, M.D.

1. A 68-year-old woman is evaluated for a 1-month history of worsening dyspnea and hoarseness. Fiberoptic laryngoscopy demonstrates left vocal cord paralysis with full mobility of the right true vocal cord. Findings on physical examination are otherwise unremarkable. Computed tomography (CT) of the chest demonstrates a large mediastinal mass. Which of the following statements is most accurate?

   A. The left recurrent laryngeal nerve (RLN) branches off of the vagus nerve and passes around the left subclavian artery back to the larynx.

   B. A nonrecurrent RLN can be associated with a retroesophageal right subclavian artery.

   C. The RLN supplies all the muscles of the larynx except the posterior cricoarytenoid muscle.

   D. The vagus nerve exits the skull through the carotid canal.

   E. The RLN enters the larynx through the thyrohyoid membrane to innervate the larynx.

ANSWER: B

COMMENTS: The left RLN separates from the vagus in the mediastinum, wraps around the aortic arch at the ductus arteriosus, and then ascends back along the tracheoesophageal groove toward the larynx. The right RLN divides off the vagus and passes around the right subclavian artery to travel to the larynx. The RLN supplies all the muscles of the larynx except the cricothyroid muscle, which is innervated by the external branch of the superior laryngeal nerve. The superior laryngeal nerve also has an internal branch that supplies sensation to the larynx above the true vocal cords. The RLN provides sensation below this area. The vagus nerve exits the skull base on both sides through the jugular foramen, not the carotid canal. The internal branch of the superior laryngeal nerve, not the RLN, enters the thyrohyoid membrane. The RLN travels along the tracheoesophageal groove and enters the larynx just superior to the cricoid cartilage. Nonrecurrent nerves occur most commonly on the right side in up to 1%–2% of patients and can be associated with a retroesophageal right subclavian vein.

Ref.: 1

2. Which of the following statements is true regarding head and neck carcinogenesis and molecular therapy?

   A. A synchronous second primary tumor is defined as the one developing within 1 year of the initial cancer.

   B. Human papillomavirus (HPV) has been shown to be a factor in the development of certain head and neck cancers.

   C. Cetuximab (IMC C225) is a monoclonal antibody therapy targeted against the transforming growth factor-β.

   D. *p53* is commonly underexpressed in head and neck cancers.

   E. The most frequently mutated tumor suppressor gene in head and neck cancers is cyclin D1.

ANSWER: B

COMMENTS: Head and neck carcinogenesis is a complex process with multiple etiologic factors and a wide variety of genetic alterations that have been identified. The incidence of second primary tumors in head and neck cancers is not insignificant (3%–7%), and they should be surveyed for in the upper aerodigestive tract, esophagus, and lung at the time of initial diagnosis. **Synchronous** versus **metachronous** lesions are defined in relation to the time of diagnosis from the initial discovery of the tumor; synchronous lesions are found within 6 months, with metachronous lesions being diagnosed after 6 months. In recent years, **HPV** has been identified as an etiologic factor in certain head and neck cancers, specifically the oropharynx. Protooncogenes are genes that produce proteins involved in the normal cell regulation and function. Mutation of these genes, including those for epidermal growth factor receptor (EGFR), cyclin D1, and vascular endothelial growth factor, occurs in head and neck cancers. Tumor suppressor genes such as *p53* and *p16-ARF* encode proteins that halt tumor growth and carcinogenesis. **Cetuximab** is a novel monoclonal antibody therapy that has been designed to target EGFR. Trials are ongoing regarding its efficacy in combination with standard treatments such as radiotherapy and chemotherapy. Mutated *p53* is poorly degraded and therefore commonly overexpressed in head and neck cancers. It is the most commonly altered tumor suppressor gene in human cancers, with *p16-ARF* being the most commonly altered gene locus in head and neck cancers.

Ref.: 1, 2

3. A 75-year-old man with T2N0M0 squamous cell carcinoma (SCC) of the lower lip undergoes primary resection of the tumor, with full-thickness resection resulting in a defect involving about 55% of the central lower lip but not involving the oral commissure. Which of the following is the best option for the reconstruction of the defect?

   A. Primary closure

   B. Abbe two-stage cross-lip transfer flap

   C. Radial forearm free flap transfer

   D. Nasolabial transposition flap

   E. Estlander flap

ANSWER: B

COMMENTS: The lip begins at the vermilion border and is a subsite of the oral cavity. Risk factors for lip carcinoma include sun exposure and tobacco use. The lower lip is by far the most common site of tumor development, with **SCC** being the most common pathology. **Basal cell carcinoma** is the most frequent pathology found on diagnosis for upper lip cancers. Initial evaluation should include testing for mental nerve involvement, evaluation for mandibular invasion, and examination of the cervical lymphatics. CT can be useful, especially in staging the mandible and cervical nodes.

Treatment of the early-stage disease can consist of either primary external beam radiation or surgical resection. Primary excision is typically the favored treatment. An elective lymph node neck dissection for a clinically negative neck is performed in patients with advanced T stage disease or in the setting of deep tumor invasion in which the risk for occult cervical lymph node disease is elevated. Therapeutic neck dissection is appropriate in patients with positive nodal disease. Indications for postoperative irradiation include advanced T stage, positive margins, perineural/perivascular invasion, multiple or bulky nodal disease, and invasion of bone. Fortunately, given its location, many lip cancers are detected early and can be treated with a high success rate. Stages I and II lesions have a 90% 5-year survival rate. The survival rate drops to about 50% in patients with cervical lymph node involvement.

Reconstructive options following the excision of carcinoma of the lip generally depend on the location of the lesion (medial versus lateral with the involvement of the oral commissure) and the size of the defect. Smaller lesions that involve less than a third to half of the lip can be closed primarily with the local advancement of the tissue. Larger defects involving between half and two-thirds of the lip will probably require donated tissue such as a pedicled two-stage cross-lip transfer flap. An **Abbe flap** is used for central defects, whereas **Estlander**-style flaps are used for lateral defects. Larger defects can be repaired with local advancement techniques, local rotational flaps, or distal free flaps.

Ref.: 1, 2

4. A 68-year-old woman with chronic respiratory failure underwent a tracheostomy for long-term ventilator support. The procedure was uneventful, and the patient was discharged to a long-term care facility after an initial tracheostomy tube change 1 week later. She is readmitted 2 weeks later with a report at the nursing facility of a 1-min episode of brisk, bright red bleeding from the tracheostomy site that resolved without intervention. Her hemoglobin concentration is 10.2 g/dL, and coagulation studies are normal. What is the most likely diagnosis?

A. Pneumonia

B. Tracheitis

C. Bleeding of granulation tissue in the stoma

D. Tracheoinnominate fistula

E. Bleeding from the anterior jugular vein

ANSWER: D

COMMENTS: This is a case of classic "**sentinel**" **bleeding** that occurs before the full rupture of the **innominate artery**. It can occur with a low tracheostomy or a high innominate artery with the erosion of the anterior tracheal wall as a result of pressure necrosis. Fiberoptic examination of the area should be performed to evaluate the situation. If there is an obvious evidence of erosion, the patient might need a sternotomy and mediastinal exploration. If the index of suspicion is lower or the examination is inconclusive, diagnostic imaging with a high-resolution CT or angiography (or both) may be appropriate. This complication carries an extremely high mortality rate if massive bleeding occurs. Attempts to control active bleeding can consist of direct digital pressure or inflation of a cuffed tube directly over the area for tamponade. Any of the other choices would not cause rapid-onset bright red bleeding. Bleeding from the anterior jugular veins usually occurs immediately in the postoperative setting if they were not ligated adequately during surgery. Other complications of tracheostomy in the early period include infection, pneumothorax, bleeding, and tube obstruction. Later complications can include wound breakdown, formation of granulation tissue, tracheal stenosis, tracheoesophageal fistula, and **tracheoinnominate fistula**, as just described.

Ref.: 1, 2

5. A 34-year-old woman is seen in the office with a 3-month history of a left-sided neck mass and pain with mastication. On examination, a 3-cm nontender mass is present at level II; it moves laterally but not in the craniocaudal direction. CT with intravenous (IV) contrast enhancement demonstrates a 3.5-cm mass at the carotid bifurcation. A follow-up angiogram is obtained. Which of the following statements is most accurate regarding this case?

A. It represents the most common paraganglioma in the head and neck.

B. The rate of malignancy is about 40%.

C. The majority of these lesions show functional secretion of catecholamines.

D. A fine-needle aspiration biopsy (FNAB) is indicated to rule out malignancy.

E. Radiation therapy is the most effective treatment for these lesions.

ANSWER: A

COMMENTS: A **carotid body tumor** is the most common **paraganglioma** in the head and neck. Other paragangliomas that occur in this region include the vagal and jugulotympanic types. The majority of paragangliomas are solitary and nonfamilial. Multicentricity is reported in about 10% of cases, with about a 6% rate of malignancy. Only about 1%–3% of them are considered functional and can be evaluated with a 24-h urine collection for the analysis of catecholamines. The "**Fontaine sign**" refers to mobility in only the lateral direction on palpation, whereas pain occurring with chewing is called "**first-bite syndrome**." Histopathologic evaluation of this tumor demonstrates two types of cells: type I, chief cells/granular cells, and type II, sustentacular supporting cells. Unlike most head and neck tumors, malignancy is not diagnosed by the presence of dysplastic changes in the primary tumor. The presence of a metastatic disease either to the regional cervical lymphatics or to the distant sites is the only diagnostic criteria. Imaging is the major modality for primary diagnosis since needle biopsy is contraindicated. CT will show a hypervascular mass at the carotid bifurcation, with magnetic resonance imaging (MRI) demonstrating a classic "salt and pepper" appearance on T2-weighted sequences because of hemorrhage and flow voids. On angiography, the internal and external carotid arteries will be bowed apart, a finding referred to as the "**lyre sign**." These tumors are best treated surgically, and vascular reconstruction may be necessary. Radiation therapy can stop the growth of these lesions but not shrink their size. Patients should be aware of the potential risk of injury to the vagus.

Ref.: 1, 2

6. Which statement is the most accurate regarding the histology of the head and neck?

A. The pharynx is lined exclusively by nonkeratinizing stratified squamous epithelium.

B. The minor salivary glands lie in the submucosa of the oral cavity and pharynx.

C. The Waldeyer ring consists of only two structures: the palatine tonsils and adenoids.

D. The adenoids have crypts lined by stratified squamous epithelium.

E. The nasal cavity consists entirely of ciliated respiratory epithelium.

ANSWER: B

COMMENTS: The pharynx is lined by both nonkeratinizing stratified squamous epithelium and ciliated respiratory epithelium. The **Waldeyer ring** consists of the palatine tonsils, adenoids, and the lingual tonsils, which lie along the base of the tongue. The palatine tonsils have crypts lined by stratified squamous epithelium. The adenoids are covered by pseudostratified ciliated columnar epithelium with surface folds but, unlike the tonsils, do not have crypts. The tonsillar crypts are designed to trap foreign antigens for presentation to the lymphoid follicles. The nasal cavity is composed primarily of respiratory epithelium but also contains specialized sensory olfactory epithelium along the roof. Hundreds of minor salivary glands lie in the submucosa of the oral cavity and pharynx.

Ref.: 1, 2

7. A 22-year-old man is brought to the emergency department by ambulance with a 2-day history of lower tooth pain and neck swelling. He was prescribed antibiotics by his primary care physician yesterday, but his condition had not improved overnight. This morning he felt his "throat beginning to close" and called the emergency medical service. He is febrile at 102°F with a heart rate of 105 beats/min, blood pressure of 110/70 mmHg, and respiratory rate of 20 breaths/min. His white blood cell count is 38,000/mm^3. On examination, he is noted to have firm tender swelling of the submental region with skin erythema. In addition, severe edema of the floor of the mouth and tongue is present. His Sao_2 is 100% on 40% O_2 by face tent, and he is ventilating well, anxious, and sitting forward drooling. Flexible laryngoscopy shows no laryngeal edema. What is the next appropriate step in the management?

A. IV antibiotics and steroids with close observation of the airway in the intensive care unit

B. High-resolution CT of the neck with dye

C. Immediate cricothyrotomy in the emergency department under local anesthesia

D. Immediate transfer to the operating room (OR) for awake fiberoptic intubation and be prepared for tracheostomy if needed

E. Incision and drainage of a suspected neck abscess at the bedside

ANSWER: D

COMMENTS: This patient has **Ludwig angina**, probably secondary to an odontogenic infection given the history of tooth pain. This condition involves a rapidly evolving soft tissue cellulitis that spreads through the fascial planes of the sublingual space, submandibular space, and anterior aspect of the neck. It can cause severe swelling of the floor of the mouth and tongue and possibly airway obstruction. Initial management in this patient should involve securing his airway. An emergency cricothyrotomy would be appropriate in the emergency department if the patient was currently decompensating and exhibiting obstruction and needed an airway immediately. He is ventilating well but drooling and posturing forward. This patient should be taken to the OR expediently to perform fiberoptic intubation and a possible tracheostomy under controlled circumstances. At that point, CT could be performed to evaluate for an abscess collection. Exploration of the neck at the bedside, especially without securing the airway, is unsafe and not appropriate. Tonsillitis is the most frequent cause of deep tissue neck infections in children with odontogenic sources, and an IV drug injection is a more common cause in adults. **Peritonsillar abscesses** are the most commonly encountered sequelae. Classic signs and symptoms include drooling, hot potato voice, otalgia [from irritation of cranial nerve (CN) IX], and unilateral swelling of the soft palate with uvular deviation to the opposite side. Treatment includes drainage by transoral needle aspiration or incision and drainage with a scalpel blade. A **parapharyngeal space abscess** can manifest in a similar fashion to a peritonsillar abscess as severe throat and neck pain but without the appearance of soft palate/peritonsillar swelling. The tonsil may appear medially. It is adjacent to many of the other spaces and can allow spread along the carotid sheath ("Lincoln highway of the neck") or damage to CNs IX to XII. Drainage is generally performed in a transcervical fashion if necessary. **Retropharyngeal space abscesses** are more common in young children and require some clinical suspicion to detect. Initial signs may include fever, lack of appetite, cervical adenopathy, and torticollis. This area can usually be approached transorally if the infection is limited but may require transcervical drainage. CT is mandatory to define its extent and to aid in planning access. The retropharyngeal space extends from the skull base to the mediastinum. The retropharyngeal space has a midline raphe that causes unilateral shifting, whereas the prevertebral space does not, with these collections appearing more midline.

Ref.: 2

8. A 75-year-old man with a long history of tobacco use comes to the office with a newly discovered tongue mass. A 3-cm ulcerated lesion is noted on the right anterior aspect of the tongue. Biopsy of the lesion demonstrates SCC. CT of the neck with IV contrast enhancement shows an enlarged 2-cm lymph node in the level II region on the left side. Findings on chest radiography are clear. How would you stage this patient's disease?

A. T1N1M0

B. T2N1M1

C. T4N2cM0

D. T2N3M0

E. T2N2cM0

TABLE 30.1 Regional Lymph Nodes (N)

NX	Regional lymph nodes cannot be assessed
N0	No regional lymph node metastasis
N1*	Metastasis in a single ipsilateral lymph node, 3 cm or less in greatest dimension
N2*	Metastasis in a single ipsilateral lymph node, more than 3 cm but not more than 6 cm in greatest dimension; or in multiple ipsilateral lymph nodes, none more than 6 cm in greatest dimension; or in bilateral or contralateral lymph nodes, none more than 6 cm in greatest dimension
N2a*	Metastasis in a single ipsilateral lymph node more than 3 cm but not more than 6 cm in greatest dimension
N2b*	Metastasis in multiple ipsilateral lymph nodes, none more than 6 cm in greatest dimension
N2c*	Metastasis in bilateral or contralateral lymph nodes, none more than 6 cm in greatest dimension
N3*	Metastasis in a lymph node more than 6 cm in greatest dimension

*Note: A designation of "U" or "L" may be used for any N stage to indicate metastasis above the lower border of the cricoids (U) or below the lower border of the cricoids (L). Similarly, clinical/radiological extracapsular spread (ECS) should be recorded as E− or E+, and histopathologic ECS should be designated as En, Em, or Eg.

Used with the permission of the American Joint Committee on Cancer (AJCC), Chicago, Illinois. The original source for this material is the *AJCC Cancer Staging Manual*, Seventh Edition (2010) published by Springer Science and Business Media LLC, www.springer.com.

ANSWER: E

COMMENTS: The **T classification** as defined by the American Joint Committee on Cancer (AJCC) refers to the primary tumor. Carcinoma of the oral cavity is staged according to size. T2 lesions are 2 to 4 cm, as in this patient. Oral cavity T staging is as follows: T1, less than 2 cm; T2, 2 to 4 cm; T3, greater than 4 cm; and T4, invasion of adjacent structures. Clinical staging of the neck has been made more accurate by high-resolution imaging (CT). Had this node been ipsilateral, it would have been staged as N1. However, since it is contralateral to the primary disease, it is classified as N2c. Table 30.1 applies to primary tumors of the oral cavity, oropharynx, hypopharynx, and larynx.

Ref.: 1, 3

9. Which of the following statements is true regarding FNAB?

A. It is contraindicated for the diagnosis of parotid masses due to the risk of tumor seeding.

B. Rates of false-negative and false-positive diagnoses are low, and the accuracy of detecting malignant lesions is high.

C. FNAB is not effective in the diagnosis of lymphoma.

D. FNAB should be done using an 18- to 21-gauge needle.

E. Once an FNAB specimen is obtained, it should be placed in saline for transport to pathology.

ANSWER: B

COMMENTS: FNAB is not contraindicated for parotid mass diagnosis. Large-bore needle biopsies have an increased risk of tumor seeding. FNAB has low false-negative and -positive rates, and malignancy detection is high. It is effective in lymphoma diagnosis and should be performed with a 21- to 25-gauge needle. FNAB specimens should not be placed in saline as it is a nonphysiologic medium.

FNAB has become the standard technique for the initial office evaluation of a neck mass due to the technique's high diagnostic accuracy. The technique reliably can differentiate between reactive and inflammatory processes not requiring surgery from neoplasia as well as between benign and malignant tumors. The overall diagnostic accuracy is approximately 95% for all masses in the head and neck including 95% for benign lesions and 87% for malignant lesions. If the result is nondiagnostic, which occurs approximately 10% of the time, the FNAB can easily be performed again or an excisional biopsy can be performed if indicated.

FNAB is additionally useful in the diagnosis of lymphoma. Immunotyping can be performed on FNAB specimens that can detect surface antigens and cell lineage (T cell or B cell) and can confirm the presence of monoclonal light or heavy chains. Even if the FNAB cannot absolutely confirm lymphoma, it typically still rules out SCC and thus would lead the surgeon to a possible open biopsy of the mass to further evaluate for lymphoma rather than pursue a workup of head and neck SCC, which would include laryngoscopy and esophagoscopy to search for a primary tumor.

The FNAB technique is typically performed in the office setting under local anesthesia, with the application of 1% lidocaine with epinephrine. A 21- to 25-gauge needle on a 10- to 20-mL syringe is then inserted into the mass and moved in and out of the mass in short vibratory strokes of 2 to 3 mm while aspirating on the syringe. These vibratory strokes continue until cellular material enters the needle hub at which point the needle is removed from the mass. This process is repeated at least twice and as many as four times according to the literature. Pressure should then be held on the mass to stop bleeding and a bandage applied.

The aspirated material can either be expelled directly onto slides and taken to a pathologist or fixed directly in CytoLyt. The advantage of placing the material directly on slides is that the specimen does not need to be spun down, and analysis with microscopy can begin immediately.

Ref: 1, 3

10. A 47-year-old male immigrant from southern China has a complaint of right-sided hearing loss for the past 3 weeks. He has no history of a recent upper respiratory infection or chronic ear disease. His clinical history is otherwise unremarkable. Serous otitis media is noted in his right ear. In addition, a 1.5-cm level V lymph node is palpated on the left side of the neck. The rest of the physical examination is within normal limits. What is the next step in management?

A. Treatment with amoxicillin for 10 days

B. Flexible nasopharyngoscopic examination

C. Ototopical antibiotic drops

D. Oral and topical decongestants for 2 weeks with reexamination

E. Observation with follow-up in 2 weeks if the symptoms do not resolve

ANSWER: B

COMMENTS: Any adult patient with a new onset of unilateral middle ear effusion and no related history of recent upper respiratory illness should undergo evaluation of the nasopharynx. Another clinical clue in this patient is the presence of a level V node, which is a common location for cervical metastasis from **nasopharyngeal cancer**. This is especially true in this patient given his history of a southern Chinese background. This area, particularly the Guangdong Province, has an increased incidence of nasopharyngeal carcinoma. The etiologic factors are multifactorial and include genetic and environmental factors. Infection with **Epstein-Barr virus (EBV)** has been shown to have an etiologic role. In addition, dietary factors, including the intake of salted fish, have a strong association with the development of this disease. Nasopharyngeal carcinoma is divided by the World Health Organization into two groups, keratinizing and nonkeratinizing carcinoma, with the second group including both differentiated and undifferentiated subtypes. The diagnosis of nasopharyngeal carcinoma is made using nasopharyngoscopy and biopsy. High serologic levels of immunoglobulin (Ig)A to EBV viral capsid antigen and early antigen are seen in patients with this disease. Nasopharyngoscopy and biopsy has been advocated as a screening tool in high-risk populations based on a study showing a 5.4% diagnosis rate of subclinical nasopharyngeal cancer in patients with elevated IgA levels to EBV who live in the Guangdong Province. Treatment consists mainly of chemotherapy and radiation therapy. Surgery has a limited role in treating nasopharyngeal cancer in patients with limited primary site recurrence and nodal recurrence.

Ref.: 1–3, 4

11. Which of the following statement is most accurate regarding the use of chemoradiation therapy for head and neck cancers?

A. Chemotherapy can be used as a single-modality primary therapy with an intent to cure in many head and neck cancers.

B. Induction chemotherapy plus radiation therapy has superior overall survival results when compared with surgery plus radiation therapy for the treatment of advanced-stage laryngeal cancer.

C. Postoperative concomitant chemotherapy with radiation therapy improves overall survival compared with postoperative radiation therapy alone in high-risk, locally advanced head and neck cancers.

D. Chemotherapy has no role in the palliative setting for metastatic head and neck cancers.

E. Chemotherapy in the postoperative adjuvant setting in conjunction with radiation therapy has the advantage of improving survival while not increasing mucosal and overall toxicity.

ANSWER: C

COMMENTS: Chemotherapy has developed an increasing role over the past two decades in the treatment of head and neck SCCs. For early-stage patients, treatment consists of either radiation therapy or surgery, with chemotherapy having little to no role in the treatment. It is never used as a primary single-modality treatment for head and neck cancers with an intent to cure. For patients with advanced metastatic or recurrent disease, chemotherapy can be used in the palliative setting to inhibit tumor growth for a limited effective period. Its main role is in the treatment of locoregionally advanced stage III/IV cancer. A second role of chemotherapy in this group of patients is for organ preservation. Patients with an advanced primary T stage are best served by total laryngectomy. For advanced-stage **unresectable tumors**, concurrent chemoradiation therapy, compared with radiation therapy alone, has shown an improved locoregional control with a questionable overall survival benefit.

Ref.: 1, 5–9

12. A 66-year-old man with T3N2bM0 SCC on the base of the tongue undergoes concomitant chemotherapy and external beam irradiation for a total of 6 weeks. At the end of the treatment, he is noted to have a persistently enlarged, left neck level II lymph node about 5 cm in size, for which salvage surgical therapy and standard radical neck dissection are planned. Which of the following is true?

A. The phrenic nerve is commonly injured during surgery.

B. Radical neck dissection includes removing the internal jugular vein, sternocleidomastoid (SCM) muscle, and vagus nerve.

C. The patient will probably need postoperative physical therapy for his shoulder.

D. Resection of the internal carotid artery is a common component of this surgery.

E. Level VI is a part of a radical neck dissection.

ANSWER: C

COMMENTS: Neck dissection involves the removal of the cervical lymphatic tissue and related structures for the treatment of head and neck cancers. **Radical neck dissection** involves removing all of the cervical lymphatic tissue in neck levels I through V, in addition to removing the internal jugular vein, SCM muscle, and spinal accessory nerve. A **modified radical neck dissection** is performed for the same clinical indications as a radical neck dissection. The differentiating feature is that it preserves at least one of the following: the internal jugular vein, SCM muscle, or spinal accessory nerve. Levels I through V lymph nodes are removed as for a traditional radical neck dissection. However, it is frequently possible to preserve one of the major structures just listed, especially when it is not involved with tumor. Particularly in the case of the spinal accessory nerve, this is preferable to prevent postoperative shoulder dysfunction from denervation of the trapezius muscle. The patient in this scenario will most certainly need postoperative physical therapy due to CN XII resection.

Selective neck dissection is used for removing a limited number of lymph node levels, as opposed to resecting levels I through V. Furthermore, the internal jugular vein, SCM muscle, and CN XII are preserved. The philosophy behind performing this type of dissection is to remove the clinically uninvolved lymphatic groups thought to be most at risk for future metastatic disease. Therefore the type of dissection is predicated on where the primary tumor is located. Oral cavity cancers typically metastasize to levels I, II, and III. These levels would be included in what is termed a **supraomohyoid selective neck dissection**. Laryngeal, hypopharyngeal, and oropharyngeal cancers commonly spread to levels II, III, and IV, which would be incorporated into a **lateral selective neck dissection**. **Posterolateral neck dissection** (levels II, III, IV, and V) is most commonly used in the setting of cutaneous malignancies involving the posterior region of the scalp.

Sentinel lymph node biopsy is under investigation for its efficacy in SCC of the head and neck. It is currently used in the management of cutaneous melanoma of the head and neck. However, the internal carotid artery is not considered a standard part of the routine neck dissection, and there is controversy regarding the utility and benefit of resection. The phrenic nerve is at risk when dissecting along the floor of the neck. A level VI or central compartment dissection is not part of a standard radical neck dissection. It is typically used in patients with thyroid tumors, tracheal tumors, or laryngeal cancers with extensive subglottic extension.

Therapeutic neck dissection has been used to treat positive metastatic cervical disease (N+) through either a radical or a modified radical neck dissection. Currently, some surgeons are beginning to advocate the use of a more limited selective neck dissection if the patient has limited N1 disease. In addition to being used as primary treatment, it also can be used as salvage treatment after failed nonsurgical therapy, such as external beam radiation. For patients with clinically negative disease in the neck (N0), **elective**

neck dissection can be performed to target the most likely sites of metastatic drainage. Such dissection is based on the primary site of the tumor. Sentinel lymph node biopsy in the treatment of SCC of the head and neck is currently under investigation and not yet advocated widely as a proven standard of care.

Ref.: 1, 2, 10

13. A 55-year-old man with an advanced-stage SCC of the larynx is undergoing a total laryngectomy with bilateral modified radical neck dissection. While dissecting on the right side, you inadvertently enter the internal jugular vein and proceed to clamp the vessel with the intention of ligating it for hemostasis. Shortly thereafter, the patient is noted to be hypotensive. Bilateral breath sounds are auscultated, but a mill-wheel murmur is heard over the precordium. What is the next step in management?

A. Place the patient in the left lateral decubitus position and insert a central venous catheter.

B. Place the patient in the right lateral decubitus position and insert a central venous catheter.

C. Place the patient in the reverse Trendelenburg position.

D. Call for an intraoperative chest radiograph.

E. Pack the wound and place the patient in the prone position.

ANSWER: A

COMMENTS: This patient has a **venous air embolism** as a result of the internal jugular vein being inadvertently opened. With all surgeries above the heart, there is a risk for air embolism. This is especially true in neurosurgical procedures, where there is significant elevation of the wound relative to the heart. In head and neck surgery, patients are typically placed in the reverse Trendelenburg position, which places them at an additional risk for entrance of air into the venous system. A "**mill-wheel murmur**" is the traditional finding on cardiac examination and may be detected on precordial Doppler ultrasound. The clinical manifestations can include cardiovascular, pulmonary, and neurologic findings. Cardiac findings can include tachyarrhythmias, right-sided heart strain, and myocardial ischemia. Pulmonary findings can include hypercapnia with decreased O_2 saturation. A decreased cardiac output results in decreased cerebral perfusion, but a direct air embolism to the central nervous system can occur through a patent foramen ovale. Initial treatment involves placing the patient in the **left lateral decubitus position** (**Durant position**) to try to force the air to stay in the right side of the heart in an attempt to prevent it from traveling into the pulmonary circulation. Placement of a central venous catheter with aspiration of air from the right atrium can also be attempted. Other supportive efforts may need to include cardiopulmonary resuscitation if the situation deteriorates. Hyperbaric oxygen therapy has been shown to be of benefit in some studies.

Ref.: 11

14. A 53-year-old male with a history of diffuse large B-cell lymphoma is admitted with neutropenic fevers and started on broad-spectrum IV antibiotics. Over the next 2 days, he complains of a progressive left-sided vision loss, decreased sensation in the left V2 distribution, nasal congestion, and epistaxis. Nasal endoscopy is significant for a blackened eschar on the left middle turbinate. He is not sensate in this region, and the tissue does not bleed. Which of the following is true regarding an invasive fungal sinusitis?

A. The causative organism is most frequently *Candida albicans*.

B. This disease process is rarely lethal.

C. The pathophysiology of this disease is characterized by the organism invading soft tissue, bone, and vessel walls, which results in vascular occlusion, infarction, and tissue necrosis.

D. This disease requires a quantitative neutrophil deficit as a precursor.

E. The gold standard for diagnosis is fungal culture.

ANSWER: C

COMMENTS: The causative organisms are most commonly ***Mucor***, characterized by **nonseptate hyphae** with a **90-degree** branching pattern, and ***Aspergillus***, characterized by **septate** hyphae with a **45-degree** branching pattern. This disease is fatal in 50%–80% of patients. The pathophysiology is characterized by the fungal organism invading the soft tissues and bone, causing vascular occlusion, infarction, and tissue necrosis. This disease occurs almost exclusively in **immunocompromised** patients (those with diabetic ketoacidosis, undergoing chemotherapy, with bone marrow transplant) and can occur in those with qualitative deficiency (e.g., diabetic ketoacidosis) as well as quantitative deficiency (chemotherapy, acquired immunodeficiency syndrome). The gold standard for diagnosis is histopathology.

Invasive fungal sinusitis is characterized by mucosal invasion of mycotic organisms and by **angioinvasion,** leading to tissue necrosis and potential for invasion into nearby structures such as the orbit and brain. The population at risk includes immunocompromised patients. Typical presenting symptoms include neutropenic fever, nasal congestion, vision change, V2 numbness, and soft tissue swelling. Physical examination may yield periorbital skin necrosis or blackened eschar of the hard or soft palate. Nasal endoscopy is characterized by mucosal changes of nasal structures such as the septum and middle turbinate. The mucosa can appear pale or may be covered by a gray or black eschar. Nasal mucosa is often insensate in these patients and does not bleed.

Treatment requires an urgent surgical debridement, often coupled with a long-term IV antifungal therapy. Histopathology is the gold standard for diagnosis. Fungal culture can be used as an adjunct, but it is less sensitive and may take weeks to provide a diagnosis, which results in decreased utility in such an acute and life-threatening disease process.

Ref.: 1, 12

15. A 65-year-old male undergoes parotidectomy for a parotid neoplasm. Which of the following is true regarding parotidectomy?

A. The facial nerve is typically found 3-cm anterior, inferior, and deep to the tragal cartilage.

B. Frey's syndrome is caused by injury to the greater auricular nerve and presents with sweating and reddening of the skin during meals.

C. A common complication of parotidectomy is injury to the greater auricular nerve, which causes perioral numbness.

D. Frey's syndrome is the result of an aberrant innervation of cutaneous sweat glands by postganglionic parasympathetic fibers.

E. The parotid gland is divided into superficial and deep lobes by the facial vein.

ANSWER: D

COMMENTS: The facial nerve is found 1 cm anterior, inferior, and deep to the tragal cartilage (tragal pointer). Frey's syndrome is the result of an injury to the auriculotemporal nerve, which results in an aberrant innervation of cutaneous sweat glands by postganglionic parasympathetic fibers. Injury to the greater auricular nerve causes numbness to the skin overlying the mastoid bone and portions of the pinna. The parotid gland is divided into superficial and deep lobes by the retromandibular vein.

Facial nerve identification is crucial while performing parotidectomy in order to preserve its integrity and function. The facial nerve can be identified by utilizing multiple landmarks.

- **Tragal pointer**: The facial nerve is 1 cm anterior, inferior, and deep to the tragal cartilage.
- **Tympanomastoid suture line**: The facial nerve is 6 to 8 mm deep to the inferior edge of the tympanomastoid suture line.
- **The digastric tendon insertion point** onto the digastric ridge defines the plane of the facial nerve.
- The facial nerve main trunk can additionally be identified exiting the skull base at **the stylomastoid foramen** or, alternatively, can be found by performing **retrograde dissection** after finding a distal branch.

There are numerous potential complications of parotidectomy. First, facial nerve injury can occur and would result in facial paresis or paralysis on the affected side. If this is identified intraoperatively, the nerve should be immediately repaired. Second, greater auricular nerve hypoesthesia can be the result of a traction injury or transection. This results in periauricular numbness and typically resolves within 9 months if not deliberately transected. Third, salivary fistulas can occur and typically resolve in 2 to 3 weeks. Fourth, Frey's syndrome occurs as a result of injury to the auriculotemporal nerve (which contains sympathetic fibers) and results in an aberrant innervation of cutaneous sweat glands by postganglionic parasympathetic fibers. It presents as sweating and reddening of the skin during meals. Other complications include hematoma, infection, and flap necrosis.

Ref.: 1, 13

16. Which of the following is true regarding a cutaneous malignant melanoma of the head and neck?

A. The most powerful predictor of survival is the depth of invasion and the presence or absence of ulceration of the primary lesion.

B. The most powerful predictor of survival is the regional nodal status.

C. The Clark level of invasion is a key portion of the tumor-node-metastasis (TNM) staging system.

D. An elective neck dissection is the recommended way to initially evaluate the regional nodal status.

E. The mitotic rate is not included in the TNM staging system.

ANSWER: B

COMMENT: The depth of invasion and ulceration are key factors of the TNM staging system, but the regional nodal status is the most powerful predictor of survival for patients with malignant melanoma of the head and neck. T staging takes into account the depth of invasion, not Clark levels. Sentinel lymph node biopsy has become the approach to the initial evaluation of the regional nodal status, not elective neck dissection. Mitotic rate plays a role in TNM staging.

The classic finding that raises suspicion for malignant melanoma is the presence of a pigmented lesion that changes over the course of weeks to months. Change in diameter, border irregularity, color change, ulceration, itching, pain, and bleeding are all signs that should raise suspicion for melanoma.

Excisional biopsies are the favored method to elucidate diagnosis, while incisional or punch biopsies are acceptable alternatives if there are anatomic or cosmetic constraints. If biopsy is positive for an invasive melanoma, even if accomplished by an excisional biopsy with negative margins, further resection of the primary site with larger margins is necessary.

T staging is based on thickness, presence of ulceration, and mitotic rate. N status is based on the regional nodal status, which, as previously stated, is the most powerful predictor of survival in patients with malignant melanoma of the head and neck. The decision to evaluate the regional nodes is based on the characteristics of the primary tumor and the risk of nodal metastasis. Patients with T1 lesions have a 3% risk of metastasis to a sentinel lymph node; T2, 8%–12%; T3, 23%–27%; and T4, 24%–44%.

Patients with lesions that are 0.75 mm or less in depth do not require evaluation of regional nodes, and observation is appropriate for them. Patients with lesions between 0.76 and 1.0 mm in depth without ulceration and less than 1 mitosis/mm^2 should consider sentinel lymph node biopsy. Patients with lesions between 0.76 and 1 mm in depth with ulceration or greater than 1 mitosis/mm^2 or with lesions greater than 1 mm in depth should be recommend a sentinel lymph node biopsy.

Ref.: 1, 13

17. A 10-year-old girl presents to your office with a history of a recurrent painful right lateral neck mass. She has required multiple rounds of antibiotics, which successfully resolve the pain and overlying skin erythema; however, the mass has always persisted. You obtain imaging that is consistent with a second branchial cleft cyst. Which of the following is true regarding branchial cleft anomalies (BCAs)?

A. The spinal accessory nerve is at risk during the excision of the first BCA.

B. The second BCA is characterized by a neck mass at the anterior border of the SCM with a tract that runs between the internal and external carotid arteries and terminates at the ipsilateral tonsillar fossa.

C. Third BCAs are the most common branchial cleft lesion.

D. The second BCA can be differentiated from the third and fourth BCAs by its position anterior to the SCM.

E. 90% of the third BCAs occur on the right side.

ANSWER: B

COMMENT: The facial nerve is at risk during the excision of the first BCA. The second BCA is characterized by a neck mass at the anterior edge of the SCM and has a tract that runs between the internal and external carotid arteries, passes superior to the glossopharyngeal and hypoglossal nerves, and finally ends at the tonsillar fossa. Second BCAs are the most common anomaly. The second BCA cannot be differentiated from the third and fourth BCAs on the basis of position of SCM alone. All three anomalies have a lesion anterior to the SCM. They are differentiated based on the path of their tracts. Moreover, 90% of the third BCAs occur on the left side.

BCAs are common in the pediatric population and are a result of the failure of involution of embryonic structures. These anomalies may remain asymptomatic, not appreciable on physical examination, and often do not require treatment. Alternatively, these anomalies can enlarge, which can raise concern for neoplastic process; can become secondarily infected; or can cause cosmetic deformity. These are all possible indications for surgical excision. There are four types of BCAs. Each may be associated with a characteristic deep tract. If the deep tract is incompletely excised, there is an increased risk for recurrence.

The first BCA is not common. It characteristically has a mass located near the lobule of the ear. A CT or MRI is critical to differentiate this lesion from dermoid cysts, lymphatic malformations, parotid masses, or other tumors. The first BCAs typically appear as fluid-filled cystic lesions on CT. During a surgical excision, it is vital to remember that the cyst may have a deep component that may pass either lateral or **medial to the facial nerve**, which must be identified in the entire first BCA lesion, and is to be safely removed.

The second BCA is the most common of the brachial cleft lesions, and it is characterized by a lesion at the **anterior border of the SCM**. Its deep tract runs between the internal and external carotid arteries, superior to the glossopharyngeal and hypoglossal nerves, and ends in the **tonsillar fossa**.

The third BCA is also characterized by a lesion at the **anterior border of the SCM**. Its associated tract passes posterior to the internal and external carotid arteries, between the glossopharyngeal and hypoglossal nerves, and terminates at the apex of the **pyriform sinus.**

The fourth BCA additionally presents as a lesion at the **anterior border of the SCM**. Its tract runs from the apex of the **pyriform sinus** and travels inferiorly in the tracheoesophageal groove; then, it runs posterior to the thyroid gland and into the thorax where it loops below the aorta on the left and below the subclavian artery on the right. It then ascends posterior to the common carotid artery and loops over the hypoglossal nerve, ending at the anterior border of the SCM.

The spinal accessory nerve exits the skull base via the jugular foramen and enters level II by passing anterior to the jugular vein but deep to the posterior belly of the digastric muscle and the SCM. The nerve heads in a posteroinferior direction and gives off a branch to the SCM before entering the substance of the SCM and exiting deep to Erb's point (the point where the greater auricular nerve sweeps around from the posteroinferior aspect of the SCM) and traverses level V in a superficial plane before innervating the trapezius muscle. For these reasons, CN XI injury risk is the highest while dissecting lesions deep to the SCM and during a level V dissection.

Ref.: 1, 13

18. A patient is extubated after undergoing a total thyroidectomy. The patient is immediately noted to be stridorous; however, the patient's voice is normal and strong. The patient requires a 4-L nasal cannula and is saturating 100%. Which of the following statements is true?

A. The patient likely has unilateral true vocal cord paralysis with the vocal cord in a lateralized position. The second true vocal cord has a normal movement.

B. The patient likely has unilateral paralysis with the true vocal cord in the paramedian position. The second true vocal cord has a normal movement.

C. The patient likely has bilateral vocal cord paralysis with bilateral true vocal cords in the paramedian position.

D. Stridor is expected after thyroidectomy.

E. A flexible fiberoptic laryngoscopy is contraindicated in this patient.

ANSWER: C

COMMENTS: The patient likely has a bilateral vocal cord paralysis with both true vocal cords found in the paramedian position due to a bilateral RLN injury sustained during a thyroidectomy. The patient is saturating well on nasal cannula; therefore a flexible laryngoscopy would not be contraindicated.

The laryngeal neuromuscular anatomy is key to understanding the vocal cord position. The laryngeal musculature can be classified into two groups: abductors and adductors. Adductors include lateral cricoarytenoid muscle, thyroarytenoid muscle, cricothyroid muscle, and the interarytenoid muscle. There is only one abducting muscle: the posterior cricoarytenoid muscle.

There are only two nerves that supply motor innervation to these muscles: the RLN and the external branch of the superior laryngeal nerve.

The RLN is responsible for innervating each one of the aforementioned muscles, except the cricothyroid muscle, which is supplied by the external branch of the superior laryngeal nerve. Therefore when a vocal cord is paralyzed due to iatrogenic trauma to the RLN, innervation to all the muscles except the cricothyroid, an adductor, is lost. Therefore the true vocal cord sits in an "adducted" position just lateral to midline. This position is called the paramedian position.

When there is bilateral true vocal cord paralysis, both cords sit in a paramedian position, which creates a slit-like airway. This results in a significant stridor. However, as the true cords are in proximity to each other, the voice can still be normal. The unilateral vocal cord paralysis typically presents with normal breathing and a normal, breathy, or hoarse voice.

Ref.: 1, 13

19. A 47-year-old patient presents with a slowly enlarging right parotid mass. You are suspicious for a neoplastic process and perform a fine-needle aspiration (FNA). Which of the following is true regarding parotid neoplasms?

A. Approximately 75%–80% of parotid gland tumors are malignant.

B. The most common parotid tumor is mucoepidermoid carcinoma.

C. Pleomorphic adenoma is seen bilaterally in 50% of patients.

D. An open biopsy of a parotid mass is the preferred method of obtaining a diagnosis and providing treatment.

E. Warthin's tumor is the second most common benign salivary gland tumor. Smoking is an etiologic risk factor.

ANSWER: E

COMMENTS: Around 75%–80% of parotid tumors are benign. The most common parotid tumor is pleomorphic adenoma. Warthin's tumor, not pleomorphic adenoma, is seen bilaterally in 12% of patients with a Warthin's tumor. A surgical biopsy is not recommended due to a high risk of recurrence. Warthin's tumor is the second most common benign salivary gland tumor and is associated with smoking as a risk factor.

Salivary glands are divided into major and minor glands. The major glands include the parotid, submandibular, and sublingual glands. These glands are paired. The minor glands include 600 to 1000 glands found throughout the upper aerodigestive tract.

About 70% of salivary gland tumors occur in the parotid gland, of which 75%–80% are benign. The most common benign parotid tumor is pleomorphic adenoma followed next in incidence by **Warthin's tumor**, which is associated with smoking and an increased rate of being found bilaterally (12%).

The most common malignant neoplasm of the parotid is the **mucoepidermoid carcinoma** followed by the adenoid cystic carcinoma. Facial paralysis related to a parotid mass should be seen as a concerning sign that the mass is malignant. In malignant neoplasms, pain is typically indicative of neural invasion by the tumor and portends a worse prognosis. However, pain itself is not a predictable indicator of malignancy because benign neoplasms can be associated with pain in the setting of a secondary infection, cystic enlargement, or intralesional hemorrhage.

FNA is an accurate and safe aid for diagnosis. It is primarily used to help guide which patients need surgery, rather than to provide a definitive diagnosis. It is very effective in helping to avoid surgery in patients with reactive lymph nodes, lymphoma, or nonneoplastic disorders. Surgical biopsies are not recommended because excisional biopsies and capsule violations are associated with an increased risk of recurrence, even with benign masses like pleomorphic adenoma. The standard surgical approach is to perform a lateral parotidectomy with a cuff of tissue around the mass in addition to the facial nerve dissection and preservation in order to avoid facial nerve injury.

Ref.: 1, 13

20. Which of the following statements about the larynx is true?

A. Laryngeal cancer is the most common type of head and neck cancer worldwide.

B. The HPV status has overtaken smoking and drinking as the greatest risk factor for the development of laryngeal SCC.

C. The glottis is a subunit of the larynx that consists of the false and true vocal cords.

D. Sensation of the larynx is supplied completely by the RLN.

E. Lymphatic drainage from the supraglottis goes to levels II, III, and IV and can be bilateral.

ANSWER: E

COMMENTS: Laryngeal cancer is the second most common cancer worldwide. The greatest risk factor for laryngeal cancer remains smoking and drinking; the HPV status is the most important risk factor pertaining to oropharyngeal SCC (OPSCC). The glottis contains the true cords and extends 1 cm inferiorly. The false cords are a supraglottic structure. Sensation to the larynx is supplied by both the internal branch of the superior laryngeal nerve and the RLN. The supraglottis lymphatic drainage tends to be bilateral and to levels II, III, and IV.

Epidemiologically, laryngeal cancer is the second most common cancer of the head and neck worldwide, after oropharyngeal cancer. There is a male-to-female preponderance of 6:1.

The most important risk factors for the development of laryngeal SCC are **smoking and drinking**, and these have a multiplicative effect. **HPV** has also been associated with the development of laryngeal SCC (**HPV types 16 and 18**) but not as strongly as in OPSCC. Occupational exposure to wood dust, polycyclic hydrocarbons, and asbestos is an additional risk factor.

Anatomically, the larynx consists of three subunits: the **supraglottis, glottis, and subglottis**. The supraglottis extends from the epiglottis to the ventricular apices and encompasses the false cords, aryepiglottic folds, arytenoids, and laryngeal surface of the epiglottis. The glottis consists of the true vocal cords, the anterior commissure, the interarytenoid region, and the floor of the ventricles and extends 1 cm inferiorly below the apex of the ventricle. The subglottis extends from 1 cm below the ventricle to the inferior border of the cricoid cartilage.

The blood supply to the supraglottis is delivered via the superior laryngeal artery, which is a branch of the superior thyroid artery. The blood supply to the glottis and subglottis is supplied by the inferior laryngeal branch of the inferior thyroid artery. Lymphatic drainage of the supraglottis is supplied by a rich network. The supraglottis tends to drain to level II but can extend to levels III and IV. Bilateral drainage can occur. The glottis has essentially no lymphatic drainage. The subglottis drains primary to level VI.

Sensation above the true cords is supplied by the internal branch of the superior laryngeal nerve, while the sensation of the true cords is supplied by the RLN. The external branch of the superior laryngeal nerve provides motor innervation to the cricothyroid muscle. The RLN is responsible for the motor innervation to the remainder of the laryngeal musculature.

Ref.: 1, 13

21. Which of the following statements is true about neck dissection?

A. A radical neck dissection removes all nodal levels in the cervical neck as well as the SCM muscle, external jugular vein, and spinal accessory nerve.

B. An important landmark for finding the hypoglossal nerve during neck dissection is the transverse process of C2.

C. The spinal accessory nerve most frequently passes anteriorly to the jugular vein in level II before giving off a branch to the SCM muscle.

D. The hypoglossal nerve exits the base of the skull and passes posterior to both the internal jugular vein and the external carotid artery and its branches before passing deep to the posterior belly of the digastric muscle to enter the submandibular triangle.

E. Level III extends from the hyoid bone to the level of the thyroid cartilage.

ANSWER: C

COMMENTS: A **radical neck dissection** is defined as the removal of all nodal levels in addition to the SCM, internal jugular vein, and spinal accessory nerve. The transverse process of C2 is an important landmark for the identification of the spinal accessory nerve. The spinal accessory nerve most frequently passes anteriorly to the internal jugular vein in level II. The hypoglossal nerve passes posterior to the internal jugular vein but anterior to the external carotid and its branches. Level III extends from the hyoid bone to the inferior border of the cricoid cartilage. Radical neck dissection is rarely performed today due to significant morbidity such as shoulder droop, an increased risk of facial swelling due to the sacrifice of the internal jugular vein, and an increased risk of carotid blowout due to less superficial tissue coverage after removal of the SCM muscle. It is still performed if there are clinically positive modes with the involvement of the SCM muscle, CN XI, and internal jugular vein.

A **modified radical neck dissection** is defined as the removal of nodes but spares CN IX in type I or CN IX and the internal jugular vein in type II.

The **selective neck dissection**, which is the most commonly performed, does not remove all nodal levels, but specifically those at most risk depending on the site of the primary tumor. The SCM muscle, CN IX, and internal jugular vein are spared.

Nodal levels have specific boundaries. Level IA includes the submental triangle and is bound by the anterior belly of the digastric muscle bilaterally, the mandible anteriorly, and the hyoid inferiorly. Level IB includes the submandibular triangle and is bound by the anterior belly of the digastric medially, the mandible superiorly, the stylohyoid ligament laterally, and the hyoid bone inferiorly. Level II includes the jugular digastric region from the level of the posterior belly of the digastric down to the hyoid bone. Level II is further divided into B and A segments by the spinal accessory nerve—level IIB is the segment superior and level IIA is the segment inferior. Level III extends from the hyoid bone to the inferior border of the cricoid cartilage. Level IV nodes extend from the inferior border of the cricoid cartilage to the clavicle. Level V is bound by the posterior border of the SCM anteriorly and the anterior border of the trapezius posteriorly. Level IV contains the pretracheal and paratracheal nodes found inferior to the thyroid gland.

Ref.: 1, 3, 13

22. Which of the following statements about the oral cavity is true?

A. The upper lip demonstrates significant lymphatic crossover. As a result, upper lip neoplasms tend to metastasize to bilateral level IB, periparotid lymph nodes, and level II lymph nodes.

B. The floor of the mouth is composed of a series of muscles. From inferior to superior these include anterior belly of the digastric, the mylohyoid muscle, and the geniohyoid muscle.

C. The intrinsic muscles of the tongue are responsible for gross tongue movement while the extrinsic muscles of the tongue are responsible for intricate mobility required for speech and deglutition.

D. The lingual nerve supplies motor innervation to the tongue.

E. Taste and sensation from the anterior two-thirds of the tongue are supplied via the mandibular division of the trigeminal nerve.

ANSWER: B

COMMENTS: The upper lip tends to drain ipsilaterally, not bilaterally. The floor of the mouth is composed of the anterior belly of the digastric, the mylohyoid muscle, and the geniohyoid muscle from inferior to superior. The extrinsic muscles of the tongue are responsible for gross tongue movements, while the intrinsic muscles of the tongue are responsible for intricate mobility. The hypoglossal nerve supplies tongue motor innervation. Taste to the anterior two-thirds of the tongue is supplied by the facial nerve via chorda tympani and the lingual nerve while sensation to this part of the tongue is supplied by the mandibular division of the trigeminal nerve.

The **oral cavity** is a complex anatomic space composed of seven distinct subunits. These subunits are important to understand as distinct entities because they each have specific lymphatic drainage pathways and different propensities for local invasion. The oral cavity extends from the vermilion borders of the lips anteriorly to its posterior limit, which is demarcated by the vertical line drawn from the junction of the hard and soft palate to the circumvallate papillae. Laterally, the boundary is the buccal mucosa. The seven subunits are the lips, alveolar ridge, floor of the mouth, oral tongue, hard palate, retromolar trigone, and the lateral buccal mucosa.

The arterial supply to the lips is provided by the labial arteries, which are a branch off the facial artery. The lower lip drains to levels IA and IB and tends to have contralateral drainage. The upper lip tends to drain ipsilaterally to level IB, periparotid lymph nodes, and level II lymph nodes.

The **lower alveolar ridge** contains the tooth-bearing component of the mandible. This is a thin bone that tends to involute when dentition is lost. The alveolar ridge blood supply is provided by endosteal and periosteal vessels. Lymphatic drainage is based on the anatomic position. Anterior lesions drain to level I and have bilateral drainage, while lateral lesions tend to drain to the ipsilateral levels IB and II.

The **floor of the mouth** extends from the attached gingiva of the medial alveolar ridge to the muscular tongue and extends posteriorly to the palatoglossus muscle. The primary vascular supply is via the lingual artery and branches of the facial system. The floor of the mouth lymphatic system has superficial and deep drainage pathways. The superficial system drains bilaterally while the deep system drains to ipsilateral level I and the upper jugular chain.

The **oral tongue** consists of three paired extrinsic muscle groups that achieve gross tongue movement: genioglossus, hypoglossus, and styloglossus. The intrinsic musculature includes the lingual muscles as well as the vertical and transverse muscular units, which work together to perform high-fidelity tongue movements that assist in speech and swallow. Motor innervation is supplied via the hypoglossal nerve. Taste from the oral tongue is supplied by way of the chorda tympani/lingual nerve system. Lymphatic drainage depends on the anatomic position. Lesions on the tip of the tongue and midline dorsum tend to spread bilaterally as well as to level IA. Lateral oral tongue lesions tend to spread to the ipsilateral level IB and level II.

The **upper alveolar** ridge receives blood supply from the facial artery and internal maxillary artery system. Lymphatic drainage tends to be to ipsilateral level IB, periparotid lymph nodes, and level II.

The **hard palate** tends to drain to levels I and II. It contains three paired foramina that allow for potential tumor spread: the greater palatine, the lesser palatine, and the incisive foramen.

The **retromolar trigone** is a mucosally covered triangular area overlying the ascending ramus of the mandible. The retromolar trigone mucosa is tightly adherent to the mandible; therefore even small mucosal lesions can easily spread to the mandible. Lymphatic drainage is to ipsilateral levels I and II. The lateral buccal mucosa lymphatics drain to levels I and II and periparotid lymph nodes.

Ref.: 1, 3, 13

23. A 68-year-old male presents with the lesion pictured in Fig. 30.1. An FNA in the office is performed and is consistent with SCC. A CT soft tissue neck is obtained, which shows the lesion has a depth of invasion of 4.5 mm. There is no radiographic or clinical neck lymphadenopathy, and the remainder of the metastatic workup is negative. What is the appropriate management for this patient?

A. Partial glossectomy with ipsilateral radical neck dissection

B. Total glossectomy only

C. Radiation only

D. Hemiglossectomy with ipsilateral radical neck dissection

E. Partial glossectomy with ipsilateral selective neck dissection

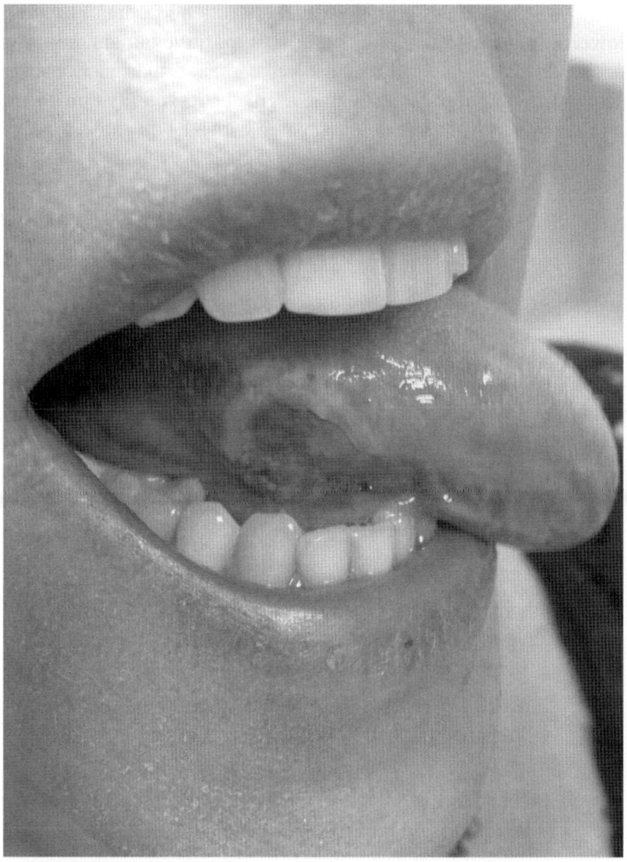

Fig. 30.1 *(Used with permission of Dr. Samer Al-Khudari.)*

ANSWER: E

COMMENTS: The patient has a lateralized tongue SCC with an invasion of 4 mm in depth. Adequate margins should be attainable with a partial glossectomy rather than a hemiglossectomy or total glossectomy. This will preserve articulation and swallow function. The patient, even though currently with an N0 neck, is at a high risk of developing cervical metastasis due to a depth of invasion of 4.5 mm. An ipsilateral selective neck dissection is recommended.

SCC of the tongue tends to occur in middle-aged males with a history of tobacco and alcohol use. However, there is a subset of patients who tend to be 20 to 40 years of age with no known risk factors. Cancer in this group tends to be more aggressive and carries a poor prognosis despite appropriate therapy.

The rate of cervical node metastasis is high, even in T1 or T2 primary cancers. Multiple studies have found that the increasing rate of metastasis is seen in tumors that have a vertical depth of invasion greater than 4 mm.

The initial treatment can be surgical or with radiation. A surgical excision is favored for most patients due to the ability to obtain adequate margins while still preserving articulation and the ability to swallow. T1 and T2 cancers can be treated with a partial glossectomy with the goal of attaining a 1-cm cuff of normal tissue around the lesion in all directions. T3 and T4 lesions tend to involve adjacent structures such as the floor of the mouth or mandible. These lesions tend to require a hemiglossectomy or total glossectomy to achieve an adequate margin. Further, these patients may require a segmental mandibulectomy or floor of the mouth resection to adequately resect the tumor.

Management of the clinically/radiographically N0 neck tends to be more aggressive in even T1/T2 cancers. The reason for this is that even early-stage cancer tends to have a high rate of nodal metastasis, with some studies reporting a rate as high as 30%. If the depth of invasion is 4 mm, a selective neck dissection should be recommended in the clinically/radiographically N0 neck and should even be considered if the depth of invasion is at least 3 mm. Selective neck dissection should include levels I–IV in a clinically/radiographically negative neck. Level IIB does not need to be dissected unless metastasis is evident intraoperatively.

Ref.: 3, 13

24. A 58-year-old female develops an increased work of breathing and stridor 10 h after undergoing a C3–5 anterior cervical diskectomy and fusion. Multiple attempts at intubation with GlideScope and fiberoptic technique fail, and a bedside cricothyroidotomy is performed. Which of the following is true regarding cricothyroidotomy?

A. Surgical revision to a formal tracheotomy should be performed within 48 h, if clinically acceptable, due to increased risk of subglottic stenosis with prolonged cricothyroidotomy.

B. Surgical revision to a formal tracheotomy should be performed due to increased risk of supraglottic stenosis with prolonged cricothyroidotomy.

C. Surgical revision to a formal tracheotomy should be performed due to the increased risk of laryngotracheal separation with prolonged cricothyroidotomy.

D. Cricothyroidotomy is accomplished by incising the thyroid cartilage in the midline to create enough space for tube placement.

E. Cricothyroidotomy is indicated in neonates and children.

ANSWER: A

COMMENTS: Surgical revision to a formal tracheotomy should be performed due to an increased risk of subglottic stenosis. Laryngotracheal separation is not associated with cricothyroidotomy. Cricothyroidotomy is accomplished by making an incision through the cricothyroid membrane, not the thyroid cartilage. It is contraindicated in children due to a high risk of cricoid injury and subglottic stenosis as well as a low likelihood of successfully entering the airway.

Cricothyroidotomy is an important maneuver when intubation is not possible in an emergent setting. It is performed by placing the patient in a supine position with shoulder roll to assist with neck extension. A skin preparation solution is used if time permits. The thyroid cartilage is then grasped between the thumb and second and third fingers of the nondominant hand. A vertical incision is then made with a number 11 or 15 blade to expose the cricothyroid membrane. A vertical incision is made to avoid injury to the anterior jugular veins. Further, it will allow for more exposure of the airway. Once exposed, a horizontal incision is made through the membrane, staying closer to the superior border of the cricoid to avoid injury to the cricothyroid vessels. If available, a tracheal dilator or clamp (Kelly, hemostat, mosquito) can be used to dilate the cricothyroidotomy. If available, a cuffed tracheostomy tube can then be placed through the cricothyroidotomy and a ventilating device attached. Once breath sounds are confirmed, the tracheostomy tube should be secured with sutures, tracheostomy tube ties if available. If no tracheostomy tube is available, any tube that will keep the airway patent and attach to a ventilating system (such as an endotracheal tube) is appropriate.

Once secured, the cricothyroidotomy should then be converted to a formal tracheostomy within 48 h due to an increased risk of subglottic stenosis. There is an increased risk because the cricothyroid space is 7 mm in vertical dimension. Since the cricothyroid space is usually smaller than the outer diameter of most tracheostomy tubes (6 Shiley disposable cuffed trach tube (DCT) is 10 mm in outer diameter), the risk of cartilage injury is high. A combination of pressure against the cricoid cartilage, shearing forces from the cricothyroid muscle tensing, and concomitant infection create a favorable environment for chondritis, necrosis, and, ultimately, subglottic stenosis.

Ref.: 3, 13, 14

25. Which of the following statements about the oropharynx is true?

A. Major risk factors for the development of OPSCC do not include smoking and drinking.

B. The anatomic subunits within the oropharynx include the soft palate, the palatine tonsillar fossa and pillars, the base of tongue, and the epiglottis.

C. HPV 23 and 40 are the most strongly associated HPV subtypes in an oropharyngeal cancer.

D. HPV-positive OPSCC is rarely identified.

E. Patients diagnosed with HPV-positive oropharyngeal carcinoma are more responsive to treatment and have a survival advantage.

ANSWER: E

COMMENTS: The major risk factors for OPSCC include HPV status, smoking, and drinking. The anatomic subunits of the oropharynx include the soft palate, the tonsillar fossa and pillars, the base of tongue, and the pharyngeal walls, while the epiglottis is a part of the larynx. HPV 16 is the most strongly associated subtype with OPSCC. HPV-positive SCC is commonly identified in OPSCC. Patients with HPV-positive SCC are more responsive to treatment and have a survival advantage.

The oropharynx is the middle third of the pharynx and connects with the nasopharynx superiorly and hypopharynx inferiorly. Its superior and inferior limitations are defined by horizontal lines drawn through the hard palate and hyoid bone, respectively, while its anterior border is a vertical line drawn through the hard palate/soft palate junction through the circumvallate papillae. Its posterior border is the posterior pharyngeal wall, which lies anterior to the prevertebral fascia. Its lateral boundary includes the tonsillar fossa and pillars as well as the lateral pharyngeal walls.

The oropharynx consists of four subunits: the soft palate, tonsillar fossa and pillars, base of tongue, and pharyngeal walls.

Historically, the most important risk factor for the development of OPSCC was exposure to tobacco and alcohol. Smokers have a 5 to 25 times greater risk of developing head and neck cancer than nonsmokers. The relative risk of developing SCC rises to 8.8 in those who consume 30 alcoholic beverages per week compared with a relative risk of 1.2 in those who consume 1 to 4 drinks per week. Smoking and drinking have a cumulative effect: for instance, a patient who has a 40-pack-year smoking history and drinks 5 alcoholic beverages daily has a relative risk of 40.

In the last three decades, there has been a demographic shift in the etiologic agent in the development of SCC. HPV is now the most common cause. HPV 16 is the most common detected subtype. HPV-positive tumors are more likely to originate in the oropharynx, be poorly differentiated, and have basaloid features. They tend to occur in younger and healthier patients and tend to present with a lower T stage but a higher N stage. HPV-positive tumors are independently associated with sexual behavior and marijuana use in some studies. These patients have a greater response to treatment and have a survival advantage compared with HPV-negative tumors.

Ref.: 1, 13, 15

26. A 64-year-old male with a 50-pack-year smoking history presents with right ear pain, odynophagia, and hoarseness for a duration of 3 months. He initially presented to his primary care physician, who prescribed a course of Augmentin for suspected upper respiratory tract infection with acute otitis media. He reports this treatment helped for a while, but his symptoms quickly returned. On examination, the patient has inspiratory stridor, prolonged inspiratory phase, and dysphonia. A flexible laryngoscopy shows a right glottic mass, causing fixation of the right true vocal cord and near-complete obstruction of the airway. What is the next best step in management?

A. Perform an office biopsy of the lesion in order to obtain diagnosis.

B. Obtain CT soft tissue neck and chest with IV contrast and have the patient follow up in clinic as soon as the scans are complete to discuss further management.

C. Proceed to the OR for standard bag mask induction with GlideScope intubation followed by a direct laryngoscopy, a biopsy of the laryngeal mass, and a tracheotomy.

D. Proceed to the OR to perform an awake tracheotomy followed by a direct laryngoscopy and a biopsy of the laryngeal mass.

E. Proceed to the OR for a rapid sequence induction flexible fiberoptic intubation followed by a direct laryngoscopy and a biopsy of the laryngeal mass, selective neck dissection, and tracheotomy.

ANSWER: D

COMMENTS: The patient has a history and physical examination consistent with SCC of the larynx. The diagnosis should be obtained with a biopsy. Furthermore, CT scans must be obtained to determine the extent of the patient's disease and to determine staging. However, the primary act in management must be to secure the patient's airway in as safe a manner as possible. The best option for this patient is to undergo an awake tracheotomy. Putting the patient to sleep prior to an attempted intubation would not be recommended as his obstructing laryngeal mass would likely prevent him from being ventilated via bag mask ventilation. Further, an obstructing mass would make it very difficult to pass an endotracheal tube successfully.

Laryngeal cancer commonly presents with dysphonia and odynophagia. Clinicians must also be suspicious if an adult patient presents with odynophagia or ear pain that is present for more than 2 to 3 weeks. Ear pain is a common presenting sign due to referred pain from the throat via Jacobson's nerve and Arnold nerve.

Jacobson's nerve, a branch of CN IX, directly innervates the ear but also has pharyngeal, lingual, tonsillar, parapharyngeal space, and retropharyngeal space innervation. Any pathologic process involving these areas can result in referred otalgia.

Arnold nerve, a branch of CN X, supplies the vallecula, lingual, and laryngeal surfaces of the epiglottis, supraglottic larynx, and pyriform sinuses. The Arnold nerve also directly innervates the ear, which can result in referred otalgia.

Ref.: 3, 13, 16

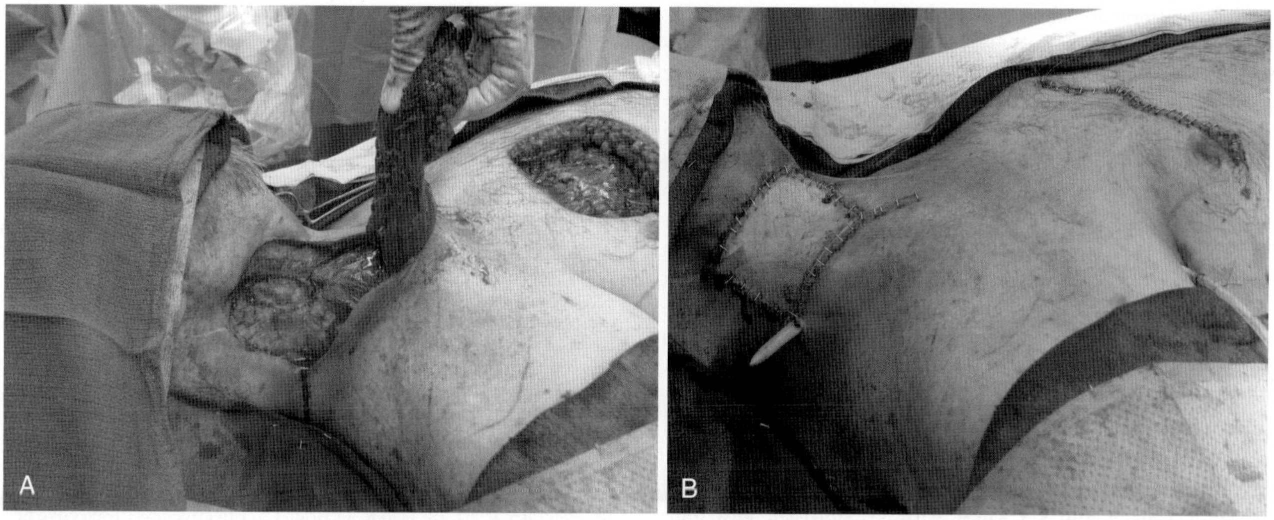

Fig. 30.2 *(Used with permission of Dr. Samer Al-Khudari.)*

27. A patient with a history of laryngeal cancer initially treated with radiation therapy presents with a T4 recurrence. A total laryngectomy is performed. The patient's pharyngeal defect is closed using the myocutaneous regional pedicled flap shown in Fig. 30.2. What is the blood supply to this flap?

A. Branch from the thoracoacromial artery

B. Thoracodorsal artery

C. Perforating vessels from the occipital artery

D. Superficial temporal artery

E. Perforating vessels of the internal mammary artery

ANSWER: A

COMMENTS: The image is of a pectoralis myocutaneous flap based on the pectoral branch of the thoracoacromial artery. The thoracodorsal artery supplies the latissimus dorsi myocutaneous flap. The perforating vessels of the occipital artery supply the superior one-third of an SCM myocutaneous flap. The superficial temporal artery supplies the temporoparietal fasciocutaneous flap. The perforating vessels of the internal mammary artery supply the deltopectoral fasciocutaneous flap.

Patients undergoing a total laryngectomy require a pharyngeal closure. In patients who have not previously received radiation, this can typically be done primarily. However, in patients who have received radiation, the local vasculature is tenuous and these patients are at a higher risk of breakdown of the pharyngeal closure without bolstering the pharyngeal closure with healthy tissue.

The **pectoralis major flap** is a regional pedicled flap that is used frequently for its reliability and excellent reach (can reach up to midface, some report to lateral canthus). Its blood supply is from the pectoral branch of the thoracoacromial artery.

Ref.: 1, 3, 17

28. A patient with a SCC of the left lower alveolus undergoes a segmental mandibulectomy of a 6-cm segment of bone. Which reconstructive option is the most appropriate?

A. Radial forearm osseocutaneous free flap

B. Latissimus dorsi myocutaneous free flap

C. Anterolateral thigh fasciocutaneous free flap

D. Gracilis muscle free flap

E. Fibula osseocutaneous free flap

ANSWER: E

COMMENTS: In the reconstruction of a segmental mandibulectomy, the surgeon must reconstruct the mandible using the strong bone. A radial forearm osseocutaneous flap provides a bone, but the bone is thin. The latissimus, anterolateral thigh, and gracilis flaps cannot be harvested with a bone and cannot be used to repair a mandibular defect. The best option for reconstruction is the fibula osseocutaneous free flap.

The free fibular graft provides the longest possible segment of revascularized bone (up to 25 cm). It can span nearly any mandibular defect. The flap is supplied by the **peroneal artery and accompanying veins.**

Ref.: 1, 3, 17

29. A 52-year-old male with no other medical history presents with a 4-cm right level II neck mass. An office FNA is performed and is consistent with SCC. A thorough physical examination including a flexible laryngoscopy does not indicate an obvious primary tumor. The P16 status is pending. Which of the following is true?

A. An appropriate next step in the management would be to perform a direct laryngoscopy and esophagoscopy with a biopsy of any suspicious lesions. A right tonsillectomy should be performed if no clear lesions are found elsewhere, and a left-sided tonsillectomy should be considered.

B. Esophagoscopy is unnecessary.

C. Bilateral tonsillectomy and base of tongue resection are indicated for the initial diagnostic workup.

D. A positron emission tomography (PET) scan is the only indicated imaging.

E. The P16 status will not provide prognostic information.

ANSWER: A

COMMENTS: A direct laryngoscopy and esophagoscopy would be the next appropriate step. Any suspicious lesions should be biopsied.

If no obvious primary site is found during this examination, a right tonsillectomy should be performed and a left tonsillectomy considered. A base of tongue resection would not be indicated at this stage in the patient's workup. However, a PET scan can be useful; anatomic studies such as CT soft tissue neck or MRI neck should be obtained to fully evaluate for any suspicious lesions. A CT chest with IV contrast should also be obtained to assess for any metastatic disease. P16 positivity would indicate the HPV status.

Patients presenting with a head and neck cancer of unknown primary make up about 2%–9% of all patients with head and neck cancer. The diagnosis of a primary tumor is of crucial significance because surgical and oncologic management of the primary lesion may be efficiently coordinated with the management of the neck disease that has improved the survival rates from 44% up to 100%. Further, the type and degree of treatment change based on whether a primary tumor is found.

The typical diagnostic protocol includes a **physical examination, CT neck and CT chest with IV contrast, and panendoscopy in the OR under general anesthesia** (including **laryngoscopy and esophagoscopy**) with **tonsillectomy** and **biopsies of suspicious mucosal areas**. The CT/MRI detection rate for a primary tumor varies from 9% to 23%. The likelihood of discovering a primary tumor by an endoscopy and random biopsies is low. Without suspicious findings in clinical or radiologic examinations, a successful result can be obtained in 20%–29% of cases in some studies. When an endoscopic biopsy can be directed according to a suspicious clinical or radiologic finding, a detection rate of up to 60% has been reported. Ipsilateral tonsillectomy yields an 18%–44% rate in primary tumor. Some authors and institutions support bilateral tonsillectomy, because bilateral or contralateral tumors have been found in up to 10%–23% of cases.

Ref.: 13, 18

REFERENCES

1. Lorenz RR, Netterville JL, Burkey BB. Head and neck. In: Townsend CM, Beauchamp RD, Evers BM, et al., eds. *Sabiston Textbook of Surgery: The Biological Basis of Modern Surgical Practice*. 18th ed. Philadelphia: WB Saunders; 2008.
2. Cummings CW, Haughey BH, Thomas JR, et al. *Cummings Otolaryngology: Head and Neck Surgery*. 4th ed. Philadelphia: CV Mosby; 2005.
3. Myers EN, Suen JY, Myers JN, et al. *Cancer of the Head and Neck*. 4th ed. Philadelphia: WB Saunders; 2003.
4. Al-Sarraf M, LeBlanc M, Giri PG, et al. Chemoradiotherapy versus radiotherapy in patients with advanced nasopharyngeal cancer: phase III randomized Intergroup Study 0099. *J Clin Oncol*. 1998;16:1310–1317.
5. The Department of Veterans Affairs Laryngeal Cancer Study Group. Induction chemotherapy plus radiation compared with surgery plus radiation in patients with advanced laryngeal cancer. *N Engl J Med*. 1991;324:1685–1690.
6. Forastiere AA, Goepfert H, Maor M, et al. Concurrent chemotherapy and radiotherapy for organ preservation in advanced laryngeal cancer. *N Engl J Med*. 2003;349:2091–2098.
7. Bernier J, Domenge C, Ozsahin M, et al. Postoperative irradiation with or without concomitant chemotherapy for locally advanced head and neck cancer. *N Engl J Med*. 2004;350:1945–1952.
8. Cooper JS, Pajak TF, Forastiere AA, et al. Postoperative concurrent radiotherapy and chemotherapy for high-risk squamous cell carcinoma of the head and neck. *N Engl J Med*. 2004;350:1937–1944.
9. Bailey BJ, Johnson JT, Newlands SD. *Head and Neck Surgery: Otolaryngology*. 4th ed. Philadelphia: Lippincott Williams & Wilkins; 2006.
10. Patel RS, Clark JR, Gao K, O'Brien CJ. Effectiveness of selective neck dissection in the treatment of the clinically positive neck. *Head Neck*. 2008;30:1231–1236.
11. Mirski MA, Lele AV, Fitzsimmons L, Toung TJK. Diagnosis and treatment of vascular air embolism. *Anesthesiology*. 2007;106:164–177.
12. Taxy JB, El-Zayaty S, Langerman A. Acute fungal sinusitis, natural history and the role of frozen section. *Am J Clin Pathol*. 2009;132(1):86–93.
13. Johnson JT, Rosen CA, eds. *Bailey's Head and Neck Surgery: Otolaryngology Review*. 5th ed. Philadelphia: Lippincott Williams & Wilkins; 2014.
14. Kuriloff DB, Setzen M, Portnoy W, Gadaleta D. Laryngotracheal injury following cricothyroidotomy. *Laryngoscope*. 1989;99(2):125–130.
15. Deschler DG, Richmon JD, Khariwala SS, Ferris RL, Wang MB. The "new" head and neck cancer patient—young, nonsmoker, nondrinker, and HPV positive. *Otolaryngol Head Neck Surg*. 2014;15(3):375–380.
16. Fang CH, Friedman R, White PE, Mady LJ, Kalyoussef E. Emergent awake tracheostomy—the five-year experience at an urban tertiary care center. *Laryngoscope*. 2015;125(11):2476–2479.
17. Papel I, Frodel J, Holt G, et al. *Facial Plastic and Reconstructive Surgery*. 2nd ed. New York: Thime; 2002.
18. Koivunen P, Bäck L, Laranne J, Irjala H. Unknown primary: diagnostic issues in the biological endoscopy and positron emission tomography scan era. *Curr Opin Otolaryngol Head and Neck Surg*. 2015;23(2):121–126.

CHAPTER 31

PEDIATRIC SURGERY

Jamie Harris, M.D., Bill Chiu, M.D., Srikumar Pillai, M.D., and Ami Shah, M.D.

1. Which of the following statements is true regarding daily fluid requirements?

A. Premature infants weighing less than 2 kg require only up to 80 mL/kg per day of fluid.

B. Neonates and infants weighing 2 to 10 kg require 200 mL/kg per day of fluid.

C. Infants and children weighing 10 to 20 kg require 1000 mL/day plus 50 mL/kg per day of fluid for every kilogram over 10 kg.

D. Children heavier than 20 kg require 1500 mL/day plus 30 mL/kg per day of fluid for every kilogram over 20 kg.

E. All of the above.

ANSWER: C

COMMENTS: Infants weighing less than 1500 g require 130 to 150 mL/kg per day of fluid. Those weighing 1500 to 2000 g require 110 to 130 mL/kg per day, 2 to 10 kg require 100 mL/kg per day, 10 to 20 kg require 1000 mL for the first 10 kg and an additional 50 mL/kg for each additional kilogram, and those weighing more than 20 kg require 1500 mL plus 20 mL/kg for each additional kilogram over 20 kg. Daily electrolyte requirements include sodium at 2 to 5 mEq/kg and potassium at 2 to 3 mEq/kg. Dextrose is administered to provide a glucose substrate at a minimum rate of 4 to 6 mg/kg/min. Fat infusions are started at 0.5 g/kg per day and advanced up to 2.5 to 3 g/kg per day. Protein requirements are 2 to 3.5 g/kg per day in infants, as opposed to requirements of about 1 g/kg per day in adults.

Ref.: 1–3

2. What is the daily energy requirement for an 8-month-old healthy baby?

A. 90 to 120 kcal/kg

B. 80 to 100 kcal/kg

C. 75 to 90 kcal/kg

D. 50 to 75 kcal/kg

E. 30 to 50 kcal/kg

ANSWER: B

COMMENTS: Energy requirements are important to consider in the pediatric population. For premature infants, 90 to 120 kcal/kg are required. Infants <6 months of age require 85 to 105 kcal/kg, 6 to 12 months require 80 to 100 kcal/kg, 1 to 7 years require 75 to 90 kcal/kg, 7 to 12 years require 50 to 75 kcal/kg, and >12 years up until 18 years of age require 30 to 50 kcal/kg. Periods of active growth have higher caloric requirements. Breast milk provides 0.64 to 0.67 kcal/mL. When feasible, it is advisable that children have breast milk until 1 year of age. Breast milk additionally helps provide passive immunity with the transmission of both humoral and cellular factors to the baby. However, breast milk must be supplemented with vitamin D to prevent vitamin D deficiency that is often seen in breastfed infants.

Ref.: 4

3. A 5-week-old boy has a 5-day history of nonbilious vomiting and weight loss of 0.4 kg (from 4.0 to 3.6 kg). His anterior fontanelle is flattened, and his mucous membranes are dry. Laboratory data are as follows (in mEq/L): sodium 132, potassium 3.2, chloride 91, and bicarbonate 28. Which of the following statements about this infant is true?

A. Characterization of the emesis as nonbilious is crucial to aid in the diagnosis.

B. Palpation of the abdomen will not help with the diagnosis.

C. Ultrasound imaging of the abdomen will not add to the diagnosis.

D. This condition is more likely to affect females.

E. Laboratory results are likely to demonstrate a metabolic acidosis.

ANSWER: A

COMMENTS: The differential diagnoses in this child include intestinal stenosis, pyloric stenosis, intussusception, and malrotation. Age is important in sorting out the differential diagnoses in children. Duodenal atresia is seen in newborns since it is congenital. This child has hypertrophic pyloric stenosis, which typically produces symptoms in infants between 3 and 12 weeks of age and is more common in males. Intussusception most commonly occurs in children between 3 and 18 months of age.

Infants with pyloric stenosis usually present with nonbilious vomiting that progressively becomes projectile since the blockage is proximal to the ampulla of Vater. Duodenal atresia most commonly occurs distal to the ampulla of Vater, and therefore the vomitus is bilious in about 80% of cases. Duodenal stenosis distal to the ampulla may present in a similar manner. Malrotation also presents with bilious emesis. The extent of dehydration and electrolyte imbalance depends on the duration of the symptoms. Early in the course, fluid and electrolyte levels may be normal. If the condition is diagnosed late, infants are more likely to have severe metabolic derangements and dehydration. Palpation during physical examination may reveal the pathognomonic olive-sized mass of the thickened pylorus in the upper mid to right abdomen. Sometimes gastric waves are seen through the epigastrium. If the pyloric mass cannot be palpated by an experienced examiner, ultrasound is the first choice for diagnostic imaging. Correction of fluid and electrolyte abnormalities takes precedence over surgery, which can be undertaken once electrolyte imbalances are corrected.

Ref.: 1–3

4. For the infant in Question 3, which of the following is the most common electrolyte abnormality?

A. Hypokalemia

B. Hyperkalemia

C. Hypocalcemia

D. Hyperchloremia

E. Hypercalcemia

ANSWER: A

COMMENTS: Infants with a gastric outlet obstruction due to hypertrophic pyloric stenosis typically present with hypokalemia, hypochloremic metabolic alkalosis, and paradoxical aciduria. The electrolyte abnormalities reflect the extensive loss of gastric contents from emesis in hypertrophic pyloric stenosis. Paradoxical aciduria and hypokalemia result from the urinary loss of acid (H+) and potassium at the expense of sodium and water retention to preserve the fluid volume. Hypochloremia is secondary to the loss of bicarbonate from emesis with resulting contraction alkalosis. Disturbances in calcium are not common in this setting. Correction of fluid and electrolyte imbalances is essential before proceeding to surgery.

Ref.: 1

5. This patient with hypertrophic pyloric stenosis presented with laboratory values of sodium 132 mEq/L, potassium 3.2 mEq/L, chloride 91 mEq/L, and bicarbonate 28 mEq/L. Which of the following intravenous fluids administered prior to surgery can decrease the risk of respiratory distress?

A. Dextrose 5% and water with 20 mEq of potassium chloride (KCl)

B. Lactated Ringer's

C. 1 unit of packed red blood cells

D. Dextrose 5% with one-half normal saline and 20 mEq of KCL

E. Dextrose 5% with one-half normal saline

ANSWER: D

COMMENTS: Hypertrophic pyloric stenosis presents with a hypochloremic, hypokalemic, and metabolic alkalosis. A serum bicarbonate < 25 mEq/L is a slight deficit, 26 to 35 mEq/L is a moderate deficit, and >35 mEq/L is severe. This deficit guides resuscitation as well as operative timing. It is important to correct alkalosis so that the serum bicarbonate level is <30mEq/L prior to operative intervention. If uncorrected, this can lead to respiratory insufficiency and prolonged intubation as the baby's system attempts to correct the acid–base balance by hypoventilation. In addition to alkalosis, these patients also have hypokalemia. Therefore adding potassium to the intravenous fluid is essential, making the optimal resuscitative fluid D5 with one-half normal saline and 20 mEq of KCL. If electrolyte abnormalities are severely deranged at presentation, very close intensive care unit monitoring and gradual resuscitation should be performed to prevent rapid shifts in electrolytes that could lead to seizures and other serious complications.

Ref.: 4

6. Which of the following statements concerning pediatric trauma is true?

A. Trauma is the second leading cause of death in children between 1 and 15 years of age.

B. Computed tomography (CT) is indicated when there is a painful distracting injury, significant head injury, or an unclear examination.

C. Indications for operative intervention include documentation of injury to the spleen or liver on CT.

D. Intraosseous access is the preferred means for delivering fluids or blood in a child younger than 10 years of age.

E. Surgical cricothyroidotomy is an acceptable means of airway control for a child younger than 12 years.

ANSWER: B

COMMENTS: Trauma is the leading cause of death in children between the ages of 1 and 15 years. Motor vehicle accidents, falls, bicycle accidents, and child abuse are the most common causes of traumatic death. The priorities of resuscitation are airway, breathing, and circulation. Fluid resuscitation is given as 20 mL/kg boluses. Intravenous access is the preferred method of fluid administration. However, if intravenous access cannot be obtained in a timely manner, a specially designed needle can be used to deliver fluids or blood through an intraosseous route in children younger than 6 years, most commonly via the tibia. The needle is placed 1 to 2 cm below the tibial tuberosity through the anteromedial surface of the tibia under sterile conditions. If hypovolemic shock is refractory to two crystalloid boluses, blood transfusion should be initiated as a 10 mL/kg bolus. CT is commonly used to evaluate pediatric trauma patients. CT, which can include chest, abdomen, and pelvis, is indicated when there is an injury elsewhere causing pain, a significant head injury precluding a reliable examination, or if there is an equivocal examination in general. Although injuries to the liver and spleen are common, the need for operative intervention is not absolute and many patients may be managed nonoperatively if stable. Surgical cricothyroidotomy should not be attempted in a child younger than 12 years because of the risk of inadvertent airway injury. If an airway is needed, needle cricothyroidotomy can be performed.

Ref.: 1, 2

7. What anatomic abnormality is present in an inguinal hernia in an infant?

A. Patent processus vaginalis

B. Weakness in the inguinal floor

C. Obliteration of the inguinal floor

D. Congenital absence of both the external and internal rings

E. Direct hernia

ANSWER: A

COMMENTS: Inguinal hernias in the pediatric population occur most frequently in males (3:1), with right inguinal hernias being more common (60%). Prematurity is strongly associated with an increased risk for having a hernia. In contrast to hernias seen in the adult population, pediatric hernias are the result of a patent processus vaginalis, which leads to an indirect hernia. Frequently, the diagnosis is made by identifying an inguinal bulge on examination. Surgical correction is indicated as these hernias will not resolve with time, and there is a risk of incarceration. Incarceration risk is highest within the first year of life. The average rate of incarceration is between 12% and 17%, but it may be as high as 30% in 2- to 3-month-old babies. Early repair is recommended because of the progressive rate of incarceration. The ovary is commonly encountered when there is incarceration in females. In young children, surgical correction consists primarily of a high ligation of the hernia sac. The use of laparoscopy to look at the contralateral side for a synchronous patent processus and hernia is variable. Factors associated with bilateral hernias include female gender, age less than 1 year, and the size of the index hernia. On the basis of these criteria, some surgeons recommend contralateral exploration. However, there is no consensus currently.

Ref.: 4

8. Patients with an undescended testicle:

A. Should have an orchiopexy done within the first 3 months of life

B. Need orchiopexy to decrease the incidence of testicular cancer in the future

C. Are not at increased risk for testicular torsion if unrepaired

D. Have no difference in fertility compared with the normal population if the other testicle is in normal position

E. Can be successfully treated with hormone therapy alone.

ANSWER: D

COMMENTS: Undescended testes are found in up to 4.5% of infants, but drop to less than 1% by the age of 1 year. For this reason, surgical correction of undescended testes is deferred until 6 to 9 months of age. The rate of undescended testes in premature infants is significantly higher. Undescended testes are at an increased risk for developing cancer in the future, whether or not they are surgically corrected. However, orchiopexy makes examining the testicle for abnormalities easier. The risk for torsion of a nonrepaired undescended testicle is as high as 20%. Fertility rates are decreased compared with the general population if bilateral undescended testes are present; however, a unilateral undescended testicle with a normally positioned opposite testicle is normal. Hormonal therapy with agents such as testosterone, beta-human chorionic gonadotropin (β-hCG), and luteinizing hormone-releasing hormone has been attempted, but the success rates remain low. Therefore if an undescended testis is present after 6 to 9 months of age, surgical correction should be offered.

Ref.: 4

9. A 1-month-old boy presents to the emergency room with an inconsolable pain and left scrotal swelling for the past 6 h. An ultrasound demonstrates no blood flow to the testicle. Which of the following is true of management in this condition?

A. The contralateral testicle does not need any intervention.

B. The testicle can almost never be salvaged after 2 h.

C. This is a surgical emergency.

D. The likely cause is epididymitis.

E. A bell clapper deformity is rarely the cause of this condition in adolescence.

ANSWER: C

COMMENTS: This infant has testicle torsion. The lack of testicular blood flow on ultrasound and a painful hemiscrotum on examination make the diagnosis. This is a surgical emergency and must be corrected immediately. Irreversible necrosis usually occurs by 24 h but has been described as early as 2 h after the onset. Surgical correction involves orchiopexy of not only the affected side but also the contralateral testicle to prevent torsion from occurring in the future. In the neonatal period, torsion is the result of either a bell clapper deformity or extratunical torsion; however, beyond this period, it is almost always associated with a bell clapper deformity. A bell clapper deformity is the horizontal positioning of the testicle within the scrotum resulting from a failure of normal anchoring of the gubernaculum, epididymis, and testis to the tunica vaginalis. Other presentations of acute scrotum include epididymitis, mumps orchitis, and fat necrosis; however, testicle torsion should always be considered when a patient presents with an acute scrotum to avoid prolonged ischemia and possible necrosis to the testicle.

Ref.: 4

10. Which of the following is the indicated treatment for a noncommunicating hydrocele in a 2-month-old infant?

A. Observation

B. Needle aspiration

C. Hydrocelectomy through a groin incision

D. Hydrocelectomy through a scrotal incision

E. Repair of the hernia and hydrocelectomy

ANSWER: A

COMMENTS: Most noncommunicating hydroceles in young children are asymptomatic and will resolve as the fluid is absorbed. If the hydrocele persists past 12 months of age, peritoneal communication is likely, and hydrocelectomy with ligation of the patent processus vaginalis is indicated. In children, these operations are performed through the groin. Aspiration of the hydrocele is not recommended. If the hydrocele is noncommunicating, it will resolve and thus make aspiration unnecessary. If the hydrocele is communicating, the fluid will reaccumulate and an operation will be required.

Ref.: 1–3

11. An infant presents with a draining sinus on the anterior border of the sternocleidomastoid. What is the most likely diagnosis?

A. Second brachial cleft anomaly

B. Third brachial cleft anomaly

C. Thyroglossal duct cyst

D. Cystic hygroma

E. Dermoid cyst

ANSWER: A

COMMENTS: Embryologic development of the head and neck arises from the brachial arches. Failure of complete closure results in fistulas, cysts, and sinuses. The most common brachial cleft anomaly is from the second brachial cleft and generally presents in infancy with a draining sinus anterior to the sternocleidomastoid. In adolescence, this same anomaly will more commonly present as a cyst. Once diagnosed, these should be resected since there is a risk of infection, enlargement, and malignant transformation. These abnormalities often present as infected sinuses or cysts, and management is initial incision and drainage with definitive resection later. Remnants from the third brachial pouch are very rare. Thyroglossal duct cysts present as a midline mass that moves superiorly with tongue protrusion. Cystic hygromas are congenital lymphangiomatous malformations that present in the posterior neck. Dermoid cysts of the head and neck arise from elements trapped during fusion of the brachial arches. They are usually found in the midline, are well-circumscribed, and are filled with sebaceous material that can become infected.

Ref.: 4

12. A 7-year-old premenarchal female presents with left lower quadrant pain. On ultrasound, she is found to have a 7-cm complex cyst arising from her left ovary. What is the appropriate management for this cyst?

A. Close observation, with ultrasound every 6 months
B. Fenestration
C. Surgical excision of the cyst, leaving the left ovary in situ
D. Ten days of antibiotics
E. Reassurance since this is a normal finding

ANSWER: C

COMMENTS: The clinical presentations of ovarian masses are highly variable. Symptoms may include acute pain often due to torsion, intermittent pain, an abdominal mass, or "acute appendicitis." It is important to assess the menstrual status and sexual history. Initial evaluation generally includes ultrasound, which may show a simple cyst, a complex cyst, a solid mass, and blood flow to the ovary. Lab tests for tumor markers such as CA-125, alpha-fetoprotein (AFP), hCG, and inhibin should be performed. The most common benign lesions are unilateral follicular cysts (50%). The most simple cysts are likely to regress. However, if they are larger than 5 cm in diameter, the risk of torsion is much higher, and cyst resection should be considered. Complex cysts could represent cysts that have already torsed or an ovarian neoplasm. Complex cysts should be resected in all premenarchal females. Excision of the cyst with preservation of the ovary should be performed whenever possible. Fenestration would be inappropriate in this scenario. There is an increased incidence of neoplasms in complex cysts, so fenestration could seed the intraabdominal cavity. In an adolescent, a complex cyst could be the result of hemorrhage into a functional cyst. Therefore surgical excision is not necessary at the time of diagnosis of an isolated complex cyst. Careful clinical and ultrasound follow-up for symptom resolution as well as involution of the cyst should be performed. If the cyst persists, it should be resected.

Ref.: 4, 5

13. An 8-year-old female presents as the restrained passenger after a head-on collision. On the secondary survey, a seatbelt sign is noted. In the pediatric population, what is an associated injury?

A. Chance fracture
B. Duodenal hematoma
C. Colonic perforation
D. Splenic hematoma
E. Hepatic hematoma

ANSWER: A

COMMENTS: Seatbelts in a motor vehicle collision are lifesaving. A "seatbelt sign" is abdominal wall ecchymosis that is in the pattern of a lap belt across the abdomen. When observed on physical examination, this has been shown to have an increased rate of both solid and hollow organ injury. In the pediatric population, the triad of abdominal wall hematoma, chance fracture, and jejunal or ileal perforations has been well described. A chance fracture is a flexion–distraction type injury that involves the anterior, posterior, and transverse portion of the vertebral body of the lumbar spine. Patients with a seatbelt sign should have a thorough evaluation for intraabdominal injuries as well as vertebral injuries. These patients should undergo initial imaging with either a CT scan or a focused assessment with sonography for trauma (FAST) examination and should be admitted for serial abdominal examinations, even with normal initial imaging studies.

Ref.: 4

14. Which of the following correctly describes a pulmonary sequestration?

A. Vascular connections are to the pulmonary artery and vein
B. Is a result of air trapping due to minimal expulsion of air with exhalation
C. Can be located both extralobar and intralobar
D. Communicates with the bronchial tree
E. Has minimal risk of infectious complications

ANSWER: C

COMMENTS: Bronchopulmonary sequestration (BPS) is characterized by nonfunctional pulmonary tissue that has an anomalous systemic vascular supply and does not communicate with the bronchopulmonary tree. BPSs can be either intralobar, within the actual lung parenchyma, or extralobar, which are completely separate from the lung. In fact, BPS may be found anywhere within the chest or even below the diaphragm. It is often identified on prenatal ultrasound as a well-defined mass. If it is not detected prenatally, the typical presentation is with recurrent pneumonia within the BPS. There is an increased risk for malignant transformation. Surgical resection is generally recommended.

Other lung malformations include congenital pulmonary airway malformation (CPAM) and congenital lobar emphysema (CLE). Congenital cystic lung lesions are usually CPAM. This entity was formally termed congenital cystic adenomatoid malformation (CCAM) but was renamed because cystic components are not always present. There are five subtypes of CPAM: 0, affecting the proximal lung; 1 to 3, varying sizes of cysts from large to smallest; and 4, peripheral lung cysts. A CPAM is connected to the bronchopulmonary tree, and its blood supply is from the pulmonary arteries and veins. These lesions most commonly arise from the lower lobes of the lungs and can be identified on prenatal ultrasound. As with BPS, CPAMs may become infected and present as recurrent pneumonia and have a risk for malignant transformation. Surgical resection is generally recommended.

CLE is the third lung abnormality in this group. Normal lung parenchyma becomes hyperinflated because of impaired expulsion of air on exhalation. This is due to either an obstruction of the feeding bronchus from dysplastic bronchial cartilages or extrinsic compression. Management is lobar resection.

Ref.: 4

15. Which of the following is the most common congenital chest wall deformity?

A. Pectus carinatum

B. Poland's syndrome

C. Convex chest wall deformity

D. Pigeon chest

E. Pectus excavatum

ANSWER: E

COMMENTS: Pectus excavatum is the most common chest wall deformity in children, accounting for 88% of all chest wall deformities. It is characterized by a concave chest wall deformity, with the sternum angled posteriorly toward the spine. There is a male prevalence (3:1). The defect may be present at birth but often becomes prominent during puberty due to rapid growth. Symptoms can include dyspnea and exercise intolerance. Surgical correction usually results in symptomatic relief, and there may be a slight improvement in pulmonary function tests. Surgical repair will improve cosmetic appearance and the common psychosocial anxiety. The Haller index should be calculated from an axial CT scan to determine the severity. It is the ratio of the widest transverse diameter within the ribs to the greatest length from the inner table of the sternum to the anterior surface of the vertebrae. A ratio of >3.2 is considered as a severe defect. Surgical repair may be performed with the open Ravitch procedure or with the minimally invasive Nuss procedure. The Nuss procedure is currently favored due to less perioperative pain and smaller scars. Pectus carinatum, also known as pigeon chest, is the next most common chest wall abnormality. It is characterized by a protrusion of the sternum. Management is initially nonsurgical with bracing. When worn appropriately, bracing can correct up to 75% of the deformities over time. However, noncompliance and discomfort are common. Surgical correction is done via the open Ravitch procedure. An osteotomy is made in the sternum, allowing it to be flattened to its normal position and contour. Other congenital chest wall deformities exist, but are very rare. Poland's syndrome is characterized by the congenital absence of the pectoralis major, syndactyly, and occasionally missing ribs.

Ref.: 4, 6, 7

16. Where is the most common location of the defect in a patient with congenital diaphragmatic hernia (CDH)?

A. Right-side posterolateral

B. Left-side posterolateral

C. Right-side anterolateral

D. Left-side anterolateral

E. Retrosternal

ANSWER: B

COMMENTS: The most common type of CDH is the Bochdalek hernia, which is located in the posterolateral portion of the diaphragm. This results from a failure of fusion of the lumbar and costal muscle groups in this location. This accounts for 80% of CDHs. A Morgagni hernia is an anteromedial defect that is usually retrosternal or parasternal and is far more rare. This usually does not present until later in life, while CDH is generally diagnosed in utero on ultrasound. At the time of birth, a plain radiograph will identify herniated intestinal contents within the chest or the nasogastric tube terminating within the chest. There is associated hypoplasia of the lung on the affected side, which often results in respiratory distress. Although the lung hypoplasia plays a role in the pathogenesis of respiratory compromise, the major cause is pulmonary hypertension due to pulmonary vasoconstriction. Management begins with cardiorespiratory stabilization of the infant at birth. Interventions may include nitric oxide, high-frequency ventilation, and extracorporeal membrane oxygenation (ECMO) followed by surgical correction. Survival rates for CDH range between 60% and 90%. Outcomes have improved over the last decade with the introduction of gentle ventilation strategies. Repair can be performed via either a subcostal abdominal approach or a thoracotomy. Open and thoracoscopic and laparoscopic methods have been described; however, there are higher hernia recurrence rates at 1 year with open approaches.

Ref.: 4

17. Which of the following is the most common malignancy found in childhood?

A. Lymphoma

B. Leukemia

C. Neuroblastoma

D. Nephroblastoma

E. Rhabdomyosarcoma

ANSWER: B

COMMENTS: Malignancy is second only to trauma as the leading cause of childhood death. In infants, it is the third most frequent cause of death after prematurity and congenital anomalies. Approximately 40% of childhood malignancies are leukemia. The most common solid tumor in children younger than 2 years is neuroblastoma, which accounts for 6%–10% of all childhood cancers. In children older than 2 years, the most common solid tumor is Wilms tumor.

Ref.: 1–3

18. Which of the following is associated with a good prognosis in neuroblastoma?

A. *MYC-N* amplification

B. Age > 13 years

C. Age < 1 year

D. Stromal poor tumor cells on histology

E. High mitotis–karyorrhexis index (MKI)

ANSWER: C

COMMENTS: Neuroblastoma is the most common solid extracranial tumor in the pediatric population. The tumor arises from neural crest cells and is most commonly found in the adrenal medulla. However, it may also be found anywhere along the sympathetic chain. The presentation is generally insidious. Commonly, a large abdominal mass is found. Masses within the thoracic cavity can present with Horner syndrome (miosis, ptosis, anhidrosis, and occasionally enophthalmos). Workup should include evaluating urinary vanillylmandelic acid (VMA) and homovanillic acid (HVA). CT scans most frequently demonstrate a mass with calcifications. Metaiodobenzylguanidine (MIBG) scanning may be used to help identify the metastatic disease. The tumor should be biopsied. Unfavorable findings associated with a poor prognosis include stroma-poor tumors, *MYC-N* amplification, and high MKI. Patients diagnosed at less than 1 year of age have significantly improved outcomes compared with older children. Survival is largely based on age at diagnosis, histologic subtype, *MYC-N* status, and extent of the disease. Management is often multimodal and includes surgical excision, systemic chemotherapy, and occasional immunotherapy. Stage 4S is a unique group of patients <18 months of age with a small primary tumor and metastatic disease limited to the liver, skin, or bone marrow, but not the lymph nodes. Many of these patients experience spontaneous regression of their disease. Some require aggressive therapy, but the overall survival rates are fairly high.

Ref.: 4, 8

19. Which of the following tumor markers is elevated in the most common pediatric liver tumor?

A. β-hCG

B. Urinary VMA

C. AFP

D. Carcinoembryonic antigen (CEA)

E. Ferritin

ANSWER: C

COMMENTS: The most common *liver tumor* in children is hepatoblastoma, comprising about 80% of all pediatric liver tumors. Hepatoblastoma generally affects children aged 3 years or younger. Liver tumors in the pediatric population usually present as enlarged abdominal masses. When a liver mass is encountered, laboratory tests can be extremely helpful in narrowing the differential diagnosis. AFP is elevated in about 90% of patients with hepatoblastomas. The second most common liver tumor in the pediatric population is the hepatocellular carcinoma (HCC). These tumors generally affect older children. Patients do not have an elevated AFP; however, they can have an elevated ferritin. Hepatoblastomas are usually solitary lesions, whereas HCC may be multifocal. Management of hepatoblastoma is based on the PRETEXT staging system, which takes into account the degree of involvement of the liver. Surgical resection remains the only curative treatment. Unfortunately, many of these tumors are not resectable at the time of diagnosis. Hepatoblastomas are chemosensitive, and neoadjuvant therapy before resection has been shown to increase resectability and improve overall outcomes. If the tumor remains unresectable, transplantation is another treatment option. CEA is generally associated with colorectal cancers, and when elevated in the setting of a liver tumor, metastatic colorectal disease should be considered. β-hCG is a tumor marker for germline tumors and not hepatoblastoma. VMAs are elevated in patients with neuroblastomas.

Ref.: 4, 9

20. Which one of the following statements concerning biliary atresia is true?

A. Without treatment, the average survival is 5 years.

B. The hallmark pathologic findings are giant cell transformation and hepatocellular necrosis.

C. There is a higher incidence in Europe and North America.

D. Ultrasound of the liver and gallbladder is an integral part of the diagnostic workup.

E. Biliary atresia is the third most common indication for pediatric liver transplantation.

ANSWER: D

COMMENTS: Biliary atresia is characterized by progressive, irreversible fibrosis of the extrahepatic and intrahepatic bile ducts. There is no proved effective medical therapy. If surgical correction is not performed, the obliterative process progresses. Biliary cirrhosis and portal hypertension develop, followed by death by 2 years of age. Severe cholestasis, bile duct proliferation, and inflammatory cell infiltration are pathologic findings in biliary atresia. Hepatocellular necrosis and giant cell transformation are seen with neonatal hepatitis. Biliary atresia is the number one indication for pediatric liver transplantation. Biliary atresia should be suspected in an infant with persistent neonatal jaundice and elevated conjugated bilirubin. It occurs in 1/10,000 live births and is most prevalent in Asia. The workup for suspected biliary atresia includes ultrasound imaging of the liver and gallbladder, hepatobiliary iminodiacetic acid (HIDA) scanning, and percutaneous liver biopsy. Typically, the extrahepatic bile ducts cannot be seen on ultrasound imaging, and the gallbladder is diminutive or absent. However, even with these tests, the final diagnosis often is made at surgical exploration. An intraoperative cholangiogram will demonstrate a lack of opacification of the intrahepatic biliary tree. When identified, a Kasai procedure is indicated. The goals of the Kasai procedure are to restore biliary flow by performing a Roux-en-Y portojejunostomy after the resection of the gallbladder, extrahepatic bile ducts, and the fibrotic portal plate.

Ref.: 1, 2

21. With regard to the Kasai procedure for the treatment of biliary atresia, which of the following statements is true?

A. It is most successfully performed after 3 months of age.

B. Cholangitis rarely complicates a successful procedure.

C. Portal hypertension remains problematic despite a successful operation.

D. If hepatic transplantation is needed, an initial Kasai enterostomy is not indicated.

E. Cholangitis is an infrequent late complication.

ANSWER: C

COMMENTS: Biliary atresia occurs as a part of a spectrum of anomalies of infantile obstructive cholangiopathy. Variable patterns of ductal involvement of the intrahepatic and extrahepatic biliary tree are seen, with 10% of patients initially having an extrahepatic disease only. The goals of treatment are to establish biliary flow and prevent the late complications of biliary cirrhosis and hepatic failure. Hepatoportoenterostomy, the Kasai procedure, is most successful in establishing biliary drainage when performed during the patient's first 2 months of life. The success rate falls dramatically after 3 months of age. Cholangitis, biliary cirrhosis, hepatic failure, and portal hypertension remain late problems despite the fact that bile drainage is achieved. Attempts to reduce later cholangitic complications include prolonged use of antibiotics and steroids to minimize inflammation and infection. One-third of patients undergoing a Kasai procedure for biliary atresia will have a successful biliary drainage and require no further intervention. One-third will initially have adequate drainage but will eventually progress to hepatic fibrosis and require transplantation. The final third will never have adequate drainage and will require liver transplantation to survive. Hepatic transplantation has been successful in the treatment of this problem but has not replaced biliary-enteric anastomosis as the initial procedure. An unsuccessful hepatoportoenterostomy does not preclude later hepatic transplantation and is therefore the initial surgical management of biliary atresia.

Ref.: 1–3

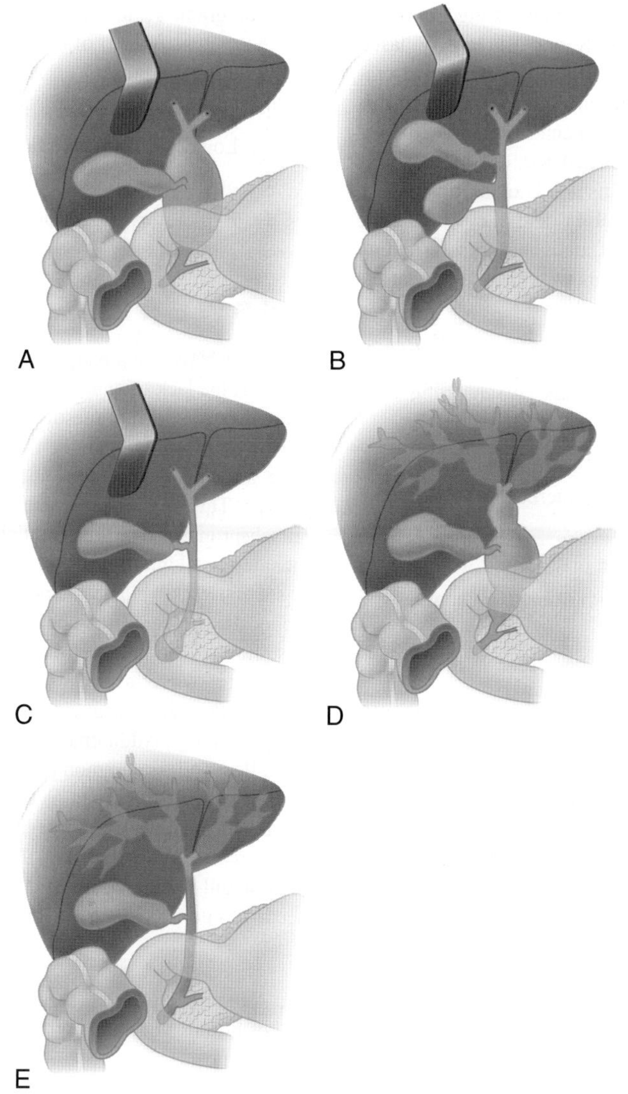

Fig. 31.1 (Question 22). Choledochal cysts: (A) Type I: Simple cystic dilation of the common bile duct. (B) Type II: Diverticulum off of the common bile duct without biliary dilatation. (C) Type III: Intraduodenal or intrapancreatic biliary dilatation. (D) Type IV: Intra- and extrahepatic ductal dilatation and cysts. (E) Type V (Caroli disease): Intrahepatic ductal dilation only. *(Source: Goldstein S, Salman B. Barish H. Goldstein S, Salman B, Barish HE, eds. Cystic disorders of the bile ducts. In:* Current Surgical Therapy, *Cameron JL & Cameron AM, eds. Philadelphia, PA. Elsevier; 2014.)*

22. What is the appropriate surgical repair for the most common type of choledochal cyst?

A. Hepaticojejunostomy

B. Choledochojejunostomy

C. Cyst resection alone

D. Observation only

E. Cholecystectomy

ANSWER: A

COMMENTS: Although it is possible to diagnose choledochal cysts in utero, more often they present by the age of 10 with right upper quadrant pain, jaundice, and occasionally a palpable mass. Ultrasound is the appropriate first diagnostic step, examining both the intra- and extrahepatic biliary systems. When there is a concern for biliary atresia versus a cyst, a HIDA scan can be performed to delineate the anatomy. There are five major types of choledochal cysts (Fig. 31.1). Type I is the most common, representing about 90% of cases. This is a fusiform dilatation of the common bile duct but does not involve the intrahepatic biliary system. Surgical management of type I cysts includes resection of the affected portion of the common bile duct with a hepaticojejunostomy and Roux-en-Y limb. Type II cysts are a diverticulum off of the side of the common bile duct, and there is no intra- or extrahepatic ductal dilation. This is managed with a simple cyst resection. Often, this may be done laparoscopically. A type III cyst is dilatation of the very distal common bile duct and is usually either intrapancreatic or intraduodenal. These cysts are also known as choledochoceles. There is no dilatation of the proximal common bile duct or intrahepatic ducts. These cysts may be managed with either marsupialization or with endoscopic retrograde cholangiopancreatography (ERCP) and sphincterotomy. A type IV disease is defined as multiple cysts that may be intrahepatic, extrahepatic, or both. It is recommended that the common bile duct cyst be resected up to the hepatic ducts with a hepaticojejunostomy and Roux-en-Y limb. Type V, also known as Caroli disease, is multiple exclusively intrahepatic biliary cysts. The operative management of this disease is not straightforward and ranges from segmental resection to liver transplantation. Cyst excision is advocated not only to avoid a biliary obstruction leading to pancreatitis and cholangitis but also to reduce the risk of malignancy. Types I, IV, and V cysts have the highest malignant potential. This risk of malignant transformation increases with incomplete cyst excision as well as older age at the time of resection.

Ref.: 4

23. Which of the following is true concerning Hirschsprung's disease?

A. More common in females
B. Absent ganglion cells in both the Auerbach and Meissner plexuses
C. Failure to pass meconium in the first 72 h of life
D. Best diagnosed by lower-gastrointestinal (GI) contrast-enhanced study
E. Atrophy of submucosal nerve endings seen in rectal biopsy specimens

ANSWER: B

COMMENTS: Hirschsprung's disease is a congenital abnormality wherein the normal ganglion nerves within the bowel wall have failed to migrate all the way down to the anus. Nerves are missing or abnormally start at the anus and extend to a variable distance up the bowel. The involved bowel does not exhibit normal motility and is contracted. As a result, the normal bowel above this dilates, resulting in megacolon. Hirschsprung's disease is more common in males than in females. The primary clinical manifestation of Hirschsprung's disease is intestinal obstruction with failure to pass meconium in the first 48 h of life or chronic constipation in older infants and children. Affected infants are prone to developing enterocolitis, which carries a high mortality rate if not recognized and treated promptly. Evaluation may include contrast enema radiographs, anorectal manometry, and rectal wall biopsy. Barium enema studies typically show a narrow low rectal segment and marked dilation above. In newborns, the barium enema may be normal since dilation of the bowel proximal to the aganglionic segment may not have developed yet. During anorectal manometry, the rectoanal inhibitory reflex is tested by distending the low rectum with a small balloon and observing a decrease in the anal canal resting pressure. Absence of the rectoanal inhibitory reflex is pathognomonic for Hirschsprung's disease. Definitive diagnosis is based on a deep rectal biopsy, which will show submucosal hypertrophied nerve endings, absent ganglion cells in the Auerbach and Meissner plexuses, and acetylcholinesterase staining. Full-term infants with Hirschsprung's disease but without enterocolitis may be treated by a single-stage pull-through operation. The remaining patients are managed mostly by a serial intestinal biopsy to determine the level of normal ganglionated intestine and a leveling colostomy acutely followed by a pull-through procedure 3 to 6 months later. Anastomosis of the normally innervated colon to the anus is the basis of all of the three classically described procedures (Swanson, Duhamel, and Soave).

Ref.: 2, 3

24. A newborn infant has failed to pass meconium by 48 h of life. The anus appears to be normally formed. An abdominal radiograph demonstrates dilated bowel loops with no air in the rectum. Which of the following tests is most likely to yield the diagnosis?

A. Upper GI study
B. Lower GI study
C. Suction rectal biopsy
D. Exploratory laparotomy
E. CT scan

ANSWER: C

COMMENTS: This baby most likely has Hirschsprung's disease, which is the lack of ganglion cells in the myenteric and submucosal plexuses of the distal intestine. The typical presentation is a failure to pass meconium within the first 48 h of life. The patients may also have abdominal distention and dilated loops of bowel on radiographs. This is the presentation for 50%–90% of all cases of Hirschsprung's. The differential diagnosis of this presentation includes distal intestinal atresia, meconium ileus, or meconium plug. A suction rectal biopsy demonstrating a lack of ganglion cells is diagnostic. Lower GI can be helpful in the diagnosis and will demonstrate a transition zone from the normal intestine to the aganglionic portions. However, a normal lower GI does not rule out Hirschsprung's disease, as a short segment could be present and not result in the classic findings. Additionally, the lower GI can help resolve a meconium ileus. A less common presentation of Hirschsprung's disease is chronic constipation in an older infant or even in an adult. Many of these patients have a short segment involvement, and once weaned from breastfeeding, they tend to develop constipation. In older children, a full-thickness biopsy rather than a suction rectal biopsy is needed to get an adequate sampling to make the diagnosis.

Ref: 4

25. A previously well 3-week-old infant exhibits a sudden onset of bilious vomiting. Which of the following is the most likely diagnosis?

A. Pyloric stenosis
B. Duodenal atresia
C. Malrotation of the midgut
D. Intussusception
E. Tracheoesophageal fistula (TEF), H type

ANSWER: C

COMMENTS: See Question 26.

Ref: 1–3

26. For the scenario described in Question 25, which would be the most appropriate initial diagnostic test?

A. Upper GI contrast study
B. Abdominal ultrasound
C. Barium enema
D. Abdominal radiograph
E. CT scan

ANSWER: A

COMMENTS: Infants with intestinal obstruction distal to the ampulla of Vater exhibit bilious emesis. Fifty percent of children with malrotation have bilious emesis during the first few weeks of life. Infants with malrotation are at a risk for midgut volvulus and possible ischemia. Infants with a previous history of normal feedings in whom a sudden onset of bilious vomiting develops should be immediately evaluated for midgut volvulus. Midgut volvulus is best demonstrated by an upper GI series showing an abrupt cutoff from failure of contrast material to pass beyond the distal duodenum or a corkscrew pattern of a partial obstruction from the torsed intestines (or both), whereas malrotation is demonstrated by an aberrant course of the duodenum and duodenal–jejunal junction. A barium enema can be misleading in the diagnosis of malrotation because the position of the cecum cannot be relied on to rule in or rule out malrotation. As soon as a diagnosis is made, the infant should be taken immediately to surgery. If for some reason the patient is unable to get an upper GI series in a timely fashion, he or she should proceed to the operating room for immediate exploration to avoid complications from volvulus. Pyloric stenosis or TEF is not accompanied by bilious vomiting. The symptoms of infants with H-type TEF are usually feeding difficulties and recurrent pneumonia. The main symptoms associated with intussusception are colicky abdominal pain and bloody stools. Duodenal atresia may mimic malrotation in the first 24 to 48 h of life, but at 3 weeks of age, duodenal atresia should already have been diagnosed and treated. Importantly, malrotation of the midgut is frequently associated with duodenal atresia and should be searched for at the time of repair of duodenal atresia.

Ref.: 1–3

27. A 2-month-old otherwise healthy male presents with a 10-h history of bilious vomiting. An upper GI shows a corkscrew appearance of the duodenum that does not cross back over to the left side of the abdomen. Which of the following is correct regarding the management of this patient?

A. Orogastric tube should be placed, and the patient should have serial abdominal examinations over the next 24 h.

B. If intestinal volvulus is found at operation, the bowel should be rotated clockwise to reduce the volvulus.

C. Appendectomy should never be performed during surgery for this problem.

D. There is a high risk that this could recur even after surgery.

E. Surgery includes lysis of Ladd's bands and positioning the duodenum along the right abdominal gutter.

ANSWER: E

COMMENTS: The radiologic finding described in combination with the clinical presentation of bilious emesis in an otherwise normally growing infant is diagnostic of intestinal malrotation. Although malrotation itself does not cause significant morbidity, midgut volvulus, the most feared complication, does. This can be catastrophic, resulting in complete necrosis of the intestine if not treated promptly. Once the diagnosis of malrotation is made, an emergent laparotomy and correction should be performed. If intestinal volvulus is found, the intestine should be rotated counterclockwise until the mesentery is straightened ("turn back the hands of time"). Bowel viability should be determined, and any ischemic and necrotic areas have to be resected. If areas that appear ischemic and do not pink up after the reduction of the volvulus are present, either resection should be performed or a second-look procedure in 24 h should be planned. Ladd's bands, which are peritoneal bands that extend across the duodenum causing an obstruction, are transected. An appendectomy is performed since the cecum will usually be positioned in the left abdomen, making the diagnosis of acute appendicitis difficult. The duodenum and small intestine are positioned in the right abdominal gutter; the colon is placed on the left. Surgical fixation of the cecum and small bowel to attempt to prevent future volvulus is actually associated with an increased risk of obstruction and internal hernia. The risk of revolvulus after a Ladd's procedure is exceedingly low. The laparoscopic approach to this procedure is being investigated. Theoretically, there is less adhesion formation with laparoscopy; therefore there is a concern for inadequate postoperative fixation of the bowel and a higher risk of recurrence. Further outcome studies with good follow-up are needed.

Ref.: 4

28. Which bowel segment is the most common site of intestinal duplication?

A. Esophagus

B. Stomach

C. Duodenum

D. Ileum

E. Rectum

ANSWER: D

COMMENTS: Intestinal duplication is a common finding at autopsy, with an incidence of 1 in 4500. Duplications have been described throughout the entire GI tract; however, the most frequent sites are the jejunum and ileum. The exact etiology of these duplications is unknown. Several theories including twinning, disorders of recanalization, and environmental factors have been proposed. Duplications are often identified as large intraabdominal cystic structures on prenatal ultrasound. After birth, large intestinal duplications, especially blind pouch duplications, should be resected within the first few months of life. If the duplication causes symptoms such as obstruction or jaundice, resection should be performed sooner. Small duplications may present later in life or may never become symptomatic.

Ref.: 4

29. Which of the following is a criterion in the Alvarado scoring system for appendicitis?

A. C-reactive protein

B. Nausea and vomiting

C. Rovsing's sign

D. Diffuse peritonitis

E. Sick contacts

ANSWER: B

COMMENTS: Appendicitis is the most common cause of surgical emergency in the pediatric population. Appendicitis is generally felt to be the result of an obstruction of the appendiceal lumen by either inflammation or appendicolith. The classic presentation for appendicitis is initial periumbilical pain that then localizes to the right lower quadrant and anorexia. Scoring systems to better predict the likelihood of appendicitis have been created. The Alvarado scoring system includes localized right lower quadrant tenderness, leukocytosis, pain migration, left shift, fever, nausea and vomiting, anorexia, and peritoneal irritation. A score of at least 6 has a 90% specificity for appendicitis. Ultrasound may improve the diagnostic accuracy with findings such as a thickened appendix, thickened appendiceal walls, appendix diameter of >7 mm, and a noncompressible appendix with palpation. Once the diagnosis of appendicitis is made, antibiotics should be initiated, and an appendectomy should be completed within 12 h of presentation to minimize the risks of perforation. Although there is some literature supporting antibiotics and observation without surgery, the persistence and recurrence rates are substantial, and the morbidity of a laparoscopic appendectomy is very low. Therefore most surgeons in the United States continue to treat acute appendicitis with surgery.

Ref.: 4, 10

30. A 1-month-old neonate has an umbilical hernia with a palpable 1-cm defect. Which of the following statements is true?

A. The likelihood of spontaneous closure is low, and the hernia should be repaired.

B. Indications for the early repair of an umbilical hernia include a history of incarceration, a large skin proboscis, and the presence of a ventriculoperitoneal shunt.

C. Repair of the hernia defect should include the placement of a mesh.

D. Complete closure of the umbilical ring may be expected in 30% of children by the age of 4 to 6 years.

E. All of the above.

ANSWER: B

COMMENTS: Umbilical hernias occur as a result of persistence of the umbilical ring. By the age of 4 to 6 years, the closure of this ring can be expected in 80% of children. In patients with umbilical hernias with greater than a 2-cm defect, spontaneous closure is less likely. Umbilical hernias are usually repaired early if the defect is greater than 2 cm, there is a history of incarceration, or a large skin proboscis or a ventriculoperitoneal shunt is present. Repair of an umbilical hernia involves an infraumbilical semicircular incision, separation of the hernia sac from the overlying skin, repair of the fascial defect, fixation of the base of the umbilicus to the fascia, and closure of the skin. The fascial closure is rarely under tension and does not require a prosthetic mesh.

Ref.: 1

31. The most common cause of duodenal obstruction at birth is:

A. Malrotation

B. Duodenal atresia

C. Annular pancreas

D. Choledochal cyst

E. Midgut volvulus

ANSWER: B

COMMENTS: Vomiting within the first 24 h of life in the absence of abdominal distention suggests duodenal atresia in a neonate. Malrotation with midgut volvulus is the most common and the most devastating cause of a duodenal obstruction beyond the neonatal period. In malrotation, the duodenal obstruction may be caused by extrinsic compression by the peritoneal Ladd's bands that extend from the abdominal wall to the anomalously located cecum in the right upper quadrant. Alternatively, the catastrophic complication of malrotation is midgut volvulus and intestinal infarction from the torsion of the superior mesenteric vessels about the narrow mesenteric pedicle by which the midgut is suspended. An annular pancreas may cause duodenal obstruction as a result of duodenal stenosis. Choledochal cysts are rare and manifest as jaundice and an abdominal mass.

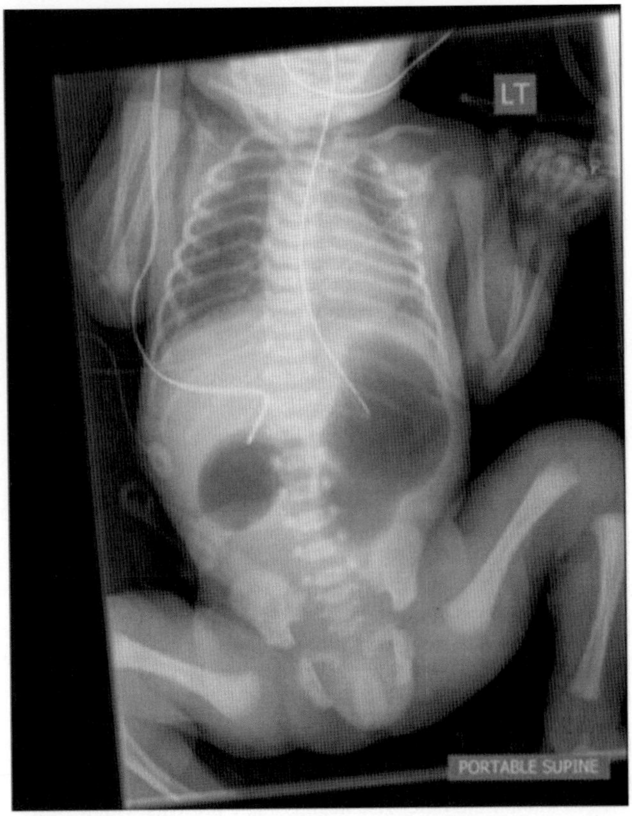

Fig. 31.2 (Question 32). Double bubble sign classically seen with duodenal atresia.

Ref.: 1–3

32. A newborn infant presents with a radiograph shown in Fig. 31.2. What is the appropriate operative intervention?

A. Duodenojejunostomy

B. Duodenoduodenostomy

C. Gastrojejunostomy

D. Orogastric tube decompression alone

E. Ladd's procedure

ANSWER: B

COMMENTS: The radiograph is demonstrating a classic "double bubble" sign that is seen with duodenal atresia. This diagnosis can be made in utero with polyhydramnios as well as a double bubble seen on ultrasound. The double bubble appearance results from air swallowing that does not progress through the duodenal atresia. The stomach and proximal duodenum dilate, and there is no air in the bowel distal to the atresia. There are three types of duodenal atresia. Type 1, by far the most common, is a web or septum obstructing the duodenal lumen. It is thought to be the result of a failure to recanalize the lumen during development. This is most commonly located in the second portion of the duodenum. Type 2 is a solid cord between the two lumens of the affected portion of the duodenum. Type 3 is two blind-ending duodenal loops, proximal and distal, without a connection between them. Duodenal atresia is associated with a congenital heart disease, trisomy 21,

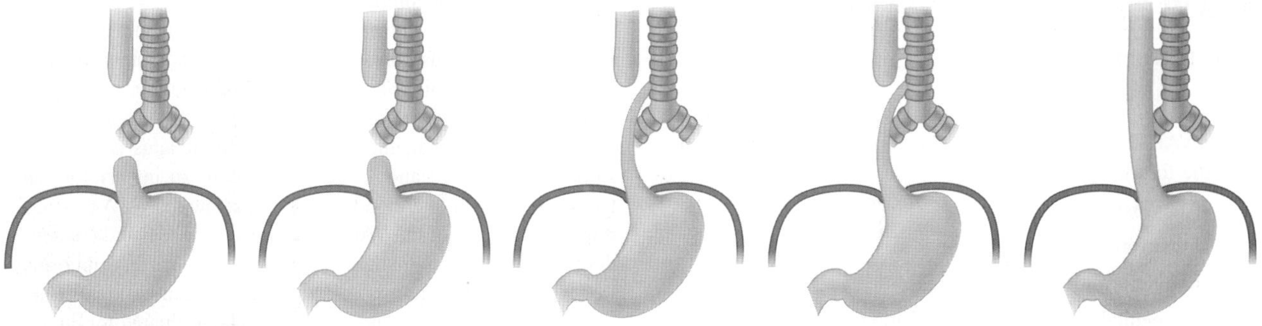

Fig. 31.3 (Question 33). Tracheal esophageal fistulas. *(Source: Chung DH. Pediatric surgery. In:* Sabiston Textbook of Surgery. *Philadelphia, PA. Elsevier; 2012. Copyright © 2012 Elsevier Inc. All rights reserved.)*

and annular pancreas. Prior to a surgical correction, it is important to evaluate the infant with an echocardiogram to look for cardiac abnormalities. The child may be managed with orogastric tube decompression and intravenous fluids until optimization for surgery. At surgery, a right upper quadrant incision is made. The entire length of the duodenum is evaluated. Most of the time, a duodeno-duodenostomy is created to join the two segments of bowel. If an annular pancreas or preduodenal portal vein is identified, the anastomosis should be made anterior to this. Although it is possible that a Ladd's band and an intestinal malrotation could cause duodenal obstruction, it is a much less common reason for a double bubble sign than duodenal atresia.

Ref.: 4

33. What is the best surgical approach to repair the most common type of TEF?

A. Left thoracotomy
B. Right thoracotomy
C. Left cervicotomy
D. Right cervicotomy
E. Midline laparotomy

ANSWER: B

COMMENTS: Five types of TEFs exist (Fig. 31.3). Type C, esophageal atresia with a distal TEF, is the most common type accounting for 80%–90% of all TEFs. Radiographs will show a coiled orogastric tube in the proximal esophagus and air within the stomach. The best access to the esophagus for repair of this fistula is through a right thoracotomy. As part of the preoperative workup, an echocardiogram should be obtained to evaluate for congenital cardiac anomalies as well as a right-sided aortic arch. If identified, repair can be performed through a left-sided thoracotomy. Type A (5%–10%) is pure atresia without a fistulous connection. Radiographs will also show a coiled orogastric tube in the proximal esophagus, but there is no air within the stomach. Type E (4%), or H type, is a TEF without atresia. This often presents in the first few days of life with repeated choking with attempted feeds and cyanotic events as the baby aspirates into the lungs. However, this can be missed in the newborn period and may present later in life with recurrent aspirations or pneumonias. These fistulas are located at the thoracic inlet, and a right cervicotomy allows for the best access for fistula ligation. The final two types of TEF, type B atresia with both a proximal and distal TEF and type D atresia with a proximal TEF, are both extremely rare. The surgical approach should be through a right thoracotomy.

Ref.: 4

34. Which of the following is a complication after the repair of a TEF?

A. Anastomotic leak
B. Esophageal stricture
C. Recurrent fistula
D. Gastroesophageal reflux
E. All of the above

ANSWER: E

COMMENTS: All of the options are potential complications following the repair of a TEF. The early complications include anastomotic leak, esophageal stricture, and recurrent fistula, while late complications include gastroesophageal reflux disease (GERD) and tracheomalacia. Esophageal stricture is the most common early complication and may occur in up to 80% of cases. This complication is managed with serial esophageal dilations. If the stricture fails to respond, resection of the anastomosis with a new anastomosis is warranted. Anastomotic leak is another early complication, occurring in about 15% of repairs. The majority of these leaks are not clinically significant and may be managed with continuous drainage and parenteral nutrition until the leak has sealed. Large leaks within the first few days of repair are generally the result of a technical error or ischemia of the anastomosis; surgical revision is advised to avoid development of a tension pneumothorax and mediastinitis. GERD is by far the most common late complication and is thought to be related to shortening of the intraabdominal portion of the esophagus.

Ref.: 4

35. An 8-h-old newborn has mild respiratory distress and excessive drooling. An abdominal radiograph shows a complete lack of air in the GI tract. What is the most likely diagnosis?

A. Bilateral choanal atresia
B. Pyloric atresia
C. Duodenal atresia
D. Esophageal atresia with a distal TEF
E. Esophageal atresia without a TEF

ANSWER: E

COMMENTS: See Question 34.

Ref.: 1–3

36. The VACTERL association most commonly includes which of the following?

A. Ankylosis
B. Imperforate anus
C. Eye deformities
D. Congenital cystic lung malformation
E. Choanal atresia

ANSWER: B

COMMENTS: Neonates have a gasless GI tract at birth. They start to swallow soon after birth, and air reaches the colon within 6 to 12 h. In pure esophageal atresia without an associated fistula, swallowed air has no access to the GI tract, and so abdominal films show a gasless abdomen. Esophageal atresia is also suggested when an infant drools excessively because of an esophageal obstruction or spits up during attempted feedings. When an orogastric tube is passed in an infant with esophageal atresia, a chest radiograph shows the tube coiled in a blind pouch in the chest. About 85%–90% of patients with a tracheoesophageal malformation have a blind proximal pouch with a distal TEF, also known as TEF type C. Respiratory symptoms are secondary to aspiration from the esophageal pouch or retrograde reflux of gastric contents through the fistula into the lungs. In esophageal atresia with a TEF, the inspired air reaches the stomach and small bowel through the TEF. Contrast-enhanced studies and a bronchoscopy may be useful in select cases to confirm the diagnosis and demonstrate the location of the fistula. Recognition of the anatomy of the anomaly is important for establishing appropriate initial treatment and definitive repair.

Air fills the stomach but fails to pass into the duodenum and small bowel in neonates with pyloric atresia, a rare congenital anomaly. Radiographic studies show extreme distention of the stomach with air-fluid levels. Choanal atresia is narrowing or blockage of the posterior nasal airway by soft or boney tissue. It is a congenital condition that is due to the failure of the recanalization of the nasal airway during embryologic development. Neonates, being obligatory nasal breathers, have major respiratory problems when born with bilateral choanal atresia but do not have difficulty swallowing air.

The VACTERL association refers to a group of commonly associated congenital defects: vertebral anomalies, imperforate anus, cardiac defects, tracheoesophageal fistula, radial and renal malformations, and limb defects.

Ref.: 1

37. A newborn male is born without an anus. If a fistula is present, what is the most likely location?

A. Rectovestibular
B. Rectourethral
C. Rectoperineal
D. Rectovesicular
E. Rectoenteric

ANSWER: B

COMMENTS: The most common site of a fistula associated with imperforate anus in males is rectourethral, while rectovestibular fistulas are the most common in females. Only 5% of patients with imperforate anus do not have a fistula. If meconium is passed in the urine, a fistulous connection to the urinary system should be suspected. If meconium is found on the perineum, a rectoperineal fistula is likely.

The initial management of an imperforate anus is to evaluate for other associated anomalies. Babies with an imperforate anus have a 50%–60% likelihood of associated anomalies. An imperforate anus is a part of the VACTERL group of associated congenital defects (vertebral anomalies, imperforate anus, cardiac abnormalities, TEFs, renal abnormalities, and limb abnormalities). Babies born with any of these conditions should be evaluated for the presence of the others within the first 24 h of life. Next, the level of the lower end of the rectal pouch must be determined. Imperforate anus is usually divided into high and low types, and this will guide treatment. Within 24 h of birth, gas will make its way through the GI tract and into the rectal pouch. A cross-table radiograph of the infant will show the gas in the rectal pouch. The high imperforate anus is diagnosed when air fails to pass below the level of the coccyx, and it is associated with more secondary anomalies compared with the low imperforate anus.

Once an imperforate anus is found, a fistula should be sought. If a perineal fistula is present, the rectal pouch is usually low, and a perineal anoplasty can be performed in the perinatal period for definitive management. If there is rectal gas below the coccyx but no fistula, a posterior sagittal anorectoplasty, or posterior sagittal anorectoplasty (PSARP), during the neonatal period could be considered. However, if the level is high or if the infant has other significant defects and is not clinically stable, a colostomy should be constructed and definitive repair postponed.

Ref.: 4

38. A 3000-g infant is born with esophageal atresia and a distal TEF. If the infant does not exhibit respiratory distress and associated anomalies are not present, which of the following is the preferred treatment?

A. Gastrostomy, cervical esophagostomy, and delayed repair
B. Gastrostomy, sump tube drainage of the proximal pouch, and delayed repair
C. Fistula ligation and delayed esophageal repair
D. Division of the fistula with primary esophageal anastomosis
E. Primary repair with colonic interposition

ANSWER: D

COMMENTS: The timing and type of surgical intervention for esophageal atresia and TEF depend on the maturity of the infant and associated cardiorespiratory problems or other congenital anomalies. Medically stable infants weighing more than 2500 g are treated by primary repair with fistula division, closure of its tracheal end, and end-to-end anastomosis of the esophageal segments. Unstable infants with respiratory issues are treated by gastrostomy and sump drainage of the blind proximal pouch until they are ready for repair. A distal TEF often results in the loss of ventilatory pressure or retrograde aspiration of gastric contents into the lungs, further exacerbating respiratory compromise. Therefore some infants may benefit from primary fistula ligation without esophageal repair, with or without gastrostomy placement. The final esophageal repair is performed after cardiorespiratory recovery.

Ref.: 1–3

39. Necrotizing enterocolitis (NEC) is characterized by which of the following statements?

A. It generally occurs in infants on parenteral nutrition who have not yet had enteral feeding.

B. A single spontaneous perforation occurs, most commonly in the jejunum.

C. It is associated with an immature GI tract, which allows for an increased permeability and bacterial translocation.

D. It almost always requires surgical intervention.

E. It affects premature and term infants with the same frequency.

ANSWER: C

COMMENTS: Although the exact etiology of NEC is unknown, it is likely that it is multifactorial. It is thought to be related to an unbalanced inflammatory reaction within an immature GI tract that results in the disruption of intestinal integrity. Translocation of intestinal bacteria follows. It is directly related to prematurity and low-to-very low birth weights. Infants at the highest risk for developing NEC are those born before 28 weeks or those having a birth weight less than 1000 g. Hypoxia is also clearly associated with the disease. Most infants who develop NEC have already had enteral feeding. NEC may be limited to a single segment of bowel or multiple segments. The terminal ileum is the most frequent site.

Spontaneous intestinal perforation (SIP) is a similar entity that is characterized by a single perforation in an infant who has never had enteral feeding. SIP also occurs most commonly in the terminal ileum. It is thought to be caused by ischemia and has been associated with postnatal indomethacin use. Radiographs will demonstrate pneumoperitoneum, as in perforated NEC, but will not show portal venous gas or pneumatosis, as is often found in NEC. Long-term morbidity and mortality are significantly better with SIP than with NEC.

Ref.: 4

40. A premature infant with a history of neonatal respiratory distress requiring ventilatory support is being fed oral formula. Abdominal distention develops, and blood-streaked stool is passed. Appropriate management includes which of the following?

A. Anoscopy and addition of Karo syrup for a probable neonatal fissure

B. Immediate barium enema to rule out intussusception

C. Restriction of oral intake to clear liquids to prevent mucosal injury

D. Nasogastric drainage, IV antibiotics, total parenteral nutrition (TPN), and serial abdominal examinations and radiographs

E. Antibiotic-directed treatment of specific pathogens cultured from the stool

ANSWER: D

COMMENTS: This patient has NEC. See Question 41.

Ref.: 1–3

41. Which of the following are indications for surgery in an infant with NEC?

A. Pneumatosis intestinalis

B. Portal venous gas

C. Pneumoperitoneum

D. Bloody stools

E. All of the above

ANSWER: C

COMMENTS: NEC affects premature infants who have received oral feedings. Clinical manifestations are initial intolerance of formula, abdominal distention, and/or blood-streaked stool and then progression to systemic sepsis, metabolic acidosis, and thrombocytopenia.

Bell's classification categorizes NEC into three groups:

Stage 1. Suspected NEC. Findings may include gastric residuals, abdominal distension, occult or gross blood in the stool, temperature instability, apnea, and bradycardia. Radiographs are either normal or show bowel dilation consistent with ileus.

Stage 2. Definite NEC with mild-to-moderate systemic illness. Additional findings include absent bowel sounds, abdominal tenderness, metabolic acidosis, and decreased platelets. Radiographs may show intestinal dilatation, pneumatosis intestinalis, portal venous gas, and ascites.

Stage 3. Advanced NEC. Severe systemic illness with marked distension, signs of peritonitis and sepsis, and hypotension. Radiographs show all of the above and pneumoperitoneum when there is a perforation.

Initial treatment is directed at the prevention of further mucosal injury and septic complications. Oral feedings are stopped, nasogastric tube decompression is instituted, broad-spectrum antibiotics are administered, and fluid and electrolyte support is provided. Close monitoring with physical examination, serial radiographs, and biochemical assessment for signs of deterioration are mandatory. Pneumatosis intestinalis is a pathognomonic radiographic finding of NEC that is caused by the invasion of the bowel wall by gas-forming organisms. This may be seen in stage 2. Portal venous gas indicates the presence of gas-forming organisms translocated to the portal circulation. Neither of these radiographic findings is an absolute indication for surgery. Surgical intervention is necessary when there are progressive clinical deterioration, sepsis, and/or shock, usually due to perforation, persistent intestinal ischemia or necrosis with worsening metabolic acidosis, thrombocytopenia, and hemodynamic instability. At surgery, the necrotic bowel is resected, and the ends of the retained bowel are brought out as enterostomies. Bowel preservation is a high priority during surgery to avoid complications associated with the short-bowel syndrome (SBS). A second-look operation in 24 h can be performed if bowel viability is questionable at the first operation.

Ref.: 1–3

42. Which of the following is the most common cause of SBS in the pediatric population?

A. NEC

B. Gastroschisis

C. Malrotation with volvulus

D. Intestinal atresias

E. Long-segment Hirschsprung's disease

ANSWER: A

COMMENTS: The common causes of SBS in the pediatric population, from most frequent to least, are NEC, intestinal atresias, gastroschisis, volvulus, and, rarely, Hirschsprung's disease. A purely functional definition of SBS is a failure to wean from parenteral nutrition after 3 months. Studies have shown that the presence of at least 35 cm of functional small bowel in neonates is associated with weaning from TPN in 50% of cases. Patients with SBS require TPN to survive. Complications of TPN include catheter-associated infections, liver disease, and bacterial overgrowth in the remaining intestine. TPN-related liver disease occurs in 40%–60% of infants who require long-term TPN. This may include cholestasis, cholelithiasis, and hepatic fibrosis that may result in biliary cirrhosis, portal hypertension, and liver failure.

The management of SBS is aimed at minimizing these complications and restoring enteral feeding whenever possible. Medical management includes careful fluid and electrolyte replacement, early enteral therapy to stimulate intestinal adaptation, suppression of early gastric hypersecretion, antibiotics for bacterial overgrowth, and cholestyramine to control bile acid–induced diarrhea. Surgical-lengthening procedures, such as the serial transverse enteroplasty (STEP) procedure, may improve absorption. Intestinal transplant, often performed with synchronous liver transplant, is indicated when medical management fails. The management of SBS is often done with a multidisciplinary approach to promote the best adaptation of the remaining intestine. A long-term survival may be expected in up to 90% of patients; however, they may require extensive medical care.

Ref.: 4

Kelly DA. Liver complications of pediatric parenteral nutrition—epidemiology. *Nutrition.* 1998;14(1):153–157. Review. PubMed PMID: 9437702.

Spencer AU, Neaga A, West B, et al. Pediatric short bowel syndrome: redefining predictors of success. *Ann Surg.* 2005;242(3):403–412. http://dx.doi:10.1097/01.sla.0000179647.24046.03.

43. With regard to neonatal defects of the abdominal wall, which statement is correct?

A. In gastroschisis, the herniated bowel contents are covered by a membrane.

B. Gastroschisis is frequently associated with cardiac malformations.

C. Chromosomal abnormalities are often present with omphalocele.

D. Treatment of abdominal wall defects is the immediate surgical closure of the fascial defect.

E. In omphalocele, a silo bag is placed to cover the exposed intestine.

ANSWER: C

COMMENTS: Both omphalocele and gastroschisis are neonatal abdominal wall defects. In omphalocele, the defect is a failure of abdominal wall formation and contraction of the umbilical sac. The extraabdominal contents are covered by layers of peritoneum and amnion. In contrast, in gastroschisis, the abdominal wall is complete, but there is a hernial defect to the right of the umbilical ring with external herniation of the intestines. Approximately 50% of infants born with omphalocele have other malformations, including cardiac and chromosomal abnormalities. Anomalies associated with gastroschisis are rare, with the major exception being intestinal atresia.

The initial management of patients with abdominal wall defects consists of nasogastric decompression, intravenous fluids, broad-spectrum antibiotics, and protection of the protruding abdominal contents. In omphalocele, the sac is covered with a sterile occlusive dressing, and a workup for associated anomalies is initiated. In gastroschisis, a silo bag is placed to cover the exposed intestines. A complete medical evaluation and resuscitation of the infant with the protection of the abdominal contents take precedence over a surgical closure. A surgical repair of omphalocele depends on the size. Small omphaloceles may be treated with serial attempts to reduce the intestinal contents into the abdominal cavity. Once the cavity is large enough to accept the contents, a definitive fascial closure can be performed. Surgical management of large omphaloceles is difficult and not standardized. Options include painting the sac with an antiseptic to encourage epithelialization, skin grafting, use of Gore-Tex or other meshes, or wound vacs.

Definite closure of gastroschisis also depends on the size of the abdominal cavity and the extent of herniation. Early closure after birth with primary reduction and fascial repair is performed when possible. If not, a silo bag is placed to cover the intestines and serially reduce them into the abdominal cavity over time.

Ref.: 1, 4

44. An asymptomatic 3-year-old boy is found to have a large palpable abdominal mass on routine examination. Imaging demonstrates a large mass originating from the kidney with a "claw sign." Which of the following is true regarding the most likely diagnosis in this child?

A. The current overall survival rate of these patients is about 50%.

B. The hereditary form of this tumor is more aggressive and more common.

C. Common metastatic foci are in the lungs and liver.

D. There is no role for preoperative chemotherapy in the treatment of this childhood tumor.

E. Measurement of serotonin metabolites in the urine aids in the diagnosis and in monitoring the course of the disease.

ANSWER: C

COMMENTS: The differential diagnosis for this mass is Wilms tumor and neuroblastoma. The most common solid tumor in children younger than 2 years is neuroblastoma, which accounts for 6%–10% of all childhood cancers. In children older than 2 years, the most common solid tumor is Wilms tumor. This patient has a Wilms tumor that is an embryonal tumor of renal origin. It commonly presents as an asymptomatic abdominal mass. Abdominal and thoracic CT, magnetic resonance imaging (MRI), or both are used preoperatively to distinguish Wilms tumor from neuroblastoma and to stage the tumor. Wilms tumors may be bilateral and may metastasize to the liver or lungs. The "claw sign" is useful in determining whether a mass arises from a solid structure or if it is located adjacent to it. With Wilms tumor, the affected kidney is concave, splayed out, and appears to be cupping or grasping the tumor mass. Vascular extension with tumor thrombus within the inferior vena cava is not uncommon. Urine examination for VMA also helps distinguish Wilms tumor from neuroblastoma since it is produced by neuroblastomas and not by Wilms tumor.

The most common germline mutation is the *Wilms tumor gene-1*. Hereditary Wilms tumor is uncommon. Wilms tumor is associated with the Denys-Drash syndrome, WAGR syndrome, and Beckwith-Wiedemann syndrome. Denys-Drash syndrome is gonadal dysgenesis, nephropathy, and Wilms tumor. WAGR syndrome is Wilms tumor, aniridia, genitourinary abnormalities, and mental retardation. Beckwith-Wiedemann syndrome is a combination of some of these: macroglossia, macrosomia (gigantism), abdominal wall defects (omphalocele, umbilical hernia, diastasis recti), ear creases or ear pits, neonatal hypoglycemia, and childhood solid tumors (Wilms tumor, hepatoblastoma, others). Patients with these syndromes need to be screened for Wilms tumor.

Treatment is neoadjuvant chemotherapy followed by surgical resection. The overall survival rate after resection exceeds 85%.

Ref.: 1

45. Progressive abdominal distention and bilious vomiting develop in a newborn. Radiographic studies reveal distended bowel loops of various sizes with air-fluid levels and a "soap suds" appearance in the right lower quadrant. Which of the following procedures should be performed next?

A. Laparotomy

B. Paracentesis

C. Gastrografin lower GI radiographic studies

D. Gastrografin upper intestinal radiographic studies

E. Sweat chloride test

ANSWER: C

COMMENTS: Meconium ileus is likely in patients with a postnatal distal intestinal obstruction and the classic radiographic findings of "soap bubbles." Nearly all affected infants have cystic fibrosis. Abnormalities in salt and water exchange across the intestinal lumen lead to a thick inspissated meconium plug, causing a distal ileal obstruction. Newborns are routinely screened for cystic fibrosis with a blood test for pancreatic immunoreactive trypsinogen (IRT). When elevated, the test is diagnostic for cystic fibrosis. A sweat test cannot be performed until the baby is out of the newborn period. Paracentesis and lavage have no role in the workup or treatment of meconium ileus.

With uncomplicated meconium ileus, a Gastrografin enema may be both diagnostic and therapeutic. The detergent and hyperosmolar effects of the contrast material may loosen the thick meconium and relieve the obstruction. Surgery is indicated if the obstruction does not respond to the Gastrografin enema or if complications arise such as perforation or peritonitis. Operative treatment includes enterotomies, with or without enterostomy, to allow postoperative irrigation of the inspissated meconium with a water-soluble agent or *N*-acetylcysteine.

Ref.: 1–3

46. A 13-month-old male presents to the emergency room with 13 h of colicky abdominal pain, emesis, a palpable sausage-like abdominal mass, and blood-tinged stools. Which test is most appropriate to determine the diagnosis?

A. Plain radiograph

B. MRI

C. Upper GI

D. Ultrasound

E. Complete blood count with differential

ANSWER: D

COMMENTS: Intussusception most commonly presents in children aged 2 years or younger. Ultrasound will demonstrate a 3- to 5-cm diameter mass with the typical target or doughnut sign. Most pediatric intussusceptions occur at the ileocolic junction; therefore it is common for the mass to be found in the right lower quadrant. Ultrasound has been described to have as high as 100% accuracy with experienced sonographers. It is often the first-line imaging study due to its portable nature, high accuracy, and lack of radiation. Plain abdominal radiograph generally does not provide enough information to exclude or confirm the diagnosis of intussusception and is therefore not used. An upper GI would be helpful if malrotation were high on the differential; however, given the combination of symptoms, the most likely diagnosis is intussusception. There is no role for MRI.

Ref.: 4

47. Select the true statement regarding the operative management of intussusception.

A. After successful reduction by barium enema, exploration is indicated to rule out the associated pathologic processes.

B. After successful reduction by barium enema in a 1-year-old child, delayed surgery should be performed because of the risk for recurrence.

C. If barium enema reduction is not successful, a resection should be performed without an attempt at intraoperative manual reduction, whether or not the bowel appears to be viable.

D. If resection is necessary, a primary ileocolic anastomosis may be performed.

E. Appendectomy should never be performed after successful operative manual reduction since this introduces an additional risk.

ANSWER: D

COMMENTS: See Question 48. Most pediatric intussusceptions occur at the ileocolic junction. Unlike in adults, there is rarely a lead point causing the intussusception. Reduction with a hydrostatic or barium enema is often successful. If this fails, surgical reduction is warranted. Incidental appendectomy has a very low complication rate, and in the future clinicians may assume that an appendectomy was performed when there is a laparotomy scar.

Ref.: 1

48. Contraindications to attempted reduction of an intussusception with a hydrostatic or barium enema in a child include which of the following?

A. Pneumoperitoneum

B. Presentation after 48 h of symptoms

C. Recurrence after prior hydrostatic reduction

D. Age older than 5 years

E. Recurrent symptoms in the immediate postreduction period

ANSWER: A

COMMENTS: Ileocolic intussusception should be strongly suspected in a child between the ages of 3 and 18 months with colicky abdominal pain and guaiac-positive stools. A barium, hydrostatic, or air enema should be performed for an attempted nonoperative reduction of the intussusception via hydrostatic or pneumatic pressure. In approximately 80% of children, a successful radiologic reduction is the only therapy needed. An attempt at nonoperative reduction is contraindicated in children with perforation or peritonitis. In such cases, prompt surgery is required. When nonviable bowel is encountered at the time of exploration, resection is carried out without an attempt at reduction.

Otherwise, reduction by gentle digital pressure on the intussusceptum is attempted. Resection is performed if the intussusception is not manually reducible. Primary anastomosis may be performed. After a successful operative manual reduction, an appendectomy is usually performed. Recurrence is not considered to be an absolute indication for surgery, and a second and third attempt may be successful. A 1-year-old child most likely has "idiopathic" intussusception with no anatomic leading point. Children older than 5 years are more likely to have surgical lead points such as an intestinal polyp, Meckel's diverticulum, or tumor such as lymphoma. If these are encountered, they should be resected. Further workup and appropriate surgery to prevent recurrences are needed. Intussusception recurs in 5%–10% of patients regardless of whether the intussusception has been reduced radiographically or operatively. Treatment involves repeated barium, hydrostatic, or air enema, which is successful in most cases.

Ref.: 1

49. A 13-month-old child is admitted to the hospital with lower GI bleeding. Which of the following is correct regarding the most common cause of lower GI bleeding in this patient?

A. Heterotopic pancreatic mucosa is likely to be the cause of bleeding.

B. The bleeding source is most commonly found on the mesenteric side of the intestine.

C. The most common location of the bleeding source is in the jejunum.

D. This problem is not likely to be confused with acute appendicitis.

E. It is a result of an incomplete closure of the omphalomesenteric duct.

ANSWER: E

COMMENTS: Meckel's diverticulum results from an incomplete closure of the omphalomesenteric duct during development, resulting in a true diverticulum, which contains all layers of the intestinal wall. Meckel's diverticula account for 50% of lower GI bleeding in the pediatric population. They are located on the antimesenteric side of the intestine. There is an equal distribution among genders. The rule of 2's states that Meckel's diverticulum usually presents by the age of 2, is 2 ft from the ileocecal valve, occurs in 2% of the population, and may contain 1 of the 2 types of heterotopic mucosa. Gastric mucosa is the most common heterotopic mucosa present. It may lead to ulcer formation just distal to the diverticulum with painless bleeding. It has been estimated that 80% of bleeding Meckel's diverticula contain heterotopic gastric mucosa. Pancreatic mucosa is the next most common; however, it is not as commonly associated with bleeding. Other manifestations of Meckel's include an obstruction or intussusception, with the diverticulum acting as the lead point. Symptomatic Meckel's should be surgically excised, either with a diverticulectomy or bowel resection and anastomosis. Diverticulitis within a Meckel's can mimic acute appendicitis. During a negative exploration for presumed appendicitis, the small bowel should be run to rule out a Meckel's diverticulum, other small bowel diverticulosis, and Crohn's disease.

Ref.: 4

50. A 2-year-old boy is seen in your office with a midline neck mass that has been present for 2 months. On examination, the mass is 2 cm in size, is not tender or pulsatile, and moves with the protrusion of his tongue. Ultrasound of the neck demonstrates a midline cystic lesion sitting deep to the strap muscles with no surrounding lymphadenopathy or other pathology. The thyroid gland is noted in the normal location. Findings on thyroid function studies are normal. Which of the following statements is true regarding this mass?

A. Simple excision of the mass is sufficient.

B. This mass most likely represents ectopic thyroid tissue.

C. The rate of recurrence is very high after an appropriate therapy.

D. These lesions can be found along the base of the tongue and hyoid bone.

E. Most lesions are associated with a draining cutaneous fistula tract.

ANSWER: D

COMMENTS: The most likely diagnosis is a thyroglossal duct cyst. The differential diagnosis for a midline neck mass in a child would also include a dermoid cyst, lymphadenopathy, ectopic thyroid, thymic cyst, or a ranula (a mucocele of a salivary gland). Thyroglossal duct cysts arise from remnants of the thyroid gland that descended from the foramen cecum at the tongue base down to its anatomic position in the neck. The hyoid bone contains the tract from the foramen cecum, and the cyst is superficial to this. Most do not have a draining fistula tract, as is common with branchial cleft remnants. If a normal thyroid is not palpated, an ultrasound and thyroid function tests should be performed prior to surgical resection. Surgical treatment involves removal of the cyst tract along with the central hyoid bone—the Sistrunk procedure. Simple cyst excision alone results in high rates of recurrence, whereas a Sistrunk procedure has reported recurrence rates of less than 5%.

Ref.: 11–13

REFERENCES

1. Warner BW. Pediatric surgery. In: Townsend CM, Beauchamp RD, Evers BM, et al., eds. *Sabiston Textbook of Surgery: The Biological Basis of Modern Surgical Practice*. 18th ed. Philadelphia: WB Saunders; 2008.
2. Hackman D, Grikscheit TC, Wang KS, et al. Pediatric surgery. In: Brunicardi FC, Andersen DK, Billiar TR, et al., eds. *Schwartz's Principles of Surgery*. 9th ed. New York: McGraw-Hill; 2010.
3. Rowe MI, O'Neill IA, Grosfied IL, et al., eds. *Essentials of Pediatric Surgery*. St. Louis: CV Mosby; 1995.
4. Coran AG, Adzick NS, Krummel TM, et al. *Pediatric Surgery*. 7th ed. Philadelphia: Saunders; 2012.
5. Fowler DJ, Gould SJ. The pathology of congenital lung lesions. *Semin Pediatr Surg*. 2015;24(4):176–182.
6. Obermeyer RJ, Goretsky MJ. Chest wall deformities in pediatric surgery. *Surg Clin North Am*. 2012;92(3):669–684.
7. Banever GT, Konefal SH, Gettens K, Moriarty KP. Nonoperative correction of pectus carinatum with orthotic bracing. *J Laparoendosc Adv Surg Tech A*. 2006;16(2):164–167.
8. Maris JM. Recent advances in neuroblastoma. *New Engl J Med*. 2010;362(23):2202–2211.
9. Agarwala S. Primary malignant liver tumors in children. *Indian J Pediatr*. 2012;79(6):793–800.
10. Dingemann J, Ure B. Imaging and the use of scores for the diagnosis of appendicitis in children. *Eur J Pediatr Surg*. 2012;22(3):195–200.
11. Lorenz RR, Netterville JL, Burkey BB. Head and neck. In: Townsend CM, Beauchamp RD, Evers BM, et al., eds. *Sabiston Textbook of Surgery: The Biological Basis of Modern Surgical Practice*. 18th ed. Philadelphia: WB Saunders; 2008.
12. Bailey BJ, Johnson JT, Newlands SD. *Head and Neck Surgery—Otolaryngology*. 4th ed. Philadelphia: Lippincott Williams & Wilkins; 2006.
13. Cummings CW, Haughey BH, Thomas JR, et al. *Cummings Otolaryngology: Head and Neck Surgery*. 4th ed. Philadelphia: CV Mosby; 2005.

CHAPTER 32

PLASTIC & RECONSTRUCTIVE SURGERY

Emilie Robinson, M.D., James Kong, M.D., Vicky Kang, B.S., and Anuja Antony, M.D., M.P.H.

A. Skin Grafts

1. Which of the following is ***false*** regarding the blood supply of skin grafts?
   A. Full-thickness skin grafts (FTSGs) revascularize faster because they are transferred with their own blood supply.
   B. For the first 48 h, a skin graft derives nutrients from passive diffusion from capillaries in the recipient bed.
   C. Inosculation is revascularization of the graft through the formation of connections between vessels in the graft and vessels in the wound bed.
   D. Arterial blood flow in the new graft is established before venous flow.
   E. Mature circulation is established by days 5 to 7.

ANSWER: A

COMMENTS: A. ***False***. Split-thickness skin grafts (STSGs) are composed of the epidermis and a portion of the dermis, whereas FTSGs include the epidermis and the entire dermis. An FTSG is not transferred with its own blood supply, and both STSGs and FTSGs undergo the same steps of revascularization. To successfully achieve good blood flow, the graft must be placed in a well-vascularized wound bed. Vascularization ***takes longer*** in an FTSG because there is more tissue to be traversed for vascular connections to be established and a more robust vascular supply is needed to support the higher volume of tissue. Similarly, a thinner STSG revascularizes more quickly than a thicker STSG.

B. *True*. During the first 48 h, serum diffuses into the graft from capillaries in the wound bed, a process called plasmatic imbibition.

C. *True*. Revascularization occurs after 48 h through a process called inosculation where vessels from the wound bed align with vessels within the graft. These connections mature with time but are initially tenuous and prone to blood pooling and pendulum-like flow. Neovascularization, or the growth of new blood vessels from the wound bed into the graft, also takes place.

D. *True*. The arterial vascularization happens faster than venous vascularization. The practice of elevating a newly grafted extremity to reduce venous congestion is based on this delayed development of venous outflow.

E. *True*. By days 5 to 7, the vasculature is mature and has established proper afferent and efferent flow. A fibrin layer initially forms, which holds the graft in place; by day 7, it is replaced by fibroblasts; and by days 10 to 14, the graft is firmly adherent. The donor site is typically treated with a moist occlusive dressing for promotion of epithelialization or with primary closure in the case of FTSGs. A split-thickness donor site maintains dermal appendages that provide stem cells for reepithelialization of the donor site. The donor site for an FTSG must be primarily closed as the dermal appendages are removed along with the graft.

Skin grafts are prone to shearing forces and failure secondary to hematoma or seroma. A bolster dressing or splint must be applied to immobilize the graft to prevent shearing of the immature vasculature and to provide compression to prevent the formation of seroma or hematoma that lifts the graft off the wound bed and interferes with revascularization.

Sensation returns to the graft over time, with reinnervation beginning at 4 to 5 weeks and completed by 1 to 2 years. Sensation does not return to that of normal skin, but protective sensation is typically attained. Pain returns first, with light touch and temperature following.

Ref: 1, 2

2. Which of the following is ***not*** an advantage of FTSGs over STSGs?
   A. Less secondary contracture at the recipient site
   B. Ability to cover greater surface area
   C. Maintains texture and appearance of normal skin
   D. More durability when subject to trauma
   E. More mobility at graft site, allowing for use over a joint

ANSWER: B

COMMENTS: A. *Advantage*. STSGs are harvested by a dermatome, a machine that shaves off the epidermis and a variable portion of dermis at a set width and depth. Split-thickness grafts undergo more secondary contracture compared with STSGs. (In contrast, FTSGs undergo more primary contracture, while STSGs have less primary contracture allowing them to cover larger areas.)

B. ***Not Advantage for FTSG***. STSGs can be meshed to increase the width and allow for additional coverage over a larger surface area. Additionally, the availability and size of STSGs are not limited by donor sites as they can be taken from almost anywhere on the body including legs and trunk. FTSGs are harvested by direct excision and are limited in size as the donor site must be closed primarily. Donor sites for an FTSG are typically areas in which the skin can be spared; frequent sites include posterior auricular crease, groin, supraclavicular area, upper eyelids, and elbow crease.

C. *Advantage*. Because FTSGs retain all dermal appendages, they grow hair and secrete sebum to lubricate the skin and have the texture and appearance of normal skin. This feature makes FTSGs preferable for sites of cosmetic importance such as the face.

D. *Advantage*. The greater thickness of the FTSGs results in a more durable graft that is less subject to failure from external trauma.

E. *Advantage*. FTSGs undergo less scarring and secondary contracture, making them preferable for use over joints and on the hands to preserve mobility.

Ref: 1, 2

3. Which of the following is ***not*** a suitable wound bed for a skin graft?

A. Muscle without overlying fascia

B. Muscle with overlying fascia

C. Tendon devoid of paratenon

D. Bowel with a layer of granulation tissue

E. Bone with overlying periosteum

ANSWER: C

COMMENTS: A., B., D., and E. *Suitable*. As described in the previous question, wound beds that support skin grafts must be well vascularized with a healthy blood supply. Muscle is well vascularized and serves as an excellent site for skin grafts, with or without overlying fascia. Bone, tendon, and nerve all can support a skin graft, provided the periosteum, paratenon, and perineurium, respectively, are all intact. Skin grafts can be used to cover the bowel as a last resort for loss of abdominal domain. When the wound bed is suboptimal, STSGs are preferred because FTSGs have a higher failure rate in compromised sites as they are more susceptible to hematoma, vascular insufficiency, and infection.

C. ***Not Suitable***. The paratenon must be present if the tendon is used as a wound bed for a skin graft.

Ref: 1, 3–5

B. Flaps

1. Which of the following free flaps is ***incorrectly*** paired to its dominant blood supply?

   A. Latissimus dorsi myocutaneous flap—thoracodorsal artery

   B. Transverse rectus abdominus myocutaneous flap (TRAM)—superior epigastric artery

   C. Fibular osteocutaneous flap—peroneal artery

   D. Dorsalis pedis fasciocutaneous flap—anterior tibial artery

   E. Tensor fascia lata flap—lateral femoral circumflex artery

ANSWER: B

COMMENTS: A., C., D., and E. *Correct.* A surgical flap involves the movement of a segment of tissue from one area to another to aid in closure of a wound or to provide soft tissue coverage. This segment of tissue contains a vascular supply that may either be kept intact with its original inflow and advanced or rotated as a pedicle or the vascular supply may be transected and anastomosis performed at the new site; this is a free flap. An island pedicle involves further skeletonizing and mobilizing the blood supply and allows for the tissue to be transferred to a site further away. Free flaps can be supplied by a dominant pedicle, smaller multiple pedicles, or a combination of the two. This question refers to muscle, fascial, or osseous flaps that are harvested utilizing a dominant vascular pedicle.

B. ***Incorrect.*** All are correctly matched to their dominant blood supply except for the TRAM flap. When performed as a pedicle flap, the superior epigastric artery is utilized; however, when the free TRAM flap is used, the vascular supply is the deep inferior epigastric artery, which is the dominant blood supply.

Ref: 1, 2

2. Which of the following is ***incorrect*** regarding flaps?

   A. Random skin flaps rely on blood supply from dermal and subdermal vascular plexus supplied by perforating arteries.

   B. Axial flaps are named as such because the blood supply is a dominant vessel that runs longitudinally along the axis of the flap.

   C. In practice, there are relatively few axial skin flaps as the majority of these are better described as fasciocutaneous flaps.

   D. Random skin flaps involve geometric rearrangement and advancement of tissue and include examples such as rotation flap, Z-plasty, V-Y advancement, and rhomboid flap.

   E. Fasciocutaneous flaps are the preferred choice of flap for a contaminated or osteomyelitic wound.

ANSWER: E

COMMENTS: A. and B. *Correct.* Blood supply to a flap can be classified into random or axial. Random skin flaps derive blood supply from dermal and subdermal vascular plexus. Axial flaps are supplied by a dominant vessel that runs longitudinally along the axis of the flap. Because of this, random flaps are prone to necrosis at the distal extent of the flap, whereas axial flaps provide a more reliable blood supply for a greater length.

C. *Correct.* Tissue transferred via an axial flap may be skin, muscle, fascia, bone, nerves, bowel, or omentum. Axial skin flaps are more accurately characterized as fasciocutaneous flaps because they are supplied by vascular pedicles that originate from the deep fascia, emerge between the muscles, and travel in the intermuscular septum. These vessels, termed septocutaneous perforators, give off branches to an overlying cutaneous territory, and these territories dictate the design of fasciocutaneous flaps.

D. *Correct.* Random skin flaps include numerous types of local rearrangement and advancement of skin and subcutaneous tissue. V-Y advancement flaps advance skin on each side of a V-shaped incision to close a wound with a Y-shaped closure. Rotation flaps are semicircular flaps of skin in which the advancement is along the arc of the semicircle. Transposition flaps transpose skin around a pivot point to cover an adjacent defect, typically with an intervening segment of tissue. Z-plasty transposes two triangular flaps oriented as a Z-shaped design along a scar to lengthen or change the direction of the final resultant scar.

E. ***Incorrect.*** Myocutaneous flaps have an enhanced ability to eradicate infection and thus are the flap of choice in a wound with contamination or osteomyelitis.

Ref: 2

3. Which of the following would most likely require free flap reconstruction?

   A. Open wound at the knee with exposed total knee prosthesis

   B. Open wound with exposed sternum following coronary artery bypass

   C. Tumor excision involving full-thickness resection of the chest wall with exposed lung

   D. Fracture of the distal third of the tibia with an open wound and exposed bone

   E. Open fracture of the mid-humerus

ANSWER: D

COMMENTS: A., B., C., and E. *Incorrect.* Wounds described in these choices require muscle coverage but can be treated with a local muscle flap unless the flap has been used previously and failed. In that case, a free flap could be performed as a salvage procedure. For example, the knee can be covered with a pedicled gastrocnemius flap; the sternum can be covered with turnover or advancement pectoralis major flaps, pedicled rectus flap, or omental flap; the chest wall can be treated with a number of pedicled flaps from the trunk depending on the location of the wound; and the mid-humerus can be treated with fasciocutaneous flaps from the ipsilateral extremity.

D. ***Correct.*** Open tibial fractures have a high incidence of infection and nonunion, and thus tissue coverage is a critical component of treatment. Local muscle flaps are not dependable for defects on the distal third of the lower leg because they are usually involved in the zone of injury, and there may not be adequate uninjured tissue available for local flap coverage. For this reason, free tissue transfer of muscle, skin, or both is the treatment of choice for defects of the distal third of the lower extremity.

Ref: 1, 5, 6

4. A 65-year-old woman with insulin-dependent diabetes mellitus develops sternal wound infection and dehiscence after coronary artery bypass that utilized the left internal mammary artery. Which of the following flaps is ***not*** an appropriate choice for coverage?

A. Bilateral pectoralis flaps

B. Omental flap based on left gastroepiploic vessel

C. Pedicle bilateral rectus abdominis flaps

D. Latissimus dorsi flap

E. Omental flap based on right gastroepiploic vessel

ANSWER: C

COMMENTS: A., B., D., and E. *Appropriate*. Pectoralis flaps are often used for sternal coverage and involve dissection of bilateral pectoralis muscles and advancement of the muscle bellies to the midline. Omental flaps can also be utilized, and some studies advocate omental flaps to have lower morbidity and mortality rates than myocutaneous flaps. These can be based off either the left or the right gastroepiploic artery. The latissimus dorsi flap can also be used and is especially useful for covering large anterolateral chest wounds or in cases where pectoralis flaps have been performed and failed.

C. ***Inappropriate Choice***. All the flaps listed above are potential options for tissue coverage for a sternal wound. However, in this patient, the left internal mammary artery has been transected and used for coronary artery bypass. This disrupts blood flow to the superior epigastric artery, the vascular pedicle for a rectus abdominis flap therefore making bilateral rectus flaps a poor choice.

Ref: 1, 7

5. What is the most common cause of free flap necrosis?

A. Arterial thrombosis

B. Venous thrombosis

C. Arterial vasospasm

D. Arterial insufficiency secondary to technical error at the anastomosis

E. Infection

ANSWER: B

COMMENTS: A., C., D., and E. *Incorrect*. In experienced hands, free flap success rates approach 95%. A well-controlled postoperative environment including a warm patient room and avoidance of tobacco (nicotine), caffeine, and vasoconstrictive medications are essential for success. Care must be taken for close postoperative monitoring of the flap typically in an intensive care unit setting, and identification of vascular compromise should be followed by prompt intervention. Arterial insufficiency is a less common cause of flap ischemia and manifests as a pale flap with the loss of capillary refill and reduction in temperature.

Compromise of vascular flow may be secondary to technical errors at the anastomosis, traction or kinking of the vessels, or compression by hematoma or edema. Return to the operating room (OR) is usually warranted with early intervention, allowing for the highest likelihood of flap salvage. Routine postoperative administration of antiplatelet agents or anticoagulants has not demonstrated superiority in the literature and is not a standard practice.

B. ***Correct***. Venous thrombosis is the most common cause of free flap failure. A dusky-appearing flap with swelling, congestion, and rapid capillary refill are early signs of venous congestion.

Ref: 1, 3, 8–10

C. Wound

1. Which of the following is ***false*** regarding the sequence of events in wound healing?

A. The initial vascular response is vasoconstriction, followed by vasodilation.

B. The phases of wound healing are inflammatory, proliferative, and remodeling.

C. The dominant cells of the inflammatory phase are macrophages.

D. The proliferative phase is mediated by fibroblasts.

E. The content of collagen in the wound continues to increase throughout the remodeling phase.

ANSWER: E

COMMENTS: A., B., C., and D. *True*. Please see Comments of Question 2.

E. ***False***. There is no net increase in collagen during the remodeling phase, only an increase in collagen cross-linking and conversion from type III to type I.

Ref: 1

2. Which cell type is ***incorrectly*** matched to its role in the phases of wound healing?

A. Platelets—hemostasis and activation of inflammatory cells

B. Neutrophils—decontamination of the wound bed and amplification of the cellular response

C. Macrophages—phagocytosis and release of inflammatory factors

D. Lymphocytes—blood progenitor cells for tissue repair

E. Fibroblasts—collagen synthesis

ANSWER: B

COMMENTS: A. *Correct*. The initial response to injury is targeted at hemostasis and clot formation. This is achieved by platelet plug formation and activation of the coagulation cascade. To minimize blood loss, the tissue undergoes 5 to 10 min of vasoconstriction while the initial clot is formed. After this, mast cells and endothelial cells, through mediators such as histamine, prostaglandin E_2, prostacyclin, and vascular endothelial growth factor, initiate vasodilation to usher in the cells of the inflammatory response. Inflammatory cells are first recruited via platelet degradation and release of platelet-derived growth factor and transforming growth factor-beta (TGF-β).

B. ***Incorrect***. Neutrophils are the first to respond, the role of which is decontamination of the wound. However, neutrophils are not responsible for amplification of the cellular response; this is accomplished by macrophages.

C. *Correct*. Unless there is significant contamination, the macrophages become the dominant cells of the inflammatory response by days 2 to 3. The release of subsequent inflammatory factors and recruitment of cells to amplify the cellular response are mediated by macrophages, not neutrophils. The macrophages recruit additional macrophages besides endothelial cells and fibroblasts. This increase in cellular activity brings the wound healing into the proliferative phase.

D. *Correct*. Lymphocytes have a more active role in chronic wounds; however, in an acute wound, the contribution of blood progenitor cells aids in tissue repair.

E. *Correct*. Beginning around day 5, the main events of the proliferative phase are collagen deposition by fibroblasts and angiogenesis by endothelial cells. The collagen in the wound bed is primarily type I, with a more minor component of type III.

The remodeling phase begins around 3 weeks and continues up to a year after the injury. This phase involves prolonged synthesis and degradation of collagen but is marked by a steady state of collagen content. During the remodeling phase, the amount of type III collagen decreases and type I collagen increases, with the final ratio of type I:type III being 4:1. The density of capillaries in the wound decreases, and the scar becomes pale.

Ref: 1

3. Which of the following statements is ***false*** regarding pressure ulcers?

A. Of all the layers of a wound, the subcutaneous tissue is the most susceptible to pressure necrosis due to its poor blood supply.

B. Stage I ulcers are defined by intact but erythematous skin that does not resolve after 1 h of pressure relief.

C. Stage II ulcers involve a partial-thickness loss of dermis with skin breaks or blistering, and stage III ulcers involve a full-thickness loss of dermis with exposed subcutaneous tissue.

D. Stage IV ulcers expose underlying muscle, tendon, or bone.

E. Ulcers where examination of the wound bed is obscured by a layer of slough or eschar are defined as unstageable.

ANSWER: A

COMMENTS: A. ***False***. The skin is more resistant to ischemia than the underlying tissues, which means that often the necrosis is more extensive than what is immediately apparent on examination. Muscle, though well vascularized, is most sensitive to ischemia. Therefore muscle is the most susceptible to pressure necrosis compared with skin and subcutaneous fat.

B., C., D., and E. *True*. Pressure ulcers occur when an unrelenting external force of compression rises above the pressure generated by the capillaries, resulting in ischemia. Capillary perfusion pressure is approximately 32 mmHg, and a recumbent body results in >80 mmHg in dependent areas. The areas at risk for developing pressure ulcers are scalp, sacrum, calcaneus when supine, ischium, and greater trochanter when sitting.

The stages described above are based on the staging system defined by the National Pressure Ulcer Advisory Panel. Stage I ulcers are defined by intact but erythematous skin that does not resolve after 1 h of pressure relief. Stage II ulcers involve a partial-thickness loss of dermis with skin breaks or blistering, and stage III ulcers involve a full-thickness loss of dermis with exposed subcutaneous tissue. Stage IV ulcers expose underlying muscle, tendon, or bone.

The treatment of pressure ulcers is a correction of causative factors as well as debridement and procedures for tissue coverage when necessary. The Braden Scale for Predicting Pressure Sore Risk is a commonly used nursing tool and accounts for extrinsic and intrinsic factors that are most commonly the cause of pressure ulcers. It includes sensory perception, moisture, activity, mobility, nutrition, and friction and shear. When feasible, optimization of these risk factors is the first step in healing pressure ulcers. Stage I and II ulcers typically heal with local wound care. Stage III ulcers have the potential to heal, but this phase is often short lived and progresses rapidly to stage IV, which often requires excision of bony prominences and definitive reconstructive flap closure.

Ref: 1

4. Which of the following statements is ***false*** regarding the formation of scars?

A. Hypertrophic scars are excessive scar tissue that remains within the boundaries of the initial tissue injury, whereas keloids extend beyond the area of injury.

B. A more cosmetic scar is achieved with incisions perpendicular to the lines of Langer or relaxed skin tension lines.

C. Relaxed skin tension lines usually run at right angles to the long axis of the underlying muscles.

D. Incisions on flexor surfaces usually heal well, whereas incisions over extensor joints heal with significant scarring.

E. In the remodeling phase of wound healing, collagen fibers become more organized, but they never achieve the precisely parallel arrangement seen in uninjured tissue.

ANSWER: B

COMMENTS: A. *True*. Hypertrophic scar and keloid scars are distinguished by the presence or absence of extent outside the confines of the initial incision or tissue injury. Hypertrophic scars generally regress with time and are treated with silicone gels and compression. Keloid scars are more difficult to treat, and some advocate the use of steroid injections or radiation to lessen the excessive scar tissue. Despite optimal treatment, keloid scars tend to recur.

B. ***False***. Lines of Langer, also known as relaxed skin tension lines or wrinkle lines, represent the line of minimal skin tension, and thus incisions parallel to these lines have less tension on their closure and result in the most cosmetic scar.

C. *True*. If you were to excise a circular area of skin, this wound heals in the shape of an ellipse; the long axis of this ellipse defines a line of Langer. These lines typically run perpendicular to the long axis of the underlying muscle. To better understand this, imagine the transverse lines that form on the forehead and deepen when the frontalis muscle contracts. These lines are perpendicular to the long axis of the muscle, and incisions along these lines are under minimal tension.

D. *True*. Incisions over extensor surfaces are subject to increased tension with the movement of the joint, resulting in significant scarring. On the other hand, incisions on flexor surfaces are in areas of relaxed tension and heal with less scarring.

E. *True*. In the remodeling phase of wound healing, collagen fibers reorganize in a parallel arrangement, but they never achieve the same parallel arrangement seen in uninjured tissue.

Ref: 1

5. A 35-year-old male is evaluated 24 h after a provoked dog bite to his left forearm. There is no suspicion for rabies. The wound is stellate and 2 cm deep. There is devitalized tissue as well as dirt at the base. His last tetanus booster was 7 years ago. Which of the following is the appropriate medical treatment?

A. Tetanus toxoid and antibiotic coverage for *Eikenella corrodens*

B. Antibiotic coverage for *Pasteurella multocida* only

C. Tetanus toxoid and antibiotic coverage for *P. multocida*

D. Tetanus toxoid, tetanus immune globulin, and antibiotic coverage for *P. multocida*

E. Tetanus toxoid only

ANSWER: C

COMMENTS: A., B., D., and E. *Inappropriate*. To determine the appropriate treatment, the wound must be divided into tetanus prone and non–tetanus prone. The characteristics of tetanus-prone wounds include the following: older than 6 h; stellate configuration or avulsion; depth greater than 1 cm; gross contamination or infection; devitalized tissue or necrosis; or the result of crush injury, burn, or frostbite. If the patient has previously received an initial tetanus and diptheria toxoids vaccine and at least three doses of tetanus toxoid or booster, an additional tetanus booster is required only if his last dose was more than 5 years ago. If the patient has not completed the initial vaccine and three boosters, or his immunization status is unknown, he should receive tetanus immune globulin and tetanus toxoid.

For non–tetanus-prone wounds, tetanus immune globulin is not indicated. Tetanus toxoid is indicated only if the patient did not previously complete the vaccine and three boosters, completed the immunization course but the last booster was more than 10 years ago, or the immunization status is unknown.

C. ***Appropriate***. This patient requires a tetanus booster because his last dose was more than 5 years prior to injury. Antibiotics prophylaxis is usually administered for animal and human bites, especially if there is delayed presentation for more than 12 h; the patient is diabetic or otherwise immunosuppressed; or there is involvement of face, hands, or feet. Although bite wounds are often polymicrobial, *P. multocida* is the major pathogen in dog and cat bites. Human bites are often contaminated with *E. corrodens, Staphylococcus aureus, S. epidermidis*, α- and β-hemolytic *Streptococcus* sp., and *Corynebacterium*. Amoxicillin–clavulanate is the drug of choice for most bite wounds because it has aerobic and anaerobic coverage, including that for *Pasturella* sp. and *Eikenella* sp.

Ref: 11, 12

6. A 60-year-old diabetic woman currently being treated for right lower extremity cellulitis is brought to the emergency room from her nursing home. She has an exquisitely tender erythematous right leg with bullae formation. She has tenderness that extends beyond the area of erythema. Her body temperature is 38.9°C, blood pressure is 82/43 mmHg, and heart rate is 128 beats/min. After initiating fluid resuscitation, what is the next best step in management?

A. Admission to the intensive care unit (ICU), blood cultures, broad-spectrum antibiotics, and serial examinations

B. Computed tomography (CT) scan of the right lower extremity

C. Admission to the ICU, blood cultures, broad-spectrum antibiotics, and bedside debridement of the bullae of the right lower extremity

D. Blood cultures, broad-spectrum antibiotics, and immediate transfer to the OR for debridement of the right lower extremity

E. Blood cultures, broad-spectrum antibiotics, and IV hydrocortisone

ANSWER: D

COMMENTS: A., B., C., and E. *Incorrect.* The clinical scenario is suggestive of a necrotizing soft tissue infection of the extremity, which is often characterized by erythema and severe pain out of proportion to physical examination findings. Additional signs include tenderness beyond the area of erythema, crepitus, bullae, and skin necrosis. Patients often demonstrate signs of sepsis with fevers, tachycardia, hypotension, changes in mental status, and oliguria/anuria. In stable patients or in cases where the diagnosis is not clear, imaging with CT, magnetic resonance imaging (MRI), or plain films may be useful and may demonstrate subcutaneous edema or emphysema and inflammation and fat stranding. Soft tissue gas confirms a necrotizing infection, but its absence does not exclude the diagnosis.

D. ***Correct.*** The appropriate treatment is the initiation of resuscitation, blood cultures, broad-spectrum antibiotics, and immediate operative debridement. In the OR, all necrotic and infected tissue should be aggressively debrided, and consent should be obtained from patients or families for possible amputation when applicable. Wide drainage with Penrose drains may also be appropriate. Often, multiple debridements are required, leading to large debilitating wounds requiring extensive reconstruction.

Ref: 13–15

7. In addition to broad-spectrum antibiotics, such as vancomycin, and a carbapenem, piperacillin/tazobactam, or an aminoglycoside, what other antibiotic should be given to the above patient?

A. Metronidazole

B. Clindamycin

C. Azithromycin

D. Cefazolin

E. Cefepime

ANSWER: B

COMMENTS: A., C., D., and E. *Incorrect.* For necrotizing soft tissue infections, antibiotic therapy should include coverage for gram-positive, gram-negative, and anaerobic bacteria. There are many acceptable regimens such as a carbapenem, piperacillin/tazobactam, or tigecycline. An appropriate multidrug regimen is high-dose penicillin and a fluoroquinolone or aminoglycoside. Vancomycin should be included until methicillin-resistant *S. aureus* (MRSA) is excluded as a causative organism. Metronidazole, azithromycinn, cefazolin, and cefepime would not provide complete coverage.

B. ***Correct.*** Clindamycin should also be administered. Clindamycin is a protein synthesis inhibitor and thus is useful for inhibition of toxic production, especially in *Clostridium* sp. and group A β-hemolytic *Streptococcus* sp. Once adequate source control is achieved with debridement and the patient clinically stabilizes, antibiotic administration can be discontinued.

Ref: 16

8. Which of the following is an acceptable wound environment for a negative-pressure wound dressing or vacuum-assisted wound closure?

A. Dehiscence after inguinal lymph node dissection with exposed femoral vessels

B. Sternal dehiscence and mediastinitis following cardiac surgery

C. Stage IV sacral decubitus ulcer with untreated sacral osteomyelitis

D. Lower extremity wound with necrotic muscle in base

E. Lower extremity wound with exposed prosthetic graft

ANSWER: B

COMMENTS: A. and E. *Incorrect.* Negative-pressure wound therapy (NPWT) is contraindicated in wounds with exposed vasculature, vascular grafts, or prosthetic grafts that may cause erosion leading to hemorrhage or infection. However, NPWT can be used in wounds with vessels or grafts that have adequate tissue coverage.

B. ***Correct.*** Vacuum-assisted wound closure involves the application of a porous sponge and occlusive dressing to the wound followed by a device to generate negative pressure over the wound surface. NPWT accelerates wound healing and granulation tissue formation by increasing blood flow, removing exudate, and providing mechanical forces to draw the wound edges together. NPWT may be used successfully for chest coverage in cases of sternal dehiscence after adequate debridement as the primary treatment or a bridge to definitive therapy with flap coverage.

C. and D. *Incorrect.* NPWT should only be utilized on wounds that have been properly debrided and are free of necrotic or infected tissue. Therefore NPWT is inappropriate in osteomyelitis if antibiotic therapy and possible debridement have not been completed.

Ref: 17–19

D. Breast

1. When counseling a young woman about breast surgery, she states that she has been doing some Internet research, and she voices many concerns about implants. Which of the following statements is ***true***?
   A. Women with breast implants are at an increased risk of developing breast cancer.
   B. When a woman with breast implants is diagnosed with breast cancer, it is more likely to be at a more advanced stage compared with women without breast implants.
   C. Thoroughly evaluating the breast tissue in a breast with an implant is more difficult using standard mammography.
   D. The concentration of silicone in breast milk is higher in women with breast implants than in those without implants.
   E. Studies have demonstrated a causal relationship between breast implants and connective tissue disorders such as lupus and rheumatoid arthritis.

ANSWER: C

COMMENTS: A. *False*. No evidence exists to suggest that breast implants impart a higher risk of breast cancer.

B. *False*. There is no significant difference in size or stage of tumor at the time of detection between women with and without implants.

C. ***True***. In women with implants, standard mammography is able to evaluate only 75% of the breast tissue, with the remaining tissue obscured by the implant. This requires specialized views utilizing displacement techniques called Eklund views to obtain additional images. Studies demonstrate that this does not result in delayed detection or poorer prognosis in women with implants.

D. *False*. Depending on the location of the implant, breastfeeding with implants may still be possible. Investigations indicate no significant difference in the concentration of silicone in breast milk in women with implants.

E. *False*. Case reports published in the 1980s generated concern about a relationship between breast implants and the development of connective tissue disorders. Over 2000 peer-reviewed studies were analyzed and demonstrated no definitive evidence of a link between implants and connective tissue disorders or that women with implants were more likely than the general population to develop these diseases.

Ref: 1

2. Regarding postmastectomy reconstruction, which of the following is false regarding the advantages and disadvantages of implant reconstruction?
   A. Although single-stage implant reconstruction allows for a single operation, implant size is often limited by the skin envelope.
   B. Tissue expanders allow for a larger size of the final implant but require frequent office visits for expansion and a second operation.
   C. Two-stage implant reconstruction often requires 4 to 6 months for completion of the process.
   D. Excessive scar tissue may form around an implant. This is termed capsular contracture and may result in deformity and pain.
   E. Because it is placed under sterile conditions and bacteria is not typically present in breast tissue, there is virtually no risk of implant infection.

ANSWER: E

COMMENTS: A. *True*. Single-stage implant reconstruction involves the placement of the final implant at the time of mastectomy. With this technique, the size of the skin envelope at the conclusion of the mastectomy dictates the maximum size of the implant. Placing too large an implant with an inadequate skin envelope leads to excess tension on the closure and increases the risk for wound dehiscence and skin necrosis.

B. *True*. Two-stage implant reconstruction is performed in two operations. The first stage involves placement of a temporary tissue expander, often at the time of mastectomy, and the second stage involves removal of the expander and placement of the final implant. Tissue expansion allows a larger size of the final implant than that allowed by the single-stage implant reconstruction.

C. *True*. The tissue expander consists of a silicone envelope with an injection port that can be accessed percutaneously and is expanded with saline over time. This typically requires weekly office visits until the skin achieves the desired size of the final implant. Surgeons often delay the second stage of the operation until 1 to 4 months after the completion of expansion.

D. *True*. Capsular contracture occurs in approximately 15% of patients and is usually apparent by 6 months after placement of the implant, although it may occur at any time over the lifetime of the implant. The incidence is lower with the use of a textured implant than with the use of a smooth shell implant. Implant massage exercises in the early postoperative period may reduce the risk of contracture development. If the fibrous tissue is significant, it may result in a painful or esthetically deformed breast often requiring surgical correction.

E. ***False***. Like all prosthetic materials, implants are subject to infection, although this is an uncommon occurrence. Bacteria present in the breast ducts are similar to normal skin flora. A meticulous aseptic technique must be utilized to reduce the risk of implant infection. In some cases, IV antibiotics can salvage the implant, but infection of the implant may ultimately necessitate removal of the implant. The implant may be replaced after adequate resolution of the infection.

Ref: 1, 2

3. You are counseling a young breast cancer patient regarding her options for reconstruction after mastectomy. She states that she does not want any artificial implants and would prefer the use of only her own tissues for reconstruction. Which of the following statements is ***false***?

A. If the patient has adequate abdominal tissue, a TRAM flap is an excellent option and has the added benefit of a modified abdominoplasty.

B. A TRAM flap offers the benefit of increasing or decreasing the volume accordingly if the patient gains or loses weight.

C. A disadvantage of the pedicle TRAM flap is the potential risk for abdominal hernias and abdominal wall laxity.

D. A latissimus dorsi myocutaneous flap is a reasonable option for this patient and has the benefit of avoiding abdominal donor site morbidity.

E. Deep inferior epigastric perforator flap is a reasonable option for this patient and has the benefit of avoiding abdominal donor site morbidity.

ANSWER: D

COMMENTS: A. *True*. TRAM flap reconstruction is the most commonly performed autologous tissue breast reconstruction. The rectus muscle and supplying superior epigastric artery serve as a vascular pedicle, and a flap of lower abdominal skin and fat is transferred to the mastectomy defect to reconstruct the breast. The muscle remains attached at the proximal origin and is tunneled superiorly to reach the chest. The abdominal defect is closed by reapproximation of the anterior rectus sheath and advancing the superior skin edge of the abdominal skin inferiorly for closure. This results in a modified abdominoplasty that many surgeons and patients regard as an added benefit. This flap generally provides more than adequate volume for reconstruction of the breast and can be utilized for unilateral or bilateral breast reconstruction.

In contrast to tissue expander and implant reconstruction, the TRAM flap is a single-stage operation that can be performed at the time of mastectomy. However, this is a considerably longer operation than either stage in the two-stage technique and requires a longer recovery time.

B. *True*. Both the TRAM and deep inferior epigastric perforator (DIEP) flaps are composed of native abdominal tissue and maintain proportionality to the overall body mass and contralateral breast and expand or decrease in volume when a patient gains or loses a significant amount of weight.

C. *True*. The resulting muscle defect does carry a potential risk for abdominal hernia and abdominal wall laxity, resulting in an undesirable bulge of the lower abdomen. The incidence of this is up to 5%. Often, the abdominal fascia is reinforced with the acellular dermal matrix or prosthetic mesh. This complication may be avoided with DIEP free flap reconstruction.

D. ***False***. A latissimus dorsi myocutaneous flap is a pedicle flap based on the thoracodorsal vessels and is tunneled anteriorly for chest wall coverage. It is particularly useful for providing coverage in patients who have a pectoralis muscle defect after radical mastectomy or when mastectomy skin flaps are inadequate. This flap often has insufficient volume to fully reconstruct the breast and is used in combination with either single- or two-stage implant reconstruction.

E. *True*. In the DIEP free flap reconstruction, a flap of lower abdominal skin and fat is harvested based on the deep inferior epigastric artery with little to no rectus abdominis muscle. This flap is then transferred to the chest with free tissue transfer. The DIEP flap is anastomosed to a recipient vessel, usually thoracodorsal, subscapular, or internal mammary. This technique allows for adequate breast reconstruction with autologous tissue but minimizes the abdominal wall morbidity at the donor site.

Ref: 1, 2

4. A 35-year-old woman who underwent augmentation mammoplasty with silicone breast implants notices a flattening of her left breast and is worried about the rupture of her implant. Which modality is the most sensitive and specific for detection of implant rupture?

A. Physical examination

B. Ultrasound

C. CT scan

D. Mammography

E. MRI

ANSWER: E

COMMENTS: A. *Incorrect*. Many implant ruptures are clinically silent and detected only at the time of implant exchange or with routine imaging.

E. ***Correct***. MRI has a sensitivity and specificity of greater than 90% for detecting implant rupture. Intracapsular rupture is identified on MRI by the so-called linguine sign in which multiple low-density lines represent the implant shell folding on itself. Extracapsular rupture is diagnosed by high-intensity focus outside the capsule, representing extravasation of the silicone gel into the tissues surrounding the capsule. Because the cohesive gel often remains in the vicinity of the ruptured implant, it may be clinically silent. It is thus recommended to undergo regular imaging surveillance of the implant, and current recommendations advise MRI 3 years after the implant placement and then every 3 to 5 years for the life of the implant. If rupture occurs, removal of the implant with or without replacement is recommended. Rupture of a saline implant is clinically easier to detect with deflation of the implant.

B., C., and D. *Incorrect*. Mammography, ultrasound, and CT scan have all been used but are less reliable for detection.

Ref: 20–22

E. Abdominal Wall

1. When performing a component separation for a large abdominal wall defect, which of the following describes the location of the relaxing incision?

A. The aponeurosis of the internal abdominal oblique, at the linea semilunaris

B. The aponeurosis of the external abdominal oblique, 1 to 2 cm lateral to the linea semilunaris

C. The anterior rectus sheath, 1 to 2 cm medial to the linea semilunaris

D. The aponeurosis of the internal abdominal oblique, 1 to 2 cm lateral to the linea semilunaris

E. The aponeurosis of the external abdominal oblique, 1 to 2 cm medial to the linea semilunaris

ANSWER: B

COMMENTS: B. ***Correct***. Separation of components is a technique that utilizes a series of abdominal fascial releases to achieve adequate mobilization of the tissues to close a large midline musculofascial defect of the anterior abdominal wall. Via a vertical midline incision, the skin and subcutaneous fat are dissected off the muscular wall.

The aponeurosis of the external abdominal oblique is transected longitudinally, 1 to 2 cm lateral to the semilunaris, and this incision is extended from the pubis onto the chest wall, at least 5 to 7 cm cranial to the costal margin. A plane of dissection is carried out laterally between the external and internal abdominal obliques as far lateral as possible, ideally to the posterior axillary line. In order to avoid wound complications and necrosis of skin flaps, care should be taken to preserve large perforating vessels that supply the skin and subcutaneous tissue.

The neurovascular supply to the muscle is not endangered by this technique as it runs between the internal oblique and the transversus abdominis. The relaxation and dissection allow for medial mobilization of the rectus and the internal oblique and primary closure of the two rectus muscles in the midline. When needed, an additional 2 to 4 cm of mobilization can be gained by separating the rectus from the posterior rectus sheath through an incision of the posterior sheath while taking care to preserve the blood supply that enters posterolaterally between the internal oblique and the transversus abdominis. Separation of components on both sides of the abdominal wall in conjunction with relaxing incisions in the posterior rectus sheath can yield up to 20 cm of medial advancement.

A., C., D., and E. *Incorrect*. Further relaxing incisions to the internal oblique or transversus abdominis have been described, but this can result in lateral bulge or herniations. Many surgeons advocate the use of biologic or prosthetic mesh as either an underlay or an onlay to reinforce the repair and reduce the rate of recurrence. Minimally invasive separation and laparoscopic/endoscopic separation of components have also been described.

Ref: 1, 2

2. A 45-year-old male is recovering on postoperative day 1 in the surgical ICU following a large separation of components operation. Due to the prolonged length of the operation, he received a high volume of intravenous fluids in the OR and was left intubated at the conclusion of the case. Which of the following is ***inconsistent*** with the diagnosis of abdominal compartment syndrome?

A. Oliguria or anuria

B. Bladder pressures exceeding 20 to 25 mmHg

C. Peak airway pressures > 45 cmH_2O

D. Intraabdominal pressure greater than 16 mmHg

E. Elevated central venous and pulmonary artery pressures

ANSWER: D

COMMENTS: A. *Consistent*. Resultant renal dysfunction occurs from both decreased renal perfusion and venous congestion from compression of the renal vein. This combination of increased parenchymal pressure and decreased renal blood flow decreases the pressure gradient across the glomerular membrane and therefore reduces the glomerular filtration rate (GFR). The same effects of decreased perfusion and increased venous congestion result in mucosal ischemia of other visceral organs and lactic acidosis.

B. *Consistent*. The most widely used method for monitoring abdominal pressures is the measurement of bladder pressures via a transducer on a Foley catheter. Under normal conditions, bladder pressure and thus the intraabdominal pressure in a supine adult are less than 10 mmHg. Following abdominal surgery, pressures range from 3 to 15 mmHg. Pressures exceeding 20 to 25 mmHg, along with other signs, should raise concern for abdominal compartment syndrome.

Recognition of abdominal compartment syndrome is critical, and management includes judicious administration of IV fluids, adequate sedation, and neuromuscular paralytics. When conservative management fails, a decompressive laparotomy is indicated.

C., E. *Consistent*. As the pressure in the abdominal cavity increases, the diaphragm is elevated and results in the transmission of the high pressure into the thoracic cavity and significant reduction in pulmonary compliance. This is manifested by an increase in the peak inspiratory pressures required for adequate ventilation with peak airway pressures > 45 cmH_2O. The increased intrathoracic pressure results in decreased venous return, which, compounded by increased systemic vascular resistance from mechanical compression of capillary beds, reduces cardiac output. The high thoracic pressures are reflected in elevated central venous and pulmonary artery pressures.

D. ***Inconsistent***. Following large abdominal wall reconstruction, the decreased volume of the abdominal cavity (decreased abdominal domain) can lead to the development of increased intraabdominal pressures. This is exacerbated by high-volume fluid resuscitation and edema, resulting in decreased compliance. Normal intraabdominal pressure is 5 to 7 mmHg in critically ill adults. Abdominal hypertension is defined as sustained pressures greater than 12 mmHg, and abdominal compartment syndrome is a sustained pressure greater than 20 mmHg with associated organ dysfunction.

Ref: 1, 23

F. Craniofacial

1. You are called to evaluate a 25-year-old female who has sustained a lip laceration from a dog bite. Both the lip mucosa and the adjacent skin are involved. Which of the following statements is ***false*** regarding the repair?

A. The most critical steps are exact alignment of the vermilion border and repair of the orbicularis oris muscle.

B. If the defect results in loss of up to one-third of the lip, it can be repaired primarily.

C. If the defect is large and to the upper lip, it can be repaired with a tissue flap from the lower lip.

D. If the defect is large and to the lower lip, it can be repaired with a tissue flap from the upper lip.

E. If the repair results in microstomia, this is often temporary.

ANSWER: D

COMMENTS: A. *True*. Repair of a lip laceration that disrupts the vermilion, or mucocutaneous junction of the lip, requires precise alignment as even small irregularities in the border will be noticeable. Repair of injury to the orbicularis oris muscle is necessary to maintain the competence of the lip.

B. *True*. Primary repair is usually possible for defects up to one-third of the lip, and if full thickness, it should be performed in three layers from deep to superficial: mucosa, muscle, and skin.

C. *True*. For large defects of the upper lip, a tissue flap from the lower lip can be used. An example of this is the Abbe flap, which is a pedicle flap of the lower lip based on the labial artery. The flap is rotated to the upper lip, and the pedicle is divided 2 to 3 weeks later, after the flap has established a new blood supply. The lower lip is well suited to this purpose because it does not have any anatomic landmarks nor central structure. Therefore its appearance is not affected by the loss of tissue or asymmetry.

D. ***False***. The upper lip, however, has the so-called Cupid's bow and central tubercle, and loss or displacement of these midline structures results in significant asymmetry. Because of this, the upper lip cannot be used as a flap donor site for repair of a defect of the lower lip. In the case of large defects of the lower lip, cheek advancement flaps can be utilized to gain enough mobility to close the defect. For the full loss of the lower lip, free flap reconstruction using the free radial forearm flaps with palmaris longus tendon can be used.

E. *True*. The flaps are full thickness up to the commissures, where the flaps become superficial to the muscles to preserve the labial vessels and nerve. This preserves oral competence but often results in microstomia, which is typically temporary as the tissues stretch over time.

Ref: 1,26

2. A 12-month-old boy with cleft lip and palate presents to the clinic for evaluation. The child underwent repair of a cleft lip at the age of 3 months. On examination, the palatal cleft involves both the hard and soft palate and is continuous with an alveolar defect. There is also asymmetry of the widened nose and deviation of the nasal septum. What is the best operative plan for this child's next surgery?

A. Closure of the palatal defect

B. Alveolar bone graft

C. Closure of the palatal defect and alveolar bone graft

D. Correction of the septal deviation

E. Correction of the septal deviation and rhinoplasty

ANSWER: A

COMMENTS: A. ***Correct***. The overall incidence of cleft lip and palate is 1 in 750 children, with a higher incidence, 1 in 300, in the Asian population. The deformity can be isolated cleft lip (21%), isolated cleft palate (33%), and combined cleft lip and palate (46%). The defect has a complex genetic inheritance pattern, and the pathophysiology remains incompletely understood. The repair of cleft lip and palate is performed in a multistaged fashion and typically requires three to four operations, with additional operations to correct persistent anomalies.

The deformity can be bilateral or unilateral and is considered complete if it extends into the nose and results in an absence of the nasal floor. The cleft can extend into the gum and through the alveolus, resulting in a bony defect. The cleft can involve only the soft palate, a result of the abnormal insertion of the levator palatini muscle on the posterior surface of the hard palate, or involve the hard palate as well. In some cases, the mucosa over the palate may be intact, and there is a separation of the underlying musculature (submucous cleft).

The first operation is repair of the cleft lip. There is no exact consensus on when this should be performed, but this operation is typically performed between 3 and 6 months of age. This allows for safer administration of anesthesia due to the weight gain in these first 3 months. The next step in reconstruction is the closure of the palatal defect. This may involve simple reapproximation of the muscle and closure of the palatal mucosa. However, wide unilateral clefts and bilateral clefts often require relaxing incisions and release of the mucosa from the underlying bone. Delay in this phase allows for the better growth of the midface and palate as dissection of the mucosal tissue off the bone restricts growth. However, early repair of the palate improves speech development. Therefore a balance must be found between the two. Palate repair is most often performed around 1 year to 18 months of age.

B. and C. *Incorrect*. Bone grafting is often performed at 7 to 10 years of age at mixed dentition stage. Correction of an alveolar cleft must be undertaken with a multidisciplinary approach that includes an orthodontist. Bone grafting to the alveolar cleft restores the dental arch, which is necessary for tooth emergence. The orthodontist monitors for tooth eruption and may initiate early therapies to align the teeth in preparation for bone grafting. The operation involves excision of the oral–nasal fistula, reconstruction of the adjacent nasal floor, placement of a bone graft in the alveolar defect, and placement of gingival flaps over the graft. The bone graft consists of cancellous bone and can be harvested from the iliac crest or the cranial diploe, which is the layer of cancellous bone between the inner and outer layers of the cranium.

D. and E. *Incorrect*. The last operation is septorhinoplasty, and this is usually performed in the teenage years, after maturation of dentition and completion of the orthodontic work. A deviated septum is almost always a component of cleft lip and palate and is straightened in this operation. Rhinoplasty is tailored to each particular patient but often involves repositioning and trimming of nasal cartilage, in-fracture of the nasal bones to correct a widened nose, and tacking of the lower nasal cartilage to improve the projection of the nose.

Ref: 1, 2

3. The mother of a 4-year-old boy with a history of cleft lip and palate repair brings her child to the clinic due to concerns regarding his speech. The child underwent lip closure at 3 months of age and palate closure at 12 months. He has been participating in speech therapy since the palatal closure but continues to have speech difficulties and produces squeaks and snorts through his nose with attempted speech. On examination, you note an alveolar cleft. The mother states she is agreeable to another operation if it exists. What is the best plan to correct the problem for this patient?

A. Continued speech therapy as there are no operative methods for correction

B. An operation to close the persistent oral–nasal fistula

C. Placement of a bone graft at the alveolar defect

D. An operation to place tissue near the velopharyngeal port

E. Operative correction of the septal deviation and rhinoplasty

ANSWER: D

COMMENTS: A. *Incorrect*. Primary repair of the palatal cleft normalizes speech in only approximately 80% of children, and the remaining 15%–20% continue to demonstrate velopharyngeal insufficiency. This is the result of an inability of the velum, or soft palate, to seal off the connection to the nasal cavity during speech. This causes hypernasality of the speech and escape of air through the nose during attempted pronunciation of certain consonants. Speech therapy may be inadequate to correct this, and operative intervention may be indicated.

B. *Incorrect*. The persistent oral–nasal fistula is at the site of the alveolar defect and is not the cause of the speech abnormalities described.

C. and E. *Incorrect*. Both alveolar bone grafting with the closure of the oral–nasal fistula and correction of the deviated septum are performed later in life and would not result in correction of the problems with speech.

D. ***Correct***. The surgery aims to correct the velopharyngeal insufficiency. A number of techniques exist (superior pharyngeal flap, sphincter pharyngoplasty, augmentation pharyngoplasty), but the objective is to improve closure of the velopharyngeal port to aid in the regulation of airflow and the ability to impede the movement of air into the nasopharynx.

The timing of this operation must be early enough to have maximum impact on speech development but late enough to give adequate time for speech therapy to attempt correction of the problem. The consensus is operative intervention after 3 years of age. Prior to an operation, the dynamics of the child's speech should be thoroughly evaluated via nasoendoscopy and functional measures obtained with nasometry to determine the best treatment approach.

Ref: 1, 2

4. Which of the following statements is ***true*** regarding vascular anomalies?

A. Newborns with capillary malformations (port wine stains) in the ophthalmic distribution of the trigeminal nerve should undergo MRI of the head.

B. A 3-year-old with a stable hemangioma on the forehead that has failed to regress should be treated with surgical excision.

C. Hemangiomas are typically present at birth.

D. Most venous malformations regress and therefore should be observed until age 5 to 7 years.

E. Sclerotherapy is usually effective for the treatment of arteriovenous malformations.

ANSWER: A

COMMENTS: A. ***True***. When a capillary malformation occupies the ophthalmic trigeminal nerve distribution, MRI of the head should be obtained to evaluate for Sturge-Weber syndrome, which is associated with ipsilateral leptomeningeal and ocular anomalies.

Vascular anomalies are divided into two groups: tumors and malformations. Vascular tumors arise as a result of increased proliferation of endothelium and include hemangiomas (most common), hemangioendotheliomas, tufted angiomas, and hemangiopericytomas. Malignant vascular tumors, such as angiosarcomas, are rare in infancy.

In contrast, vascular malformations result from abnormal arterial, capillary, venous, or lymphatic components. These malformations may consist of a single component or a combination of components and may be high flow, low flow, or mixed.

B. and D. *False*. There is typically complete regression of hemangiomas in 50% of cases by the age of 5 years and in 70% of cases by the age of 7 years. Observation is appropriate unless the tumor affects the vision or involves the airway; in such cases intervention is indicated. A course of injected or systemic steroids may induce involution, but if this fails, operative resection should be performed. Beta-blockers have shown to be effective in decreasing the proliferative phase of hemangiomas and may be utilized topically or systemically.

Lymphatic malformations, also known as lymphangiomas or cystic hygromas, are the most difficult to treat because they are diffuse and often adjacent to vital structures in the head and neck. Lymphangiomas expand and contract with alterations in the flow of lymphatic fluid. If functionally impairing, these are to be removed via a series of staged partial excisions.

C. *False*. Hemangiomas are not present at birth and typically develop in the first 2 weeks of life; these are commonly referred to as strawberry angiomas. They are typically characterized by a rapid growth phase followed by slow spontaneous involution.

On the other hand, vascular malformations are usually present at birth and often grow in proportion with the child. Initially a flat lesion, these malformations can become thick and verrucous as they enlarge and there is no spontaneous regression. Early treatment is indicated and depends on the vascular components involved. Small capillary malformations, such as port wine stains, are well treated with pulse dye laser, and large lesions may require combined laser and operative therapy.

E. *False*. Sclerotherapy is the standard treatment for venous malformations and may be a useful adjunct in arteriovenous malformations. However, due to the development of collaterals, sclerotherapy alone is often insufficient for arteriovenous malformations and surgical resection should be performed after sclerotherapy and embolization.

Ref: 1, 2

5. A concerned father brings his 7-month-old female to the clinic for evaluation. He is concerned that her skull is misshapen and not growing properly. On examination, the brow above the baby's right eye is recessed, and the left brow is overly protuberant. You suspect she has craniosynostosis. Which suture is most likely affected in this patient?

A. Sagittal suture

B. Metopic suture

C. Right coronal suture

D. Left coronal suture

E. Bilateral coronal sutures

ANSWER: C

COMMENTS: A. *Incorrect.* Fusion of the sagittal suture, which is the most commonly affected by craniosynostosis, develops a long oval-shaped head, which is often described as boat or keel shaped or scaphocephaly.

B. *Incorrect.* Synostosis of the metopic suture results in a triangular forehead and is known as trigonocephaly.

C. ***Correct.*** Craniosynostosis is characterized by premature fusion of one or more cranial sutures and resultant restriction in the growth of the skull. Although the fontanelles are obliterated early in life, the sutures remain open to allow for expansion of the brain and skull. With the exception of the metopic suture that closes around the age of 3 to 9 months, the remaining sutures do not fuse until adulthood.

When early synostosis occurs, the growth of the skull is restricted in the direction perpendicular to the affected suture and compensatory growth occurs in a parallel direction to the suture. Multiple sutures can be affected and produce a combination of the shapes described. This syndrome may result in solely a physical deformity or may cause enough restriction to cause increased intracranial pressure, and brain development may be affected. Unilateral coronal suture involvement produces a recessed supraorbital bar on the affected side and compensatory growth of ***the contralateral brow***; this is referred to as frontal plagiocephaly.

Surgical treatment aims to correct the deformity, restore projection to the brow for the protection of the eyes, and relieve or prevent increased intracranial pressure. This is most often performed within the first year of life. The operation is typically performed through a sinusoidal coronal incision, and although many operative techniques exist, the objective is release or excision of the fused suture. In the first 2 years of life, the dura is osteogenic and gaps in the skull from the operation slowly ossify over time.

D. *Incorrect.* Premature fusion of the left coronal suture results in compensatory growth of the right brow, resulting in a recessed left eye and protuberant right brow.

E. *Incorrect.* Bilateral coronal synostosis results in a shortened and flattened forehead, termed brachycephaly.

Deformational plagiocephaly should be included in the differential diagnosis and is caused by supine sleeping. This does not require operative intervention and will often "self-correct" as the child grows and is able to turn during sleep. Helmet molding therapy can be considered in these children to improve cosmesis.

Ref: 2

6. A 15-year-old female presents to the clinic for evaluation. She has a history of bilateral cleft lip and palate and has undergone all stages of repair, including alveolar bone grafting. She has completed orthodontic therapy and has all of her permanent teeth. She is concerned because the middle of her face is recessed and her upper and lower teeth do not align well, with the lower teeth projecting further than the upper ones. What is the best management of this condition?

A. Refer her back to the orthodontist for realignment of the teeth.

B. Refer her to physical and occupational therapy for techniques to maximize function.

C. Perform fat grafting to the midface to fill in the recessed areas and reshape the face.

D. Perform an operation to advance the maxilla forward.

E. Correct the recessed midface with a local advancement flap or a free flap.

ANSWER: D

COMMENTS: A. *Incorrect.* The growth of the midface may be compromised by palatal closure, especially if there is an extensive dissection of the mucosa from the bone as is necessary for large clefts. Midface hypoplasia is characterized by a recessed maxilla, which is especially apparent in lateral views of the patient's face. This can result in an overly projectile appearance of the eyes and malocclusion of the mandible.

If there is an esthetic or functional impairment to the patient, operative intervention can restore normal occlusion. This operation should be delayed until the orthodontic work is complete, skeletal maturity has been reached, and the dentition is in its final position. This is most commonly performed in the teenage years. This patient has already completed orthodontic work; referral back to the orthodontist will not correct this condition.

B., C., and E. *Incorrect.* Physical therapy, occupational therapy, fat grafting, and flap reconstruction will not correct the patient's midface hypoplasia.

D. ***Correct.*** The most common operative correction is a Le Fort I osteotomy, where the maxilla is incised horizontally above the level of the tooth roots and below the zygomatic body with or without repositioning of the mandible. The bones of the midface are separated from the cranial base, and the maxilla is advanced into the proper position. Preoperative planning should be undertaken with the orthodontist to determine the amount of advancement needed for proper occlusion and where the maxilla should be placed.

A splint is fashioned preoperatively so that intraoperatively, the maxilla can be advanced and placed into the splint. The maxilla is reaffixed to the cranium with plates and screws. In severe cases, if occlusion cannot be achieved with only the advancement of the maxilla, the mandible may also require operative adjustment to attain proper occlusion.

Ref: 1, 2, 24

7. Which of the following is ***true*** regarding nasal trauma?

A. A septal hematoma should not be disturbed and should be left to absorb on its own.

B. Diagnosis of nasal fractures requires a dedicated maxillofacial CT.

C. Naso-orbitoethmoid fractures are usually managed with closed reduction and splinting.

D. Patients with telecanthus usually require reattachment of the medial canthus tendons.

E. Nasolacrimal duct stenting is avoided.

ANSWER: D

COMMENTS: A. *False*. When evaluating a patient with nasal trauma, the nasal septum should be examined for signs of a septal hematoma. If undiagnosed, a septal hematoma can lead to necrosis and erosion of the nasal septum and result in a saddle nose deformity. A septal hematoma should be incised and drained, and either quilting sutures with absorbable suture or a nasal stent should be placed to prevent reaccumulation.

B. *False*. Fractures of the nasal bones are diagnosed clinically, and dedicated radiography is rarely necessary. Nasal fractures are usually treated by closed reduction, splinting, and intranasal packing. If nasal packing is used, antibiotics should be initiated as cases of toxic shock have been described with intranasal packing.

C. *False*. Naso-orbitoethmoid fractures result from high-impact injuries and are associated with fractures of the nasal bones, ethmoid complex, medial orbital walls, nasofrontal junction, and nasal septum. The nasolacrimal duct may also be injured. Closed reduction is not sufficient to repair these injuries.

D. ***True***. Telecanthus is the increased distance between the medial canthi of the eyes, and repair involves reattachment of the medial canthus tendons or repositioning of the bony segments to which the medial canthal tendons are attached.

E. *False*. Naso-orbitoethmoid fractures may involve disruption of the nasolacrimal ducts, especially if telecanthus is present. These injuries should be repaired over a stent to avoid stricture.

Ref: 25

8. Which of the following statements regarding the facial nerve is ***true***?

A. The three major branches of the facial nerve are the ophthalmic, maxillary/buccal, and mandibular.

B. Injury to the buccal branch of the facial nerve medial to the lateral canthus should be tagged or reapproximated within 72 h.

C. A sural nerve graft may be used when a gap between the cut ends of the facial nerve precludes primary repair.

D. Injury to the marginal mandibular branch of the facial nerve results in no significant functional sequelae.

E. Gold upper eyelid implants are used sometimes in early reconstruction.

ANSWER: C

COMMENTS: A. *False*. The facial nerve, cranial nerve VII, has five major branches—the frontal/temporal, zygomatic, buccal, marginal mandibular, and cervical. The frontal branch runs just deep to the superficial temporal fascia. The zygomatic, buccal, and marginal mandibular branches run deep to the superficial musculoaponeurotic system after traversing the substance of the parotid gland. The ophthalmic (V1), maxillary (V2), and mandibular (V3) branches are the three major branches of the trigeminal nerve, which supplies sensory innervation to the face.

B. *False*. Repair or identification plus tagging of facial nerve injuries is generally undertaken within the first 72 h following transection. After transection, stimulation of the nerve branches with contraction of the facial muscles occurs for up to 72 to 96 h after the injury, aiding in facial nerve branch identification. Generally, injuries to the zygomatic and buccal branches medial to the lateral canthus are not repaired because of difficulty in identifying these small branches and because of multiple interconnections with cross-innervation, which make the sacrifice of a peripheral branch insignificant most of the time.

C. ***True***. Early reconstruction involves approximation of the cut nerve ends or reconstruction with a nerve graft (usually the sural nerve) to span a defect that cannot be approximated in a tension-free manner. For proximal facial nerve injuries, a cross-face nerve graft to the contralateral facial nerve may be undertaken.

D. *False*. Injury to peripheral branches of the frontal and marginal mandibular branches should be repaired whenever possible because injury results in a significant functional loss. Bell palsy is the most common cause of facial paralysis, followed by facial trauma. Reconstruction for facial paralysis can be divided into early and late reconstruction.

E. *False*. About 18 months after the initial injury, the facial muscles atrophy and lose function. Once this happens, reconstruction with muscle transfers is usually undertaken (e.g., gracilis muscle transfer with or without a cross-face nerve graft). Static reconstructions with gold upper eyelid implants, browlifts, and blepharoplasty are also options for delayed reconstruction.

Ref: 1, 3

9. Which of the following statements regarding frontal sinus fractures is ***true***?

A. Frontal sinus fractures usually occur in isolation as a result of blast injuries.

B. Nondisplaced fractures of the anterior wall of the frontal sinus require operative exploration, mucosal stripping of the sinus, and rigid fixation.

C. Treatment of frontal sinus fractures with significant disruption of the posterior wall and associated cerebrospinal fluid (CSF) leak involves cranialization of the sinus.

D. Anterior wall fractures involving the nasofrontal duct require stenting the nasofrontal duct with a Silastic stent for 2 weeks.

E. Cranialization involves decompressing the sinus into the peri-cavernous lymphatics.

ANSWER: C

COMMENTS: A. *False*. Frontal sinus fractures are usually the result of a high-energy impact. The majority of frontal sinus fractures are associated with other maxillofacial and intracranial injuries. CT is generally used to diagnose frontal sinus fractures. All patients suspected of having a frontal sinus injury should be evaluated for signs of CSF rhinorrhea, which indicates a dural tear. This will clinically present as clear persistent nasal drainage or salty discharge.

B. *False*. Some advocate the observation of nondisplaced or isolated posterior wall fractures without evidence of CSF leak, whereas others advocate exploration of all posterior wall fractures. Antibiotics should be considered in patients with suspected CSF rhinorrhea. Nondisplaced anterior table fractures without posterior table involvement typically do not require operative intervention.

C. ***True***. Treatment of a frontal sinus fracture depends on the number of walls involved, the status of the nasofrontal duct, and the degree of displacement.

D. *False*. Isolated fractures of the anterior wall are treated only if there is considerable displacement or esthetic defect. If the nasofrontal duct is involved in the fracture, the frontal sinus is demucosalized, the nasofrontal duct is plugged with a bone graft or other material, and the sinus is obliterated with cancellous bone or fat. Fractures of the posterior wall raise suspicion for a dural laceration.

E. *False*. For displaced fractures of the posterior wall, a team approach with a neurosurgeon is preferred. If there is a significant loss of the posterior wall, the sinus is cranialized. Cranialization involves removing the posterior wall, plugging the nasofrontal duct with bone graft or other material, demucosalizing the sinus, and replacing the sinus with a pericranial flap.

Ref: 1, 25

10. Which of the following is ***true*** regarding the repair of orbital floor fractures?

A. Cosmetically unacceptable enophthalmos is not an indication for surgical repair.

B. Diplopia is an indication for surgical exploration.

C. Exposure of the orbital floor via a subciliary incision is associated with less risk for lower lid retraction than is exposure via a transconjunctival incision.

D. Marked periorbital swelling is an indication for urgent surgical exploration.

E. Treatment of complex bone fractures take precedence over that of globe injuries.

ANSWER: B

COMMENTS: The diagnosis of an orbital floor fracture is suspected when periorbital ecchymosis and subconjunctival hematoma are present. Patients may also exhibit anesthesia in the sensory distribution of the infraorbital nerve, which lies beneath the orbital floor. Orbital floor fractures may also be manifested as diplopia and enophthalmos. Diplopia may result from the restriction of extraocular movement because of contusion or entrapment of the inferior rectus or inferior oblique muscles in the fracture segment. Enophthalmos, or posterior displacement of the globe, results from increased orbital volume (as the floor is displaced inferiorly) or is caused by disruption of the ligamentous support of the globe. Initial evaluation of a patient with a suspected orbital fracture includes testing for visual acuity, extraocular muscle movement, and pupillary reflexes. A forced duction test whereby the insertion of the inferior rectus is grasped with forceps and manually rotated (after a topical anesthetic is instilled) helps identify extraocular muscle entrapment. If visual acuity is affected or globe rupture is suspected, ophthalmologic consultation is mandatory.

A. *False*. Cosmetically unacceptable enophthalmos is one of the indications for surgical repair.

B. ***True***. The indications for surgical repair of orbital floor fractures include diplopia, entrapment of extraocular muscles, and enophthalmos. Surgery may be performed immediately or delayed until the edema has resolved, usually within a 2- to 3-week period from the time of injury. Exposure is usually achieved with either a transconjunctival incision or subciliary or subtarsal incisions. Subciliary and subtarsal incisions carry a greater risk for lower lid retraction or ectropion. Many materials have been used to reconstruct the orbital floor, including titanium mesh, polyethylene sheets, and bioresorbable mesh.

C. *False*. Exposure of the orbital floor via a subciliary incision is associated with ***a higher*** risk for lower lid retraction than is exposure via a transconjunctival incision.

D. *False*. Marked periorbital swelling is ***not*** an indication for urgent surgical exploration.

E. *False*. Globe injury always takes precedence over bone repair. Fine-cut maxillofacial CT is performed with both axial images and coronal reconstructions to better characterize the nature of the fracture and aid in the identification of an entrapped extraocular muscle.

Ref: 1, 25

G. Hand

1. An 8-year-old child is taken to the emergency department after slamming his right index finger in a door. There is a laceration on the pulp of the finger and a subungual hematoma. A radiograph shows a tuft fracture. Your treatment plan should include which of the following:

A. Leave the laceration open, dress the finger with antibiotic ointment, and place it in a finger splint.

B. Perform a finger block, remove the nail plate, repair any nail bed laceration, and repair the pulp laceration.

C. Use Kirschner wire fixation of the fracture, remove the nail plate, and repair the nail bed.

D. Perform operative exploration with internal fixation of the tuft fracture and repair the nail bed and pulp lacerations.

E. Place the eponychial fold over the nail plate.

ANSWER: B

COMMENTS: A., C., D., and E. *Incorrect.* These choices do not describe the correct treatment plan. Distal phalangeal fractures are among the most common fractures seen in the hand, and of these, tuft fractures are the most common. These fractures are often comminuted and are frequently associated with a nail bed injury.

B. ***Correct.*** Treatment involves removal of the nail plate, irrigation, repair of the nail bed with absorbable suture, replacement of the nail plate under the eponychial fold to prevent scarring or synechiae formation of the fold to the nail plate, and use of a hand or finger splint. If the nail plate is not available, an alternative material can be used to splint the proximal eponychial fold. Such management allows a new nail to grow out from under the eponychial fold. Most of these fractures can be reduced at the time of nail bed repair and protected with a splint for 3 to 4 weeks. Kirschner wire fixation and operative repair are rarely indicated.

Ref: 1, 5

2. Which of the following statements regarding the placement of hand incisions is *true*?

A. Palm incisions should be placed in the skin creases.

B. It is better to err on the volar aspect than on the dorsal aspect when placing incisions on the side of the digit.

C. Incisions on the volar side of the digit must cross the interphalangeal (IP) flexion creases transversely.

D. Dorsal skin incisions should cross skin creases transversely or obliquely.

E. The key principle in planning hand incisions is to maximize motion to avoid contractures.

ANSWER: D

COMMENTS: A. and C. *False.* There are several key principles in planning hand incisions. Oblique incisions connecting these points (Bruner), or volar zigzag incisions, are also an excellent approach that provides full exposure to the entire palmar side of the digit. A line marking the change in character between the dorsal and volar skin of the digit is also a useful landmark.

Those on the palm should run parallel to the skin creases or across them obliquely because the blood supply in this region comes straight upward into the skin. Digital incisions should be placed dorsal to the midlateral line through the midaxial line, which is exactly neutral between flexion and extension. This line is determined by connecting the most dorsal points of the IP joint creases when the finger is in a flexed position.

B. *False.* Given a choice, it is far better to err in placing an incision dorsally than on the volar aspect of the side of the digit because the volar incisions may form a bridging scar.

D. ***True.*** Skin incisions on the dorsum of the hand and digits should cross skin creases transversely, obliquely, or over the mid-dorsum when between joints. In a rheumatoid hand, incisions that cross the skin of the dorsal surface of the wrist should be longitudinal or minimally curved to avoid slough of a distally based flap.

E. *False.* Whenever possible, the incision should be designed along lines that undergo no change in length with motion.

Ref: 1, 5, 27

3. A surgeon is called to examine a 30-year-old painter who cut the palm of his right hand with a dirty razor blade. Examination reveals a 2-cm clean laceration at the base of the long finger. Metacarpophalangeal (MCP) joint flexion is intact, but the patient cannot flex either IP joint in that finger. The injury is 1 h old. What is the diagnosis?

A. Lacerated flexor digitorum superficialis (FDS) tendon

B. Lacerated flexor digitorum profundus (FDP) tendon

C. Combined FDS and FDP laceration

D. Laceration of the intrinsic muscles to the long finger

E. Median nerve transection

ANSWER: C

COMMENTS: A. *Incorrect.* Lacerated FDS tendon would not affect the ability to flex at the distal interphalangeal (DIP) joint.

B. *Incorrect.* Lacerated FDP tendon would not affect the ability to flex at the proximal interphalangeal (PIP) joint.

C. ***Correct.*** The patient's laceration at the base of the long finger is within zone II, where the FDS and FDP are within the same tendon sheath and vulnerable to simultaneous injury. The patient has also lost flexion at both the DIP and PIP joints, demonstrating an injury to both the FDS and FDP tendons.

D. *Incorrect.* This patient is able to flex the MCP of his injured finger, demonstrating that the lumbricals are intact. Injury to other intrinsic muscles of the hand would not result in the loss of IP joint flexion.

E. *Incorrect.* Transection of the median nerve at the hand may result in numbness of the thumb and first two fingers or the loss of thumb adduction and opposition. However, a distal median nerve injury would not result in loss of the IP joints as is seen with a proximal median nerve injury.

Ref: 1, 5, 27

4. The immediate treatment plan for the patient described in Question 345 should include which of the following?

A. Plans for immediate tendon repair (within 6 h) to avoid the hazards of delayed tendon anastomosis

B. Wrist block anesthesia, extension of the skin wound along proper incision lines, and exploration to confirm the diagnosis

C. Careful cleansing and irrigation of the wound, placement of an appropriate dressing or simple sutures, and hand immobilization before definitive primary surgical repair within 2 weeks

D. Cleansing of the wound, primary skin closure, hand immobilization, and outpatient follow-up visits because this injury will require free tendon graft reconstruction 6 weeks after injury

E. Cleansing of the wound, closure, and then physical therapy starting 2 weeks after the injury

ANSWER: C

COMMENTS: A., B., D., and E. *Incorrect.* These choices do not describe the correct treatment plan. Flexion of the MCP joint is a function of the intrinsic muscles and can persist in the face of extrinsic flexor muscle and tendon injury. The goal of flexor tendon repair is the restoration of IP joint flexion. Flexor tendon repair demands meticulous attention to detail and, whenever possible, should be performed by a hand surgeon. The character of the wound, the nature of the injury, the degree of contamination, and the time between injury and definitive treatment determine whether primary or delayed repair is performed.

C. ***Correct.*** Proper wound cleansing, dressing, immobilization, and prophylactic antibiotics allow delay of primary repair if a hand surgeon is not immediately available. The hand should be immobilized in a neutral or slightly flexed position. If there is a question about the degree of contamination or if the initial wound treatment has been delayed beyond several hours thus making primary closure hazardous, delayed repair after 2 to 14 days may be performed. This allows the presence or absence of infection to be clearly established. Many experts believe that this type of delay does not significantly alter the ultimate outcome of the repair.

Tendon injuries with grossly contaminated wounds, those with significant tendon loss, or wounds with significant associated injuries to the soft tissue, bone, nerve, or blood vessels should be treated by secondary repair in 3 to 6 weeks—after the wounds have stabilized, the infection has cleared, and edema formation has subsided.

Ref: 1, 5, 27

5. Which of the following statements regarding the most common metacarpal fractures is true?

A. They are commonly known as Bennett fractures.

B. They are commonly known as boxer's fractures.

C. They most often involve the distal metacarpal of the index and long fingers.

D. Physical examination is the most effective means of assessing the degree of angulation.

E. They usually require open reduction and internal fixation.

ANSWER: B

COMMENTS: A. *False.* A Bennett fracture is a fracture at the base of the thumb metacarpal and not the most common metacarpal fracture.

B. ***True.*** Metacarpal fractures commonly result from hitting an object with a clenched fist. They usually involve the distal metacarpal of the fifth and occasionally the fourth fingers and are known as "boxer's fractures." The metacarpal head is displaced palmward, and pain, swelling, and some loss of knuckle prominence are the usual physical findings. Associated lacerations should be treated as human bites until proved otherwise, and early exploration, with the administration of intravenous antibiotics, is recommended.

D. *False.* Physical examination would not be sufficient to evaluate the injury because swelling usually masks the degree of angulation. A lateral radiograph is needed for accurate evaluation. Each finger should be individually flexed to the palm to assess the degree of rotational deformity. During flexion, the fingers normally point to the scaphoid tubercle. Deviation from this alignment allows estimation of the rotational deformity.

E. *False.* The usual treatment is closed reduction followed by immobilization of the involved and adjacent digits, with the MCP joint placed in 65 to 90 degrees of flexion and the IP joints placed in full extension in the intrinsic plus position.

Unstable or multiple metacarpal fractures often require open reduction and internal fixation. Metacarpal shaft fractures require reduction and immobilization. Percutaneous Kirschner wires or a plate and screws for internal fixation are frequently required if the fracture is unstable, particularly if the fracture is oblique or comminuted.

Ref: 1, 5, 27, 28

6. Which of the following statements regarding tenosynovitis is ***true***?

A. Infections of the flexor sheath of the little finger more often extend to the thumb than to the adjacent ring finger.

B. A flexor tendon sheath infection causes the involved finger to assume a position of mild extension at all joints.

C. The involved digit is rarely swollen and often exhibits little pain.

D. By definition, deep palmar space infections involve the flexor tendons.

E. Because of potential for contracture, conservative management without drainage is contraindicated.

ANSWER: A

COMMENTS: A. ***True.*** The flexor sheath of the little finger communicates with the ulnar bursa. The flexor sheath of flexor pollicis longus communicates with the radial bursa. An infection in the ulnar bursa and radial bursa at the level of the wrist can lead to a "horseshoe" abscess involving both radial and ulnar bursae.

B. and C. *False.* The cardinal signs of suppurative flexor tenosynovitis are known as Kanavel's signs. These include fusiform swelling of the digit, digit held in mid-flexed position, severe pain with passive extension of the digit, and tenderness along the entire flexor tendon sheath. Pain with passive extension of the digit is considered the most sensitive sign for flexor tenosynovitis.

D. *False.* In the palm, the deep spaces are divided into the thenar space and the midpalmar space at the level of the third metacarpal, where a vertical septum extends between the metacarpal and sheath of the long finger flexor tendons. Infection here is manifested as localized, tender swelling and must be drained with an appropriate incision.

E. *False.* Infection of the synovial sheaths of the flexor tendons is a serious problem that requires prompt appropriate treatment including proper drainage and antibiotics. The tendons are relatively avascular and are characterized by poor natural resistance to infection. This may be compounded in patients with diabetes mellitus or in those who are immunocompromised.

Ref: 1, 5 27, 28

7. Which of the following statements regarding replantation of the hand is ***false***?

A. Single digits (other than the thumb) are uncommonly replanted except in children.

B. The amputated part may tolerate cool ischemia for up to 24 h if there is no significant avascular muscle mass.

C. Bleeding from the proximal part is ideally treated with pressure rather than with clamping.

D. A history of heavy smoking, diabetes mellitus, hypertension, and Raynaud phenomenon are relative contraindications to replantation.

E. Replantation above the elbow is contraindicated.

ANSWER: E

COMMENTS: A. *True*. Replantation is a highly specialized procedure that is best performed by a team of replantation surgeons. Single digits are less frequently replanted, except in children or if there is a sharp noncrushing cut at the level of the middle phalanx distal to the splitting of the superficialis tendon.

The hand and thumb are always considered for replantation unless definite contraindications exist or the extremity was not properly preserved. The thumb is the most important digit, and as much of its length as possible should be preserved. An index finger amputated proximal to the PIP joint loses its ability to pinch, and the brain naturally switches the pinching to the long finger. Attempts to preserve length distal to the PIP joint should be made, but if the digit is painful, is insensate, or "gets in the way," the patient may best be served by transection through the metacarpal (ray amputation) because the long finger can assume the role of primary pinch. Loss of little finger length proximal to the PIP joint may also best be treated by ray amputation.

B. *True*. Distal amputations properly cooled immediately after injury may be viable for up to 24 h. Central finger amputations (long and ring fingers) near the MCP joint can cause bothersome spaces in the clenched fist that can be treated by transfer of the adjacent peripheral finger with its metacarpal to fill the space.

C. *True*. Bleeding should be controlled with pressure. Clamping or ligating the bleeding vessels should not be attempted.

D. *True*. Relative contraindications to replantation include medically unstable patients (i.e., history of smoking, diabetes mellitus, and hypertension), prolonged ischemia time with avascular muscle mass, and tissue contamination.

E. ***False***. Amputations above the elbow are considered for replantation (particularly in children) because even partial success can convert an above-elbow to a below-elbow stump for future rehabilitation. Guillotine amputations are the injuries that are most favorable for replantation.

Ref: 1, 5, 27

8. Which of the following statements regarding peripheral nerve injury is ***false***?

A. Nerve repair is progressively less effective if delayed beyond 2 months after surgery.

B. Nerve repair is best performed under 4 to 15 times magnification.

C. Nerve repair is best performed in a fashion that minimizes tension across the repair.

D. Regeneration may be followed clinically by observing the distal progression of the Tinel sign.

E. The use of conduits can assist in nerve regeneration.

ANSWER: A

COMMENTS: A. ***False***. Nerve injuries do not need to be repaired at the time of injury, but it is believed that the results are progressively worse if the repair is delayed beyond 6 months, when the distal nerve tubules have contracted and the new axons can no longer grow distally. Occasionally, repair delayed for up to 2 years has been successful, particularly in children.

B. and C. *True*. Nerve injuries result from stretching or compression (neurapraxia) or from transection. Neurapraxic injuries carry a better prognosis than do transection injuries. Most surgeons perform a careful epineural repair at 4 to 15 times magnification with minimal tension. However, repair of the individual fascicular bundle may be required in large, mixed peripheral nerves. Recovery after repair begins with the return of function starting proximally. Regenerating axons grow down the distal nerve sheath at the rate of approximately 1 mm/day.

D. *True*. Distal progression of the Tinel sign (tingling felt after percussion over the growing nerve) usually follows the start of regeneration.

E. *True*. Recently, successful nerve regeneration with healing has been achieved with vein grafts, synthetic tubes, and cadaver allograft, which act as conduits for nerve growth across the repair.

Ref: 1, 27, 28

9. A 70-year-old mechanic sustains a "pinching" amputation when his dominant long finger is caught between a garage door pulley and the belt. There is loss of the volar two-thirds of the pulp skin, along with exposed subcutaneous tissue. Select the most appropriate reconstruction:

A. Sterile dressing changes with topical antibiotics and closure by contracture and epithelialization

B. Full-thickness hypothenar skin graft

C. STSG

D. V-Y advancement flap

E. Replantation

ANSWER: B

COMMENTS: A. *Incorrect*. Sterile dressing changes with topical antibiotics and closure by contracture and epithelialization would not be appropriate to reconstruct this defect.

B. ***Correct***. In this particular case, a hypothenar skin graft is best. It provides glabrous skin (the unique non–hair-bearing skin found on the volar aspect of the digits and palms, as well as the soles), which matches the other digits and resists contracture and hypersensitivity. Sensibility, an important factor with all hand grafts, is similar to that achieved with flaps.

Fingertip amputation is one of the most common hand injuries. The mechanism of injury; the orientation and location of the amputation; and the age, gender, general condition, and hand dominance of the patient are integral to decision making and planning of the reconstruction. Reconstructions that require prolonged immobilization in "unsafe" positions, such as a thenar flap or a cross-finger flap, are not recommended in older individuals due to the risk of immobilization. If properly cared for and free of crush-avulsion injury, the amputated part can be defatted, meticulously sutured back, and used for a salvage procedure.

C. *Incorrect.* An STSG would be too thin, and allowing the wound to heal by contracture and epithelialization is a good option when there is only soft tissue loss, but the orientation should be such that the tissues can contract to cover the defect. The broad surface area described here would not be satisfactory for this method of healing.

D. *Incorrect.* The V-Y advancement flap is best used with straight transverse amputations.

E. *Incorrect.* Microvascular replantations have been successful even as far distal as the mid-nail but are not generally performed for fingertip injuries.

Ref: 1, 5, 27

10. Which of the following statements is ***false***?

A. Jersey finger refers to an intraarticular fracture of the DIP joint.

B. Mallet finger results from traumatic avulsion of the extensor tendon insertion into the distal phalanx.

C. Skier's (ski pole injury) thumb results from disruption of the ulnar collateral ligament at the thumb MCP joint.

D. Kienböck disease refers to idiopathic lunatomalacia.

E. Rolando and Bennett fractures are fractures of the base of the thumb metacarpal.

ANSWER: A

COMMENTS: A. ***False.*** There are numerous common names for disorders of the hand. Understanding the cause of the disorder sheds light on the common name. Jersey finger refers to a traumatic avulsion of the FDP at the DIP level. It is an injury sustained most commonly by rugby and football players as the tendon avulses from the bone with forceful gripping, such as when grabbing a jersey most commonly affecting the ring digit.

B. *True.* Mallet finger is the extensor counterpart of jersey finger and is a traumatic disruption of the extensor mechanism at its insertion into the distal phalanx that is usually caused by forced flexion at the joint, such as the one that occurs when "jamming" one's long finger while catching a softball. Injuries to the extensor insertion into the dorsum of the distal phalanx result in the mallet deformity. Frequently, no fracture can be seen.

If such an injury is associated with no fracture or is associated with a fracture and the fragment is small, dorsal splinting with the joint in 0 to 10 degrees of hyperextension for 6 to 8 weeks provides good results. If more than one-third of the articular surface is displaced with the avulsed tendon and volar subluxation of the distal phalanx occurs, open reduction plus internal fixation is advised.

A boutonnière deformity results from disruption of the central extensor tendon at its insertion into the dorsum of the base of the middle phalanx. Immobilization of the PIP joint at zero degrees of extension with dynamic extension splinting for 6 to 8 weeks is recommended whenever possible. The name gamekeeper's thumb is derived from Scottish gamekeepers' practice of breaking the necks of rabbits by twisting their necks. The repetitive trauma of this type tended to weaken the ulnar collateral ligament of the thumb and cause both pain and laxity of the thumb at the MCP joint in this area.

C. *True.* Skier's (ski pole injury) thumb is specifically an acute traumatic avulsion of the ulnar collateral ligament, although gamekeeper's thumb is sometimes used incorrectly to describe this situation.

D. *True.* Robert Kienböck, an Austrian professor of radiology, was the first to describe a syndrome of idiopathic lunatomalacia in 1910—Kienböck disease. It is most commonly manifested as a stiff, painful, and weak wrist in a young adult male.

E. *True.* A Bennett fracture is a fracture at the base of the thumb metacarpal. It is inherently unstable, but its management tends to be less complicated and its prognosis much better than that of a Rolando fracture. The latter is a comminuted, intraarticular fracture at the base of the thumb metacarpal that exhibits a T or Y fracture pattern in which the articular surface is split at the base of the first metacarpal.

Ref: 1, 5

REFERENCES

1. Townsend CM, Beauchamp RD, Evers BM, et al. *Sabiston Textbook of Surgery: The Biological Basis of Modern Surgical Practice.* 19th ed. Philadelphia: Saunders; 2012.
2. Mulholland MW, Greenfield LJ. *Greenfield's Surgery: Scientific Principles & Practice.* 5th ed. Philadelphia, PA: Wolters Kluwer/Lippincott Williams & Wilkins; 2010.
3. Losee JE, Gimbel M, Rubin JP, et al. Plastic and reconstructive surgery. In: Brunicardi FC, Andersen DK, Billiar TR, et al., eds. *Schwartz's Principles of Surgery.* 9th ed. New York: McGraw-Hill; 2010.
4. Senchenkov A, Valerio IL, Manders EK. Grafts. In: Guyuron B, Eriksson E, Persing JA, et al., eds. *Plastic Surgery: Indications and Practice.* Philadelphia: WB Saunders; 2009.
5. Thorne CH. Techniques and principles in plastic surgery. In: Thorne CH, Beasley RW, Aston SJ, et al., eds. *Grabb and Smith's Plastic Surgery.* 6th ed. Philadelphia: Lippincott Williams & Wilkins; 2007.
6. Shaw WW, Hidalgo DA, eds. *Microsurgery in Trauma.* Mount Kisco, NY: Futura; 1987.
7. Agnese DM, Povoski SP, Souba WW. Benign breast disease. In: Ashley SW, Barie PS, Cance WG, et al., eds. *ACS Surgery: Principles & Practice.* New York: WebMD; 2007.
8. Kwei SL, Weiss DD, Pribaz JJ. Microsurgery and free flaps. In: Guyuron B, Eriksson E, Persing JA, et al., eds. *Plastic Surgery: Indications and Practice.* Philadelphia: WB Saunders; 2009.
9. Bui DT, Cordeiro PG, Hu QY, et al. Free flap reexploration: indications, treatment, and outcomes in 1193 free flaps. *Plast Reconstr Surg.* 2007;119:2092–2100.
10. Trussler AP, Rohrich RJ. Blepharoplasty. *Plast Reconstr Surg.* 2008;121:1–10.
11. Norris RL, Auerbach PS, Nelson EE. Bites and stings. In: Townsend Jr CM, Beauchamp RD, Evers BM, et al., eds. *Sabiston Textbook of Surgery: The Biological Basis of Modern Surgical Practice.* 18th ed. Philadelphia: WB Saunders; 2008.
12. Sullivan SR, Engrav LH, Klein MB. Acute wound care. In: Ashley SW, Barie PS, Cance WG, et al., eds. *ACS Surgery: Principles & Practice.* New York: WebMD; 2007.
13. Anaya DA, Dellinger EP. Surgical infections and choice of antibiotics. In: Townsend Jr CM, Beauchamp RD, Evers BM, et al., eds. *Sabiston Textbook of Surgery: The Biological Basis of Modern Surgical Practice.* 18th ed. Philadelphia: WB Saunders; 2008.
14. Manahan MA, Milner SM, Freeswick P, et al. Necrotizing skin and soft tissue infections. In: Cameron JL, ed. *Current Surgical Therapy.* 9th ed. Philadelphia: CV Mosby; 2008.
15. Malangoni MA, McHenry CR. Soft tissue infection. In: Ashley SW, Barie PS, Cance WG, et al., eds. *ACS Surgery: Principles & Practice.* New York: WebMD; 2007.
16. Anaya DA. Necrotizing soft-tissue infection: diagnosis and management. *Clin Infect Dis.* 2016;44(5):705–710.
17. Disa JJ, Halvorson EG, Hidalgo DA. Open wound requiring reconstruction. In: Ashley SW, Barie PS, Cance WG, et al., eds. *ACS Surgery: Principles & Practice.* New York: WebMD; 2007.
18. Argenta LC, Morykwas MJ, Mark MW, et al. Vacuum-assisted closure: state of clinic art. *Plast Reconstr Surg.* 2006;117(suppl 7):127S–142S.
19. V.A.C. Therapy Clinical Guidelines: a reference source for clinicians (July 2007).
20. Agnese DM, Povoski SP, Souba WW. Benign breast disease. In: Ashley SW, Barie PS, Cance WG, et al., eds. *ACS Surgery: Principles & Practice.* New York: WebMD; 2007.

21. Khosla RK. Augmentation mammoplasty. In: Kenkel JM, ed. *Selected Readings in Plastic Surgery, Inc*. Texas; 2008.
22. U.S. Food and Drug Administration. Breast implant questions & answers. Available at: http://www.fda.gov/MedicalDevices/ProductsandMedicalProcedures/ImplantsandProsthetics/BreastImplants/UCM063719.
23. Saggi BH, Ivatury R, Sugerman HJ. *Surgical Treatment: Evidence-Based and Problem-Oriented.* Munich: Zuckschwerdt; 2001.
24. Felemovicius J, Taylor JA. Midface hypophasic and the Le Fort I osteotomy in cleft lip and palate patients: a classification scheme and treatment protocol. *Cleft Palate Craniofac J*. 2009;46(6):613–620.
25. Manson PN. Facial injuries. In: Cameron JL, ed. *Current Surgical Therapy*. 9th ed. Philadelphia: CV Mosby; 2008.
26. Malard O, Corre P. Surgical repair of labial defect. *Eur Ann Otorhinolaryngol, Head Neck Dis*. 2010;127(2):49–62.
27. Boyer MI, Taras JS, Kaufmann RA. Flexor tendon injuries. In: Green DP, Hotchkiss RN, Pederson WC, et al., eds. *Green's Operative Hand Surgery*. 5th ed. Philadelphia: Churchill-Livingstone; 2005.
28. Jobe MT, Calandruccio JH. In: Canale ST, ed. *Campbell's Operative Orthopaedics*. 10th ed. St. Louis: CV Mosby; 2003.

SECTION IX

PRACTICE OF SURGERY

CHAPTER 33

SPECIAL CONSIDERATIONS IN SURGERY: PREGNANT, GERIATRIC, AND IMMUNOCOMPROMISED PATIENTS

Michelle A. Kominiarek, M.D., and Edward F. Hollinger, M.D., Ph.D.

1. A 22-year-old woman who is 8 weeks pregnant arrives at the emergency department with persistent nausea and vomiting. She has not been able to tolerate any liquids for the past 3 days. On physical examination, she is afebrile, her pulse is 110 beats/min, and her blood pressure is 120/70 mmHg. Her abdomen is soft, nontender, and nondistended. Moderate ketones are found on urinalysis. The next step in her evaluation includes:

A. Intravenous hydration

B. Liver function tests

C. Right upper quadrant ultrasound

D. Parenteral nutrition

E. Abdominal computed tomography (CT)

ANSWER: A

COMMENTS: See Question 3.

Ref.: 1–3

2. The differential diagnosis of nausea and vomiting in pregnancy includes all of the following except:

A. Appendicitis

B. Pyelonephritis

C. Diabetic ketoacidosis

D. Drug toxicity

E. Renal insufficiency

ANSWER: E

COMMENTS: See Question 3.

Ref.: 1–3

3. What is the first-line medication for the treatment of nausea and vomiting in pregnancy?

A. Ondansetron

B. Doxylamine and vitamin B_6

C. Metoclopramide

D. Diphenhydramine

E. Prochlorperazine

ANSWER: B

COMMENTS: Approximately 70%–85% of pregnant women experience nausea and vomiting of varying intensity and for various lengths of time in pregnancy. Symptoms usually start 5 to 6 weeks after the last menstrual period. The severity and frequency of symptoms generally peak at approximately 9 weeks and then begin to subside. The diagnosis of **nausea and vomiting of pregnancy** (NVP) can be difficult to make in early pregnancy because many other conditions can cause nausea and vomiting. An important distinguishing feature of NVP is that it usually begins before 10 weeks' gestation. Nausea and vomiting that begin after 10 weeks are most likely caused by a different etiology. The differential diagnosis includes gastroenteritis, gastroparesis, diabetic ketoacidosis, achalasia, biliary tract disease, hepatitis, intestinal obstruction, peptic ulcer disease, pancreatitis, and appendicitis. Mildly elevated liver enzymes (usually <300 U/L) and serum bilirubin (<4 mg/dL) are encountered in 20%–30% of pregnant women. Similarly, high serum concentrations of amylase and lipase (up to five times higher than normal levels) are seen in 10%–15% of women with NVP.

The first-line treatment of NVP consists of conservative measures (dietary modifications and vitamin supplementation) along with patient reassurance. Medications effective in reducing nausea and vomiting without an increased risk for teratogenicity include antihistamines, hydroxyzine, meclizine, dopamine antagonists (chlorpromazine, metoclopramide, perphenazine, prochlorperazine, promethazine, trifluoperazine, trimethobenzamide), and pyridoxine. Treatment of NVP with 10 mg vitamin B_6 or 10 mg vitamin B_6 plus 10 mg doxylamine (Diclegis ®) is safe and effective and should be considered the first-line pharmacotherapy. The U.S. Food and Drug Administration (FDA) approved doxylamine–vitamin B_6 in 2013 in the United States for treatment of NVP in women who do not respond to dietary and lifestyle changes. A multicenter randomized controlled trial of doxylamine and pyridoxine for NVP found that a delayed-release formulation of doxylamine and pyridoxine significantly improved NVP compared with placebo. Patients with severe dehydration should be admitted to the hospital and treated with isotonic crystalloid solutions that contain glucose and supplemental potassium chloride.

Ref.: 4, 5

4. A surgical consultation is requested on a patient who had a cesarean delivery 5 days earlier. On examination, her Pfannenstiel incision shows separated skin and subcutaneous tissue with an intact fascia. There are no signs of infection, and the probable diagnosis is a seroma. The next step in management is:

   A. Open the fascia.
   B. Close the wound with interrupted sutures immediately.
   C. Place a vacuum-assisted closure device.
   D. Instruct the patient on wet-to-dry dressing changes with iodine solution.
   E. Debride the fascia and subcutaneous tissues.

ANSWER: C

COMMENTS: In the United States, more than 30% of all deliveries are by cesarean delivery. Disruption of the skin incision is a major source of postoperative morbidity after cesarean delivery and occurs after 2.5%–16% of procedures. **Pfannenstiel incisions** are the most common transverse incisions used in obstetrics and gynecology. **Hematomas** and **seromas**, common problems after cesarean delivery, require the manual opening of the wounds to allow drainage and proper healing. An open wound can be managed in three ways: secondary closure, secondary intention with serial dressing changes, and secondary intention using negative pressure wound therapy. **Secondary closure** can be performed once a wound is free of infection or necrotic tissue and has started to granulate. This procedure, which may be performed at the bedside with the patient under local anesthesia or sedation (or both), is performed within 1 to 4 days after the wound separates or the hematoma or seroma is evacuated. **Negative pressure wound therapy**, also known as vacuum-assisted closure, received FDA approval in 1995. In this system, controlled levels of negative pressure help accelerate wound healing by evacuating localized edema. Negative pressure treatment results in faster healing times with fewer associated complications and can be used for noninfected wounds. If **a wet-to-dry approach** is used, the solution should be nontoxic in as much as studies have shown that povidone-iodine, iodophor gauze, and hydrogen peroxide are cytotoxic to white blood cells (WBCs) and other vital wound-healing components. Use of these products can delay wound healing.

Ref.: 6

5. Which of the following measures has been shown to decrease wound complications in women with a subcutaneous thickness > 2 cm?

   A. Subcutaneous drain
   B. Irrigation of the subcutaneous tissue with an antibiotic solution
   C. Closure of the subcutaneous tissue
   D. Supplemental oxygen
   E. Skin closure with staples

ANSWER: C

COMMENTS: Risk factors for **wound breakdown** after cesarean section include prolonged duration of surgery, obesity, diabetes, patient age, coincident infection, and poor nutrition. **Obesity** increases the risk probably as a result of the poor vascularity of subcutaneous fat and the propensity for serous fluid collections and hematoma formation. Suture closure of subcutaneous fat during cesarean delivery results in a 34% decrease in the risk of wound disruption in women with the fat thickness greater than 2 cm. Other methods (antibiotic solutions, subcutaneous drains) have not been shown to be effective in preventing wound complications. The explanation for the difference in **diabetic wound healing** is complex but is probably related to alterations in the inflammatory response and differences in enzyme secretion and growth factor production. Recommendations to improve wound healing in diabetics are to avoid hyperglycemia and regulate insulin doses. **Corticosteroids** increase the risk of infection by suppressing inflammation, inhibiting leukocyte function, slowing wound contraction, decreasing collagen matrix deposition, and delaying epithelialization. **Chorioamnionitis** is an infection of the membranes (chorion, amnion) surrounding the fetus. The presence of chorioamnionitis increases the risk of wound infection tenfold. Preterm labor is not a risk factor for impaired wound healing.

Ref.: 6–8

6. A 32-year-old gravida 4 who is 29 weeks pregnant reports left leg pain and swelling for 3 days. A diagnosis of deep venous thrombosis (DVT) is suspected. What is the most appropriate test to diagnose DVT during pregnancy?

   A. D dimer
   B. Contrast-enhanced venography
   C. Impedance plethysmography
   D. Compression duplex ultrasound
   E. Spiral CT of the chest

ANSWER: D

COMMENTS: There is a predisposition for **DVT** to occur in the left leg (approximately 70%–90% of cases). This is probably attributed to an exacerbation of the compressive effects of the uterus on the left iliac vein because of it being crossed by the right iliac artery. Clinical suspicion is critical for the diagnosis of DVT. However, many of the classic signs and symptoms of DVT and pulmonary embolism, such as leg swelling, tachycardia, tachypnea, and dyspnea, may be associated with a normal pregnancy. In nonpregnant patients, **D-dimer levels** have a high negative predictive value and can reliably exclude the diagnosis of DVT. However, in pregnancy, the D-dimer level gradually increases, and therefore its value is not reliable in the evaluation of DVT. **Contrast-enhanced venography** should not be used in pregnant patients because it is invasive and involves a high radiation dose. Although **impedance plethysmography** has been evaluated in pregnancy and has proven accuracy in excluding DVT, it has been replaced by **duplex ultrasound** because of its higher sensitivity and specificity and wider availability.

Ref.: 9

7. Venous thromboembolism occurs four times more often in pregnant patients than in the general population. Physiologic changes that occur during pregnancy include:

   A. Decreased fibrin generation
   B. Increased fibrinolytic activity
   C. Decreased levels of coagulation factors II, VII, VIII, and X
   D. Resistance to activated protein C
   E. Improved venous flow velocity

ANSWER: D

COMMENTS: Pregnancy is classically believed to be a **hypercoagulable state**. Fibrin production is increased; fibrinolytic activity is decreased; levels of coagulation factors II, VII, VIII, and X are all increased; free protein S levels are decreased; and acquired resistance to activated protein C is common. These physiologic changes, including increased markers of coagulation activation such as prothrombin fragment and D dimer, occur in all pregnancies. In addition, a 50% reduction in venous flow velocity occurs in the legs by 25 to 29 weeks of gestation and lasts until approximately 6 weeks after delivery.

Ref.: 10

8. The best treatment of acute venous thromboembolism in pregnancy is:
   - A. Warfarin
   - B. Low-molecular-weight heparin
   - C. Unfractionated heparin bridge to a therapeutic international normalized ratio with warfarin
   - D. Aspirin
   - E. Vena cava filter

ANSWER: B

COMMENTS: Treatment and prophylaxis of **DVT** in pregnancy center on the use of unfractionated heparin or low-molecular-weight heparin because of the teratogenicity associated with **warfarin**, which is known to cross the placenta. **Warfarin-induced embryopathy** is characterized by fetal midface hypoplasia, stippled chondral calcifications, scoliosis, short proximal limbs, and short phalanges. It occurs in 5% of fetuses exposed to the drug between 6 and 9 weeks of gestation. Because neither **unfractionated heparin** nor **low-molecular-weight heparin** crosses the placenta in a significant amount, there is no possibility of teratogenesis or fetal hemorrhage with these medications. The use of retrievable **vena cava filters** should be considered only for patients in whom anticoagulation is contraindicated or in whom extensive DVT develops 2 weeks before delivery.

Ref.: 10, 11

9. Which of the following is true about appendicitis complicating pregnancy?
   - A. Delayed diagnosis is most likely to occur in the first trimester.
   - B. The presence of pyuria suggests a urinary tract infection rather than appendicitis as a cause for abdominal pain.
   - C. If a pregnant patient presents with perforation and peritonitis, the fetal loss rate is more than 50%.
   - D. Appendicitis complicates 1% of pregnancies.
   - E. Pregnant women with appendicitis present with perforation in more than 40% of cases.

ANSWER: E

COMMENTS: **Appendicitis** is the most common nonobstetric cause of acute abdominal pain leading to exploratory laparotomy. It occurs in 1 in 1500 pregnancies. **Urinary tract problems** are often the initial diagnosis because up to 20% of pregnant patients with appendicitis have pyuria, hematuria, or both. If a perforation or peritonitis occurs, the **fetal loss rate** is 10%–35% because of preterm labor and fetal demise. Preterm labor usually occurs within 5 days of the perforation. **Delayed diagnosis** is more likely to occur in the second (18%) and third (75%) trimesters. **Perforation rates** as high as 55% in pregnant patients have been reported, as opposed to 4%–19% in the general population.

Ref.: 12

10. For the evaluation of appendicitis, an abdominal CT with oral and intravenous contrast is typically NOT the first-line imaging modality in pregnancy and lactation because of:
    - A. Fetal risks due to oral contrast
    - B. Fetal risks due to intravenous contrast
    - C. Excretion of intravenous contrast into breast milk
    - D. Higher radiation exposure than magnetic resonance imaging (MRI) or ultrasound
    - E. Higher rates of nonvisualization of the appendix compared with ultrasound

ANSWER: D

COMMENTS: **Ultrasonography** with a graded compression technique is the imaging modality of choice in pregnant patients with right lower quadrant pain because of its availability and lack of ionizing radiation. This approach has some limitations. **Graded compression ultrasound** may not be feasible because of the size of the enlarged gravid uterus, particularly in the third trimester. Furthermore, a normal appendix is visualized in only 13%–50% of patients who are not pregnant. The negative predictive value of a nonvisualized appendix is, at best, 90%. Consequently, if the appendix is not visualized and no other cause of the pain can be found, further evaluation is warranted. **CT**, which is often the modality of choice in the evaluation of acute appendicitis in patients who are not pregnant, delivers an estimated radiation dose as high as 30 mGy (3 rad) to the uterus with conventional protocols. Oral contrast agents are not absorbed and are not associated with any maternal or fetal risks. Iodinated media is the most common form of intravenous contrast for CT studies. Although it can cross the placenta and enter the amniotic fluid, no studies have shown that it increases maternal or fetal risk. Less than 1% of iodinated contrast is excreted into breast milk; less than 1% of this amount is absorbed through the gastrointestinal track of an infant. As such, it is recommended to continue breastfeeding after receiving iodinated contrast. A **barium enema** is also associated with significant radiation exposure and has generally been supplanted by other imaging tests for the evaluation of acute appendicitis. MRI can be performed during pregnancy and is often preferred over ultrasound because the rates of nonvisualization are lower. Gadolinium use during pregnancy should be limited and used only if it improves the diagnostic performance of the test and ultimately improves fetal and maternal outcomes.

Ref.: 12–16

11. A 34-year-old woman pregnant with twins at 26 weeks' gestation presents with abdominal pain and low-grade fevers. Labs are remarkable for leukocytosis (13×10^3 cells/mm^3) and mild anemia. The urinalysis shows hematuria, but the urine culture is negative. Which of the following is true?
    - A. An appendectomy during pregnancy increases the risk for congenital malformations and stillbirth.

B. Hematuria is a normal finding during pregnancy.
C. Negative laparotomy rates of up to 35% are considered acceptable in the pregnant population when appendicitis is suspected.
D. To decrease the risk for congenital malformations, antibiotics should not be given to pregnant patients.
E. Laparoscopic appendectomy is contraindicated during pregnancy.

ANSWER: C

COMMENTS: In pregnancy, an elevated leukocyte count is normal (9–15 × 10^3 cells/mm^3). In most cases, there is a gradual upward displacement of the appendix as the pregnancy progresses; however, some more recent studies suggest that there is no change in the location of the appendix during pregnancy. Hemoglobin levels decrease during pregnancy, and hematuria is not a normal finding in a pregnant patient. An appendectomy does not increase the risk for stillbirth or congenital malformations. A higher negative laparotomy rate (up to 35%) is acceptable in the pregnant population (15% for the nonpregnant population) because of the serious consequences of delayed diagnosis. Perioperative antibiotics are appropriate in the pregnant population but should be tailored to the use of antibiotics with minimal risk for birth defects. A laparoscopic approach during pregnancy is appropriate in most gestations of less than 24 weeks.

Ref.: 1, 12, 13

12. A 39-year-old gravida 3 para 2 at 32 weeks' gestation is evaluated for a 3-day history of nausea, vomiting, and anorexia. She also reports abdominal pain, primarily located in the right upper quadrant and epigastric areas. Her blood pressure is 120/60 mmHg with a pulse of 110 beats/min and a temperature of 98.6°F. After completing the physical examination, the diagnosis of cholelithiasis is suggested. Which of the following conditions must also be considered in the differential diagnosis?

A. Acute fatty liver of pregnancy (AFLP)
B. Syndrome of hemolysis, elevated liver enzymes, and low platelets (HELLP)
C. Appendicitis
D. Pyelonephritis
E. All of the above

ANSWER: E

COMMENTS: See Question 13.

Ref.: 1, 12, 17

13. The patient's pain improves with nonoperative management, including intravenous hydration, bowel rest, and analgesics. Her liver function tests, amylase, and lipase are normal. A right upper quadrant ultrasound confirms cholelithiasis without evidence of cholecystitis or obstruction. What is the safest plan for her management?

A. Laparoscopic cholecystectomy during this admission
B. Endoscopic retrograde cholangiopancreatography (ERCP)
C. Supportive care, plan for postpartum cholecystectomy
D. Induction of labor followed by postpartum cholecystectomy
E. Open cholecystectomy during this admission

ANSWER: C

COMMENTS: Biliary tract diseases are the second most common gastrointestinal disorders that require surgery during pregnancy. Pregnancy predisposes to gallstone formation because of increased bile lithogenicity and decreased gallbladder contractility caused by the effects of progesterone. Gallstones occur in approximately 3%–12% of pregnant women, but most patients are asymptomatic. The incidence of **acute cholecystitis** is 1 to 8 per 10,000 pregnancies. Early surgery is recommended to avoid biliary complications because recurrent symptoms are common during pregnancy. **Cholecystectomy** should be deferred until the **second trimester** whenever possible. The rationale behind this recommendation is an increased rate of fetal loss with surgery in the first trimester and a greater risk for preterm labor during the third trimester. When symptoms are mild or the patient is in the third trimester, cholecystectomy can often be delayed until after delivery. An operation may need to be performed early for patients with gallstone pancreatitis, choledocholithiasis, or unresolving acute cholecystitis, regardless of gestational age.

Ref.: 1, 12, 17

14. When performing laparoscopic surgery in a pregnant patient, which of the following is recommended?

A. Antibiotic prophylaxis with a fluoroquinolone (e.g., levofloxacin)
B. Right lateral decubitus positioning
C. Limiting carbon dioxide pneumoperitoneum to 12 mmHg for laparoscopy
D. Using an umbilical entry site for laparoscopy for gestational ages beyond 24 weeks
E. Performing open rather than laparoscopic procedures after 24 weeks' gestation

ANSWER: C

COMMENTS: The major general consideration when performing abdominal surgery on a pregnant woman is to maintain adequate perfusion to the uterus and fetus and decrease maternal risks. To improve venous return, the patient should always be placed in a slight left lateral position. One should also use caution with a Veress needle because the gravid uterus is located closer and closer to the umbilical site with increasing gestational age. Accordingly, one may consider a **left upper quadrant entry** (**Palmer point**) at the midclavicular line 1 to 2 cm below the costal margin, open (Hassan) entry techniques, or placing the trocars under direct visualization. Carbon dioxide pneumoperitoneum should be **limited to 12 mmHg**. During laparotomy, retractors should not come in contact with the uterus because this could lead to uterine irritability and preterm labor.

Ref.: 1, 12, 17

15. A 17-year-old gravida 1 at 25 weeks' gestation is brought to the emergency department after a motor vehicle accident with direct abdominal trauma. She complains of abdominal pain. Initial management should include all of the following except:

A. Establishment of the airway
B. Maintenance of oxygenation
C. Fluid resuscitation
D. Administration of corticosteroids for fetal lung maturity
E. Left lateral displacement of the uterus

ANSWER: D

COMMENTS: Management of a **pregnant trauma patient** parallels that of a nonpregnant patient—the initial evaluation includes the establishment of the airway, maintenance of oxygenation, and fluid resuscitation. Because the gravid uterus can compress the inferior vena cava in the supine position in the late second and third trimesters, turning the patient to the left side can displace the uterus and increase cardiac output up to 30%. Although this maneuver contradicts the principle of maintaining the patient in a supine position, spinal stabilization precautions can still be taken. For example, the patient may be transported in the left lateral decubitus position or the backboard rotated to the right. Early and rapid fluid resuscitation is important even in a pregnant patient who is normotensive. Corticosteroids are important for fetal lung maturation in the event of preterm delivery; however, they can be administered after the patient is stabilized.

Ref.: 1

16. What is typically the earliest sign of intravascular volume depletion (hypovolemia) in a young pregnant woman?

A. Decreased systolic blood pressure

B. Increased respiratory rate

C. Increased heart rate

D. Decreased heart rate

E. Decreased capillary refill

ANSWER: C

COMMENTS: Trauma complicates approximately 6%–7% of all pregnancies. Regardless of the injury, resuscitation of the mother with treatment of **hypovolemia and hypoxia** is emphasized during the initial evaluation. Because blood volume expands during pregnancy, a third of the blood volume may be lost without a noticeable change in blood pressure or heart rate. Clinically significant blood loss of up to 2 L, or 30% of the total blood volume, may not be readily apparent. The clinician must be aware of a falsely reassuring hemodynamic state masking ongoing hemorrhage.

Ref.: 1

17. Which of the following radiologic examinations poses the greatest radiation exposure to a fetus?

A. Chest radiograph (two views)

B. Abdominal film (single view)

C. CT of the head

D. CT of the abdomen/pelvis

E. CT pelvimetry

ANSWER: D

COMMENTS: The primary concern with X-ray procedures during pregnancy relates to the risks to the fetus from ionizing radiation. These risks depend on the gestational age and radiation dose. Most plain-film x-rays are associated with relatively low fetal doses. For chest radiographs and single-view abdominal films, fetal doses are estimated at <0.01 mGy and 0.5-3mGy, respectively. Fluoroscopy studies provide higher doses, ranging from 1-20 mGy for studies like barium enema or IV pyelogram. New developments in CT technology and image processing continue to reduce fetal (and maternal) doses required to obtain these exams. CT of the head/neck or CT chest are associated with fetal doses of less than 10mGy. CT of the abdomen (1- 35mGy) and pelvic CT (10-50mGy) are associated with the highest fetal doses. However, fetal anomalies, growth restriction, and miscarriage have not been reported with radiation exposures less than 50 mGy which is higher than the exposure for most single diagnostic procedures.

Ref.: 18, 19

18. Which of the following agents is appropriate to use in conjunction with radiographic studies in pregnancy?

A. Gadolinium

B. Iodine-131

C. Technetium-99m

D. Superparamagnetic iron oxide

E. Iridium-192

ANSWER: C

COMMENTS: Technetium-99m is a commonly used radioisotope for brain, bone, renal, and cardiovascular nuclear medicine imaging. For the evaluation of pulmonary embolism with ventilation–perfusion studies, the total radiation exposure with technetium-99m is estimated at 5 mGy, an acceptable dose during pregnancy. Gadolinium contrast increases the specificity of MRI, but its use is controversial during pregnancy for several reasons. Gadolinium is water soluble and can cross the placenta and enter the fetal circulation and amniotic fluid. If gadolinium is administered during pregnancy, the fetus swallows the gadolinium in the amniotic fluid, and it continues to reenter the fetal circulation. As such, the duration of fetal exposure cannot be reliably calculated. Furthermore, gadolinium agents are teratogenic at high and repeated doses in animal studies. Given these theoretical concerns, gadolinium use is primarily recommended for studies where there is a clear benefit to its administration. Iodine-131 also crosses the placenta and can impair the growth of the fetal thyroid, so it is not used during pregnancy for either diagnostic or therapeutic purposes. There are no animal or human studies regarding the safety of superparamagnetic iron oxide contrast in pregnancy.

Ref.: 16

19. A 25-year-old gravida 1 at 37 weeks' gestation is being evaluated for right upper quadrant abdominal pain. On examination, she is found to be afebrile with a blood pressure of 130/70 mmHg, pulse of 110 beats/min, and respiratory rate of 18 breaths/min. She has scleral icterus. Her laboratory results are shown in Table 33.1. What is the most likely diagnosis for this patient?

A. AFLP

B. Viral hepatitis

TABLE 33.1

Test	Value	Normal Range for Pregnancy
Hemoglobin	12	10.5–12 g/dL
WBCs	20,000	3200–15,000/mL
Platelets	111,000	150,000–350,000/mm^3
Prothrombin time	40	9.5–13.5 s
Blood urea nitrogen	29	7–18 mg/dL
Creatinine	2.8	0.6–0.9 mg/dL
Aspartate transaminase	317	7–27
Alanine transaminase	297	1–21
Total and direct bilirubin	7.8, 4.6	<1.0 mg/dL, <0.4 mg/dL
Glucose	48	70–110 mg/dL

C. Thrombotic thrombocytopenic purpura

D. Hemolytic-uremic syndrome

E. HELLP syndrome

ANSWER: A

COMMENTS: AFLP is rare (1 in 7000 to 16,000 deliveries). It occurs more commonly in male fetuses and twins. It is related to an autosomally inherited mutation that causes a deficiency of long-chain 3-hydroxyacyl coenzyme A dehydrogenase, a fatty acid β-oxidation enzyme. AFLP is usually manifested in the third trimester as nausea and vomiting, followed by right upper quadrant pain. A 7- to 10-day prodrome of a viral illness is common as well. Hepatomegaly is rare, but other findings include progressive jaundice, malaise, somnolence, and coma. Laboratory abnormalities include liver and renal dysfunction, coagulopathy, increased ammonia, leukocytosis (20,000 to 50,000), hypoglycemia, and pancreatitis. **HELLP syndrome** usually develops in patients with hypertension, and often the diagnosis of preeclampsia precedes the development of HELLP syndrome. The syndrome includes **HE**molysis, elevated **L**iver enzymes, and **L**ow **P**latelet count. HELLP syndrome develops in 0.1%–0.2% of all pregnancies, with an incidence as high as 10%–20% in pregnancies complicated by preeclampsia or eclampsia. Although the laboratory results may also be consistent with HELLP syndrome, hypoglycemia is one of the distinguishing factors in AFLP. Treatment consists of supportive measures to correct the coagulopathy, electrolyte abnormalities, and hypoglycemia, as well as prompt delivery. Maternal mortality is very low with early diagnosis, appropriate supportive therapy, and early delivery. The fetal mortality rate associated with AFLP is less than 15%.

Ref.: 20

20. Many unplanned pregnancies occur after bariatric surgery, in part because of improved fertility rates in patients who were infertile before the procedure. Most experts recommend waiting between bariatric surgery procedures and pregnancy. Select the most appropriate time frame:

A. 0 to 3 months

B. 6 to 9 months

C. 12 to 15 months

D. 18 to 24 months

E. >2 years

ANSWER: D

COMMENTS: Most clinicians recommend waiting at least 18 months between **bariatric surgery** and conception. In this case, the fetus is not exposed to a rapid maternal weight loss environment, and the patient can achieve full weight loss goals.

Ref.: 21

21. The leading cause of maternal morbidity and mortality in the developed world is:

A. Postpartum hemorrhage

B. Thromboembolism

C. Preeclampsia

D. Uterine rupture

E. Pneumonia

ANSWER: B

COMMENTS: In 2012, the national **maternal mortality rate** was 15.9 deaths per 100,000 live births. Maternal mortality is defined as the number of maternal deaths (direct and indirect) per 100,000 live births. "Maternal deaths" are defined by the World Health Organization as "the death of a woman while pregnant or within 42 days of termination of pregnancy, irrespective of the duration and the site of the pregnancy, from any cause related to or aggravated by the pregnancy or its management, but not from accidental or incidental causes." Direct obstetric deaths result primarily from **thromboembolic events** (19.9%), hemorrhage (18.2%), hypertensive disorders of pregnancy (15.9%), and infectious complications (13.2%). Indirect obstetric deaths arise from preexisting medical conditions, including diabetes, systemic lupus erythematosus, pulmonary disease, and cardiac disease aggravated by the physiologic changes of pregnancy.

Ref.: 22–25

22. A 27-year-old woman at 24 weeks' gestation is transferred from the antepartum unit to the intensive care unit for management of sepsis in the setting of pyelonephritis. She is receiving broad-spectrum antibiotics, but her oxygenation requirements are increasing. Her obstetrician is concerned that she is developing acute respiratory distress syndrome. Which of the following physiologic changes in pregnancy do you consider in her evaluation?

A. Decreased cardiac output

B. Increased blood pressure

C. Increased heart rate

D. Increased systemic vascular resistance

E. Decreased erythrocyte sedimentation rate

ANSWER: C

COMMENTS: See Question 23.

Ref.: 22, 23

23. A 32-year-old woman in the first trimester of her second pregnancy comes to the emergency department because of epigastric pain, anorexia, vomiting, and low-grade fever. Which of the following findings would be considered normal in a pregnant patient?

A. WBC count of 20,500 cells/mm^3

B. Respiratory rate of 40 breaths/min

C. Pco_2 of 32 mmHg on arterial blood gas analysis

D. Amylase concentration of 500 U/L

E. Serum creatinine level of 1.6 mg/dL

ANSWER: C

COMMENTS: During pregnancy, a number of **physiologic changes** occur, such as increases in plasma volume and red blood cell mass. The platelet count is generally normal or slightly decreased, whereas the WBC counts increase from 3000 to 15,000 cells/mm^3 in the first trimester and to 6000 to 16,000 cells/mm^3 during the second and third trimesters. Progesterone and increased CO_2 production contribute to the hyperpnea of pregnancy. There is a reduction in arterial Pco_2 from the usual 40 mmHg to 28 to 35 mmHg and an increase in arterial oxygen tension (Po_2) from 60 mmHg to 100 mmHg. This facilitates efficient exchange of gases between the mother and fetus. A respiratory alkalosis with compensatory metabolic acidosis is normal in pregnancy. Hemodynamic changes include increased cardiac output by as high as 50%, decreased systemic vascular resistance by approximately 20%, and increased heart rate to 15 to 20 beats/min above normal. Since the blood pressure is a product of the cardiac output and systemic vascular resistance, changes in blood pressure are noted throughout pregnancy, with a nadir in the second trimester. The glomerular filtration rate increases, with a concomitant decrease in normal serum creatinine levels. Serum osmolality is also decreased. Serum amylase values remain normal to slightly elevated during pregnancy. A significant elevation in amylase along with abdominal pain suggests pancreatitis; in pregnancy, the most common causes of pancreatitis are gallstones and hypertriglyceridemia. Markers of inflammation such as C-reactive protein and erythrocyte sedimentation rate typically increase during pregnancy.

Ref.: 1, 12, 26

24. A 37-year-old gravida 1 at 31 weeks is taken to the emergency department with complaints of midepigastric pain, nausea, and vomiting that began 30 min after eating a fatty meal. Her surgical history is significant for a Roux-en-Y gastric bypass 2 years earlier. Her body mass index is currently 32 kg/m^2. On examination, the patient's temperature is 39°C, and her abdomen is diffusely tender with rebound and guarding. The fetal heart rate was slightly tachycardic (170 beats/min), and the cervix was not dilated. The differential diagnosis should include all of the following except:

A. Cholelithiasis

B. Chorioamnionitis

C. Internal hernia

D. Pancreatitis

E. Preterm labor

ANSWER: E

COMMENTS: See Question 25.

Ref.: 1, 12, 21

25. The patient's amylase and lipase levels are normal. Right upper quadrant ultrasonography shows a normal gallbladder and liver. Her abdominal pain worsens, and she is tachycardic to 130 beats/min. The fetal heart rate also continues to be tachycardic (170 beats/min). What is the next step in management?

A. Laparotomy

B. Cesarean delivery

C. Intravenous methylprednisolone to induce fetal lung maturity

D. Tocolysis to prevent preterm delivery

E. ERCP

ANSWER: A

COMMENTS: The number of bariatric surgery procedures performed annually in the United States was 179,000 in 2013. More than 80% of these patients are female, and as of 2004, one-half of the bariatric procedures were performed in women of reproductive age with a mean age of 40 years. Evaluation of abdominal pain in pregnancy is complicated by difficulty in differentiating symptoms of pathology from normal, pregnancy-associated symptoms. The evaluation becomes even more difficult in a pregnant patient who has undergone bariatric surgery. Confusion regarding the cause of symptoms can lead to a critical delay in the diagnosis of **bariatric surgery complications**, including anastomotic leaks, bowel obstruction, internal hernias, ventral hernias, band erosion, and band migration. All gastrointestinal complaints such as nausea, vomiting, and abdominal pain, which occur commonly during pregnancy, should be thoroughly evaluated in a bariatric surgery patient. This patient has an acute abdomen, which is concerning for bowel obstruction or an internal hernia. Although her pregnancy may have an impact on anesthesia and postoperative care, immediate treatment should focus on her abdominal complaints. **Cesarean delivery** is not indicated. Corticosteroids (betamethasone or dexamethasone) are administered to patients between 24 and 34 weeks' gestation if delivery is anticipated within 7 days. They promote fetal lung maturity and decrease the risk for interventricular hemorrhage. Other steroids such as prednisone or methylprednisolone do not cross the placenta. The patient is not in labor (the cervix is not dilated), so **tocolytic agents** will not be helpful. **ERCP** can be performed during pregnancy; fluoroscopy should be limited and the fetus should be shielded, but some radiation exposure will occur. ERCP is unlikely to be helpful in this patient.

Ref.: 1, 12, 27

26. A 24-year-old woman was treated for papillary thyroid cancer with a total thyroidectomy 3 months ago. Her postoperative course has been uncomplicated, and she takes 150 μg of levothyroxine daily. She states that her home pregnancy test was positive 1 week ago. Which of the following would you advise?

A. Discontinue levothyroxine until she sees her obstetrician.

B. Increase the levothyroxine dose to 300 μg daily as thyroid replacement requirements increase in pregnancy.

C. Order a thyroid ultrasound to evaluate for residual tissue.

D. Order thyroid-stimulating hormone (TSH) and free T4 level tests.

E. Immediately terminate the pregnancy.

ANSWER: D

COMMENTS: After treatment with either surgery or radioiodine or both for thyroid cancer, T4 is typically given to suppress the TSH and prevent stimulation of residual thyroid tissue. For the treatment of thyroid cancer, radioactive iodine can only be given after delivery and after breastfeeding has been completed. One recommendation is to delay pregnancy for 1 year after thyroid cancer that was treated with radioactive iodine because of the increased risk for congenital anomalies. Levothyroxine is classified in FDA pregnancy risk category A (Adequate research has been done with the conclusion that drugs in this category are not likely to cause any harm to the fetus in the first trimester as well as later in pregnancy). As such, it is appropriate to continue its use during pregnancy. Thyroid requirements typically increase during pregnancy and one suggested goal TSH is 0.5 to 5.0 μU/mL, but alterations in levothyroxine doses are typically done in conjunction with thyroid function tests.

Ref.: 28

27. A 32-year-old woman is 18 weeks pregnant in her third pregnancy. She reports increased fullness in her neck, and her obstetrician suspects there is a thyroid nodule. The thyroid ultrasound shows a single 4-cm solid nodule. What is the next best step in her management?

A. Defer evaluation until after delivery

B. Complete thyroidectomy

C. Radioactive iodine

D. Fine-needle aspiration

E. Core-needle biopsy

ANSWER: D

COMMENTS: Thyroid nodules are common and occur in 1%–2% of reproductive-age women. Thyroid nodules are found in 2% of pregnant women, and one study suggests there is an increased incidence of malignancy in pregnancy. Nodules that are suspicious for malignancy require further evaluation and/or treatment during pregnancy. Radioactive iodine can distinguish between "hot" and "cold" nodules, but this approach is contraindicated in pregnancy due to teratogenic risks of radioactive iodine. Ultrasound is the next alternative to the evaluation of a suspected nodule in pregnancy. The indications for fine-needle aspiration do not alter in the presence of a pregnancy and should not be delayed on account of pregnancy. In this case, the dimensions of the nodule warrant further investigation with a fine-needle aspiration. If there is concomitant hyperthyroidism, it is appropriate to treat with antithyroid drugs during pregnancy. Surgery should not be delayed on account of pregnancy unless the patient is close to term.

Ref.: 29

28. Which of the following values would you expect in an otherwise uncomplicated pregnancy at 24 weeks?

A. Normal TSH, normal total T4

B. Elevated TSH, normal total T4

C. Normal TSH, elevated total T4

D. Decreased TSH, elevated total T4

E. Decreased TSH, decreased total T4

ANSWER: C

COMMENTS: Not only does thyroid volume increase by 30% by the third trimester, but thyroid hormone levels and thyroid function also vary throughout pregnancy. Table 33.2 shows how thyroid function tests change in a normal pregnancy and in relation to overt and subclinical thyroid disease. In pregnancy, total thyroid hormone levels increase because the concentration of thyroid-binding globulin increases. TSH initially decreases in pregnancy due to stimulation of TSH receptors by human chorionic gonadotropin (hCG), which shares a common α-subunit with TSH. This results in increased thyroid hormone secretion, and consequently free T4 levels increase initially. TSH values return to baseline values after the first trimester but progressively increase in the third trimester due to placental growth and production of placental deiodinase.

These physiologic changes should be considered when interpreting thyroid function test results during pregnancy.

Ref.: 30

TABLE 33.2 Thyroid Function Tests in Pregnancy

Maternal Status	TSH	Free T_4
Pregnancy	Varies by trimester	No change
Overt hyperthyroidism	Decrease	Increase
Subclinical hyperthyroidism	Decrease	No change
Overt hypothyroidism	Increase	Decrease
Subclinical hypothyroidism	Increase	No change

29. A 32-year-old woman who is 23 weeks pregnant finds a 1.5-cm firm mass during a breast self-examination. An ultrasound-guided core-needle biopsy shows infiltrating ductal carcinoma. Which of the following would be the most appropriate treatment option?

A. Lumpectomy, axillary dissection, and immediate radiation therapy and chemotherapy

B. Lumpectomy, axillary dissection, immediate chemotherapy, and radiation therapy after delivery

C. Lumpectomy, axillary dissection, immediate radiation therapy, and chemotherapy after delivery

D. Immediate radiation therapy and chemotherapy followed by surgery after delivery

E. Termination of the pregnancy followed immediately by treatment of breast cancer

ANSWER: B

COMMENTS: Breast cancer that is diagnosed during pregnancy or within 1 year after delivery is known as **pregnancy-associated breast cancer**. Breast cancer represents the most common nongynecologic malignancy associated with pregnancy, and it occurs in 0.01%–0.03% of pregnancies. It has been associated with delayed diagnosis (mean delay of 1 to 2 months). When compared with matched, nonpregnant patients, women with pregnancy-associated breast cancer have a similar stage-related prognosis but overall worse prognosis because on average, they have larger primary tumors and a higher risk for lymph node involvement. **Mammography** can be performed with the fetus appropriately shielded; however, the increased density of the fibroglandular breast tissue limits its specificity. **Ultrasound imaging** is useful both for assessing the tumor and for guiding the biopsy. Although **MRI** can be used during pregnancy, gadolinium crosses the placenta and may be associated with a risk for fetal abnormalities. As with breast masses in a nonpregnant patient, a tissue diagnosis is imperative. Either core-needle or fine-needle aspiration biopsy may be used. Surgical resection represents the most important component of treatment. Classically, **modified radical mastectomy** was considered the standard therapy. More recent data suggest that patients in whom breast cancer is diagnosed later in pregnancy can be treated with immediate **breast-conserving lumpectomy** and **axillary dissection**, followed by **radiation therapy** after delivery. Axillary dissection rather than sentinel lymph node biopsy has been recommended because of the more aggressive nature of pregnancy-associated breast cancer and because no radioisotope is required. Most **chemotherapeutic regimens** can be administered safely after the first trimester, although changes in plasma volume, protein content, and the volume of distribution associated with chemotherapeutic agents crossing the placenta may complicate dosing. Radiation therapy should be avoided until after delivery because of the risk to the fetus. **Pregnancy termination** to allow the full gamut of therapeutic options for breast cancer is not recommended because it has not been shown to increase patient survival.

Ref.: 1

30. A 36-year-old gravida 3 para 2 is now 12 weeks pregnant. She received a living-donor kidney transplant 2 years ago. Which of the following is most likely to complicate her pregnancy?

A. Graft loss

B. Acute rejection

C. Hypertension

D. Diabetes

E. High birth weight

ANSWER: C

COMMENTS: Successful pregnancy is possible after solid organ transplantations such as kidney transplants. In 1963, Murray et al. reported the first pregnancy to occur in a kidney transplant recipient. The woman received a kidney from her identical twin, and she subsequently delivered a healthy neonate in 1958. The voluntary National Transplantation Pregnancy Registry (NTPR) was established in 1991 to study the safety of pregnancy and pregnancy outcomes for North American transplant recipients; the outcomes of pregnancies fathered by transplant recipients; and the long-term implications of pregnancy on the recipient, graft, and offspring. Pregnancy does not appear to influence the long-term renal graft survival according to case reports and cohort studies. Biopsy-proven acute rejection complicates only 2%–4% of pregnancies, and the occurrence depends on calcineurin inhibitor exposure. Many women with solid organ transplants have preexisting diabetes or develop diabetes as a side effect of immunosuppressant treatment, but diabetes developing during a pregnancy is estimated at 5%–12% for kidney transplants. Chronic hypertension and preeclampsia most frequently complicate pregnancies after kidney transplants, estimated at 57%–69% and 29%, respectively. Low birth weight (less than 2500 g) is more common in pregnancies after organ transplantation, and this may result from either the underlying maternal disease or the immunosuppressive therapy.

Ref.: 24, 31

31. Which of the following agents do you advise your patient to discontinue when she informs you that she is 6 weeks pregnant and has had a kidney transplant?

A. Tacrolimus

B. Mycophenolate mofetil (MMF)

C. Sirolimus

D. Prednisone

E. Cyclosporine

ANSWER: B

COMMENTS: In pregnancy, no medication is without risks to a developing fetus. The **antimetabolite drugs**, MMF or mycophenolic acid (MPA), have greater risks for teratogenicity based on reproductive toxicity studies in animals. These risks include malformations and fetal growth restriction. The specific pattern of malformation is microtia (an ear deformity) and other facial malformations, such as cleft lip and palate. The package inserts for these medications state that women of reproductive age must use contraception while taking MMF or MPA, and this is reinforced by a patient-education program mandated by the FDA. Based on data from the NTPR and other large cohorts, there has not been an increase in the incidence of malformations or any recurrent pattern of malformations among fetuses exposed to tacrolimus, sirolimus, or cyclosporine. Studies regarding corticosteroid use in pregnancy are mixed with respect to fetal malformations, but, overall, when used in therapeutic dosages, prednisone poses minimal risks to a developing fetus.

Ref.: 32

32. A 46-year-old woman undergoing chemotherapy for acute myeloid leukemia presents to the emergency department with right lower quadrant pain, guarding, and rebound tenderness. Vital signs include a temperature of 103.4°F, pulse of 82 beats/min, and blood pressure 118/84 mmHg. Her WBC count is 0.44 K/uL. An abdominal x-ray shows an enlarged, fluid-filled cecum with adjacent dilated loops of small bowel. The radiologist suspects that there is localized pneumatosis in the cecum. What is the most appropriate next step in the management of this patient?

A. Barium enema

B. Colonoscopy

C. Exploratory laparoscopy

D. CT scan of the abdomen

E. Exploratory laparotomy

ANSWER: D

COMMENTS: See Question 33.

Ref.: 33, 34

33. Abdominal CT scan in the aforementioned patient demonstrates marked thickening and edema of the cecum with localized pneumatosis. The appendix is not inflamed. The adjacent small bowel is thickened and mildly dilated. Which of the following would be least appropriate?

A. Rectal tube decompression of the colon

B. Broad-spectrum intravenous antibiotics

C. Administration of granulocyte colony-stimulating factor (G-CSF)

D. Stool evaluation for *Clostridium difficile* toxin

E. Nasogastric decompression of the stomach

ANSWER: A

COMMENTS: Neutropenic enterocolitis (or **typhlitis**) is a necrotizing colitis seen in patients with profound neutropenia that often occurs after myelosuppressive chemotherapy. It can also occur in patients with aplastic anemia, human immunodeficiency virus (HIV) infection, and acute leukemia or after immunosuppressive therapy for solid tumors or organ transplants. The pathogenesis appears to include mucosal injury, bacterial translocation, intramural infection, and bowel wall ischemia with eventual necrosis. **Typhlitis** is typically characterized by thickening and edema of the cecum, although the distal ileum and ascending colon may also be involved. Typical symptoms include fever and abdominal pain, usually in the right lower quadrant. Other symptoms may include nausea, vomiting, distention, and watery or bloody diarrhea. Abdominal CT is useful in differentiating typhlitis from other causes of abdominal pain, such as appendicitis, abscess, Ogilvie syndrome, or pseudomembranous colitis. Operative findings include cecal wall thickening with edema or air, a soft tissue mass, hemorrhage, or perforation. Ultrasound imaging can also be used, although it is less specific. Barium enema or colonoscopy should be avoided because of the risk for perforation or additional bacterial translocation.

Prompt surgical intervention is required for patients with peritonitis, free perforation, or persistent gastrointestinal bleeding. If surgery is required, a right hemicolectomy and diversion should be performed, with reanastomosis reserved for a later procedure when the patient has stabilized and the neutropenia has resolved. Treatment of patients who do not meet the criteria for surgery includes bowel rest, nasogastric decompression, intravenous hydration, nutritional support, and broad-spectrum antibiotics. G-CSF can be used to accelerate normalization of the leukocyte count. Anticholinergic, antidiarrheal, and opioid analgesics should be avoided because of their propensity to worsen the ileus. Blood and stool cultures and ***C. difficile*** **toxin** assays should be obtained. In patients who do not improve after a short course of antibiotics, antifungal therapy should be added. Rectal tube decompression should be avoided in neutropenic patients because of the risk for mucosal compromise and bacterial translocation.

Ref.: 33, 34

34. A 62-year-old woman with long-standing end-stage renal disease who is being maintained on **peritoneal dialysis** (PD) has had several months of intermittent abdominal pain and difficulty obtaining normal dwell volumes for her peritoneal catheter. She goes to the emergency department because she was unable to adequately drain her peritoneal fluid. Review of her medical records reveals that her creatinine level has slowly been increasing for the last several months without any change in her dialysis regimen. Abdominal CT shows ascites; shortened, thickened small bowel mesentery; and diffusely thickened small bowel with areas of luminal narrowing. There are punctate calcifications throughout the peritoneum. Which of the following is least appropriate?

A. Trial of tamoxifen therapy
B. Oral steroid pulse
C. Replacement of the PD catheter
D. Immunosuppressive therapy with azathioprine
E. Exploratory laparoscopy and enterolysis

ANSWER: C

COMMENTS: Encapsulating peritoneal sclerosis (EPS, sclerosing peritonitis) is one of the most dreaded complications of **PD**. EPS is characterized by a decrease in the efficacy of PD and the development of extensive intraperitoneal fibrosis, mesenteric shortening, and encasement of the bowel. It can progress to bowel obstruction. Radiologic features include mesenteric, bowel, and peritoneal thickening, often with calcifications. Loculated ascites, adherent bowel loops, and luminal narrowing of the bowel may also be visualized. The etiology of EPS is not well understood. Risk factors include the duration of PD therapy, episodes of peritonitis, and acetate dialysis. Treatment is often unsuccessful. Most patients with EPS are switched to hemodialysis (although such a switch can sometimes precipitate EPS). Steroid therapy, tamoxifen, and immunosuppressive regimens, including azathioprine or cyclosporine, have all been used to treat EPS. When bowel obstruction is present, total parenteral nutrition may be required. The role of surgical therapy for EPS remains controversial. Early results with enterectomy and anastomosis have shown high mortality, but more recent studies suggest a role for early enterolysis.

Ref.: 35, 36

35. A 54-year-old woman with end-stage renal disease treated by PD complains of abdominal pain and fever. When performing her exchanges she has noted turbid fluid for the last several days. She has been undergoing PD for 3 years and has never had any complications. Which of the following statements is correct?

A. She should undergo immediate peritoneal exploration with removal of the dialysis catheter.
B. Fungal peritonitis requires long-term antifungal therapy through the PD catheter.
C. PD-associated peritonitis from coagulase-negative staphylococci can be cured with antibiotics alone in more than 80% of cases.
D. She will need to resume hemodialysis while the infection is treated.
E. Broad-spectrum empirical antibiotic therapy is required because peritoneal fluid cultures have little value.

ANSWER: C

COMMENTS: Peritonitis is a common complication of **PD** and occurs about 1.4 times per patient-year of PD. It is one of the most important reasons for failure of PD and accounts for nearly one-half of all technical failures. Typically, patients have abdominal pain and tenderness (75%), fever (33%), and cloudy dialysate. The diagnosis is confirmed by a fluid leukocyte count of greater than 100/mL with more than one-half of the cells being neutrophils. Most infections are caused by gram-positive organisms, but gram-negative bacilli and fungi can also be responsible. Initial treatment should consist of intraperitoneal antibiotics, most commonly vancomycin or a first-generation cephalosporin. About 75% of infections are cured with culture-directed antibiotic therapy without discontinuation of PD. Persistent or recurrent infection may require removal of the PD catheter and a switch to hemodialysis. Cure rates with antibiotics alone are best for coagulase-negative staphylococci (90%) and less for *Staphylococcus aureus* (66%) or gram-negative bacilli (56%). **Fungal infections** require prompt removal of the catheter. Prompt treatment of peritoneal infections is important to reduce the formation of adhesions and the loss of peritoneal area, which can limit the patient's ability to continue with PD.

Ref.: 37

36. A 76-year-old man with cardiac, liver, and renal disease is admitted to the intensive care unit with fever, hypotension, and abdominal distention. An abdominal ultrasound reveals ascites. His serum albumin level is 2.8 g/dL, and the albumin concentration in the ascites fluid is 3.6 g/dL. This serum-ascites albumin gradient (SAAG) is most supportive of which of the following diagnoses?

A. Lymphatic leak
B. Cirrhosis
C. Tuberculous peritonitis
D. Nephrotic syndrome
E. Pancreatic ascites

ANSWER: B

COMMENTS: The most useful tests for characterizing **ascites** are cell counts, differential count, and total protein and albumin concentrations of the fluid. If the fluid has a high neutrophil concentration, an acute inflammatory process is suggested. The **SAAG** provides one of the most useful tools for characterizing the cause

TABLE 33.3 Classification of Ascites by Serum-Ascites Albumin Gradient

High Gradient (≥1.1 g/dL)
Cirrhosis
Alcoholic hepatitis
Cardiac ascites
Massive liver metastases
Fulminant hepatic failure
Budd-Chiari syndrome
Portal vein thrombosis
Myxedema
Low Gradient (<1.1 g/dL)
Peritoneal carcinomatosis
Tuberculous peritonitis
Pancreatic ascites
Biliary ascites
Nephrotic syndrome
Postoperative lymphatic leak
Serositis in connective tissue disease

From Runyon B. Ascites: spontaneous bacterial peritonitis. In: Sleisenger MH, Feldman M, Friedman LS, eds. *Sleisenger and Fordtran's Gastrointestinal and Liver Disease: Pathophysiology, Diagnosis, Management*. 7th ed. Philadelphia: WB Saunders; 2002:1523.

of ascites (Table 33.3). SAAG is calculated by subtracting the albumin concentration of the ascites fluid from that of serum. **High-SAAG ascites** (SAAG ≥ 1.1 g/dL) is associated with portal hypertension. Causes include cirrhosis, alcoholic or cardiac ascites, liver metastases, fulminant hepatic failure, Budd-Chiari syndrome, myxedema, and portal vein thrombosis. **Low-SAAG ascites** (SAAG < 1.1 g/dL) is associated with tuberculous peritonitis, pancreatic or biliary ascites, nephrotic syndrome, and lymphatic leaks.

Ref.: 37

37. A 64-year-old man with end-stage renal disease is visiting from Mexico. He is evaluated in the emergency department for worsening vague abdominal pain, occasional vomiting, and abdominal swelling. The pain has been present intermittently for several months but has worsened over the last few weeks. He has lost about 30 lbs. and has no appetite or energy. A purified protein derivative (PPD) skin test is positive, and the patient gives a history of being successfully treated for tuberculosis (TB) several years ago. Ultrasound shows moderate ascites with echogenic material within the fluid and no dilated bowel. Which of the following tests would be most helpful in making a diagnosis?

A. CT of the abdomen and pelvis

B. Percutaneous peritoneal biopsy

C. Microscopic examination of peritoneal fluid

D. Mycobacterial cultures of peritoneal fluid

E. Diagnostic laparoscopy and peritoneal biopsy

ANSWER: E

COMMENTS: Tuberculous peritonitis was commonly associated with individuals with **acquired immunodeficiency syndrome (AIDS)**; however, it can also occur in the setting of cirrhosis (especially alcoholic) and chronic renal failure. Most cases result from reactivation of latent peritoneal disease in patients with previous pulmonary TB. Typical complaints include abdominal distention from ascites and generalized abdominal discomfort. Constitutional symptoms, including fever, night sweats, anorexia, and malaise, may also be present. Most patients have a positive PPD skin test. In the absence of cirrhosis, the ascites has a **low SAAG**, high glucose, high protein, and high fluid WBCs, mainly lymphocytes. Abdominal ultrasound may show echogenic material within the ascites, whereas CT shows a thickened, nodular mesentery, lymphadenopathy, and omental thickening. **Laparoscopic peritoneal biopsy** is diagnostic. Most commonly the peritoneum is studded with multiple small whitish nodules, which on biopsy contain caseating granulomas. Blind peritoneal biopsy has much lower sensitivity than directed biopsy. Microscopic examination of the ascites for acid-fast bacteria is rarely positive, and cultures are relatively insensitive (20%) and require several weeks of incubation. Tuberculous peritonitis can be manifested as a pelvic mass with elevated cancer antigen (CA) 125, which can lead to an incorrect diagnosis of metastatic ovarian cancer. Treatment consists of 6 to 9 months of antituberculous drugs; regimens typically include rifampin, isoniazid, and pyrazinamide.

Ref.: 38–40

38. A 48-year-old man underwent human leukocyte antigen (HLA)–matched allogeneic bone marrow transplantation for myelofibrosis with myeloid metaplasia. One month after discharge, he returned to the clinic with a 2-week history of anorexia, malaise, low-grade fevers, and difficulty swallowing. His tongue was chalky white. Esophagogastroduodenoscopy revealed white plaques throughout the esophagus, and colonoscopy showed linear, well-demarcated ulcers in the terminal ileum and cecum. He was prescribed oral nystatin and treated for his neutropenia. Two days later, severe abdominal pain develops, and CT shows a perforation at the distal ileum. Which of the following is the most likely cause of the ileal perforation?

A. Epstein-Barr virus (EBV)

B. Cytomegalovirus (CMV)

C. Parvovirus

D. *Candida albicans*

E. Herpes simplex virus

ANSWER: B

COMMENTS: CMV infection can result in serious complications in patients who are immunosuppressed, including patients with HIV infection, organ transplants, or cancer, or in those receiving immunosuppressive therapy. The most common site of CMV disease is the eye, and **CMV retinitis** can result in blindness. Gastrointestinal involvement can occur anywhere from the mouth to the anus, although the colon is most commonly involved. Clinical symptoms include fever, malaise, anorexia, nausea, diarrhea, abdominal pain, ileus, and bleeding. Endoscopic evaluation shows well-defined, "punched-out" ulcers. Lesions are usually limited to a segment of the gastrointestinal tract, with diffuse involvement being less common. Biopsies usually show mucosal inflammation, tissue necrosis, and vascular endothelial involvement. Visualization of **viral inclusions** by light microscopy remains the standard of diagnosis. CMV typically causes gastritis, enteritis, or colitis, but in rare cases, it can result in perforation and significant gastrointestinal bleeding. Viral serology and quantitative polymerase chain reaction (PCR) may be helpful in diagnosing CMV enteritis, but endoscopy with biopsy remains the gold standard. EBV can be associated with viral syndromes and lymphomas but rarely causes perforation. Parvovirus causes anemia. Invasive ***Candida*** infections very rarely cause perforation, although this patient did have findings of superficial esophageal candidiasis (probably suggesting that he is very immunosuppressed). **Herpes simplex virus** has cutaneous manifestations and may result in proctitis, but perforation does not usually occur.

Ref.: 41, 42

39. Which of the following should not be included in the initial approach to a profoundly neutropenic patient with fever?

A. Skin, mucous membrane, and ophthalmoscopic examination

B. Inspection and cultures from central venous access

C. Digital rectal examination

D. Chest radiograph

E. Initiation of empirical antibiotic therapy

ANSWER: C

COMMENTS: Determining the cause of a fever in a **neutropenic** patient requires careful attention to detail because signs of infection or inflammation are often subtle or absent in patients with profound neutropenia. The skin, mucous membranes, and ocular fundi should be carefully examined for an infectious source. All access sites, including intravenous and central lines, should be checked for soft tissue infection or thrombophlebitis. Mucous membranes should be examined for signs of viral or fungal infection. All indwelling catheters should be cultured. Laboratory studies should include urine and blood cultures from peripheral sites and all indwelling lines. Stool should be sent for study if there are any changes in bowel habits. Lumbar puncture should be performed in patients who have altered mental status or localizing symptoms. A chest radiograph should be performed; however, the findings may be subtle or absent even with pneumonia. **Chest CT** may demonstrate evidence of infection not revealed on radiography. Empiric antibiotic therapy should be initiated promptly and modified on the basis of the results of examination, imaging, and culture. Anorectal infection can be very subtle in immunosuppressed patients. Routine digital rectal examination should be avoided because of the risk of provoking bacteremia. However, if prostatitis or a perirectal abscess is suspected, gentle digital rectal examination can be performed after antibiotic therapy is initiated.

Ref.: 43

40. A 39-year-old HIV-positive man who is noncompliant with his antiretroviral medications wishes a second opinion because of 1 month of progressive abdominal pain, diarrhea, low-grade fever, and malaise. He has a history of *Pneumocystis carinii* pneumonia. At initial presentation, his abdominal CT showed thickening of the terminal ileum with a small amount of surrounding fluid. Colonoscopy showed circumferential ulcers and inflamed mucosa; biopsy of the cecum and terminal ileum showed granulomas. Therefore a diagnosis of Crohn's disease was made, and the patient was treated with steroids. However, 1 month later his symptoms are worse, and repeated CT shows increased cecal and peritoneal thickening, ascites, and large mesenteric lymph nodes with hypodense centers. Suspecting that the initial diagnosis may have been in error, which of the following conditions is the most likely diagnosis?

A. Crohn's disease

B. Cecal carcinoma

C. Tuberculous enteritis

D. Intestinal amebiasis

E. Small bowel lymphoma

ANSWER: C

COMMENTS: The differential diagnosis for ileocecal thickening or a mass includes **neoplasms** such as lymphoma, sarcoma, and adenocarcinoma; **Crohn's disease**; and **infectious causes** such as amebiasis, histoplasmosis, actinomycosis, *Yersinia*, or intestinal TB. Because the symptoms of many of these conditions overlap, a careful diagnostic approach is needed. Commonly, evaluation includes imaging and colonoscopy with biopsy. Many of these conditions may result in ulcers. However, the finding of granulomas on biopsy led to the diagnosis of Crohn's disease. Carcinoma or lymphoma biopsy specimens should show malignant cells. A biopsy specimen revealing **intestinal amebiasis** should show trophozoites, and stool studies and serologic evaluation should confirm the diagnosis. **Tuberculous enteritis** can be confused with Crohn's disease because both have granulomas, although the granulomas in Crohn's disease are infrequent, small, nonconfluent, and noncaseating. Tuberculous granulomas are larger and confluent, often with caseating necrosis. Imaging of TB may show large lymph nodes with characteristic central caseous liquefaction. Many patients will have pulmonary manifestations of previous TB infection, although active disease is often not present. Culture results may take several weeks to become positive, and it is being supplanted by PCR testing of biopsy specimens. **Treatment** of intestinal TB consists of antituberculosis drugs, with surgery being reserved for patients with an abscess or fistula, uncontrolled bleeding, perforation, or complete obstruction. Misdiagnosis of TB as Crohn's disease is particularly unfortunate because immunosuppressive therapy can result in miliary dissemination.

Ref.: 39, 40

41. Which of the following strategies is least useful for improving surgical outcomes in geriatric patients?

A. Preoperative evaluation of medical physiologic status

B. Optimization of physical and cognitive function

C. Minimization of perioperative nutritional deficiency

D. Postoperative assessment for rehabilitation options

E. Surgical risk assessment based on a specific diagnosis

ANSWER: E

COMMENTS: There are several important factors in achieving positive surgical outcomes in geriatric patients. Assessment of a patient's preoperative physical and cognitive function, along with optimization of these variables, is critical in elderly patients. Failure to recognize preoperative risk factors may result in more aggressive surgical procedures and poor outcomes. As the risks associated with surgical therapy increase, elderly patients may opt for palliative procedures, which allow resumption of preoperative independence and activities of daily life, as opposed to more radical procedures, which entail a prolonged convalescence and questionable quality of life. Elderly patients may be at risk for **malnutrition** because of physical and cognitive disabilities, poverty, and lack of awareness of the importance of a balanced diet. Patients with more than 10% weight loss and serum albumin level less than 2.5 g/dL should be considered to have **protein-energy malnutrition** and may benefit from a minimum of 7 to 10 days of nutritional repletion before surgery. Proper **preoperative rehabilitation planning** has been shown in patients with hip fractures to result in the quicker resumption of independent living. Surgical risk assessment is **multifactorial** and **not based on a specific diagnosis**. Physical fitness, cognitive fitness, and social factors (e.g., family and financial support), in addition to a specific diagnosis and surgical plan, are part of a thorough preoperative risk assessment.

Ref.: 44–48

42. Regarding the following several scenarios, which one of the operations can proceed as scheduled?

A. An 80-year-old scheduled for cataract surgery who has a pulse of 60 beats/min and a blood pressure of 180/110 mmHg and is completely asymptomatic

B. A 67-year-old scheduled for left total hip arthroplasty who has a pulse of 80 beats/min and blood pressure of 180/110 mmHg, is asymptomatic, and takes metoprolol

C. A 65-year-old hypertensive scheduled for bilateral total knee arthroplasty who has a pulse of 94 beats/min and a blood pressure of 104/68 mmHg and who takes an angiotensin-converting enzyme (ACE) inhibitor

D. An 80-year-old scheduled for bilateral laparoscopic hernia repair who has a pulse of 42 beats/min and a blood pressure of 100/60 mm Hg and who has a pacemaker and takes metoprolol

E. None of these operations should proceed

ANSWER: A

COMMENTS: Management of **hypertension** in the perioperative period remains controversial. However, several studies have consistently shown that a preoperative diastolic blood pressure higher than 110 mmHg confers increased risk for major morbidity. Aggressive perioperative normalization may not reduce the risk. However, the patient in scenario A is scheduled for a low-risk operation, unlike the patient in scenario B. Therefore the operation in scenario A can be performed safely as long as the patient has adequate follow-up. **ACE inhibitors** have been associated with severe perioperative hypotension during major surgery, especially in patients who receive an epidural catheter as part of their management. The patient in scenario D may have a pacemaker malfunction that needs to be evaluated. **Beta-blockers** have been shown to decrease intraoperative ischemia and should be continued. **Calcium channel blockers** and **diuretics** may be continued.

Ref.: 47–49

43. A 73-year-old man undergoes open cholecystectomy. His return of gastrointestinal function is delayed, so he has a nasogastric tube for 2 days. On postoperative day 4, he has fever, productive cough, and an infiltrate on chest x-ray. Which of the following is true?

A. The risk of aspiration in an 80-year-old is nearly double that of a 25-year-old patient.

B. Prolonged nasogastric suction eliminates the risk for aspiration pneumonia.

C. Older patients with dementia or delirium are at increased risk for aspiration.

D. While the risk for aspiration events increases with age, the incidence of aspiration pneumonia actually decreases because the immune response to chemical pneumonitis is less vigorous.

E. Resumption of oral feeds should be delayed for all patients over 60 years old to reduce the risk for aspiration.

ANSWER: C

COMMENTS: Aspiration is common in elderly patients, with an 80-year-old patient being 9 to 10 times more likely to have aspiration than a patient aged 18 to 29 years. Risk factors include diseases (stroke, dementia, neuromuscular disorders), iatrogenic factors (nasogastric tube, prolonged intubation), or medications (such as sedatives). Older patients may be at greater risk for developing pneumonia following aspiration because of impaired immune response and decreased respiratory clearance. Aspiration risk can be assessed preoperatively and may guide the need for postoperative precautions. Interventions such as monitoring of gastric residuals for tube feeds, upright position following meals, and keeping the head of the bed elevated 30 to 45 degrees can decrease the risk for aspiration events.

Ref.: 49, 50

44. Which of the following is incorrect when comparing geriatric patients with younger patients?

A. Elderly patients have lower creatinine values.

B. The risk for hypothermia is greater in elderly patients.

C. Fever is a less reliable sign of infection in elderly patients.

D. Colon pathology is the most common indication for surgery in elderly patients.

E. Cardiac complications are the leading cause of perioperative complications in the elderly.

ANSWER: D

COMMENTS: When obstetric procedures are excluded, more than 40% of operations are performed in patients older than 65 years. Elderly surgical patients represent a heterogeneous group, and **physiologic age** is generally of greater importance than chronologic age. To optimize the care of older patients, it is critical to understand age-related changes in physiology. Because muscle mass decreases with aging, baseline serum **creatinine** levels may decrease in the elderly despite the progressive loss of renal function. Geriatric patients are at increased risk for **hypothermia** because of impaired mechanisms of heat conservation, especially during operative procedures. Decreased muscle mass and metabolic heat production, malnutrition, and increased heat loss as a result of thinning skin all contribute to this phenomenon. **Fever** is not a reliable indicator of infection in elderly patients and may be absent in up to one-third of patients with serious infections. It is important to evaluate the patient's baseline temperature, with fever being suspected with an elevation in temperature of greater than 2°C above baseline. Malnourished geriatric patients or the extremely old are especially unlikely to mount a febrile response to infection. **Biliary tract disease**, including acute cholecystitis, is the most common indication for abdominal surgical intervention in elderly patients. This may be related to the increased lithogenicity of bile and increased prevalence of cholelithiasis. **Cardiac complications** are the leading cause of perioperative problems and death in all age groups but are of particular importance in elderly patients because of the prevalence of preexisting cardiac dysfunction and poor functional reserve.

Ref.: 49

45. Following cholecystectomy, an 82-year-old patient has an oxygen saturation of 88% on 2 L of oxygen by nasal cannula. Which of the following is not a probable explanation for this phenomenon?

A. Maximal breathing capacity is 50% of what the patient had at age 30.

B. The cough mechanism is less effective in elderly patients.
C. The pulse oximetry reading is spurious.
D. The patient was recently repositioned from supine to a sitting position.
E. The patient required conversion from laparoscopic to open cholecystectomy.

ANSWER: D

COMMENTS: Pulmonary complications represent some of the most common adverse events in elderly surgical patients; they account for up to 50% of postoperative complications and 20% of preventable deaths. Decreased strength and endurance of respiratory muscles, decreased lung volumes, and decreased compensatory responses to hypoxia or hypercapnia make tachypnea a less reliable sign of impending respiratory failure. Furthermore, changes in the respiratory system limit the maximal breathing capacity at the age of 70 years to about one-half of that present at the age of 30 years. Decreased airway sensitivity, dysfunctional mucociliary clearance, and decreased muscle strength all contribute to a decreased cough mechanism. **Shivering**, a common postoperative phenomenon, dramatically increases oxygen consumption, which could cause hypoxia. In addition, movement of the patient could result in a spurious pulse oximetry reading. The patient's positioning has a direct effect on a ventilation–perfusion mismatch and the alveolar–arterial oxygen gradient. In contrast to sitting, a supine position results in closure of small airways in the dependent portion of the lung. This leads to ventilation–perfusion mismatch and may contribute to hypoxemia. Therefore placing a patient in a sitting position should improve oxygenation. Unlike laparoscopic cholecystectomy, open cholecystectomy entails an upper abdominal incision, which results in decreased tidal volume, impaired diaphragmatic excursion with resultant hypoxemia, and an increased risk for atelectasis and pneumonia.

Ref.: 44, 45, 49

46. Which of the following statements regarding age-related changes in the cardiovascular system is not correct?

A. Ventricular contractility decreases
B. Sympathetic nervous system activity decreases
C. Mean arterial pressure increases
D. Left ventricular afterload increases
E. Myocardial contraction is prolonged

ANSWER: B

COMMENTS: Aging is associated with **functional and structural changes** in the heart and blood vessels, as well as alterations in autonomic regulatory mechanisms. The myocardium becomes thicker and stiffer, with reduced conduction fiber density and a decrease in the number of cells within the sinus node. These changes lead to decreased contractility and increased filling pressures. The elastic arteries become larger and stiffer, which results in increased mean arterial pressure and pulse pressure. The larger, stiffer arteries lead to increased pulse wave velocity, which allows earlier reflection of the pulse waves from the peripheral circulation. The reflected waves may reach the heart during end-systole, thereby increasing **cardiac afterload**. Decreased ventricular compliance and increased afterload cause a compensatory prolongation of **myocardial contraction** and decreased early ventricular filling time. Because the ventricle has less time to fill, the contribution of the atrium becomes more significant. Thus elderly patients are less tolerant of arrhythmias such as atrial fibrillation. The activity of the sympathetic nervous system increases, although decreased receptor affinity and alterations in signal transduction lead to decreased β-receptor responsiveness. This impairs an elderly patient's ability to increase the heart rate and ejection fraction in response to physiologic stress and may contribute to intraoperative hemodynamic lability.

Ref.: 44, 45, 49

47. A 74-year-old man is admitted for cardiac surgery. His preoperative creatinine level is 1.6 mg/dL. Which of the following statements about renal function in elderly patients is correct?

A. Renal blood flow decreases by up to 20% from baseline by the age of 80.
B. Loss of renal mass is most pronounced in the renal medulla.
C. Nephron hypertrophy compensates for the loss of nephrons with age.
D. Simple renal cysts in older patients are frequently malignant.
E. Serum creatinine is usually elevated because of decreased glomerular filtration rate.

ANSWER: C

COMMENTS: About one-half of Americans 70 years or older have an estimated **glomerular filtration rate** (eGFR) of less than 60 mL/min per 1.73 m^2, a threshold often used to define **chronic kidney disease** (CKD) with moderate or severely decreased renal function. With age, there is a progressive loss of **renal mass** (up to 30% at 80 years), especially in the renal cortex. Micro-anatomic changes include an increase in **nephrosclerosis** (focal and global glomerulosclerosis, interstitial fibrosis, tubular atrophy, and arteriosclerosis). As the number of functional nephrons decreases, the remaining nephrons hypertrophy. Gross anatomic changes include a decline in kidney volume, increase in number and size of simple (usually benign) renal cysts, and development of renal tumors. **Renal blood flow** decreases by 5%–10% per decade, with a 50% decrease being common in elderly patients. Despite the decrease in eGFR, progressive decline in lean body (muscle) mass may result in **serum creatinine** concentrations remaining constant or even decreasing.

Ref.: 44, 45, 49

48. Which of the following is correct when assessing the clinical impact of age-related changes in renal function?

A. Medication dosing should be based on serum creatinine rather than eGFR.
B. A decrease in the ability of the kidney to conserve chloride results in a predisposition to dehydration.
C. Most urinary tract infections are symptomatic.
D. Susceptibility to acute kidney injury (AKI) is about the same in older patients because of a decrease in lean body mass.
E. The response to increases in serum osmolarity is blunted in older adults.

ANSWER: E

COMMENTS: Changes in renal function with age have significant clinical ramifications. Decreased eGFR may impact dosing of medications cleared by glomerular filtration, and loss of functional reserve predisposes older patients to **AKI**. Because of a decline in renin–angiotensin axis activity, the kidneys' capacity to conserve **sodium** decreases, thereby leading to a propensity for sodium loss when salt intake is inadequate. There is also a marked decline in the subjective feeling of **thirst** in response to increases in serum osmolarity. The kidneys become less responsive to **antidiuretic hormone**. These changes lead to an increased risk for **dehydration**. However, mild reductions in eGFR with aging do not indicate an increased risk for end-stage renal disease, and older adults with good age-appropriate renal function can still serve as living kidney donors. Asymptomatic **urinary tract infections** are more common in elderly patients. Urinary tract infections are responsible for 30%–50% of all cases of bacteremia in older individuals. Increased collagen content causes the bladder to become less distensible. **Prostate hypertrophy** can impair bladder emptying in males, and decreased serum **estrogen** levels and impaired tissue responsiveness to estrogen in females predispose to **incontinence**.

Ref.: 44–46, 49

49. A 77-year-old man is admitted after a radical prostatectomy. On postoperative day 3, a productive cough and fever develop. A chest radiograph shows a right lower lobe infiltrate. Which of the following is correct regarding immune function in older patients?

A. WBC counts increase significantly even with mild infections.

B. The T-cell response to new antigens is impaired.

C. Normal neutrophil counts decline with age.

D. Normal acute phase protein levels are decreased.

E. Normocytic anemia is uncommon in older patients.

ANSWER: B

COMMENTS: The ability to mount an **immune response** becomes blunted with age, which leads to increased susceptibility to infections and increased **tumorigenesis**. These changes are particularly apparent under physiologic stress. Elderly patients with infections often have normal WBC counts, but the differential will show a profound left shift with many immature cells. Although baseline neutrophil counts remain relatively constant, the ability of the bone marrow to increase neutrophil production when indicated is diminished. Decreased T-cell production by the bone marrow, as well as thymic involution, impairs the production and differentiation of naïve T cells and therefore leads to a weakened response to new antigens. Chronic infection with viruses such as CMV may also alter T-cell function. **Inflammatory cytokine** levels are persistently elevated, as are levels of **acute phase proteins**. Chronic inflammation is believed to contribute to frailty, including loss of muscle mass, impaired nutrition, and decreased mobility. It may also contribute to the **normocytic anemia** commonly seen in elderly patients.

Ref.: 49

50. An 86-year-old woman with a history of complicated diverticulitis presents for colon resection. Which of the following is true?

A. The American Society of Anesthesiology (ASA) classification of physical health ("ASA score") includes an objective assessment of multiple organ systems.

B. The ASA score for a given patient would be higher for a Whipple procedure than for a laparoscopic appendectomy.

C. ASA score differentiates between emergent and elective procedures.

D. The revised Lee (Revised Cardiac Risk Index) and Eagle criteria are most useful for evaluating the risk for cardiac surgeries.

E. Low Lee and Eagle scores are associated with higher perioperative mortality.

ANSWER: C

COMMENTS: Older patients are at higher risk for perioperative complications. Several scoring systems have been developed to assess perioperative risk. The **ASA classification of physical health** is a subjective assessment of the patient's overall state of health that includes six classes:

I. Patient is a completely healthy fit patient.

II. Patient has a mild systemic disease.

III. Patient has a severe systemic disease that is not incapacitating.

IV. Patient has an incapacitating disease that is a constant threat to life.

V. A moribund patient who is not expected to live 24 h with or without surgery.

VI. A brain-dead patient who is undergoing surgery as an organ donor.

The score is appended with an "E" suffix if the surgery is deemed emergent. The risk for postoperative complications correlates with the ASA score. However, the subjective nature of the assessment as well as interoperator variability in assigning "systemic disease" and disease severity has led to a significant variation in reported outcomes.

The **Lee index (revised cardiac risk index)** is a prospectively validated model used to predict the risk of cardiac events in patients undergoing noncardiac surgery. It is calculated by assigning points in six equally weighted domains: (1) high-risk surgery, (2) history of ischemic heart disease, (3) history of congestive heart failure, (4) history of cerebrovascular disease, (5) preoperative treatment with insulin, and (6) preoperative serum creatinine > 2.0 mg/dL (>177 μmol/L). It was developed by simplifying the Goldman index. Higher Lee index scores are associated with higher rates of perioperative cardiac events; no risk factors are associated with a 0.4% risk of cardiac event while three or more risk factors are associated with a 5.4% risk. The Eagle model identifies five clinical predictors of perioperative cardiac events: age greater than 70 years, history of angina, diabetes, history of ventricular ectopy, and Q waves on an electrocardiogram (ECG). Patients with no clinical predictors had a 3% risk of perioperative ischemic events, while patients with 2 or 3 to 5 risk factors had an incidence of 16% and 50%, respectively. Typically, the stratification provided by the Eagle model is combined with radionuclide myocardial perfusion imaging to improve the sensitivity and specificity. Both the Lee (RCRI) and Eagle models were developed for risk stratification for noncardiac surgeries.

Ref.: 49, 51, 52

51. Which of the following is not true about frailty?

A. Frailty entails decreased physiologic reserve and inability to respond to stressors.

B. The concept of frailty was initially developed for perioperative risk stratification for older patients undergoing elective noncardiac surgery.

C. Unintended weight loss, decreased physical activity, and loss of muscle mass are all associated with increased operative risks in older patients.

D. Standardized assessments of frailty can be used to improve the predictive power of other perioperative risk assessment tools.

E. A higher frailty score predicts that a previously independent patient may require prolonged hospitalization or discharge to a nursing facility after surgery.

ANSWER: B

COMMENTS: The lack of standardized methods to assess decreased reserve in older patients has made it especially difficult to provide accurate perioperative risk stratification and predict complications. The concept of **frailty** as a global assessment of physiologic reserve and susceptibility to stressors has gained increasing use in the gerontology community. However, it has only more recently been applied to surgical risk assessment. One of the first validated assessments of frailty in the surgical population was the "**Hopkins Frailty Score.**" Domains assessed include **shrinking** (weight loss of at least 10 lbs. in the past year), **weakness** (assessed by grip strength adjusted based on gender and BMI), **exhaustion** (measured by responses to questions about effort and motivation), **low physical activity** (assessed by inquiring about leisure time activities), and **walking speed** (measured by the speed at which the patient could walk 15 feet). Each domain is assigned a score of 0 or 1. The presence of preoperative frailty has been shown to be predictive of postoperative complications, increased length of stay, and discharge to a nursing facility. Assessment of preoperative frailty can also be used to improve the predictive power of other preoperative risk indices such as the ASA, Eagle, and Lee scores.

Ref.: 45, 53–56

52. Which of the following is the best single-item measurement to quantify surgical risk as a surrogate for a formal assessment of frailty?

A. Shrinking (weight loss)

B. Exhaustion

C. Low physical activity

D. Walking speed

E. Dementia

ANSWER: D

COMMENTS: Multiple tools have been developed to assess frailty as a predictor of adverse surgical outcomes. These can range in complexity from assessing one item to a 90-item comprehensive evaluation. One of the simplest is a brief "**Frail scale**" assessing: F—Fatigue (are you tired); R—Resistance (can you climb one flight of stairs); A—Ambulation (can you walk one block); I—Illness (more than five total); L—Loss of weight (greater than 5%). If resources limit full implementation of frailty screening, evaluation of patients over the age of 70 years with some weight loss has been proposed as a good first step. The most reliable single measure that correlates with postoperative complications is **gait speed**.

Ref.: 56

53. An 84-year-old previously independent man undergoes a colectomy for complicated diverticulitis. One week postoperatively he remains confused and unable to independently complete activities of daily living. Which of the following is true regarding cognitive function in elderly patients following surgery?

A. Delirium presents as chronic, largely irreversible mental status decline.

B. Postoperative cognitive decline (POCD) is increased by even brief periods of interoperative hypotension in patients aged more than 60 years.

C. Hallucinations and inappropriate communication that vary over the course of the day are most typical of dementia.

D. POCD is most frequently seen with noncardiac surgery.

E. Preoperative dementia increases the risk for postoperative delirium.

ANSWER: E

COMMENTS: Delirium is an acute confusional state featuring decreased attention and awareness of the environment. Symptoms may include hallucinations, delusions, anxiety, inappropriate communication, and distress and may fluctuate during the course of the day. Delirium may be related to medications (especially anticholinergic agents, opioids, and sedatives), infection, or withdrawal from substances such as alcohol. Delirium is reversible when the underlying causes are addressed. **Dementia** encompasses chronic organic brain syndromes such as Alzheimer's disease that are typically insidious and irreversible. The presence of dementia predisposes a patient to delirium, especially in the presence of stressors such as illness, sleep deprivation, or removal from a known environment (such as a hospital admission). **POCD** is a long-term, possibly permanent, disabling deterioration in cognitive function following surgery. It is characterized by preserved orientation but with a significant decline from the patient's baseline neuropsychologic evaluation. The greatest incidence of POCD is in patients undergoing a surgery that requires cardiopulmonary bypass, but recent evidence suggests that it may present following noncardiac surgeries as well. Some studies suggest that the incidence of POCD in patients aged over 60 years may be as high as 25% at 1 week and 10% at 3 months postoperatively, with even higher incidence in older patients. Proposed preoperative patient risk factors include education level, preoperative depression or cognitive impairment, and habits such as drug or alcohol use. The etiology of POCD is not known, although the similarity to the cognitive decline observed with multiple cerebral emboli following cardiopulmonary bypass suggests this as a possible cause. Biochemical alterations such as hyponatremia, perioperative hypotension, and hypoxemia have not been shown to increase POCD.

Ref.: 49, 57

REFERENCES

1. Mikami DJ, Henry JC, Ellison EC. Surgery in the pregnant patient. In: Townsend CM, Sabiston DC, eds. *Sabiston Textbook of Surgery: The Biological Basis of Modern Surgical Practice*, 20th ed. Philadelphia, PA: Elsevier; 2016.
2. Goodwin TM. Hyperemesis gravidarum. *Obstet Gynecol Clin North Am.* 2008;35(3):401–417.
3. Herbert WNP, Goodwin TM, Koren G, Phelan ST. *Nausea and Vomiting of Pregnancy. APGO Educational Series on Women's Health Issues.* Washington, DC: Association of Professors of Gynecology and Obstetrics (APGO); 2001:1–28.
4. Koren G, Clark S, Hankins GD, et al. Effectiveness of delayed-release doxylamine and pyridoxine for nausea and vomiting of pregnancy: a randomized placebo controlled trial. *Am J Obstet Gynecol.* 2010; 203(6):571.e1–e7.

5. Practice Bulletin No. 153: Nausea and vomiting of pregnancy. *Obstet Gynecol*. 2015;126(3):e12–e24.
6. Sarsam SE, Elliott JP, Lam GK. Management of wound complications from cesarean delivery. *Obstet Gynecol Surv*. 2005;60(7):462–473.
7. Chelmow D, Rodriguez EJ, Sabatini MM. Suture closure of subcutaneous fat and wound disruption after cesarean delivery: a meta-analysis. *Obstet Gynecol*. 2004;103(5 Pt 1):974–980.
8. Hellums EK, Lin MG, Ramsey PS. Prophylactic subcutaneous drainage for prevention of wound complications after cesarean delivery—a metaanalysis. *Am J Obstet Gynecol*. 2007;197(3):229–235.
9. Scarsbrook AF, Evans AL, Owen AR, Gleeson FV. Diagnosis of suspected venous thromboembolic disease in pregnancy. *Clin Radiol*. 2006;61(1):1–12.
10. Marik PE, Plante LA. Venous thromboembolic disease and pregnancy. *N Engl J Med*. 2008;359(19):2025–2033.
11. Greer IA. Clinical practice. Pregnancy complicated by venous thrombosis. *N Engl J Med*. 2015;373(6):540–547.
12. Brooks DC, Oxford C. The pregnant surgical patient. In: A. S. W., ed. *ACS Surgery: Principles and Practice*. Philadelphia: American College of Surgeons; 2010.
13. Pastore PA, Loomis DM, Sauret J. Appendicitis in pregnancy. *J Am Board Fam Med*. 2006;19(6):621–626.
14. Hodjati H, Kazerooni T. Location of the appendix in the gravid patient: a re-evaluation of the established concept. *Int J Gynaecol Obstet*. 2003;81(3):245–247.
15. Pedrosa I, Levine D, Eyvazzadeh AD, Siewert B, Ngo L, Rofsky NM. MR imaging evaluation of acute appendicitis in pregnancy. *Radiology*. 2006;238(3):891–899.
16. Committee Opinion No. 656: Guidelines for diagnostic imaging during pregnancy and lactation. *Obstet Gynecol*. 2016;127(2):e75–e80.
17. Malangoni MA. Gastrointestinal surgery and pregnancy. *Gastroenterol Clin North Am*. 2003;32(1):181–200.
18. Cunningham FG. General considerations and maternal evaluation. In: Cunningham FG, Leveno KJ, Bloom SL, et al., eds. *Williams Obstetrics*. 24th ed. New York, NY: McGraw-Hill Education; 2013.
19. ACOG Committee Opinion. Number 299, September 2004 (replaces No. 158, September 1995). Guidelines for diagnostic imaging during pregnancy. *Obstet Gynecol*. 2004;104(3):647–651.

19a. *Committee Opinion No. 656: Guidelines for Diagnostic Imaging During Pregnancy and Lactation*. Obstet Gynecol, 2016. 127(2): p. e75-80.

19b. Chen, MM, Coakley, FV, Kaimal, A, Laros, RK, *Guidelines for Computed Tomography and Magnetic Resonance Imaging Use During Pregnancy and Lactation*, Obstetrics & Gynecology 2008, 112(2): p. 333-340.

19c. Patel, SJ, Reede, DL, Katz, DS, Subramaniam, R, *Imaging the Pregnant Patient for Nonobstetric Conditions: Algorithms and Radiation Dose Considerations*, RadioGraphics 2007, 27(6): 1705-23.

20. Cappell MS. Hepatic and gastrointestinal diseases. In: Gabbe SG, ed. *Obstetrics: Normal and Problem Pregnancies*. Philadelphia: Elsevier/Saunders: vii, 1291 p. 1291.
21. ACOG Practice Bulletin No. 105: Bariatric surgery and pregnancy. *Obstet Gynecol*. 2009;113(6):1405–1413.
22. Heron M. Deaths: leading causes for 2014. *Natl Vital Stat Rep*. 2016;65(5):1–96.
23. Creanga AA, Berg CJ, Syverson C, Seed K, Bruce FC, Callaghan WM. Pregnancy-related mortality in the United States, 2006–2010. *Obstet Gynecol*. 2015;125(1):5–12.
24. Deshpande NA, Coscia LA, Gomez-Lobo V, Moritz MJ, Armenti VT. Pregnancy after solid organ transplantation: a guide for obstetric management. *Rev Obstet Gynecol*. 2013;6(3-4):116–125.
25. Moaddab A, Dildy GA, Brown HL, et al. Health care disparity and state-specific pregnancy-related mortality in the United States, 2005–2014. *Obstet Gynecol*. 2016;128(4):869–875.
26. Practice Bulletin No. 158. Critical care in pregnancy. *Obstet Gynecol*. 2016;127(1):e21–e28.
27. Nguyen NT, Masoomi H, Magno CP, Nguyen XM, Laugenour K, Lane J. Trends in use of bariatric surgery, 2003–2008. *J Am Coll Surg*. 2011;213(2):261–266.
28. Alexander EK, Marqusee E, Lawrence J, Jarolim P, Fischer GA, Larsen PR. Timing and magnitude of increases in levothyroxine requirements during pregnancy in women with hypothyroidism. *N Engl J Med*. 2004;351(3):241–249.
29. Mazzaferri EL. Evaluation and management of common thyroid disorders in women. *Am J Obstet Gynecol*. 1997;176(3):507–514.
30. Practice Bulletin No. 148. Thyroid disease in pregnancy. *Obstet Gynecol*. 2015;125(4):996–1005.
31. Mastrobattista JM, Gomez-Lobo V. Pregnancy after solid organ transplantation. *Obstet Gynecol*. 2008;112(4):919–932.
32. Coscia LA, Constantinescu S, Davison JM, Moritz MJ, Armenti VT. Immunosuppressive drugs and fetal outcome. *Best Pract Res Clin Obstet Gynaecol*. 2014;28(8):1174–1187.
33. Sachak T, Arnold MA, Naini BV, et al. Neutropenic enterocolitis: new insights into a deadly entity. *Am J Surg Pathol*. 2015;39(12):1635–1642.
34. Sifri CD, Madoff LC. Diverticulitis and typhlitis. In: Mandell GL, Bennett JE, Dolin R, eds. *Mandell, Douglas, and Bennett's Principles and Practice of Infectious Diseases*. Philadelphia, PA: Elsevier; 2015.
35. Correa-Rotter R, Mehrotra R, Saxena A. Peritoneal dialysis. In: Taal MW, Brenner BM, Rector FC, eds. *Brenner & Rector's the Kidney*. Philadelphia, PA: Elsevier/Saunders; 2016.
36. Kawaguchi Y, Tranaeus A. A historical review of encapsulating peritoneal sclerosis. *Perit Dial Int*. 2005;25(suppl 4):S7–S13.
37. Turnage RH, Mizell J, Badgwell B. Abdominal wall, umbilicus, peritoneum, mesenteries, omentum, and retroperitoneum. In: Townsend CM, Sabiston DC, eds. *Sabiston Textbook of Surgery: The Biological Basis of Modern Surgical Practice*, 20th ed. Philadelphia, PA: Elsevier/Saunders; 2016.
38. Wyers SG, Matthews JB. Surgical peritonitis and other diseases of the peritoneum, mesentery, omentum, and diaphragm. In: Feldman M, Friedman LS, Brandt LJ, eds. *Sleisenger and Fordtran's Gastrointestinal and Liver Diseases: Pathophysiology/Diagnosis/Management*. Philadelphia, PA: Elsevier/Saunders; 2016:2. volumes.
39. Giouleme O, Paschos P, Katsaros M, et al. Intestinal tuberculosis: a diagnostic challenge—case report and review of the literature. *Eur J Gastroenterol Hepatol*. 2011;23(11):1074–1077.
40. Hassan I, Brilakis ES, Thompson RL, Que FG. Surgical management of abdominal tuberculosis. *J Gastrointest Surg*. 2002;6(6):862–867.
41. Ponticelli C, Passerini P. Gastrointestinal complications in renal transplant recipients. *Transpl Int*. 2005;18(6):643–650.
42. Keates J, Lagahee S, Crilley P, Haber M, Kowalski T. CMV enteritis causing segmental ischemia and massive intestinal hemorrhage. *Gastrointest Endosc*. 2001;53(3):355–359.
43. Castagnola E, Mikulska M, Viscoli C. Prophylaxis and empirical therapy of infection in cancer patients. In: Mandell GL, Bennett JE, Dolin R, eds. *Mandell, Douglas, and Bennett's Principles and Practice of Infectious Diseases*. Philadelphia, PA: Elsevier; 2015.
44. Yeo H, Indes J, Rosenthal RA. Surgery in the geriatric patient. In: Townsend CM, Beauchamp RD, Evers BM, et al., eds. *Sabiston Textbook of Surgery: the Biological Basis of Modern Surgical Practice*. 20th ed, Philadelphia, PA: Elsevier/Saunders; 2016.
45. Hardin RE, Zenilman ME. Surgical considerations in the elderly. In: Brunicardi FC, Andersen DK, Billiar TR, et al., eds. *Schwartz's Principles of Surgery*. 10th ed. New York, NY: McGraw-Hill Education; 2014.
46. Pavlin DJ, Pavlin EG, Fitzgibbon DR, Koerschgen ME, Plitt TM. Management of bladder function after outpatient surgery. *Anesthesiology*. 1999;91(1):42–50.
47. Fleisher LA, Fleischmann KE, Auerbach AD, et al. 2014 ACC/AHA guideline on perioperative cardiovascular evaluation and management of patients undergoing noncardiac surgery: executive summary: a report of the American College of Cardiology/American Heart Association Task Force on practice guidelines. *J Nucl Cardiol*. 2015;22(1):162–215.
48. Velasco A, Reyes E, Hage FG. Guidelines in review: comparison of the 2014 ACC/AHA guidelines on perioperative cardiovascular evaluation and management of patients undergoing noncardiac surgery and the 2014 ESC/ESA guidelines on noncardiac surgery: cardiovascular assessment and management. *J Nucl Cardiol*. 2017;24:165.
49. Sieber F, Pauldine R. Geriatric anesthesia. In: Miller RD, ed. *Miller's Anesthesia*. Philadelphia, PA: Elsevier/Saunders; 2015:2. volumes (3270, I-122 pages).
50. Kikawada M, Iwamoto T, Takasaki M. Aspiration and infection in the elderly: epidemiology, diagnosis and management. *Drugs Aging*. 2005;22(2):115–130.
51. Eagle KA, Coley CM, Newell JB, et al. Combining clinical and thallium data optimizes preoperative assessment of cardiac risk before major vascular surgery. *Ann Intern Med*. 1989;110(11):859–866.

52. Lee TH, Marcantonio ER, Mangione CM, et al. Derivation and prospective validation of a simple index for prediction of cardiac risk of major noncardiac surgery. *Circulation*. 1999;100(10):1043–1049.
53. Makary MA, Segev DL, Pronovost PJ, et al. Frailty as a predictor of surgical outcomes in older patients. *J Am Coll Surg*. 2010;210(6): 901–908.
54. Revenig LM, Canter DJ, Kim S, et al. Report of a simplified frailty score predictive of short-term postoperative morbidity and mortality. *J Am Coll Surg*. 2015;220(5):904–911.
55. Revenig LM, Canter DJ, Taylor MD, et al. Too frail for surgery? Initial results of a large multidisciplinary prospective study examining preoperative variables predictive of poor surgical outcomes. *J Am Coll Surg*. 2013;217(4):665–670.
56. Robinson TN, Walston JD, Brummel NE, et al. Frailty for surgeons: review of a National Institute on Aging Conference on Frailty for Specialists. *J Am Coll Surg*. 2015;221(6):1083–1092.
57. Tsai TL, Sands LP, Leungc JM. An update on postoperative cognitive dysfunction. *Adv Anesth*. 2010;28(1):269–284.

CHAPTER 34

EVIDENCE-BASED SURGERY AND APPLICATIONS OF BIOSTATISTICS

Vidya A. Fleetwood, M.D., and Shabirhusain S. Abadin, M.D.

1. As part of an effort to reduce the length of hospital stay, right hemicolectomy patients were placed on a clinical pathway. All of the first seven patients placed on the pathway did well except the last patient, in whom aspiration pneumonia developed and necessitated 1 month in the intensive care unit. The lengths of stay for these patients were 3, 4, 4, 5, 6, 7, and 41 days. What are the mean, median, and mode of the length-of-stay data?

    A. Mean = 10, median = 5, mode = 4

    B. Mean = 5, median = 10, mode = 5

    C. Mean = 10, median = 4, mode = 1

    D. Mean = 10, median = 5, mode = 41

    E. Mean = 5, median = 5, mode = 1

ANSWER: A

COMMENTS: The mean, median, and mode are all measures of the **central tendency** of a data set. Both mean and median summarize the center of the data set. The **mean** is calculated by summing all of the observations and dividing by the number of observations. The **median** is the data value in which one-half of the data points fall above it and one-half below it. The median can be determined by listing the data points in rank order (as in the example). The median is the middle point of the ranked data. For odd sample sizes, one-half of the remaining observations fall to the left of this value, and the other one-half fall to the right of this value. For even sample sizes, the median is the mean of the two middle values. As in this example, the mean is sensitive to outliers (the patient with a length of stay of 41 days); for these data sets, the median may more correctly represent the data. The **mode** is the most frequently occurring value in the data set. For a normal distribution, the mean, median, and mode have approximately the same values.

Ref.: 1–3

2. A patient is at postoperative day 5 from an open cholecystectomy and has a prolonged ileus. You are attempting to use the pain scales to titrate down his pain medication dosage. Which of the following data types (i.e., nominal, ordinal, interval, and ratio) correctly describe the variables (i.e., gender, respiratory rate, pain scale, and date of month)?

	Gender (M/F)	Respiratory Rate	Pain Scale (1 to 10)	Date of Month
A.	Nominal	Ordinal	Interval	Ratio
B.	Nominal	Ratio	Ordinal	Interval
C.	Interval	Ratio	Ordinal	Nominal
D.	Ordinal	Interval	Ratio	Nominal
E.	Nominal	Interval	Ordinal	Ratio

ANSWER: B

COMMENTS: Experimental data can be classified as **categorical** or **quantitative**. Categorical data can be further divided into nominal and ordinal variables. **Nominal data** are classified into groups or named categories in which the order is arbitrary, for example, a "race" variable that can take on the values of black, white, Hispanic, or other. Means and medians are not meaningful for nominal data, although the mode represents the value most commonly measured. **Ordinal data** are nonquantitative variables that are ordered by some meaningful criteria, such as cancer staging (I to IV) or Likert scales (1 = strongly agree, 2 = agree, etc.). Modes and medians most appropriately represent the ordinal data; although means can be calculated (and mean ranks form the basis for many nonparametric statistical tests), they must be used with caution. Quantitative data are represented by an ordered scale with equal distances between values. Calculations of arithmetic means and standard deviations (SDs) can be performed for quantitative data. **Interval data** have equal distance between values but with an arbitrary zero point, such as temperature scales or dates. **Ratio data** also have an ordered scale with equal intervals between values but with a meaningful zero point, for example, patient weight or blood pressure. Ratios are meaningful for ratio data but not for interval data because the ratio depends on the scale chosen. For instance, a central venous pressure (CVP) of 20 cmH_2O is twice as great as a CVP of 10 cmH_2O (ratio data), but a 60°F (15°C) day is not twice as warm as a 30°F (−1°C) day (interval data).

Ref.: 2, 4

3. A fourth-year resident is attempting to determine where his American Board of Surgery In-Training Examination score falls nationally. He is given a histogram and the

standard deviation (SD). Which of the following is true about descriptive statistics?

A. A histogram graphically depicts the means of experimental observations from a population.

B. A skewed distribution will be highly symmetrical.

C. For a normal distribution, 95% of data points will fall within 1 SD of the mean.

D. Mean, median, and mode are all approximately the same for a normal (Gaussian) distribution.

E. The 50th percentile of any data set is equivalent to the mean.

ANSWER: D

COMMENTS: A **frequency distribution** is obtained by dividing the range of observed values into intervals and then counting the number of observations that fall into each interval. Frequency data can be depicted graphically in bar charts, histograms, and frequency polygons. These graphs allow quick evaluation of the distribution of data. A distribution is **symmetrical** if the two halves are mirror images. If more observations are clumped to one end of the distribution, it is **skewed**. The flat or peaked shape of a distribution is called **kurtosis**. A **normal (Gaussian) distribution** is symmetrical (skew = 0) and graphically appears bell shaped. For normal distributions, the mean, median, and mode all have approximately the same value. Approximately 68% and 95% of data points fall within 1 and 2 SD of the mean, respectively. **Percentile ranks** are used to describe the location of a data point within a data set. A percentile is a value on a scale of 0 to 100 that specifies the percentage of a distribution that is equal to or below it. For example, an individual who scores in the 80th percentile on an examination has performed as well as or better than 80% of all examinees. The 50th percentile of any data set is equivalent to the median.

Ref.: 1, 2, 5

4. Which of the following is true?

A. Variance is the sum of the absolute differences between each sample point and the mean.

B. The sample SD will be small if the sample size is large.

C. The standard error of the mean (SEM) is independent of the sample size.

D. SEM can be obtained by dividing the sample SD by the square of the sample size (N^2).

E. SD is better than SEM for describing scatter in the data.

ANSWER: E

COMMENTS: The **distribution** of a random variable is a representation that gives the probability that the variable takes different values or ranges of values. Experimental data sets typically represent a **sample** of observations from a distribution. The characteristics of a distribution, such as population mean, population SD, and population variance, are called **parameters**. The corresponding characteristics of the sample, such as sample mean, sample SD, and sample variance, are called **statistics**. The **variance** is the sum of the squares of the difference between each sample point and the mean. The **SD** is the square root of the variance. Both variance and SD quantify how much individual data values vary from the mean. The sample SD is an estimate of the population SD calculated by using deviations from the sample mean. The sample SD is not proportional to the sample size; it will be large if the data are highly scattered, even if the sample size is large. The **SEM** is a measure of the variability in the distribution of sample means from the population mean. Because larger samples allow the sample mean to better approximate the population mean, SEM decreases as the sample size increases. SEM is calculated by dividing the sample SD by the square root of the sample size ($SEM = SD/\sqrt{N}$). If the SD is small and the sample size is large (yielding a small SEM), the sample mean is an accurate estimate of the population mean. The SD better represents the scatter of the data, whereas the SEM estimates the variability of an estimate of the sample mean.

Ref: 1, 3, 5

5. While attempting to research whether an excisional biopsy or a stereotactic core-needle biopsy is more effective at obtaining a tissue diagnosis in breast cancer, you find that the odds ratio of a true positive cancer diagnosis with a core-needle biopsy is 0.95 [95% confidence interval (CI), 0.92–10.8]. Which of the following is correct about descriptions and estimations of populations?

A. The 95% reference range will contain all of the data 95% of the time.

B. To calculate a 95% CI, the sample must contain 95% of the population.

C. Nonparametric statistics are most useful if the population distribution is normal and the sample size is large.

D. The 95% CI of the mean becomes smaller as the dispersion of the data decreases or the sample size increases.

E. The number of degrees of freedom is inversely proportional to the sample size.

ANSWER: D

COMMENTS: For data that are approximately normally distributed, the sample mean and SD can be used to calculate a **reference range**. The 95% reference range, or (mean − 1.96 SD) to (mean + 1.96 SD), will contain approximately 95% of the data. A **CI** reflects the accuracy of the sample parameter (often the mean) in estimating the value of the corresponding population parameter. In calculating CIs, two criteria must be met: the distribution of the sample parameter of interest must be approximately normal (generally valid if the sample size is large enough) and the population SD must be well approximated by the sample SD. In this case, the 95% CI of the mean can be calculated from the **normal distribution** as sample mean ± (1.96 × SEM). For small sample sizes, the assumption of a normal distribution of the sample means may not apply. If the sample size is very small and the population distribution is distinctly not normal, nonparametric statistical methods should be used. However, even if the sample size is relatively small, CIs can usually be calculated by using the ***t*-distribution** (to determine the multiplier for SEM in the CI equation) in place of the normal distribution. The *t*-distribution looks much like the bell-shaped normal distribution but has a flatter peak and more drawn-out tails. The size of the tails relative to the peak is inversely proportional to the **degrees of freedom** of the *t*-distribution, which is determined by the sample size − 1. As the number of degrees of freedom increases (with increasing sample size), the tails become smaller, and the *t*-distribution more closely approximates a normal distribution. The reference range is most useful in describing the population, whereas the CI is more useful in estimating the precision of a population value from a single sample of measurements.

Ref.: 3, 5

6. Seventy-five surgical residents are surveyed to determine whether overnight calls have an impact on their driving habits. The relative risk (RR) of having a traffic accident after calls versus before calls is found to be 2.4 with a 95% CI of 0.4 to 4.8. Which of the following are true?
   A. The null hypothesis for this study (no difference in accident rates) is an RR of 0.
   B. A P value of .05 represents a stronger association than does P = .007.
   C. The P value for this study will probably be greater than .05.
   D. CIs are not useful for hypothesis testing.
   E. This study proves that overnight calls do not increase the risk of having an automobile accident.

ANSWER: C

COMMENTS: Hypothesis testing is the process by which conclusions are drawn in an objective, probabilistic manner. The goal of hypothesis testing is to determine whether an observed difference between two groups is caused by the controlled variable or by chance. The **null hypothesis** is typically defined to be that there is *no* difference between the groups. The **alternative hypothesis** is usually the postulate that there *is* a significant difference between the two study arms. The P **value** (probability) measures how likely it is that any observed differences between groups are not caused by chance. Although P can take any value between 0 and 1, a result is termed often significant if $P < .05$; that is, the probability that the observed difference between groups was caused by chance is less than 5%. In this case the null hypothesis is rejected. If the calculation yields a nonsignificant P value, no conclusions about differences between the groups can be made and the null hypothesis is retained. Although the P value quantifies the strength of association (P = .0001 suggests a stronger association than P = .05), it does not provide any measure of the size of the effect. Thus a small P value does not necessarily imply a clinically significant effect. Providing exact P values is helpful in quantifying the strength of association (rather than simply stating $P < .05$). The **CI** gives a range of values within which it is likely that the true population value lies. If the expected value of the null hypothesis does not lie within the 95% CI, the null hypothesis can generally be rejected. For example, when examining RR, the null hypothesis is that the two groups do not have different risks for the end point of interest (RR = 1). If the 95% CI for the RR includes the value 1, the null hypothesis cannot be rejected.

Ref.: 3, 5, 6

7. You compare your laparoscopy patients who have their umbilical port sites closed in two layers to those closed in one layer to determine whether multiple layers decrease the incidence of seroma. Your sample size (*n*) is 5 in the first group and 32 in the second. You are unsure whether you have sufficient power in your study. Which of the following is true about hypothesis testing?
   A. A type I error is the probability of concluding that no difference exists when in fact it does.
   B. A type II error is the probability of concluding that a difference exists when it does not.
   C. The Bonferroni adjustment attempts to minimize the risk of incorrectly finding differences between groups when multiple comparisons are made.
   D. Power increases with the sample size and effect size but decreases as type I error (alpha) increases.
   E. Underpowered studies often show statistically significant differences when in fact none exist.

ANSWER: C

COMMENTS: A **type I error (alpha)** is the probability of falsely rejecting the null hypothesis or saying that there is a difference between groups when there actually is not. The alpha level is set a priori, or before a study is conducted. Alpha is typically set at 0.01 or 0.05 for clinical, behavioral, and basic science research. Type I error increases in proportion to the number of tests performed on the same data set. When performing multiple comparisons between two or more groups, the risk that a statistically significant difference between the groups is caused by chance increases as more variables are compared. The **Bonferroni adjustment** reduces the alpha level by dividing by the number of hypotheses that are tested. This attempts to maintain the type I error for the entire study at the preselected level. A **type II error (beta)** is the probability of failing to reject the null hypothesis when it is in fact false or, in other words, failing to observe a difference when one actually exists. A type I error is **false positive**, whereas a type II error is **false negative**. The **power** of a statistical test is the probability that the test will reject the null hypothesis when the alternative hypothesis is true (i.e., it will not make a type II error). Power is equal to 1 − beta. In other words, power is the probability of correctly identifying a difference between the study groups when one actually exists in the populations from which the samples were selected. It is best to perform a power calculation when designing a study. This usually entails selecting a level for alpha, determining the effect size (generally from previous data, clinical expertise, or both), and then calculating the necessary sample size. Power increases with larger sample sizes, greater true differences between populations, and higher acceptance of false-positive results (higher alpha). Many studies that appear to demonstrate no difference between groups may simply be underpowered.

Ref.: 3, 6, 7

8. A study is performed to determine the impact of enteric spillage on the rate of anastomotic leak for bowel anastomosis. Using the chart below, what is the RR for an anastomotic leak?

		Anastomotic Leak	
		Yes	No
Enteric Spillage	Yes	20	80
	No	10	190

   A. 1
   B. 2
   C. 4
   D. 5
   E. 8

ANSWER: C

COMMENTS: See Question 9.

Ref.: 1, 3

9. Referring to the data in Question 8, for about how many patients must enteric spillage be avoided to prevent one anastomotic leak?
   A. 2
   B. 3
   C. 5
   D. 7
   E. 10

ANSWER: D

COMMENTS: The **RR** (or risk ratio) is the likelihood of experiencing the outcome in the group with the risk factor divided by the likelihood of experiencing the outcome in the group without the risk factor. In this example, RR = (20/100)/(10/200) = 4. That is, patients with enteric spillage are four times more likely than those without to have a subsequent anastomotic leak. The **absolute risk reduction** (ARR) is the difference in the percentages of patients experiencing the outcome in the groups with and without the risk factor. In this example, ARR = (20/100) − (10/200) = 0.15, or 15%. The **number needed to treat** (NNT) represents the number of patients treated (or in this case the number of patients who must avoid the risk factor) to prevent one episode of the outcome. The NNT is the inverse of the ARR, or in this case 1/0.15 = 6.7. In this example, one needs to avoid seven episodes of enteric spillage to eliminate one anastomotic leak.

Ref.: 1, 3

10. When determining how to compare the quality of life after diagnosis between stages of lung cancer, you decide to use nonparametric statistics. Which of the following is true about nonparametric statistics?

A. They have greater power than the corresponding parametric tests.

B. They require fewer assumptions about the form of the population from which the data are obtained.

C. They are generally more sensitive to outliers.

D. They are usually less robust than corresponding parametric statistics.

E. One example is the unpaired *t* test.

ANSWER: B

COMMENTS: Traditional statistical tests are called **parametric** because they require estimation of the parameters that define the distribution. They often require assumptions about the format of the distribution. One commonly required assumption is that the underlying distribution (or a suitable transformation of the data) is normal or nearly normal. In cases in which these assumptions are not valid, **nonparametric** statistical analysis may be used. Nonparametric tests require few or no assumptions about the format of the data. They can be helpful in dealing with nominal or ordinal (categorical) data that cannot be meaningfully ordered or when there is no fixed interval between categories (e.g., cancer stages, demographic data such as race, or temperature data). They are often more robust than traditional methods (because fewer assumptions are required) and may be easier to apply. They are also usually less sensitive to **outliers** in the data. However, nonparametric tests frequently lack power compared with parametric tests; therefore a larger sample size is required. They are also generally geared toward hypothesis testing rather than estimation of effects.

Ref.: 3, 8, 9

11. A study is performed to assess the impact of weight loss surgery on diabetes. A total of 64 obese, diabetic patients undergo gastric bypass. Glycosylated hemoglobin (HbA1c) is measured for each patient 2 months before and 6 months after the surgery. For patients before surgery, the mean and SD of HbA1c were 9.2 and 2.1, respectively. After surgery, the corresponding values were 6.8 and 1.9, respectively. Which test would be most appropriate for comparing the two samples?

A. Unpaired *t* test

B. Paired *t* test

C. One-way analysis of variance (ANOVA)

D. Mann-Whitney U test

E. McNemar test

ANSWER: B

COMMENTS: See Question 12.

Ref.: 1–3, 8

12. Many of the obese diabetic patients also had gastroesophageal reflux disease (GERD). The investigators decided to assess whether gastric bypass surgery decreased the incidence of GERD. Before surgery, 46 (of 64) patients reported GERD. After surgery, only 32 patients reported GERD symptoms. What test would be most appropriate for determining whether the decrease in GERD was caused by chance?

A. Unpaired *t* test

B. Paired *t* test

C. One-way ANOVA

D. Mann-Whitney U test

E. McNemar test

ANSWER: E

COMMENTS: The choice of statistical test depends on multiple factors: the expected distribution of the population (normal, scattered), the types of outcomes measured (categorical, continuous, and time to event), the number of groups, whether the data are paired, and the number of factors that are tested. The ***t* test** is a parametric test for examining the difference between means for two independent samples. The **paired *t* test** compares the means for a single sample before and after some intervention (e.g., systolic blood pressure for the same patients before and after the administration of atenolol) or for two samples in which the patients are paired (e.g., a study patient and a matched control). **ANOVA** is a parametric test for comparing the means of three or more unpaired samples. All of these tests require the typical assumptions for parametric tests (nearly normal distribution, similar sample SDs, etc.). The **Mann-Whitney U test** (also called the Wilcoxon rank sum test) is the nonparametric analogue to the *t* test. It is more robust (in large part because it is less sensitive to deviation from population normality or outliers) and can be used for ordinal data. The **McNemar test** is a nonparametric test that can be used to compare nominal data (e.g., race, true/false, and gender). This test requires that the data be paired (e.g., same patient before and after treatment).

Ref.: 1–3, 8

13. Which of the following is true about regression and correlation?

A. The dependent variable is used to predict the independent variable.

B. Multiple regression generally refers to more than one outcome variable.

C. In logistic regression, the outcome variable is categorical.

D. Two variables are uncorrelated if they have a negative correlation coefficient.

E. Correlation usually implies causation.

ANSWER: C

COMMENTS: Regression methods are statistical models used to predict the value of a dependent variable from one or more independent variables. **Multiple regression** generally refers to models with more than one independent variable. In linear regression, the outcome variable is normally distributed, whereas in logistic regression, the outcome variable is dichotomous. Frequently, instead of predicting one variable or another, we wish to determine whether there is a relationship between two variables. A **correlation coefficient** reflects the strength of the relationship between two random variables. A positive correlation coefficient means that as one variable increases, the other variable also increases. A negative correlation means that as one variable increases, the other variable decreases. It is important to recognize that "correlation does not imply causation"; that is, an observed correlation may not reflect a causal relationship between two variables. For example, several epidemiologic studies have shown that women taking hormone replacement therapy (HRT) have a lower than average incidence of coronary artery disease (CAD), which led to postulating that HRT was protective against CAD. However, randomized controlled studies demonstrated that HRT was actually associated with a small but significantly increased risk for CAD. Reanalysis of the epidemiologic studies showed that women taking HRT were more likely to be from higher socioeconomic groups. Thus the use of HRT and the observed decrease in CAD were coincident effects of a higher socioeconomic status rather than the postulated (causal) protective effect of HRT.

Ref.: 3, 10

14. Researchers have developed a rapid bedside assay for detection of a new *Clostridium difficile* strain (*C. difficile*). The assay is applied to patients with diarrhea (group 1) and diarrhea with fever (group 2). Each patient was also tested with the "gold standard" polymerase chain reaction evaluation to determine whether the new bacterial strain is present. The results are shown in Table 34.1. Which of the following statements is not correct?

A. The prevalence of the *C. difficile* strain in group 1 is 1%.

B. The RR for *C. difficile* (patients with a positive rapid assay versus those with a negative one) in group 1 is about 75.

C. The odds ratio (assay positive versus assay negative) for having the *C. difficile* strain in group 2 is 81.

D. The incidence of the *C. difficile* strain in group 2 is 10%.

E. An RR of 1 implies that the event is equally probable in both groups.

ANSWER: D

COMMENTS: Prevalence is the number of patients in a sample who currently have a disease divided by the total number of patients sampled. The prevalence is calculated from the column totals; for group 1, it is 10/1000 = 1%. It is important to distinguish incidence from prevalence. In epidemiologic studies, it is often desirable to determine the **incidence**, which is the number of *new* cases of a disease that occur during a specified period. However, when calculating incidence, only cases newly diagnosed during the study period are counted (rather than the total number of observed cases). The **odds** of an event are defined as the probability of the event occurring divided by the probability of it not occurring. The **odds ratio** compares the odds of something occurring in two different groups. The odds of a patient in group 2 with a positive assay having influenza is 90/90 = 1; that is, the patient is equally likely to have or to not have influenza. The odds ratio for group 2 (assay positive versus assay negative) is calculated as (90/90)/(10/810) = 81. **RR** is a more intuitive concept that compares the **probabilities** of two events rather than the odds. The RR for a disease is calculated as the incidence in one population divided by the incidence in the other. If the incidence cannot be determined, we can still compare the risk for disease in two populations by using the odds ratio (the odds of disease in the exposed group divided by the odds of disease in the nonexposed group). For group 1, the RR of having influenza in patients with positive assays versus those with negative assays is given by (9/108)/(1/892) = 74.3. An RR of 1 implies that the event is equally probable in the two groups.

Ref.: 1, 3

TABLE 34.1 Evaluation of Rapid Assay for *C. difficile*

	C. difficile Present	*C. difficile* Absent	Total
Group 1: Symptoms Only			
Rapid assay +	9	99	108
Rapid assay −	1	891	892
Total	10	990	1000
Group 2: Symptoms + Fever			
Rapid assay +	90	90	180
Rapid assay −	10	810	820
Total	100	900	1000

15. Referring to Question 14, which of the following statements is not correct?

A. The sensitivity of the new *C. difficile* assay in group 1 is 90%.

B. The accuracy of the new *C. difficile* assay in group 2 is 90%.

C. The positive predictive value (PPV) of the assay in group 1 is 8%.

D. The negative predictive value (NPV) of the assay in group 2 is 50%.

E. Sensitivity and specificity are better intrinsic measures of a test than are PPV and NPV.

ANSWER: D

COMMENTS: When interpreting diagnostic tests, it is common to be able to reduce the data to a 2 × 2 grid. For each of the groups in the table, the test results can be reduced to:

	C. difficile Present	*C. difficile* Absent
Rapid assay +	True positive	False positive
Rapid assay −	False negative	True negative

The sensitivity and specificity are characteristics of tests that are independent of the population tested. **Sensitivity** represents the proportion of actual positives that are correctly identified as such. For a diagnostic test, it is the number of patients with the disease who test positive [true positive (TP)] divided by the total number of patients with the disease [TP plus false negative (FN)]: **Sensitivity = TP/(TP + FN)**. **Specificity** assesses the proportion of negatives that are correctly identified. For a diagnostic test, it is defined as the number of patients without the disease who test negative [true negative (TN)] divided by the total number of patients in the sample without the disease [TN plus false positive (FP)]: **Specificity = TN/(TN + FP)**. Sensitivity is a measure of the test's ability to detect the disease, whereas specificity is a measure of the test's ability to detect the absence of disease. For this example, the prevalence of disease in these two populations is different, but the sensitivity and specificity of the test do not change across the populations tested. In this example, the sensitivity and specificity are (coincidentally) the same (90%). In general, as one improves either the sensitivity or the specificity of a test, the other is degraded. **Accuracy** measures how closely the test value represents the true value. **Accuracy = (TP + TN)/(TP + TN + FP + FN)**. PPV and NPV are characteristics of tests that depend on the prevalence of disease in the population tested. **PPV** is the number of patients who test positive and have the disease divided by the total number who test positive in the sample: **PPV = TP/(TP + FP)**. **NPV** is defined as the number of patients who test negative and do not have the disease divided by the total number who test negative in the sample: **NPV = TN/(TN + FN)**. PPV is a measure of the test's ability to predict the presence of disease, whereas NPV is a measure of the test's ability to predict the absence of disease. It is important to realize that PPV and NPV can change dramatically as the prevalence of disease in a population changes. In this example, when prevalence changes from 1% (group 1) to 10% (group 2), PPV increases from 8% to 50%. The new assay may be a good screening test for the population in group 2 but a poor one for group 1, where most positive tests are falsely positive. This is often the case when testing low-prevalence populations (even with a highly sensitive and specific test). It is critically important to understand the population for which PPV and NPV were calculated; extrapolating these parameters to a different population with a different prevalence of disease may yield misleading results.

Ref.: 1, 3

16. You decide to conduct a study on whether magnetic resonance enterography is an effective colon cancer screening test. Which of the following is true of a screening test?

A. If the prevalence of the disease is low, the test must be highly sensitive.

B. Increasing the sensitivity of the test also usually increases its specificity.

C. Treatment before the development of the clinical disease should reduce the morbidity and mortality of the disease more than treatment initiated after clinical manifestations of the disease are present.

D. Length–time bias occurs when a new test diagnoses the disease earlier, but there is no effect on the disease outcome.

E. The best studies for assessing whether a screening test will increase a population's health are well-designed case-control studies.

ANSWER: C

COMMENTS: The PPV of a screening test improves if the test is applied to a population with a high prevalence of disease. If the prevalence of disease is low, the test must have high specificity (to avoid large numbers of false-positive results), in addition to acceptable sensitivity. Measures taken to improve specificity usually tend to reciprocally decrease sensitivity. Obviously, screening is useful only when it diminishes morbidity and mortality rates. A screening program is beneficial when early treatment (based on screening test results) improves morbidity and mortality more than a treatment initiated later does, when the disease is detected clinically. **Lead–time bias** occurs when a new test diagnoses the disease earlier, but there is no effect on the outcome of the disease. Although the survival time from diagnosis to death is longer (when compared with the old test), the actual length of survival is the same. **Length–time bias** occurs when screening overrepresents a less-aggressive disease. For example, more aggressive cancers generally have a shorter clinically occult phase than the less-aggressive tumors and consequently are less likely to be detected on fixed-interval screening. However, the aggressive tumors also have poorer outcomes; therefore although the screening test appears to improve outcomes, this improvement is in fact caused by the less-aggressive cancers being overrepresented in the population in whom cancer was identified by screening. **Selection bias** occurs when the differences in outcome seen with screening reflect the willingness of different populations to be screened rather than a true alteration of the disease process. Although expensive and time consuming, **randomized controlled trials** are the best methods for avoiding bias when evaluating screening protocols.

Ref.: 1, 11

17. You are evaluating a prospective trial in which you suspect the patients were highly selected into the treatment group. Which of the following is true?

A. Type I errors are associated mainly with tests with poor sensitivity.

B. Internal validity reflects the confidence that a study can be generalized to patients beyond the limited study group.

C. Bias is best addressed by increasing the size of each group in the study.

D. Selection bias occurs when the researcher spends more time supervising the care of patients in the treatment group than those in the control group.

E. None of the above.

ANSWER: E

COMMENTS: Good **internal validity** is defined by a statistical association that is not caused by chance, confounding with other causal factors, or bias introduced into the study design. That is, internal validity reflects the confidence that the intervention of interest is the actual cause of a study's outcome. Internal validity is subject to **chance**, **bias**, and **confounding**. There are two types of chance-related errors. **Type I errors** occur when the researcher rejects the null hypothesis when it is in fact true (an effect is observed when there is really none). Type I errors (alpha) are associated with tests with poor **specificity**. **Type II errors** occur when the null hypothesis is not rejected despite the fact that it is not true (no effect is observed when in truth one exists). Type II errors (beta) are associated with tests with poor **sensitivity**. A **confounding variable** is an effect that independently influences the measured outcome and is unevenly distributed among the two groups of patients. Confounding is addressed during the study design by randomization, although it can also be addressed during the analysis by statistical risk adjustment (usually with multivariate regression analysis). **Bias** occurs when there is a methodologic difference in the handling of the comparison groups. Bias can occur when participants are enrolled by different criteria (selection bias), when there is participant attrition, when noncomparable information is collected from various groups (observational bias), or when inaccuracies are introduced during data collection (classification bias). Efforts to control bias include blinding and prospective study design. The **external validity** of a clinical study is the degree to which its findings can be generalized to other patients in other settings. Good external validity is also required to postulate a cause-and-effect relationship. A study is considered to have good external validity if the association demonstrated is biologically credible (i.e., consistent with other observations and theories) and is generalizable to clinically relevant populations beyond the group selected for the study. Selecting the appropriate population for study can be challenging and often requires balancing internal validity against external validity.

Ref.: 1, 11

18. You are attempting to determine the odds of having a history of tobacco use in patients with pancreatic cancer. You decide to compare all patients with pancreatic cancer, smokers and nonsmokers, with healthy controls. Which of the following is true regarding observational (case-control or cohort) studies?

A. Patients with the disease of interest are randomized into treatment and nontreatment groups.

B. Case-control studies should not be used when a single disease has multiple causes.

C. Case-control studies are useful for assessing temporal relationships between causative agents and disease.

D. Incidence and RR can be measured directly in cohort studies.

E. Cohort studies are most useful for commonly occurring exposures and diseases.

ANSWER: D

COMMENTS: When properly conducted, **observational studies** can provide conclusions nearly as compelling as those drawn from **interventional studies** (randomized controlled trials). In **case-control studies**, patients with the disease of interest are selected from a population and compared with representative, nondiseased individuals from the same population. There are several advantages of case-control studies. They are generally faster and less expensive. They are useful when there is a long latent period between exposure and disease or if the disease is rare, and multiple causes of a single disease can be studied with a case-control design. However, there are several disadvantages of case-control studies. They are inefficient when the exposure is rare. The incidence of a disease or RR cannot be directly calculated (the odds ratio must be used instead). Finally, temporal relationships can be difficult to measure in case-control studies, and case-control design is prone to bias. In **cohort studies**, a population is selected and monitored for the development of exposure and disease over time. Cohort studies are more useful when exposure is rare. They can examine multiple effects of an exposure and may demonstrate temporal relationships. When performed prospectively, bias is minimized, and incidence and RR can be measured directly. Disadvantages include greater expense, inefficiency for studying rare diseases, and the need for a complete follow-up and detailed record keeping.

Ref.: 11

19. You are developing a prospective randomized control trial to establish the noninferiority of nonoperative treatment of appendicitis. Which of the following is true about interventional studies (randomized controlled trials)?

A. Randomization and large sample size generally reduce the effects of confounding variables.

B. Randomization serves to eliminate observational bias.

C. The effects of poor compliance with therapy can be eliminated with an "intention-to-treat" design.

D. Interventional studies are usually cheaper than observational studies such as case-control studies.

E. Randomized controlled trials are less subject to ethics concerns than are observational studies.

ANSWER: A

COMMENTS: Interventional studies that are designed well and conducted properly can generate a level of validity greater than that of observational studies. Interventional studies include an adequate sample of a study population, and subjects are randomly assigned to treatment or control conditions. Proper randomization not only equalizes the prevalence of known confounding factors in each group but also makes the prevalence of unknown factors equal. In a **single-blind study**, the researcher knows the details of the treatment but the patient does not. In a **double-blind study**, both the investigator and the patient are unaware of the assignment to the intervention or control conditions. Double-blind studies are preferred because they help eliminate observation bias. The **"intention-to-treat"** research design requires that a patient be assigned to the treatment group for the duration of a study, regardless of whether the treatment can be completed. This method can enhance the generalizability of a study. However, there are several problems when performing controlled trials. Poor compliance of subjects with therapy can bias the study results toward the null hypothesis. The ethical considerations of randomizing a potentially effective therapy to a treatment group are significant for researchers considering an interventional study design. Feasibility issues, such as high cost and time-intensive data collection, can make interventional studies impractical. In addition, the placebo effect—the phenomenon by which the perception of receiving a therapy tends to improve an individual's assessment of well-being—can dramatically alter results if the treatment cannot be effectively blinded.

Ref.: 11

20. A researcher decides to perform a meta-analysis to determine the best form of induction immunosuppression for living related-donor kidney transplantation. Which of the following is true with regard to meta-analysis?

A. Meta-analysis techniques cannot increase the power of an investigation.

B. Meta-analysis methods can eliminate observational or selection bias.

C. Many of the statistical techniques used in the meta-analysis are unique to it.

D. Meta-analysis can be used to assess effect sizes and CIs.

E. "File drawer" or publication bias refers to the overinclusion of studies supporting the null hypothesis.

ANSWER: D

COMMENTS: Meta-analysis is a statistical technique used to synthesize the literature on a particular topic. A meta-analysis is essentially a study of a group of studies and is conducted to increase the power of an investigation or to resolve inconsistencies among the study results. Meta-analysis methods cannot control for bias in the original studies. The steps of a meta-analysis are to (1) formulate a research question, (2) search the literature, (3) establish incorporation criteria for including studies in the meta-analysis, (4) decide which dependent variables (or summary measures) are useful, and (5) select a model as a framework for the statistical analysis on the extracted data. Statistical analyses conducted as part of a meta-analysis typically include calculations of effect size and CIs, as well as homogeneity tests. Limitations of meta-analysis include a lack of control for bias in the original studies. A good meta-analysis of badly designed studies will still result in suspect (or misleading) results. Some meta-analyses add a study-level variable that quantifies the methodologic quality of each study to examine the impact of study quality on the effect size. Furthermore, meta-analysis is often limited to published studies. **Publication bias**, or the "file drawer effect," refers to studies that remain unpublished because they do not show a statistically significant result. Many meta-analyses now include a calculation of the number of studies supporting the null hypothesis that would need to be included for an effect to no longer be reliable. The **Simpson paradox** is an apparent paradox in which the successes of groups seem reversed when the groups are combined. This can occur when frequency data are given a nonrigorous causal interpretation. The paradox disappears when a causal relationship is derived systematically. Finally, a synthesis of research studies may provide evidence about the overall effectiveness of a test or treatment protocol but not the specific details that would help guide implementation.

Ref.: 11

21. A study is initiated to determine whether the preoperative administration of an antibody directed against vascular endothelial growth factor increases the disease-free survival in patients with colon cancer treated by segmental colon resection. Which of the following is correct?

A. Survival analysis can be used only if the end point is death of the patient.

B. If a subject dies during a follow-up, the case is considered "censored."

C. The hazard function represents the probability of a subject surviving a given length of time.

D. The Kaplan-Meier estimator can be used to compare two survival curves.

E. The Cox proportional hazards model allows examination of covariates underlying the survival curves.

ANSWER: E

COMMENTS: Survival analysis involves examination of time-to-event data, that is, the elapsed time from a defined starting point (e.g., birth, disease diagnosis, and organ transplantation) until an explicit event (e.g., death, end of remission, and transplant organ failure). For example, a study may examine the longevity of patients receiving chemotherapy for lymphoma. Many of the subjects included will not have died before the study ends or they are lost to follow-up. When the terminal event has not occurred at the end of the given follow-up time, the case is considered to be **censored**. Obviously, excluding these subjects from the analysis would be misleading (e.g., in a study of chemotherapy, the subjects still alive with long follow-ups are the successful results). The **survival function** $S(t)$ represents the probability of a subject surviving until time t, whereas the **hazard function** $h(t)$ represents the conditional probability of dying at time t after having survived to that time. A graph of the survival function against time is the **survival curve**. The **Kaplan-Meier estimator** is a way to approximate the survival curve from data when some of the observations are censored. A Kaplan-Meier plot shows an estimate of the survival curve in which survival is plotted (against time) as a series of horizontal steps with decreasing magnitude. Each step represents a subject who has undergone the terminal event; survival is regarded as a constant between steps. Censored losses are represented on a Kaplan-Meier plot by vertical tic marks. As the number of observations increases, the Kaplan-Meier plot better represents the true survival curve. The **log-rank test** is a nonparametric test used to test the hypothesis that there is no difference between two survival curves. However, it does not provide any analysis of the variables underlying the difference. The **Cox proportional hazards model** (Cox regression) allows examination of additional covariates. For example, a study of cancer patient survival with and without adjuvant chemotherapy might include patient age at diagnosis, tumor size, and stage of disease as covariates.

Ref.: 2, 12

22. Which of the following represents the most effective evidence for screening or treatment modalities?

A. Randomized controlled trial

B. Controlled trial without randomization

C. Multicenter case-control study

D. Uncontrolled trial with dramatic results

E. Expert committee recommendations

ANSWER: A

COMMENTS: Evidence-based medicine attempts to rank the different types of available clinical evidence on the basis of their rigor and how well they control limitations in internal and external validity. Multiple-ranking systems have been developed. One of the simplest (and frequently quoted) is the hierarchy developed by the **U.S. Preventive Services Task Force**:

Level I: Evidence obtained from at least one properly designed randomized controlled trial.

Level II-1: Evidence obtained from well-designed controlled trials without randomization.

Level II-2: Evidence obtained from a well-designed cohort or case-control analytic studies, preferably from more than one center or research group.

Level II-3: Evidence obtained from multiple time series with or without the intervention. Dramatic results in uncontrolled trials might also be regarded as this type of evidence.

Level III: Opinions of respected authorities, based on clinical experience, descriptive studies, or reports of expert committees.

This system has been criticized for its limitations; for example, it does not account for study power, multiple institutions, blinding, and other criteria. Multiple additional grading criteria have been developed to further stratify the quality of available clinical evidence.

Ref.: 13

23. A patient with colon cancer wishes to enroll in a study of a new chemotherapeutic agent. Which of the following is not an essential element of informed consent?

A. A description of any risks or discomfort that the subject may experience

B. A review of alternative courses of treatment

C. A description of the methods for keeping the subject's medical records private

D. Disclosure of the financial support for the study

E. A statement that participation in the study is voluntary

ANSWER: D

COMMENTS: Informed consent requires that the following information be conveyed to each subject:

1. A statement that the study involves research, an explanation of the purposes of the research and the expected duration of the subject's participation, a description of the procedures to be followed, and identification of any procedures that are experimental
2. A description of any reasonably foreseeable risks or discomfort that the subject may experience
3. A description of any benefits to the subject or to others that may reasonably be expected from the research
4. Disclosure of appropriate alternative procedures or courses of treatment, if any, that might be advantageous to the subject
5. A statement describing the extent, if any, to which confidentiality of records identifying the subject will be maintained
6. For research involving more than the minimal risk, an explanation regarding whether any compensation and medical treatments are available if injury occurs and, if so, what they consist of or where further information may be obtained
7. An explanation of whom to contact for answers to pertinent questions about the research and research subjects' rights and whom to contact in the event of a research-related injury to the subject
8. A statement that participation is voluntary, that refusal to participate will involve no penalty or loss of benefits to which the subject is otherwise entitled, and that the subject may discontinue participation at any time without penalty or loss of benefits to which the subject is otherwise entitled

Ref.: 14

REFERENCES

1. Davis AT. Biostatistics. In: O'Leary JP, ed. *The Physiologic Basis of Surgery*. 4th ed. Philadelphia: JB Lippincott; 2008.
2. Shott S. *Statistics for Health Professionals*. Philadelphia: WB Saunders; 1990.
3. Guller U, DeLong ER. Interpreting statistics in medical literature: a *vade mecum* for surgeons. *J Am Coll Surg*. 2004;198:441–458.
4. Whitley E, Ball J. Statistics review 1: presenting and summarizing data. *Crit Care*. 2002;6:66–71.
5. Whitley E, Ball J. Statistics review 2: samples and populations. *Crit Care*. 2002;6:143–148.
6. Whitley E, Ball J. Statistics review 3: hypothesis testing and P values. *Crit Care*. 2002;6:222–225.
7. Norman G, Streiner D. *Biostatistics: The Bare Essentials*. Hamilton, Ontario, Canada: BC Decker; 1998.
8. Whitley E, Ball J. Statistics review 4: sample size calculations. *Crit Care*. 2002;6:335–341.
9. Whitley E, Ball J. Statistics review 6: nonparametric methods. *Crit Care*. 2002;6:509–513.
10. Rosner B. *Fundamentals of Biostatistics*. 5th ed. Belmont, CA: Wadsworth; 2000.
11. Hennekens CH, Buring JE. *Epidemiology in Medicine*. Boston: Little Brown; 1987.
12. Bewick V, Cheek L, Ball J. Statistics review 12: survival analysis. *Crit Care*. 2004;8:389–394.
13. Harris RP, Helfand M, Woolf SH, et al. Current methods of the U.S. Preventive Services Task Force: a review of the process. *Am J Prev Med*. 2001;20(suppl 3):21–35.
14. CFR 46.116(a) retrieved 10/14/09 from the U.S. Department of Health and Human Services, Office for Human Research Protections. Available at: www.hhs.gov/ohrp/humansubjects.

CHAPTER 35

CORE COMPETENCIES AND QUALITY IMPROVEMENT

Katherine Kopkash, M.D., and Shauna Sheppard, M.D.

1. How many core competencies emerged from the Accreditation Council for Graduate Medical Education (ACGME) Outcomes Project?

A. 2
B. 3
C. 4
D. 5
E. 6

ANSWER: E

COMMENTS: In 1999, the ACGME Outcomes Project identified six domains of general competencies: patient care, medical knowledge, practice-based learning and improvement, interpersonal and communication skills, professionalism, and systems-based practice. These core competencies serve as the framework for organizing resident training. Each resident is graded on the core competencies based on the milestone system, with the goal of reaching level 4 prior to graduation.

Ref.: 1

2. Which of the following specific statements is part of the patient care core competency requirement?

A. Set learning and improvement goals
B. Incorporate formative evaluation feedback into daily practice
C. Demonstrate manual dexterity appropriate for the resident's level
D. Participate in the education of patients and families
E. Communicate effectively with patients, families, and the public

ANSWER: C

COMMENTS: Demonstrating manual dexterity appropriate for the resident's level is the first component of the patient care core competency. According to ACGME, residents must be able to provide patient care that is compassionate, appropriate, and effective for the treatment of the patient's health problems and the promotion of their health. To meet the requirements of this core competency, residents should be able to complete the following: (1) demonstrate manual dexterity appropriate for the resident's level; (2) develop and execute patient care plans appropriate for the resident's level, including management of pain; and (3) participate in a program that must document a clinical curriculum that is sequential, comprehensive, and organized from basic to complex. Choices A and B are from the practice-based learning core competency. Choices D and E are from the systems-based practices core competency.

Ref.: 1

3. The ACGME medical knowledge core competency involves participation in an educational program that details the fundamentals of basic science as applied to clinical surgery. Topics include (1) wound healing; (2) homeostasis; (3) shock and circulatory physiology; (4) hematologic disorders; (5) immunobiology and transplantation; (6) oncology; (7) surgical endocrinology; (8) surgical nutrition and fluid and electrolyte balance; (9) metabolic response to injury, including burns, and:

A. Bioinformatics and information systems in health care systems
B. Wound closure techniques
C. Principles of cardiac surgery
D. Applied surgical anatomy and surgical pathology
E. Technical aspects of a cholecystectomy

ANSWER: D

COMMENTS: To achieve the medical knowledge core competency, residents must demonstrate knowledge of established and evolving biomedical, clinical, epidemiologic, and social-behavioral sciences and understand how this knowledge is applied to patient care. Therefore residents should be able to perform the following: (1) critically evaluate and demonstrate the knowledge of pertinent scientific information and (2) participate in an educational program that includes the fundamentals of basic science as applied to clinical surgery. These fundamentals include applied surgical anatomy and surgical pathology; the elements of wound healing; homeostasis, shock, and circulatory physiology; hematologic disorders; immunobiology and transplantation; oncology; surgical endocrinology; surgical nutrition and fluid and electrolyte balance; and metabolic response to injury, including burns. Choices A, B, C, and E are not relevant to fundamental basic science knowledge.

Ref.: 1

4. Residents are expected to develop certain skills and habits so that they can meet all of the following goals to satisfy the criteria of practice-based learning and improvement of core competency except:
   A. Use an evidence-based approach to patient care
   B. Participate in mortality and morbidity conferences that evaluate and analyze patient care outcomes
   C. Use information technology to optimize learning
   D. Locate, appraise, and assimilate evidence from scientific studies related to their patients' health problems
   E. Promote the participation of their patients in a clinical trial

ANSWER: E

COMMENTS: For the ACGME practice-based learning and improvement of core competencies, residents must demonstrate the ability to investigate and evaluate their care of patients, to appraise and assimilate scientific evidence, and to continuously improve patient care based on constant self-evaluation and lifelong learning. Residents are expected to develop skills and habits to be able to meet the following goals:

1. Identify strengths, deficiencies, and limits in one's knowledge and expertise
2. Set learning and improvement goals
3. Identify and perform appropriate learning activities
4. Systematically analyze practice by using quality improvement methods and implement changes with the goal of improvement in practice
5. Incorporate formative evaluation feedback into daily practice
6. Locate, appraise, and assimilate evidence from scientific studies related to their patients' health problems
7. Use information technology to optimize learning
8. Participate in the education of patients, families, students, residents, and other health care professions
9. Participate in mortality and morbidity conferences that evaluate and analyze patient care outcomes
10. Use an evidence-based approach to patient care

Ref.: 1

5. The ACGME Milestone Project developed a system for evaluating residents' developmental outcomes in the core competencies. Which of the following is correct in regard to the ACGME Milestone Project?
   A. There are six milestone levels.
   B. Milestone level should correlate with the postgraduate year.
   C. Residents are required to reach the top milestone level in order to graduate.
   D. Milestones provide a framework for assessment of the development of residents.
   E. Milestones are reviewed with residents on a bimonthly basis.

ANSWER: D

COMMENTS: The Milestone Project was developed by the ACGME in 2015 as a tool to evaluate residents' development in the key dimensions of competency in a specialty. Surgery milestones have four levels (1 to 4). At level 1, the resident demonstrates milestones expected of an incoming resident; at level 2, the resident advances and demonstrates additional milestones, but does not yet perform at a mid-residency level; at level 3, the resident continues to advance and demonstrate additional milestones and demonstrates the majority of milestones targeted for residency in this subcompetency; at level 4, the resident has advanced, so he or she now substantially demonstrates the milestones targeted for residency; this final level is designed as a graduation target. In contrast, residents can be deemed "critically deficient." If these learner behaviors are not within the spectrum of developing competence, that indicates significant deficiencies in a resident's performance. The milestone levels are not intended to correlate with the postgraduate year, and reaching level 4 is a graduation target but NOT a requirement. The results are reviewed semiannually with residents and are meant to serve as a framework for the assessment of development as the individual's progress through residency.

Ref.: 2

6. The ACGME milestones are designed to help residencies produce highly competent physicians who meet the health and health care needs of the public. What other purpose do the milestones fulfill?
   A. Milestones evaluate residents' use of the Surgical Council on Resident Education (SCORE) curriculum.
   B. Milestones provide explicit and transparent expectations of resident performance.
   C. Milestones correlate with the likelihood of passing the American Board of Surgery (ABS) qualifying exam.
   D. Milestones allow the ACGME to eliminate site visits for programs that consistently perform well.
   E. Milestones provide residency programs with an evaluation system that is independent of the program accreditation process.

ANSWER: B

COMMENTS: Milestones were developed by the ACGME and relevant American Board of Medical Specialties specialty board, along with program director association members, specialty college members, ACGME Review Committee Members, residents, and fellows. The Milestone program serves an important role in the program accreditation and provides continuous monitoring of programs and lengthening of site visit cycles. Milestones provide a descriptive developmental framework for clinical competency committees, guide curriculum development of residency programs, support better assessment practices, and enhance opportunities for early identification of struggling residents. For the residents, the milestones serve to provide more explicit and transparent expectations of performance, support better self-directed assessment and learning, and facilitate better feedback for professional development. The milestones are used by the ACGME to demonstrate the accountability of the effectiveness of Graduate Medical Education within the ACGME-accredited programs in meeting the needs of the public.

Ref.: 3

7. Residents are expected to accomplish which of the following to meet the systems-based practice core competency?

A. Understand the nuances of the health care delivery systems

B. Coordinate their patient's care even outside their clinical specialty

C. Ensure good patient outcomes regardless of cost awareness

D. Participate in identifying system errors

E. Understand the roles of other specialists only for the purposes of patient care

ANSWER: D

COMMENTS: Residents should develop an awareness and responsiveness to the larger context of the health care system and learn to call effectively on other resources in the system to provide optimal health care to achieve the ACGME systems-based practice core competency. Residents are expected to function as follows: (1) work effectively in various health care delivery settings and systems relevant to their clinical specialty; (2) coordinate patient care within the health care system relevant to their clinical specialty; (3) incorporate considerations of cost awareness and risk–benefit analysis in patient- or population-based care, or both, as appropriate; (4) advocate for quality patient care and optimal patient care systems; (5) work in interprofessional teams to enhance patient safety and improve the quality of patient care; (6) participate in identifying system errors and implementing potential systems solutions; (7) practice high-quality, cost-effective patient care; (8) demonstrate knowledge of risk–benefit analysis; and (9) demonstrate an understanding of the role of different specialists and other health care professionals in overall patient management.

Ref.: 1

8. With respect to a surgical skills laboratory, which statement is true?

A. The surgical skills laboratory improves technical skills only.

B. Currently, no standardized skills curriculum exists.

C. Acquisition of surgical skills in the laboratory should be weighted toward the senior residency years.

D. Team training should be taught in the operating room only after the junior- and senior-level resident surgical skills are learned in a surgical skills laboratory.

E. The Residency Review Committee (RRC) mandates surgical skill laboratories to maintain accreditation.

ANSWER: E

COMMENTS: As of July 2008, the RRC mandated that all surgery training programs have a surgical skills laboratory to maintain their accreditation. A surgical skills laboratory has been shown to improve technical skills and medical knowledge. The American College of Surgeons (ACS) and the Association of Program Directors in Surgery (APDS) have developed a standardized skills curriculum consisting of three phases. Phase I has modules for junior residents, phase II has modules for senior residents, and phase III has modules for team training.

Ref.: 1

9. "Never events" are errors in medical care that are clearly identifiable, preventable, and serious in their consequences for patients. Which of the following is TRUE about "never events"?

A. Retained surgical instruments can be prevented by using surgical counts.

B. Risk factors for wrong-site surgery include time pressure and morbid obesity.

C. For surgeons who work on symmetric anatomic structures, there is a 10% chance they will be involved in a wrong-site error during their career.

D. The surgical subspecialty most commonly involved in reported wrong-site surgery is neurosurgery.

E. Systems errors are the root cause of the majority of "never events."

ANSWER: B

COMMENTS: The benefit of performing surgical counts to prevent the occurrence of retained surgical items is controversial. Correct counts are reported in up to 100% of cases in which a retained instrument was found, suggesting that just performing a count does not prevent retained instruments. Risk factors for wrong-site surgery include time pressure, emergency surgery, abnormal patient anatomy, and morbid obesity. There is a one-in-four chance that surgeons who work on symmetric anatomic structures will be involved in a wrong-site error sometime during their careers. According to the Joint Commission, specialties more commonly involved in wrong-site surgeries include orthopedic surgery (40%), general surgery (20%), neurosurgery (14%), urology (11%), and others (14%). Although orthopedic surgery is the most frequently involved, this may be attributed to the higher volume of cases performed, as well as the increased opportunity for lateralization errors inherent in orthopedics. Additionally, orthopedic surgeons are more likely to report wrong-site surgery when it occurs. Communication errors are the root cause in more than 70% of wrong-site surgeries reported to the Joint Commission. Other risk factors include receiving incomplete preoperative assessment, having inadequate procedures in place to verify the correct surgical site, and having an organizational culture that lacks teamwork.

Ref.: 4

10. The ACS National Surgical Quality Improvement Program (NSQIP) collects data that provides an in-depth, insightful analysis to help surgeons and hospitals better understand their quality of care. To this end, NSQIP uses data:

A. Based on 1-year mortality

B. Gathered from insurance claims

C. That is risk-adjusted

D. Independent of the complexity of the case

E. Based on outcomes during the operative hospital stay

ANSWER: C

COMMENTS: The ACS NSQIP uses data from the patient's medical chart, as opposed to using information from his or her insurance claims or billing information. The data are risk-adjusted to help compare data between institutions in a fairer manner. The data are based on 30-day patient outcomes; studies have shown that at least half of all complications occur after the patient leaves the hospital, often leading to readmission. Following the patient for 30 days postoperatively provides a more complete picture of a patient's care. The data are case-mix adjusted, allowing hospitals to take on more complex surgical cases and still provide accurate national benchmarking.

Ref.: 5

11. Identify the four steps in practice-based learning and improvement.

A. Identify areas for improvement, engage in learning, apply the new knowledge and skills to a practice, and check for improvement.

B. Seek knowledge, identify areas of weakness in scientific knowledge, aim to add to the knowledge, and await constructive feedback.

C. Learn about new techniques, apply new techniques, refine new techniques, and individualize techniques.

D. Look for improvement in current practice, observe others with a better practice model, attempt a new model in the current paradigm, and teach others the new practice model.

E. Identify areas that are innovative, learn innovation, apply innovation, and teach innovation.

ANSWER: A

COMMENTS: The process of practice-based learning and improvement involves (1) identifying strengths, deficiencies, and limits in one's knowledge and expertise; (2) setting learning and improvement goals; (3) identifying and performing appropriate learning activities; (4) systematically analyzing practice using quality improvement methods and implementing changes with the goal of practice improvement; (5) incorporating formative evaluation feedback into daily practice; (6) locating, appraising, and assimilating evidence from scientific studies related to patients' health problems; (7) using information technology to optimize learning; (8) participating in the education of patients, families, students, residents, and other health professionals; (9) participating in morbidity and mortality conferences; and (10) utilizing an evidence-based approach to patient care.

Ref.: 1

12. Complications of central venous access catheters are relatively common. Identified steps to decrease the rate of complications include all of the following EXCEPT:

A. Exchanging central venous catheters on a routine basis

B. Using proper positioning during central venous catheter insertion

C. Using ultrasound for all internal jugular vein catheter insertions

D. Removing all central catheters as soon as possible

E. Having experienced personnel oversee all central catheter insertions

ANSWER: A

COMMENTS: Identified steps to decrease complications associated with central venous catheters include (1) ensuring central venous access is indicated, (2) having experienced personnel insert the catheter or directly supervise the insertion, (3) using proper positioning and sterile technique, (4) using ultrasound for internal jugular vein insertion, (5) assessing catheters on a daily basis and exchanging them only for specific indications (NOT as a matter of routine), and (6) removing all central catheters as soon as possible.

Ref.: 4

13. Interpersonal and communication skills allow residents to effectively exchange information with patients, their families, and other health professionals. Which of the following is NOT part of the communication core competency?

A. Act in a consultative role to other health professionals

B. Maintain timely, legible medical records

C. Document appropriately for billing and coding purposes

D. Counsel patients and families

E. Communicate with patients across a range of cultural backgrounds

ANSWER: C

COMMENTS: To achieve the interpersonal and communication skills core competency, residents are expected to (1) communicate effectively with patients, families, and the public across a broad range of socioeconomic and cultural backgrounds; (2) communicate effectively with physicians, other health professionals, and health-related agencies; (3) work effectively as a member or leader of a health care team; (4) act in a consultative role to other physicians and health professionals; (5) maintain comprehensive, timely, and legible medical records; (6) counsel and educate patients and families; and (7) effectively document practice activities.

Ref.: 1

14. According to the 2007 "Hospital Quality Improvement: Strategies and Lessons from U.S. Hospitals" report, all of the following are aspects of the pattern of hospital improvements EXCEPT:

A. Practice changes

B. Problem identification

C. A trigger for change

D. Structural changes

E. Improved transparency and accountability

ANSWER: E

COMMENTS: The quality improvement sequence is as follows: A trigger leads to organizational and structural changes that facilitate problem identification and solving. This leads to practice changes, which eventually result in better outcomes. The trigger serves as a wake-up call that begins a cultural shift. Examples of organizational and structural changes include the establishment of quality-related councils and committees, empowerment of nurses and other staff, and investment in new technology. Problem identification and solving includes involving a multidisciplinary team approach to identifying a problem area, conducting a root cause analysis, developing an action plan, and holding team leaders accountable. Examples of practice changes are including evidence-based policies and procedures, developing clinical pathways and guidelines, and using error-reducing software and patient flow management techniques. The process leads to better outcomes (i.e., reduced errors, complications, mortality, costs, and higher satisfaction).

Ref.: 6

15. According to the Joint Commission, what is the leading cause of sentinel events?

A. Training errors

B. Systems errors

C. Communication errors

D. Cognitive errors

E. Medical administration errors

ANSWER: C

COMMENTS: Effective communication is a vital aspect of patient care. Studies examining medical errors have identified communication error as one of the most common causes of medical errors. The Joint Commission identifies miscommunication as the leading cause of sentinel events. Information transfer and communication errors cause delays in patient care, waste surgeon and staff time, and cause serious adverse patient events. A strong correlation exists between communication and patient outcomes.

Ref.: 7

16. The overall goal of NSQIP is to prevent all adverse postoperative outcomes. Outcomes are assessed by looking at:

A. Percentage of adverse outcomes per 10,000 operations

B. Surgeon-specific outcomes

C. Risk-adjusted ratio of the observed to expected outcomes

D. Total number of adverse outcomes per year

E. Process-based outcomes

ANSWER: C

COMMENTS: NSQIP uses a risk-adjusted ratio of the observed to expected outcomes (focusing primarily on 30-day morbidity and mortality) to compare the performance of participating hospitals with their peers. The model used determines the hospitals' odds ratio of morbidity or mortality compared with the odds for an event at the average ACS NSQIP hospital. The ACS database was expanded from the Veterans Administration (VA) NSQIP database and has helped shift the focus from merely preventing provider errors and sentinel events, to the larger goal of preventing all adverse postoperative outcomes.

Ref.: 4

17. There are four defined types of medical errors. They include:

A. Diagnostic error, negligence, near miss, and communication error

B. Adverse event, negligence, near miss, and sentinel event

C. Human error, systems error, communication error, and technical error

D. Negligence, systems error, technical error, and sentinel event

E. Medication administration error, cognitive error, technical error, and communication error

ANSWER: B

COMMENTS: The four types of medical errors are an adverse event, negligence, a near miss, and a sentinel event. An adverse event is an injury caused by the medical management that results in prolonged hospitalization, produces a disability at discharge, or both, and can be classified as preventable or unpreventable. Negligence is defined as care that falls below the recognized standard of care (which is considered as care that a reasonable physician of similar knowledge, training, and experience would use in similar circumstances). A near miss is an event that does not result in patient harm but provides an opportunity to identify and fix systems issues before the occurrence of harm. Finally, a sentinel event is an unexpected occurrence involving death or serious injury (physical or psychologic), which requires immediate investigation and response.

Ref.: 4

18. Safety is defined, specifically, as which of the following?

A. Implementation of preventive measures

B. Freedom from harm

C. Zero tolerance for mistakes

D. Avoidance of human errors

E. Prevention of mistakes caused by a larger system

ANSWER: B

COMMENTS: Safety is defined as "freedom from harm." In the context of patient care, safety means freedom from harm associated with any medical action or treatment. In discussions about patient safety and quality improvement, it is important to differentiate between these two concepts. Quality, by contrast, is a more global term that refers to a "degree of excellence." It is theoretically possible for a hospital to be safe but of average or even poor quality.

Ref.: 8

19. Surgical Care Improvement Project (SCIP) measures are aimed at reducing surgical site infections (SSIs) and preventing cardiovascular complications and venous thromboembolism (VTE) after major surgical procedures. Which of the following is a correct list of SCIP measures?

A. Prophylactic antibiotics given within 1 h prior to surgical incision, perioperative temperature measurement, and correct ordering of the recommended VTE prophylaxis

B. Prophylactic antibiotics given within 1 h prior to surgical incision, correct documentation of wound class, and correct ordering of the recommended VTE prophylaxis

C. Prophylactic antibiotics given within 30 min prior to surgical incision, perioperative temperature measurement, and correct ordering of the recommended VTE prophylaxis

D. Prophylactic antibiotics given within 30 min prior to surgical incision, correct documentation of wound class, and correct ordering of the recommended VTE prophylaxis

E. Prophylactic antibiotics given within 30 h prior to surgical incision, correct documentation of wound class, and use of incentive spirometer within 24 h postoperatively

ANSWER: A

COMMENTS: SCIP measures aim to reduce SSIs, cardiovascular complications, and VTEs after major surgeries by focusing on process issues. SCIP measures include (1) administering prophylactic antibiotics within 1 h prior to surgical incision, (2) correct prophylactic antibiotic selection for surgical patients, (3) discontinuation of prophylactic antibiotics within 24 h of surgery, (4) cardiac surgery patients with controlled 6 am postoperative blood glucose levels, (5) appropriate hair removal on surgical patients (i.e., clippers, not razors), (6) surgical patients with preoperative temperature management, and (7) appropriate administration of the correct VTE prophylaxis.

Ref.: 9

20. In an effort to comply with the Institute of Medicine's goal of reducing medical errors, five transforming concepts have been proposed for adoption by health care organizations seeking to become "high-reliability organizations" by creating a culture of safety. These include all of the following EXCEPT:

A. Transparency must be a practice value in everything the organization does.

B. Care must be delivered by multidisciplinary teams working in integrated platforms.

C. Patients must become full partners in all aspects of health care.

D. Health care workers need to find joy and meaning in their work.

E. Reporting of all suspected medical errors is mandatory.

ANSWER: E

COMMENTS: In order to work toward preventing medical errors, health care entities should work toward becoming "high-reliability organizations" that hold themselves accountable to consistently offer safe and effective patient-centered care. The five proposed transforming concepts for adoption by health care organizations seeking cultural transformative changes include (1) transparency must be a practice value in everything the organization does, (2) care must be delivered by multidisciplinary teams working in integrated platforms, (3) patients must become full partners in all aspects of health care, (4) health care workers need to find joy and meaning in their work, and (5) medical education must be redesigned to prepare new physicians to function in this new environment.

Ref.: 9

21. The Joint Council on Accreditation of Healthcare Organizations (JCAHO) mandates that the time-out immediately preceding a procedure must be conducted in the location where the procedure will be performed. Documentation of a checklist created by each institution must be provided and must include a minimum of all of the following except:

A. Correct patient identity

B. Correct site

C. Agreement on the procedure to be performed

D. Specific confirmation of antibiotic administration

E. Availability of correct implants and any special equipment

ANSWER: D

COMMENTS: The JCAHO requires that correct patient identity, correct site and side, agreement on the procedure to be performed, correct patient position, and availability of correct implants and any special equipment or special requirements be confirmed before the procedure—the time-out. Confirmation of antibiotic administration, although useful, is not mandatory and is dependent on the institution. Each institution should have processes and systems in place for reconciling differences in staff responses during the time-out.

Ref.: 10

22. Which organization is responsible for maintaining a joint venture with the NSQIP?

A. ABS

B. ACGME

C. Association for Surgical Education (ASE)

D. RRC

E. ACS

ANSWER: E

COMMENTS: The quality of care has been examined by analyzing various indicators that can be classified into three main categories: structure, process of care, and outcomes. The NSQIP was initially administered solely in the VA but has now been implemented in many private sector hospitals through an alliance with the ACS. In part, NSQIP is designed to provide a comprehensive view of surgical quality. The ACS NSQIP focuses on the systems of care at its participating sites, not the individual provider of surgical care.

Ref.: 9

23. SCIP differs from NSQIP in what major feature?

A. SCIP does not partner with the ACS, but rather the JCAHO.

B. NSQIP focuses on individual providers of care, whereas SCIP does not.

C. NSQIP focuses primarily on process measures.

D. SCIP focuses primarily on surgical outcomes.

E. SCIP focuses primarily on process measures.

ANSWER: E

COMMENTS: SCIP is a national partnership of organizations (including the ACS) committed to improving the safety of surgical care through a reduction in postoperative complications. Initiated by the Centers for Medicare and Medicaid Service (CMS) and the Centers for Disease Control and Prevention (CDC), SCIP partnership is a multiyear national campaign to substantially reduce surgical mortality and morbidity through collaboration efforts. Although the focus of the ACS NSQIP has been the measurement of surgical outcomes, SCIP will focus primarily on process measures. SCIP partnership is targeting areas where the incidence and cost of complications are high, including SSIs, adverse cardiac events, deep venous thrombosis, and postoperative pneumonia. The program will focus on surgical process measures such as the timing, choice, and duration of prophylactic antibiotic administration. It is anticipated that as SCIP expands, additional relevant data will be included and will be in alignment with the ACS NSQIP data set. Both the ACS NSQIP and SCIP share a core mission of improvement of care for surgical patients. As a member of the SCIP partnership, the ACS NSQIP has developed a data collection tool to capture SCIP measures and enable participating sites to meet the CMS SCIP reporting requirements.

Ref.: 9

24. The American Board of Surgery In-Training Examination (ABSITE) is designed to measure the progress of residents in their knowledge of applied science and management of clinical problems related to surgery. Which of the following is TRUE regarding the ABSITE?

A. The ABSITE is required as part of the board certification process.

B. The ABSITE is aligned with SCORE curriculum.

C. The primary focus of the ABSITE is on applied science.

D. You must be affiliated with a residency program to take the ABSITE.

E. The ABSITE is the most important factor in assessing residents' knowledge.

ANSWER: B

COMMENTS: The ABSITE is a formative evaluation instrument to assess residents' progress, but it is NOT required as part of the board certification process. The content of the ABSITE is aligned with the SCORE Curriculum Outline for General Surgery Residency, which is a list of patient care and medical knowledge topics to be covered in a 5-year general surgery residency. The primary focus of the ABSITE is on clinical management, with 80% of questions addressing clinical management topics. Only approximately 20% of the test addresses applied science topics. Persons not affiliated with a residency program may take the ABSITE; however, they must find a program director willing to allow them to take the ABSITE along with the residents of their program. The ABS considers the ABSITE as one factor of many that should be used to assess a resident's knowledge and performance, and NOT as the sole or most important factor.

Ref.: 11

REFERENCES

1. ACGME Program Requirements for Graduate Medical Education in Surgery. Available at: http://www.acgme.org/Portals/0/PFAssets/ProgramRequirements/440_general_surgery_07012015.pdf. Effective July 1, 2012. Accreditation Council on Graduate Medical Education. Accessed May 2016.
2. The General Surgery Milestone Project: A Joint Initiative of the Accreditation Council for Graduate Medical Education and the American Board of Surgery. July 2015. Available at: https://www.acgme.org/Portals/0/PFAssets/ProgramRequirements/440_general_surgery_2016.pdf. Accessed May 2016.
3. The Accreditation Council for Graduate Medical Education. What we do: milestones. Available at: http://www.acgme.org/What-We-Do/Accreditation/Milestones/Overview. Accessed May 2016.
4. Chen CL, Cooper MA, Shapiro ML, Angood PB, Makary MA. Patient safety. In: Belval B, Naglieri C, eds. *Schwartz's Principles of Surgery*. 10th ed. New York: McGraw-Hill; 2015. Available at. http://accessmedicine.mhmedical.com.ezproxy.rush.edu/book.aspx?bookID=980.
5. The American College of Surgeons: ACS National Surgical Quality Improvement Program. Available at: https://www.facs.org/quality-programs/acs-nsqip. Accessed May 2016.
6. Silow-Carroll S, Alteras T, Meyer JA. *Hospital Quality Improvement: Strategies and Lessons from US Hospitals*. New York: The Commonwealth Fund; 2007.
7. Hill AL, Wu J, Girgis MD, et al. Fundamental principles of leadership training in surgery. In: Brunicardi FC, Andersen DK, Billiar TR, et al., eds. *Schwartz's Principles of Surgery*. 10th ed. New York: McGraw-Hill; 2015. Available at. http://accessmedicine.mhmedical.com.ezproxy.rush.edu/book.aspx?bookID=980.
8. Campbell Jr DA. Patient safety. In: Mulholland M, Lillemoe K, Doherty G, Maier R, Simeone D, Upchurch G, eds. *Greenfield's Surgery*. 5th ed. Philadelphia: Lippincott Williams & Wilkins; 2011. Available at. http://www.r2library.com.ezproxy.rush.edu/resource/title/1605473553.
9. Beauchamp RD, Higgins MS. Preoperative patient safety. In: Townsend CM, Beauchamp RD, Evers BM, et al., eds. *Sabiston Textbook of Surgery: The Biological Basis of Modern Surgical Practice*. 19th ed. Philadelphia: Elsevier Saunders; 2012. Available at. http://www.mdconsult.com/das/book/body/163578292-2/0/1565/113.html.
10. The Universal Protocol: Preventing Wrong Site, Wrong Procedure, and Wrong Person Surgery. The Joint Commission. Available at: http://www.jointcommission.org/assets/1/18/UP_Poster.pdf. Accessed May 2016.
11. The American Board of Surgery: Training & Certification. About the ABSITE. Available at: http://www.absurgery.org/default.jsp?certabsite. Accessed May 2016.